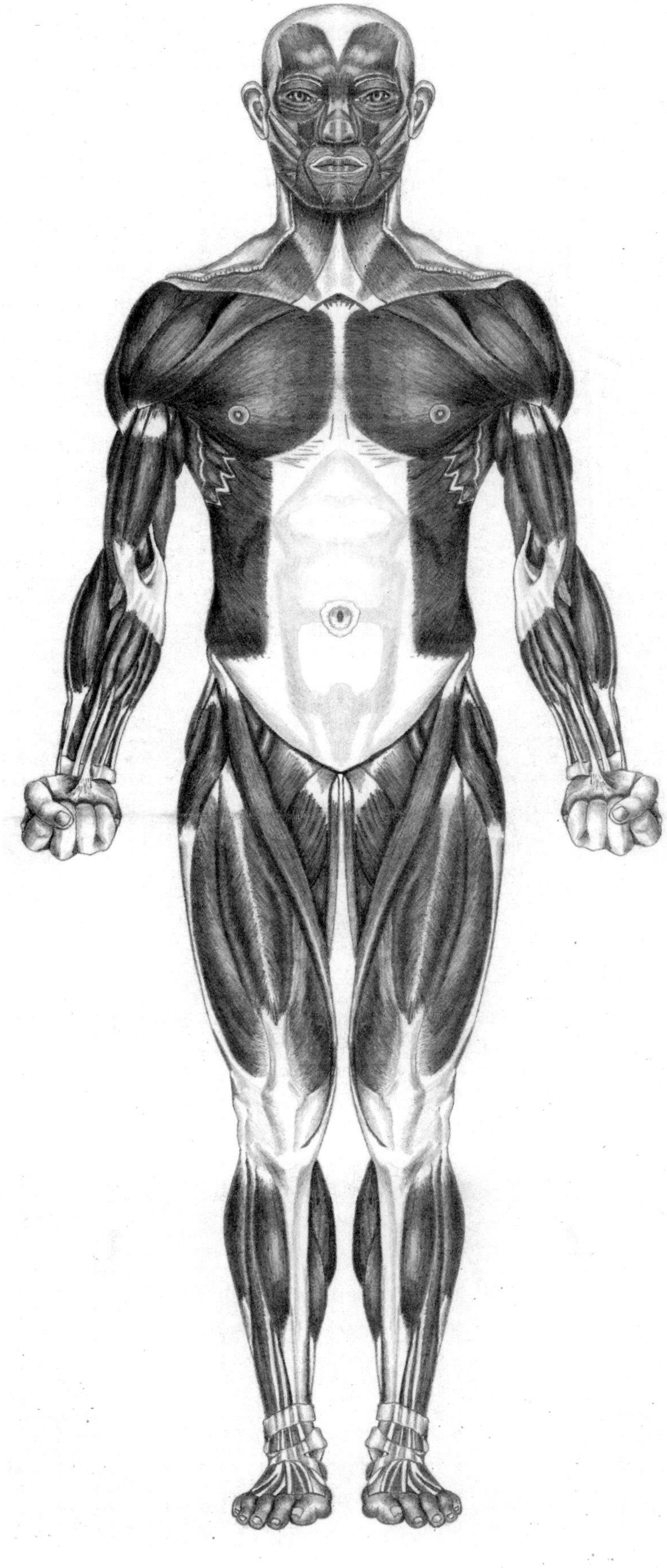

AXIAL BODY

LOWER EXTREMITY

UPPER EXTREMITY

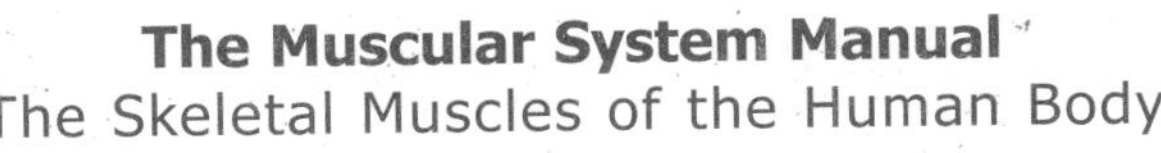
The Muscular System Manual
The Skeletal Muscles of the Human Body

SKELETAL MUSCLES OF THE BODY – ALPHABETICALLY

SKELETAL MUSCLES OF THE BODY – ALPHABETICALLY

Author: **Dr. Joseph E. Muscolino**

Art Direction and Graphic Layout: Deana LoGiudice

Illustrations: Jean Luciano

Additional Illustrations: Rosa Cervoni, Barbara Haeger, Joseph C. Muscolino

Model for Facial Expressions: Randi Muscolino

Production Work and Editing: Jane Walsh

Content Editor: David Eliot, Ph.D.

Proofreader: Joan Campbell

Arterial Supply Information Provided by: Sharon Sawitzke, Ph.D.

Mnemonics: Principal Contributor: Laura Howell

Other Contributors: Sue Backman, Tracy Bloom, Missy DeAngelis, Lori Galiotti, Tammy Martin, Gevvy Mathis, Andie Polley, Mickey Trombley, Janina Zembroski

To purchase additional copies of this book, visit our website, www.learnmuscles.com or call (203) 938-3323. Discounts available for large quantity sales.

Disclaimer

The purpose of this book is to provide information for bodyworkers on the subject of muscular anatomy and physiology. This book does not offer medical advice to the reader and should not be used as replacement for appropriate health care. For proper health care and treatment, please consult a licensed physician.

ISBN 0-9717750-0-1

The Muscular System Manual

The Skeletal Muscles of the Human Body

A WORKING TEXTBOOK AND AN ILLUSTRATED REFERENCE GUIDE OF MUSCULOSKELETAL ANATOMY

DR. JOSEPH E. MUSCOLINO

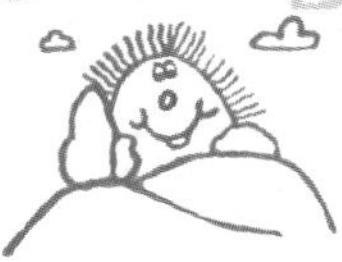

JEM Publications
Redding, Connecticut
www.learnmuscles.com

PREFACE

One day in December of 2000, I was talking with a student of mine named William after our kinesiology class. In the course of our conversation, William expressed the difficulty he had in finding certain information for a required class project. During our discussion on this particular topic of muscle physiology, William said to me, "You should write a book." Although students told this to me before, it never clicked. But that day, William's words sparked something in me. Thirty minutes later, when I walked in the door at my home, I declared to my fiancé, Simona, that I was going to write a book. What happened that day seemed to be a version of the old adage, *When the student is ready, the teacher appears.* Only in this case, perhaps, it would be changed to, *When the teacher is ready, the student appears.*

The reason I wrote this book is because I wanted to create a comprehensive, all-in-one resource that covers all the need-to-know information about muscles and more. I tried to orient this information directly toward those who do bodywork. I have also endeavored to make this book professional and well organized, yet also friendly, approachable and easy to use.

I believe that William's words resonated with me because by that point in time, I had been teaching various anatomy and physiology courses to students of massage therapy for nearly fifteen years and became increasingly frustrated with the lack of books and resources oriented directly toward students of bodywork*. In the particular field of muscular anatomy and physiology in which I have my forte, I believe that few comprehensive texts address the muscular system. There are many books that address muscle attachments and/or actions very competently at a beginning level, but tend to be overly simplistic and soon outgrown. Others, notably many fine kinesiology textbooks, cover more complex topics but often leave out the basics or are geared more toward a physics orientation with lengthy discussions of vector forces and mathematical formulas. Other books out there excel at one particular aspect of muscular anatomy and physiology, but leave other aspects out.

For this reason, I decided to write two comprehensive books that together will cover the musculoskeletal system. One book, *The Skeletal System Manual and How Muscles Function*, will cover the skeletal system of the body, bones and bony landmarks, joints and joint actions, along with the basic understanding of muscle anatomy, how muscles function and some selected advanced topics of kinesiology, all supported by first-rate graphics. The other book, *The Muscular System Manual, The Skeletal Muscles of the Human Body*, is an atlas of the skeletal muscles of the human body. Each muscle page includes attachments, actions, innervation and arterial supply, as well as a discussion of the methodology to figure out why the muscle has its particular actions, a section on the relationship of that muscle to other musculoskeletal structures, and a section on palpation. Each muscle is supported by at least two first-rate illustrations. There are also overview pages, group illustrations and appendices.

I like to say that these two books will be the best "first books" you would need in order to learn about the muscular system. I say this realizing that there are many other fine texts out there. I, myself, am an ardent book collector. Most every text currently out there has its particular area of expertise regarding the musculoskeletal system and depending upon your degree of ambition to learn and master this body of knowledge, you may want to own some or all of the texts that I have listed in my bibliography. I relied upon all these other works to create this book that you now hold. The reason I wrote this book is because I wanted to create a comprehensive, all-in-one resource that covers all the need-to-know information about muscles, and more. I tried to orient this information directly toward those who do bodywork. I have also endeavored to make this book professional and well organized, yet also friendly, approachable and easy to use.

*Whether they be massage therapists, physical therapists, occupational therapists, chiropractors, osteopaths, rolfers, acupuncturists, fitness trainers or a member of any other health or fitness field.

A strength of this book that I would like to emphasize is the approach in how to learn and understand muscles, especially their actions. This is the approach I use to teach my students, and an approach I have not seen systematically covered in other texts. A thorough understanding of how muscles function and how to understand and reason out their actions is given in *The Skeletal System Manual and How Muscles Function*. A brief synopsis of this approach is also given in this book in the appendices (appendix L). The methodology section of this book then applies that approach to each action of every muscle, so that a student can get an understanding of why a particular muscle has certain actions. Once an understanding exists, these actions can then be figured out instead of memorized.

Lastly, another concern of mine has been the utility of these books as both manuals and reference textbooks. These books are bound so that they can lie flat and the student may easily add in handwritten notes. Furthermore, the information has been laid out in an "a-la-carte" fashion by having check boxes placed next to most every piece of information. An individual using these books on his/her own can check off the amount and level of information that he/she chooses to learn. In a classroom setting, the teacher can clearly indicate to the students exactly what the students are to be responsible for. In this manner, these books could function as learning manuals for a beginning, intermediate or an advanced level course. These books can also sit on the bookshelf as reference textbooks for the future.

I hope that these two books enrich and simplify your learning of the musculoskeletal system. If you would like to send comments or constructive criticism regarding these two volumes, please e-mail me at my website, www.learnmuscles.com. I would appreciate any feedback that would improve the quality of future editions.

"I would not give a fig for the simplicity this side of complexity,

but I would give my life for the simplicity on the other side of complexity."

– Oliver Wendell Holmes Jr.

ABOUT THE AUTHOR

Dr. Joe Muscolino has been teaching musculoskeletal and visceral anatomy and physiology, kinesiology, neurology and pathology courses at the Connecticut Center For Massage Therapy (C.C.M.T.) for over 16 years. He has also been instrumental in course manual development and assisted with curriculum development at C.C.M.T. Dr. Muscolino also runs continuing education workshops on such topics as anatomy and physiology, kinesiology, deep tissue massage, as well as cadaver workshops. He is an NCBTMB approved provider of continuing education and C.E.U.s are available for Massage Therapists toward certification renewal. In 2002, Dr. Joe Muscolino participated on the NCBTMB Job Analysis Survey Task Force as well as the Test Specification Meeting as a Subject Matter Expert in Anatomy, Physiology and Kinesiology.

Dr. Joe Muscolino holds a Bachelor of Arts degree in Biology from the State University of New York at Binghamton, Harpur College. He attained his Doctor of Chiropractic Degree from Western States Chiropractic College in Portland, Oregon and is licensed in Connecticut, New York and California. Dr. Joseph Muscolino has been in private practice in Connecticut for more than 17 years and incorporates soft tissue work into his chiropractic practice for all of his patients.

If you would like further information regarding *The Muscular System Manual*, the upcoming *The Skeletal System Manual and How Muscles Function*, or workshops, or if you are an instructor and would like additional information about these books for use at your school, or information regarding the many supportive materials such as colored overheads, test-banks of questions, accompanying coloring book or flash cards, please contact Dr. Joe Muscolino at his website: www.learnmuscles.com.

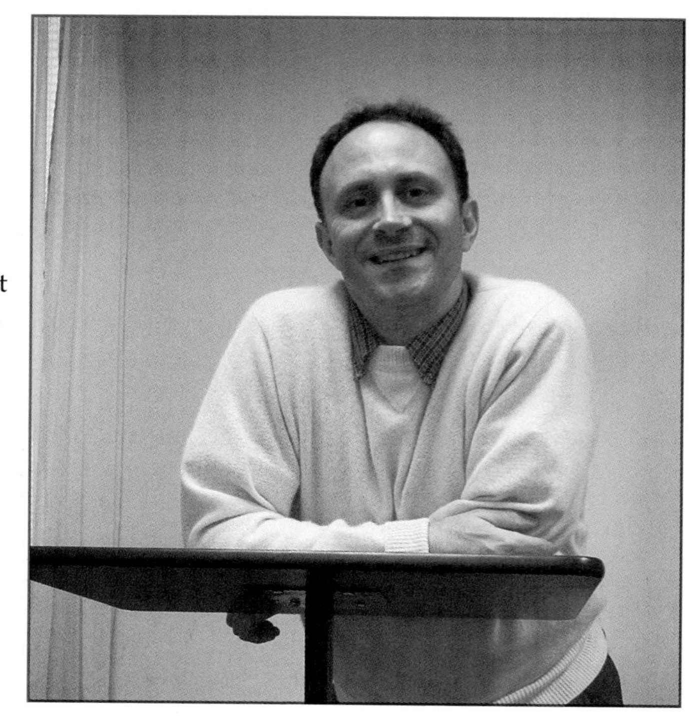

photo by Linda Biancardi

ACKNOWLEDGEMENTS

No book of this magnitude can be achieved without help. I would like to express my gratitude to so many people who aided and supported me in the production of this book. This book would not exist today if it were not for the help and support that all of you have given me. ☺

My art director, Deana LoGiudice, took my dry outline of information and created an inviting and visually pleasing book that is also professional and well organized.

Much of the beauty and success of this book rests in the beautiful, clear illustrations, which were drawn by Jean Luciano. The book was enriched by the addition of many fine graphics by Rosa Cervoni and Barbara Haeger.

Ensuring that my many grammatical mistakes and organizational inconsistencies were kept to a minimum, my editor and production assistant, Jane Walsh, read through this book countless times, reworking much of it to be clearer to the readers.

Dr. Sharon Sawitzke, Ph.D., Associate Professor, Division of Anatomical Sciences at the University of Bridgeport, College of Chiropractic lent her expertise to provide the information regarding the arterial supply to the muscles. I could not have simplified and organized this material without her.

David Elliot, Ph.D. of the Touro University College of Osteopathic Medicine, my content editor, combed through this book ensuring that the informational content was correct. He also fielded countless questions from me, helping me organize the content and provided needed information when the boundaries of my knowledge had been reached.

I would like to thank Dr. Michael Carnes, my first anatomy instructor, of Western States Chiropractic College. He first whetted my appetite for learning and understanding this material.

I would also like to thank all the anatomy and physiology students that I have had at the Connecticut Center for Massage Therapy (C.C.M.T.) over the past 15 years. As they sat in my class, I don't think they realized just how much I, their teacher, was learning along with them. I must reserve a special acknowledgement to one student, William Courtland. Talking together after class one day, he uttered the simple words, "You should write a book." That short statement provided the spark that began this entire project.

I also had the pleasure to work with so many supportive teachers and staff at the Connecticut Center for Massage Therapy. Although an institution of learning, C.C.M.T. has a heart and soul and constantly endeavors to put people first. In particular, I would like to thank the entire staff, past and present, at the Westport branch. It has always been and continues to be a pure pleasure to work with all of you. Specifically, I would like to thank Sue Scoboria and Kathy Watt who have been so supportive of this project and me. I must also thank Matt Schrier D.C.; I couldn't ask for a better Dean of Sciences and kinder human being to work for. And I would like to express my gratitude to Steve Kitts, the executive director and co-founder of CCMT, from whom the heart and soul of C.C.M.T. emanates.

I must also thank Barry Antoniow and Ron Garvock of Kiné-Concept Schools in Canada. Their enthusiasm and support for this book from the beginning helped to create much of the success this book enjoys.

I would also like to thank Tracy Walton and Sue Lourenco of M.T.I. in Cambridge for their helpful recommendations and guidance with the format of this book.

Lastly, I must express my appreciation to my entire family for their unending love, support and understanding as I sat at my computer hour after hour working on this book.

This book is dedicated to Simona Cipriani, my fiancé and angel.

TABLE OF CONTENTS

TABLE OF CONTENTS

TABLE OF CONTENTS

TABLE OF CONTENTS

ORGANIZATION OF THIS BOOK

The body of this book is divided into three parts:

PART ONE – THE AXIAL BODY

PART TWO – THE LOWER EXTREMITY

PART THREE – THE UPPER EXTREMITY

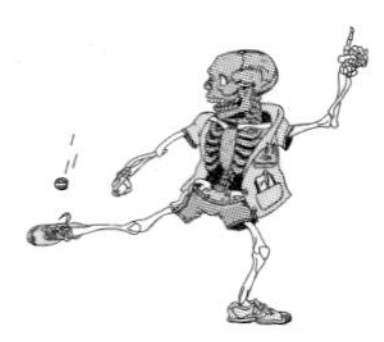

PART ONE – THE AXIAL BODY

INCLUDES THE HEAD, NECK AND THE TRUNK

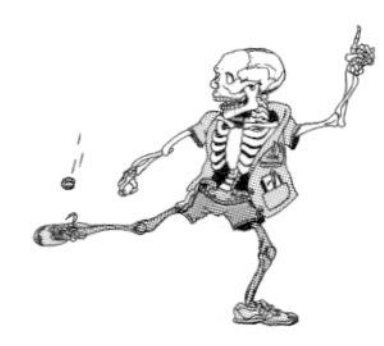

PART TWO – THE LOWER EXTREMITY

INCLUDES THE PELVIS*, THIGH, LEG AND THE FOOT

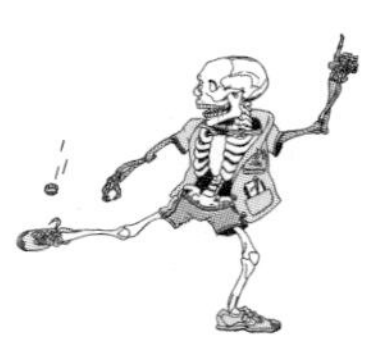

PART THREE – THE UPPER EXTREMITY

INCLUDES THE SCAPULA/ARM, FOREARM AND THE HAND

There are also nine appendices located at the end of the book.

---

*The pelvis was placed as part of the lower extremity of the appendicular body instead of including it as part of the axial body. The pelvis is a transitional region of the body and can be considered to be part of the axial body or the appendicular body. The bony pelvis, the sacrum and coccyx, are certainly part of the axial skeleton; further, the descriptive terms for movements of the pelvis are more similar to axial body part movement terminology than they are similar to appendicular movement terminology (e.g., the pelvis is described as rotating to the right and left as movements of the head, neck and trunk are described, compared to using the terms medial and lateral rotation as movements of the appendicular body parts are described). However, the pelvis also comprises the pelvic girdle, whose movements are coupled with movements of the thigh. Just as movements of the shoulder girdle (the scapula and clavicle) are coupled with movements of the arm and therefore considered to be part of the upper extremity, the pelvis can be considered to be part of the lower extremity. Therefore, given the placement of the shoulder girdle as part of the upper extremity, to stay consistent with the pelvic girdle, the pelvis is placed as part of the lower extremity of the appendicular skeleton in the book.

A NOTE FROM THE AUTHOR REGARDING THE INFORMATION IN THIS BOOK

When approaching texts on muscular anatomy and physiology, one is often confronted with what seems to be contradictory information regarding attachments, actions, innervation and arterial supply. Therefore, having an open mind and a flexible outlook can be beneficial. Below are a few examples of the varying information and a brief explanation for why it might occur.

MUSCLE ATTACHMENTS

Regarding muscle attachments, two examples are the serratus anterior and the tibialis anterior. Some sources state that the serratus anterior attaches to the first eight ribs; other sources state that it attaches to the first nine ribs. The tibialis anterior is sometimes cited as attaching to the proximal 1/2 of the tibia, and other times it is described as attaching to the proximal 2/3 instead. It is not that one source is right and the other wrong. Rather, one must appreciate that not every human body is exactly the same. Just as two people may have different heights, body builds, skin, hair and eye colorings, internal structures can also vary. Depending upon which cadaver studies are used, different books may present different muscular attachments. In this text, I have presented muscle attachments in two levels of detail. In the first level, I have tried to present the most commonly agreed upon attachments for a muscle in a simplified manner. The second level then presents more detailed attachments. Where common variations occur, that information is stated in the miscellaneous section.

MUSCLE ACTIONS

As for a muscle's actions, it can seem just as confusing; different sources often report different actions for the same muscle. Usually, the main action or main actions of a muscle are fairly reliably reported. It is usually the minor weaker actions that many sources disagree as whether to present or not. For example, I have never found a source that would disagree that the biceps brachii can perform its main actions of flexion and supination of the forearm. However, many sources may disagree about the relative importance of the biceps brachii's role in producing flexion, abduction or adduction of the arm at the shoulder joint. One source might report one of these actions and leave the other two out; another source may report two of them and leave the third out; and other sources choose to leave all three of them out. Again, not a case of clear right and wrong, but rather a case of differing priorities over which information to convey. In this text, I have endeavored to be quite comprehensive and present most every action that is recognized as being performed by the muscle being covered. The most important actions of a muscle are presented first in bold and the less important actions are presented last. Where controversy exists as to whether or not a muscle can perform an action, I have tried to present that as well in the miscellaneous section.

When a muscle action is described, it is usually described one of two ways. I will use the biceps brachii to illustrate these two methods.

The most common method is to say the biceps brachii flexes the elbow joint. This tells us that the movement occurs at or about the elbow joint but it does not tell us which body part moved. It will usually be the forearm, but the arm can move at the elbow joint if the forearm is fixed as in when a pull-up is performed. When the arm moves in this circumstance, some sources describe this action as a "reverse action" because the bone that is usually fixed does the moving. (This would be the origin moving instead of the insertion for those who use this terminology.)

The second method is to say that the biceps brachii flexes the forearm. This tells us that the forearm is the body part that is moving but does not tell us at which joint the movement is occurring. It will usually be the elbow joint but the forearm can move at the wrist joint as well. I encourage the student to use both of these methods together: "the biceps brachii flexes the forearm at the elbow joint." This tells us exactly which body part is moving at exactly which joint and avoids all possible confusion!

This book states the actions of a muscle in the action section as simply movement of the body part; the methodology section then describes the action in more detail. There are some cases where the reverse action is explicitly stated, but it usually is not. Be aware that the reverse action of a muscle is always another possible action, even if it is not explicitly stated. (This concept of "reverse actions" is addressed in appendix C on page 702)

MUSCLE INNERVATION

Regarding innervation, information can also vary. A conspicuous example is the spinal nerve contribution to the upper subscapular nerve. One source states that it is comprised of spinal nerve roots C5 and 6, another states it is C4, 5 and 6, another gives it as C5, 6 and 7, and still another gives it as C4, 5, 6 and 7. In this case, it is once again a matter of either different studies being relied upon or different priorities. All of these studies agree that C5 and 6 are part of the upper subscapular nerve. It is a matter of whether or not C4 and/or C7 are mentioned. This is usually because C4 and C7 are minor or inconsistent contributors to this nerve. In this text, innervation are presented in two levels of detail. The first level is a simple presentation. The second level will include spinal nerve root levels and other more detailed information. Where innervation information differs, I have tried to present the information that seems to be most consistently found in the literature.

MUSCLE ARTERIAL SUPPLY

Arterial supply is perhaps the most variable of all. Many sources do not even choose to include arterial supply in muscular anatomy texts because arterial supply varies so widely from individual to individual. An anastomosis may form in an individual that completely changes the main arterial supply to a muscle from one artery to another artery. In this text, I have again presented arterial supply in two tiers of information. The first tier lists the arteries usually considered to be the contributors of a muscle's arterial supply. The second tier includes arteries that are usually considered to be secondary in importance to a muscle's arterial supply. Of the four main categories of information about muscles presented in this book, attachments, actions, innervation and arterial supply, it is arterial supply that must be learned with the most open and flexible mind and a keen recognition that there is rarely one truth that fits every individual.

SUMMARY

One purpose of this discussion is to hopefully clear up what may seem to be contradictions found throughout the field of muscular anatomy and physiology. Another reason is to open the reader's mind to the tremendous variations that can exist in the human form and in human function. And lastly, we must always keep in mind that all the information is not yet in; new studies are continually shedding light on our base of knowledge. I hope that you will approach this subject matter and the material presented within this book with an open and inquisitive mind.

A NOTE REGARDING TERMINOLOGY

Medical terminology or "medicalese" is the language we use when we talk or write about human anatomy and physiology. The terms of medicalese allow us to communicate clearly and specifically and avoid ambiguities and misunderstandings. Although it is a little more work in the beginning to learn this new language, knowing how to use these terms makes life much easier in the mid to long run. If you are new to this field, a short section explaining these terms has been provided in the back of the book (see Appendix K, pages 779-785). I encourage you to embrace this terminology. ☺

Having said that, I unfortunately must also report that in certain cases, there are competing terminologies that are used, which in effect means that there are different versions or dialects of our language. If there is any doubt as to the meaning of any term found in this book, I refer the reader to *The Skeletal System and How Muscles Function*, which clearly defines all the terms used here. Regardless of which term you use in a given situation, please be aware that others may be using a different term to describe the same situation and that clear communication of one's idea is the intended goal.

HOW TO USE THIS BOOK

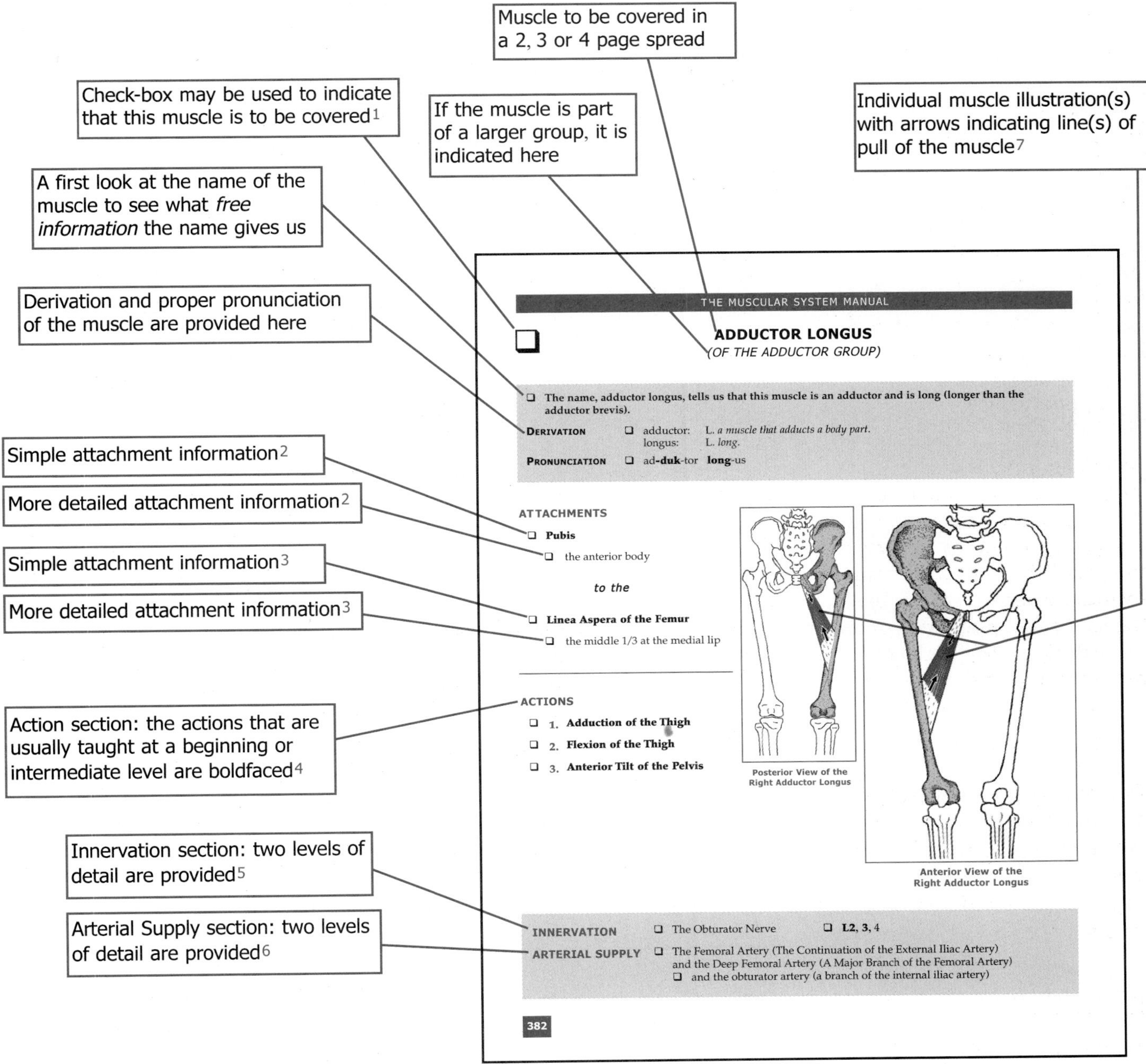

Muscle to be covered in a 2, 3 or 4 page spread
Check-box may be used to indicate that this muscle is to be covered1
If the muscle is part of a larger group, it is indicated here
Individual muscle illustration(s) with arrows indicating line(s) of pull of the muscle7
A first look at the name of the muscle to see what free information the name gives us
Derivation and proper pronunciation of the muscle are provided here
Simple attachment information2
More detailed attachment information2
Simple attachment information3
More detailed attachment information3
Action section: the actions that are usually taught at a beginning or intermediate level are boldfaced4
Innervation section: two levels of detail are provided5
Arterial Supply section: two levels of detail are provided6
THE MUSCULAR SYSTEM MANUAL
ADDUCTOR LONGUS
(OF THE ADDUCTOR GROUP)
The name, adductor longus, tells us that this muscle is an adductor and is long (longer than the adductor brevis).
DERIVATION
adductor: L. a muscle that adducts a body part.
longus: L. long.
PRONUNCIATION
ad-duk-tor long-us
ATTACHMENTS
Pubis
the anterior body
to the
Linea Aspera of the Femur
the middle 1/3 at the medial lip
ACTIONS
1. Adduction of the Thigh
2. Flexion of the Thigh
3. Anterior Tilt of the Pelvis
Posterior View of the Right Adductor Longus
Anterior View of the Right Adductor Longus
INNERVATION
The Obturator Nerve
L2, 3, 4
ARTERIAL SUPPLY
The Femoral Artery (The Continuation of the External Iliac Artery) and the Deep Femoral Artery (A Major Branch of the Femoral Artery)
and the obturator artery (a branch of the internal iliac artery)
382

Notes:

1. Check-boxes can be used throughout the layout for the muscle to indicate information to be covered.
2. For those who use *origin/insertion* terminology, this is the *origin.*
3. For those who use *origin/insertion* terminology, this is the *insertion.*
4. For illustrations of joints actions, see appendix B. For groups of muscles that do these actions, see appendix D.
5. The predominant spinal levels are in bold print.
6. Arterial supply to muscles is extremely variable. Although specific information is provided here, this variability must be kept in mind when learning this material.
7. Any bone attached to by the muscle is stippled and shaded. If a muscle is deep to (behind) a bone from this view, dashed lines are used. There will be a few times in this textbook when an arrow will be drawn with dashed lines. This will indicate that the arrow is deep to (behind) a bone from our view.

HOW TO USE THIS BOOK

Right page header indicates the chapter title

See page XXX refers the reader to the larger and more detailed version of this picture at the beginning of the chapter

Palpation section: easy-to-follow bulleted steps to palpate the muscle[8]

Relationship section: gives information regarding the muscle's anatomical relationship to other musculoskeletal structures

Group illustration depicting the muscle's anatomical relationship to other muscles of the body[11]

Methodology section: explains the reasoning behind each of the muscle's actions[9]

Key: indicating the muscles of this region[12]

Miscellaneous section: miscellaneous information about the muscle is provided[10]

MUSCLES OF THE THIGH

PALPATION AND SUPPLEMENTARY TEXT

PALPATION

- ❑ The adductor longus has the most prominent tendon in the groin region.
  - Have the client supine.
  - Place palpating hand on the proximal anteromedial thigh.
  - Ask the client to actively adduct the thigh at the hip joint and feel for the proximal tendon of the adductor longus. It will be the most prominent tendon in the proximal anteromedial thigh.
  - Once located, follow the adductor longus' tendon proximally toward the pubis.
  - Next, try to follow the adductor longus distally as far as possible. At a certain point, the adductor longus will be posterior (deep) to the sartorius.

see page 352

Anterior View of the Right Thigh (Superficial)

a. Tensor Fasciae Latae
b. Sartorius
c. Rectus Femoris
d. Vastus Lateralis
e. Vastus Medialis
f. Vastus Intermedius (not seen)
g. Pectineus
h. **Adductor Longus**
i. Gracilis
j. Adductor Magnus

RELATIONSHIP TO OTHER MUSCULOSKELETAL STRUCTURES

❑ 1. Much of the adductor longus is superficial in the proximal anteromedial thigh.

❑ 2. The adductor longus is medial to the pectineus and lateral to the gracilis.

❑ 3. From the anterior perspective, the adductor brevis is directly deep to the adductor longus. (The adductor magnus is directly deep to the adductor brevis.)

❑ 4. All three "adductors" attach distally onto the linea aspera. The attachment of the adductor longus on the linea aspera is the most medial of the three adductor muscles.

❑ 5. The vastus medialis attaches onto the medial lip of the linea aspera, medial to the adductor longus.

METHODOLOGY FOR LEARNING MUSCLE ACTIONS

❑ **1. Adduction of the Thigh at the Hip Joint:** The adductor longus crosses the hip joint medially (with its fibers running somewhat horizontally in the frontal plane); therefore, it adducts the thigh at the hip joint.

❑ **2. Flexion of the Thigh at the Hip Joint:** The adductor longus crosses the hip joint anteriorly (with its fibers running vertically in the sagittal plane); therefore, it flexes the thigh at the hip joint.

❑ **3. Anterior Tilt of the Pelvis at the Hip Joint:** With the distal attachment fixed, the adductor longus, by pulling inferiorly on the anterior pelvis, anteriorly tilts the pelvis at the hip joint.

MISCELLANEOUS

❑ 1. The adductor longus has the most prominent proximal tendon in the groin region.

❑ 2. The attachment of the adductor longus at the linea aspera often blends with the attachment of the vastus medialis.

383

Notes:

8. See *Appendix C* for general palpation guidelines.
9. The *Methodology* section numbers correspond to the *Action* section numbers. Further, a more complete description of naming the joint action is given here. For general information on "reverse actions," see appendix C, page 702.
10. Generally, anatomical information is given first, followed by physiological information, then other facts about the muscle are given.
11. Only the muscle of this two-page spread is colored for easy identification.
12. Only muscles of this chapter are labeled and indicated in the key. The name of the featured muscle is in bold print.

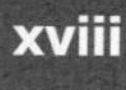

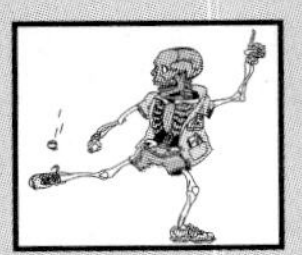

PART ONE – MUSCLES OF THE AXIAL BODY

MUSCLES OF THE HEAD
MUSCLES OF THE NECK
MUSCLES OF THE TRUNK

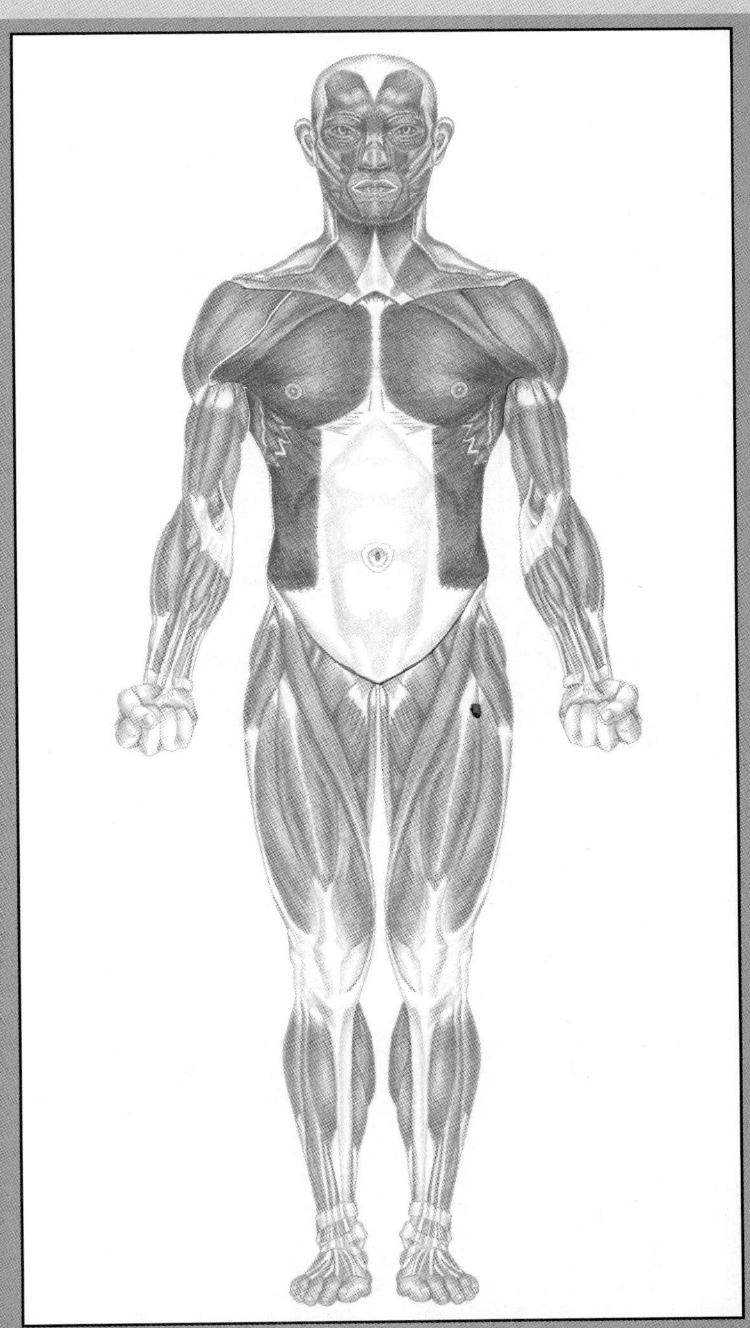

AXIAL BODY

MUSCLES OF THE HEAD

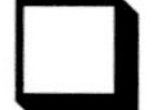

OVERVIEW OF THE MUSCLES OF THE HEAD

ANATOMICALLY, THE MUSCLES OF THE HEAD ARE USUALLY DIVIDED INTO THREE GROUPS:

Muscles of the Scalp:

- Occipitofrontalis
- Temporoparietalis
- Auricularis muscles

Muscles of Facial Expression:

Eye

- Orbicularis Oculi
- Levator Palpebrae Superioris
- Corrugator Supercilii

Nose

- Procerus
- Nasalis
- Depressor Septi Nasi

Mouth

- Levator Labii Superioris Alaeque Nasi
- Levator Labii Superioris
- Zygomaticus Minor
- Zygomaticus Major
- Levator Anguli Oris
- Risorius
- Depressor Anguli Oris
- Depressor Labii Inferioris
- Mentalis
- Buccinator
- Orbicularis Oris

Muscles of Mastication:

- Temporalis
- Masseter
- Lateral Pterygoid
- Medial Pterygoid

THE FOLLOWING MUSCLES ARE COVERED IN OTHER CHAPTERS OF THIS BOOK, BUT ARE ALSO PRESENT IN THE HEAD:

- Trapezius
- Splenius Capitis
- Rectus Capitis Posterior Major
- Rectus Capitis Posterior Minor
- Obliquus Capitis Superior
- Platysma
- Sternocleidomastoid
- Digastric
- Stylohyoid
- Mylohyoid
- Geniohyoid
- Longus Capitis
- Rectus Capitis Anterior
- Rectus Capitis Lateralis
- Erector Spinae
  - Longissimus
  - Spinalis
- Transversospinalis
  - Semispinalis

(Please see Appendix F for other muscles that attach onto the head.)

This is how the muscles of the head are usually classified. Please note the following:

- The muscles of the scalp are thin, sheet-like muscles that are located in the scalp, attaching into or near the galea aponeurotica.
- The muscles of facial expression are thin, small muscles that are primarily located in and attach to the skin and subcutaneous fascia of the face.

- The levator labii superioris alaeque nasi, levator labii superioris and the zygomaticus minor (muscles of facial expression) attach together into the lateral side of the upper lip.
- The zygomaticus major, risorius, depressor anguli oris, levator anguli oris, buccinator and orbicularis oris (muscles of facial expression) attach together into the modiolus. The modiolus is a fibromuscular mass located at the angle (corner) of the mouth.
- The muscles of mastication are muscles that are located in the face and attach onto the mandible.

Functionally, the muscles of the head are located superficially in the fascia and, therefore, move the fascia of the scalp and/or the face. They may also cross the temporomandibular joint (T.M.J.) and move the mandible at the temporomandibular joint. The following general rules regarding actions can be stated for the muscles of the head:

- The muscles of the scalp move the scalp, ears and eyebrows.
- The muscles of facial expression can be subdivided into muscles that move the skin around the eyes, the nose and the mouth. By their actions, these muscles create facial expressions which are important toward transmitting our moods to others.
- The levator labii superioris alaeque nasi is a facial muscle that moves the mouth and the nose.
- Since the muscles of mastication attach onto the mandible, they can move the mandible, which is necessary for chewing, i.e., mastication.

INNERVATION

- The muscles of the scalp are innervated by the facial nerve (CN VII).
- The muscles of facial expression are innervated by the facial nerve (CN VII).
- The muscles of mastication are innervated by the trigeminal nerve (CN V).

ARTERIAL SUPPLY

- The muscles of the scalp receive their arterial supply from branches of the external carotid artery (except the frontalis of the occipitofrontalis, which receives its arterial supply from branches of the internal carotid artery).
- The muscles of facial expression receive their arterial supply from the facial artery.
- The muscles of mastication receive the majority of their arterial supply from the maxillary artery.

A NOTE REGARDING REVERSE ACTIONS

As a rule, this book does not employ the terms "origin" and "insertion." However, it is useful to utilize these terms to describe the concept of "reverse actions." The action section of this book describes the action of a muscle by stating the movement of a body part that is created by a muscle's contraction. The body part that usually moves when a muscle contracts is called the insertion. The methodology section further states at which joint the movement of the insertion occurs. However, the other body part that the muscle attaches to, the origin, can also move at that joint. *This movement can be called the reverse action of the muscle.* Keep in mind that the reverse action of a muscle is always possible. The likelihood that a reverse action will occur is based upon the ability of the insertion to be fixed so that the origin moves (instead of the insertion moving) when the muscle contracts. For more information and examples of reverse actions, see page 702.

❑ ANTERIOR VIEW OF THE BONES AND BONY LANDMARKS OF THE HEAD

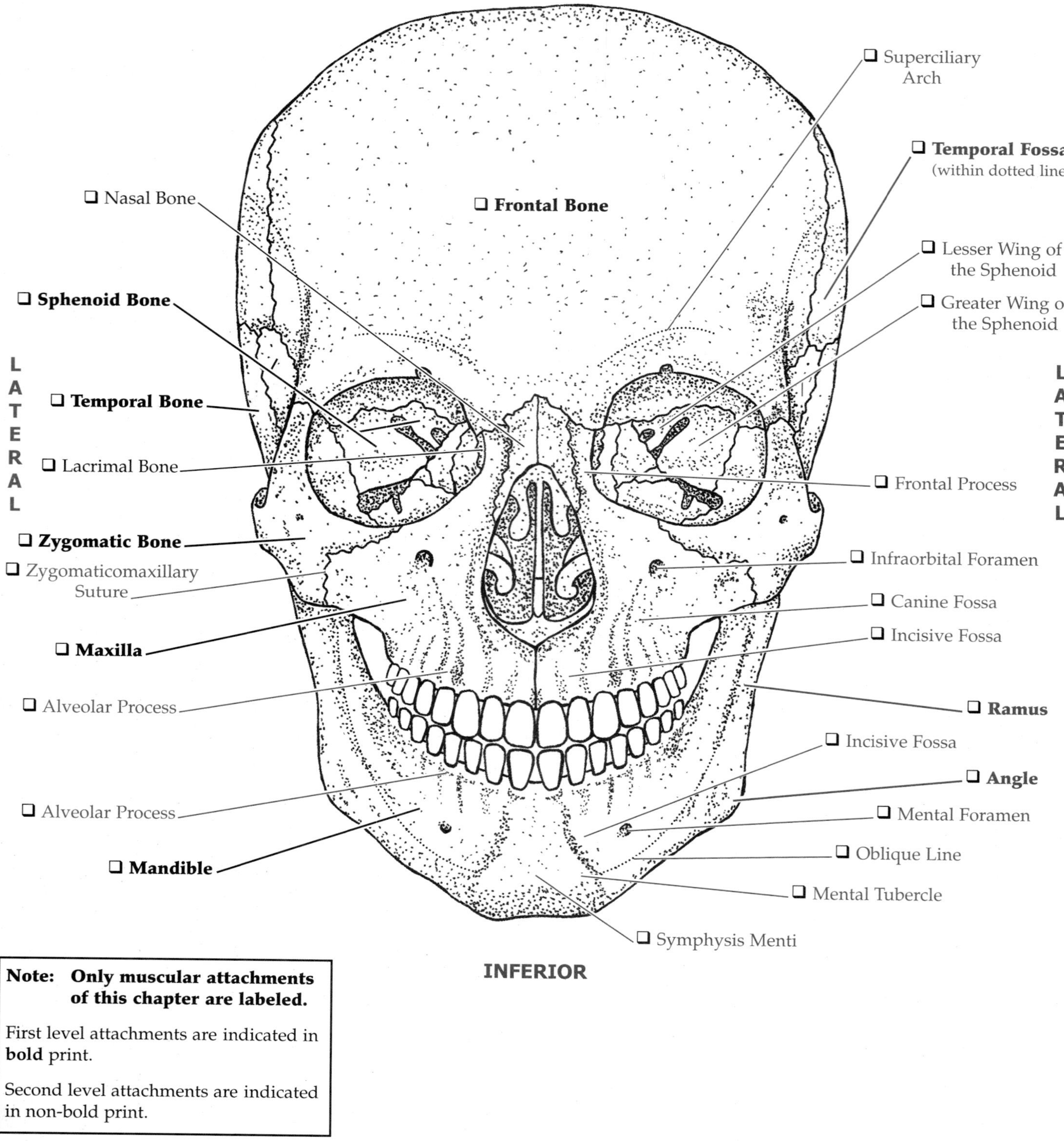

Note: Only muscular attachments of this chapter are labeled.

First level attachments are indicated in **bold** print.

Second level attachments are indicated in non-bold print.

ANTERIOR VIEW OF THE BONY ATTACHMENTS OF THE HEAD 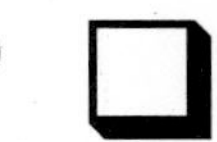

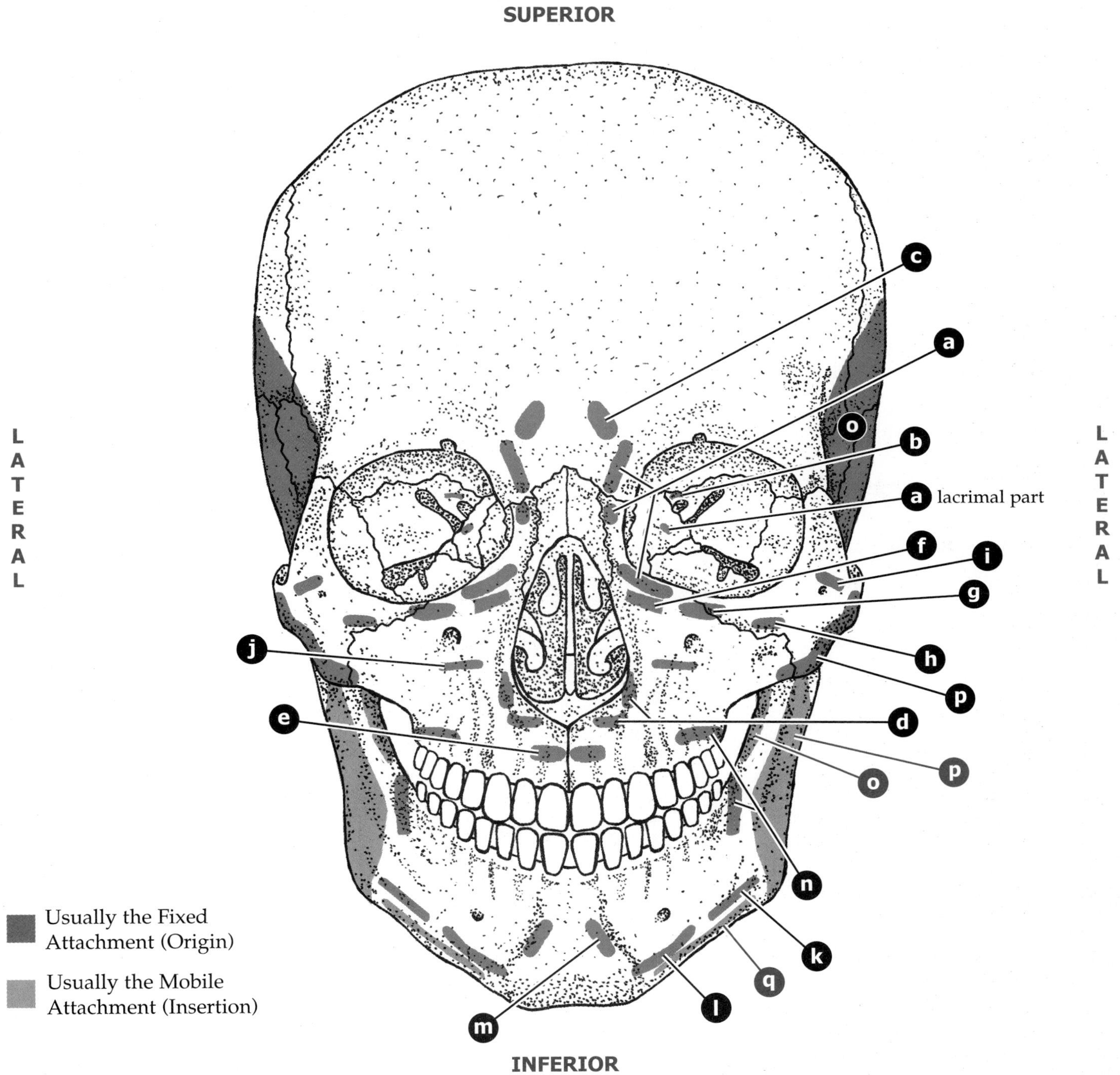

SUPERIOR

LATERAL

LATERAL

a lacrimal part

INFERIOR

Usually the Fixed Attachment (Origin)

Usually the Mobile Attachment (Insertion)

a. **Orbicularis Oculi**
b. **Levator Palpebrae Superioris**
c. **Corrugator Supercilii**
d. **Nasalis**
e. **Depressor Septi Nasi**
f. **Levator Labii Superioris Alaeque Nasi**
g. **Levator Labii Superioris**
h. **Zygomaticus Minor**
i. **Zygomaticus Major**
j. **Levator Anguli Oris**
k. **Depressor Anguli Oris**
l. **Depressor Labii Inferioris**
m. **Mentalis**
n. **Buccinator**
o. **Temporalis**
p. **Masseter**
q. Platysma

❑ LATERAL VIEW OF THE BONES AND BONY LANDMARKS OF THE HEAD

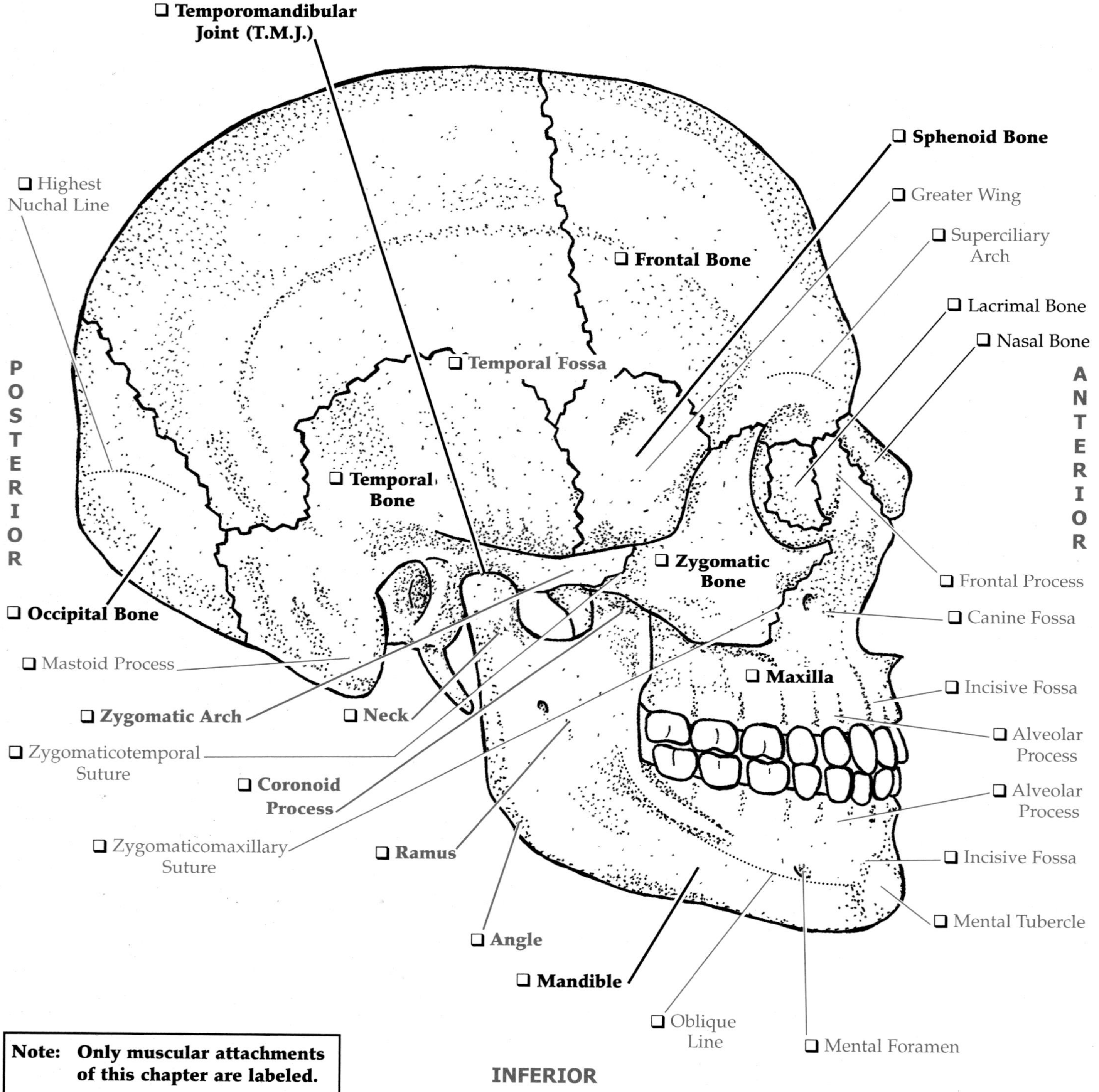

Note: Only muscular attachments of this chapter are labeled.

First level attachments are indicated in **bold** print.

Second level attachments are indicated in non-bold print.

LATERAL VIEW OF THE BONY ATTACHMENTS OF THE HEAD

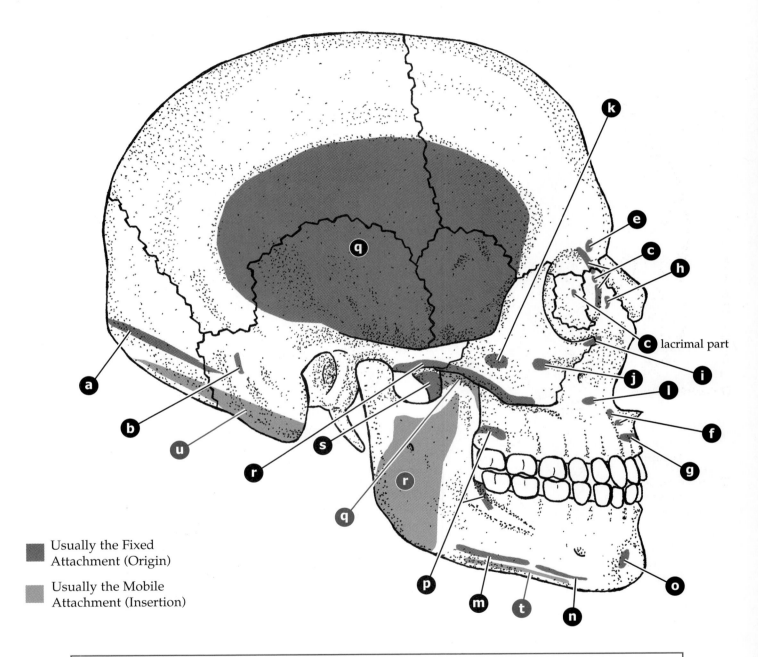

c lacrimal part

Usually the Fixed Attachment (Origin)

Usually the Mobile Attachment (Insertion)

a. Occipitofrontalis
b. Posterior Auricular
c. **Orbicularis Oculi**
d. **Levator Palpebrae Superioris** (not seen)
e. **Corrugator Supercilii**
f. **Nasalis**
g. **Depressor Septi Nasi**
h. **Levator Labii Superioris Alaeque Nasi**
i. **Levator Labii Superioris**
j. **Zygomaticus Minor**
k. **Zygomaticus Major**
l. **Levator Anguli Oris**
m. **Depressor Anguli Oris**
n. **Depressor Labii Inferioris**
o. **Mentalis**
p. **Buccinator**
q. **Temporalis**
r. **Masseter**
s. **Lateral Pterygoid**
t. Platysma
u. Sternocleidomastoid

❑ INFERIOR VIEW OF THE BONES AND BONY LANDMARKS OF THE HEAD

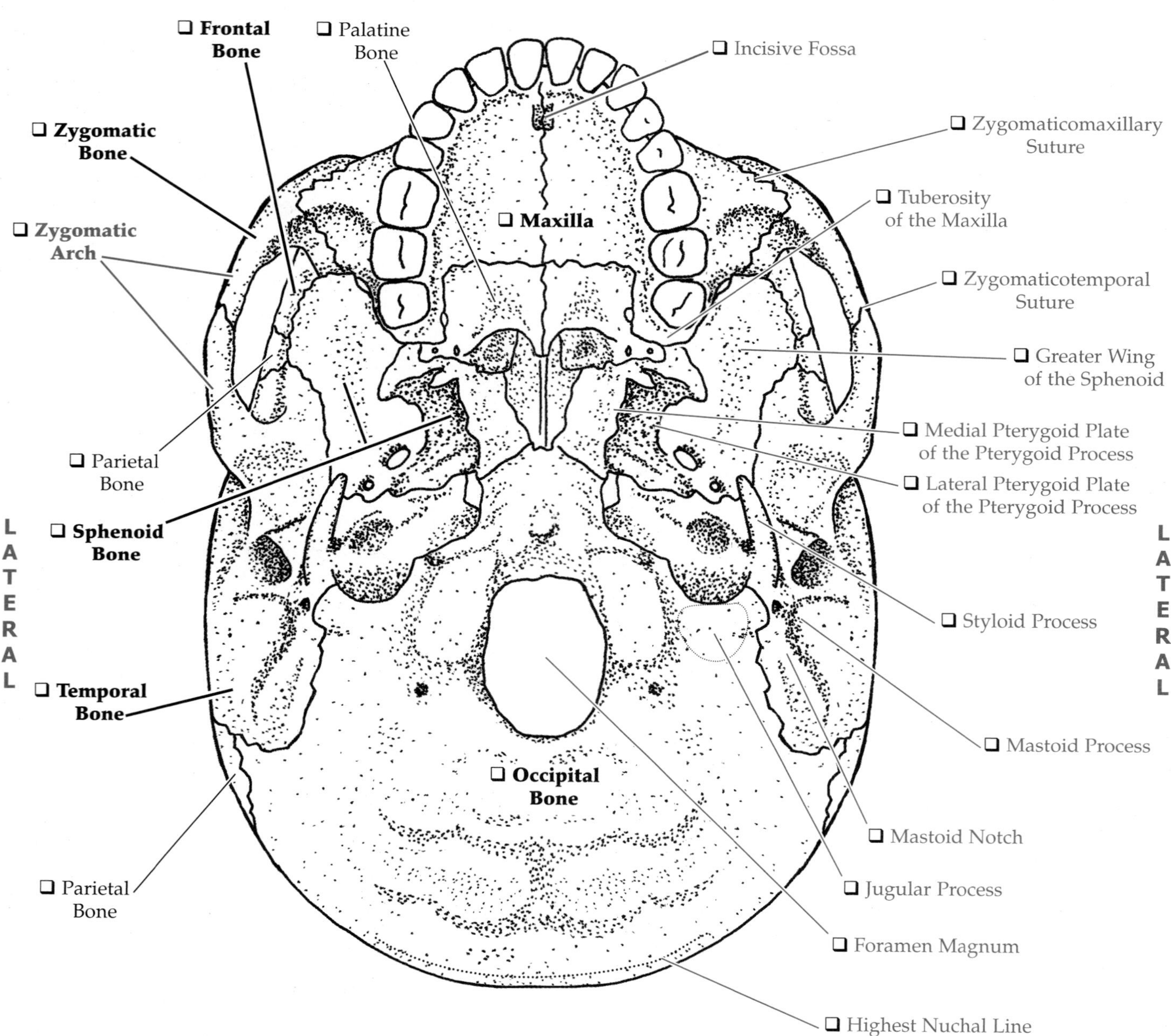

Note: The mandible has been removed.

Note: Only muscular attachments of this chapter are labeled*.

First level attachments are indicated in **bold** print.

Second level attachments are indicated in non-bold print.

*Except the mastoid notch and jugular process, which are attachment sites for the neck chapter.

INFERIOR VIEW OF THE BONY ATTACHMENTS OF THE HEAD

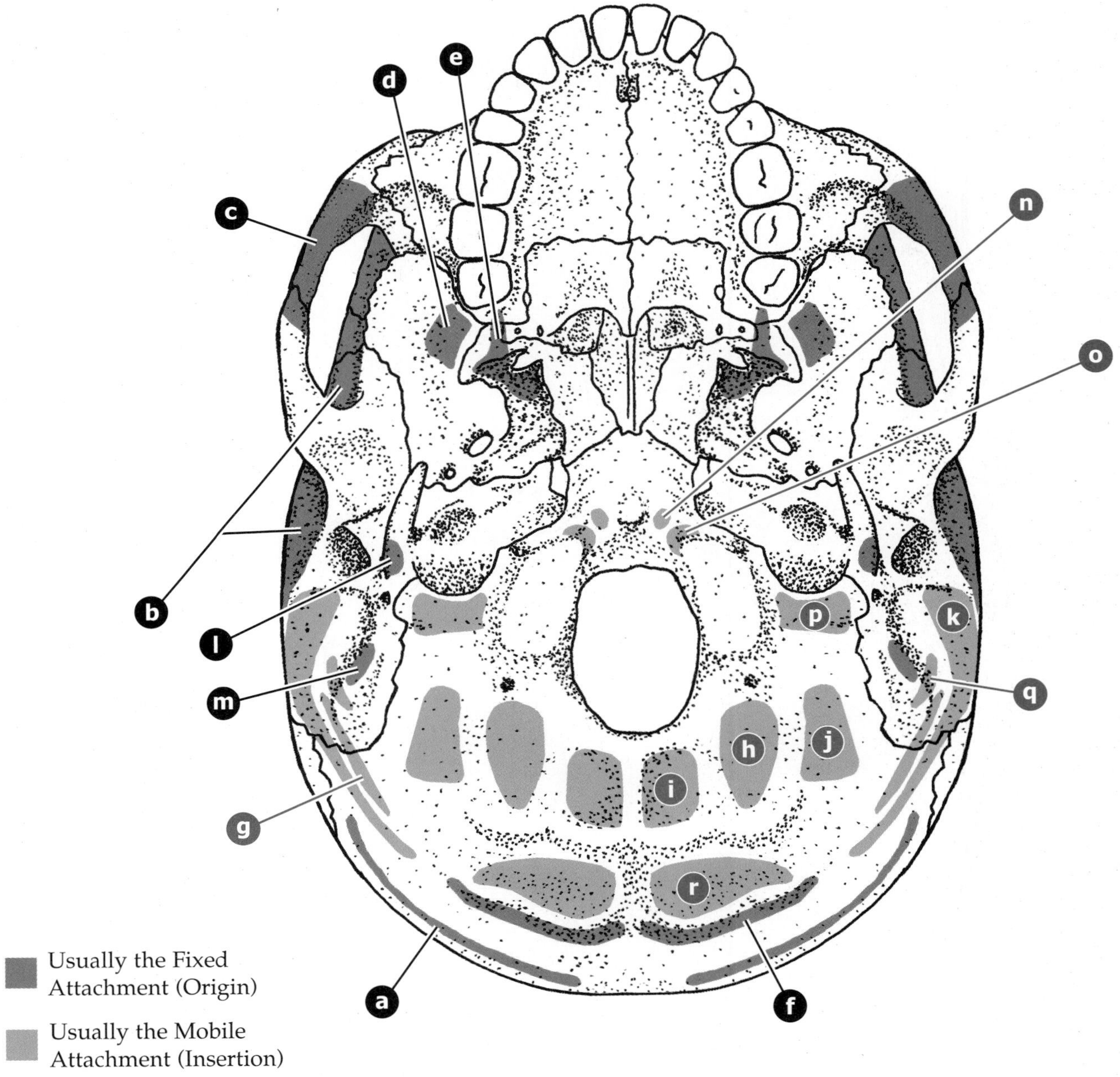

Usually the Fixed Attachment (Origin)

Usually the Mobile Attachment (Insertion)

a. Occipitofrontalis
b. Temporalis
c. Masseter
d. Lateral Pterygoid
e. Medial Pterygoid
f. Trapezius
g. Splenius Capitis
h. Rectus Capitis Posterior Major
i. Rectus Capitis Posterior Minor
j. Obliquus Capitis Superior
k. Sternocleidomastoid
l. Digastric
m. Stylohyoid
n. Longus Capitis
o. Rectus Capitis Anterior
p. Rectus Capitis Lateralis
q. Longissimus (of the Erector Spinae)
r. Semispinalis (of the Transversospinalis)

ANTERIOR VIEW OF THE HEAD

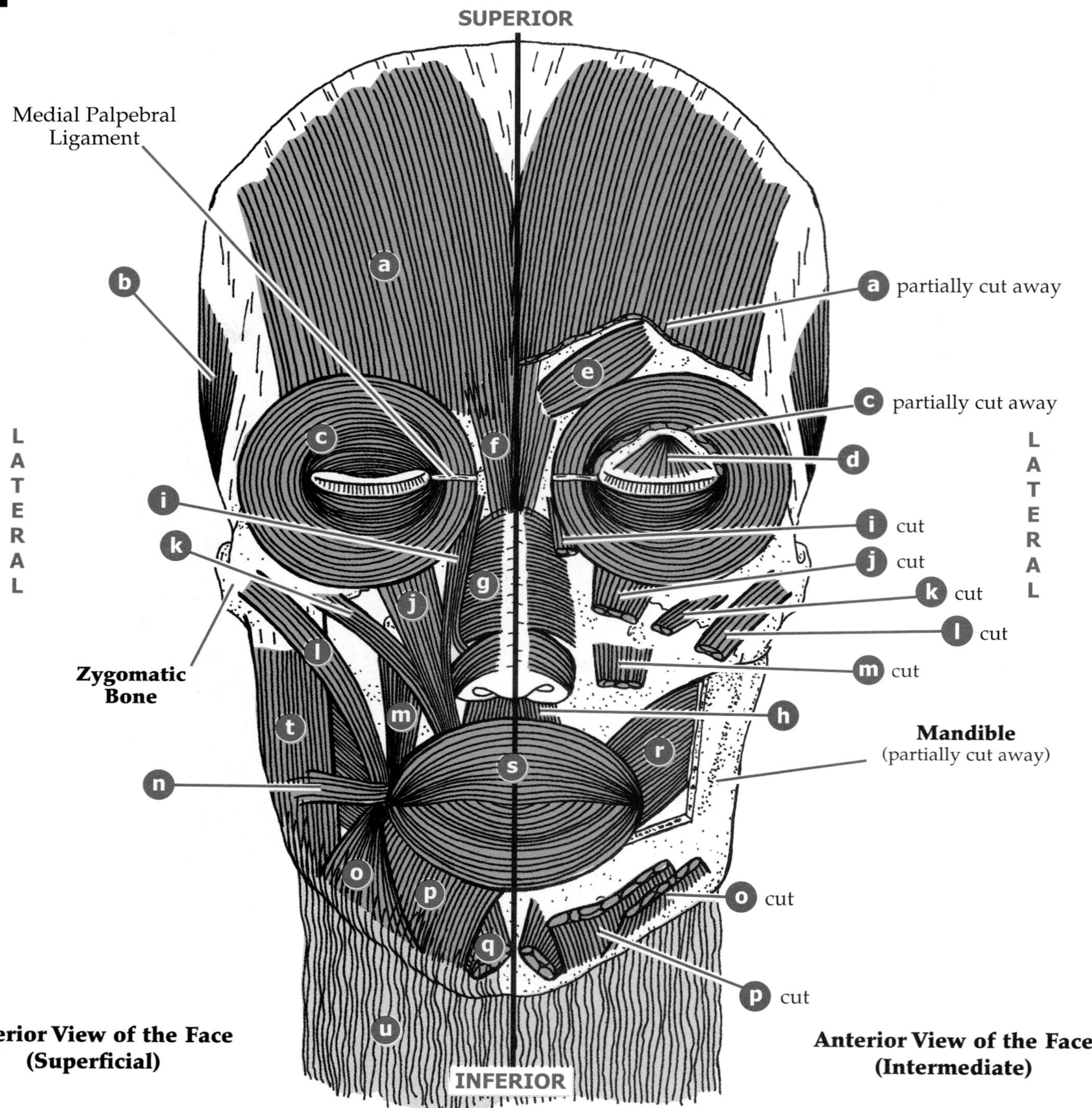

Anterior View of the Face (Superficial)

Anterior View of the Face (Intermediate)

a. **Occipitofrontalis**	j. **Levator Labii Superioris**	s. **Orbicularis Oris**
b. **Temporoparietalis**	k. **Zygomaticus Minor**	t. **Masseter**
c. **Orbicularis Oculi**	l. **Zygomaticus Major**	u. Platysma
d. **Levator Palpebrae Superioris**	m. **Levator Anguli Oris**	
e. **Corrugator Supercilii**	n. **Risorius**	
f. **Procerus**	o. **Depressor Anguli Oris**	
g. **Nasalis**	p. **Depressor Labii Inferioris**	
h. **Depressor Septi Nasi**	q. **Mentalis** (cut)	
i. **Levator Labii Superioris Alaeque Nasi**	r. **Buccinator**	

LATERAL VIEW OF THE HEAD

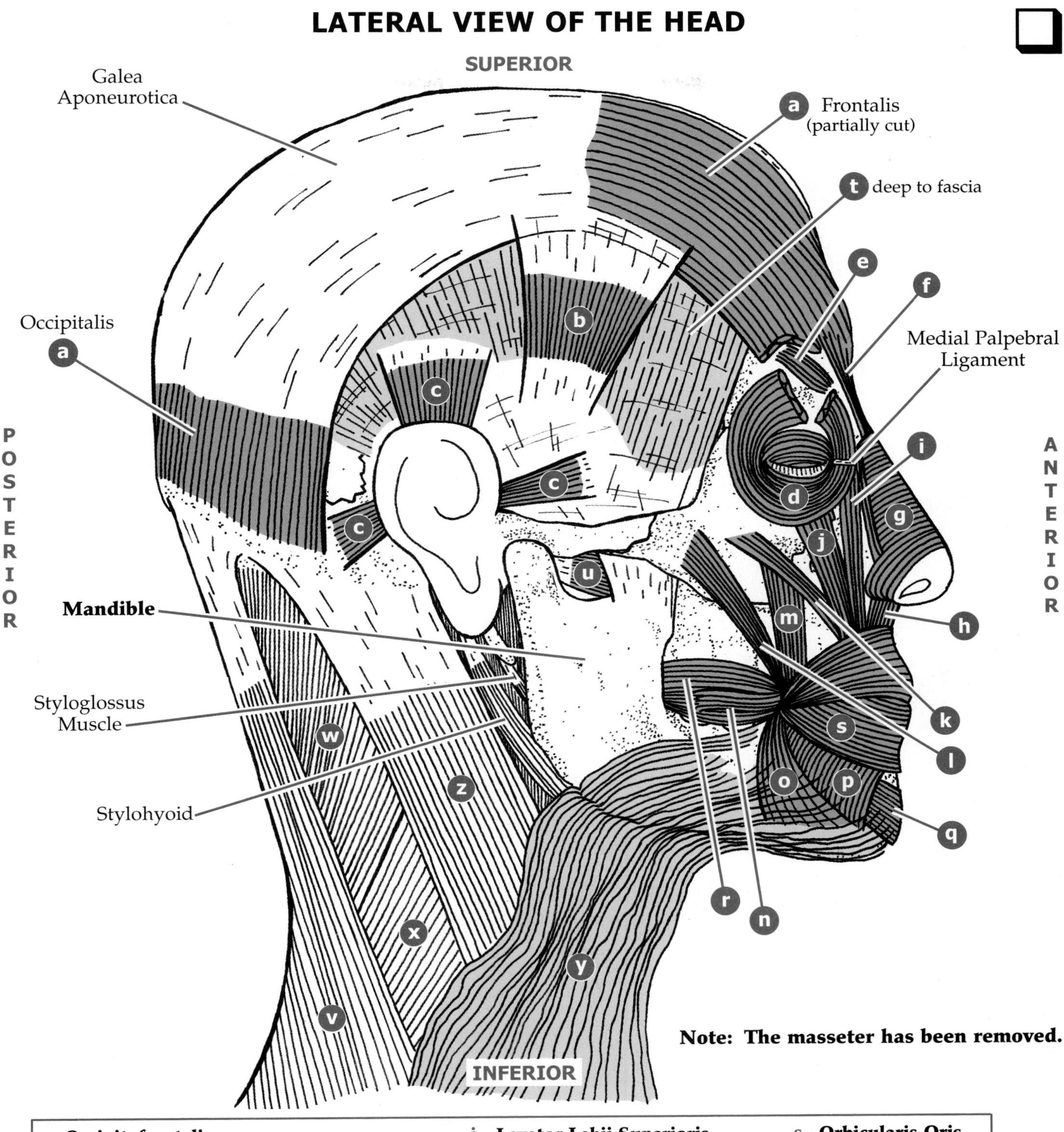

Note: The masseter has been removed.

- a. **Occipitofrontalis**
- b. **Temporoparietalis**
- c. **Auricularis Muscles**
- d. **Orbicularis Oculi** (partially cut)
- e. **Corrugator Supercilii**
- f. **Procerus**
- g. **Nasalis**
- h. **Depressor Septi Nasi**
- i. **Levator Labii Superioris Alaeque Nasi**
- j. **Levator Labii Superioris**
- k. **Zygomaticus Minor**
- l. **Zygomaticus Major**
- m. **Levator Anguli Oris**
- n. **Risorius**
- o. **Depressor Anguli Oris**
- p. **Depressor Labii Inferioris**
- q. **Mentalis** (cut)
- r. **Buccinator**
- s. **Orbicularis Oris**
- t. **Temporalis**
- u. **Lateral Pterygoid**
- v. Trapezius
- w. Splenius Capitis
- x. Levator Scapulae
- y. Platysma
- z. Sternocleidomastoid

❑

OCCIPITOFRONTALIS
(PART OF THE EPICRANIUS)

❑ **The name, occipitofrontalis, tells us that this muscle lies over the occipital and frontal bones.**

DERIVATION ❑ occipitofrontalis: L. *refers to the occiput and the frontal bone.*

PRONUNCIATION ❑ ok-**sip**-i-to-**fron**-ta-lis

ATTACHMENTS

❑ **OCCIPITALIS: Occipital Bone and the Temporal Bone**

- ❑ the lateral 2/3 of the highest nuchal line of the occipital bone and the mastoid area of the temporal bone

❑ **FRONTALIS: Galea Aponeurotica**

to the

❑ **OCCIPITALIS: Galea Aponeurotica**

❑ **FRONTALIS: Fascia and Skin Superior to the Eyes and the Nose**

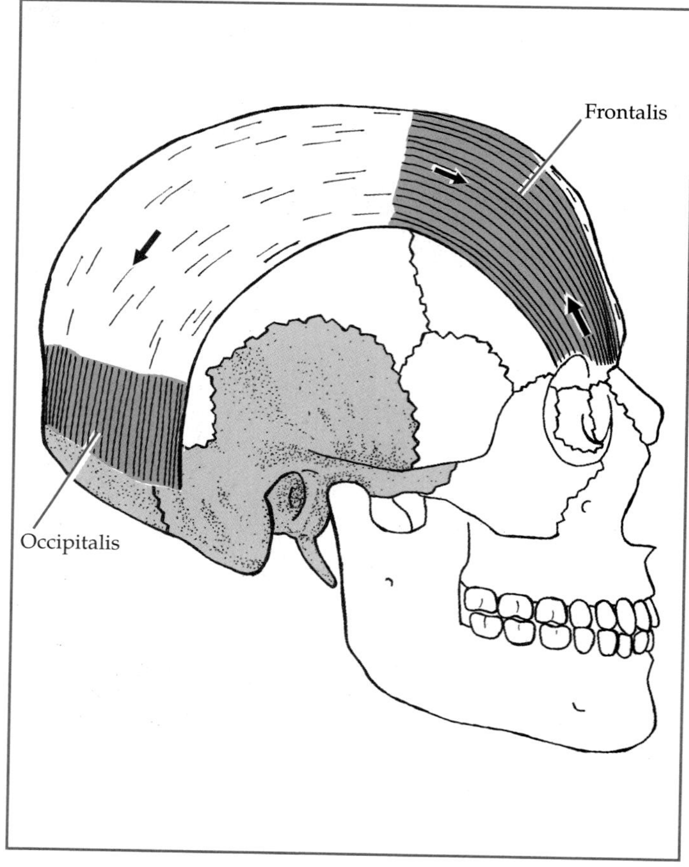

Lateral View of the Right Occipitofrontalis

ACTIONS

❑ 1. **Draws the Scalp Posteriorly (Occipitalis)**

❑ 2. **Draws the Scalp Anteriorly (Frontalis)**

❑ 3. Elevation of the Eyebrows (Frontalis)

INNERVATION ❑ The Facial Nerve (CN VII)
- ❑ occipitalis: posterior auricular branch of the facial nerve
- ❑ frontalis: temporal branches of the facial nerve

ARTERIAL SUPPLY ❑ Occipitalis: The Occipital and Posterior Auricular Arteries (Branches of the External Carotid Artery)
❑ Frontalis: Supraorbital and Supratrochlear Branches of the Ophthalmic Artery (A Branch of the Internal Carotid Artery)

PALPATION AND SUPPLEMENTARY TEXT

PALPATION

- ❑ The occipitofrontalis is superficial in the scalp and easy to palpate.
  - Have the client prone or supine.
  - Place palpating hand over the occipital bone and feel for the occipitalis.
  - Palpate over the frontal bone for the frontalis, and over the parietal bones for the galea aponeurotica.

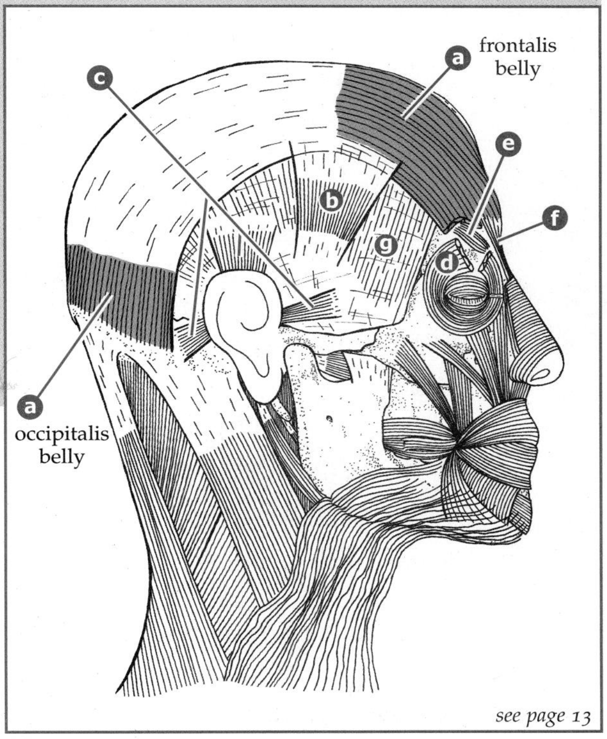

see page 13

Lateral View of the Head

a. **Occipitofrontalis** (partially cut)
b. Temporoparietalis
c. Auricularis Muscles
d. Orbicularis Oculi (partially cut)
e. Corrugator Supercilii
f. Procerus
g. Temporalis (deep to fascia)

RELATIONSHIP TO OTHER MUSCULOSKELETAL STRUCTURES

❑ 1. The occipitalis is directly superior to the most superficial muscles of the neck that attach into the superior nuchal line and the mastoid process, namely, the trapezius and the sternocleidomastoid.

❑ 2. The frontalis is superior to and even blends into the procerus, the corrugator supercilii and the orbicularis oculi.

❑ 3. Lateral to the frontalis and the galea aponeurotica is the temporoparietalis, and deep to that, the temporalis.

METHODOLOGY FOR LEARNING MUSCLE ACTIONS

❑ **1. Draws the Scalp Posteriorly (Occipitalis):** The occipitalis attaches from the occipital and temporal bones posteriorly, to the galea aponeurotica anteriorly. The posterior attachment, which is bone, is more fixed than the anterior attachment, which is soft tissue. Therefore, when the posterior attachment is fixed, and the occipitalis contracts, it pulls the anterior attachment toward the posterior attachment. When this occurs, the galea aponeurotica, and the entire scalp, will move posteriorly.

❑ **2. Draws the Scalp Anteriorly (Frontalis):** The frontalis attaches from the fascia and skin located superior to the eyes and nose anteriorly, to the galea aponeurotica posteriorly. When the anterior attachment is fixed and the frontalis contracts, it pulls the posterior attachment (the galea aponeurotica) toward the anterior attachment. Therefore, the scalp will be drawn anteriorly. When this occurs, the skin of the forehead may also wrinkle.

❑ **3. Elevation of the Eyebrows (Frontalis):** The frontalis attaches from the fascia and skin located superior to the eyes and nose anteriorly, to the galea aponeurotica posteriorly. When the posterior attachment of the frontalis (the galea aponeurotica) is fixed, and the frontalis contracts, it pulls the fascia and skin located superior to the eyes and the nose superiorly. This causes the eyebrows to elevate. When this occurs, the skin of the forehead may also wrinkle.

OCCIPITOFRONTALIS – continued

MISCELLANEOUS

- ❑ 1. The occipitofrontalis can be considered to be two separate muscles: the *occipitalis* and the *frontalis*.
- ❑ 2. The occipitofrontalis attaches into the galea aponeurotica; the temporoparietalis also attaches into the galea aponeurotica. The occipitofrontalis and the temporoparietalis together are known as the *epicranius*. (Note: The galea aponeurotica is also known as the *epicranial aponeurosis*.)
- ❑ 3. The occipitofrontalis is located within the scalp. The scalp consists of five layers: the skin, subcutaneous tissue, the epicranius and its aponeurosis (the galea aponeurotica), loose connective tissue and the pericranium. Of these layers, the skin, the subcutaneous tissue and the galea aponeurotica are firmly connected to each other.
- ❑ 4. The left and right frontalis muscles blend into each other in the midline of the head. The left and right occipitalis muscles usually have a gap between them that is filled in with an extension of the galea aponeurotica.
- ❑ 5. Elevation of the eyebrows often accompanies glancing upwards.
- ❑ 6. Although the occipitofrontalis is listed here as a muscle of the scalp and not as a muscle of facial expression, it is involved in facial expressions. The action of elevating the eyebrows is involved in the expression of surprise, shock, horror, fright or recognition.
- ❑ 7. The occipitofrontalis is often ignored or only worked lightly during bodywork. It is a muscle like any other in the body and moderate or even deeper work may be done to benefit the client. Since *tension headaches* often involve the occipitofrontalis, this muscle should be evaluated in any client complaining of headaches, especially tension headaches.

TEMPOROPARIETALIS
(PART OF THE EPICRANIUS)

❑ **The name, temporoparietalis, tells us that this muscle lies over the temporal and parietal bones.**

DERIVATION ❑ temporoparietalis: L. *refers to the temporal and parietal bones.*

PRONUNCIATION ❑ **tem**-po-ro-pa-**ri**-i-**tal**-is

ATTACHMENTS

❑ **Fascia Superior to the Ear**

to the

❑ **Lateral Border of the Galea Aponeurotica**

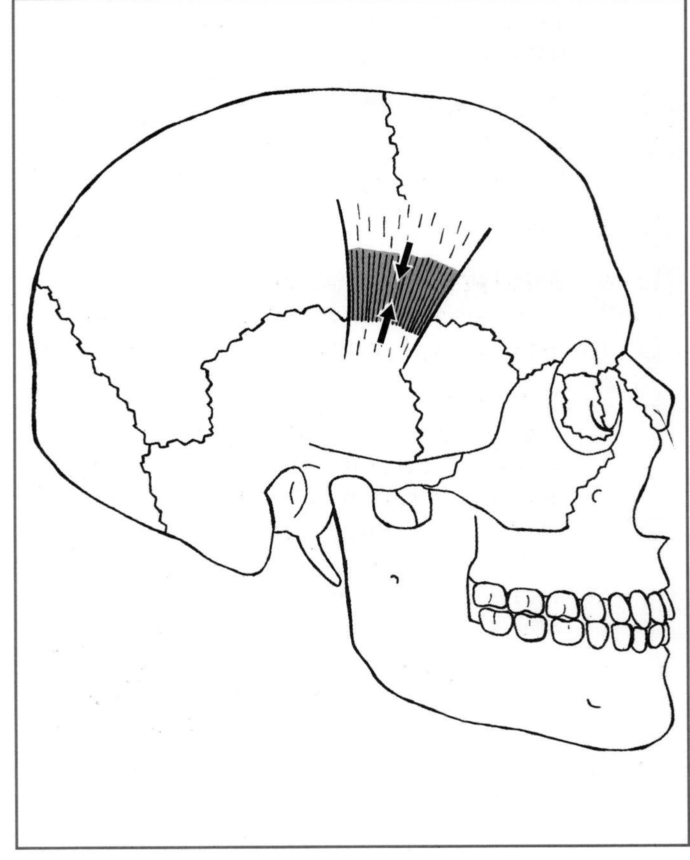

Lateral View of the Right Temporoparietalis

ACTIONS

❑ **1. Elevation of the Ear**

❑ **2.** Tightens the Scalp

INNERVATION ❑ The Facial Nerve (CN VII) ❑ temporal branch

ARTERIAL SUPPLY ❑ The Superficial Temporal and Posterior Auricular Arteries (Branches of the External Carotid Artery)

TEMPOROPARIETALIS – PALPATION AND SUPPLEMENTARY TEXT

PALPATION

- ❑ The temporoparietalis is superficial and palpable in the scalp.
  - Have the client prone or supine.
  - Place palpating hand 1-2 inches superior and slightly anterior to the ear.
  - Ask the client to contract the temporoparietalis to elevate the ear (if they are able to) and feel for the contraction of the temporoparietalis. Be sure that you are superior enough so that you are on the temporoparietalis and not on the auricularis superior (see page 19), which can also elevate the ear.

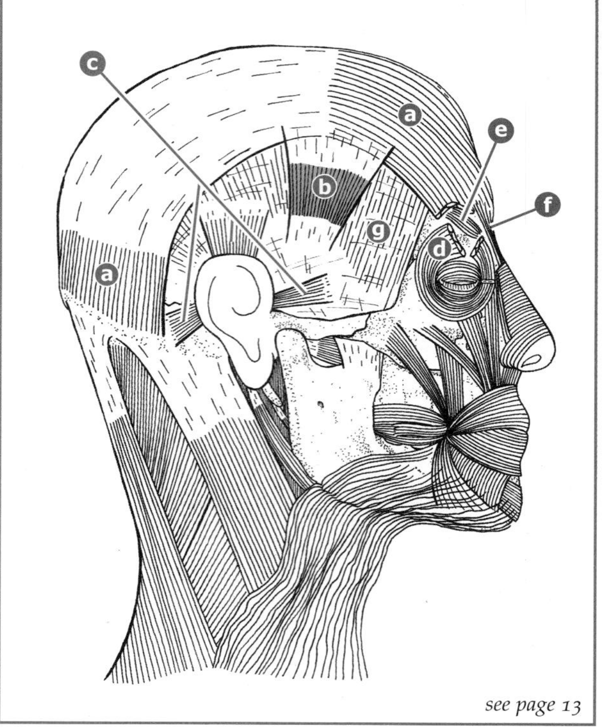

see page 13

Lateral View of Head

a. Occipitofrontalis (partially cut)
b. **Temporoparietalis**
c. Auricularis Muscles
d. Orbicularis Oculi (partially cut)
e. Corrugator Supercilii
f. Procerus
g. Temporalis (deep to fascia)

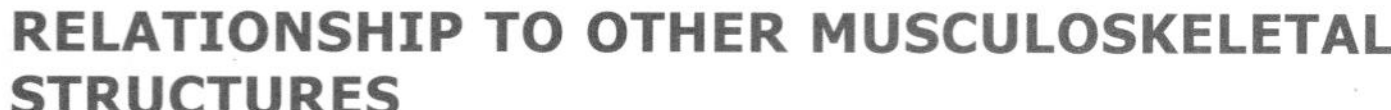

RELATIONSHIP TO OTHER MUSCULOSKELETAL STRUCTURES

- ❑ The temporoparietalis is superficial and lies between the frontalis and the auricularis anterior and auricularis superior.

METHODOLOGY FOR LEARNING MUSCLE ACTIONS

- ❑ **1. Elevation of the Ear:** The temporoparietalis attaches from the fascia superior to the ear inferiorly, to the galea aponeurotica superiorly (with its fibers running vertically). When the temporoparietalis contracts, it pulls the fascia that is superior to the ear superiorly toward the galea aponeurotica, which causes the ear to elevate.
- ❑ **2. Tightens the Scalp:** Since the fibers of the temporoparietalis attach into the galea aponeurotica, when the temporoparietalis contracts, it exerts a pull upon the galea aponeurotica which causes the scalp to tighten.

MISCELLANEOUS

- ❑ 1. The temporoparietalis is located within the scalp. The scalp consists of five layers: the skin, subcutaneous tissue, the epicranius and its aponeurosis (the galea aponeurotica), loose connective tissue and the pericranium. Of these layers, the skin, the subcutaneous tissue and the galea aponeurotica are firmly connected to each other.
- ❑ 2. The temporoparietalis attaches into the galea aponeurotica; the occipitofrontalis also attaches into the galea aponeurotica. The occipitofrontalis and the temporoparietalis together are known as the *epicranius*. (Note: The galea aponeurotica is also known as the *epicranial aponeurosis*.)
- ❑ 3. The degree of development of the temporoparietalis varies. In some individuals, it is very thin; in others, it is non-existent.
- ❑ 4. In addition to the galea aponeurotica, the temporoparietalis often attaches directly into the belly of the frontalis muscle.

AURICULARIS ANTERIOR, SUPERIOR AND POSTERIOR ❑

❑ **The name, auricularis, tells us that these muscles are involved with the ear. Anterior, superior and posterior tells us their location relative to the ear.**

DERIVATION ❑ auricularis: L. *ear.*
anterior: L. *before, in front of.*
superior: L. *upper, higher than.*
posterior. L. *behind, toward the back.*

PRONUNCIATION ❑ aw-**rik**-u-la-ris an-**tee**-ri-or, sue-**pee**-ri-or, pos-**tee**-ri-or

ATTACHMENTS

- ❑ **ANTERIOR: Galea Aponeurotica**
  - ❑ the lateral margin
- ❑ **SUPERIOR: Galea Aponeurotica**
  - ❑ the lateral margin
- ❑ **POSTERIOR: Temporal Bone**
  - ❑ the mastoid area of the temporal bone

to the

- ❑ **ANTERIOR: Anterior Ear**
  - ❑ the spine of the helix
- ❑ **SUPERIOR: Superior Ear**
  - ❑ the superior aspect of the cranial surface
- ❑ **POSTERIOR: Posterior Ear**
  - ❑ the ponticulus of the eminentia conchae

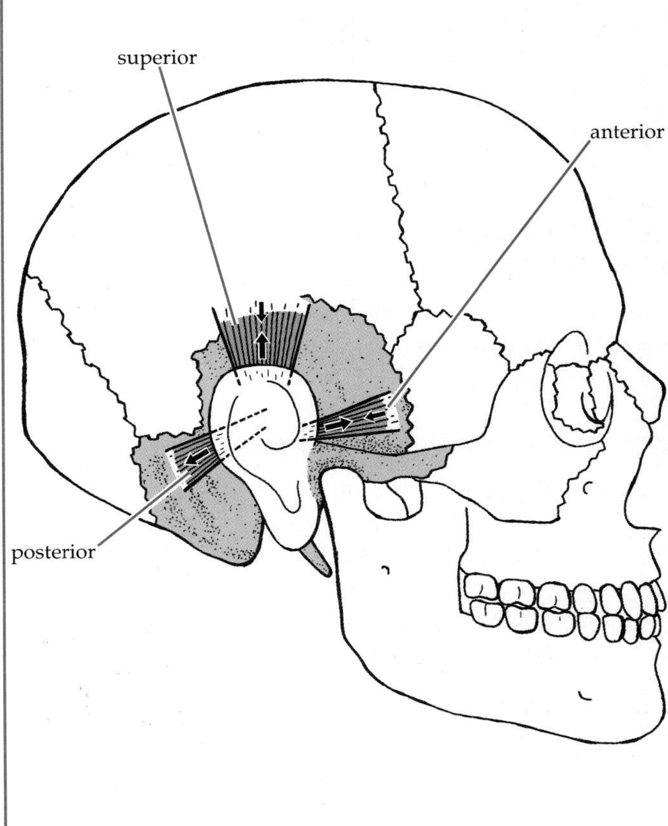

Lateral View of the Right Auricularis Muscles

ACTIONS

- ❑ 1. **Draws the Ear Anteriorly (Auricularis Anterior)**
- ❑ 2. **Elevation of the Ear (Auricularis Superior)**
- ❑ 3. **Draws the Ear Posteriorly (Auricularis Posterior)**
- ❑ 4. Tightens and Moves the Scalp (Auricularis Anterior and Superior)

INNERVATION ❑ The Facial Nerve (CN VII)
❑ auricularis anterior and superior: temporal branches
❑ auricularis posterior: posterior auricular branch

ARTERIAL SUPPLY ❑ The Superficial Temporal and Posterior Auricular Arteries (Branches of the External Carotid Artery)

AURICULARIS ANTERIOR, SUPERIOR AND POSTERIOR PALPATION AND SUPPLEMENTARY TEXT

PALPATION

❑ The auricularis anterior, superior, and posterior are located anterior, superior and posterior to the ear respectively. They are superficial in the scalp and easy to palpate if the client is able to contract them.

- Have the client prone or supine.
- Place palpating fingers directly anterior, superior, or posterior to the ear.
- Ask the client to move the ear anteriorly, posteriorly, or superiorly, palpating in the respective area and feel for the contraction of the corresponding muscle. Keep in mind that many people cannot consciously "will" these muscles to contract.

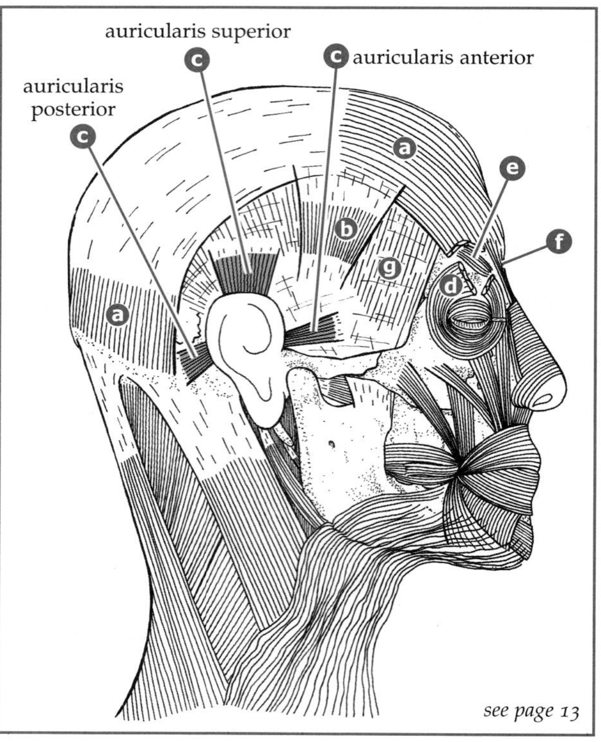

Lateral View of Head

a. Occipitofrontalis (partially cut)
b. Temporoparietalis
c. **Auricularis Muscles**
d. Orbicularis Oculi (partially cut)
e. Corrugator Supercilii
f. Procerus
g. Temporalis (deep to fascia)

RELATIONSHIP TO OTHER MUSCULOSKELETAL STRUCTURES

❑ 1. The auricularis muscles are located superficially in the scalp.

❑ 2. The auricularis anterior and superior are located inferior to the temporoparietalis.

❑ 3. The auricularis posterior is located just superior to the cranial attachment of the sternocleidomastoid.

METHODOLOGY FOR LEARNING MUSCLE ACTIONS

❑ **1. Draws the Ear Anteriorly:** The auricularis anterior attaches from the ear posteriorly, to the galea aponeurotica anteriorly (with its fibers running horizontally). When the auricularis anterior contracts, it pulls the ear toward the more anterior attachment. Therefore, the auricularis anterior draws the ear anteriorly.

❑ **2. Elevation of the Ear:** The auricularis superior attaches from the ear inferiorly, to the galea aponeurotica superiorly (with its fibers running vertically). When the auricularis superior contracts, it pulls the ear toward the more superior attachment; therefore, the auricularis superior elevates the ear. (Note: The auricularis anterior also has a slight vertical orientation to its fibers and therefore, it can also help to elevate the ear.)

❑ **3. Draws the Ear Posteriorly:** The auricularis posterior attaches from the ear anteriorly, to the temporal bone posteriorly (with its fibers running horizontally). When the auricularis posterior contracts, it pulls the ear toward the more posterior attachment. Therefore, the auricularis posterior draws the ear posteriorly.

AURICULARIS ANTERIOR, SUPERIOR AND POSTERIOR – continued

- ❑ **4. Tightens and Moves the Scalp:** If the auricular (ear) attachment is more fixed, the auricularis anterior and superior could pull on the galea aponeurotica, thereby tightening and moving the scalp.

MISCELLANEOUS

- ❑ 1. The auricularis anterior is the smallest of the three auricular muscles; the auricularis superior is the largest.
- ❑ 2. One, two or all three of the auricularis muscles are nonfunctional in many people.
- ❑ 3. The spine of the helix is the cartilage in the helix of the ear.
- ❑ 4. The eminentia conchae is the cartilage in the concha of the ear, which forms an eminence on the cranial surface of the ear. The ponticulus of the eminentia conchae is a ridge found on the eminentia conchae that is the attachment site for the posterior auricular muscle.

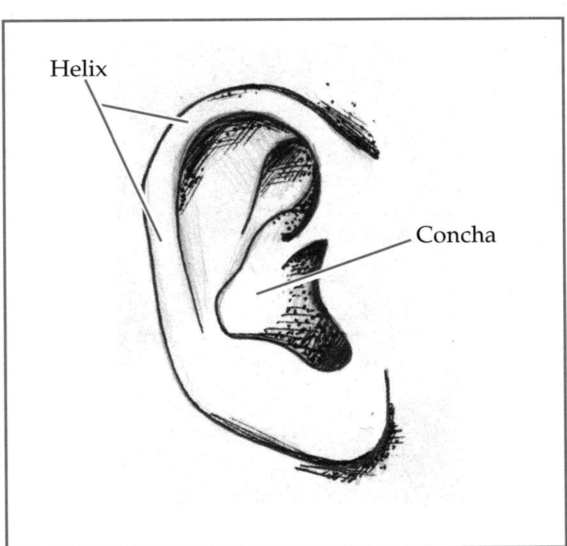

Lateral View of the Right Ear

THE MUSCLES OF FACIAL EXPRESSION

THE MUSCLES OF FACIAL EXPRESSION CAN BE SUBDIVIDED INTO THREE GROUPS:		
Muscles of the Eye: Levator Palpebrae Superioris Corrugator Supercilii Orbicularis Oculi **Muscles of the Nose:** Procerus Nasalis Depressor Septi Nasi	**Muscles of the Mouth:** Levator Labii Superioris Alaeque Nasi Levator Labii Superioris Zygomatic Minor Zygomatic Major Levator Anguli Oris Risorius Depressor Anguli Oris Depressor Labii Inferioris	 Mentalis Buccinator Orbicularis Oris

Attachments:

- The orbicularis oris encircles the mouth. All the other muscles of the mouth radiate out from the mouth like spokes of a wheel.
- The modiolus is a fibromuscular condensation approximately 1/4 inch (1/2 cm) lateral to the angle of the mouth. Six muscles of the mouth attach into the modiolus: zygomaticus major, levator anguli oris, risorius, depressor anguli oris, buccinator and the orbicularis oris.

Actions:

- The levator labii superioris alaeque nasi, levator labii superioris, levator anguli oris, and the zygomaticus minor and major all elevate the upper lip.
- The zygomaticus minor, zygomaticus major, risorius, depressor anguli oris and the depressor labii inferioris all draw the lip(s) and/or the angle (corner) of the mouth laterally.
- The depressor anguli oris, depressor labii inferioris and the mentalis all depress the lower lip.
- All the facial muscles move the fascia and/or skin of the face. Therefore, they all contribute to facial expressions, which are important for displaying emotions. Although there is certainly some universality of facial expressions expressing emotions, there can be variations from one culture to another. Further, many of these muscles may act in concert with others to add to the spectrum of facial expressions displayed.

Miscellaneous:

- The frontalis of the occipitofrontalis of the cranium is also involved with facial expression.
- The levator labii superioris alaeque nasi is a muscle of both the mouth and the nose.

INNERVATION The facial muscles (except the levator palpebrae superioris) are innervated by the facial nerve (CN VII).

♥ ARTERIAL SUPPLY The muscles of facial expression receive the majority of their arterial supply from the facial artery.

VIEWS OF THE MUSCLES OF FACIAL EXPRESSION

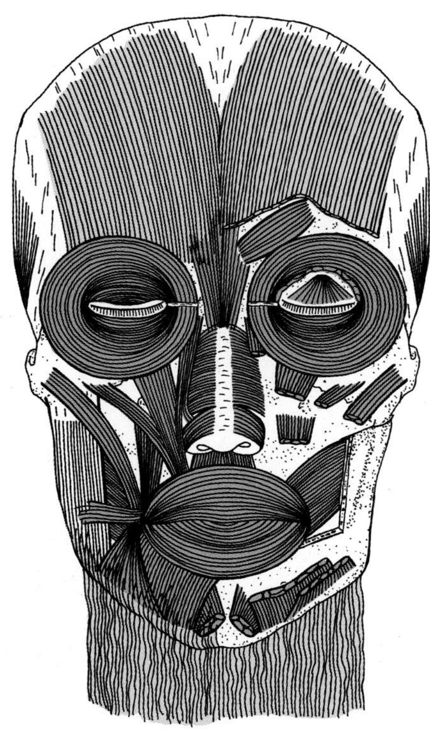

Anterior View of the Muscles of Facial Expression
(superficial on our left; intermediate on our right)
(see page 12)

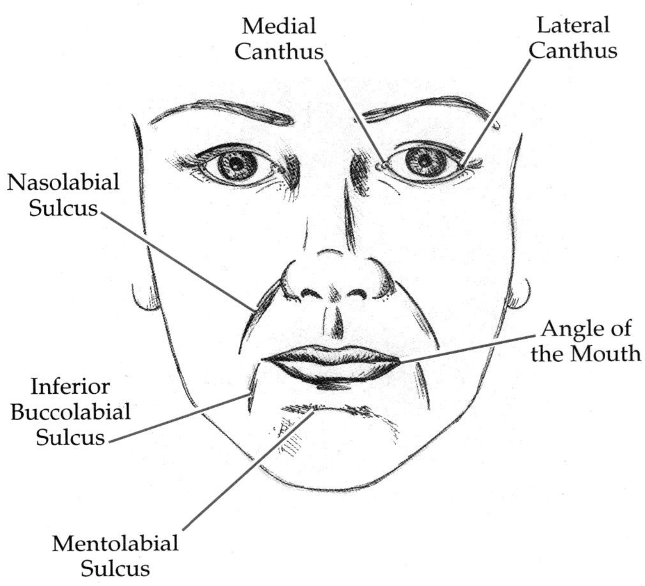

Anterior View of the Face

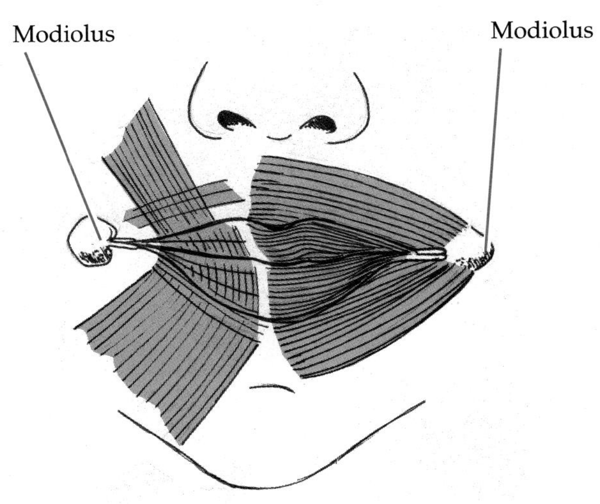

Anterior View of the Modiolus
(with and without orbicularis oris attached)

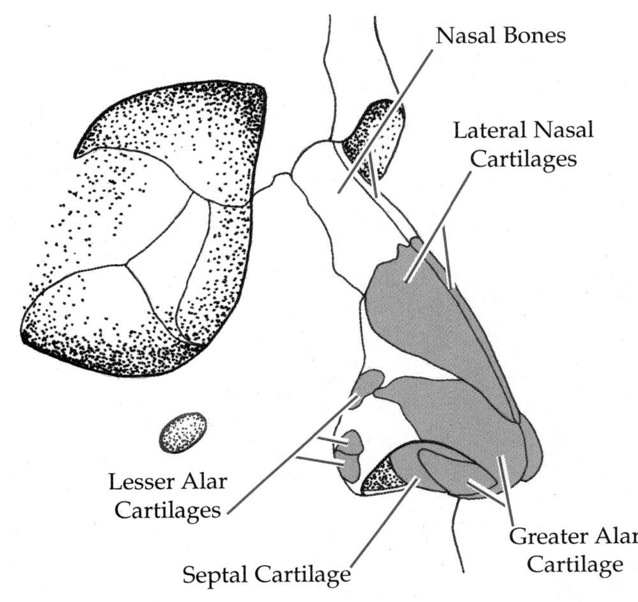

Anterolateral View of the Nose

FACIAL EXPRESSIONS CREATED BY THEIR CORRESPONDING MUSCLES

❑ ORBICULARIS OCULI

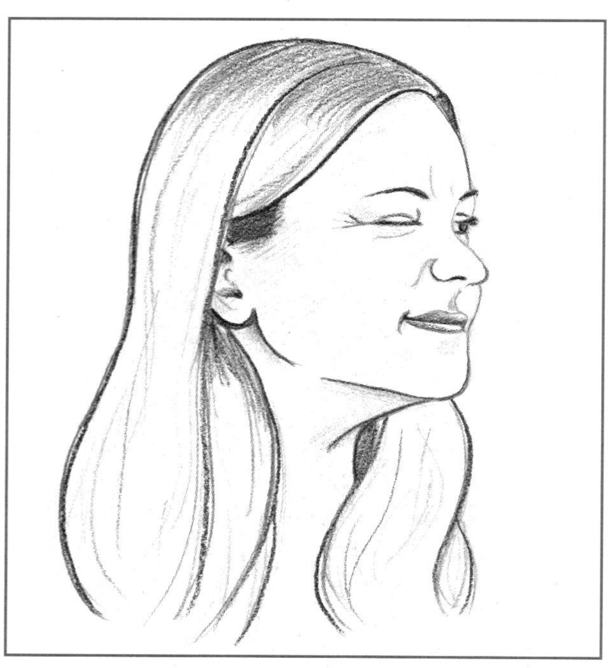

1. **Closes and Squints the Eye**
2. **Depression of the Upper Eyelid**
3. **Elevation of the Lower Eyelid**

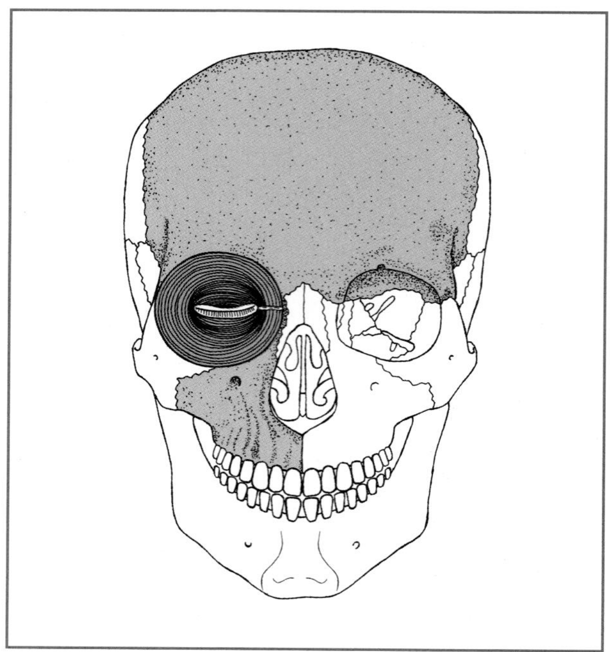

Anterior View of the Right Orbicularis Oculi

❑ LEVATOR PALPEBRAE SUPERIORIS

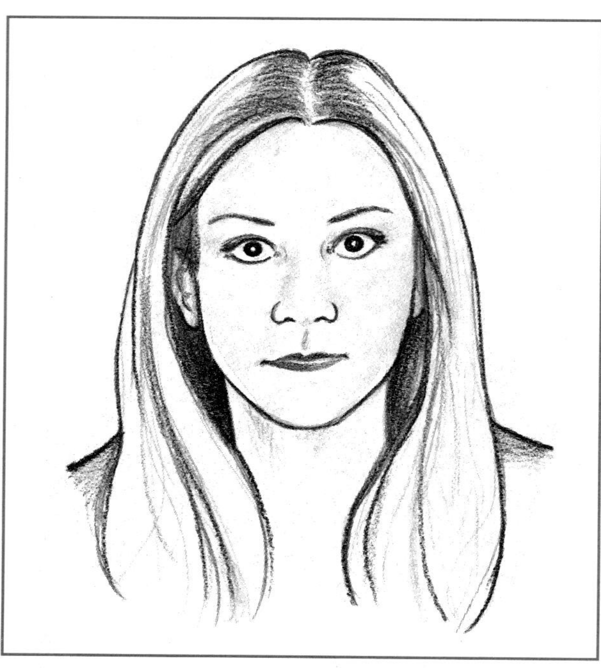

Elevation of the Upper Eyelid

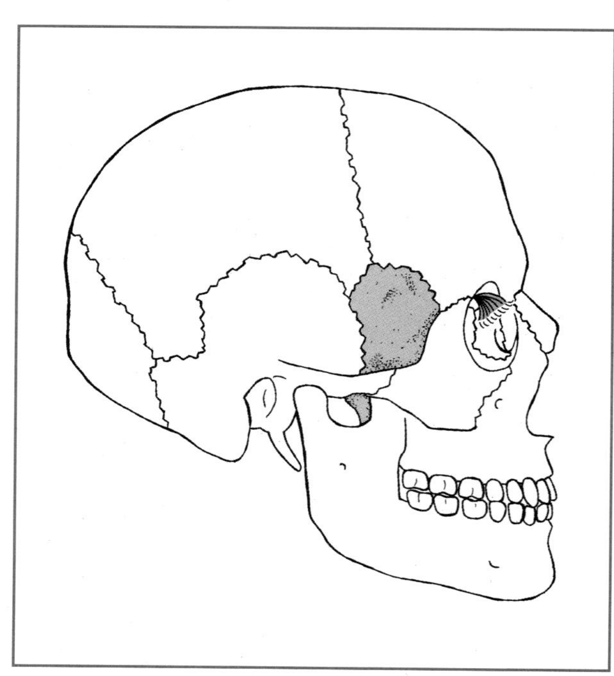

Lateral View of the Right Levator Palpebrae Superioris

FACIAL EXPRESSIONS CREATED BY THEIR CORRESPONDING MUSCLES

❑ CORRUGATOR SUPERCILII

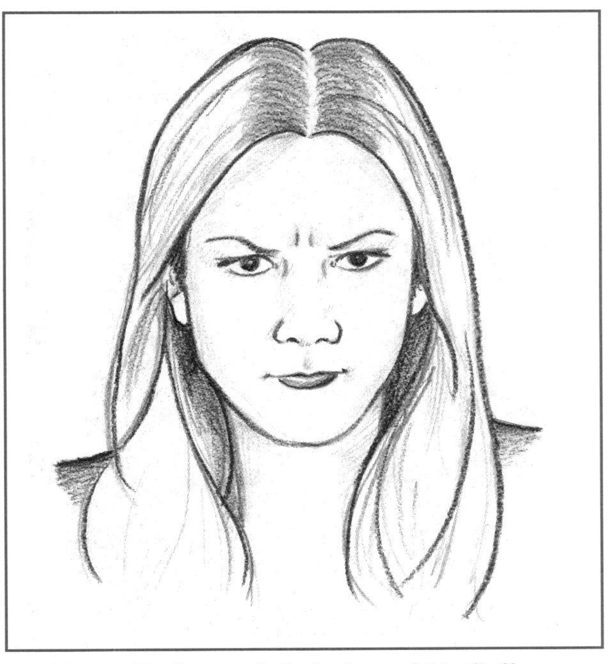

Draws Eyebrows Inferiorly and Medially

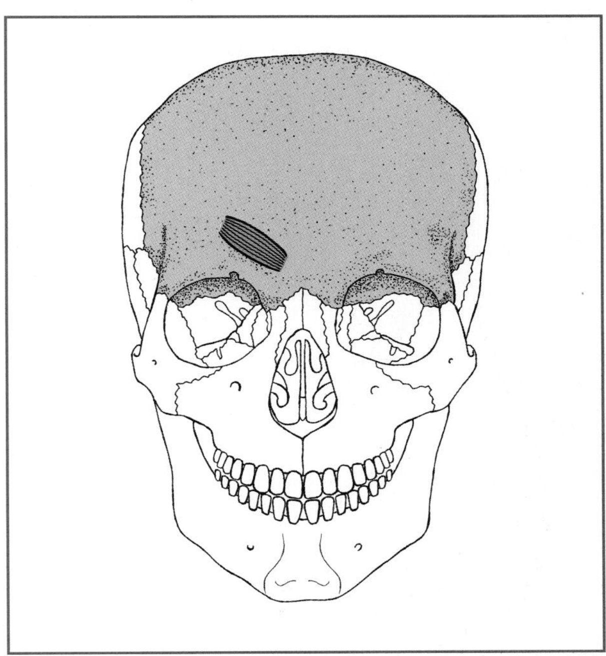

Anterior View of the Right Corrugator Supercilii

❑ PROCERUS

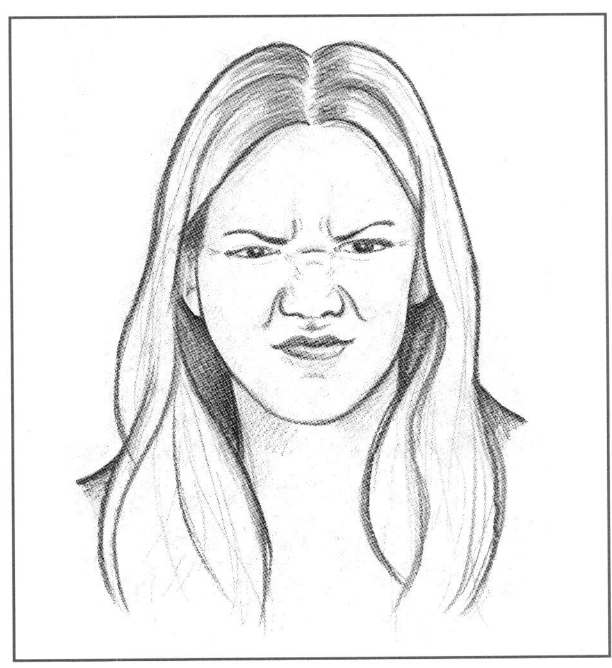

1. **Draws Down the Medial Eyebrows**
2. **Wrinkles the Skin of the Nose**

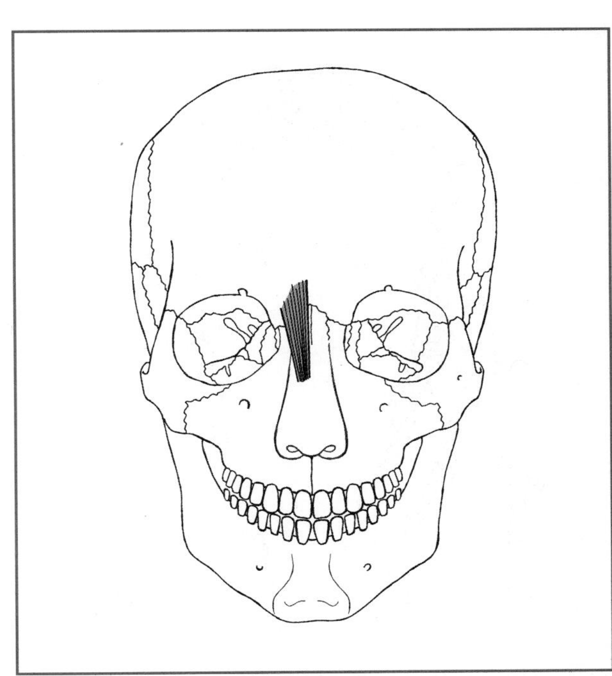

Anterior View of the Right Procerus

FACIAL EXPRESSIONS CREATED BY THEIR CORRESPONDING MUSCLES

❑ NASALIS

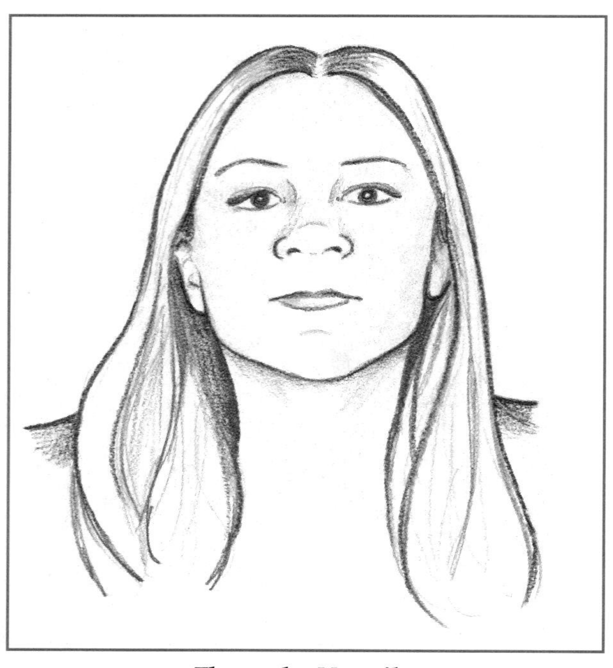

Flares the Nostril

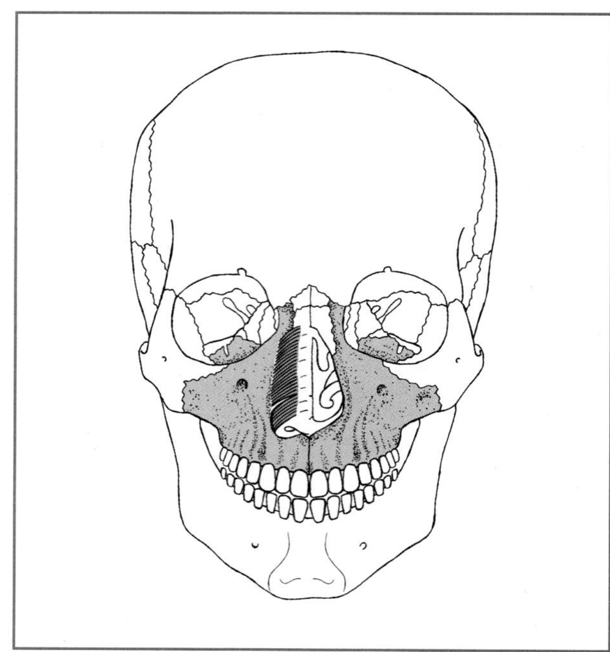

Anterior View of the Right Nasalis

❑ DEPRESSOR SEPTI NASI

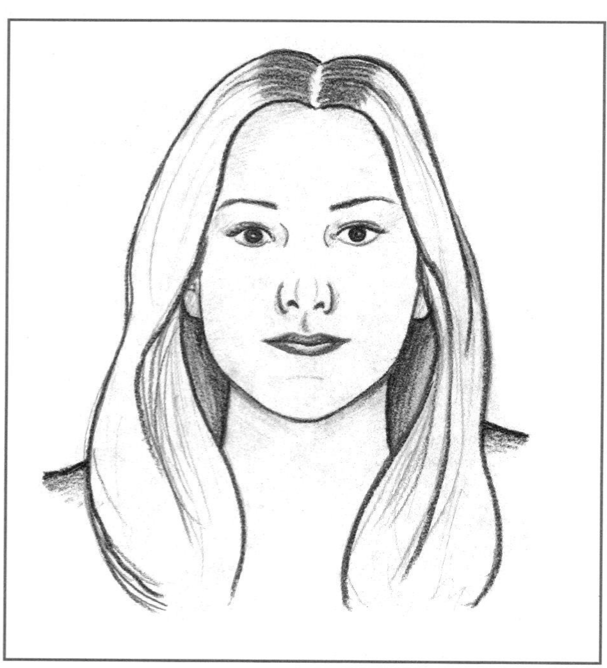

Constricts the Nostril

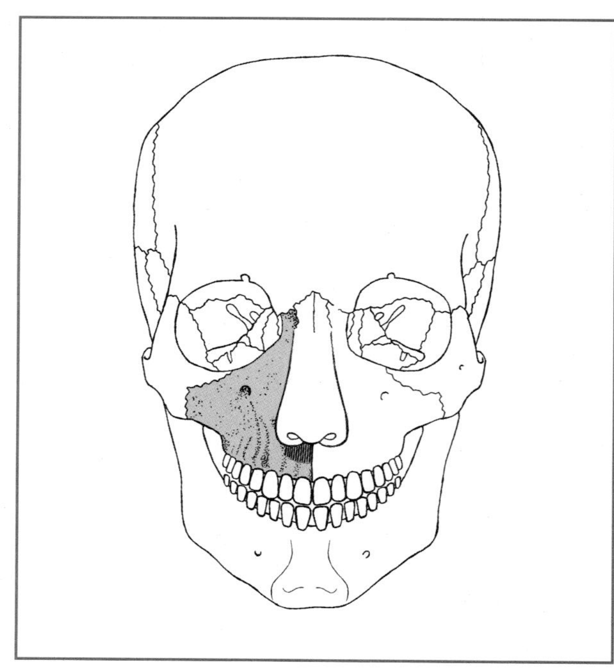

Anterior View of the Right Depressor Septi Nasi

FACIAL EXPRESSIONS CREATED BY THEIR CORRESPONDING MUSCLES

❑ LEVATOR LABII SUPERIORIS ALAEQUE NASI

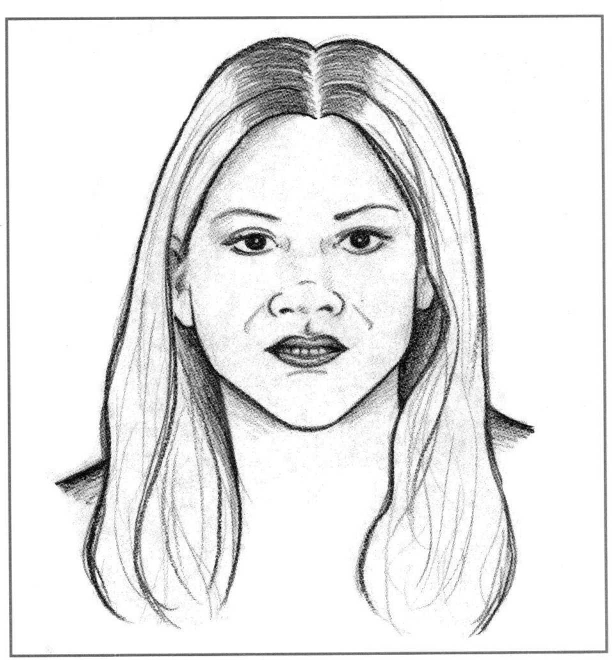

1. **Elevation of the Upper Lip**
2. **Eversion of the Upper Lip**
3. **Flares the Nostril**

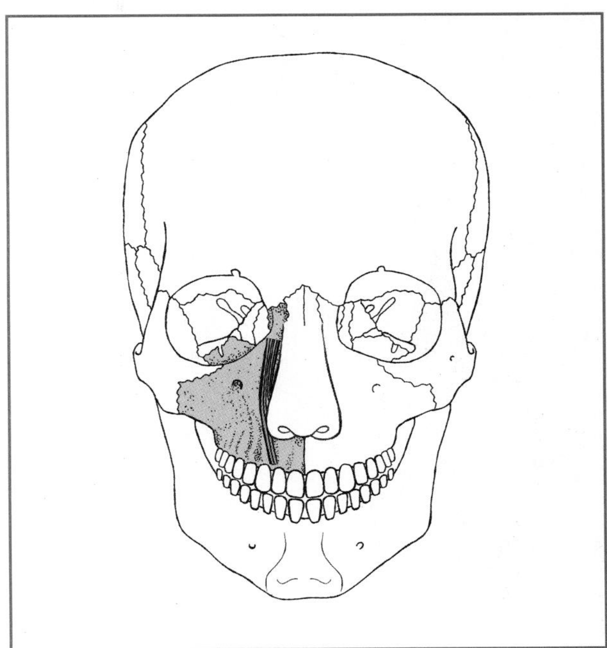

Anterior View of the Right Levator Labii Superioris Alaeque Nasi

---

❑ LEVATOR LABII SUPERIORIS

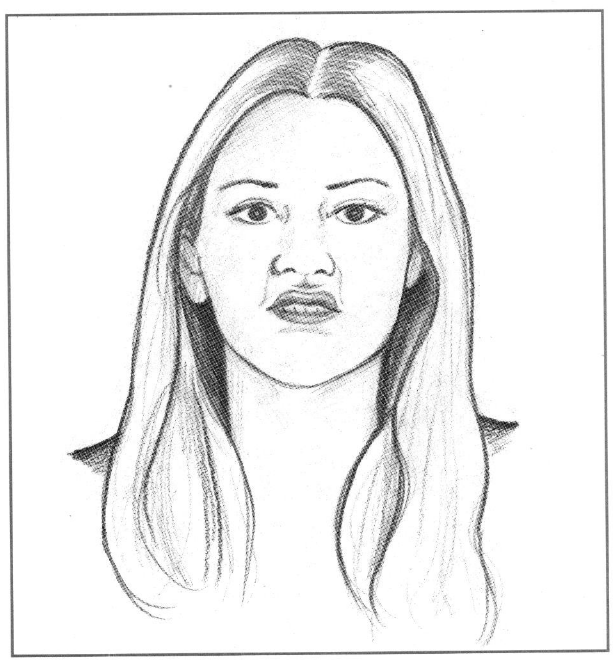

1. **Elevation of the Upper Lip**
2. **Eversion of the Upper Lip**

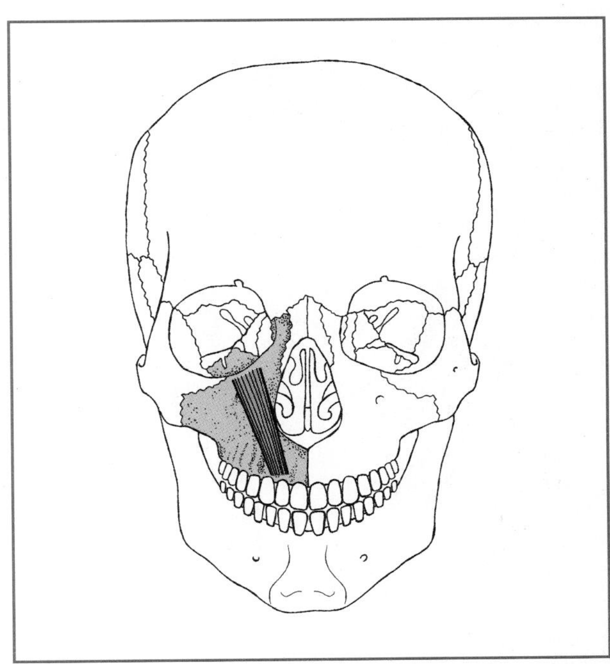

Anterior View of the Right Levator Labii Superioris

FACIAL EXPRESSIONS CREATED BY THEIR CORRESPONDING MUSCLES

❑ ZYGOMATICUS MINOR

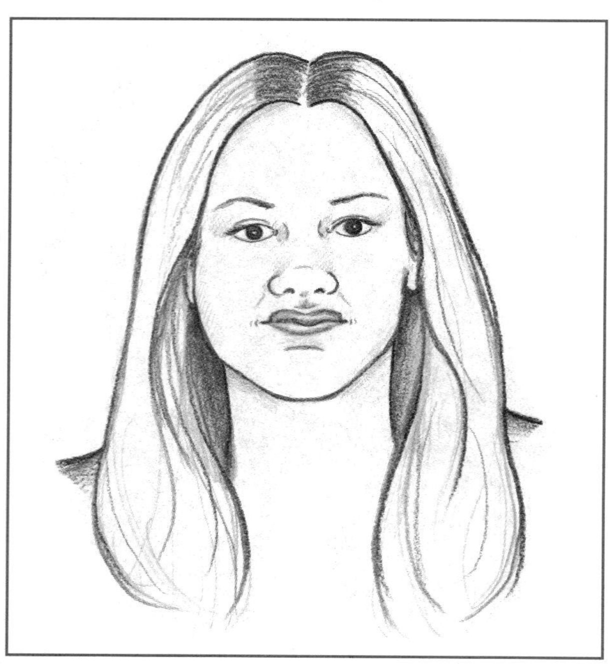

1. **Elevation of the Upper Lip**
2. **Eversion of the Upper Lip**

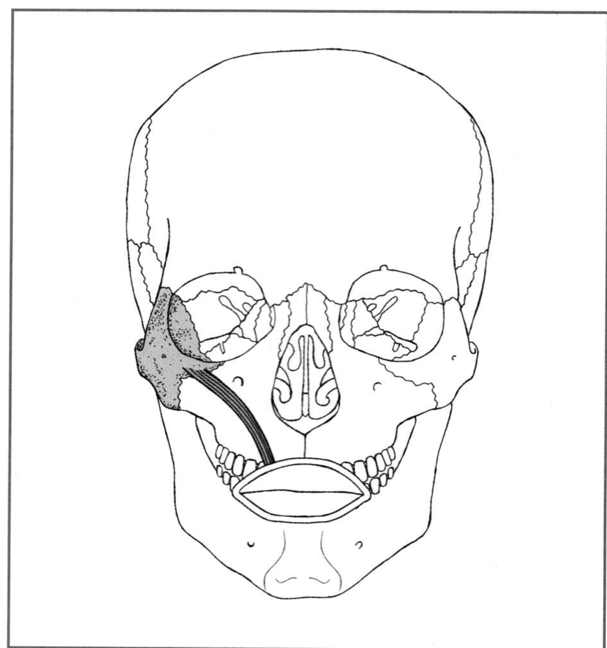

Anterior View of the Right Zygomaticus Minor

❑ ZYGOMATICUS MAJOR

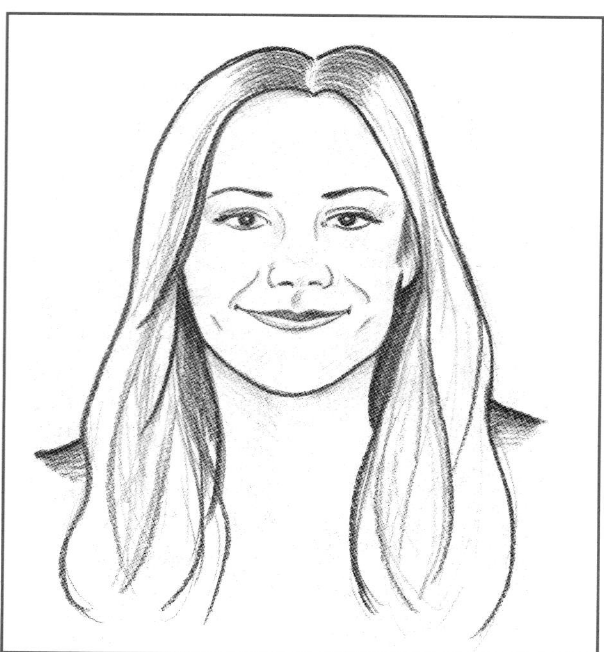

1. **Elevation of the Angle of the Mouth**
2. **Draws Laterally the Angle of the Mouth**

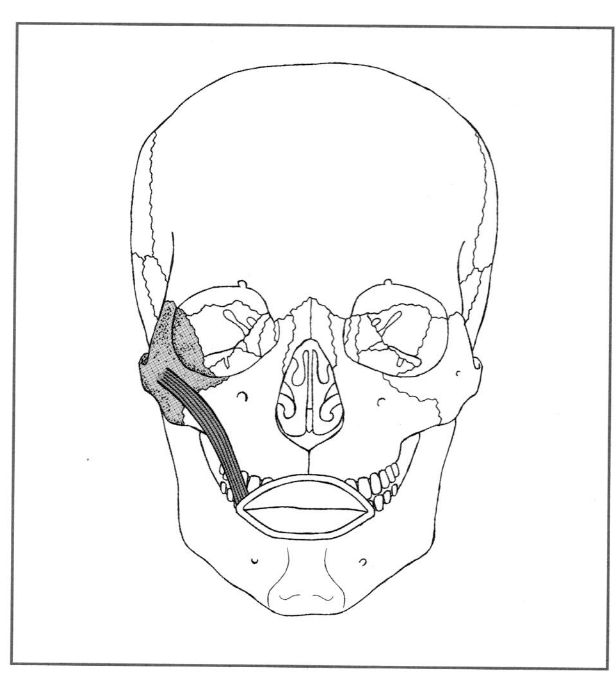

Anterior View of the Right Zygomaticus Major

FACIAL EXPRESSIONS CREATED BY THEIR CORRESPONDING MUSCLES

❑ LEVATOR ANGULI ORIS

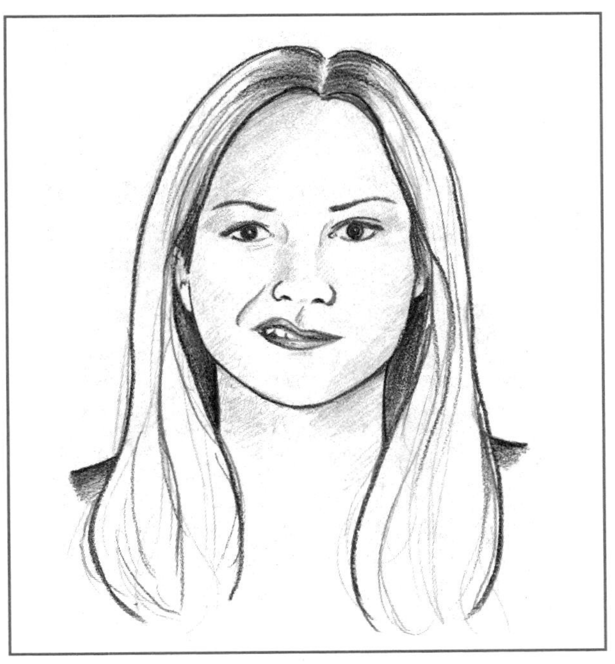

Elevation of the Angle of the Mouth

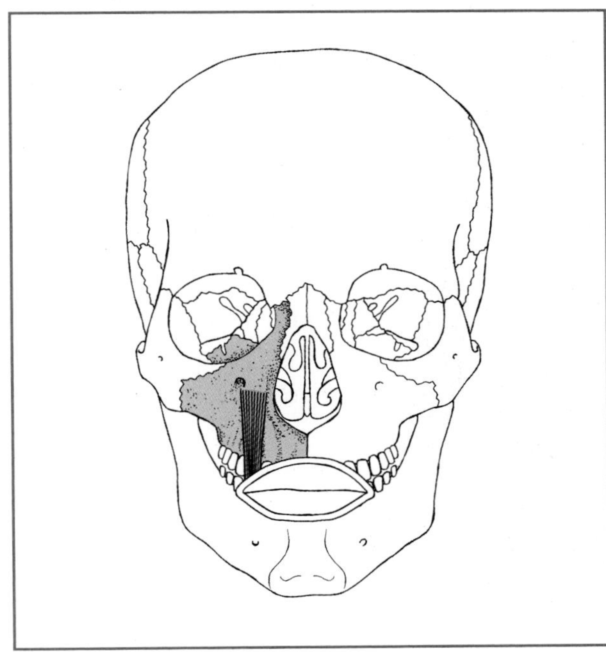

Anterior View of the Right Levator Anguli Oris

❑ RISORIUS

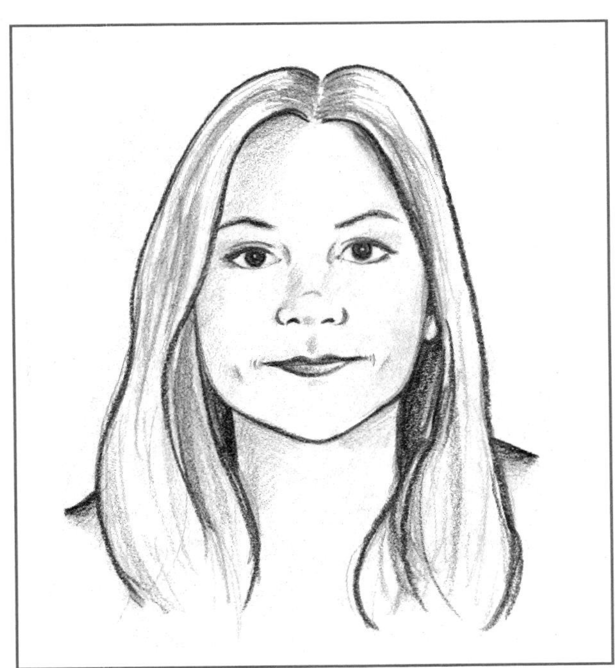

Draws Laterally the Angle of the Mouth

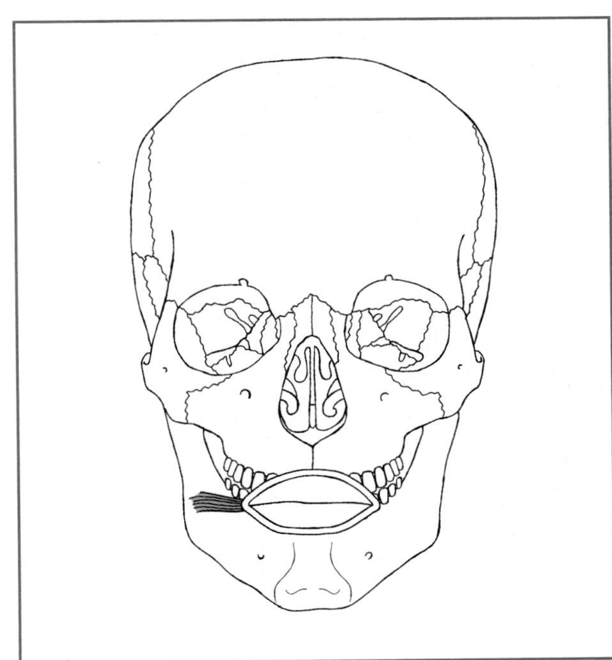

Anterior View of the Right Risorius

FACIAL EXPRESSIONS CREATED BY THEIR CORRESPONDING MUSCLES

❑ DEPRESSOR ANGULI ORIS

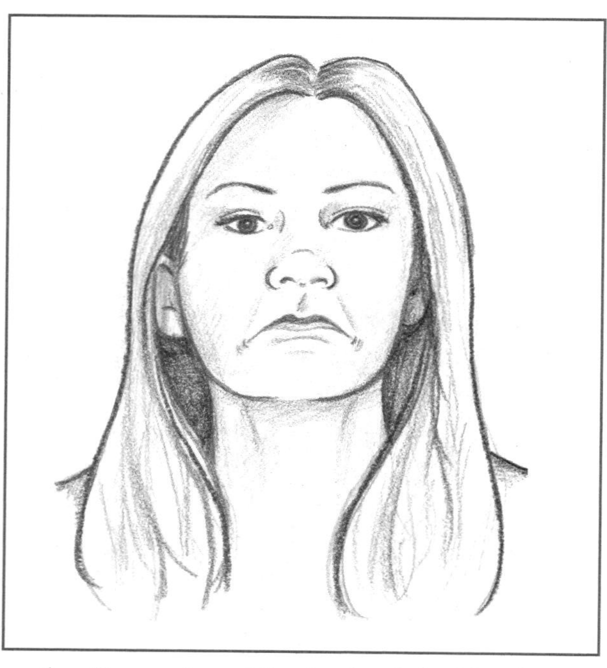

1. Depression of the Angle of the Mouth
2. Draws Laterally the Angle of the Mouth

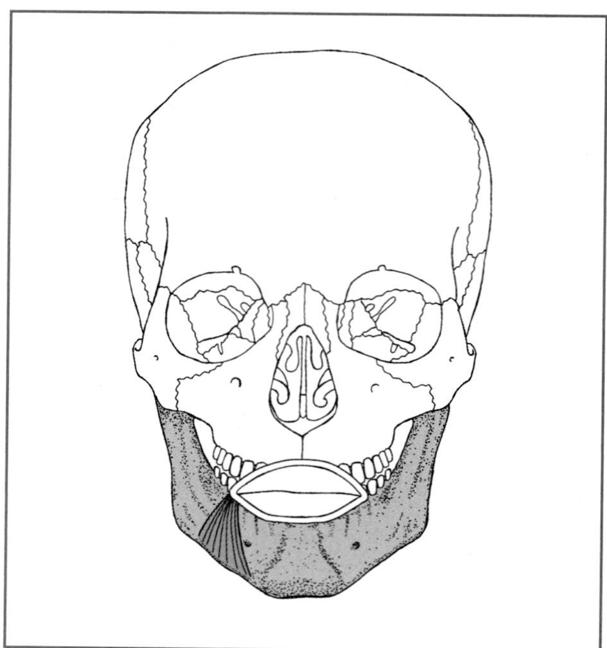

Anterior View of the
Right Depressor Anguli Oris

❑ DEPRESSOR LABII INFERIORIS

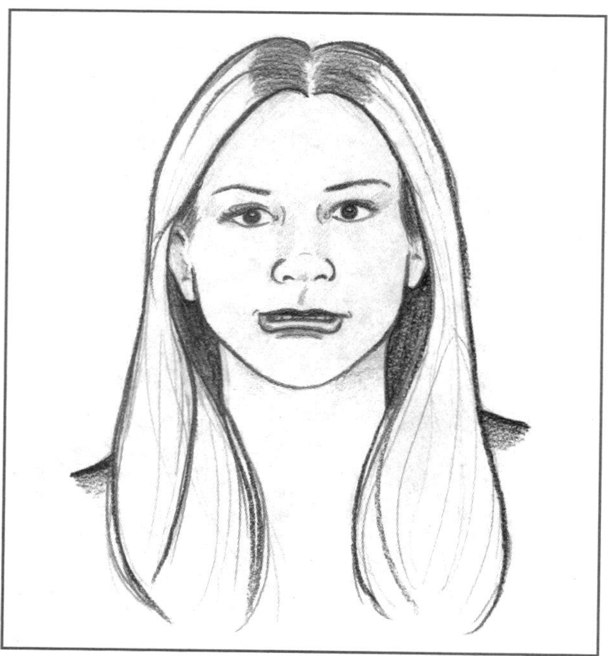

1. Depression of the Lower Lip
2. Draws Laterally the Lower Lip
3. Eversion of the Lower Lip

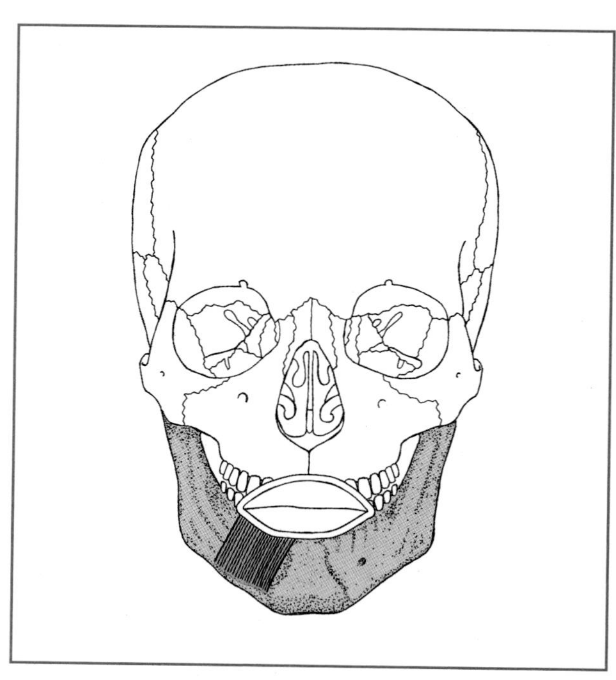

Anterior View of the
Right Depressor Labii Inferioris

FACIAL EXPRESSIONS CREATED BY THEIR CORRESPONDING MUSCLES

❑ MENTALIS

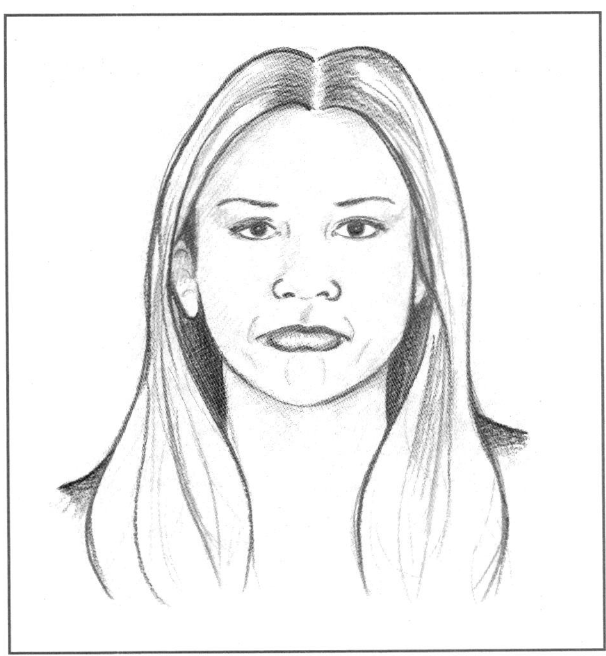

1. Elevation of the Lower Lip
2. Eversion and Protraction of the Lower Lip
3. Wrinkles the Skin of the Chin

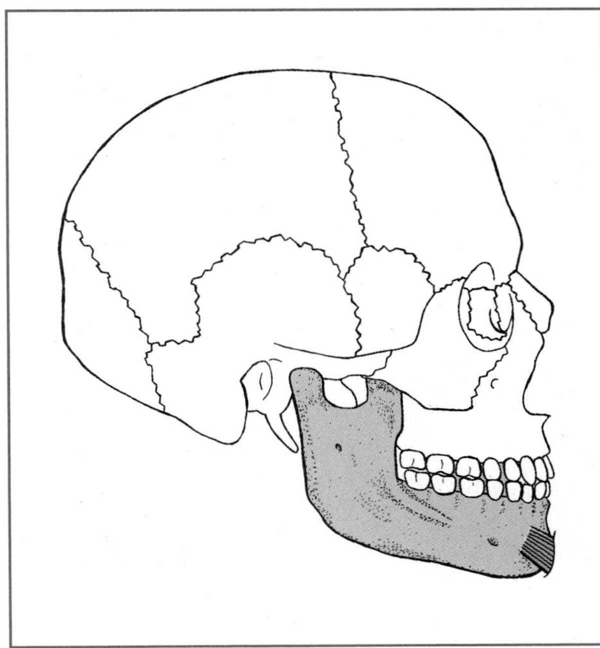

Lateral View of the Right Mentalis

❑ BUCCINATOR

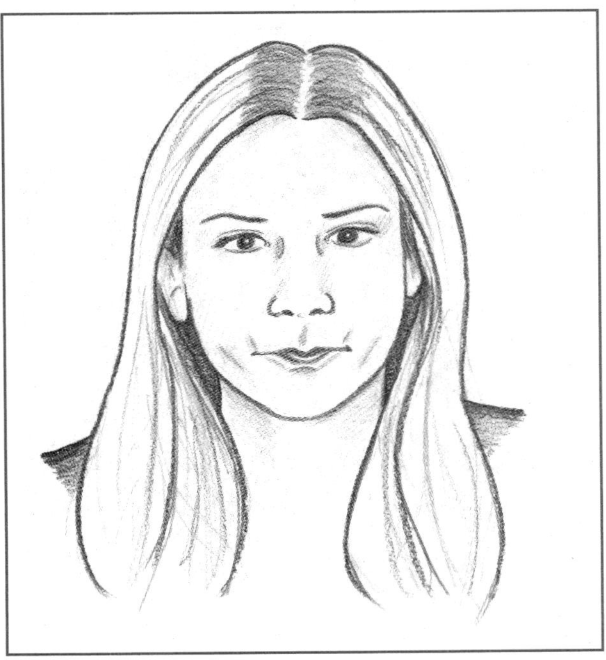

Compression of the Cheeks (Against the Teeth)

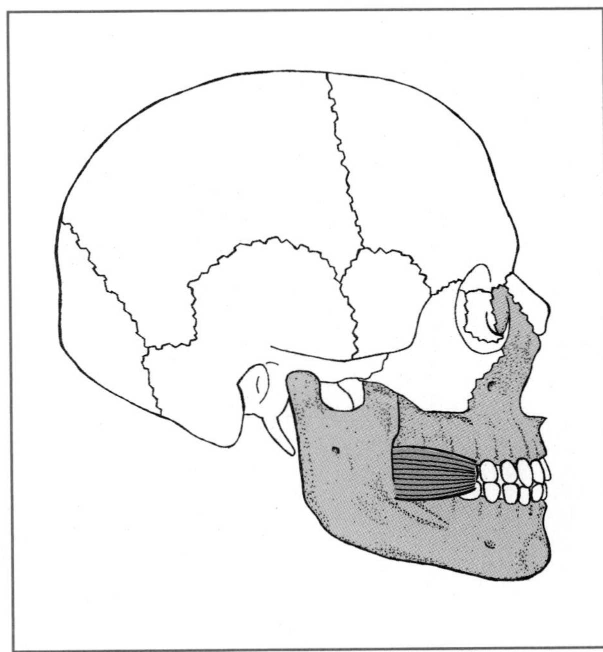

Lateral View of the Right Buccinator

FACIAL EXPRESSIONS CREATED BY THEIR CORRESPONDING MUSCLES

❑ **ORBICULARIS ORIS**

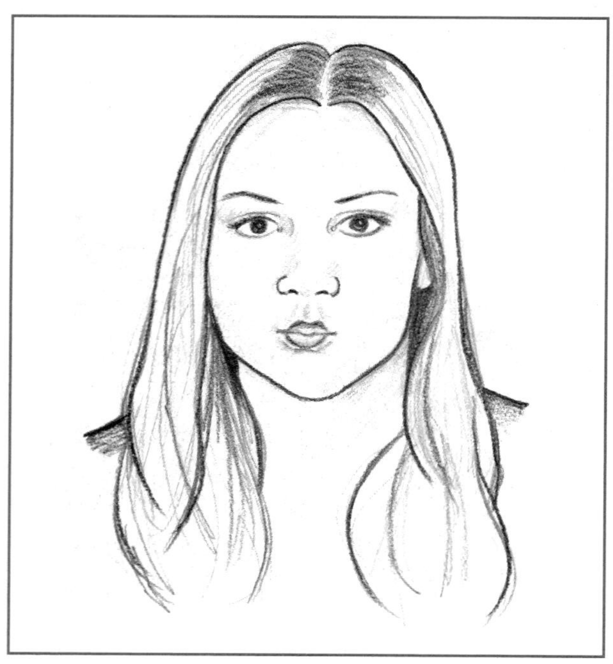

1. **Closes the Mouth**
2. **Protraction of the Lips**

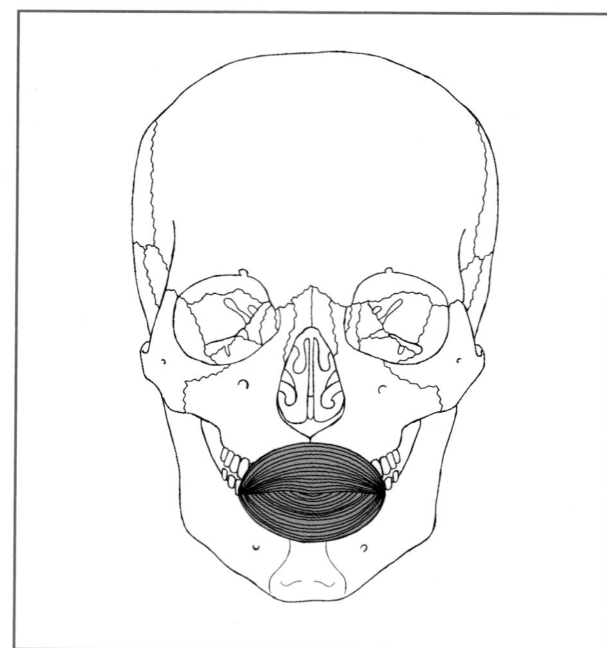

Anterior View of the Orbicularis Oris

FACIAL EXPRESSIONS CREATED BY THEIR CORRESPONDING MUSCLES

❑ OCCIPITOFRONTALIS (of the head chapter – see pages 14-16)

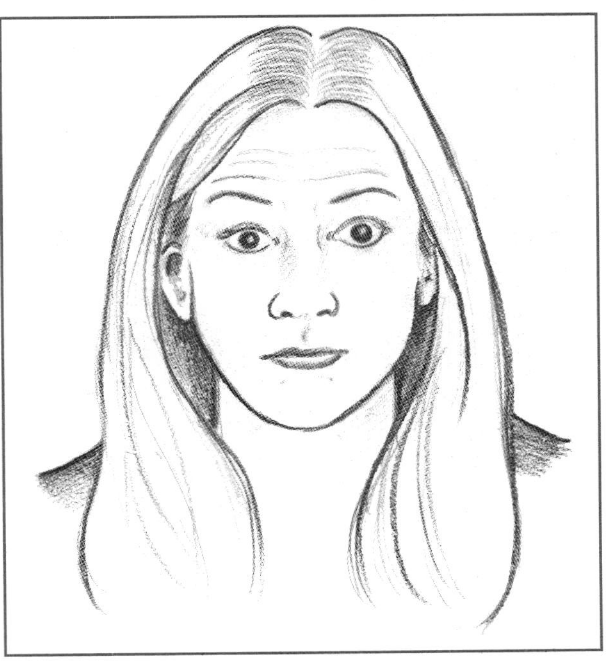

1. Draws the Scalp Posteriorly
2. Draws the Scalp Anteriorly
3. Elevation of the Eyebrows

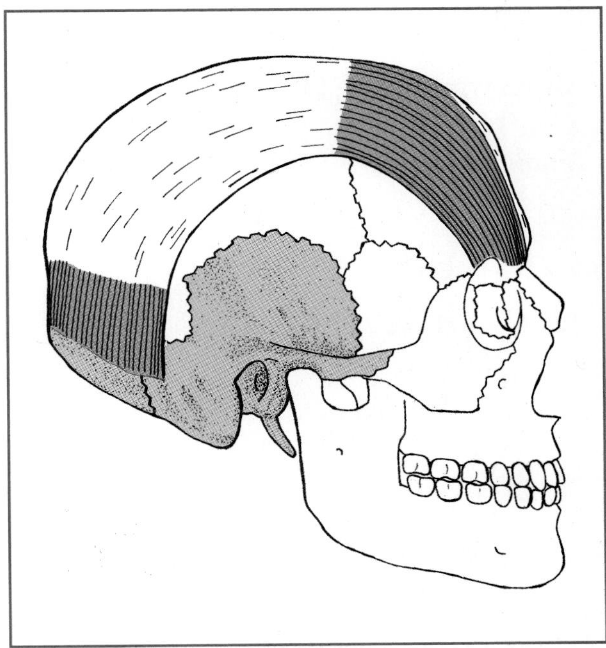

Lateral View of the Right Occipitofrontalis

❑ PLATYSMA (of the neck chapter – see pages 137-9)

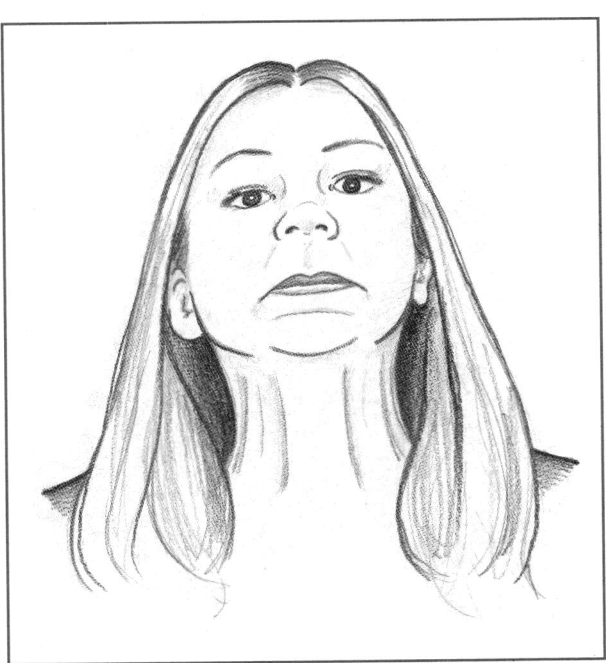

1. Draws Up the Skin of the Superior Chest and the Neck, Creating Ridges of Skin in the Neck
2. Depresses and Draws the Lower Lip Laterally

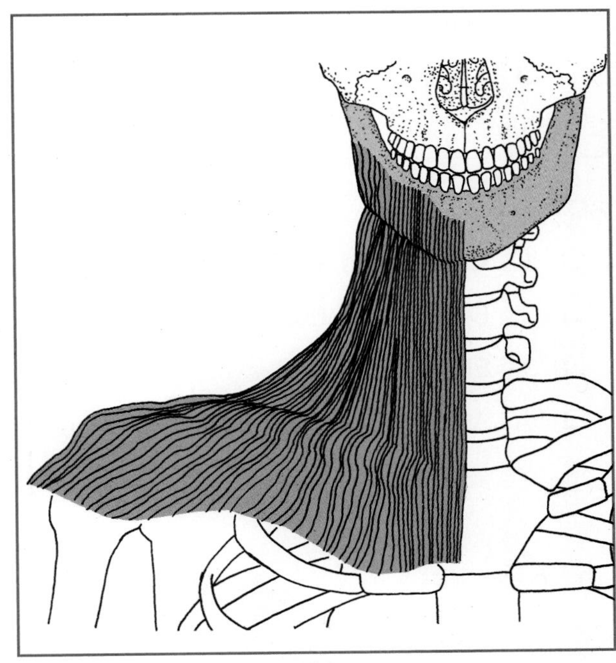

Anterior View of the Right Platysma

ORBICULARIS OCULI

❑ **The name, orbicularis oculi, tells us that this muscle encircles the eye.**

DERIVATION ❑ orbicularis: L. *a small circle.*
oculi: L. *refers to the eye.*

PRONUNCIATION ❑ or-**bik**-you-la-ris **ok**-you-lie

ATTACHMENTS

❑ **Medial Side of the Eye**

- ❑ ORBITAL PART: the nasal part of the frontal bone, the frontal process of the maxilla, and the medial palpebral ligament
- ❑ PALPEBRAL PART: the medial palpebral ligament
- ❑ LACRIMAL PART: the lacrimal bone

to the

❑ **Medial Side of the Eye (returns to the same attachment, encircling the eye)**

- ❑ ORBITAL PART: returns to the same attachment (these fibers encircle the eye)
- ❑ PALPEBRAL PART: the lateral palpebral ligament (these fibers run through the connective tissue of both eyelids)
- ❑ LACRIMAL PART: the medial palpebral raphe (these fibers are deeper in the eye socket)

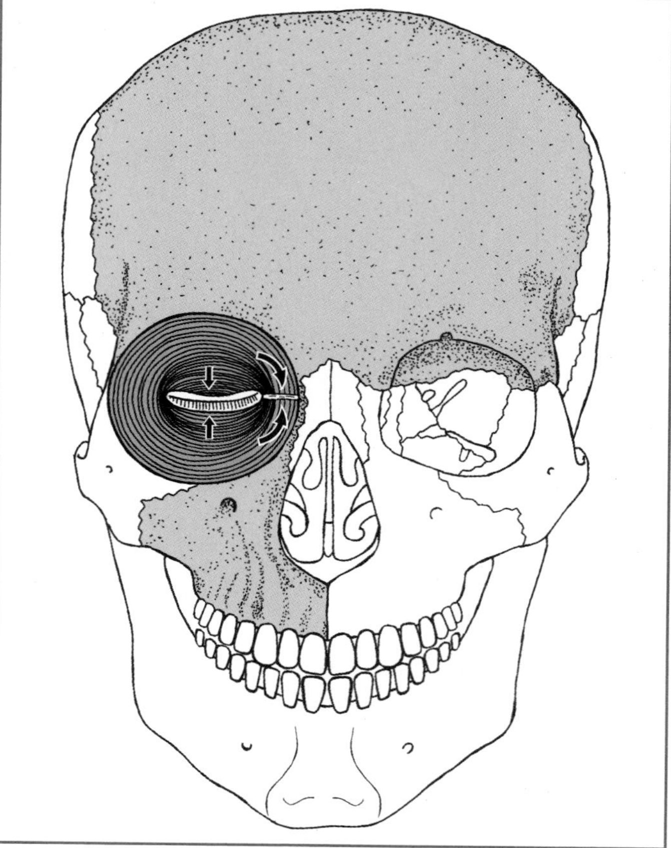

Anterior View of the Right Orbicularis Oculi

ACTIONS

❑ 1. **Closes and Squints the Eye (Orbital Part)**

❑ 2. Depression of the Upper Eyelid (Palpebral Part)

❑ 3. Elevation of the Lower Eyelid (Palpebral Part)

❑ 4. Assists Tear Transport and Drainage (Lacrimal Part)

INNERVATION ❑ The Facial Nerve (CN VII) ❑ temporal and zygomatic branches

ARTERIAL SUPPLY ❑ The Branches of the Facial Artery and Superficial Temporal Artery (Both Branches of the External Carotid Artery)

PALPATION AND SUPPLEMENTARY TEXT

PALPATION

Of the three parts of the orbicularis oculi, only the orbital and palpebral parts are palpable.

- Have the client supine.

❑ **To palpate the orbital part:**

- Place palpating hand inferior, lateral, or superior to the eye.
- Ask the client to forcefully close the eye and feel for the contraction of the orbicularis oculi.

❑ **To palpate the palpebral part:**

- Place palpating fingers gently on the upper and lower eyelids.
- Ask the client to gently close the eye and feel for the contraction of the orbicularis oculi.

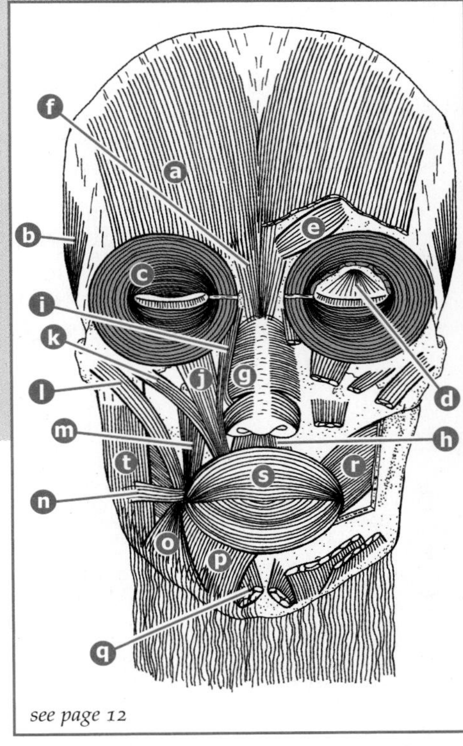

see page 12

Anterior View of the Head

a. Occipitofrontalis
b. Temporoparietalis
c. **Orbicularis Oculi**
d. Levator Palpebrae Superioris
e. Corrugator Supercilii
f. Procerus
g. Nasalis
h. Depressor Septi Nasi
i. Levator Labii Superioris Alaeque Nasi
j. Levator Labii Superioris
k. Zygomaticus Minor
l. Zygomaticus Major
m. Levator Anguli Oris
n. Risorius
o. Depressor Anguli Oris
p. Depressor Labii Inferioris
q. Mentalis
r. Buccinator
s. Orbicularis Oris
t. Masseter

RELATIONSHIP TO OTHER MUSCULOSKELETAL STRUCTURES

❑ The orbicularis oculi is superficial and encircles the eye. The orbicularis oculi is inferior to the frontalis and the corrugator supercilii and superior to the levator labii superioris alaeque nasi, levator labii superioris, zygomaticus minor and the zygomaticus major. It is lateral to the procerus and nasalis and medial to the temporoparietalis and the temporalis.

METHODOLOGY FOR LEARNING MUSCLE ACTIONS

❑ 1. **Closes and Squints the Eye:** The fiber direction of the orbital part of the orbicularis oculi is circular around the eye. When the orbital part of the orbicularis oculi contracts, it acts as a circular sphincter muscle that closes in around the eye, not only forcing the two eyelids together, but also closing in the tissue above and below the eye. This is often termed *forceful closure* of the eye, or more commonly, squinting. (Note: To understand how a circular sphincter muscle works, the following reason applies: If a linear muscle shortens, its length clearly and obviously decreases. When that same linear muscle is arranged in a circular fashion and shortens, the length of the line you have to make the circle decreases and therefore the size of the circle lessens, which can close in on whatever structure is being surrounded by this circular muscle.)

ORBICULARIS OCULI – continued

- ❑ **2. Depression of the Upper Eyelid:** The palpebral part of the orbicularis oculi has fibers that are arranged in an arc-like fashion in the upper eyelid. (The direction of the fibers is a horizontal arc with the convexity oriented superiorly.) When the fibers of the palpebral part contract, the arc flattens down and the upper eyelid is depressed, gently closing the eye from above.
- ❑ **3. Elevation of the Lower Eyelid:** The palpebral part of the orbicularis oculi has fibers that are arranged in an upside-down, arc-like fashion in the lower eyelid. (The direction of the fibers is a horizontal arc with the convexity oriented inferiorly.) When the fibers of the palpebral part contract, the arc flattens upwards and the lower eyelid is elevated, gently closing the eye from below.
- ❑ **4. Assists Tear Transport and Drainage:** The lacrimal part of the orbicularis oculi is located deeper in the eye socket (with its fibers running horizontally from anterior to posterior). When the lacrimal part contracts, it pulls on the medial palpebral raphe, causing the lower eyelid to be pulled against the surface of the eye (thus preventing eversion of the lower eyelid). Holding the lower eyelid against the surface of the eye helps to direct (transport) tear fluid toward the medial corner of the eye where it can be drained into the lacrimal sac. When the lacrimal part of the orbicularis oculi contracts, it also exerts a pulls on the lacrimal sac that dilates it and increases its ability to drain tears from the surface of the eye.

MISCELLANEOUS

- ❑ 1. The palpebral part of the orbicularis oculi is under both conscious and unconscious control and may contract reflexly to close the eye (for protection and as part of blinking).
- ❑ 2. Some fibers of the levator palpebrae superioris pierce through the palpebral part of the orbicularis oculi to attach into the skin of the upper eyelid.
- ❑ 3. Superiorly, the orbital part of the orbicularis oculi blends in with fibers of the frontalis and the corrugator supercilii. Inferiorly, the orbital part of the orbicularis oculi blends in with fibers of the zygomaticus minor, levator labii superioris and the levator labii superioris alaeque nasi.
- ❑ 4. Some fibers of the orbital part may blend into the skin deep to the eyebrows creating the *depressor supercilii* muscle.
- ❑ 5. If the entire orbicularis oculi contracts, not only will the eye close forcefully (i.e., the eyelids and the surrounding tissue closing in around the eye), but the skin of the eyelids and surrounding area (forehead, temple and cheek) will be drawn medially toward the attachment at the medial eye. This action creates a facial expression in which the amount of light entering the eye decreases and wrinkles radiating out from the lateral eye (*crow's feet*) form.
- ❑ 6. The medial and lateral palpebral raphes are where the tissue from the upper and lower eyelids come together at the corners (canthi) of the eye. The medial and lateral palpebral ligaments are small ligaments located directly next to the raphes in the corners of the eye. (A raphe is a seam of tissue formed by the union of the halves of a part.)
- ❑ 7. When the tissue located superior to the eye is pulled down around the eye by the contraction of the orbicularis oculi, it helps to shield the eye from bright sunlight. The corrugator supercilii and the procerus can also assist with this function of shielding the eye from bright sunlight.
- ❑ 8. Given that the lacrimal part of the orbicularis oculi helps to drain tears from the surface of the eye into the lacrimal sac, weakness or flaccid paralysis of the lacrimal part of the orbicularis oculi results in excessive spilling of tears over the lower eyelid (crying).

LEVATOR PALPEBRAE SUPERIORIS

❑ **The name, levator palpebrae superioris, tells us that this muscle elevates the upper eyelid.**

DERIVATION ❑ levator: L. *lifter.*
palpebrae: L. *eyelid.*
superioris: L. *upper.*

PRONUNCIATION ❑ **le**-vay-tor pal-**pee**-bree su-**pee**-ri-**or**-is

ATTACHMENTS

❑ **Sphenoid Bone**

❑ the anterior surface of the lesser wing of the sphenoid

to the

❑ **Upper Eyelid**

❑ the fibrous tissue and the skin of the upper eyelid

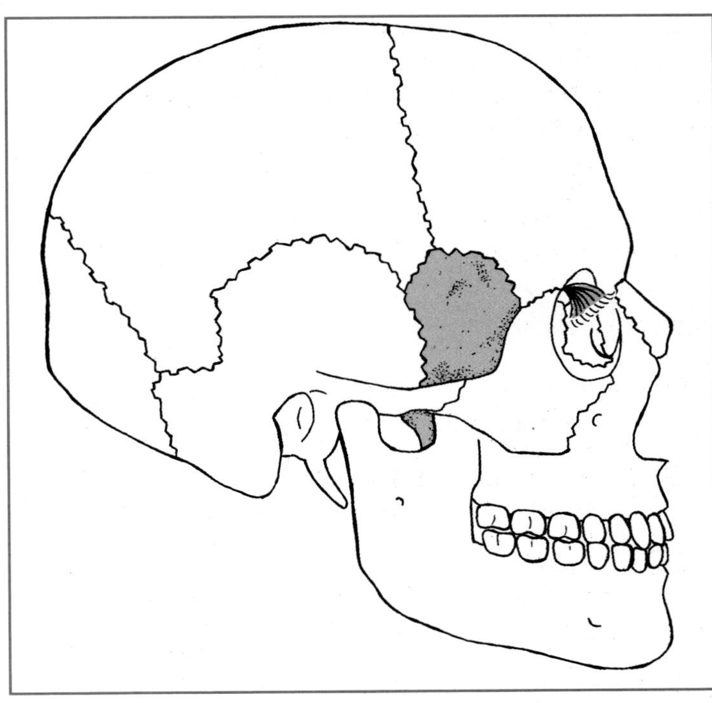

Lateral View of the
Right Levator Palpebrae Superioris

ACTION

❑ **Elevation of the Upper Eyelid**

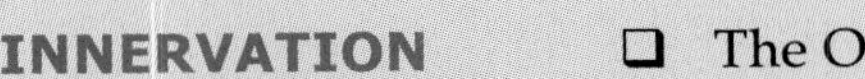

INNERVATION ❑ The Oculomotor Nerve (CN III)

ARTERIAL SUPPLY ❑ The Ophthalmic Artery
(A Branch of the Internal Carotid Artery)

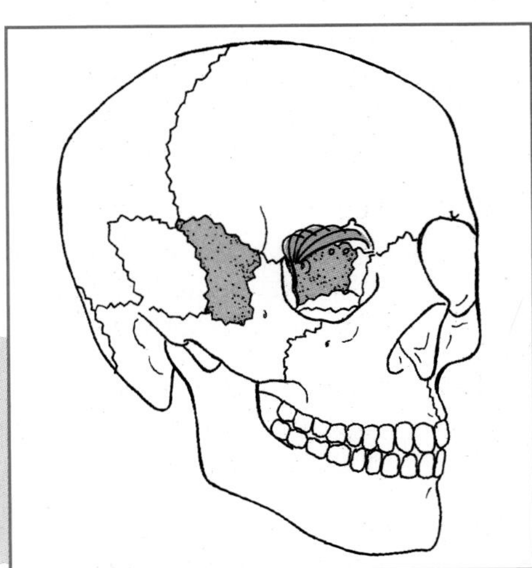

Anterolateral View of the
Right Levator Palpebrae Superioris

LEVATOR PALPEBRAE SUPERIORIS PALPATION AND SUPPLEMENTARY TEXT

PALPATION

- ☐ Most of the levator palpebrae superioris is deep within the orbital socket and not accessible to palpation. However, the part of the muscle that attaches into the eyelid itself is palpable.
  - Have the client supine.
  - Ask the client to close the eye.
  - Gently place your palpating finger on the client's upper eyelid.
  - Ask the client to open the eye and feel for the contraction of the levator palpebrae superioris.

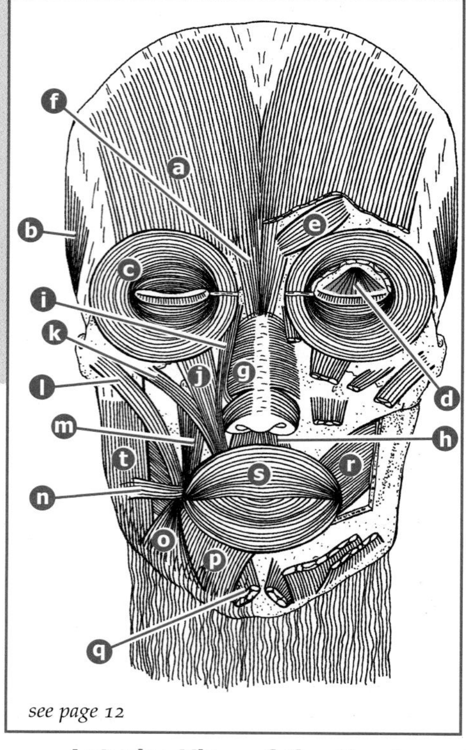

see page 12

Anterior View of the Head

RELATIONSHIP TO OTHER MUSCULOSKELETAL STRUCTURES

☐ 1. The levator palpebrae superioris begins in the orbital socket, deep to the orbicularis oculi. Some of its fibers pierce through the orbicularis oculi to attach into the skin of the eyelid, superficial to the orbicularis oculi.

☐ 2. The levator palpebrae superioris is superior to, and somewhat conjoined to, the superior rectus muscle of the eye.

METHODOLOGY FOR LEARNING MUSCLE ACTIONS

☐ **Elevation of the Upper Eyelid:** The levator palpebrae superioris attaches from the sphenoid bone superiorly, to the upper eyelid inferiorly. When the levator palpebrae superioris contracts, it pulls the upper eyelid superiorly toward the sphenoid bone. Therefore, the levator palpebrae superioris elevates the eyelid.

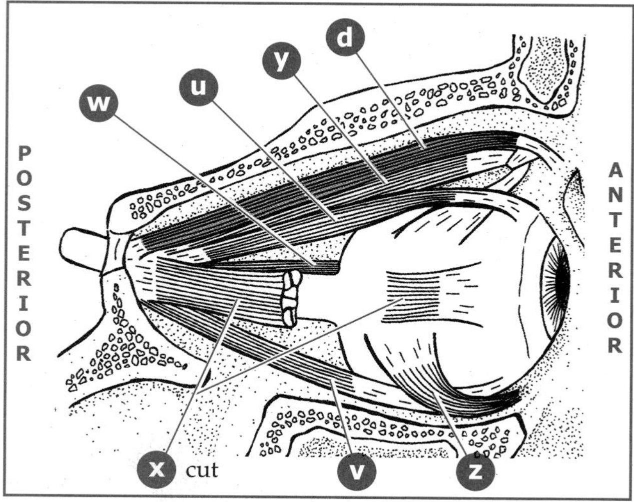

Lateral View of the Eye

a. Occipitofrontalis
b. Temporoparietalis
c. Orbicularis Oculi
d. **Levator Palpebrae Superioris**
e. Corrugator Supercilii
f. Procerus
g. Nasalis
h. Depressor Septi Nasi
i. Levator Labii Superioris Alaeque Nasi
j. Levator Labii Superioris
k. Zygomaticus Minor
l. Zygomaticus Major
m. Levator Anguli Oris
n. Risorius
o. Depressor Anguli Oris
p. Depressor Labii Inferioris
q. Mentalis
r. Buccinator
s. Orbicularis Oris
t. Masseter
u. Superior Rectus
v. Inferior Rectus
w. Medial Rectus
x. Lateral Rectus
y. Superior Oblique
z. Inferior Oblique

CORRUGATOR SUPERCILII ❑

❑ **The name, corrugator supercilii, tells us that these muscles wrinkle the skin of the two eyebrows together.**

DERIVATION ❑ corrugator: L. *to wrinkle together.*
supercilii: L. *eyebrows.*

PRONUNCIATION ❑ **kor**-u-gay-tor su-per-**sil**-i-eye

ATTACHMENTS

❑ **Inferior Frontal Bone**

❑ the medial end of the superciliary arch of the frontal bone

to the

❑ **Skin Deep to the Medial Portion of the Eyebrow**

ACTION

❑ **Draws Eyebrow Inferiorly and Medially**

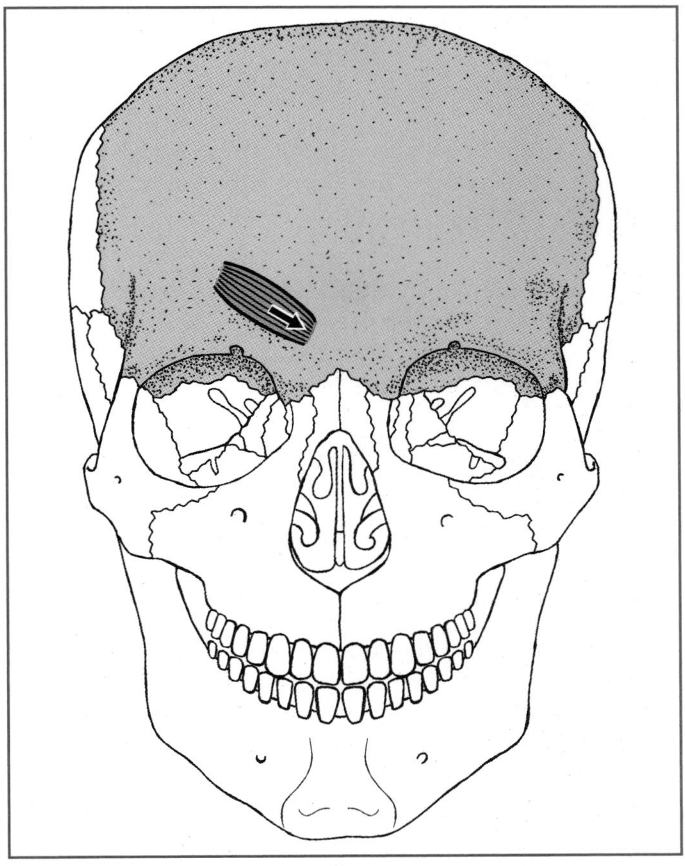

Anterior View of the Right Corrugator Supercilii

INNERVATION ❑ The Facial Nerve (CN VII) ❑ temporal branch

ARTERIAL SUPPLY ❑ The Supratrochlear and Supraorbital Arteries (Branches of the Ophthalmic Artery)

CORRUGATOR SUPERCILII – PALPATION AND SUPPLEMENTARY TEXT

PALPATION

- [ ] The corrugator supercilii is superficial in the face and located deep to the medial portion of the eyebrows.
  - Have the client supine.
  - Place palpating fingers over the medial portion of the eyebrows.
  - Ask the client to frown, drawing the eyebrows medially and inferiorly and feel for the contraction of the corrugator supercilii. (Be sure to isolate the corrugator supercilii from the orbicularis oculi, which can also help to draw the eyebrows medially and inferiorly, by making sure that the eye is not being closed at the same time.)
  - Continue palpating the corrugator supercilii superolaterally toward its frontal bone attachment.

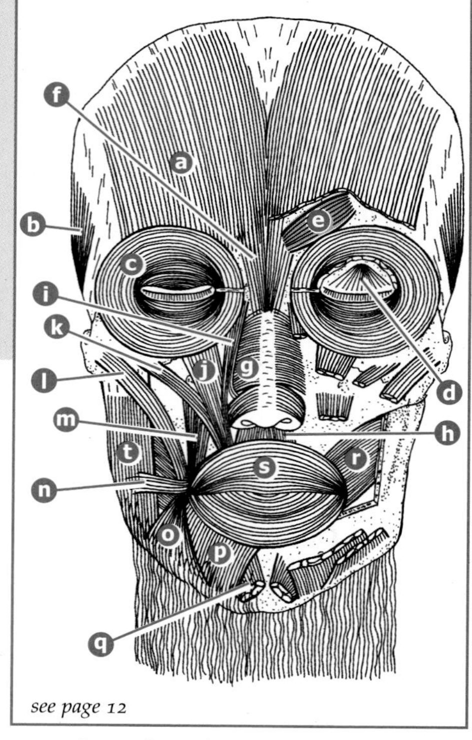

see page 12

Anterior View of the Head

a. Occipitofrontalis
b. Temporoparietalis
c. Orbicularis Oculi
d. Levator Palpebrae Superioris
e. **Corrugator Supercilii**
f. Procerus
g. Nasalis
h. Depressor Septi Nasi
i. Levator Labii Superioris Alaeque Nasi
j. Levator Labii Superioris
k. Zygomaticus Minor
l. Zygomaticus Major
m. Levator Anguli Oris
n. Risorius
o. Depressor Anguli Oris
p. Depressor Labii Inferioris
q. Mentalis
r. Buccinator
s. Orbicularis Oris
t. Masseter

RELATIONSHIP TO OTHER MUSCULOSKELETAL STRUCTURES

- [ ] 1. The corrugator supercilii is lateral to the procerus.
- [ ] 2. The corrugator supercilii is deep to the frontalis.
- [ ] 3. The corrugator supercilii lies toward the superior end of the orbicularis oculi. Where these two muscles overlap, the corrugator supercilii is deep to the orbicularis oculi.

METHODOLOGY FOR LEARNING MUSCLE ACTIONS

- [ ] **Draws Eyebrow Inferiorly and Medially:** The corrugator supercilii attaches to the region of the frontal bone next to the nasal bone. From there, its fibers run superiorly and laterally to attach into the skin deep to the medial end of the eyebrow. Since the frontal bone attachment is more fixed, when the corrugator supercilii contracts, it pulls the skin deep to the eyebrow inferiorly and medially toward the frontal bone attachment (the other eyebrow). When both corrugator supercilii muscles contract, both eyebrows are pulled inferiorly and medially toward each other.

MISCELLANEOUS

- [ ] 1. Some fibers of the corrugator supercilii blend in with fibers of the frontalis and the orbicularis oculi.
- [ ] 2. The action of drawing the eyebrows inferiorly and medially is involved in frowning. It is also useful in shielding the eyes from bright sunlight. (Note: The orbicularis oculi and the procerus can also assist with this function of shielding the eyes from bright sunlight.)
- [ ] 3. When the corrugator supercilii contracts, it causes vertical wrinkles superior and medial to the eyes.

PROCERUS

❑ **The name, procerus, tells us that this muscle helps to create the expression of superiority of a nobleman or prince.**

DERIVATION ❑ procerus: L. *a chief noble, prince* **PRONUNCIATION** ❑ pro-**se**-rus

ATTACHMENTS

❑ **Fascia over the Nasal Bone**

to the

❑ **Skin between the Eyebrows**

ACTIONS

❑ **1. Draws Down the Medial Eyebrows**

❑ **2.** Wrinkles the Skin of the Nose

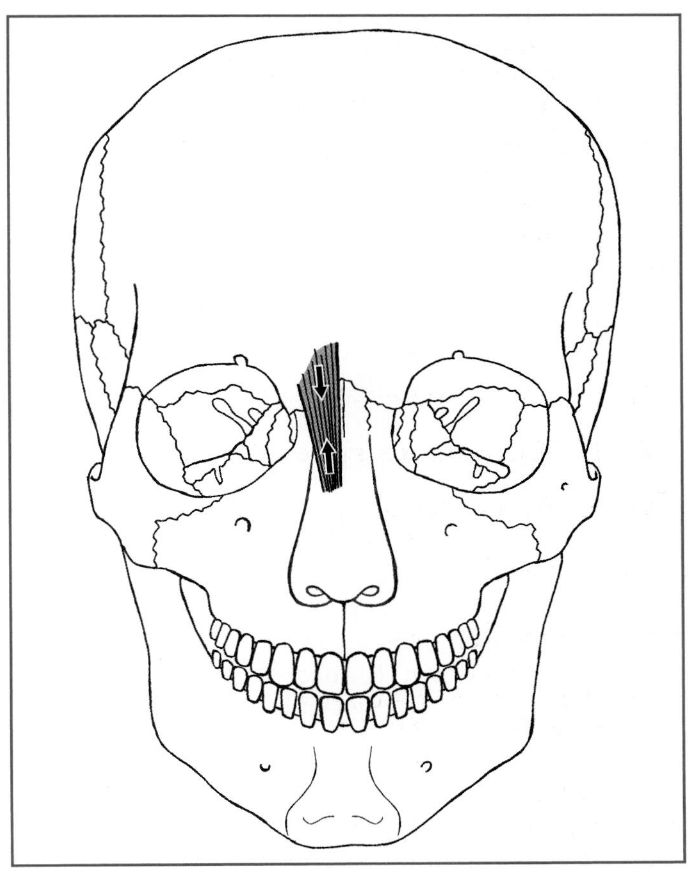

Anterior View of the Right Procerus

INNERVATION ❑ The Facial Nerve (CN VII) ❑ superior buccal branches

ARTERIAL SUPPLY ❑ The Facial Artery (A Branch of the External Carotid Artery)

PROCERUS – PALPATION AND SUPPLEMENTARY TEXT

PALPATION

- ❑ The procerus is superficial in the face and located superior to the nose.
  - Have the client supine.
  - Place palpating fingers directly superior to the bridge of the nose.
  - Ask the client to draw the medial eyebrows down and/or wrinkle the nose upward with a look of disdain as in frowning and feel for the contraction of the procerus.
  - Continue palpating the procerus superiorly until you reach the border of the procerus with the frontalis, and inferiorly until the attachment into the fascia of the nose is felt.

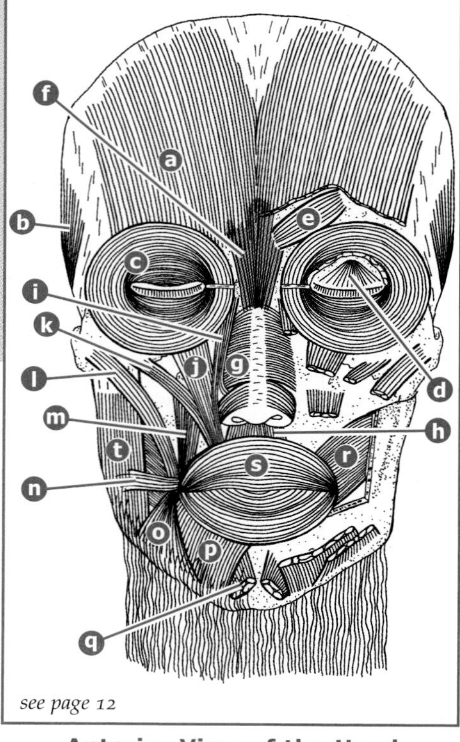

see page 12

Anterior View of the Head

a. Occipitofrontalis
b. Temporoparietalis
c. Orbicularis Oculi
d. Levator Palpebrae Superioris
e. Corrugator Supercilii
f. **Procerus**
g. Nasalis
h. Depressor Septi Nasi
i. Levator Labii Superioris Alaeque Nasi
j. Levator Labii Superioris
k. Zygomaticus Minor
l. Zygomaticus Major
m. Levator Anguli Oris
n. Risorius
o. Depressor Anguli Oris
p. Depressor Labii Inferioris
q. Mentalis
r. Buccinator
s. Orbicularis Oris
t. Masseter

RELATIONSHIP TO OTHER MUSCULOSKELETAL STRUCTURES

- ❑ The procerus is located superior to the nasalis, inferior to the frontalis, and medial to the corrugator supercilii and the orbicularis oculi.

METHODOLOGY FOR LEARNING MUSCLE ACTIONS

❑ 1. **Draws Down the Medial Eyebrow:** The procerus attaches from the fascia over the nose to the skin between the eyebrows (with its fibers running vertically). When the inferior attachment is fixed and the procerus contracts, it pulls the medial eyebrow inferiorly (downward) toward the nose. Therefore, the procerus draws down the medial eyebrow.

❑ 2. **Wrinkles the Skin of the Nose:** The procerus attaches from the fascia over the nose to the skin between the eyebrows (with its fibers running vertically). When the superior attachment is fixed and the procerus contracts, it pulls the fascia of the nose superiorly, which causes skin of the nose to wrinkle.

MISCELLANEOUS

❑ 1. The procerus often blends with the frontalis superiorly and the nasalis inferiorly.

❑ 2. Bringing the medial eyebrows down is part of the facial expression of frowning, but it also helps to shield the eyes from bright sunlight. (Note: The orbicularis oculi and the corrugator supercilii can also assist with this function of shielding the eyes from bright sunlight.)

❑ 3. When the procerus draws down the medial eyebrow, it also causes wrinkling of the skin above the nose.

❑ 4. The action of wrinkling the skin of the nose and/or drawing down the medial eyebrows can create the look of frowning or disdain that a person may make to convey an air of superiority (hence the name "procerus" meaning chief, noble or prince).

NASALIS

❑ **The name, nasalis, tells us that this muscle is involved with the nose.**

DERIVATION ❑ nasalis: L. *nose.* **PRONUNCIATION** ❑ nay-**sa**-lis

ATTACHMENTS

❑ **Maxilla**

- ❑ TRANSVERSE PART: the maxilla, lateral to the nose
- ❑ ALAR PART: the maxilla, inferior and medial to the attachment of the transverse part of the nasalis

to the

❑ **Cartilage of the Nose and the Opposite Side Nasalis Muscle**

- ❑ TRANSVERSE PART: the opposite side nasalis over the upper cartilage of the nose
- ❑ ALAR PART: the alar cartilage of the nose

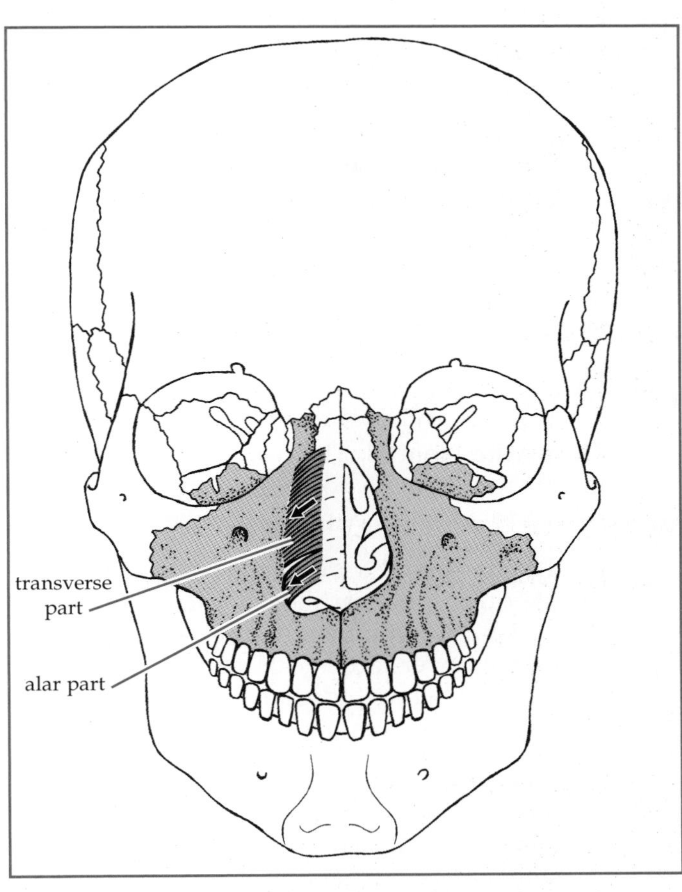

Anterior View of the Right Nasalis

ACTION

❑ **Flares the Nostril**

INNERVATION ❑ The Facial Nerve (CN VII) ❑ superior buccal branches

ARTERIAL SUPPLY ❑ The Facial Artery (A Branch of the External Carotid Artery)

NASALIS – PALPATION AND SUPPLEMENTARY TEXT

PALPATION

- ❑ The nasalis is superficial in the face and located over the superior part of the nose.
  - Have the client supine.
  - Place palpating fingers over the cartilage of the nose as well as the skin just lateral to the cartilage of the nose.
  - Ask the client to flare the nostrils as if taking in a deep breath and feel for the contraction of the nasalis.

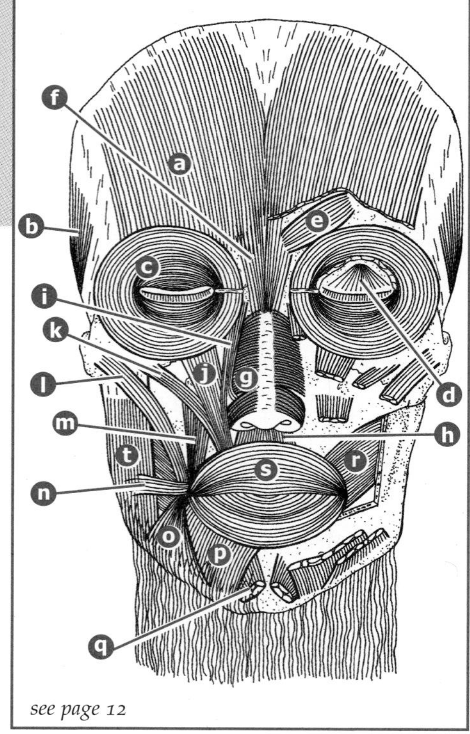

see page 12

Anterior View of the Head

- **a.** Occipitofrontalis
- **b.** Temporoparietalis
- **c.** Orbicularis Oculi
- **d.** Levator Palpebrae Superioris
- **e.** Corrugator Supercilii
- **f.** Procerus
- **g.** **Nasalis**
- **h.** Depressor Septi Nasi
- **i.** Levator Labii Superioris Alaeque Nasi
- **j.** Levator Labii Superioris
- **k.** Zygomaticus Minor
- **l.** Zygomaticus Major
- **m.** Levator Anguli Oris
- **n.** Risorius
- **o.** Depressor Anguli Oris
- **p.** Depressor Labii Inferioris
- **q.** Mentalis
- **r.** Buccinator
- **s.** Orbicularis Oris
- **t.** Masseter

RELATIONSHIP TO OTHER MUSCULOSKELETAL STRUCTURES

- ❑ The nasalis is inferior to the procerus, medial to the levator labii superioris alaeque nasi, superior to the orbicularis oris and superolateral to the depressor septi nasi.

METHODOLOGY FOR LEARNING MUSCLE ACTIONS

- ❑ **Flares the Nostril:** The two parts of the nasalis muscles act together to flare the nostril (open up the aperture for breathing). Each part contributes in its own way.
  - The transverse parts of the nasalis muscles attach into each other over the upper cartilage of the nose. When they contract, they pull at their common midline attachment, causing compression on the upper cartilage of the nose. This results in a widening of the nose, which aids flaring of the nostrils to increase the aperture for breathing.
  - The alar parts of the nasalis muscles pull directly on the lower part of the alar cartilage of the nose from the maxillary attachment, which is more lateral (the fibers are running somewhat horizontally). Therefore, the two alae of the nose are pulled laterally, flaring the nostrils and increasing the aperture for breathing.

MISCELLANEOUS

- ❑ 1. The transverse part of the nasalis is sometimes called the *compressor naris*. The alar part of the nasalis is sometimes called the *dilatator naris.*
- ❑ 2. The maxillary attachments of the transverse part of the nasalis and the alar part of the nasalis often partially blend together.
- ❑ 3. Superiorly, the nasalis often blends in with the procerus.
- ❑ 4. The muscle directly inferior to the nasalis, the depressor septi nasi, is sometimes considered to be a part of the alar portion *(dilatator nasi)* of the nasalis.
- ❑ 5. The action of flaring the nostrils to increase the aperture for breathing in is important for deep inspiration. This action can also be associated with facial expressions during emotional states.

DEPRESSOR SEPTI NASI ❑

❑ **The name, depressor septi nasi, tells us that this muscle depresses the nasal septum. (The septum is the midline cartilage of the nose.)**

DERIVATION ❑ depressor: L. *depressor.*
septi: L. *refers to the nasal septum.*
nasi: L. *refers to the nose.*

PRONUNCIATION ❑ dee-**pres**-or **sep**-ti **nay**-zi

ATTACHMENTS

❑ **Maxilla**

❑ the incisive fossa of the maxilla

to the

❑ **Cartilage of the Nose**

❑ the septum and the alar cartilage of the nose

ACTION

❑ **Constricts the Nostril**

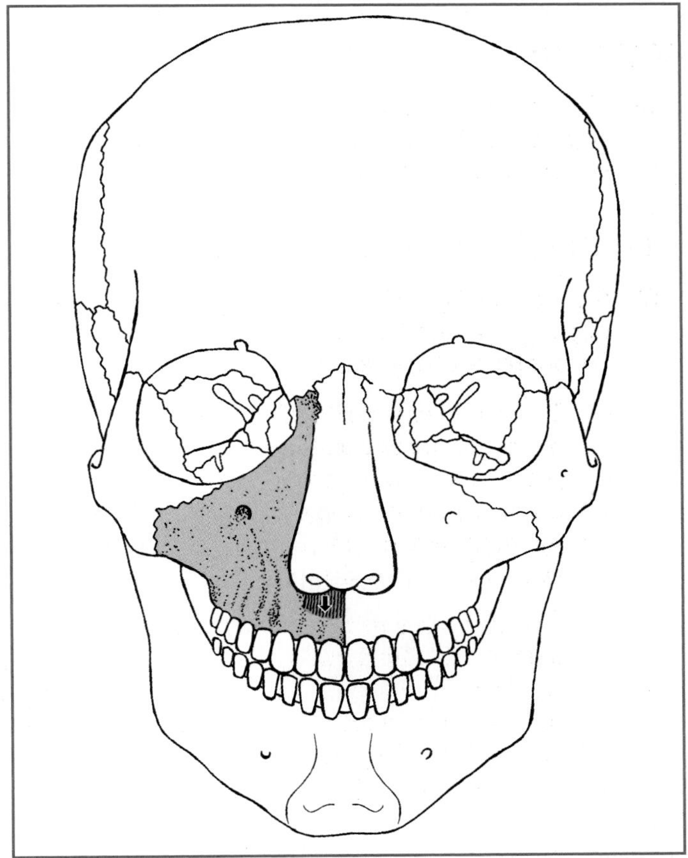

Anterior View of the Right Depressor Septi Nasi

INNERVATION ❑ The Facial Nerve (CN VII) ❑ superior buccal branches

ARTERIAL SUPPLY ❑ The Facial Artery (A Branch of the External Carotid Artery)

DEPRESSOR SEPTI NASI – PALPATION AND SUPPLEMENTARY TEXT

PALPATION

- ❑ The depressor septi nasi is superficial in the face and located directly inferior to the nose.
  - Have the client supine.
  - Place palpating fingers directly inferior to the nose.
  - Ask the client to try to pull the middle of the nose down toward the mouth and/or to constrict the nostrils and feel for the contraction of the depressor septi nasi. If the client does either or both these actions, the contraction should be easily felt.

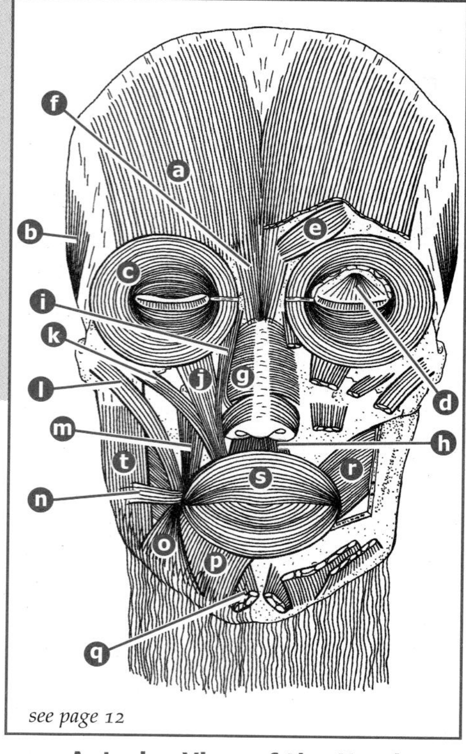

see page 12

Anterior View of the Head

a. Occipitofrontalis
b. Temporoparietalis
c. Orbicularis Oculi
d. Levator Palpebrae Superioris
e. Corrugator Supercilii
f. Procerus
g. Nasalis
h. **Depressor Septi Nasi**
i. Levator Labii Superioris Alaeque Nasi
j. Levator Labii Superioris
k. Zygomaticus Minor
l. Zygomaticus Major
m. Levator Anguli Oris
n. Risorius
o. Depressor Anguli Oris
p. Depressor Labii Inferioris
q. Mentalis
r. Buccinator
s. Orbicularis Oris
t. Masseter

RELATIONSHIP TO OTHER MUSCULOSKELETAL STRUCTURES

❑ 1. The depressor septi nasi is superior to the orbicularis oris, and where they overlap, the depressor septi nasi is deep to the orbicularis oris.

❑ 2. The depressor septi nasi is inferior and medial to the nasalis (alar part).

METHODOLOGY FOR LEARNING MUSCLE ACTIONS

❑ **Constricts the Nostril:** The depressor septi nasi attaches from the maxilla inferiorly, to the cartilage of the nose superiorly (with its fibers running vertically). Given that the maxillary attachment is fixed, when the depressor septi nasi contracts, it pulls the cartilage of the nose inferiorly toward the maxillary attachment. More specifically, the septum of the nose will be depressed and the alar cartilage will be depressed and pulled medially. These actions cause the nostril to constrict.

MISCELLANEOUS

❑ 1. The depressor septi nasi muscle is sometimes simply known as the *depressor septi.*

❑ 2. The depressor septi nasi is sometimes considered to be a part of the alar portion of the nasalis.

❑ 3. The action of constricting the nostrils can be associated with facial expressions during emotional states.

LEVATOR LABII SUPERIORIS ALAEQUE NASI

❑ **The name, levator labii superioris alaeque nasi, tells us that this muscle elevates the upper lip and is involved with the alae (cartilages of the nostrils of the nose).**

DERIVATION ❑
levator: L. *lifter.*
labii: L. *refers to the lips.*
superioris: L. *upper.*
alaeque: L. *refers to the ala* (alar cartilage).
nasi: L. *refers to the nose.*

PRONUNCIATION ❑ le-**vay**-tor **lay**-be-eye soo-**pee**-ri-**o**-ris a-**lee**-kwe **nay**-si

ATTACHMENTS

❑ **Maxilla**

- ❑ the frontal process of the maxilla near the nasal bone

to the

❑ **Upper Lip and the Nose**

- ❑ LATERAL SLIP: the muscular substance of the lateral part of the upper lip
- ❑ MEDIAL SLIP: the alar cartilage and the skin of the nose

ACTIONS

❑ 1. **Elevation of the Upper Lip**

❑ 2. **Flares the Nostril**

❑ 3. Eversion of the Upper Lip

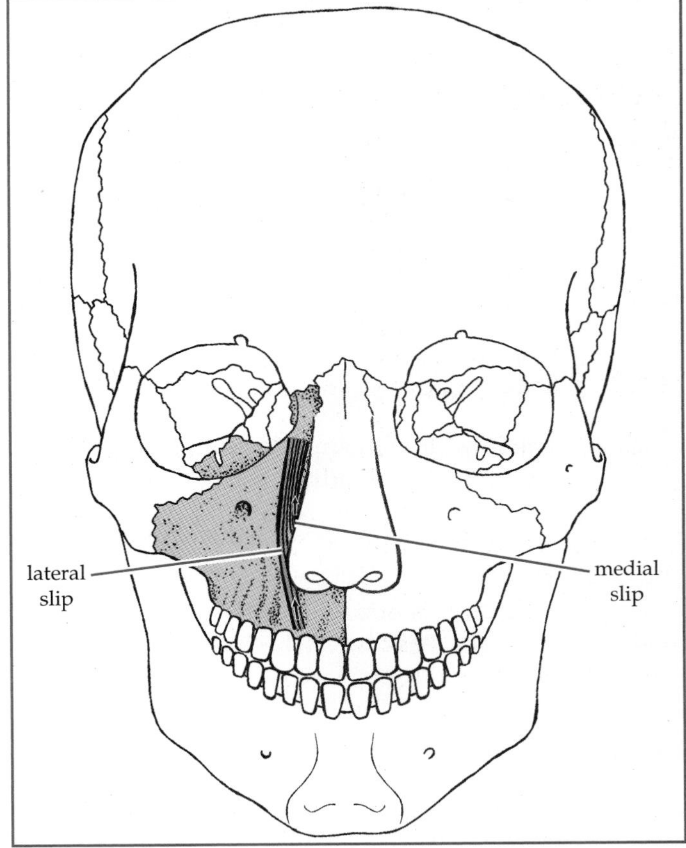

Anterior View of the Right Levator Labii Superioris Alaeque Nasi

INNERVATION ❑ The Facial Nerve (CN VII) ❑ buccal branches

ARTERIAL SUPPLY ❑ The Infraorbital Artery (A Branch of the Maxillary Artery)

LEVATOR LABII SUPERIORIS ALAEQUE NASI PALPATION AND SUPPLEMENTARY TEXT

PALPATION

- ❑ While the levator labii superioris alaeque nasi is superficial, it is a bit difficult to palpate with precision and to distinguish from the adjacent musculature. It is located medial and superficial to the levator labii superioris and the levator anguli oris, and medial to the zygomaticus minor, all of which can also elevate the upper lip. The levator labii superioris alaeque nasi is located lateral to the nasalis, which can also flare the nostril.
  - Have the client supine.
  - Place palpating fingers just lateral to the nose.
  - Ask the client to flare the nostrils and/or elevate the upper lip to show you the upper teeth and feel for the contraction of the levator labii superioris alaeque nasi. Try to distinguish the levator labii superioris alaeque nasi from the nasalis medially and the levator labii superioris laterally.

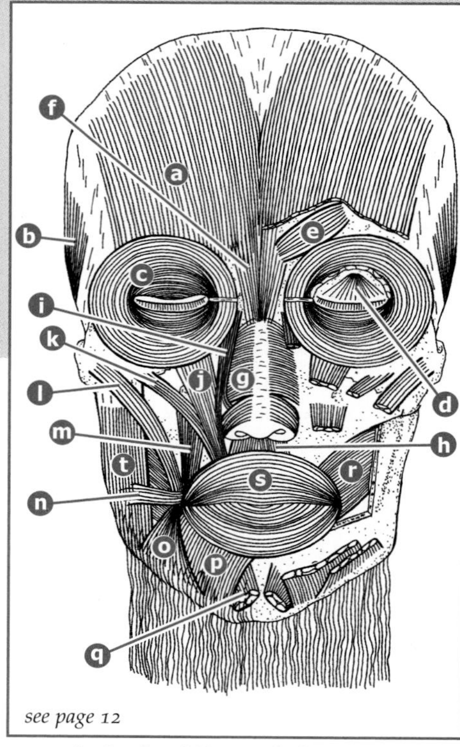

see page 12

Anterior View of the Head

a. Occipitofrontalis
b. Temporoparietalis
c. Orbicularis Oculi
d. Levator Palpebrae Superioris
e. Corrugator Supercilii
f. Procerus
g. Nasalis
h. Depressor Septi Nasi
i. **Levator Labii Superioris Alaeque Nasi**
j. Levator Labii Superioris
k. Zygomaticus Minor
l. Zygomaticus Major
m. Levator Anguli Oris
n. Risorius
o. Depressor Anguli Oris
p. Depressor Labii Inferioris
q. Mentalis
r. Buccinator
s. Orbicularis Oris
t. Masseter

RELATIONSHIP TO OTHER MUSCULOSKELETAL STRUCTURES

❑ 1. The levator labii superioris alaeque nasi is located lateral to the nasalis and medial (and somewhat superficial) to the levator labii superioris. The levator labii superioris alaeque nasi is also medial to the zygomaticus minor.

❑ 2. The levator labii superioris alaeque nasi is medial and inferior to the orbicularis oculi

❑ 3. The levator labii superioris alaeque nasi is superior to the orbicularis oris.

METHODOLOGY FOR LEARNING MUSCLE ACTIONS

❑ 1. **Elevation of the Upper Lip:** The lateral slip of the levator labii superioris alaeque nasi attaches from the upper lip inferiorly, and has a bony attachment near the eye superiorly (with its fibers running vertically). Since the superior attachment is into bone, it is more fixed than the other soft tissue attachment. When the levator labii superioris alaeque nasi contracts, it pulls the upper lip superiorly toward the other attachment. Therefore, the levator labii superioris alaeque nasi elevates the upper lip.

LEVATOR LABII SUPERIORIS ALAEQUE NASI – continued

- ☐ 2. **Flares the Nostril:** The medial slip of the levator labii superioris alaeque nasi attaches from the alar cartilage and the skin of the nose medially, to attach onto the maxilla laterally (with its fibers running somewhat horizontally). Since the lateral attachment is into bone, it is more fixed than the other soft tissue attachment. When the levator labii superioris alaeque nasi contracts, it pulls the skin and alar cartilage of the nose toward the other attachment. Therefore, the cartilage of the nose is pulled laterally, flaring the nostril and increasing the aperture for breathing.

- ☐ 3. **Eversion of the Upper Lip:** When the inferior attachment of the lateral slip of the levator labii superioris alaeque nasi is pulled superiorly toward the superior attachment, the lower margin of the upper lip will not only be pulled superiorly (see methodology #1), but will also be pulled away from the mouth, curling the upper lip. This curling or pulling away of the upper lip from the face is called eversion of the upper lip.

MISCELLANEOUS

- ☐ 1. Some sources consider the levator labii superioris alaeque nasi muscle to be the *angular head* of the levator labii superioris.

- ☐ 2. The three main elevators of the upper lip are the levator labii superioris alaeque nasi, levator labii superioris and the zygomaticus minor. These three muscles were once considered to be three individual heads (named *angularis, infraorbitalis* and *zygomaticus* respectively) of the *musculus quadratus labii superioris.*

- ☐ 3. The levator labii superioris alaeque nasi blends into the levator labii superioris and the orbicularis oris.

- ☐ 4. Flaring the nostrils by the medial slip of the levator labii superioris alaeque nasi, in addition to increasing the aperture for breathing, can also be part of the look of anger.

- ☐ 5. Contraction of the lateral slip of the levator labii superioris alaeque nasi alone will elevate the upper lip, as in showing someone your upper teeth. However its action, along with other facial muscles, can contribute to the facial expression of a smile or expressing smugness, contempt or disdain.

❑ LEVATOR LABII SUPERIORIS

❑ **The name, levator labii superioris, tells us that this muscle elevates the upper lip.**

DERIVATION ❑ levator: L. *lifter.*
labii: L. *refers to the lip.*
superioris: L. *upper.*

PRONUNCIATION ❑ le-**vay**-tor **lay**-be-eye soo-**pee**-ri-**o**-ris

ATTACHMENTS

❑ **Maxilla**

❑ at the inferior orbital margin of the maxilla

to the

❑ **Upper Lip**

❑ the muscular substance of the lateral part of the upper lip

ACTIONS

❑ **1. Elevation of the Upper Lip**

❑ 2. Eversion of the Upper Lip

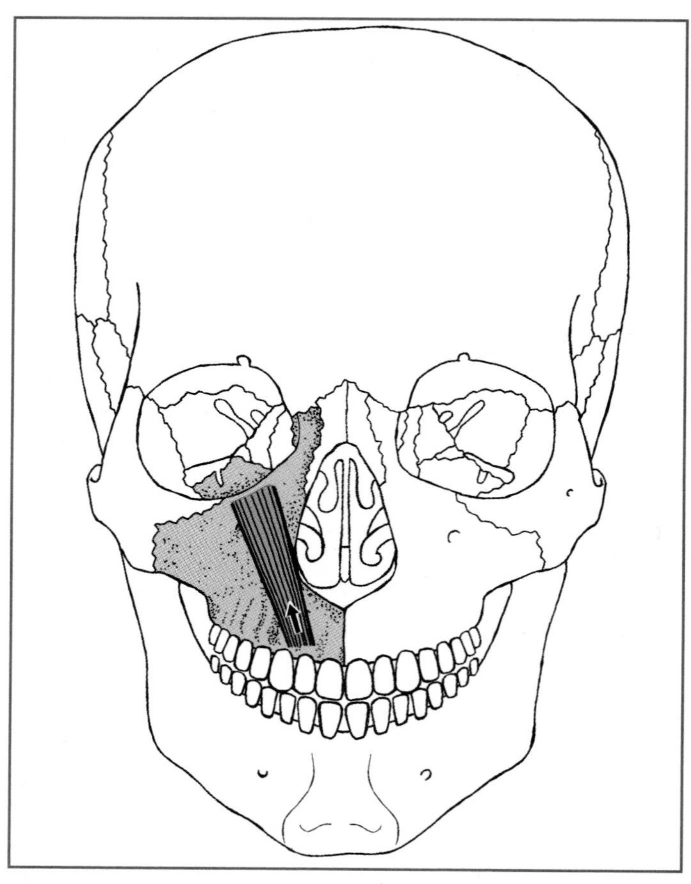

Anterior View of the Right Levator Labii Superioris

INNERVATION ❑ The Facial Nerve (CN VII) ❑ buccal branches

ARTERIAL SUPPLY ❑ The Facial Artery (A Branch of the External Carotid Artery)

PALPATION AND SUPPLEMENTARY TEXT

PALPATION

- ❑ While the levator labii superioris is superficial, it is difficult to palpate with precision and to distinguish from the adjacent musculature. It is located lateral to the levator labii superioris alaeque nasi and medial to the zygomaticus minor, both of which can also elevate the upper lip.
  - Have the client supine.
  - Place palpating fingers just superior to the upper lip approximately 1/2 - 1 inch (2 cm) medial to the corner of the mouth.
  - Ask the client to elevate the upper lip to show you the upper gums and feel for the contraction of the levator labii superioris. Try to distinguish it from the levator labii superioris alaeque nasi medially and the zygomaticus minor laterally.

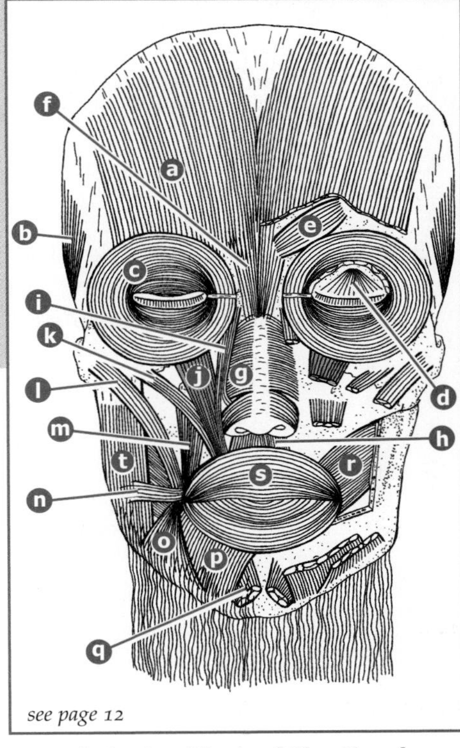

see page 12

Anterior View of the Head

a. Occipitofrontalis
b. Temporoparietalis
c. Orbicularis Oculi
d. Levator Palpebrae Superioris
e. Corrugator Supercilii
f. Procerus
g. Nasalis
h. Depressor Septi Nasi
i. Levator Labii Superioris Alaeque Nasi
j. **Levator Labii Superioris**
k. Zygomaticus Minor
l. Zygomaticus Major
m. Levator Anguli Oris
n. Risorius
o. Depressor Anguli Oris
p. Depressor Labii Inferioris
q. Mentalis
r. Buccinator
s. Orbicularis Oris
t. Masseter

RELATIONSHIP TO OTHER MUSCULOSKELETAL STRUCTURES

❑ 1. The levator labii superioris is between the levator labii superioris alaeque nasi (medially) and the zygomaticus minor (laterally).

❑ 2. The levator labii superioris is inferior to the orbicularis oculi, and where they overlap, the levator labii superioris is deep to the orbicularis oculi.

❑ 3. The levator labii superioris is superior to the orbicularis oris. When the levator labii superioris meets the orbicularis oris, the fibers of the levator labii superioris run deep to and blend into the orbicularis oris.

METHODOLOGY FOR LEARNING MUSCLE ACTIONS

❑ **1. Elevation of the Upper Lip:** The levator labii superioris attaches from the upper lip inferiorly, to attach onto bone superiorly (with its fibers running vertically). The superior attachment is into bone and is therefore more fixed than the other attachment, which is into soft tissue. When the levator labii superioris contracts, it pulls the upper lip superiorly toward the other attachment. Therefore, the levator labii superioris elevates the upper lip.

❑ **2. Eversion of the Upper Lip:** When the inferior attachment of the levator labii superioris is pulled superiorly toward the superior attachment, the lower margin of the upper lip is not only pulled superiorly (see methodology #1), but is also pulled away from the mouth, curling the upper lip. This curling or pulling away of the upper lip from the face is called eversion of the upper lip.

LEVATOR LABII SUPERIORIS – continued

MISCELLANEOUS

- ☐ 1. Some sources consider the levator labii superioris alaeque nasi muscle to be the *angular head* of the levator labii superioris.
- ☐ 2. The three main elevators of the upper lip are the levator labii superioris alaeque nasi, levator labii superioris and the zygomaticus minor. These three muscles were once considered to be three individual heads (named *angularis, infraorbitalis* and *zygomaticus* respectively) of the *musculus quadratus labii superioris.*
- ☐ 3. The levator labii superioris blends in with the levator labii superioris alaeque nasi and the orbicularis oris.
- ☐ 4. Contraction of the levator labii superioris alone will elevate the upper lip, as in showing someone your upper teeth. However, its action, along with other facial muscles, can contribute to the facial expression of a smile or expressing smugness, contempt, or disdain.

ZYGOMATICUS MINOR

❑ **The name, zygomaticus minor, tells us that this muscle attaches to the zygomatic bone and is small (smaller than the zygomaticus major).**

DERIVATION ❑ zygomaticus: Gr. *refers to the zygomatic bone.*
minor: L. *smaller.*

PRONUNCIATION ❑ **zi**-go-**mat**-ik-us **my**-nor

ATTACHMENTS

❑ **Zygomatic Bone**

- ❑ near the zygomaticomaxillary suture of the zygomatic bone

to the

❑ **Upper Lip**

- ❑ the muscular substance of the lateral part of the upper lip

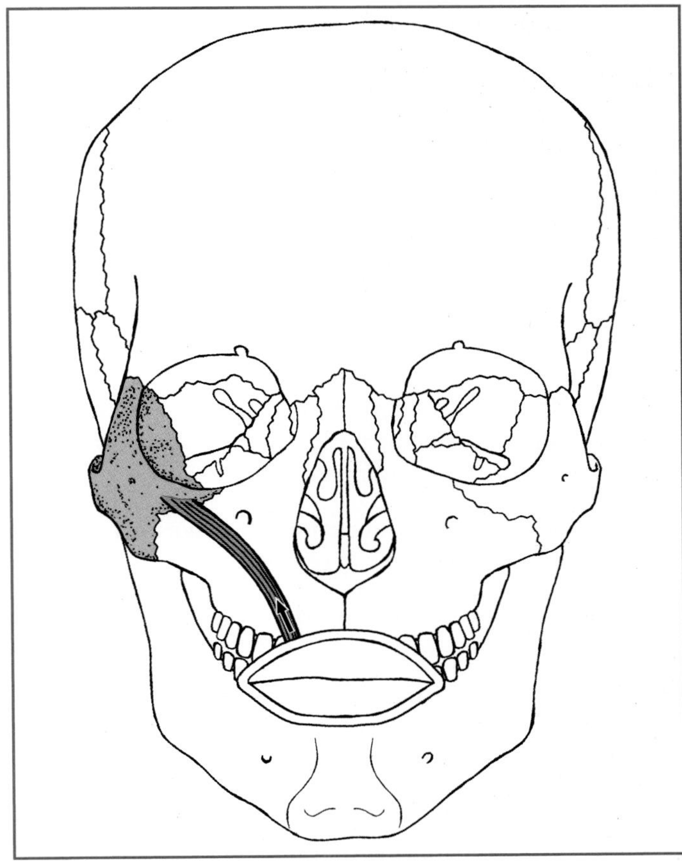

Anterior View of the Right Zygomaticus Minor

ACTIONS

❑ 1. **Elevation of the Upper Lip**

❑ 2. Eversion of the Upper Lip

INNERVATION ❑ The Facial Nerve (CN VII) ❑ buccal branches

ARTERIAL SUPPLY ❑ The Facial Artery (A Branch of the External Carotid Artery)

ZYGOMATICUS MINOR – PALPATION AND SUPPLEMENTARY TEXT

PALPATION

- ❑ While the zygomaticus minor is superficial, it is difficult to palpate with precision and to distinguish from the adjacent musculature. It is located lateral to the levator labii superioris and the levator labii superioris alaeque nasi and medial to the zygomaticus major, all of which can also elevate the upper lip.
  - Have the client supine.
  - Place palpating fingers just superior to the upper lip, approximately 1/2 -1 inch (2 cm) medial to the angle of the mouth.
  - Ask the client to elevate the upper lip to show you the upper teeth and feel for the contraction of the zygomaticus minor. Try to distinguish it from the levator labii superioris and the levator labii superioris alaeque nasi medially, and the zygomaticus major laterally.

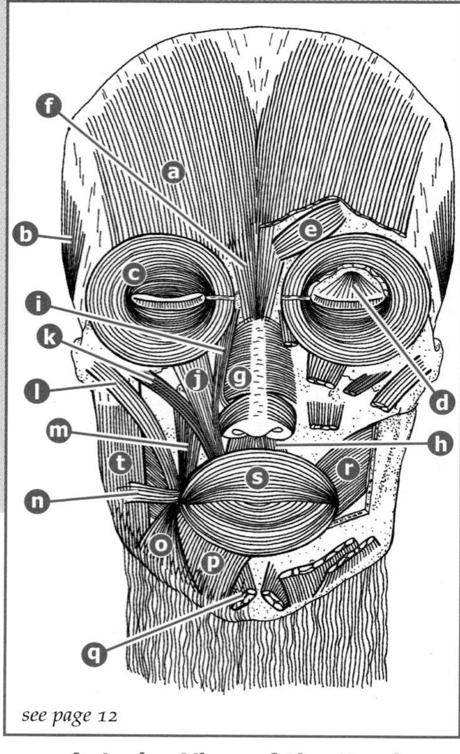

see page 12

Anterior View of the Head

- **a.** Occipitofrontalis
- **b.** Temporoparietalis
- **c.** Orbicularis Oculi
- **d.** Levator Palpebrae Superioris
- **e.** Corrugator Supercilii
- **f.** Procerus
- **g.** Nasalis
- **h.** Depressor Septi Nasi
- **i.** Levator Labii Superioris Alaeque Nasi
- **j.** Levator Labii Superioris
- **k. Zygomaticus Minor**
- **l.** Zygomaticus Major
- **m.** Levator Anguli Oris
- **n.** Risorius
- **o.** Depressor Anguli Oris
- **p.** Depressor Labii Inferioris
- **q.** Mentalis
- **r.** Buccinator
- **s.** Orbicularis Oris
- **t.** Masseter

RELATIONSHIP TO OTHER MUSCULOSKELETAL STRUCTURES

- ❑ 1. The zygomaticus minor is lateral to the levator labii superioris alaeque nasi and the levator labii superioris and medial to the zygomaticus major.
- ❑ 2. The zygomaticus minor is superior to the orbicularis oris and inferior to the orbicularis oculi.
- ❑ 3. The zygomaticus minor is superficial to the levator anguli oris.

METHODOLOGY FOR LEARNING MUSCLE ACTIONS

- ❑ **1. Elevation of the Upper Lip:** The zygomaticus minor attaches from the upper lip inferiorly, to the zygomatic bone superiorly (with its fibers running vertically). The maxillary attachment is into bone and is therefore more fixed than the other attachment, which is into soft tissue. When the zygomaticus minor contracts, it pulls the upper lip superiorly toward the zygomatic bone. Therefore, the zygomaticus minor elevates the upper lip.
- ❑ **2. Eversion of the Upper Lip:** When the inferior attachment of the zygomaticus minor is pulled superiorly toward the superior attachment, the lower margin of the upper lip is not only pulled superiorly (see methodology #1), but is also pulled away from the mouth, curling the upper lip. This curling or pulling away from the face is called eversion of the upper lip.

ZYGOMATICUS MINOR – continued

MISCELLANEOUS

- ❑ 1. The zygomaticus minor blends with the levator labii superioris.
- ❑ 2. The three main elevators of the upper lip are the levator labii superioris alaeque nasi, levator labii superioris and the zygomaticus minor. These three muscles were once considered to be three individual heads (named *angularis, infraorbitalis* and *zygomaticus* respectively) of the *musculus quadratus labii superioris.*
- ❑ 3. Contraction of the zygomaticus minor alone will elevate the upper lip, as in showing someone your upper teeth. However, its action, along with other facial muscles, can contribute to the facial expression of a smile or expressing smugness, contempt, or disdain.
- ❑ 4. Contraction of the zygomaticus minor will also increase the nasolabial sulcus.

ZYGOMATICUS MAJOR

❑ **The name, zygomaticus major, tells us that this muscle attaches to the zygomatic bone and is large (larger than the zygomaticus minor).**

DERIVATION ❑ zygomaticus: Gr. *refers to the zygomatic bone.*
major: L. *larger.*

PRONUNCIATION ❑ **zi**-go-**mat**-ik-us **may**-jor

ATTACHMENTS

❑ **Zygomatic Bone**

❑ near the zygomaticotemporal suture

to the

❑ **Angle of the Mouth**

❑ the modiolus, just lateral to the angle of the mouth

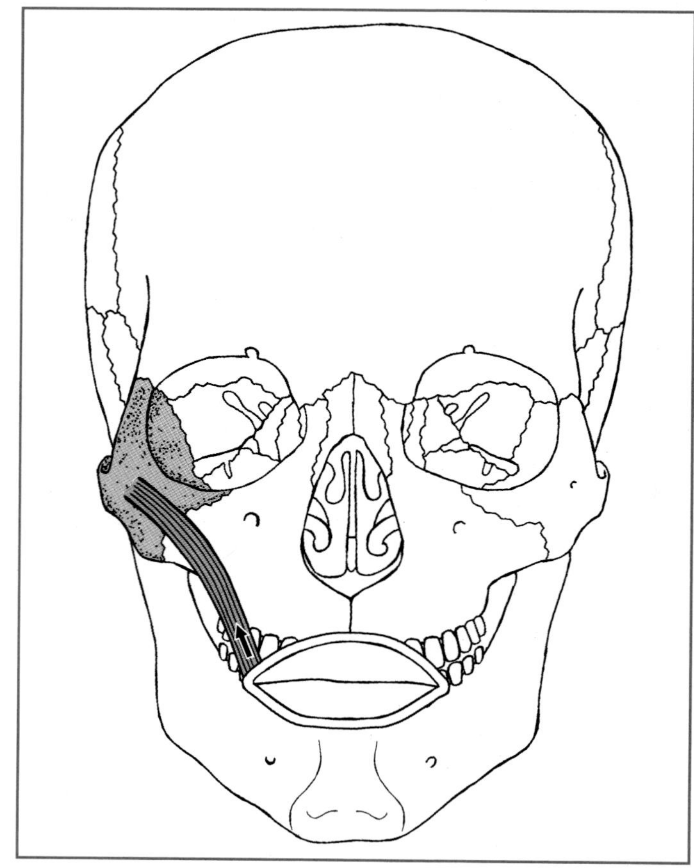

Anterior View of the Right Zygomaticus Major

ACTIONS

❑ **1. Elevation of the Angle of the Mouth**

❑ **2.** Draws Laterally the Angle of the Mouth

INNERVATION ❑ The Facial Nerve (CN VII) ❑ buccal branches

ARTERIAL SUPPLY ❑ The Facial Artery (A Branch of the External Carotid Artery)

PALPATION AND SUPPLEMENTARY TEXT

PALPATION

While the zygomaticus major is superficial, it can be difficult to palpate with precision and distinguish from the adjacent musculature. It is located between the zygomaticus minor and the risorius. The inferomedial attachment of the zygomaticus major can be palpated at the modiolus, a common attachment site for many facial muscles.

❑ **To palpate the belly:**

- Have the client supine.
- Place palpating fingers superior and lateral to the angle of the mouth.
- Ask the client to smile by drawing the angle of the mouth both superiorly and laterally and feel for the contraction of the belly of the zygomaticus major.

❑ **To palpate the inferomedial attachment at the modiolus:**

- Wearing a finger cot or glove, place the thumb of your palpating hand outside the client's mouth just lateral to the angle of the mouth, and the index finger inside the mouth.
- Compress the skin and mucosa of the cheek between your thumb and index finger and feel for the modiolus. Many muscles attach into the modiolus and it is not easy to differentiate them.

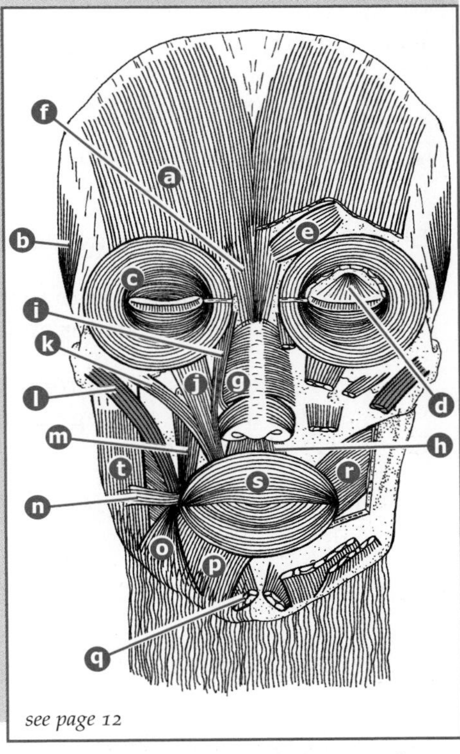

see page 12

Anterior View of the Head

a. Occipitofrontalis
b. Temporoparietalis
c. Orbicularis Oculi
d. Levator Palpebrae Superioris
e. Corrugator Supercilii
f. Procerus
g. Nasalis
h. Depressor Septi Nasi
i. Levator Labii Superioris Alaeque Nasi
j. Levator Labii Superioris
k. Zygomaticus Minor
l. **Zygomaticus Major**
m. Levator Anguli Oris
n. Risorius
o. Depressor Anguli Oris
p. Depressor Labii Inferioris
q. Mentalis
r. Buccinator
s. Orbicularis Oris
t. Masseter

RELATIONSHIP TO OTHER MUSCULOSKELETAL STRUCTURES

❑ 1. The zygomaticus major is lateral to the zygomaticus minor and superior to the risorius. The zygomaticus major is also superior to the orbicularis oris.

❑ 2. The zygomaticus major is superficial to the buccinator and the masseter.

METHODOLOGY FOR LEARNING MUSCLE ACTIONS

❑ **1. Elevation of the Angle of the Mouth:** The zygomaticus major attaches from the zygomatic bone superiorly, to the angle of the mouth inferiorly (with its fibers running vertically). The zygomatic attachment is into bone and is therefore more fixed than the other attachment, which is into soft tissue. When the zygomaticus major contracts, it pulls the angle of the mouth superiorly toward the zygomatic bone. Therefore, the zygomaticus major elevates the angle of the mouth.

ZYGOMATICUS MAJOR – continued

- ❑ 2. **Draws Laterally the Angle of the Mouth:** The zygomaticus major attaches from the zygomatic bone laterally, to the angle of the mouth medially (with its fibers running somewhat horizontally). The zygomatic attachment is into bone and is therefore more fixed than the other attachment, which is into soft tissue. When the zygomaticus major contracts, it pulls the angle of the mouth toward the zygomatic bone. Therefore, the zygomaticus major draws laterally the angle of the mouth.

MISCELLANEOUS

- ❑ 1. The zygomaticus major blends in with the levator anguli oris and the orbicularis oris.
- ❑ 2. The action of elevating the angle of the mouth and drawing it laterally contributes to smiling and laughing.
- ❑ 3. Contraction of the zygomaticus major also increases the nasolabial sulcus.
- ❑ 4. Six muscles attach into the modiolus: the zygomaticus major, levator anguli oris, risorius, depressor anguli oris, buccinator and the orbicularis oris.
- ❑ 5. The modiolus is a fibromuscular condensation approximately 1/4 inch (1/2 cm) lateral to the angle of the mouth (see page 23).

LEVATOR ANGULI ORIS

❑ **The name, levator anguli oris, tells us that this muscle elevates the angle (corner) of the mouth.**

DERIVATION ❑ levator: L. *lifter.*
anguli: L. *angle.*
oris: L. *mouth.*

PRONUNCIATION ❑ le-**vay**-tor **ang**-you-lie **o**-ris

ATTACHMENTS

❑ **Maxilla**

❑ the canine fossa of the maxilla (just inferior to the infraorbital foramen)

to the

❑ **Angle of the Mouth**

❑ the modiolus, just lateral to the angle of the mouth

ACTION

❑ **Elevation of the Angle of the Mouth**

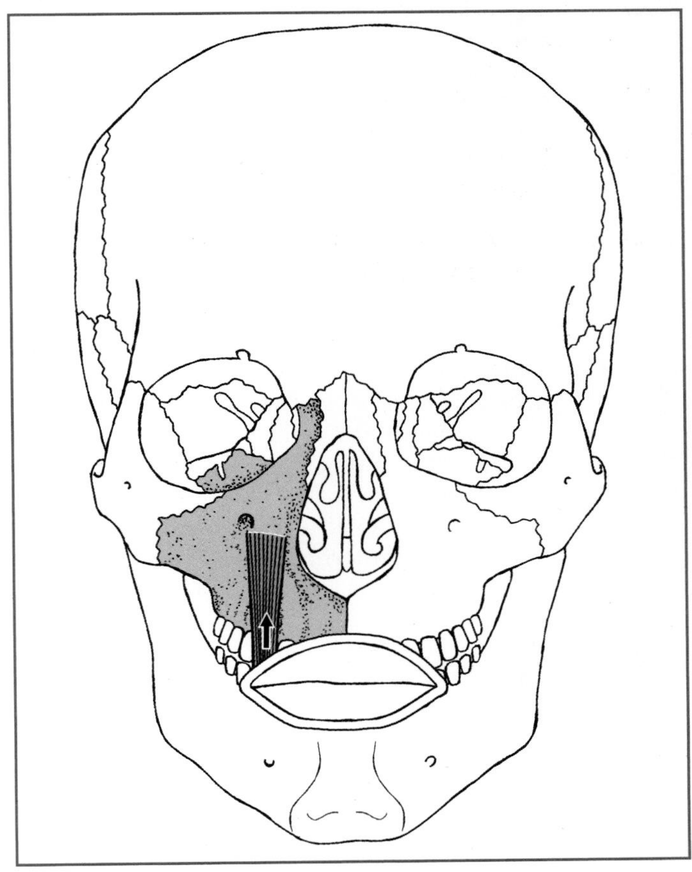

Anterior View of the Right Levator Anguli Oris

INNERVATION ❑ The Facial Nerve (CN VII) ❑ buccal branches

ARTERIAL SUPPLY ❑ The Facial Artery (A Branch of the External Carotid Artery)

LEVATOR ANGULI ORIS – PALPATION AND SUPPLEMENTARY TEXT

PALPATION

While the levator anguli oris is deep to other facial muscles, it is superficial between the zygomaticus minor and the zygomaticus major. The inferior attachment of the levator anguli oris can be palpated at the modiolus, a common attachment site for many facial muscles.

❑ **To palpate the belly:**

- Have the client supine.
- Place palpating fingers just superior to the angle (corner) of the mouth.
- Ask the client to elevate the angle of the mouth straight superiorly, attempting to show you the canine tooth, and feel for the contraction of the belly of the levator anguli oris. Try to distinguish it from the levator labii superioris, zygomaticus major, and the zygomaticus minor.

❑ **To palpate the inferior attachment at the modiolus:**

- Wearing a finger cot or glove, place the thumb of your palpating hand outside the client's mouth just lateral to the angle of the mouth, and the index finger inside the mouth.
- Compress the skin and mucosa of the cheek between your thumb and index finger and feel for the modiolus. Many muscles attach into the modiolus and it is not easy to differentiate them.

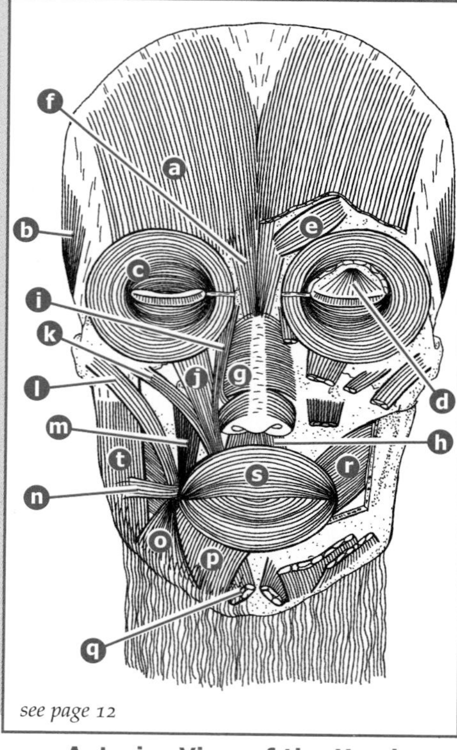

see page 12

Anterior View of the Head

a. Occipitofrontalis
b. Temporoparietalis
c. Orbicularis Oculi
d. Levator Palpebrae Superioris
e. Corrugator Supercilii
f. Procerus
g. Nasalis
h. Depressor Septi Nasi
i. Levator Labii Superioris Alaeque Nasi
j. Levator Labii Superioris
k. Zygomaticus Minor
l. Zygomaticus Major
m. Levator Anguli Oris
n. Risorius
o. Depressor Anguli Oris
p. Depressor Labii Inferioris
q. Mentalis
r. Buccinator
s. Orbicularis Oris
t. Masseter

RELATIONSHIP TO OTHER MUSCULOSKELETAL STRUCTURES

❑ 1. The levator anguli oris is deep to the levator labii superioris, zygomaticus minor and the zygomaticus major. The levator anguli oris is superficial between the zygomaticus minor and the zygomaticus major.

❑ 2. The inferior attachment of the levator anguli oris is superficial to the buccinator.

❑ 3. The levator anguli oris is superior to the orbicularis oris and inferior to the orbicularis oculi.

LEVATOR ANGULI ORIS – continued

METHODOLOGY FOR LEARNING MUSCLE ACTIONS

- ❑ **Elevation of the Angle of the Mouth:** The levator anguli oris attaches from the maxilla superiorly, to the tissue at the angle (corner) of the mouth inferiorly (with its fibers running vertically). The maxillary attachment is into bone and is therefore more fixed than the other attachment, which is into soft tissue. When the levator anguli oris contracts, it pulls the angle of the mouth superiorly toward the maxilla. Therefore, the levator anguli oris elevates the angle of the mouth.

MISCELLANEOUS

❑ 1. The levator anguli oris is also known as the *caninus* (kay-**ni**-nus). This name is given because the contraction of the levator anguli oris can result in the teeth, especially the canine tooth, becoming visible.

❑ 2. At the attachment near the angle of the mouth (the modiolus), fibers of the levator anguli oris blend in with the orbicularis oris, zygomaticus major and the depressor anguli oris.

❑ 3. Although the action of the levator anguli oris may contribute to a smile, its action alone (unilaterally or bilaterally) can manifest a sneer. Bilateral contraction of this muscle can also reproduce the typical "Dracula" expression wherein the canine teeth are exposed.

❑ 4. Contraction of the levator anguli oris also increases the nasolabial sulcus.

❑ 5. Six muscles attach into the modiolus: the zygomaticus major, levator anguli oris, risorius, depressor anguli oris, buccinator and the orbicularis oris.

❑ 6. The modiolus is a fibromuscular condensation approximately 1/4 inch (1/2 cm) lateral to the angle of the mouth (see page 23).

RISORIUS

❑ **The name, risorius, tells us that this muscle is involved with laughing.**

DERIVATION ❑ risorius: L. *laughing*.

PRONUNCIATION ❑ ri-**so**-ri-us

ATTACHMENTS

❑ **Fascia Superficial to the Masseter**

to the

❑ **Angle of the Mouth**

- ❑ the modiolus, just lateral to the angle of the mouth

ACTION

❑ **Draws Laterally the Angle of the Mouth**

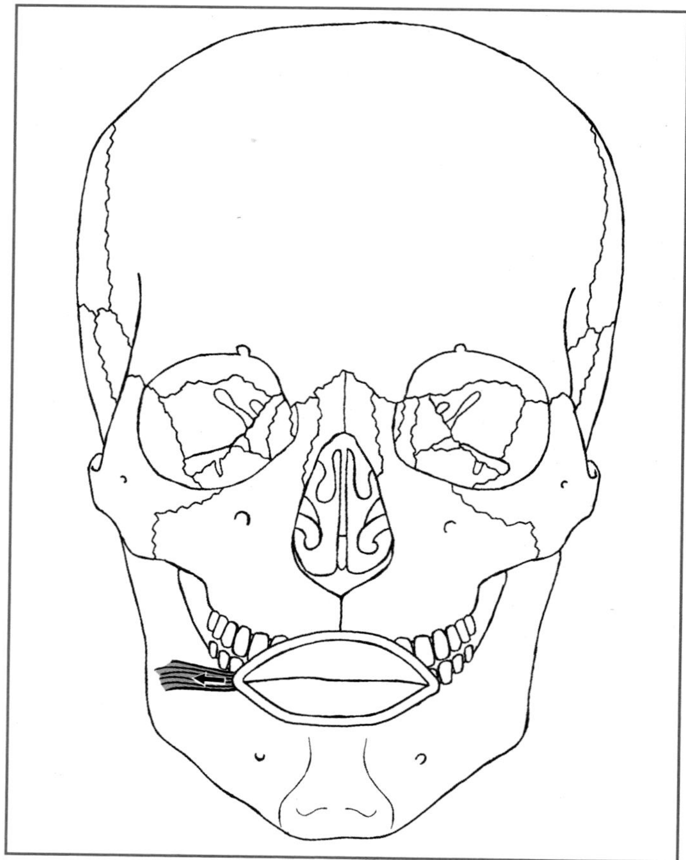

Anterior View of the Right Risorius

INNERVATION ❑ The Facial Nerve (CN VII) ❑ buccal branches

ARTERIAL SUPPLY ❑ The Facial Artery (A Branch of the External Carotid Artery)

PALPATION AND SUPPLEMENTARY TEXT

PALPATION

While the risorius is superficial in the face and located lateral to the angle of the mouth, it is a thin muscle and can be difficult to palpate with precision and distinguish from adjacent musculature. The medial attachment of the risorius can be palpated at the modiolus, a common attachment site for many facial muscles.

❑ **To palpate the belly:**

- Have the client supine.
- Place palpating fingers directly lateral to the angle of the mouth.
- Ask the client to draw the angle (corner) of the mouth directly lateral and feel for the contraction of the belly of the risorius. (Be sure that you are not palpating too superiorly onto the zygomaticus major, which can also help to draw the angle of the mouth laterally.)

❑ **To palpate the medial attachment at the modiolus:**

- Wearing a finger cot or glove, place the thumb of your palpating hand outside the client's mouth just lateral to the angle of the mouth, and the index finger inside the mouth.
- Compress the skin and mucosa of the cheek between your thumb and index finger and feel for the modiolus. Many muscles attach into the modiolus and it is not easy to differentiate them.

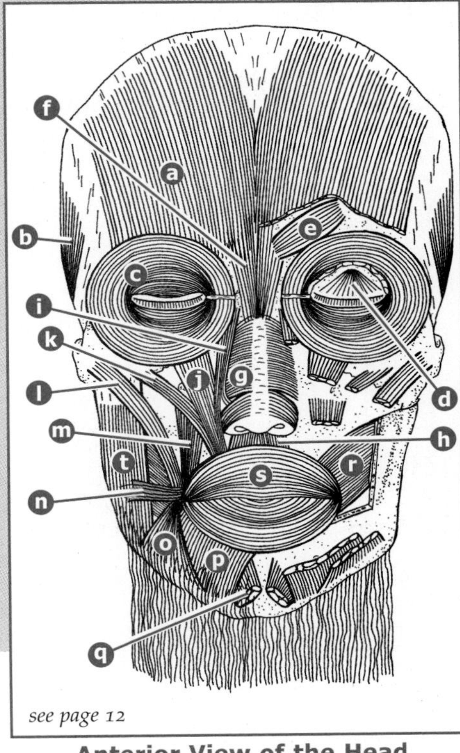

see page 12

Anterior View of the Head

a. Occipitofrontalis
b. Temporoparietalis
c. Orbicularis Oculi
d. Levator Palpebrae Superioris
e. Corrugator Supercilii
f. Procerus
g. Nasalis
h. Depressor Septi Nasi
i. Levator Labii Superioris Alaeque Nasi
j. Levator Labii Superioris
k. Zygomaticus Minor
l. Zygomaticus Major
m. Levator Anguli Oris
n. **Risorius**
o. Depressor Anguli Oris
p. Depressor Labii Inferioris
q. Mentalis
r. Buccinator
s. Orbicularis Oris
t. Masseter

RELATIONSHIP TO OTHER MUSCULOSKELETAL STRUCTURES

❑ 1. The risorius is inferior to the zygomaticus major and lateral to the orbicularis oris.

❑ 2. The risorius is superior to the depressor anguli oris and the platysma. Where these muscles overlap, the risorius is superficial.

❑ 3. The risorius is superficial to the buccinator.

METHODOLOGY FOR LEARNING MUSCLE ACTIONS

❑ **Draws Laterally the Angle of the Mouth:** The risorius attaches from the fascia superficial to the masseter laterally, to the angle of the mouth medially (with its fibers running somewhat horizontally). If the lateral attachment is the more fixed attachment, and the risorius contracts, it pulls the angle of the mouth laterally toward the more lateral attachment. Therefore, the risorius draws laterally the angle of the mouth.

RISORIUS – continued

MISCELLANEOUS

- ❑ 1. The lateral attachment of the risorius varies greatly in its presentation.
- ❑ 2. The medial attachment of the risorius also varies, often attaching approximately 1/4 inch (1/2 cm) inferior to the angle of the mouth.
- ❑ 3. Drawing the angle of the mouth laterally is involved with grinning, smiling and laughing.
- ❑ 4. Six muscles attach into the modiolus: the zygomaticus major, levator anguli oris, risorius, depressor anguli oris, buccinator and the orbicularis oris.
- ❑ 5. The modiolus is a fibromuscular condensation approximately 1/4 inch (1/2 cm) lateral to the angle of the mouth (see page 23).

DEPRESSOR ANGULI ORIS

❑ **The name, depressor anguli oris, tells us that this muscle depresses the angle of the mouth.**

DERIVATION ❑ depressor: L. *depressor.*
anguli: L. *angle.*
oris: L. *mouth.*

PRONUNCIATION ❑ dee-**pres**-or **ang**-you-lie **o**-ris

ATTACHMENTS

❑ **Mandible**

❑ the oblique line of the mandible, inferior to the mental foramen

to the

❑ **Angle of the Mouth**

❑ the modiolus, just lateral to the angle of the mouth

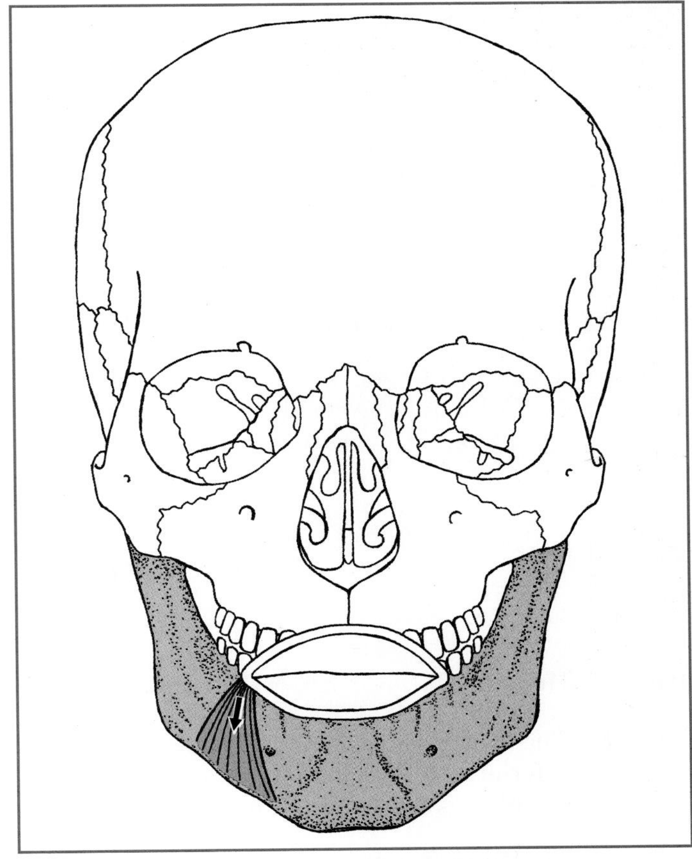

Anterior View of the Right Depressor Anguli Oris

ACTIONS

❑ 1. **Depression of the Angle of the Mouth**

❑ 2. Draws Laterally the Angle of the Mouth

INNERVATION ❑ The Facial Nerve (CN VII) ❑ mandibular branch

ARTERIAL SUPPLY ❑ The Facial Artery (A Branch of the External Carotid Artery)

DEPRESSOR ANGULI ORIS – PALPATION AND SUPPLEMENTARY TEXT

PALPATION

The depressor anguli oris is superficial in the face and is located slightly lateral and inferior to the mouth. The superomedial attachment of the depressor anguli oris can be palpated at the modiolus, a common attachment site for many facial muscles.

❑ **To palpate the belly:**

- Have the client supine.
- Place palpating fingers slightly lateral and inferior to the angle of the mouth.
- Ask the client to draw the angle of the mouth inferiorly (and perhaps pull the angle of the mouth slightly laterally) and feel for the contraction of the belly of the depressor anguli oris. It may be difficult to precisely distinguish this muscle from the nearby depressor labii inferioris.

❑ **To palpate the superomedial attachment:**

- Wearing a finger cot or glove, place the thumb of your palpating hand outside the client's mouth just lateral to the angle of the mouth, and the index finger inside the mouth.
- Compress the skin and mucosa of the cheek between your thumb and index finger and feel for the modiolus. Many muscles attach into the modiolus and it is not easy to differentiate them.

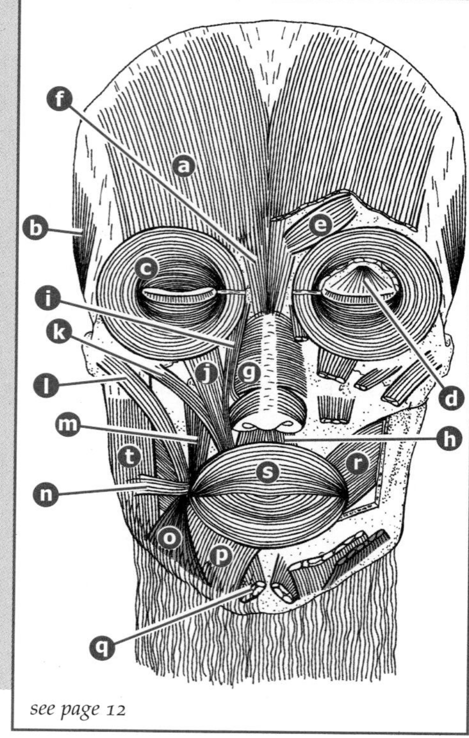

see page 12

Anterior View of the Head

a. Occipitofrontalis
b. Temporoparietalis
c. Orbicularis Oculi
d. Levator Palpebrae Superioris
e. Corrugator Supercilii
f. Procerus
g. Nasalis
h. Depressor Septi Nasi
i. Levator Labii Superioris Alaeque Nasi
j. Levator Labii Superioris
k. Zygomaticus Minor
l. Zygomaticus Major
m. Levator Anguli Oris
n. Risorius
o. **Depressor Anguli Oris**
p. Depressor Labii Inferioris
q. Mentalis
r. Buccinator
s. Orbicularis Oris
t. Masseter

RELATIONSHIP TO OTHER MUSCULOSKELETAL STRUCTURES

❑ 1. The depressor anguli oris is lateral to the depressor labii inferioris. Where these two muscles overlap, the depressor anguli oris is superficial to the depressor labii inferioris.

❑ 2. The depressor anguli oris is inferior to the orbicularis oris and the risorius.

❑ 3. The depressor anguli oris is superior to the platysma.

DEPRESSOR ANGULI ORIS – continued

METHODOLOGY FOR LEARNING MUSCLE ACTIONS

❑ 1. **Depression of the Angle of the Mouth:** The depressor anguli oris attaches from the mandible inferiorly, to the tissue at the angle (corner) of the mouth superiorly (with its fibers running vertically). The mandibular attachment is into bone and is therefore more fixed than the other attachment, which is into soft tissue. When the depressor anguli oris contracts, it pulls the angle of the mouth inferiorly toward the mandible. Therefore, the depressor anguli oris depresses the angle of the mouth.

❑ 2. **Draws Laterally the Angle of the Mouth:** The depressor anguli oris attaches from the mandible laterally, into the angle of the mouth medially (with its fibers running somewhat horizontally). The mandibular attachment is into bone and is therefore more fixed than the other attachment, which is into soft tissue. When the depressor anguli oris contracts, it pulls the angle of the mouth laterally toward the mandible. Therefore, the depressor anguli oris draws laterally the angle of the mouth.

MISCELLANEOUS

❑ 1. The depressor anguli oris blends into the platysma.

❑ 2. Sometimes, some fibers of the depressor anguli oris blend into the opposite-sided depressor anguli oris and/or the same-sided levator anguli oris.

❑ 3. Both the depressor anguli oris and the depressor labii inferioris arise from the oblique line of the mandible. On the oblique line, the depressor anguli oris attaches more laterally than the depressor labii inferioris.

❑ 4. The actions of the depressor anguli oris contribute to the facial expression of sadness or uncertainty.

❑ 5. Six muscles attach into the modiolus: the zygomaticus major, levator anguli oris, risorius, depressor anguli oris, buccinator and the orbicularis oris.

❑ 6. The modiolus is a fibromuscular condensation approximately 1/4 inch (1/2 cm) lateral to the angle of the mouth (see page 23).

❑ DEPRESSOR LABII INFERIORIS

❑ **The name, depressor labii inferioris, tells us that this muscle depresses the lower lip.**

DERIVATION ❑ depressor: L. *depressor.*
labii: L. *refers to the lips.*
inferioris: L. *lower.*

PRONUNCIATION ❑ dee-**pres**-or **lay**-be-eye in-**fee**-ri-**o**-ris

ATTACHMENTS

❑ **Mandible**

❑ the oblique line of the mandible, between the symphysis menti and the mental foramen

to the

❑ **Lower Lip**

❑ the midline of the lower lip

ACTIONS

❑ **1. Depression of the Lower Lip**

❑ 2. Draws Laterally the Lower Lip

❑ 3. Eversion of the Lower Lip

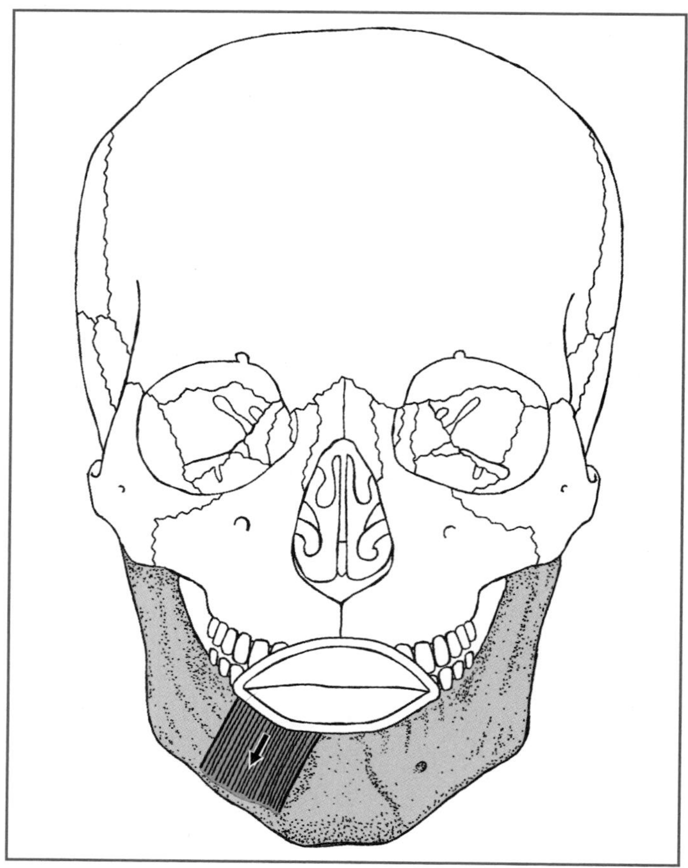

Anterior View of the Right Depressor Labii Inferioris

INNERVATION ❑ The Facial Nerve (CN VII) ❑ mandibular branch

ARTERIAL SUPPLY ❑ The Facial Artery (A Branch of the External Carotid Artery)

PALPATION AND SUPPLEMENTARY TEXT

PALPATION

❑ While the lateral portion of the depressor labii inferioris is deep to the depressor anguli oris, the medial portion is superficial between the mentalis and the depressor anguli oris.

- Have the client supine.
- Place palpating fingers inferior to the lower lip, slightly lateral from the center.
- Ask the client to draw the lower lip inferiorly and laterally and feel for the contraction of the medial portion of the depressor labii inferioris. It may be difficult to precisely differentiate the depressor labii inferioris from the nearby mentalis and the depressor anguli oris.

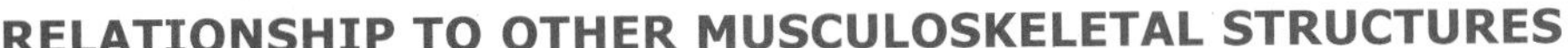

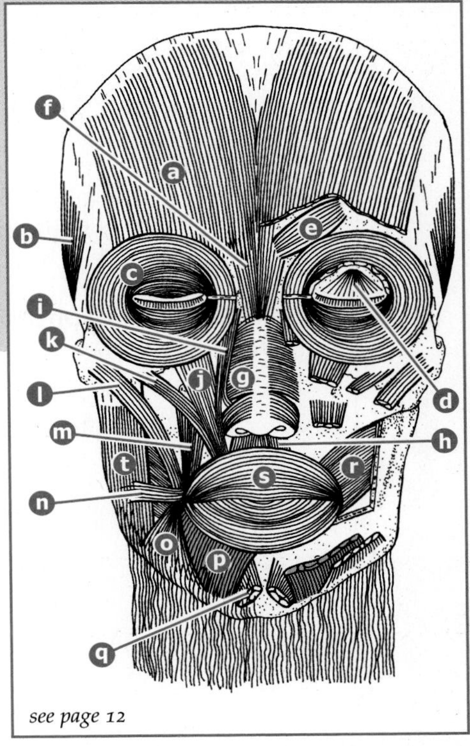

see page 12

Anterior View of the Head

a. Occipitofrontalis
b. Temporoparietalis
c. Orbicularis Oculi
d. Levator Palpebrae Superioris
e. Corrugator Supercilii
f. Procerus
g. Nasalis
h. Depressor Septi Nasi
i. Levator Labii Superioris Alaeque Nasi
j. Levator Labii Superioris
k. Zygomaticus Minor
l. Zygomaticus Major
m. Levator Anguli Oris
n. Risorius
o. Depressor Anguli Oris
p. **Depressor Labii Inferioris**
q. Mentalis
r. Buccinator
s. Orbicularis Oris
t. Masseter

RELATIONSHIP TO OTHER MUSCULOSKELETAL STRUCTURES

❑ 1. The depressor labii inferioris is lateral to the mentalis. Where these two muscles overlap, the depressor labii inferioris is superficial.

❑ 2. The depressor labii inferioris is medial to the depressor anguli oris. Where these two muscles overlap, the depressor labii inferioris is deeper.

❑ 3. The depressor labii inferioris is inferior to the orbicularis oris and superior to the platysma.

METHODOLOGY FOR LEARNING MUSCLE ACTIONS

❑ **1. Depression of the Lower Lip:** The depressor labii inferioris attaches from the mandible inferiorly, into the lower lip superiorly (with its fibers running vertically). The mandibular attachment is into bone and is therefore more fixed than the other attachment, which is into soft tissue. When the depressor labii inferioris contracts, it pulls the lower lip inferiorly toward the mandible. Therefore, the depressor labii inferioris depresses the lower lip.

❑ **2. Draws Laterally the Lower Lip:** The depressor labii inferioris attaches from the mandible laterally, into the lower lip medially (with its fibers running somewhat horizontally). The mandibular attachment is into bone and is therefore more fixed than the other attachment, which is into soft tissue. When the depressor labii inferioris contracts, it pulls the lower lip laterally toward the mandible. Therefore, the depressor labii inferioris draws laterally the lower lip.

DEPRESSOR LABII INFERIORIS – continued

❑ 3. **Eversion of the Lower Lip:** When the superior attachment of the depressor labii inferioris is pulled inferiorly toward the inferior attachment, the lower margin of the lower lip will not only be pulled inferiorly, but will also be pulled away from the mouth, curling the lower lip. This curling or pulling away from the face is called eversion of the lower lip.

MISCELLANEOUS

❑ 1. The depressor labii inferioris blends with the opposite side depressor labii inferioris and the orbicularis oris at the lip. Inferiorly, the depressor labii inferioris blends with the platysma.

❑ 2. Both the depressor labii inferioris and the depressor anguli oris arise from the oblique line of the mandible. On the oblique line, the depressor labii inferioris attaches more medially than the depressor anguli oris.

❑ 3. The actions of the depressor labii inferioris can contribute to the facial expressions of sorrow, doubt and irony.

MENTALIS

❑ **The name, mentalis, tells us that this muscle is related to the chin.**

DERIVATION ❑ mentalis: L. *refers to the chin.*

PRONUNCIATION ❑ men-**ta**-lis

ATTACHMENTS

❑ **Mandible**

❑ the incisive fossa of the mandible

to the

❑ **Skin of the Chin**

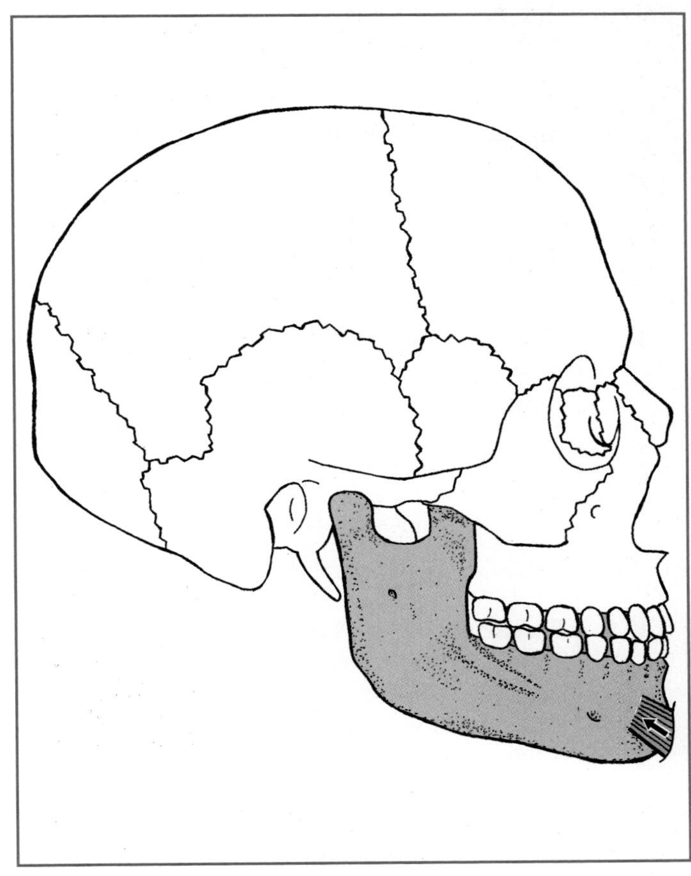

Lateral View of the Right Mentalis

ACTIONS

❑ 1. **Elevation of the Lower Lip**

❑ 2. **Eversion and Protraction of the Lower Lip**

❑ 3. Wrinkles the Skin of the Chin

INNERVATION ❑ The Facial Nerve (CN VII) ❑ mandibular branch

ARTERIAL SUPPLY ❑ The Facial Artery (A Branch of the External Carotid Artery)

MENTALIS – PALPATION AND SUPPLEMENTARY TEXT

PALPATION

- ❑ While the lateral portion of the mentalis is deep to the depressor labii inferioris, the medial portion of the mentalis is superficial and medial to the depressor labii inferioris.
  - Have the client supine.
  - Place palpating fingers inferior to the midline of the lower lip, just slightly lateral from the center. (Be sure that you are inferior to the orbicularis oris and medial to the depressor labii inferioris.)
  - Ask the client to stick out the lower lip as if pouting and feel for the contraction of the mentalis.

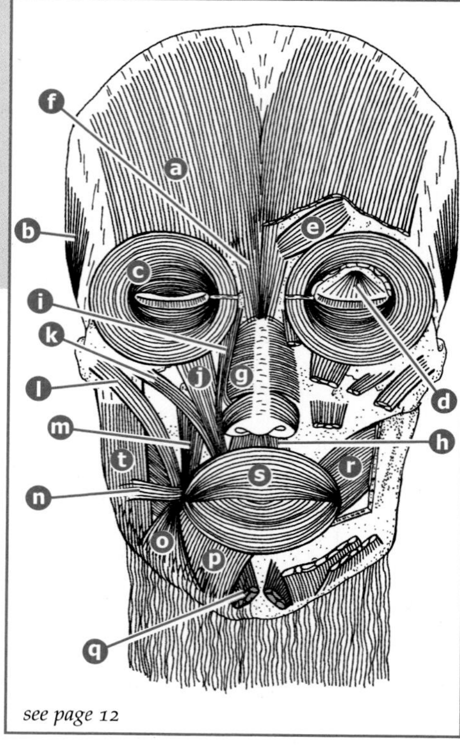

see page 12

Anterior View of the Head

a. Occipitofrontalis
b. Temporoparietalis
c. Orbicularis Oculi
d. Levator Palpebrae Superioris
e. Corrugator Supercilii
f. Procerus
g. Nasalis
h. Depressor Septi Nasi
i. Levator Labii Superioris Alaeque Nasi
j. Levator Labii Superioris
k. Zygomaticus Minor
l. Zygomaticus Major
m. Levator Anguli Oris
n. Risorius
o. Depressor Anguli Oris
p. Depressor Labii Inferioris
q. **Mentalis**
r. Buccinator
s. Orbicularis Oris
t. Masseter

RELATIONSHIP TO OTHER MUSCULOSKELETAL STRUCTURES

❑ 1. The mentalis is medial to the depressor labii inferioris. Where these two muscles overlap, the mentalis is deeper. The mentalis is also medial to the depressor anguli oris.

❑ 2. The mentalis is inferior to the orbicularis oris and superior to the platysma.

METHODOLOGY FOR LEARNING MUSCLE ACTIONS

❑ 1. **Elevation of the Lower Lip:** The mentalis attaches from the mandible superiorly, and attaches into the skin of the chin inferiorly (with its fibers running vertically). The mandibular attachment is into bone and is therefore more fixed than the other attachment, which is into soft tissue. When the mentalis contracts, it pulls the skin of the chin superiorly toward the mandible. When this occurs, the skin of the chin is pulled into the lower lip, pushing the lower lip superiorly. Therefore, the mentalis elevates the lower lip.

❑ 2. **Eversion and Protraction of the Lower Lip:** When the mentalis pulls superiorly on the skin of the chin, the lower lip is elevated (see methodology #1). As the mentalis continues to contract, the upper margin of the lower lip is forced away from the mouth anteriorly. This action is called eversion of the upper lip. As the mentalis continues to contract, the entire lower lip is forced away from the mouth. This action is called protraction (or protrusion) of the lower lip. Therefore, the mentalis everts and protracts the lower lip.

❑ 3. **Wrinkles the Skin of the Chin:** When the mentalis contracts and pulls superiorly on the skin of the chin, the lower lip is elevated and/or protracted (see methodology #2), and the skin of the chin is wrinkled.

MENTALIS – continued

MISCELLANEOUS

- ❑ 1. The actions of the mentalis are involved in manifesting the facial expressions of doubt, pouting or disdain.
- ❑ 2. Elevating, everting and protracting the lower lip are also useful when drinking.
- ❑ 3. When the mentalis contracts, it also raises the mentolabial sulcus (see page 23).

BUCCINATOR

❑ **The name, buccinator, tells us that this muscle is found in the cheek region.**

DERIVATION ❑ buccinator: L. *refers to the cheek.*

PRONUNCIATION ❑ **buk**-sin-**a**-tor

ATTACHMENTS

❑ **Maxilla and the Mandible**

❑ the external surfaces of the alveolar processes of the mandible and the maxilla, opposite the molars, and the pterygomandibular raphe

to the

❑ **Lips**

❑ deeper into the musculature of the lips and the modiolus, just lateral to the angle of the mouth

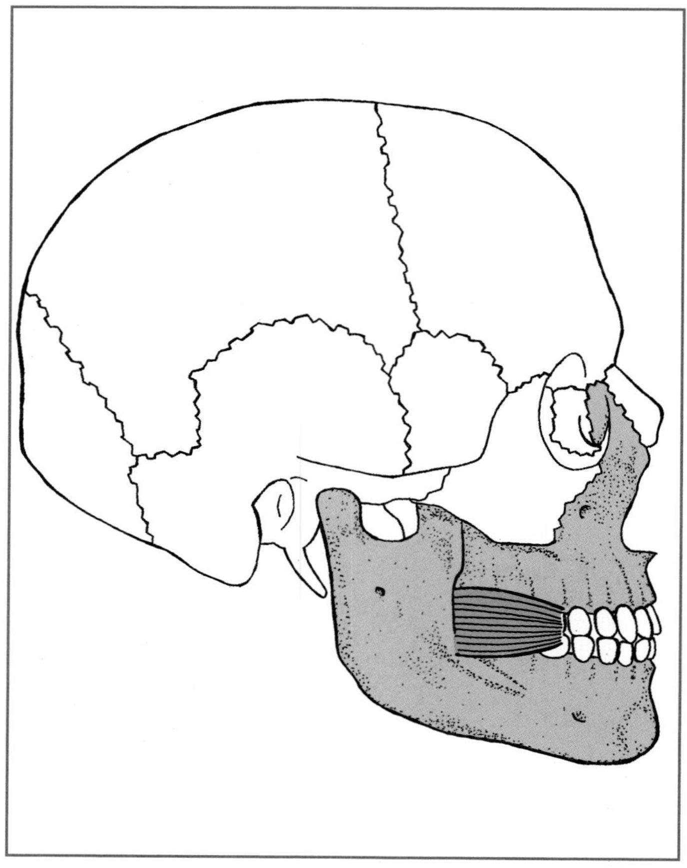

Lateral View of the Right Buccinator

ACTION

❑ **Compression of the Cheeks (Against the Teeth)**

INNERVATION ❑ The Facial Nerve (CN VII) ❑ buccal branches

ARTERIAL SUPPLY ❑ The Maxillary and Facial Arteries (Branches of the External Carotid Artery)

PALPATION AND SUPPLEMENTARY TEXT

PALPATION

- ❑ The buccinator is located in the cheek, deep to more superficial muscles of facial expression.
  - Have the client supine.
  - Place palpating fingers on the cheek, anterior to the ramus of the mandible.
  - Ask the client to take in a breath, purse the lips, and press the lips against the teeth as if they were expelling air to play the trumpet, and feel for the contraction of the buccinator.

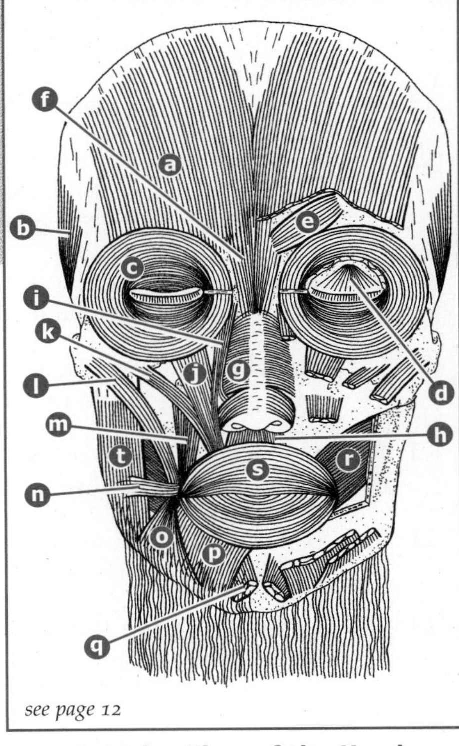

Anterior View of the Head

a. Occipitofrontalis
b. Temporoparietalis
c. Orbicularis Oculi
d. Levator Palpebrae Superioris
e. Corrugator Supercilii
f. Procerus
g. Nasalis
h. Depressor Septi Nasi
i. Levator Labii Superioris Alaeque Nasi
j. Levator Labii Superioris
k. Zygomaticus Minor
l. Zygomaticus Major
m. Levator Anguli Oris
n. Risorius
o. Depressor Anguli Oris
p. Depressor Labii Inferioris
q. Mentalis
r. **Buccinator**
s. Orbicularis Oris
t. Masseter

RELATIONSHIP TO OTHER MUSCULOSKELETAL STRUCTURES

- ❑ 1. The anterior part of the buccinator is superficial and located in the tissue of the cheek. The posterior part of the buccinator is deeper and located posterior to the ramus of the mandible.
- ❑ 2. The anterior part of the buccinator is deep to the levator anguli oris, zygomaticus major, risorius and the depressor anguli oris.
- ❑ 3. Deep to the buccinator is the mucosa of the cheek.

METHODOLOGY FOR LEARNING MUSCLE ACTIONS

- ❑ **Compression of the Cheeks (Against the Teeth):** Posteriorly, the fibers of the buccinator arise from the maxilla and the mandible (and the pterygomandibular raphe between the maxilla and the mandible). From there, the buccinator fibers travel anteriorly through the tissue of the cheek (running horizontally) to attach into the lips. The posterior attachments are into bone and are therefore more fixed than the anterior attachment, which is into soft tissue. When the buccinator contracts, the tissue of the cheek and the lips is pulled posteriorly and compressed against the teeth.

MISCELLANEOUS

- ❑ 1. The buccinator has three parts posteriorly that all converge into the anterior attachment. These three parts come from the maxilla, the mandible and the pterygomandibular raphe.
- ❑ 2. The buccinator's central attachment is to the pterygomandibular raphe. (A raphe is a seam of tissue formed by the union of the halves of a part.) Essentially, the pterygomandibular raphe is composed of fibrous connective tissue that bridges the pterygoid process of the sphenoid bone to the mandible, hence, its name.

BUCCINATOR – continued

- ❑ 3. The pterygomandibular raphe is located deep near the sphenoid bone, posterior to the maxilla. More specifically, the pterygomandibular raphe runs from the hamulus of the medial pterygoid plate of the sphenoid bone to the posterior end of the mylohyoid line of the mandible. (The pterygomandibular raphe [see illustration on page 737] also serves as an attachment site for the superior pharyngeal constrictor muscle [see page 738]. The pterygomandibular raphe can be thought of as the intersection of the buccinator and the superior pharyngeal constrictor muscle.)
- ❑ 4. The parotid duct pierces through the buccinator to enter the mouth.
- ❑ 5. The action of compressing the cheeks against the teeth by the two buccinators working bilaterally is important for forcefully expelling air from the mouth. If one is forcefully expelling air through tightly closed lips, it is the buccinator that expels the air and keeps the cheeks from distending.
- ❑ 6. The buccinator is the muscle that contracts when a musician blows air into a brass or woodwind instrument. In fact, the latin word for trumpeter is "buccinator."
- ❑ 7. The buccinators are also important with whistling, blowing up a balloon and with helping to keep food from lingering in the vestibule of the mouth (between the teeth and the cheeks).
- ❑ 8. The buccinators are the muscles responsible for the expression made (puckering the cheeks) when a person eats something sour, like biting into a lemon.
- ❑ 9. Six muscles attach into the modiolus: the zygomaticus major, levator anguli oris, risorius, depressor anguli oris, buccinator and the orbicularis oris.
- ❑ 10. The modiolus is a fibromuscular condensation approximately 1/4 inch (1/2 cm) lateral to the angle of the mouth (see page 23).

ORBICULARIS ORIS

❑ **The name, orbicularis oris, tells us that this muscle encircles the mouth.**

DERIVATION ❑ orbicularis: L. *a small circle.*
oris: L. *mouth.*

PRONUNCIATION ❑ or-**bik**-you-**la**-ris **o**-ris

ATTACHMENTS

❑ **Orbicularis Oris is a muscle that, in its entirety, surrounds the mouth**

- ❑ In more detail, there are four parts to the orbicularis oris: two on the left (upper and lower) and two on the right (upper and lower). Therefore, there is one part in each of the four quadrants. Each of these four parts of the orbicularis oris anchors to the modiolus on that side. From there, the fibers traverse through the tissue of the upper or the lower lips. At the midline, the fibers on each side interlace with each other, thereby attaching into each other.

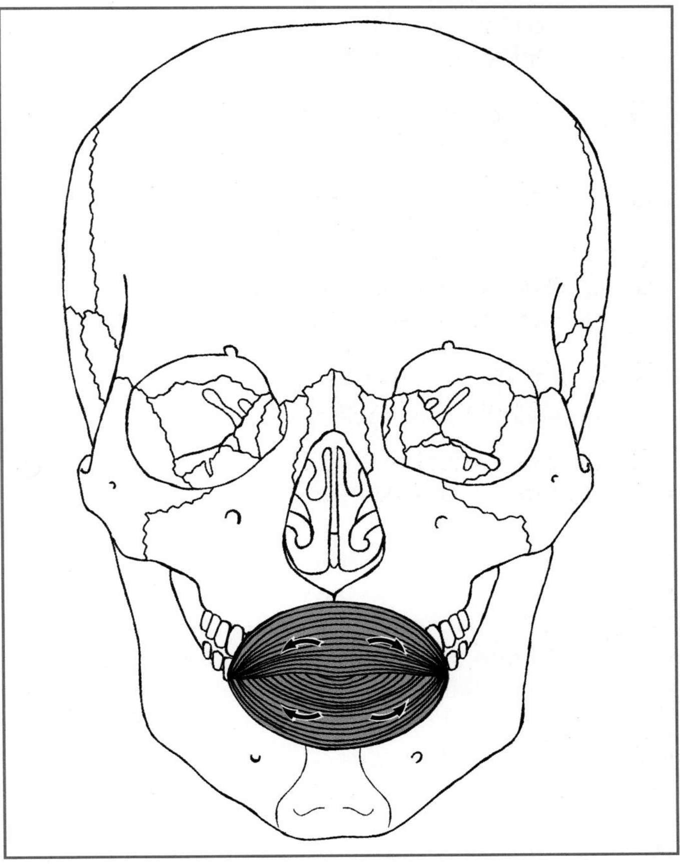

Anterior View of the Orbicularis Oris

ACTIONS

❑ **1. Closes the Mouth**

❑ **2. Protraction of the Lips**

INNERVATION ❑ The Facial Nerve (CN VII) ❑ buccal and mandibular branches

ARTERIAL SUPPLY ❑ The Facial Artery (A Branch of the External Carotid Artery)

ORBICULARIS ORIS – PALPATION AND SUPPLEMENTARY TEXT

PALPATION

- ❑ The orbicularis oris is superficial in the face and surrounds the mouth.
  - Have the client supine.
  - Wearing a finger cot or glove, place palpating fingers on the tissue of the lips.
  - Ask the client to pucker up the lips and feel for the contraction of the orbicularis oris. (Note: It is important that you do not palpate too far from the lips or you may be feeling the contraction of muscles other than the orbicularis oris.)

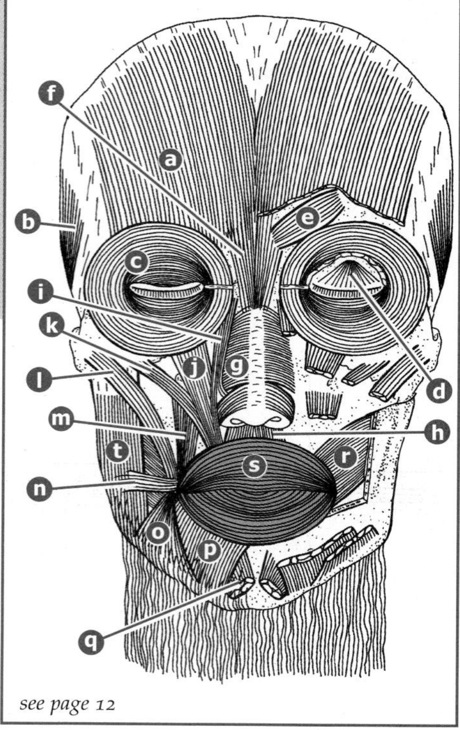

see page 12

Anterior View of the Head

- **a.** Occipitofrontalis
- **b.** Temporoparietalis
- **c.** Orbicularis Oculi
- **d.** Levator Palpebrae Superioris
- **e.** Corrugator Supercilii
- **f.** Procerus
- **g.** Nasalis
- **h.** Depressor Septi Nasi
- **i.** Levator Labii Superioris Alaeque Nasi
- **j.** Levator Labii Superioris
- **k.** Zygomaticus Minor
- **l.** Zygomaticus Major
- **m.** Levator Anguli Oris
- **n.** Risorius
- **o.** Depressor Anguli Oris
- **p.** Depressor Labii Inferioris
- **q.** Mentalis
- **r.** Buccinator
- **s.** **Orbicularis Oris**
- **t.** Masseter

RELATIONSHIP TO OTHER MUSCULOSKELETAL STRUCTURES

- ❑ The orbicularis oris surrounds the mouth. The following muscles radiate outward from the orbicularis oris like spokes from a wheel: the depressor septi nasi, levator labii superioris alaeque nasi, levator labii superioris, zygomaticus minor, levator anguli oris, zygomaticus major, risorius, buccinator, depressor anguli oris, depressor labii inferioris, mentalis and the platysma.

METHODOLOGY FOR LEARNING MUSCLE ACTIONS

❑ 1. **Closes the Mouth:** The fiber direction of the orbicularis oris is circular around the mouth. When the orbicularis oris contracts, it acts like a circular sphincter muscle that closes in around the mouth, forcing the two lips together. (Note: To understand how a circular sphincter muscle works, the following reasoning applies: If a linear muscle shortens, its length clearly and obviously decreases. When that same linear muscle is arranged in a circular fashion and shortens, the length of the line you have to make the circle decreases and therefore the size of the circle lessens, which can close in on whatever structure is being surrounded by this circular muscle.)

❑ 2. **Protraction of the Lips:** After closure of the mouth occurs, if the orbicularis oris continues to contract, the lips are pushed against each other harder and may push out anteriorly. This action is called protraction (or protrusion) of the lips.

MISCELLANEOUS

❑ 1. In even more detail, the orbicularis oris has two layers, the *pars peripheralis* and the *pars marginalis*, in each of the four quadrants. Therefore, the orbicularis oris actually has eight parts to it.

❑ 2. The orbicularis oris in humans is particularly well developed. This is necessary for the intricacies of speech.

ORBICULARIS ORIS – continued

- ❑ 3. The fibers of the orbicularis oris are reinforced by fibers of other muscles that blend into it at the angles of the mouth. The levator labii superioris alaeque nasi, levator labii superioris, levator anguli oris, zygomaticus major, buccinator, depressor anguli oris and the depressor labii inferioris all blend into the orbicularis oris at the angles of the mouth.
- ❑ 4. The contraction of the orbicularis oris causes the lips to close and protrude as in puckering the lips or whistling.
- ❑ 5. Six muscles attach into the modiolus: the zygomaticus major, levator anguli oris, risorius, depressor anguli oris, buccinator and the orbicularis oris.
- ❑ 6. The modiolus is a fibromuscular condensation approximately 1/4 inch (1/2 cm) lateral to the angle of the mouth (see page 23).

THE MUSCLES OF MASTICATION

Mastication is the act of chewing. Therefore, the muscles of mastication are those that move the mandible.

THERE ARE FOUR MUSCLES OF MASTICATION:	
Temporalis Masseter	Lateral Pterygoid Medial Pterygoid

Attachments:

- All muscles of mastication attach onto the mandible.
- The temporalis and the masseter are superficial and the two pterygoids are deeper.

Actions:

- The temporalis, masseter and the medial pterygoid all elevate the mandible.
- The temporalis and the masseter both retract the mandible.
- Both pterygoids protract the mandible.
- Both pterygoids laterally deviate (side-to-side motion) the mandible.

Miscellaneous:

- The act of chewing (mastication) involves the jaw opening and closing. Opening the jaw can be called depression of the mandible. Opening the jaw can occur in more than one way. This action can be pure *downward rotation* of the mandible at the temporomandibular joint (T.M.J.), in which the condyle of the mandible stays in exactly the same place and the anterior mandible moves inferiorly. Opening the jaw can also involve protraction of the mandible, in which the entire mandible moves anteriorly (along with downward rotation of the mandible) at the temporomandibular joint. Opening the jaw may even involve some side-to-side movement, which is called lateral deviation of the mandible at the temporomandibular joint. Although a combination of downward rotation and protraction of the mandible is usually considered to be optimal, there is some controversy as to which movement(s) constitutes the healthy manner for opening the jaw. Closing the jaw would be comprised of the reverse action(s) of opening the jaw. Improper balance and coordination of the muscles of mastication during opening and closing the jaw (especially the lateral pterygoid due to its attachment directly into the capsule and articular disc of the temporomandibular joint) may lead to dysfunction of the temporomandibular joint, known as *T.M.J. Syndrome*.
- Other muscles can move the mandible, but the four muscles listed above are considered to be the primary muscles of mastication. (For a complete listing of muscles that can move the mandible, see Appendix F.)

INNERVATION The muscles of mastication are innervated by the trigeminal nerve (CN V).

ARTERIAL SUPPLY The muscles of mastication receive the majority of their arterial supply from the maxillary artery.

VIEWS OF THE MUSCLES OF MASTICATION

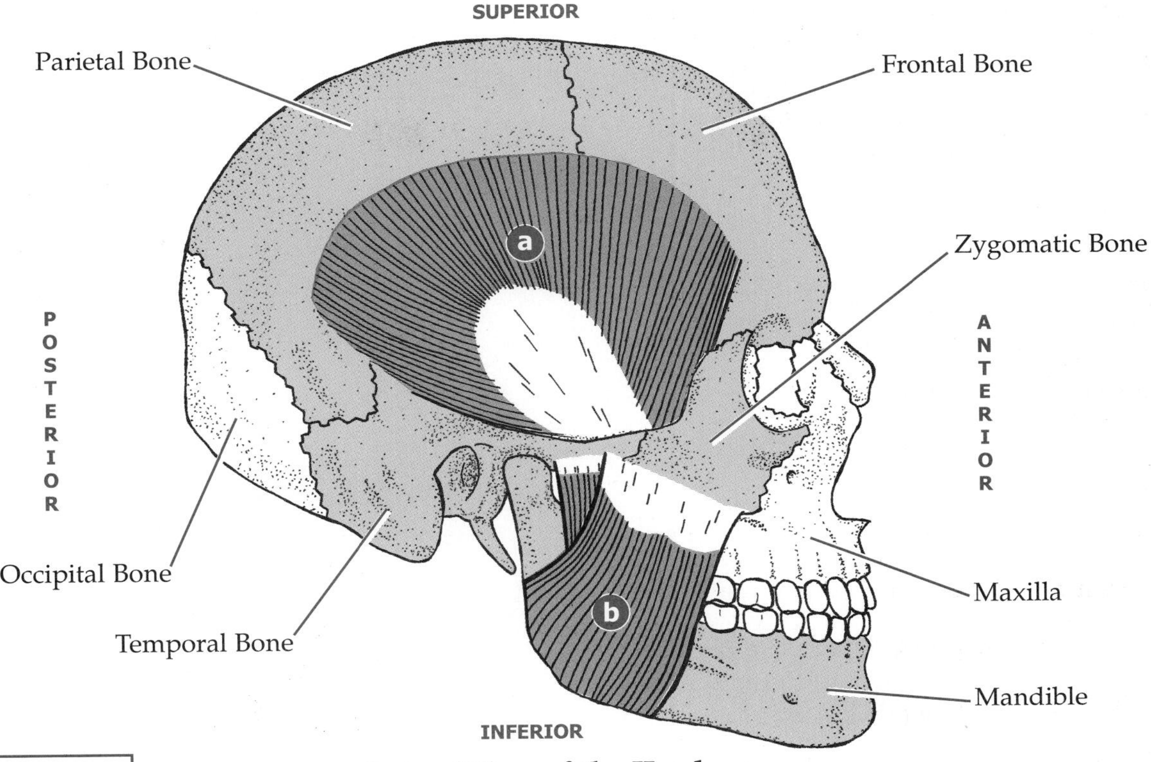

Lateral View of the Head

a. **Temporalis**
b. **Masseter**
c. **Lateral Pterygoid**
d. **Medial Pterygoid**

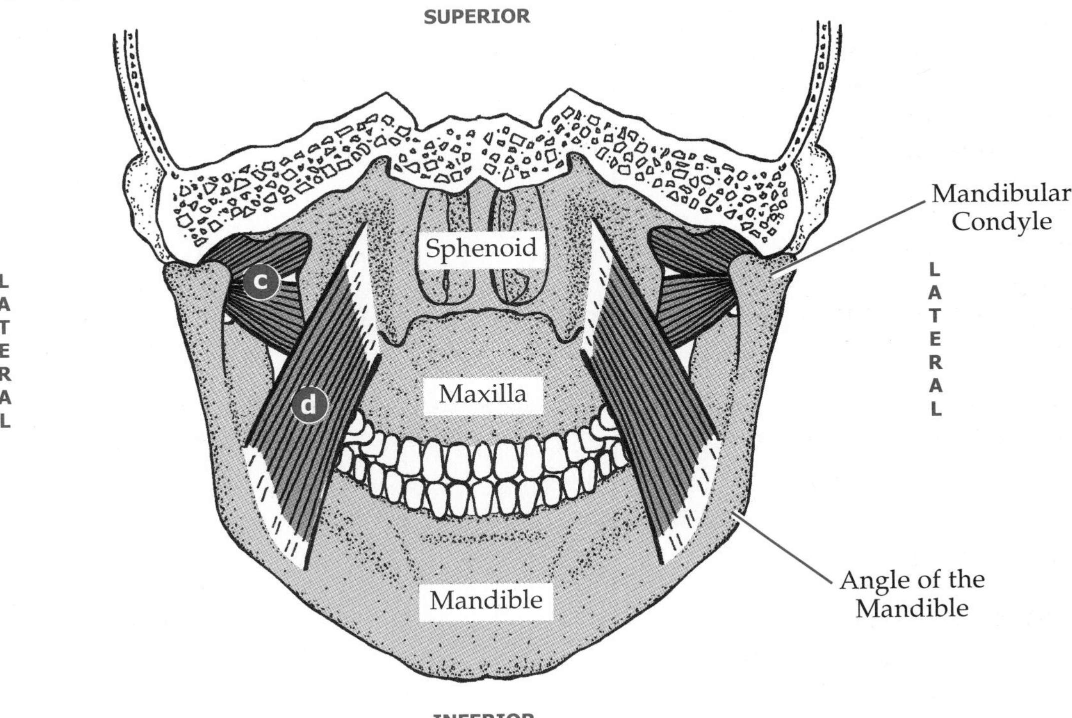

Posterior View of the Internal Face

❑ TEMPORALIS

❑ **The name, temporalis, tells us that this muscle attaches into the temporal bone.**

DERIVATION ❑ temporalis: L. *refers to the temple.* **PRONUNCIATION** ❑ tem-po-**ra**-lis

ATTACHMENTS

❑ **Temporal Fossa**

- ❑ the entire temporal fossa except the portion on the zygomatic bone

to the

❑ **Coronoid Process and the Ramus of the Mandible**

- ❑ the anterior border, apex, posterior border and the medial surface of the coronoid process of the mandible, and the anterior border of the ramus of the mandible

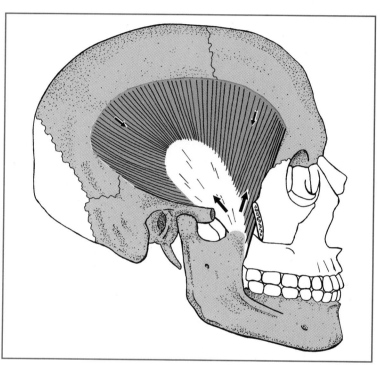

Lateral View of the
Right Temporalis
(the zygomatic arch has been cut)

ACTIONS

❑ 1. **Elevation of the Mandible**

❑ 2. Retraction of the Mandible

INNERVATION ❑ The Trigeminal Nerve (CN V)
- ❑ deep temporal branches of the anterior trunk of the mandibular division of the trigeminal nerve

ARTERIAL SUPPLY ❑ The Maxillary and Superficial Temporal Arteries (Branches of the External Carotid Artery)

PALPATION AND SUPPLEMENTARY TEXT

PALPATION

- ❑ The temporalis is superficial in the temple region of the face and scalp.
  - Have the client supine.
  - Place palpating fingers on the temporal fossa.
  - Ask the client to alternately elevate and depress the mandible (clench and relax the teeth) and feel for the contraction and relaxation of the temporalis. In this manner, the majority of the temporalis superior to the zygomatic arch can be easily palpated. However, the portion of the temporalis that is inferior to the zygomatic arch is difficult to palpate and distinguish from the more superficial masseter because the masseter will also contract with elevation of the mandible.
  - The inferior attachment of the temporalis on the coronoid process of the mandible can be palpated if the client opens the mouth wide (depresses the mandible) but again, it will be difficult to distinguish from the masseter.

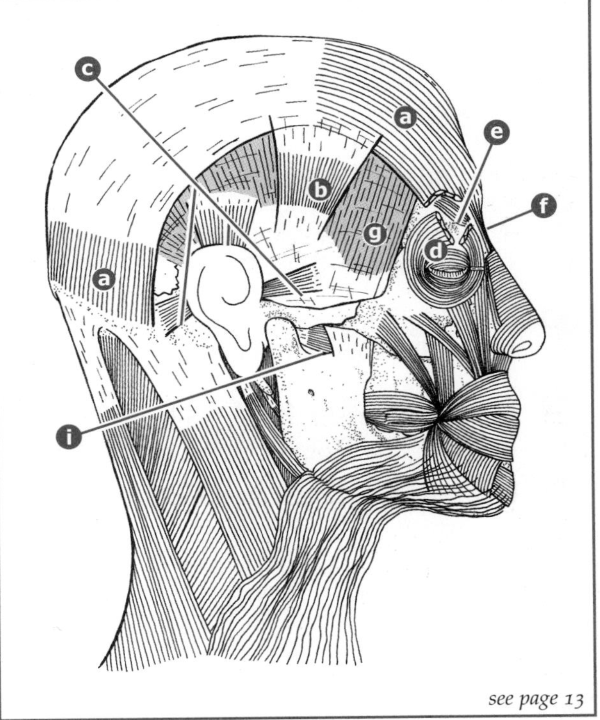

see page 13

Lateral View of the Head

a. Occipitofrontalis (partially cut)
b. Temporoparietalis
c. Auricularis Muscles
d. Orbicularis Oculi (partially cut)
e. Corrugator Supercilii
f. Procerus
g. **Temporalis** (deep to fascia)
h. Masseter (removed)
i. Lateral Pterygoid

RELATIONSHIP TO OTHER MUSCULOSKELETAL STRUCTURES

❑ 1. The superior portion of the temporalis is superficial (except for the auriculares anterior and superior, which are superficial to it). The inferior portion of the temporalis runs deep to the zygomatic arch. Inferior to the zygomatic arch, the temporalis is deep to the masseter.

❑ 2. Deep to the superior portion of the temporalis are the cranial bones (frontal, parietal, temporal and the sphenoid).

❑ 3. Deep to the inferior portion of the temporalis are the lateral pterygoid, the superficial head of the medial pterygoid and a small part of the buccinator.

METHODOLOGY FOR LEARNING MUSCLE ACTIONS

❑ **1. Elevation of the Mandible at the Temporomandibular Joint:** The anterior fibers of the temporalis are oriented in a vertical fashion from the cranium superiorly, to the mandible inferiorly. When the temporalis contracts, it pulls the mandible superiorly toward the cranium. Therefore, the temporalis elevates the mandible at the temporomandibular joint.

TEMPORALIS – continued

- ❑ 2. **Retraction of the Mandible at the Temporomandibular Joint:** The posterior fibers of the temporalis are oriented in a horizontal fashion from the cranium posteriorly, to the mandible anteriorly. When the temporalis contracts, it pulls the mandible posteriorly toward the cranium. Therefore, the temporalis retracts the mandible at the temporomandibular joint.

MISCELLANEOUS

- ❑ 1. The temporalis muscle is deep to thick fibrous fascia called the *temporalis fascia*.
- ❑ 2. The more superficial fibers of the temporalis actually attach into the temporal fascia.
- ❑ 3. Some sources state that the temporalis also contributes to side-to-side grinding (lateral deviation) of the mandible.
- ❑ 4. A tight temporalis may be involved with *tension headaches* and with dysfunction of the temporomandibular joint (*T.M.J. Syndrome*).
- ❑ 5. The temporal fossa is a fossa (depression) that overlies not only the temporal bone, but also the frontal, parietal, zygomatic and sphenoid bones.
- ❑ 6. The superficial temporal artery is superficial to the temporalis muscle and the pulse of the temporal artery can be palpated.

MASSETER

❑ **The name, masseter, tells us that this muscle is involved with chewing.**

DERIVATION ❑ masseter: Gr. *chewer.*

PRONUNCIATION ❑ **ma**-sa-ter

ATTACHMENTS

❑ **Inferior Margins of Both the Zygomatic Bone and the Zygomatic Arch of the Temporal Bone**

- ❑ SUPERFICIAL LAYER: the inferior margin of the zygomatic bone and the zygomatic arch
- ❑ DEEP LAYER: the inferior margin and the deep surface of the zygomatic arch

to the

❑ **Angle, Ramus and Coronoid Process of the Mandible**

- ❑ SUPERFICIAL LAYER: the angle and the inferior 1/2 of the external surface of the ramus of the mandible
- ❑ DEEP LAYER: the lateral surface of the coronoid process and the superior 1/2 of the external surface of the ramus of the mandible

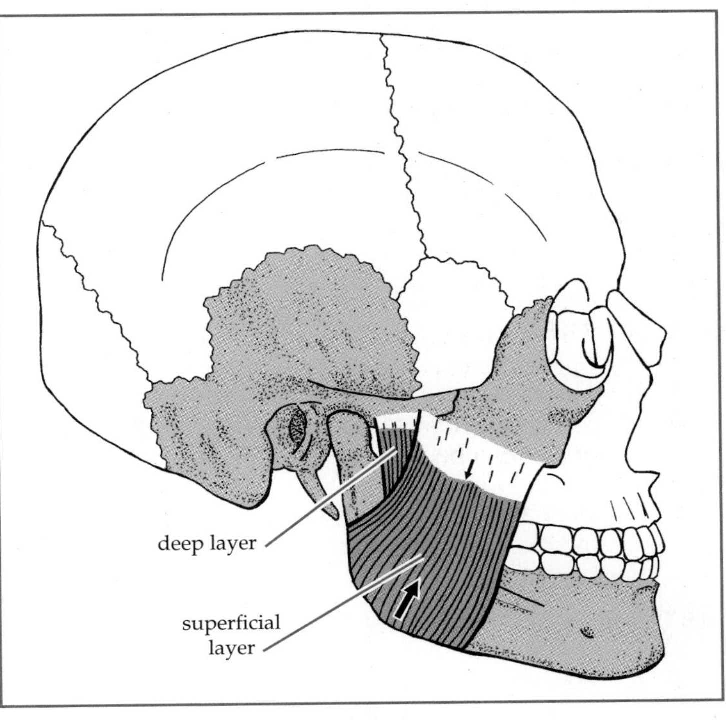

Lateral View of the Right Masseter

ACTIONS

❑ 1. **Elevation of the Mandible**

❑ 2. Protraction of the Mandible

❑ 3. Retraction of the Mandible

INNERVATION ❑ The Trigeminal Nerve (CN V)
- ❑ anterior trunk of the mandibular division of the trigeminal nerve

ARTERIAL SUPPLY ❑ The Maxillary Artery (A Branch of the External Carotid Artery)
- ❑ and the transverse facial artery (a branch of the superficial temporal artery)

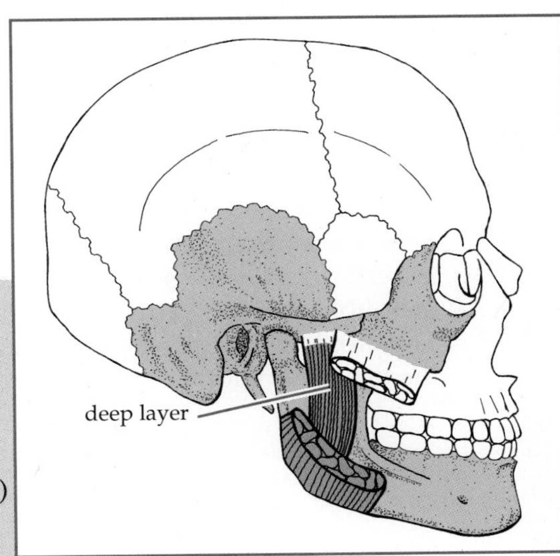

Lateral View of the Right Masseter
(the superficial layer has been cut)

MASSETER – PALPATION AND SUPPLEMENTARY TEXT

PALPATION

- ❑ The masseter is easily palpable in the face, superficial to the ramus of the mandible.
  - Have the client supine.
  - Place palpating fingers between the zygomatic arch and the angle of the mandible.
  - Ask the client to alternately elevate and depress the mandible (clench and relax the teeth) and feel for contraction and relaxation of the masseter. (When the masseter contracts, the muscle may visibly bulge out.)

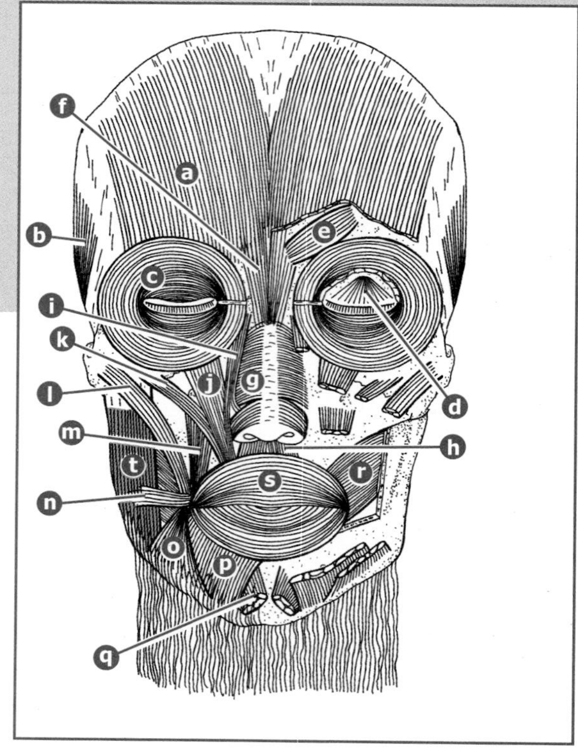

Anterior View of the Head

- **a.** Occipitofrontalis
- **b.** Temporoparietalis
- **c.** Orbicularis Oculi
- **d.** Levator Palpebrae Superioris
- **e.** Corrugator Supercilii
- **f.** Procerus
- **g.** Nasalis
- **h.** Depressor Septi Nasi
- **i.** Levator Labii Superioris Alaeque Nasi
- **j.** Levator Labii Superioris
- **k.** Zygomaticus Minor
- **l.** Zygomaticus Major
- **m.** Levator Anguli Oris
- **n.** Risorius
- **o.** Depressor Anguli Oris
- **p.** Depressor Labii Inferioris
- **q.** Mentalis
- **r.** Buccinator
- **s.** Orbicularis Oris
- **t.** **Masseter**

RELATIONSHIP TO OTHER MUSCULOSKELETAL STRUCTURES

❑ 1. The masseter is superficial in the cheek except for the platysma, risorius and the zygomaticus major (muscles of facial expression).

❑ 2. Deep to the masseter are the temporalis, part of the buccinator and the ramus of the mandible.

METHODOLOGY FOR LEARNING MUSCLE ACTIONS

❑ **1. Elevation of the Mandible at the Temporomandibular Joint:** The fibers of the masseter are oriented in a vertical fashion from the zygomatic bone and zygomatic arch superiorly, to the mandible inferiorly. When the masseter contracts, it pulls the mandible superiorly toward the zygomatic bone and arch. Therefore, the masseter elevates the mandible at the temporomandibular joint.

❑ **2. Protraction of the Mandible at the Temporomandibular Joint:** The superficial layer of the masseter is somewhat oriented in a horizontal fashion from the zygomatic bone anteriorly, to the mandible posteriorly. When the superficial layer of the masseter contracts, it pulls the mandible anteriorly toward the zygomatic bone. Therefore, the masseter protracts the mandible at the temporomandibular joint.

MASSETER – continued

❑ 3. **Retraction of the Mandible at the Temporomandibular Joint:** The deep layer of the masseter is somewhat oriented in a horizontal fashion from the zygomatic arch posteriorly, to the mandible anteriorly. When deep layer of the masseter contracts, it pulls the mandible posteriorly toward the zygomatic arch. Therefore, the masseter retracts the mandible at the temporomandibular joint. (Note: If it is difficult to visualize the action of retraction of the mandible, keep in mind that retraction can only occur if the mandible is first protracted. When the mandible is first protracted, the horizontal orientation of the fibers of the deep layer of the masseter becomes accentuated.)

MISCELLANEOUS

❑ 1. The masseter is a square-shaped muscle.

❑ 2. The masseter is usually divided into two layers: a superficial layer and a deep layer.

❑ 3. Some sources further subdivide the deep layer of the masseter into two layers, and therefore, state that overall, the masseter has three layers: a *superficial* layer, a *middle* layer and a *deep* layer.

❑ 4. The superficial layer of the masseter is the largest.

❑ 5. Some sources state that the masseter can also laterally deviate the mandible (side-to-side grinding) and protract the mandible at the temporomandibular joint (T.M.J.).

❑ 6. The masseter is the prime mover of elevation of the mandible at the temporomandibular joint (T.M.J.).

❑ 7. The large parotid gland and parotid duct are superficial to the masseter.

❑ 8. The masseter may be involved with dysfunction of the temporomandibular joint (*T.M.J. Syndrome*).

❑ 9. Proportional to its size, the masseter is the strongest muscle in the human body.

LATERAL PTERYGOID

❑ **The name, lateral pterygoid, tells us that this muscle attaches to the sphenoid bone (the pterygoid process) and is lateral (lateral to the medial pterygoid muscle).**

DERIVATION ❑ lateral: L. *side.*
pterygoid: Gr. *wing shaped.*

PRONUNCIATION ❑ **lat**-er-al **ter**-i-goyd

ATTACHMENTS

❑ **ENTIRE MUSCLE: Sphenoid Bone**

- ❑ SUPERIOR HEAD: the greater wing of the sphenoid
- ❑ INFERIOR HEAD: the lateral surface of the lateral pterygoid plate of the pterygoid process of the sphenoid

to the

❑ **Mandible and the Temporomandibular Joint (T.M.J.)**

- ❑ SUPERIOR HEAD: the capsule and articular disc of the temporomandibular joint
- ❑ INFERIOR HEAD: the neck of the mandible

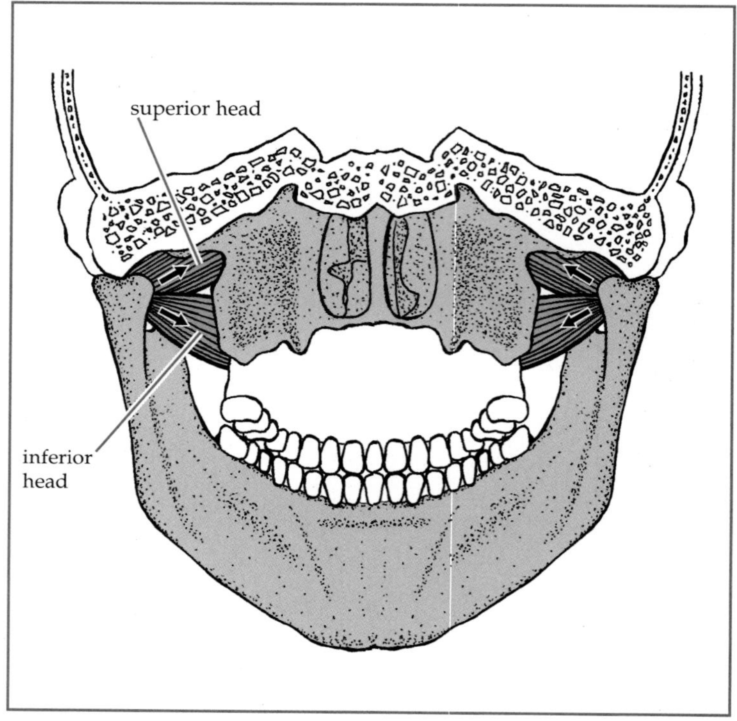

Posterior View of the Lateral Pterygoids

ACTIONS

❑ 1. **Protraction of the Mandible**

❑ 2. Contralateral Deviation of the Mandible

INNERVATION ❑ The Trigeminal Nerve (CN V)
❑ lateral pterygoid nerve from the anterior trunk of the mandibular division of the trigeminal nerve

ARTERIAL SUPPLY ❑ The Maxillary Artery (A Branch of the External Carotid Artery)

PALPATION AND SUPPLEMENTARY TEXT

PALPATION

The lateral pterygoid is deep to the masseter and temporalis and can be difficult to palpate from outside the mouth. From inside the mouth, it is easier to palpate.

❑ **To palpate from inside the mouth:**

- Have the client seated or supine.
- Wearing a finger cot or glove, place palpating fingers along the internal surfaces of the upper teeth until you reach the back molars.
- Press posteriorly and superiorly against the inside wall of the mouth.
- Ask the client to laterally deviate the mandible to the opposite side and feel for the contraction of the lateral pterygoid.

❑ **To palpate from outside the mouth:**

- Have the client seated or supine.
- Place palpating fingers inferior to the zygomatic arch between the condyle and coronoid process of the mandible.
- Ask the client to laterally deviate the mandible to the opposite side and feel for the contraction of the lateral pterygoid. However, the masseter and temporalis may also be involved in this action, which makes distinguishing the lateral pterygoid from these muscles difficult.

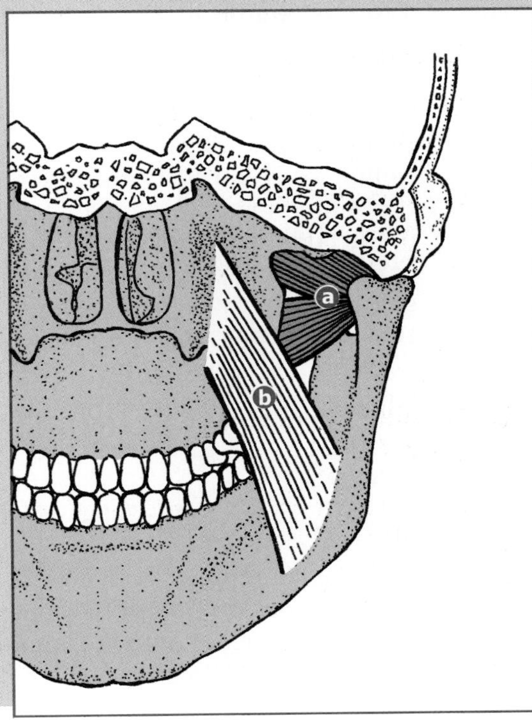

Posterior View of the Right Pterygoids

a. **Lateral Pterygoid**
b. Medial Pterygoid

RELATIONSHIP TO OTHER MUSCULOSKELETAL STRUCTURES

❑ 1. Of the two pterygoid muscles, the lateral pterygoid is named lateral because its attachment onto the pterygoid process of the sphenoid bone is more lateral than the attachment of the medial pterygoid onto the pterygoid process of the sphenoid bone. Regarding the gross location of the bellies of these two muscles, the lateral pterygoid is generally lateral and superior in location relative to the medial pterygoid.

❑ 2. The majority of the lateral pterygoid is deep to the zygomatic arch of the temporal bone and the coronoid process of the mandible. The lateral pterygoid is also deep to the masseter muscle and the inferior tendon of the temporalis.

❑ 3. The superior part of the deep head of the medial pterygoid is deep to the lateral pterygoid.

LATERAL PTERYGOID – continued

METHODOLOGY FOR LEARNING MUSCLE ACTIONS

❑ 1. **Protraction of the Mandible at the Temporomandibular Joint:** The lateral pterygoid attaches from the mandible posteriorly, to the sphenoid anteriorly (with its fibers running horizontally in the sagittal plane). When the lateral pterygoid contracts, it pulls the mandible anteriorly toward the sphenoid. Therefore, the lateral pterygoid protracts the mandible at the temporomandibular joint.

❑ 2. **Contralateral Deviation of the Mandible at the Temporomandibular Joint:** The lateral pterygoid attaches from the mandible laterally, to the sphenoid medially (with its fibers running horizontally in the frontal plane). When the lateral pterygoid contracts, it pulls the mandible medially toward the sphenoid. By pulling one side of the mandible toward the sphenoid, the entire mandible is pulled toward the opposite side of the body. This movement is called lateral deviation of the mandible. Because the lateral pterygoid on one side of the body pulls the mandible toward the opposite side of the body, this action is called contralateral deviation of the mandible, and it occurs at the temporomandibular joints.

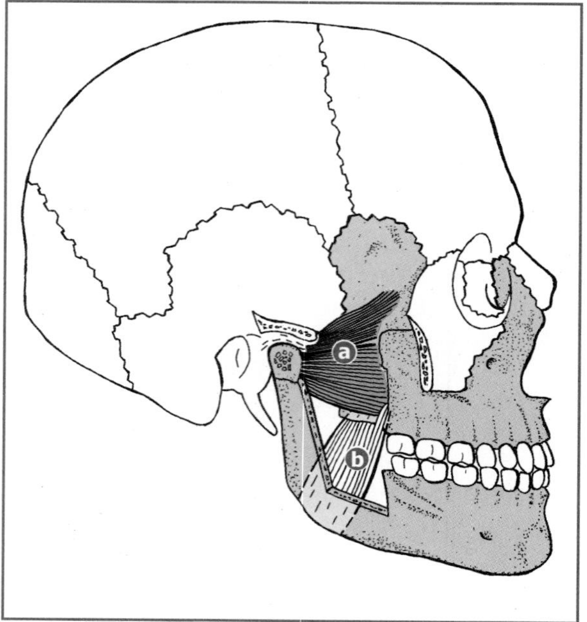

Lateral View of the Right Lateral Pterygoid (and the medial pterygoid - part of the mandible has been cut away)

a. Lateral Pterygoid
b. Medial Pterygoid

MISCELLANEOUS

❑ 1. The lateral pterygoid is sometimes known as the *external pterygoid*.

❑ 2. Both the lateral pterygoid and the medial pterygoid attach onto the lateral pterygoid plate of the pterygoid process of the sphenoid bone. The two pterygoids are so named because the lateral pterygoid attaches onto the lateral surface of the lateral pterygoid plate and the medial pterygoid attaches onto the medial surface of the lateral pterygoid plate.

❑ 3. Lateral deviation of the mandible is important for grinding and chewing food.

❑ 4. Some sources report that the inferior belly of the lateral pterygoid is active during jaw opening. From its line of pull relative to the axis of mandibular motion (usually considered to be lingula of the internal surface of the mandible) the inferior belly of the lateral pterygoid can depress the mandible. It may also serve to pull the condyle of the mandible anteriorly (an action that usually accompanies opening of the jaw), and/or contribute to protraction of the entire mandible (which may accompany opening the jaw).

❑ 5. If any protraction of the mandible occurs with opening the jaw (see page 80), then the articular disc of the temporomandibular joint (T.M.J.) must also protract to stay in proper alignment between the mandibular condyle and the mandibular fossa of the temporal bone. Given its attachment into the articular disc, the lateral pterygoid guides this movement of the articular disc. Therefore, if the contraction of the lateral pterygoid is not precisely coordinated with the other muscles that move the mandible, the articular disc may become jammed between the two bones of the joint and dysfunction of the temporomandibular joint (*T.M.J. Syndrome*) may occur.

❑ 6. Although all four muscles of mastication (temporalis, masseter, and the lateral and medial pterygoids) may be involved in *T.M.J. syndrome*, given the attachments of the lateral pterygoid directly into the capsule and articular disc of the temporomandibular joint (T.M.J.), it is clear that hypertonicity of a lateral pterygoid could excessively pull on the temporomandibular joint structures and therefore cause dysfunction of the temporomandibular joint (*T.M.J. Syndrome*).

MEDIAL PTERYGOID

❑ **The name, medial pterygoid, tells us that this muscle attaches to the sphenoid bone (the pterygoid process) and is medial (medial to the lateral pterygoid muscle).**

DERIVATION ❑ medial: L. *middle.*
pterygoid: Gr. *wing shaped.*

PRONUNCIATION ❑ **mee**-dee-al **ter**-i-goyd

ATTACHMENTS

❑ **ENTIRE MUSCLE: Sphenoid Bone**

- ❑ DEEP HEAD: the medial surface of the lateral pterygoid plate of the pterygoid process of the sphenoid, the palatine bone and the tuberosity of the maxilla
- ❑ SUPERFICIAL HEAD: the palatine bone and the maxilla

to the

❑ **Internal Surface of the Mandible**

- ❑ at the angle and the inferior border of the ramus of the mandible

Posterior View of the Medial Pterygoids

ACTIONS

❑ 1. **Elevation of the Mandible**

❑ 2. Protraction of the Mandible

❑ 3. Contralateral Deviation of the Mandible

INNERVATION ❑ The Trigeminal Nerve (CN V)
❑ medial pterygoid nerve from the mandibular division of the trigeminal nerve

ARTERIAL SUPPLY ❑ The Maxillary Artery (A Branch of the External Carotid Artery)

MEDIAL PTERYGOID – PALPATION AND SUPPLEMENTARY TEXT

PALPATION

From the outside of the mouth, the mandibular attachment of the medial pterygoid onto the inner surface of the angle of the mandible can be palpated. The medial pterygoid can also be palpated from inside the mouth.

❑ **To palpate from outside the mouth:**

- Have the client seated or supine.
- Place palpating fingers on the angle of the mandible and then hook them under onto the internal surface of the mandible.
- Ask the client to clench the teeth (elevate the mandible) and feel for the contraction of the medial pterygoid.

❑ **To palpate from inside the mouth:**

- Have the client seated or supine.
- Wearing a finger cot or glove, place palpating finger along the internal surfaces of the lower teeth until you reach the back molars.
- Press posterolaterally against the inside wall of the mouth.
- Ask the client to clench the teeth (elevate the mandible) against an object and feel for the contraction of the medial pterygoid. (Note: This object must be secure in its placement because your palpating finger is vulnerable in this situation.)

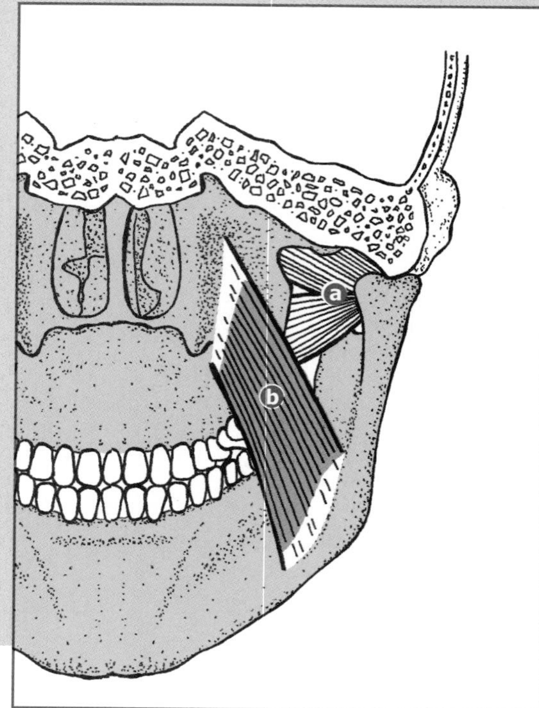

Posterior View of the Right Pterygoids

a. Lateral Pterygoid
b. Medial Pterygoid

RELATIONSHIP TO OTHER MUSCULOSKELETAL STRUCTURES

❑ 1. Of the two pterygoid muscles, the medial pterygoid is named medial because its attachment onto the pterygoid process of the sphenoid bone is more medial than the attachment of the lateral pterygoid onto the pterygoid process of the sphenoid bone. Regarding the gross location of the bellies of these two muscles, the medial pterygoid is generally medial and inferior in location relative to the lateral pterygoid.

❑ 2. The medial pterygoid is deep to the coronoid process, ramus and the angle of the mandible (and the zygomatic arch as well). The medial pterygoid is also deep to the masseter and the inferior tendon of the temporalis.

❑ 3. From the lateral perspective, the majority of the medial pterygoid is deep to the lateral pterygoid.

❑ 4. Deep to the medial pterygoid is the internal wall of the mouth.

❑ 5. A number of small muscles of the palate and the pharynx lie close to the medial attachment of the medial pterygoid.

MEDIAL PTERYGOID – continued

METHODOLOGY FOR LEARNING MUSCLE ACTIONS

- ❑ 1. **Elevation of the Mandible at the Temporomandibular Joint:** The fibers of the medial pterygoid are oriented in a vertical fashion from the sphenoid superiorly, to the mandible inferiorly. When the medial pterygoid contracts, it pulls the mandible superiorly toward the sphenoid. Therefore, the medial pterygoid elevates the mandible at the temporomandibular joint.
- ❑ 2. **Protraction of the Mandible at the Temporomandibular Joint:** The medial pterygoid attaches from the mandible posteriorly, to the sphenoid anteriorly (with its fibers running somewhat horizontally in the sagittal plane). When the medial pterygoid contracts, it pulls the mandible anteriorly toward the sphenoid. Therefore, the medial pterygoid protracts the mandible at the temporomandibular joint.
- ❑ 3. **Contralateral Deviation of the Mandible at the Temporomandibular Joint:** The medial pterygoid attaches from the mandible laterally, to the sphenoid medially (with its fibers running somewhat horizontally in the frontal plane). When the medial pterygoid contracts, it pulls the mandible medially toward the sphenoid. By pulling one side of the mandible toward the sphenoid, the entire mandible is pulled toward the opposite side of the body. This movement is called lateral deviation of the mandible. Because the medial pterygoid on one side of the body pulls the mandible toward the opposite side of the body, this action is called contralateral deviation of the mandible, and it occurs at the temporomandibular joints.

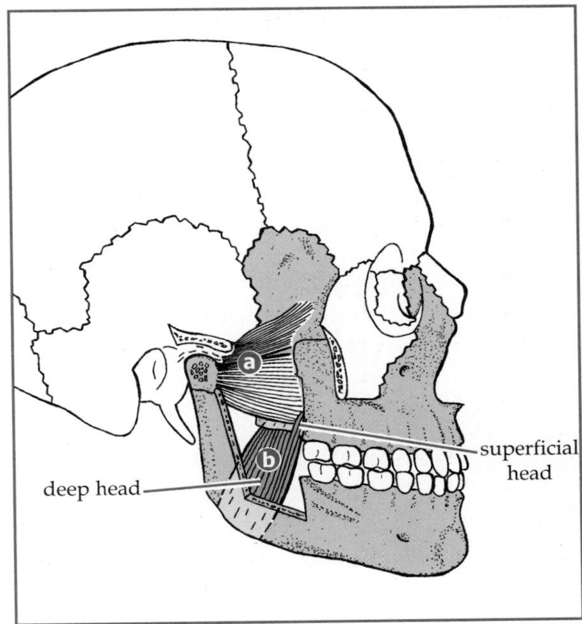

Lateral View of the Right Medial Pterygoid
(and the lateral pterygoid - part of the mandible has been cut away)

a. Lateral Pterygoid
b. Medial Pterygoid

MISCELLANEOUS

- ❑ 1. The medial pterygoid is sometimes known as the *internal pterygoid.*
- ❑ 2. The medial pterygoid is a fairly thick, quadrilateral (square) muscle.
- ❑ 3. The medial pterygoid is usually divided into a deep and superficial head.
- ❑ 4. The deep head of the medial pterygoid is the larger of the two heads.
- ❑ 5. The direction of fibers of the medial pterygoid is essentially identical to the direction of the fibers of the masseter; in fact, these two muscles occupy the same position. The difference is that the masseter is external (lateral) to the mandible, and the medial pterygoid is internal (medial) to the mandible.
- ❑ 6. Both the medial pterygoid and the lateral pterygoid attach onto the lateral pterygoid plate of the pterygoid process of the sphenoid bone. The two pterygoids are so named because the medial pterygoid attaches onto the medial surface of the lateral pterygoid plate and the lateral pterygoid attaches onto the lateral surface of the lateral pterygoid plate.
- ❑ 7. A tight medial pterygoid may be involved with dysfunction of the temporomandibular joint (*T.M.J. Syndrome*).
- ❑ 8. Lateral deviation of the mandible is important for grinding and chewing food.

MUSCLES OF THE NECK

OVERVIEW OF THE MUSCLES OF THE NECK

ANATOMICALLY, THE MUSCLES OF THE NECK CAN BE DIVIDED INTO TWO MAJOR GROUPS:

The Posterior Neck:

Superficial
- Trapezius
- Splenius Capitis
- Splenius Cervicis
- Levator Scapulae

Deep (Suboccipitals)
- Rectus Capitis Posterior Major
- Rectus Capitis Posterior Minor
- Obliquus Capitis Inferior
- Obliquus Capitis Superior

The Anterior Neck:

Superficial
- Platysma
- Sternocleidomastoid

Hyoids

Infrahyoids
- Sternohyoid
- Sternothyroid
- Thyrohyoid
- Omohyoid

Suprahyoids
- Digastric
- Stylohyoid
- Mylohyoid
- Geniohyoid

Scalenes
- Anterior Scalene
- Middle Scalene
- Posterior Scalene

Deep
- Longus Colli
- Longus Capitis
- Rectus Capitis Anterior
- Rectus Capitis Lateralis

THE FOLLOWING MUSCLES ARE COVERED IN OTHER CHAPTERS OF THIS BOOK, BUT ARE ALSO PRESENT IN THE NECK:

- The Erector Spinae Group
- The Transversospinalis Group
- The Rhomboid Minor (attaches to C7)
- The Serratus Posterior Superior (attaches to C7)
- Interspinales
- Intertransversarii
- Levatores Costarum

(Please see Appendix F for other muscles that attach to the neck.)

This is how the muscles of the neck are usually classified. Some sources divide the neck into anterior, posterior, and lateral groups and place some of the above muscles into the lateral group.

Functionally, since the muscles of the neck cross the joints of the cervical spine, these muscles can move the neck at the cervical spinal joints. If a muscle of the neck also crosses the atlanto-occipital joint between the atlas and the occiput (the head), then the muscle can move the head upon the neck at the atlanto-occipital joint. The following general rules regarding actions can be stated for muscles of the neck:

- If a muscle crosses the neck posteriorly, it can extend the neck at the cervical spinal joints.
- If a muscle crosses the neck anteriorly, it can flex the neck at the cervical spinal joints.
- If a muscle crosses the neck laterally on the right side, it can right laterally flex the neck at the cervical spinal joints.
- If a muscle crosses the neck laterally on the left side, it can left laterally flex the neck at the cervical spinal joints.
- If a muscle wraps around the neck, it can cause rotation of the neck at the cervical spinal joints.
- Note that every muscle of the neck that crosses anteriorly or posteriorly (except the interspinales, which are located directly midline in the center) also cross the neck somewhat laterally. Therefore, (except for the interspinales) every muscle of the neck can laterally flex the neck at the cervical spinal joints.

Miscellaneous

- The anterior neck may be palpated and tissue work may be done here, but care must be taken due to the presence of many structures.
  - The carotid sinus of the common carotid artery, if compressed, can cause a neurological reflex that diminishes the contraction of the heart. This is especially important to be aware of with weak and/or elderly clients.
  - The trachea, laryngeal cartilages and the thyroid gland are delicate structures.
  - The bony contours of the transverse processes of the cervical vertebrae are somewhat sharp and pointy and discomfort may occur if soft tissue is compressed into them.

Innervation and arterial supply of the neck muscles are varied so it is difficult to state one generalization. The following should be noted:

INNERVATION

- The trapezius and the sternocleidomastoid are both innervated by the spinal accessory nerve (CN XI).
- The suboccipitals are innervated by the suboccipital nerve.
- The scalenes, prevertebrals and the splenius capitis and splenius cervicis are innervated by cervical spinal nerves.
- The platysma, involved with facial expression, is innervated by the facial nerve (CN VII), which innervates all the muscles of facial expression.
- The infrahyoids are all innervated by cervical nerves and the suprahyoids are by cranial nerves.

ARTERIAL SUPPLY

- The four suboccipital muscles receive their arterial supply from the occipital artery.
- The four infrahyoid muscles receive their arterial supply from the superior thyroid artery. Arterial supply to the four suprahyoid muscles is varied.

A NOTE REGARDING REVERSE ACTIONS

As a rule, this book does not employ the terms "origin" and "insertion." However, it is useful to utilize these terms to describe the concept of "reverse actions." The action section of this book describes the action of a muscle by stating the movement of a body part that is created by a muscle's contraction. The body part that usually moves when a muscle contracts is called the insertion. The methodology section further states at which joint the movement of the insertion occurs. However, the other body part that the muscle attaches to, the origin, can also move at that joint. *This movement can be called the reverse action of the muscle.* Keep in mind that the reverse action of a muscle is always possible. The likelihood that a reverse action will occur is based upon the ability of the insertion to be fixed so that the origin moves (instead of the insertion moving) when the muscle contracts. For more information and examples of reverse actions, see page 702.

❑ ANTERIOR VIEW OF THE BONES AND BONY LANDMARKS OF THE NECK

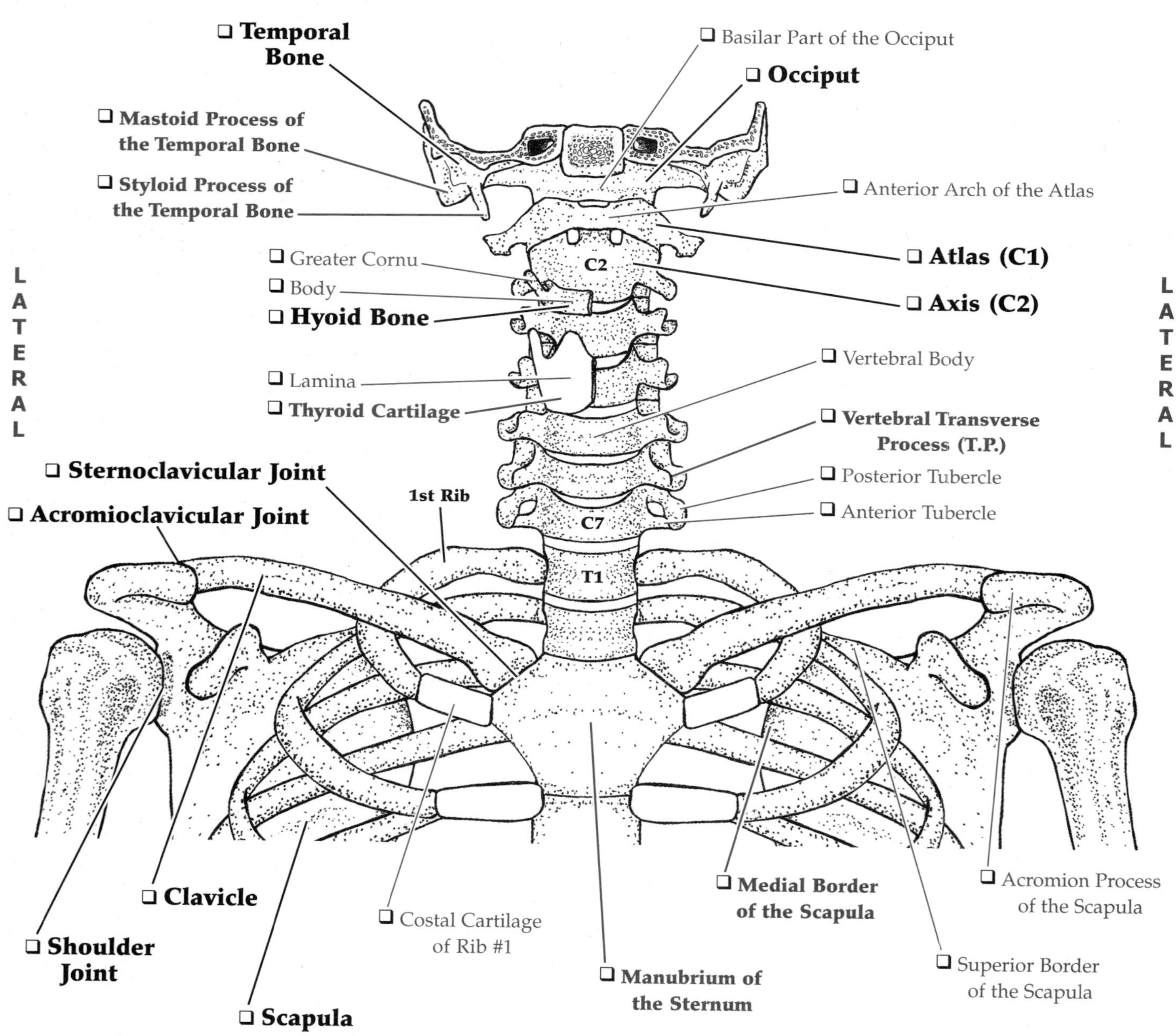

Note: Only muscular attachments of this chapter are labeled.

First level attachments are indicated in **bold** print.

Second level attachments are indicated in non-bold print.

ANTERIOR VIEW OF THE BONY ATTACHMENTS OF THE NECK

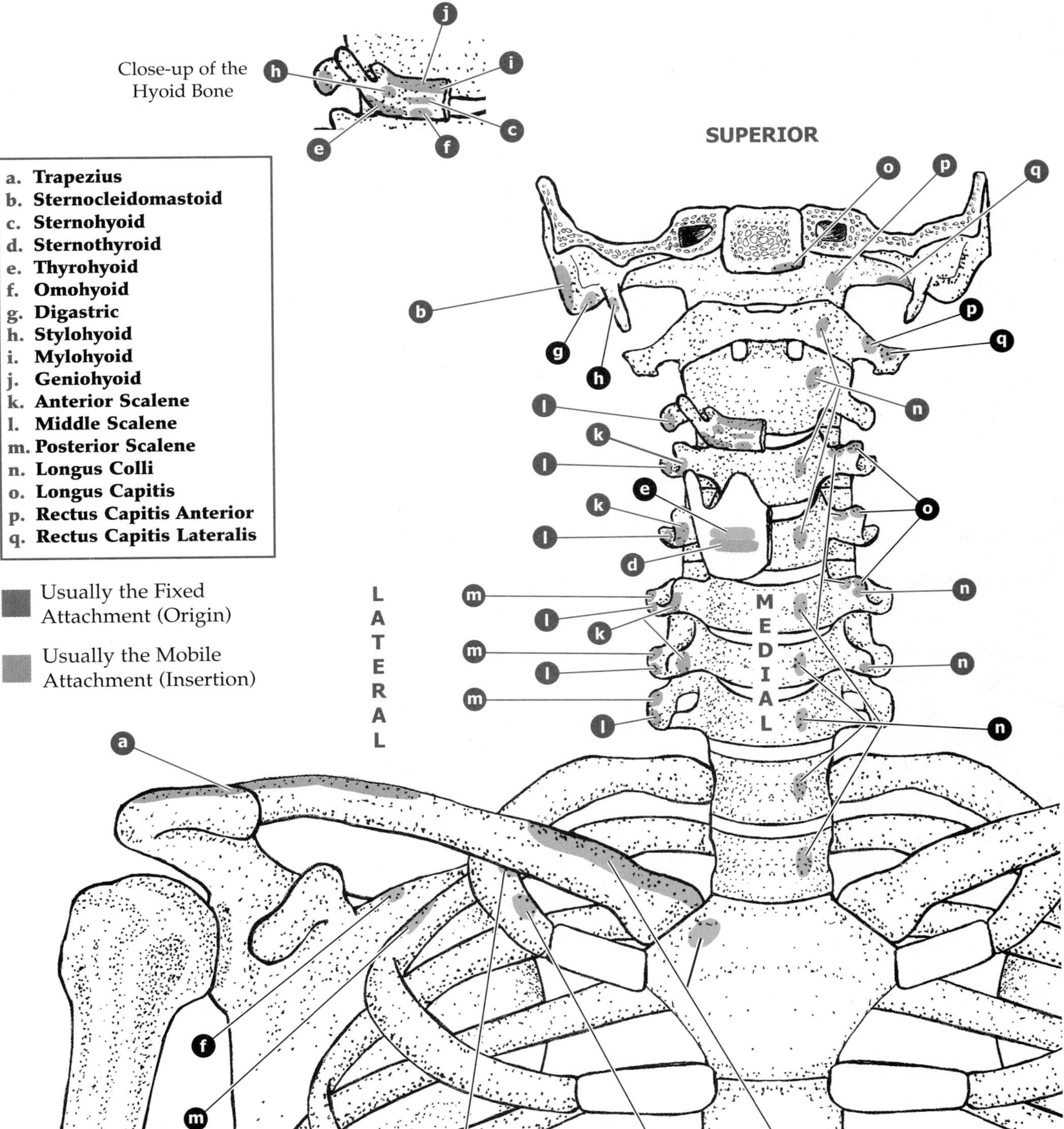

Notes:
1. The mandible and much of the skull have been removed.
2. Only the attachments of the muscles of this chapter have been shown.
3. The prevertebrals are seen on our right.

POSTERIOR VIEW OF THE BONES AND BONY LANDMARKS OF THE NECK

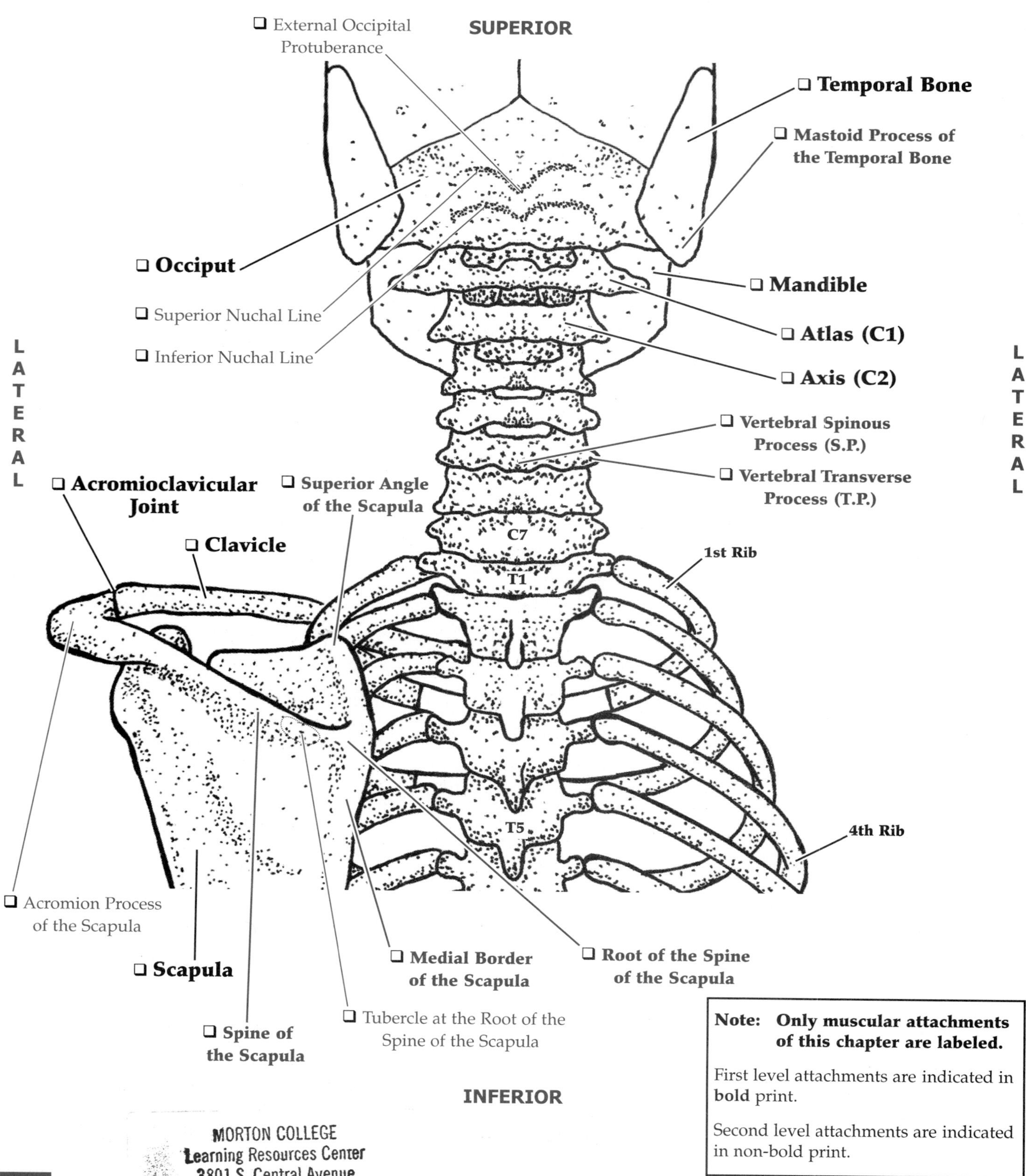

Note: Only muscular attachments of this chapter are labeled.

First level attachments are indicated in **bold** print.

Second level attachments are indicated in non-bold print.

POSTERIOR VIEW OF THE BONY ATTACHMENTS OF THE NECK 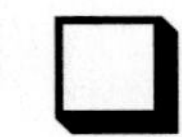

SUPERIOR

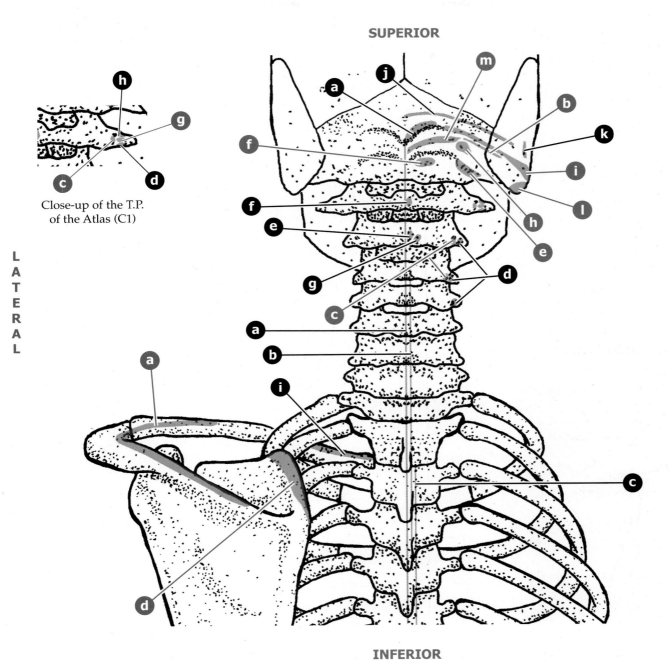

Close-up of the T.P. of the Atlas (C1)

LATERAL

LATERAL

INFERIOR

- Usually the Fixed Attachment (Origin)
- Usually the Mobile Attachment (Insertion)

a. **Trapezius**
b. **Splenius Capitis**
c. **Splenius Cervicis**
d. **Levator Scapulae**
e. **Rectus Capitis Posterior Major**
f. **Rectus Capitis Posterior Minor**
g. **Obliquus Capitis Inferior**
h. **Obliquus Capitis Superior**
i. **Sternocleidomastoid**
j. Occipitofrontalis
k. Posterior Auricular
l. Longissimus (of the Erector Spinae)
m. Semispinalis (of the Transversospinalis)

❑ ANTERIOR VIEW OF THE NECK (SUPERFICIAL)

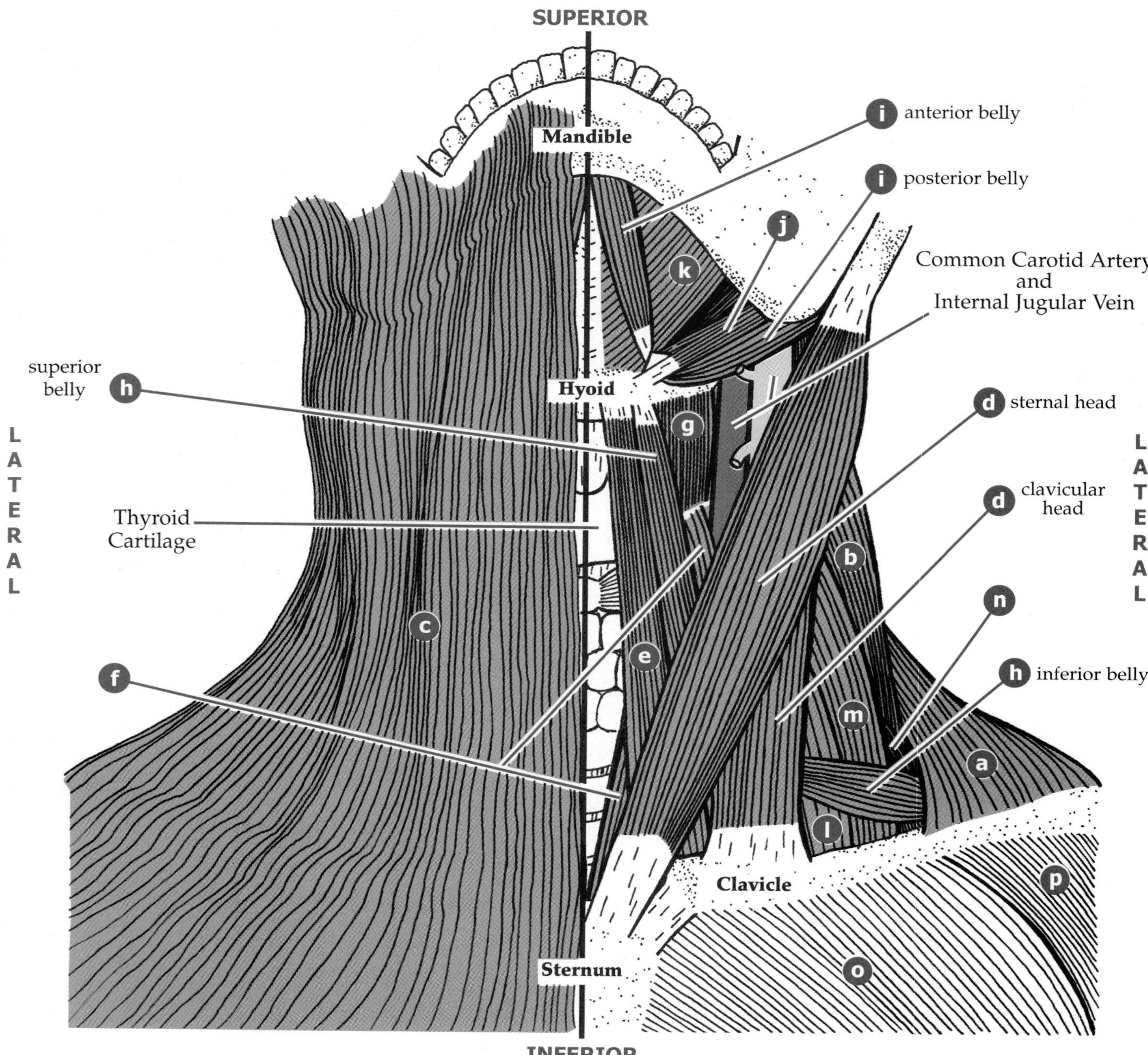

Note: The head is extended in this view.

a. **Trapezius**	i. **Digastric**
b. **Levator Scapulae**	j. **Stylohyoid**
c. **Platysma** (removed on our right)	k. **Mylohyoid**
d. **Sternocleidomastoid**	l. **Anterior Scalene**
e. **Sternohyoid**	m. **Middle Scalene**
f. **Sternothyroid**	n. **Posterior Scalene**
g. **Thyrohyoid**	o. Pectoralis Major
h. **Omohyoid**	p. Deltoid

ANTERIOR VIEW OF THE NECK (INTERMEDIATE)

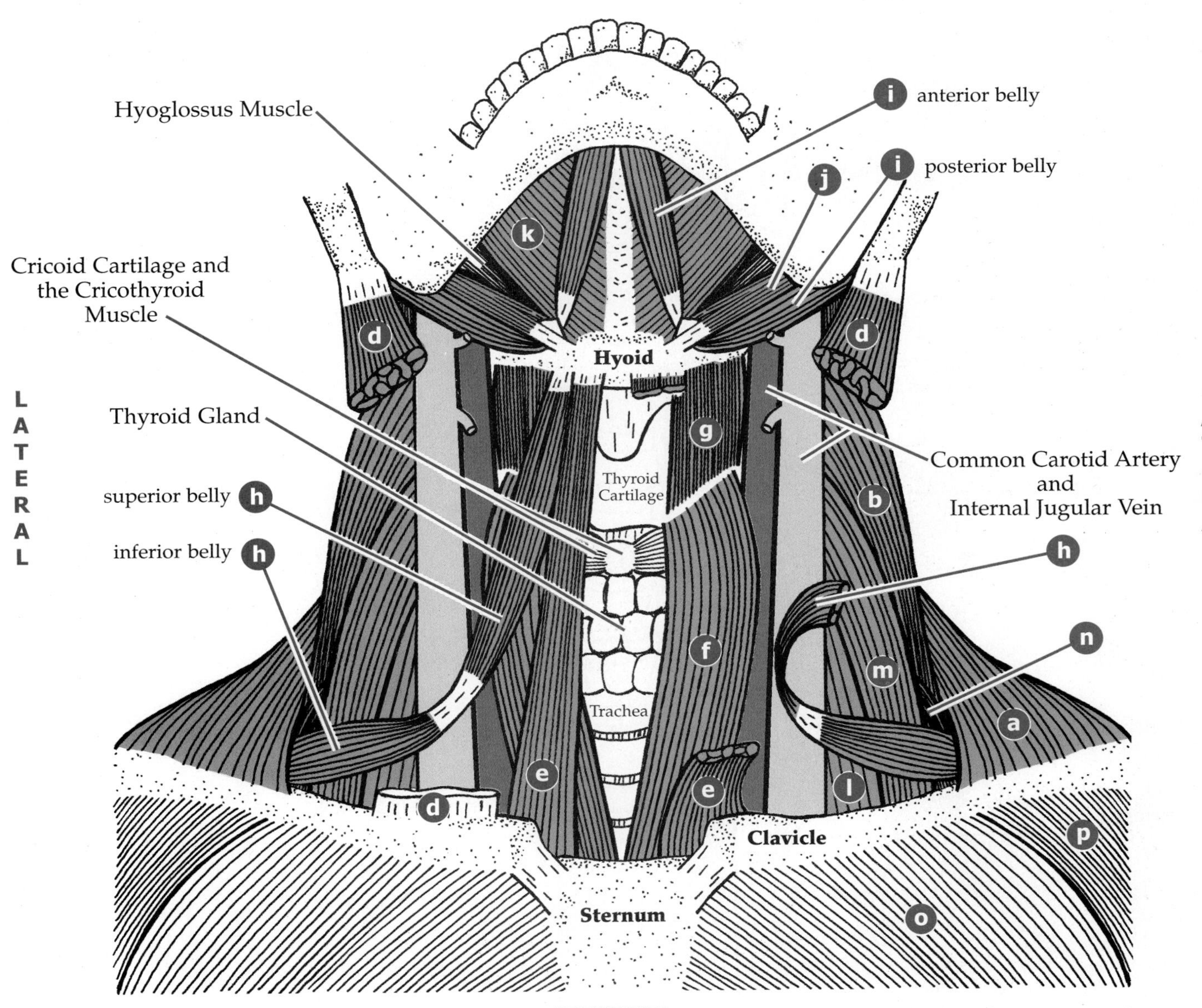

Note: The head is extended in this view.

a. **Trapezius**	i. **Digastric**
b. **Levator Scapulae**	j. **Stylohyoid**
c. **Platysma** (removed)	k. **Mylohyoid**
d. **Sternocleidomastoid** (cut)	l. **Anterior Scalene**
e. **Sternohyoid** (cut on our right)	m. **Middle Scalene**
f. **Sternothyroid**	n. **Posterior Scalene**
g. **Thyrohyoid**	o. Pectoralis Major
h. **Omohyoid** (cut and reflected on our right)	p. Deltoid

ANTERIOR VIEW OF THE NECK (DEEP)

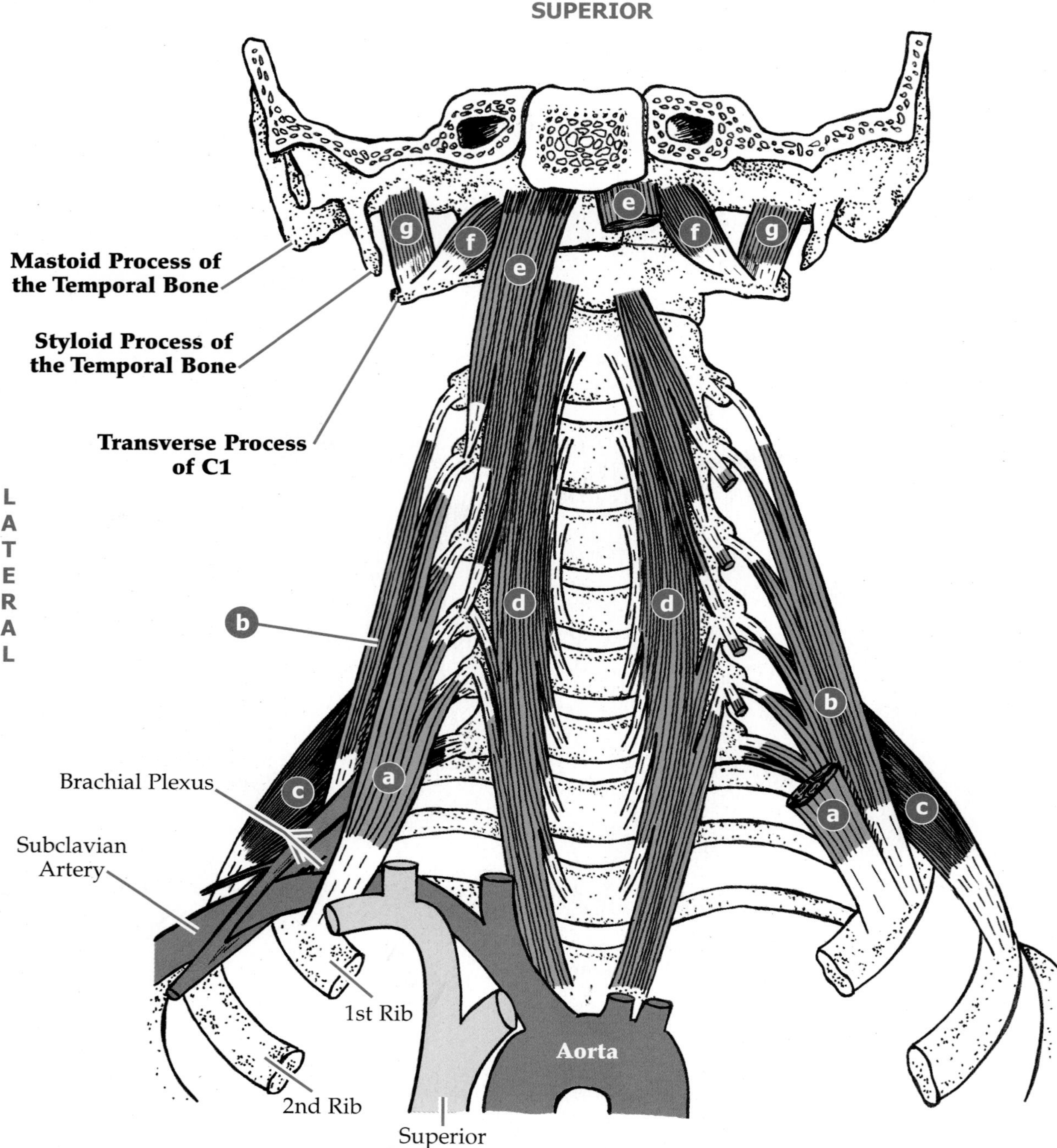

a. **Anterior Scalene** (cut on our right)
b. **Middle Scalene**
c. **Posterior Scalene**
d. **Longus Colli**
e. **Longus Capitis** (cut on our right)
f. **Rectus Capitis Anterior**
g. **Rectus Capitis Lateralis**

LATERAL VIEW OF THE NECK

a. **Trapezius**	j. **Stylohyoid**
b. **Splenius Capitis**	k. **Mylohyoid**
c. **Levator Scapulae**	l. **Anterior Scalene**
d. **Sternocleidomastoid**	m. **Middle Scalene**
e. **Sternohyoid**	n. **Posterior Scalene**
f. **Sternothyroid**	o. **Longus Capitis**
g. **Thyrohyoid**	p. Masseter (cut)
h. **Omohyoid**	q. Pectoralis Major
i. **Digastric**	r. Deltoid

POSTERIOR VIEW OF THE NECK (SUPERFICIAL AND INTERMEDIATE)

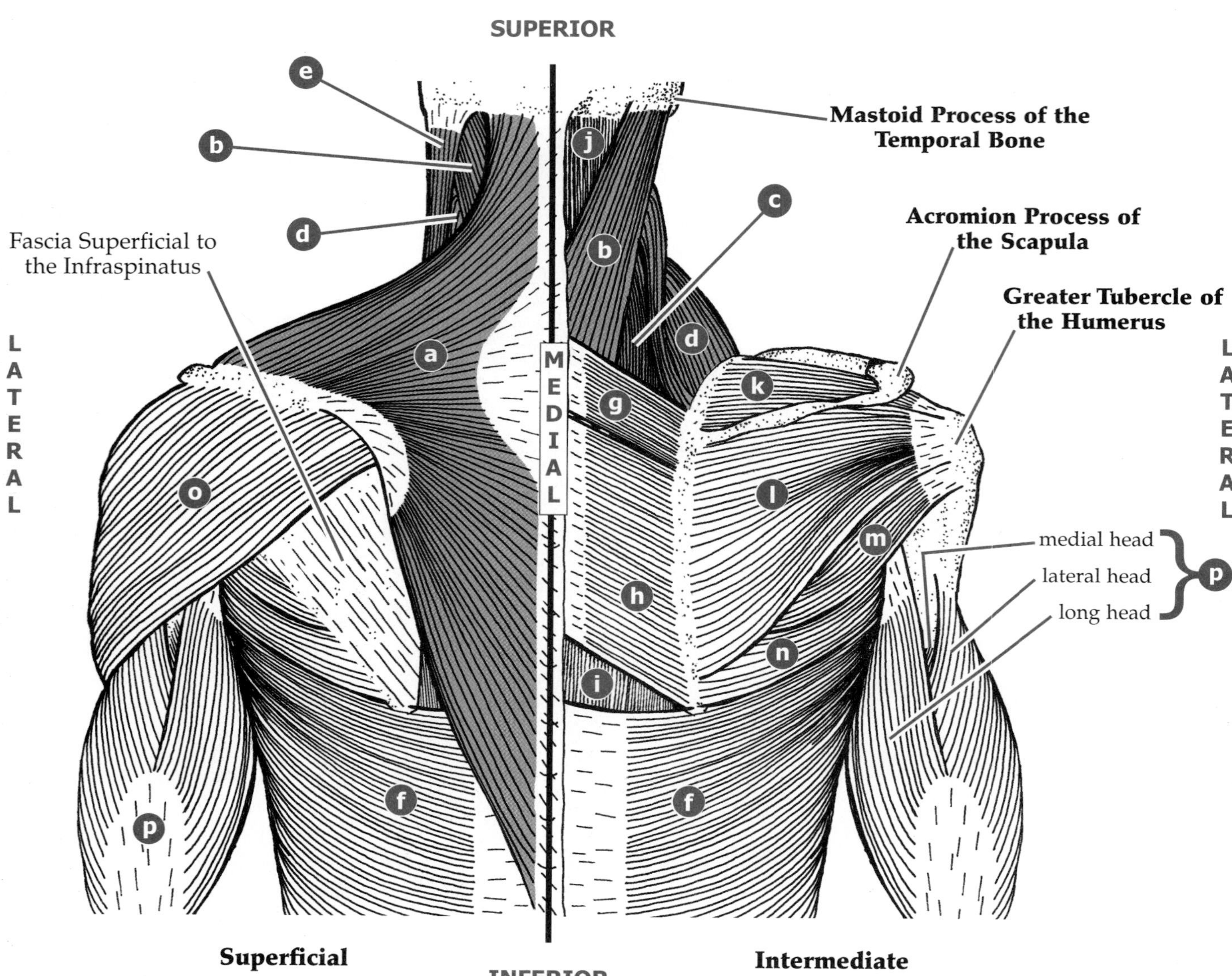

a. **Trapezius**	j. Semispinalis Capitis (of Transversospinalis)
b. **Splenius Capitis**	k. Supraspinatus
c. **Splenius Cervicis**	l. Infraspinatus
d. **Levator Scapulae**	m. Teres Minor
e. **Sternocleidomastoid**	n. Teres Major
f. Latissimus Dorsi	o. Deltoid
g. Rhomboid Minor	p. Triceps Brachii
h. Rhomboid Major	
i. Erector Spinae	

POSTERIOR VIEW OF THE NECK (INTERMEDIATE AND DEEP)

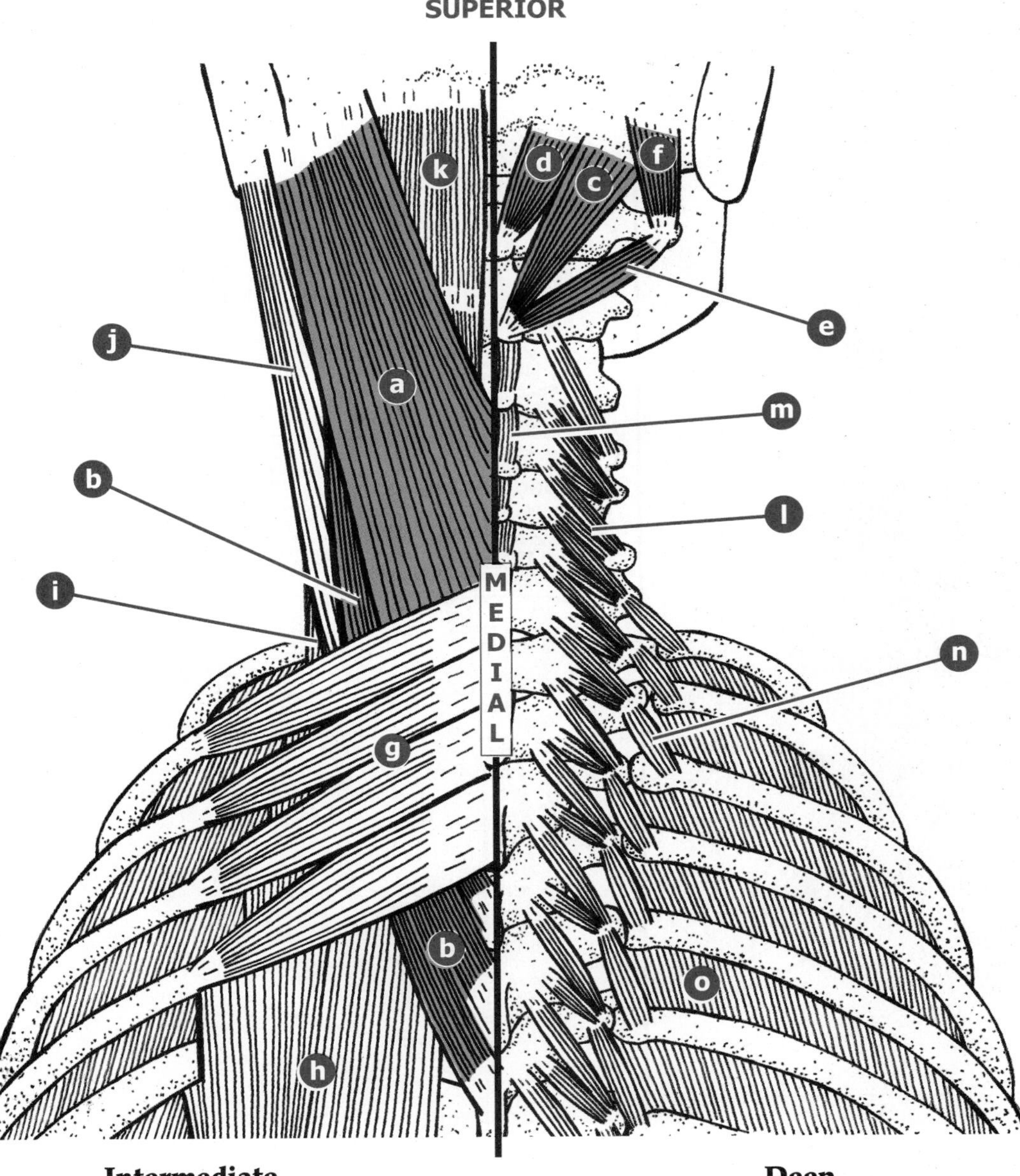

Note: In this intermediate view, the levator scapulae has been removed and the longissimus capitis is shown.

- a. **Splenius Capitis**
- b. **Splenius Cervicis**
- c. **Rectus Capitis Posterior Major**
- d. **Rectus Capitis Posterior Minor**
- e. **Obliquus Capitis Inferior**
- f. **Obliquus Capitis Superior**
- g. Serratus Posterior Superior
- h. Iliocostalis and Longissimus (of Erector Spinae)
- i. Iliocostalis Cervicis (of Erector Spinae)
- j. Longissimus Capitis (of Erector Spinae)
- k. Semispinalis Capitis (of Transversospinalis)
- l. Rotatores (of Transversospinalis)
- m. Interspinales
- n. Levatores Costarum
- o. External Intercostals

CROSS SECTION VIEW OF THE NECK

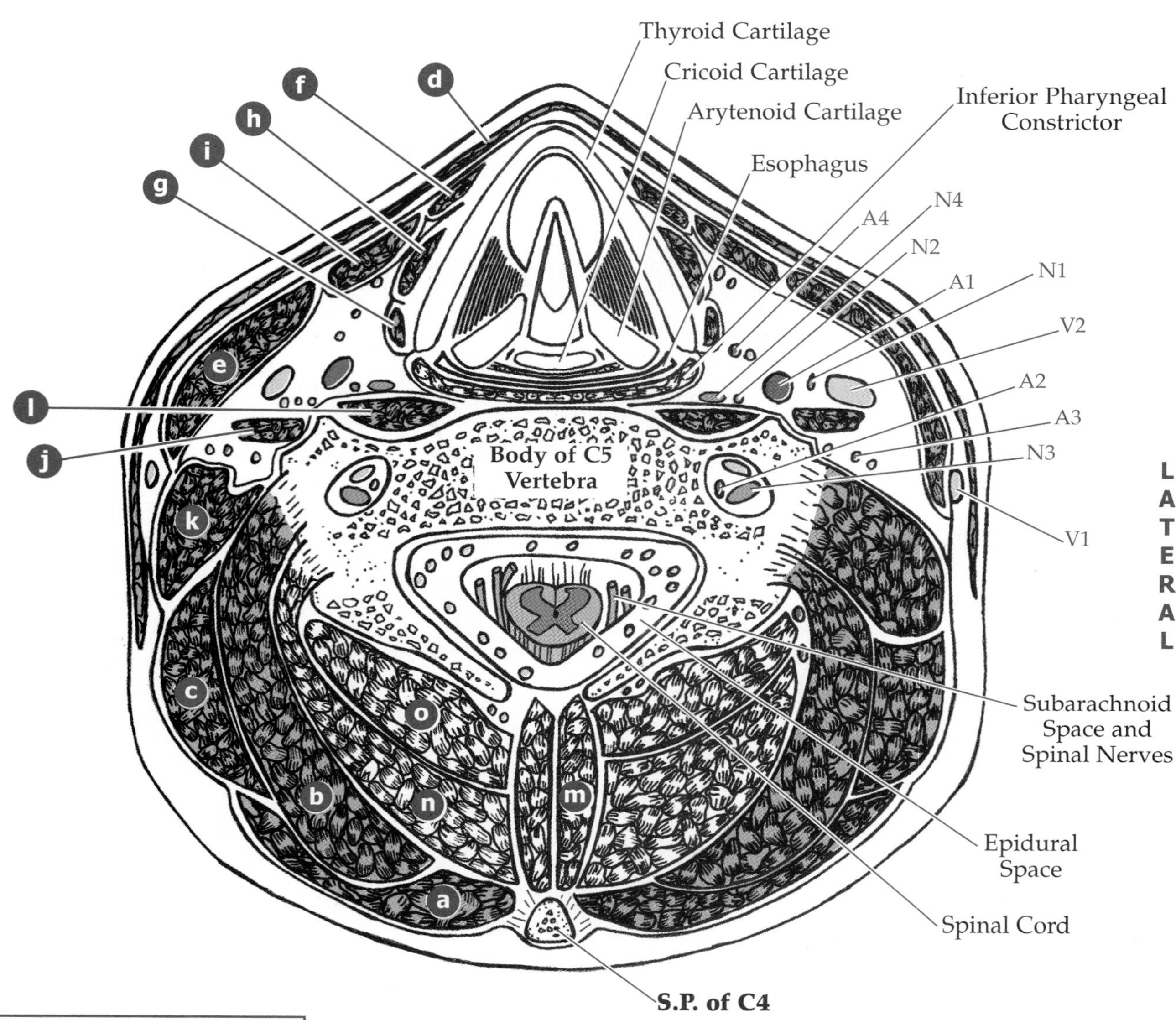

Muscles
- a. **Trapezius**
- b. **Splenius Capitis and Cervicis**
- c. **Levator Scapulae**
- d. **Platysma**
- e. **Sternocleidomastoid**
- f. **Sternohyoid**
- g. **Sternothyroid**
- h. **Thyrohyoid**
- i. **Omohyoid**
- j. **Anterior Scalene**
- k. **Middle Scalene**
- l. **Longus Colli**
- m. Spinalis (of Erector Spinae)
- n. Semispinalis (of Transversospinalis)
- o. Multifidus (of Transversospinalis)

Note: Cross section at C5vertebral level

Nerves
- N1. **Vagus (CN X)**
- N2. **Phrenic**
- N3. **C5 Spinal**
- N4. **Sympathetic Trunk**

Arteries
- A1. **Common Carotid**
- A2. **Vertebral**
- A3. **Ascending Cervical**
- A4. **Superior Thyroid**

Veins
- V1. **External Jugular**
- V2. **Internal Jugular**

❑ TRAPEZIUS (THE "TRAPS")

❑ **The name, trapezius, tells us that the left and right trapezius muscles together have the shape of a trapezoid (diamond shape).**

DERIVATION ❑ trapezius: Gr: *a little table* (or trapezoid shape). **PRONUNCIATION** ❑ tra-**pee**-zee-us

ATTACHMENTS

❑ **ENTIRE MUSCLE: Occiput, Nuchal Ligament, and S.P.s of C7-T12**

- ❑ ENTIRE MUSCLE: external occipital protuberance and the medial third of the superior nuchal line of the occiput
  - ❑ UPPER: the external occipital protuberance, the medial 1/3 of the superior nuchal line of the occiput, the nuchal ligament and the S.P. of C7
  - ❑ MIDDLE: the S.P.s of T1-T5
  - ❑ LOWER: the S.P.s of T6-T12

to the

❑ **ENTIRE MUSCLE: Lateral Clavicle, Acromion Process and the Spine of the Scapula**

- ❑ ENTIRE MUSCLE: lateral 1/3 of the clavicle
  - ❑ UPPER: lateral 1/3 of the clavicle and the acromion process of the scapula
  - ❑ MIDDLE: acromion process and spine of the scapula
  - ❑ LOWER: the tubercle at the root of the spine of the scapula

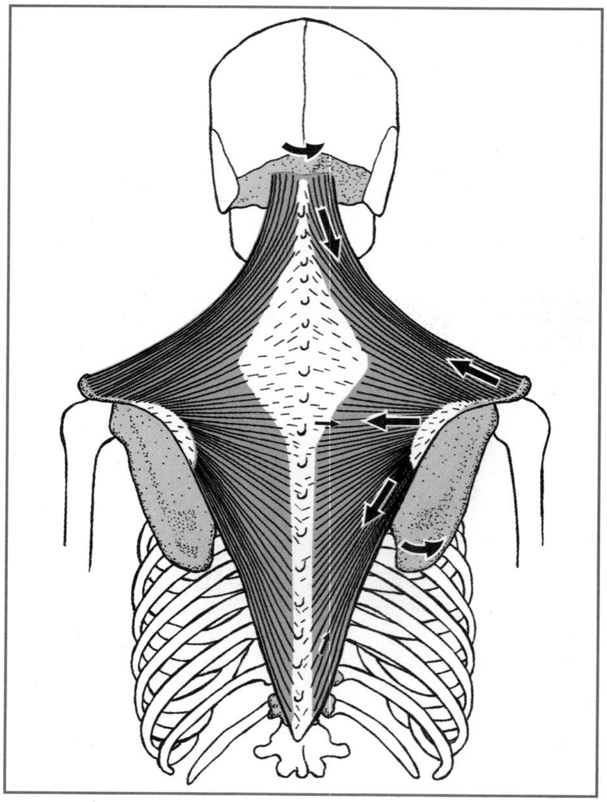

Posterior View of the Right and Left Trapezius Muscles
(arrows indicate lines of pull of the right trapezius)

ACTIONS

❑ 1. **Lateral Flexion of the Neck and the Head (upper)**

❑ 2. **Extension of the Neck and the Head (upper)**

❑ 3. **Contralateral Rotation of the Neck and the Head (upper)**

❑ 4. **Elevation of the Scapula (upper)**

❑ 5. **Retraction (Adduction) of the Scapula (entire muscle)**

❑ 6. **Depression of the Scapula (lower)**

❑ 7. Upward Rotation of the Scapula (upper and lower)

❑ 8. Extension of the Trunk (middle and lower)

INNERVATION ❑ Spinal Accessory Nerve (CN XI) ❑ and C3, **4**

ARTERIAL SUPPLY ❑ The Transverse Cervical Artery (A Branch of the Thyrocervical Trunk) and the Dorsal Scapular Artery (A Branch of the Subclavian Artery)

PALPATION AND SUPPLEMENTARY TEXT

PALPATION

- ❑ The trapezius is superficial and easy to palpate.
  - Have the client prone.
  - Place palpating hand over the upper trapezius.
  - Ask the client to actively abduct the arm at the shoulder joint and retract the scapula.
    (Abduction of the arm requires upward rotation of the scapula, thus contracting the upper and lower trapezius; retraction of the scapula causes the middle trapezius to contract.)
  - Follow the above procedure to palpate the middle and lower trapezius.
  - To further bring out the upper trapezius, have the client perform slight active extension of the head and neck

see page 106

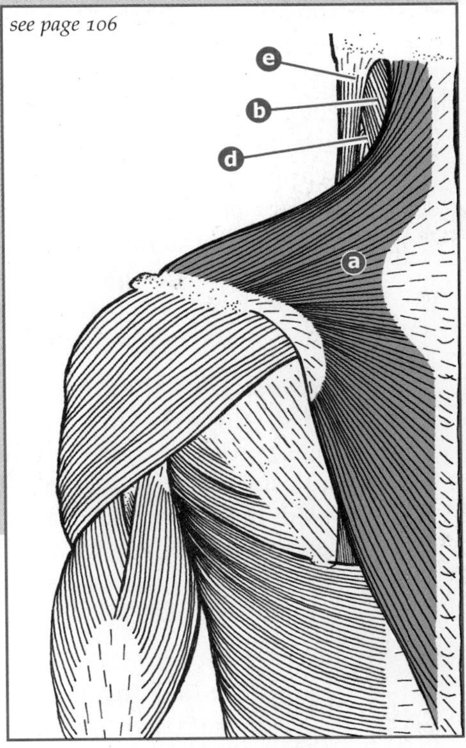

Posterior View of the Neck (Superficial)

a. **Trapezius**
b. Splenius Capitis
c. Splenius Cervicis (not seen)
d. Levator Scapulae
e. Sternocleidomastoid

RELATIONSHIP TO OTHER MUSCULOSKELETAL STRUCTURES

❑ 1. The entire trapezius is superficial in the neck and the back (except for the most anterior portion, which is deep to the platysma).

❑ 2. Directly deep to the trapezius in the neck are the semispinalis capitis, splenius capitis and the levator scapulae. Directly deep to the trapezius in the trunk are the rhomboids and the most superior part of the latissimus dorsi.

❑ 3. Directly anterior to the anterior border of the trapezius are the levator scapulae and the scalenes.

METHODOLOGY FOR LEARNING MUSCLE ACTIONS

❑ **1. Lateral Flexion of the Neck and the Head at the Spinal Joints (upper):** The upper trapezius crosses the joints of the cervical spine and the atlanto-occipital joint laterally (with fibers running vertically in the frontal plane). Therefore, the trapezius laterally flexes the neck at the cervical spinal joints and the head at the atlanto-occipital joint.

❑ **2. Extension of the Neck and the Head at the Spinal Joints (upper):** The upper trapezius crosses the joints of the cervical spine and the atlanto-occipital joint posteriorly (with fibers running vertically in the sagittal plane). Therefore, the trapezius extends the neck at the cervical spinal joints and the head at the atlanto-occipital joint.

TRAPEZIUS (THE "TRAPS") – continued

❑ 3. **Contralateral Rotation of the Neck and the Head at the Spinal Joints (upper):** The upper trapezius crosses the joints of the cervical spine and the atlanto-occipital joint posteriorly (with fibers running somewhat horizontally in the transverse plane). When the upper trapezius contracts, it pulls the more medial attachment (the spinal/occipital attachment) toward the lateral attachment (the scapula), causing the anterior surface of the neck and/or head to face the opposite side of the body from the side of the body that the trapezius is attached. Therefore, the upper trapezius contralaterally rotates the neck at the cervical spinal joints and the head at the atlanto-occipital joint.

❑ 4. **Elevation of the Scapula at the Scapulocostal Joint (upper):** The upper trapezius attaches from the scapula inferiorly, to the spine and the occiput superiorly. When the spinal/occipital attachment is fixed, and the upper trapezius contracts, it pulls the scapula superiorly toward the head and neck. Therefore, the upper trapezius elevates the scapula at the scapulocostal joint.

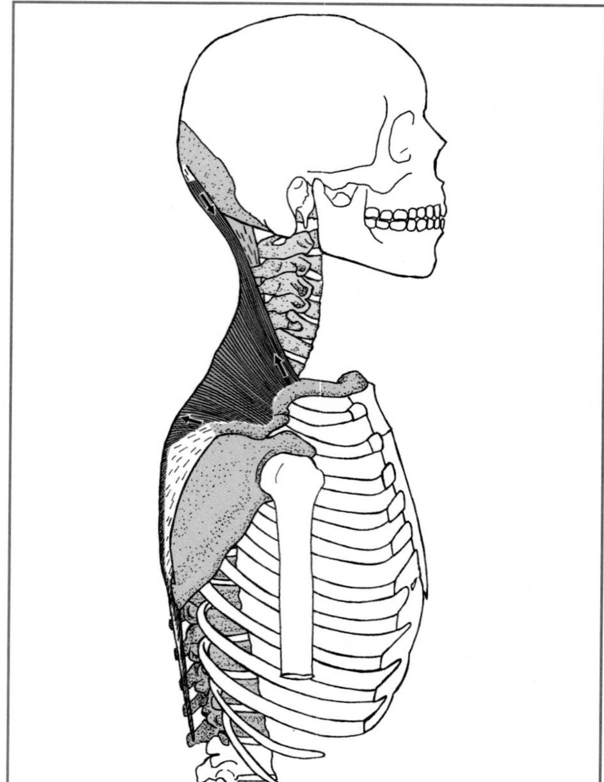

Lateral View of the Right Trapezius

❑ 5. **Retraction (Adduction) of the Scapula at the Scapulocostal Joint (entire muscle):** The entire trapezius attaches from the scapula laterally to the spine medially (with its fibers running horizontally in the frontal plane). When the spinal attachment is fixed, and the entire trapezius contracts, it pulls the scapula medially toward the spine. Therefore, the entire trapezius retracts (adducts) the scapula at the scapulocostal joint. Of the three parts, the middle trapezius is best at this action because its fibers are oriented most horizontally in the frontal plane.

❑ 6. **Depression of the Scapula at the Scapulocostal Joint (lower):** The lower trapezius attaches from the scapula superiorly to the spine inferiorly. When the spinal attachment is fixed, and the lower trapezius contracts, it pulls the scapula inferiorly toward the spine. Therefore, the lower trapezius depresses the scapula at the scapulocostal joint.

❑ 7. **Upward Rotation of the Scapula at the Scapulocostal Joint (upper and lower):** When the upper trapezius pulls at the acromion process, and the lower trapezius pulls at the tubercle of the scapula, both pull on the scapula in such a manner that the scapula rotates, orienting the glenoid fossa superiorly. Therefore, the upper and lower trapezius upwardly rotate the scapula at the scapulocostal joint.

❑ 8. **Extension of the Trunk at the Spinal Joints (middle and lower):** The middle and lower trapezius cross the joints of the thoracic spine posteriorly (with their fibers running vertically in the sagittal plane). Therefore, the trapezius extends the trunk at the thoracic spinal joints.

MISCELLANEOUS

❑ 1. The trapezius is usually considered to have three functional parts: upper, middle and lower. Some sources divide it into two parts, and others divide it into four parts.

TRAPEZIUS (THE "TRAPS") – continued

❑ 2. The trapezius' lateral attachments are the same as the proximal attachments of the deltoid, namely, the lateral clavicle, the acromion process and the spine of the scapula.

❑ 3. **Scapular Tilt Actions:** In addition to its other actions, the scapula can also tilt. If the medial border of the scapula were to move away from the body wall, contraction of the middle and lower trapezius would pull the medial border of the scapula to return to its position against the body wall. The medial border of the scapula moving toward the body wall is called medial tilt; therefore, the middle trapezius and lower trapezius medially tilt the scapula.

❑ 4. The action of medial tilt of the scapula is particularly important when the scapula is protracted because the scapula tends to laterally tilt (wing out) when it protracts. Muscles that medially tilt the scapula prevent the scapula from laterally tilting (winging out).

❑ 5. **Clavicular Actions:** Although the clavicle often moves passively by accompanying scapular movement, the clavicle can be directly acted upon by musculature and therefore actively moved. The upper trapezius attaches from the lateral clavicle to the head and neck. When the head and neck are fixed, the upper trapezius can elevate, upwardly rotate and/or retract the clavicle (at the sternocostal joint) toward the attachments on the head and neck.

❑ 6. When a person has his/her head inclined anteriorly, the center of gravity of the head is such that it would fall into flexion if it were not for the isometric contraction of head and neck extensor musculature. Since this type of posture is so often assumed, posterior cervical muscles, including the trapezius, are probably the most commonly found tight muscles in the human body.

❑ 7. Whenever a purse or any type of bag is carried upon the shoulder, the bag should slide off given the downward slope of the shoulder. However, people usually prevent this by subconsciously elevating the scapula on the side in which the bag is being carried to keep the bag on the shoulder. This posture causes elevators of the scapula (including the upper trapezius) to isometrically contract for long periods of time and therefore become tight and painful. This is another common posture that may cause tightness of the upper trapezius.

❑ 8. Whenever a phone is crimped between the head and the shoulder instead of being held by the hand, lateral flexors of the neck and/or elevators of the scapula (including the upper trapezius) on that side of the body must isometrically contract to hold the phone in place. This is true whether or not the phone has the added piece to make it larger. This posture for prolonged periods of time will cause tension and pain in the muscles involved. This is another common posture that may cause tightness of the upper trapezius.

❑ 9. *Rounded shoulders* is a common postural condition in which the scapulae are protracted (abducted) and depressed (at the scapulocostal joints) and the humeri are medially rotated (at the shoulder joints). Given the trapezius' action of retraction of the scapulae (especially the middle trapezius), when the trapezius muscles are weak, they can contribute to this condition because they are unable to efficiently oppose protraction of the scapulae. This is especially true if the protractors of the scapulae (often the pectoralis minor muscles) are tight.

❑ 10. The greater occipital nerve, which innervates the posterior half of the scalp, pierces through the upper trapezius (as well as the semispinalis capitis of the transversospinalis group). When the upper trapezius is tight, the greater occipital nerve can be compressed, causing a *tension headache* that is felt in the posterior head. (This condition is also known as *greater occipital neuralgia.*)

❑ 11. Whenever a heavy weight is held in the hand, a downward force is exerted upon the scapula and clavicle. Another important function of the trapezius is to isometrically contract to support the distal clavicle and the scapula from being pulled inferiorly by this downward force. Therefore, long periods of carrying a heavy weight in the hand can result in tension and soreness in the upper trapezius.

❑ SPLENIUS CAPITIS

❑ **The name, splenius capitis, tells us that this muscle is shaped like a bandage (a narrow rectangle) and attaches onto the head.**

DERIVATION ❑ splenius: Gr. *bandage.*
capitis: L. *refers to the head.*

PRONUNCIATION ❑ **splee**-knee-us **kap**-i-tis

ATTACHMENTS

❑ **Nuchal Ligament and the S.P.s of C7-T4**

- ❑ the nuchal ligament from the level of C3-C6

to the

❑ **Mastoid Process of the Temporal Bone and the Occipital Bone**

- ❑ the lateral 1/3 of the superior nuchal line of the occiput

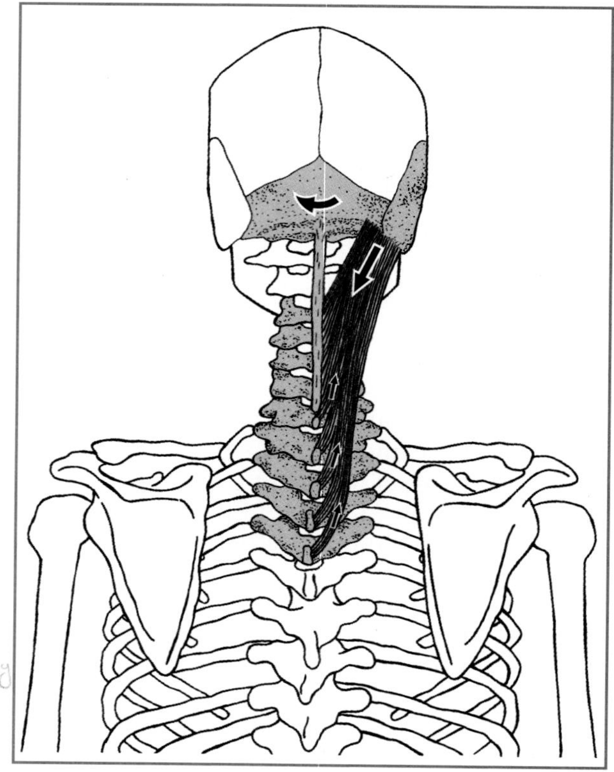

Posterior View of the Right Splenius Capitis

ACTIONS

❑ 1. **Extension of the Head and the Neck**

❑ 2. **Lateral Flexion of the Head and the Neck**

❑ 3. **Ipsilateral Rotation of the Head and the Neck**

INNERVATION ❑ Cervical Spinal Nerves
- ❑ dorsal rami of the middle cervical spinal nerves

ARTERIAL SUPPLY ❑ The Occipital Artery (A Branch of the External Carotid Artery)

PALPATION AND SUPPLEMENTARY TEXT

PALPATION

- ❑ Although there is a small portion of the splenius capitis that is superficial between the trapezius and sternocleidomastoid, most of it is deep to these two muscles.
  - Have the client seated.
  - Locate the levator scapulae (see the palpation section for this muscle on page 121).
  - Place palpating hand just superior and slightly medial to the levator scapulae on the posterior neck.
  - Ask the client to actively rotate the head and the neck (at the atlanto-occipital joint and the cervical spinal joints respectively) and feel for the contraction of the same-sided splenius capitis.
  - To further bring out the splenius capitis, resistance may be added.

see page 106

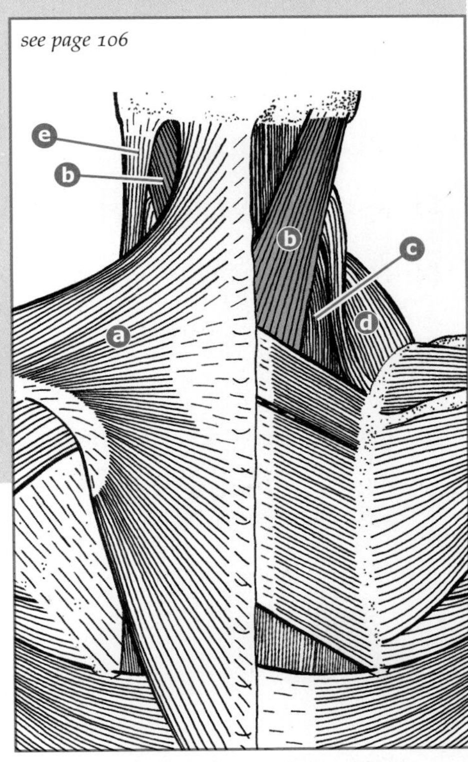

Posterior View of the Neck (Superficial and Intermediate)

- a. Trapezius
- b. **Splenius Capitis**
- c. Splenius Cervicis
- d. Levator Scapulae
- e. Sternocleidomastoid

RELATIONSHIP TO OTHER MUSCULOSKELETAL STRUCTURES

- ❑ 1. Most of the splenius capitis is deep to the trapezius inferiorly and the sternocleidomastoid superiorly.
- ❑ 2. The most inferior part of the splenius capitis is deep to the rhomboid minor and the serratus posterior superior.
- ❑ 3. The attachment of the splenius capitis onto the mastoid process is deep (anterior) to the sternocleidomastoid, but superficial (posterior) to the longissimus capitis.
- ❑ 4. There is a small part of the splenius capitis (along with the levator scapulae, which is just inferior to the splenius capitis) that is superficial between the trapezius and the sternocleidomastoid in the lateral neck.
- ❑ 5. The inferior portion of the splenius cervicis lies directly inferior to the splenius capitis.
- ❑ 6. The erector spinae lie deep to the splenius capitis.

METHODOLOGY FOR LEARNING MUSCLE ACTIONS

- ❑ **1. Extension of the Head and the Neck at the Spinal Joints:** The splenius capitis crosses the atlanto-occipital joint and the joints of the cervical spine posteriorly (with its fibers running vertically in the sagittal plane). Therefore, the splenius capitis extends the head at the atlanto-occipital joint and the neck at the cervical spinal joints.
- ❑ **2. Lateral Flexion of the Head and the Neck at the Spinal Joints:** The splenius capitis crosses the atlanto-occipital joint and the joints of the cervical spine laterally (with its fibers running vertically in the frontal plane). Therefore, the splenius capitis laterally flexes the head at the atlanto-occipital joint and the neck at the cervical spinal joints.

SPLENIUS CAPITIS – continued

- ☐ 3. **Ipsilateral Rotation of the Head and the Neck at the Spinal Joints:** The splenius capitis attaches from the nuchal ligament/S.P. attachment and then wraps around the neck anteriorly to attach onto the cranium (with its fibers running somewhat horizontally in the transverse plane). When the splenius capitis contracts, it pulls the cranial attachment posteromedially, causing the anterior surface of the head and/or the neck to face the same side of the body that the splenius capitis is attached. Therefore, the splenius capitis ipsilaterally rotates the head at the atlanto-occipital joint and the neck at the cervical spinal joints.

MISCELLANEOUS

- ☐ 1. The left and right splenius capitis muscles bilaterally form a "V" shape.
- ☐ 2. Because of their "V" shape, the left and right splenius capitis muscles are sometimes known as the *golf tee* muscles.
- ☐ 3. The inferior attachment of the splenius capitis is variable and often attaches only as far inferior as the S.P. of T3.
- ☐ 4. The mastoid attachment of the splenius capitis is sandwiched between the attachments of the sternocleidomastoid (which is posterior to it) and the longissimus capitis (which is anterior to it).

SPLENIUS CERVICIS ❑

❑ **The name, splenius cervicis, tells us that this muscle is shaped like a bandage (a narrow rectangle) and attaches onto the cervical spine (the neck).**

DERIVATION ❑ splenius: Gr. *bandage.*
cervicis: L. *refers to the cervical spine.*

PRONUNCIATION ❑ **splee**-nee-us **ser**-vi-sis

ATTACHMENTS

❑ **S.P.s of T3-T6**

to the

❑ **T.P.s of C1-C3**

- ❑ the posterior tubercles of the T.P.s

ACTIONS

❑ 1. **Extension of the Neck**

❑ 2. **Lateral Flexion of the Neck**

❑ 3. **Ipsilateral Rotation of the Neck**

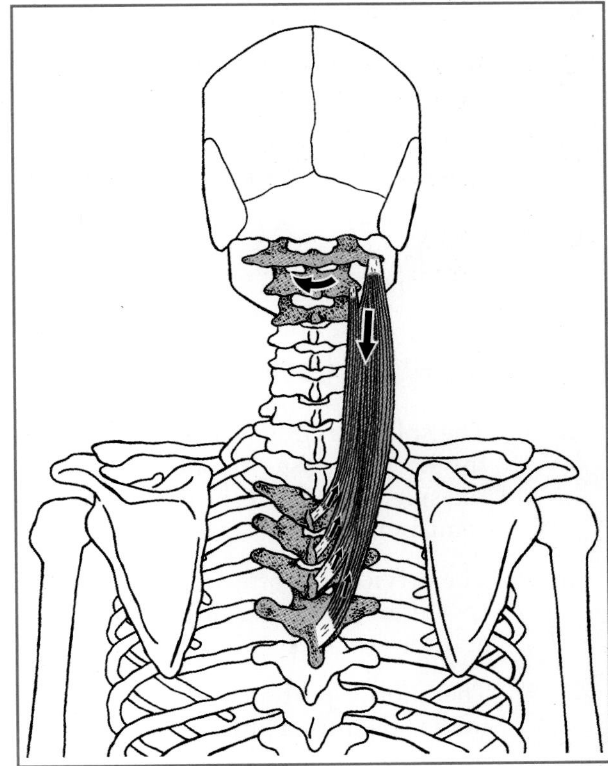

Posterior View of the Right Splenius Cervicis

INNERVATION ❑ Cervical Spinal Nerves
- ❑ dorsal rami of the lower cervical spinal nerves

ARTERIAL SUPPLY ❑ The Occipital Artery (A Branch of the External Carotid Artery) and the Dorsal Branches of the Upper Posterior Intercostal Arteries

SPLENIUS CERVICIS – PALPATION AND SUPPLEMENTARY TEXT

PALPATION

- ❑ The splenius cervicis is deep to other musculature throughout its entire course in the posterior neck and difficult to palpate. The best place to attempt to palpate it is in the lower cervical spine (C5-7 level) where it is deep only to the trapezius.
  - Have the client seated.
  - Locate the levator scapulae (see the palpation section for this muscle on page 121).
  - Place palpating hand just medial to the levator scapulae. This location will be slightly inferior to the location where the splenius capitis was palpated (see the palpation section for this muscle on page 115).
  - Ask the client to actively rotate the neck and feel for the contraction of the same-sided splenius cervicis.
  - To further bring out the splenius cervicis, resistance may be added.

see page 106

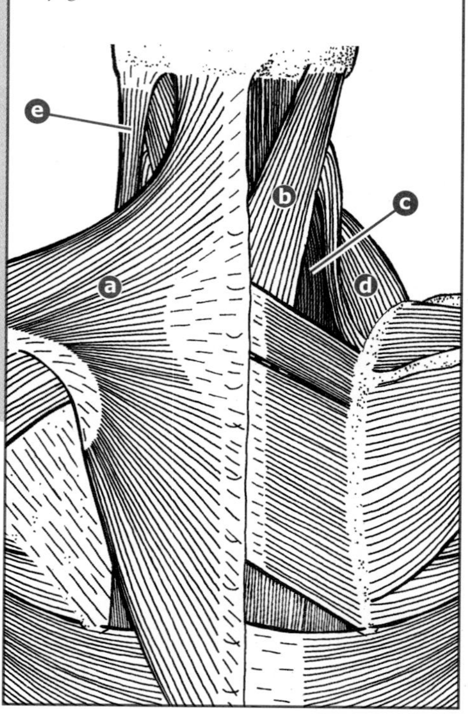

Posterior View of the Neck (Superficial and Intermediate)

a. Trapezius
b. Splenius Capitis
c. **Splenius Cervicis**
d. Levator Scapulae
e. Sternocleidomastoid

RELATIONSHIP TO OTHER MUSCULOSKELETAL STRUCTURES

❑ 1. The splenius cervicis is deep to the trapezius, the rhomboids and the serratus posterior superior. Toward its superior attachment, the splenius cervicis is also deep to the splenius capitis and the semispinalis capitis (of the transversospinalis group).

❑ 2. The cervical T.P. attachment of the splenius cervicis is superficial (posterior) to the cervical T.P. attachments of the levator scapulae and the scalenes.

❑ 3. The inferior portion of the splenius cervicis lies directly inferior to the splenius capitis.

❑ 4. The erector spinae musculature lies deep to the splenius cervicis.

METHODOLOGY FOR LEARNING MUSCLE ACTIONS

❑ **1. Extension of the Neck at the Spinal Joints:** The splenius cervicis crosses the joints of the cervical spine posteriorly (with its fibers running vertically in the sagittal plane); therefore, it extends the neck at the cervical spinal joints.

❑ **2. Lateral Flexion of the Neck at the Spinal Joints:** The splenius cervicis crosses the joints of the cervical spine laterally (with its fibers running vertically in the frontal plane); therefore, it laterally flexes the neck at the cervical spinal joints.

❑ **3. Ipsilateral Rotation of the Neck at the Spinal Joints:** The splenius cervicis attaches from the S.P. attachment in the thoracic region and then wraps around the neck anteriorly to attach onto the T.P.s of the cervical spine (with its fibers running somewhat horizontally in the transverse plane). When the splenius cervicis contracts, it pulls the T.P. attachment posteromedially, causing the anterior surface of the neck to face the same side of the body that the splenius cervicis is attached. Therefore, the splenius cervicis ipsilaterally rotates the neck at the cervical spinal joints.

SPLENIUS CERVICIS – continued

MISCELLANEOUS

- ❑ 1. The left and right splenius cervicis muscles bilaterally form a "V" shape.
- ❑ 2. The superior attachment of the splenius cervicis is variable and often attaches only onto the T.P.s of C1-2.
- ❑ 3. The cervical T.P. attachment of the splenius cervicis is sandwiched between the cervical T.P. attachment of the levator scapulae (which is posterior to it) and the scalenes (which are anterior to it).

LEVATOR SCAPULAE

❑ **The name, levator scapulae, tells us that this muscle elevates the scapula.**

DERIVATION ❑ levator: L. *lifter.*
scapulae: L. *scapula.*

PRONUNCIATION ❑ le-**vay**-tor **skap**-you-lee

ATTACHMENTS

❑ **T.P.s of C1-C4**

❑ the posterior tubercles of the T.P.s of C3 and C4

to the

❑ **Medial Border of the Scapula, from the Superior Angle to the Root of the Spine of the Scapula**

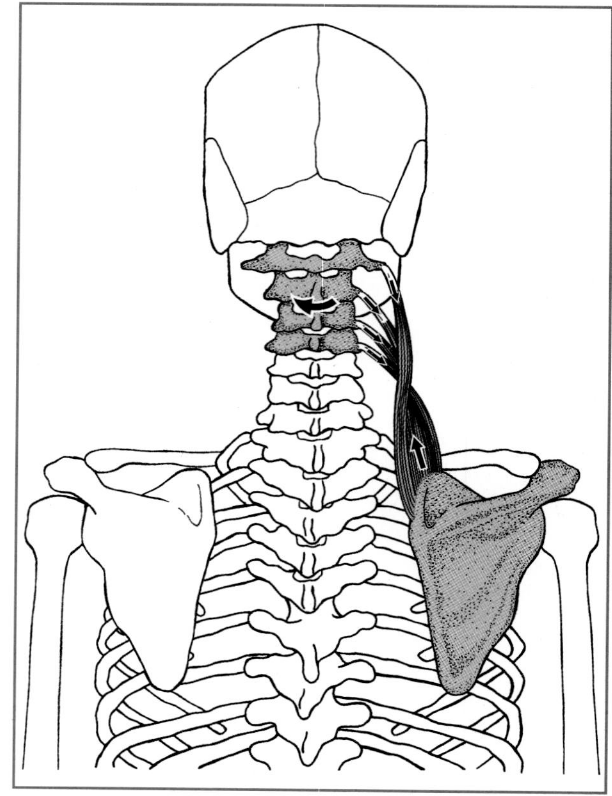

Posterior View of the Right Levator Scapulae

ACTIONS

☑ 1. **Elevation of the Scapula**

❑ 2. **Extension of the Neck**

❑ 3. **Lateral Flexion of the Neck**

❑ 4. Ipsilateral Rotation of the Neck

❑ 5. Downward Rotation of the Scapula

❑ 6. Retraction (Adduction) of the Scapula

INNERVATION ❑ Dorsal Scapular Nerve ❑ C3, 4, 5

ARTERIAL SUPPLY ❑ The Dorsal Scapular Artery (A Branch of the Subclavian Artery)

PALPATION AND SUPPLEMENTARY TEXT

PALPATION

- ❑ Most of the levator scapulae is deep to the trapezius. When palpating, it is important to have the trapezius relaxed.
  - Have the client seated with the forearm in the small of the back (causing downward rotation of the scapula, which relaxes the trapezius).
  - Place palpating hand just superior to the superior angle of the scapula.
  - Ask the client to perform a short, quick range of motion of active elevation of the scapula and feel for the contraction of the levator scapulae. (The contraction is done in this manner to prevent the trapezius from contracting.)
  - Continue palpating the levator scapulae superiorly, between the borders of the trapezius and the sternocleidomastoid.

see page 106

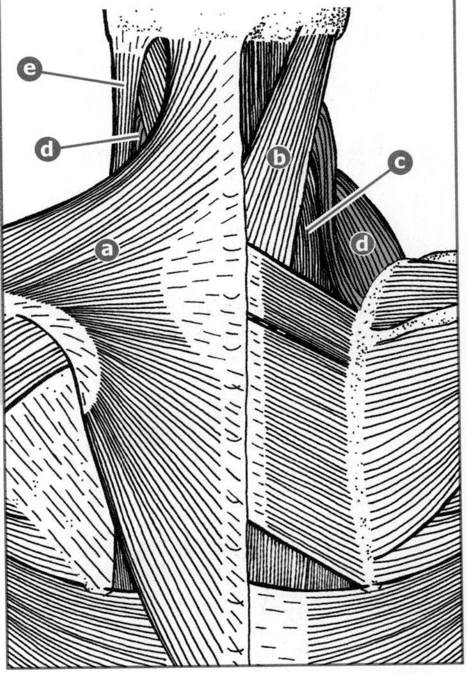

Posterior View of the Neck (Superficial and Intermediate)

a. Trapezius
b. Splenius Capitis
c. Splenius Cervicis
d. **Levator Scapulae**
e. Sternocleidomastoid

RELATIONSHIP TO OTHER MUSCULOSKELETAL STRUCTURES

❑ 1. Inferiorly, the levator scapulae is deep only to the trapezius. Superiorly, the levator scapulae is also deep to the splenius capitis and the sternocleidomastoid.

❑ 2. There is a part of the middle to upper levator scapulae that is superficial between the trapezius and splenius capitis posteriorly, and the sternocleidomastoid and scalenes anteriorly.

❑ 3. The scapular attachment of the levator scapulae is slightly superior to the attachment of the rhomboids.

❑ 4. The T.P. attachment of the levator scapulae is directly deep (anterior) to the T.P. attachment of the splenius cervicis, and directly superficial (posterior) to the T.P. attachment of the scalenes.

METHODOLOGY FOR LEARNING MUSCLE ACTIONS

❑ **1. Elevation of the Scapula at the Scapulocostal Joint:** The levator scapulae attaches from the scapula inferiorly, to the cervical spine superiorly (with its fibers running vertically). When the cervical spine is fixed and the levator scapulae contracts, it pulls the scapula superiorly toward the cervical spine. Therefore, the levator scapulae elevates the scapula at the scapulocostal joint.

❑ **2. Extension of the Neck at the Spinal Joints:** The levator scapulae crosses the cervical spine posteriorly (with its fibers running vertically in the sagittal plane). Therefore, it extends the neck at the cervical spinal joints.

LEVATOR SCAPULAE – continued

- ☐ 3. **Lateral Flexion of the Neck at the Spinal Joints:** The levator scapulae crosses the cervical spine laterally (with its fibers running vertically in the frontal plane). When the scapula is fixed, and the levator scapulae contracts, it pulls the cervical spine inferiorly and laterally toward the scapula. Therefore, the levator scapulae laterally flexes the neck at the cervical spinal joints.
- ☐ 4. **Ipsilateral Rotation of the Neck at the Spinal Joints:** The levator scapulae's fibers wrap around the cervical spine to attach onto the transverse processes (with its fibers oriented somewhat horizontally, from posterior to anterior, in the transverse plane). When the levator scapulae contracts, it pulls the transverse processes posteromedially, causing the anterior surface of the neck to face the same side of the body that the levator scapulae is attached. Therefore, the levator scapulae ipsilaterally rotates the neck at the cervical spinal joints.
- ☐ 5. **Downward Rotation of the Scapula at the Scapulocostal Joint:** When the cervical spine is fixed, and the levator scapulae contracts, it pulls the superior angle of the scapula superiorly and the inferior angle superiorly and medially. This causes the glenoid fossa to orient inferiorly. Therefore, the levator scapula downwardly rotates the scapula at the scapulocostal joint.
- ☐ 6. **Retraction (Adduction) of the Scapula at the Scapulocostal Joint:** The levator scapulae attaches from the spine medially to the scapula laterally (with its fibers running somewhat horizontally in the frontal plane). When the levator scapulae contracts, it pulls the scapula medially toward the spine. Therefore, the levator scapulae retracts (adducts) the scapula at the scapulocostal joint.

MISCELLANEOUS

- ☐ 1. At approximately the midpoint of the levator scapulae, there is a twist in the fibers that creates an increased density in the middle of the levator scapulae which is often mistaken for a trigger point. (When a trigger point is present, it is usually located more inferiorly, just superior to the superior angle of the scapula.)
- ☐ 2. Because the cervical transverse process attachment of the levator scapulae is more anterior than the scapular attachment, the levator scapulae has the ability to pull the scapula anteriorly. Therefore, the levator scapulae is able to protract (abduct) the scapula at the scapulocostal joint.
- ☐ 3. Scapular Tilt Actions: In addition to its other actions, the scapula can also tilt. When the levator scapulae pulls on the scapula, it can pull the scapula in such a manner that the scapula is pulled superiorly and the inferior angle moves superiorly and away from the posterior body wall. The inferior angle of the scapula coming away from the body wall is called upward tilt; therefore, the levator scapulae upwardly tilts the scapula at the scapulocostal joint.

THE SUBOCCIPITALS

The suboccipitals are a group of four short muscles located deep in the posterior suboccipital region.

THERE ARE FOUR SUBOCCIPITAL MUSCLES:	
Rectus Capitis Posterior Major Rectus Capitis Posterior Minor	Obliquus Capitis Inferior Obliquus Capitis Superior

Attachments:

- The names of the suboccipital muscles generally refer to their fiber direction:
  - "Rectus" means straight. The rectus capitis posterior major and minor attach from the S.P. of C2 and the posterior tubercle of C1 respectively and run straight up to the inferior nuchal line of the occiput.
  - "Obliquus" means slanted. The obliquus capitis inferior and superior run in a slanted fashion. The obliquus capitis inferior slants from the S.P. of C2 to the T.P. of C1, and the obliquus capitis superior slants from the T.P. of C1 to the occiput (between the inferior and superior nuchal lines).
- The suboccipitals are found deep to the upper trapezius, sternocleidomastoid, splenius capitis and the semispinalis capitis.

Actions:

- The major action of the suboccipital group is extension of the head upon the neck at the atlanto-occipital joint.
- The obliquus capitis inferior ipsilaterally rotates the atlas (C1) upon the axis (C2) at the atlantoaxial joint.
- The suboccipital muscles are generally thought to be more important as postural muscles, providing fine control of head posture, than as movers.

Miscellaneous:

- The suboccipital muscles are not the only muscles located in the suboccipital region. When tight muscles are palpated in this region, it is not always the suboccipital muscles, but rather it can be the superior attachments of the trapezius, splenius capitis, semispinalis capitis or perhaps even the longissimus capitis or the sternocleidomastoid.
- When the suboccipital musculature is chronically tight, tension headaches may occur.

INNERVATION The four suboccipital muscles are innervated by the suboccipital nerve.

♥ **ARTERIAL SUPPLY** The four suboccipital muscles receive their arterial supply from the occipital artery.

POSTERIOR VIEW OF THE SUBOCCIPITALS

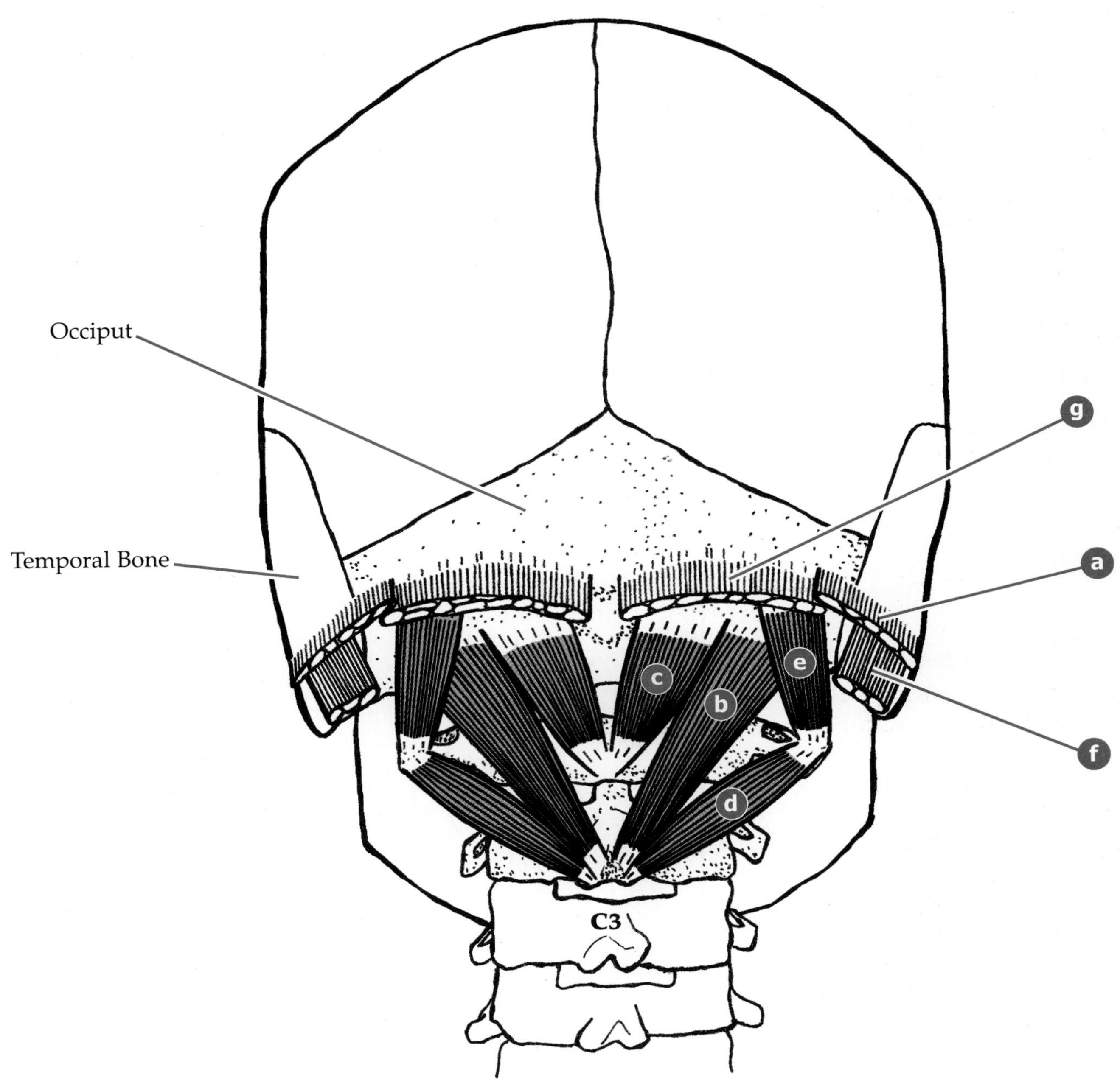

- **a.** Splenius Capitis (cut)
- **b. Rectus Capitis Posterior Major**
- **c. Rectus Capitis Posterior Minor**
- **d. Obliquus Capitis Inferior**
- **e. Obliquus Capitis Superior**
- **f.** Longissimus Capitis (cut)
- **g.** Semispinalis Capitis (cut)

Note: The trapezius and sternocleidomastoid have been removed.

RECTUS CAPITIS POSTERIOR MAJOR
(OF THE SUBOCCIPITAL GROUP)

❑ **The name, rectus capitis posterior major, tells us that the fibers of this muscle run straight (straighter than the two obliquus capitis suboccipital muscles). It also tells us that this muscle attaches to the head posteriorly and is large (larger than the rectus capitis posterior minor).**

DERIVATION ❑ rectus: L. *straight.*
capitis: L. *refers to the head.*
posterior: L. *behind, toward the back.*
major: L. *larger.*

PRONUNCIATION ❑ **rek**-tus **kap**-i-tis pos-**tee**-ri-or **may**-jor

ATTACHMENTS

❑ **The Axis (C2)**

❑ the S.P.

to the

❑ **Occiput**

❑ the lateral 1/2 of the inferior nuchal line

ACTIONS

☑ 1. **Extension of the Head**

❑ 2. Lateral Flexion of the Head

❑ 3. Ipsilateral Rotation of the Head

❑ 4. Extension and Ipsilateral Rotation of the Atlas

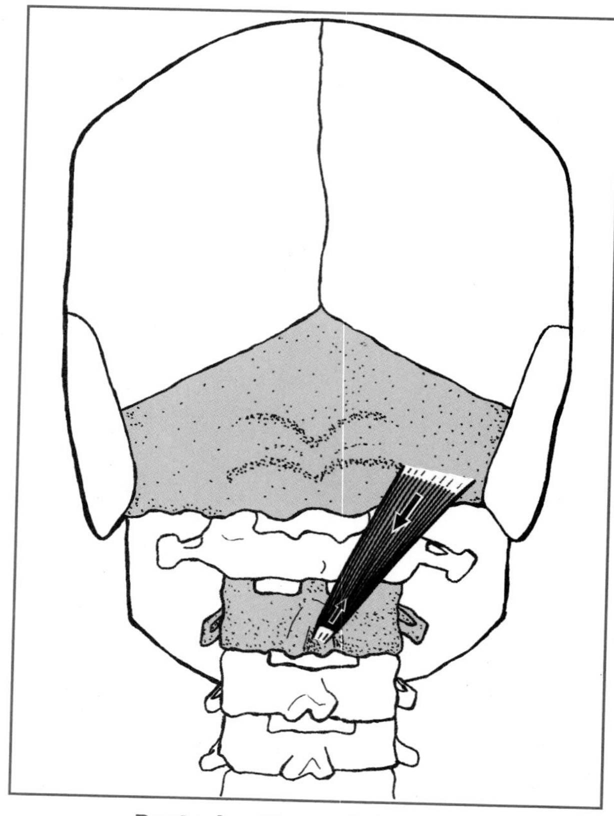

Posterior View of the Right Rectus Capitis Posterior Major

INNERVATION ❑ The Suboccipital Nerve ❑ dorsal ramus of C1

ARTERIAL SUPPLY ❑ The Occipital Artery (A Branch of the External Carotid Artery) and the Deep Cervical Artery (A Branch of the Costocervical Trunk)
❑ and the muscular branches of the vertebral artery (a branch of the subclavian artery)

PALPATION AND SUPPLEMENTARY TEXT

PALPATION

- ❑ As with all the suboccipital muscles, the rectus capitis posterior major is very deep and difficult to palpate. However, if the superficial musculature is relaxed and the rectus capitis posterior major is tight, it can be felt.
  - Have the client supine and as relaxed as possible.
  - Place palpating fingers between the S.P. of the axis (C2), which is the most prominent S.P. in the upper cervical region, and the occiput and feel for the fibers of the rectus capitis posterior major running superolaterally from the S.P. of the axis toward the occiput.

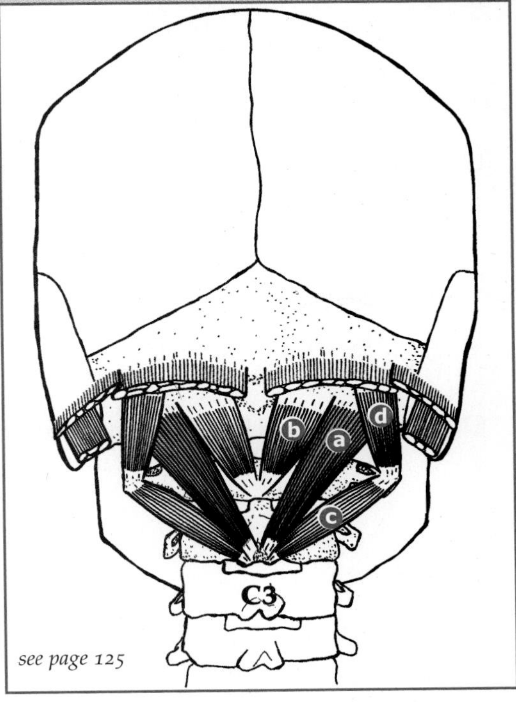

Posterior View of the Suboccipital Muscle Group

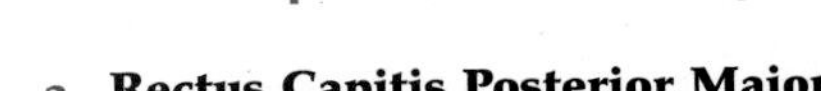

a. **Rectus Capitis Posterior Major**
b. Rectus Capitis Posterior Minor
c. Obliquus Capitis Inferior
d. Obliquus Capitis Superior

RELATIONSHIP TO OTHER MUSCULOSKELETAL STRUCTURES

❑ 1. The rectus capitis posterior major, as with all the suboccipital muscles, is very deep in the suboccipital region. The rectus capitis posterior major is deep to the trapezius and the semispinalis capitis.

❑ 2. Deep to the suboccipital muscle group are the occiput, the atlas (C1) and the axis (C2).

❑ 3. The rectus capitis posterior major lies directly lateral to the rectus capitis posterior minor.

❑ 4. The occipital attachment of the rectus capitis posterior major is deep to the occipital attachment of the obliquus capitis superior.

METHODOLOGY FOR LEARNING MUSCLE ACTIONS

❑ 1. **Extension of the Head at the Atlanto-Occipital Joint:** The rectus capitis posterior major crosses the atlanto-occipital joint posteriorly (with its fibers running vertically in the sagittal plane); therefore, it extends the head upon the atlas (C1) at the atlanto-occipital joint.

❑ 2. **Lateral Flexion of the Head at the Atlanto-Occipital Joint:** The rectus capitis posterior major crosses the atlanto-occipital joint from near the midline on the axis (C2) to more laterally on the occiput (with its fibers running vertically in the frontal plane). Therefore, the rectus capitis posterior major laterally flexes the head upon the atlas (C1) at the atlanto-occipital joint.

❑ 3. **Ipsilateral Rotation of the Head at the Atlanto-Occipital Joint:** The rectus capitis posterior major crosses the atlanto-occipital joint with its fibers wrapping around the suboccipital region from posteriorly on the axis, to more anteriorly on the occiput (with its fibers running somewhat horizontally in the transverse plane). When the rectus capitis posterior major contracts, it pulls on the occiput, causing the anterior surface of the head to face the same side of the body that the rectus capitis posterior major is attached. Therefore, the rectus capitis posterior major ipsilaterally rotates the head upon the atlas (C1) at the atlanto-occipital joint.

RECTUS CAPITIS POSTERIOR MAJOR – continued

❑ **4. Extension and Ipsilateral Rotation of the Atlas at the Atlantoaxial Joint:** The rectus capitis posterior major crosses the joint between the atlas and the axis (the atlanto-axial joint) in the same manner that it crosses the joint between the head and the atlas (the atlanto-occipital joint). Therefore, the rectus capitis posterior major should perform the same actions at the atlanto-axial joint that it performs at the atlanto-occipital joint (see methodologies #1-3), which it does except that the atlanto-axial joint does not permit lateral flexion. Therefore, the rectus capitis posterior major extends and ipsilaterally rotates the atlas (C1) upon the axis (C2) at the atlantoaxial joint.

MISCELLANEOUS

❑ 1. The rectus capitis posterior major is one of four muscles that are called the *suboccipital muscles*. They are the rectus capitis posterior major, rectus capitis posterior minor, obliquus capitis inferior and the obliquus capitis superior.

❑ 2. In addition to the four suboccipital muscles, there is a rectus capitis anterior and a rectus capitis lateralis.

❑ 3. The rectus capitis posterior major and the rectus capitis posterior minor both attach to the inferior nuchal line of the occiput.

❑ 4. The suboccipital muscles are generally thought to be more important as postural muscles, providing fine control of head posture, than as movers.

RECTUS CAPITIS POSTERIOR MINOR
(OF THE SUBOCCIPITAL GROUP)

❑ **The name, rectus capitis posterior minor, tells us that the fibers of this muscle run straight (straighter than the two obliquus capitis suboccipital muscles). It also tells us that this muscle attaches to the head posteriorly and is small (smaller than the rectus capitis posterior major).**

DERIVATION ❑ rectus: L. *straight.*
capitis: L. *refers to the head.*
posterior: L. *behind, toward the back.*
minor: L. *smaller.*

PRONUNCIATION ❑ **rek**-tus **kap**-i-tis pos-**tee**-ri-or **my**-nor

ATTACHMENTS

❑ **The Atlas (C1)**

❑ the posterior tubercle

to the

❑ **Occiput**

❑ the medial 1/2 of the inferior nuchal line

ACTION

❑ **Extension of the Head**

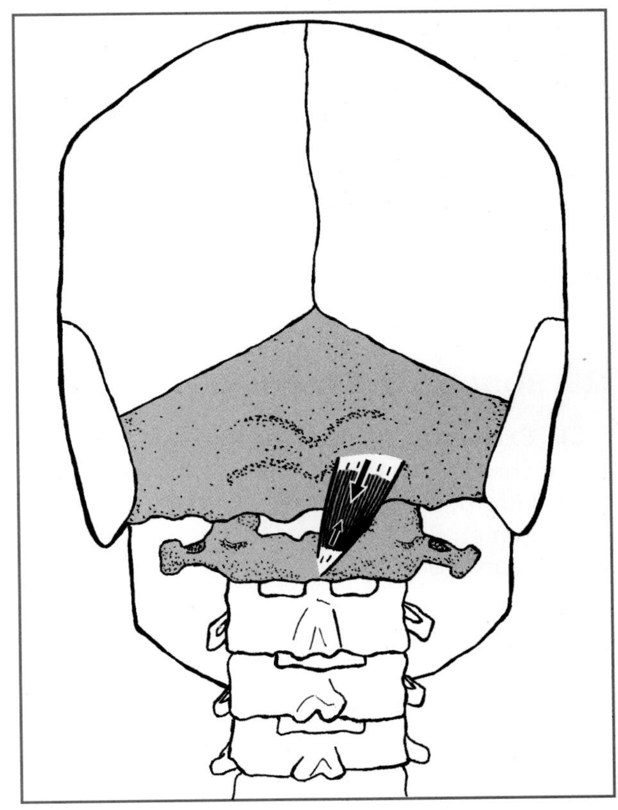

Posterior View of the Right Rectus Capitis Posterior Minor

INNERVATION ❑ The Suboccipital Nerve ❑ dorsal ramus of C1

ARTERIAL SUPPLY ❑ The Occipital Artery (A Branch of the External Carotid Artery) and Muscular Branches of the Vertebral Artery (A Branch of the Subclavian Artery)
❑ and the deep cervical artery (a branch of the costocervical trunk)

RECTUS CAPITIS POSTERIOR MINOR PALPATION AND SUPPLEMENTARY TEXT

PALPATION

- ❑ As with all the suboccipital muscles, the rectus capitis posterior minor is very deep and difficult to palpate. However, if the superficial musculature is relaxed and the rectus capitis posterior minor is tight, it can be felt.
  - Have the client supine and as relaxed as possible.
  - Place palpating fingers just inferior to the occiput and feel for the fibers of the rectus capitis posterior minor running superiorly from the posterior tubercle of the atlas (C1) toward the occiput.

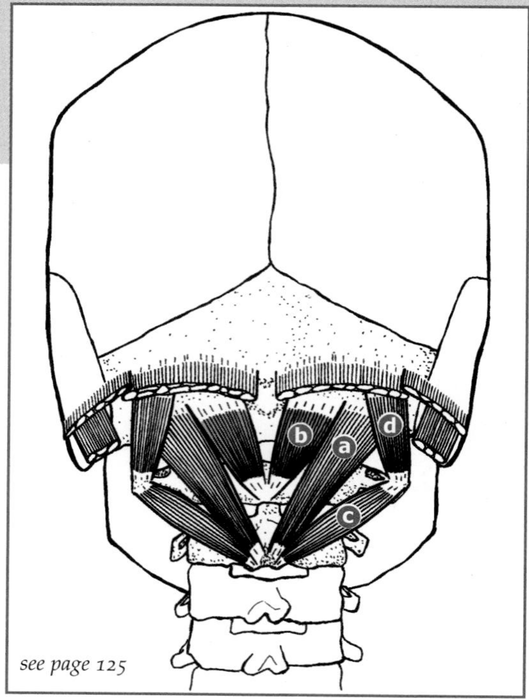

see page 125

Posterior View of the Suboccipital Muscle Group

a. Rectus Capitis Posterior Major
b. Rectus Capitis Posterior Minor
c. Obliquus Capitis Inferior
d. Obliquus Capitis Superior

RELATIONSHIP TO OTHER MUSCULOSKELETAL STRUCTURES

❑ 1. The rectus capitis posterior minor, as with all the suboccipital muscles, is very deep in the suboccipital region. The rectus capitis posterior minor is deep to the trapezius and the semispinalis capitis.

❑ 2. Deep to the suboccipital muscle group are the occiput, the atlas (C1) and the axis (C2).

❑ 3. The rectus capitis posterior minor lies directly medial to the rectus capitis posterior major.

METHODOLOGY FOR LEARNING MUSCLE ACTIONS

❑ **Extension of the Head at the Atlanto-Occipital Joint:** The rectus capitis posterior minor crosses the atlanto-occipital joint posteriorly (with its fibers running vertically in the sagittal plane); therefore, it extends the head upon the atlas (C1) at the atlanto-occipital joint.

MISCELLANEOUS

❑ 1. The rectus capitis posterior minor is one of four muscles that are called the *suboccipital muscles*. They are the rectus capitis posterior major, rectus capitis posterior minor, obliquus capitis inferior and the obliquus capitis superior.

❑ 2. In addition to the four suboccipital muscles, there is a rectus capitis anterior and a rectus capitis lateralis.

❑ 3. The rectus capitis posterior major and the rectus capitis posterior minor both attach to the inferior nuchal line of the occiput.

❑ 4. The suboccipital muscles are generally thought to be more important as postural muscles, providing fine control of head posture, than as movers.

❑ 5. In addition to the inferior nuchal line attachment, the rectus capitis posterior minor also attaches more inferiorly onto the occiput between the inferior nuchal line and the foramen magnum. A connective tissue attachment of the rectus capitis posterior minor has been discovered which attaches directly into the dura mater. Although tightness of any of the posterior cervical musculature in the suboccipital region may cause *tension headaches*, given this dura mater attachment, tightness of the rectus capitis posterior minor may more easily precipitate a tension headache than the other muscles in the region.

OBLIQUUS CAPITIS INFERIOR

(OF THE SUBOCCIPITAL GROUP)

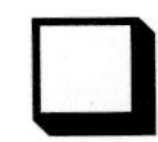

❑ **The name, obliquus capitis inferior, tells us that the fibers of this muscle run obliquely (in comparison to the two rectus capitis posterior suboccipital muscles). It also tells us that this muscle attaches near the head (this is the only one of the four suboccipital muscles that does not attach directly onto the head) and is located inferiorly (inferior to the obliquus capitis superior).**

DERIVATION ❑ obliquus: L. *oblique.*
capitis: L. *refers to the head.*
inferior: L. *below.*

PRONUNCIATION ❑ ob-**lee**-kwus **kap**-i-tis in-**fee**-ri-or

ATTACHMENTS

❑ **The Axis (C2)**

- ❑ the S.P.

to the

❑ **Atlas (C1)**

- ❑ the T.P.

ACTION

❑ **Ipsilateral Rotation of the Atlas**

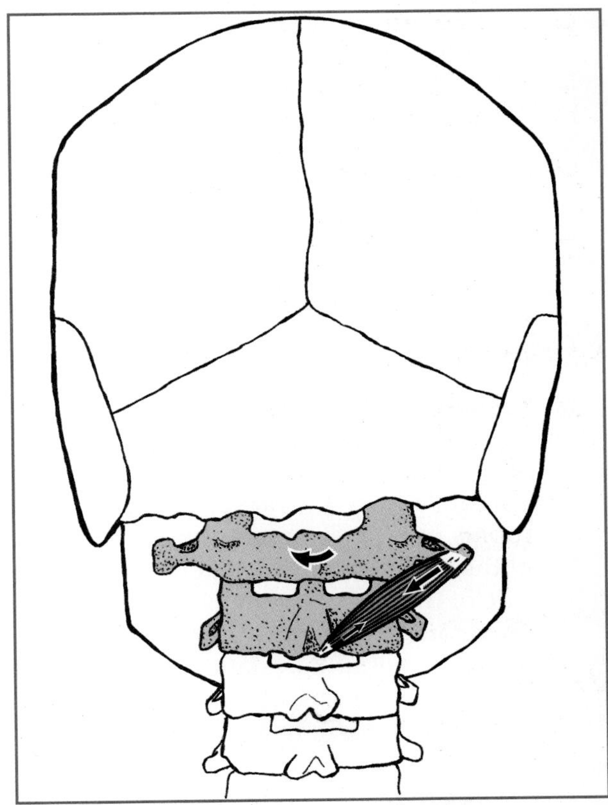

Posterior View of the Right Obliquus Capitis Inferior

INNERVATION ❑ The Suboccipital Nerve ❑ dorsal ramus of C1

ARTERIAL SUPPLY ❑ The Deep Cervical Artery (A Branch of the Costocervical Trunk) and the Descending Branch of the Occipital Artery (A Branch of the External Carotid Artery)
❑ and the muscular branches of the vertebral artery (a branch of the subclavian artery)

OBLIQUUS CAPITIS INFERIOR
PALPATION AND SUPPLEMENTARY TEXT

PALPATION

- ❑ As with all the suboccipital muscles, the obliquus capitis inferior is very deep and difficult to palpate. However, if the superficial musculature is relaxed and the obliquus capitis inferior is tight, it can be felt.
  - Have the client supine and as relaxed as possible.
  - Place palpating fingers on the S.P. of the axis (C2), which is the most prominent S.P. in the upper cervical region and feel for the fibers of the obliquus capitis inferior running laterally and slightly superiorly from the S.P. of the axis toward the T.P. of the atlas (C1).

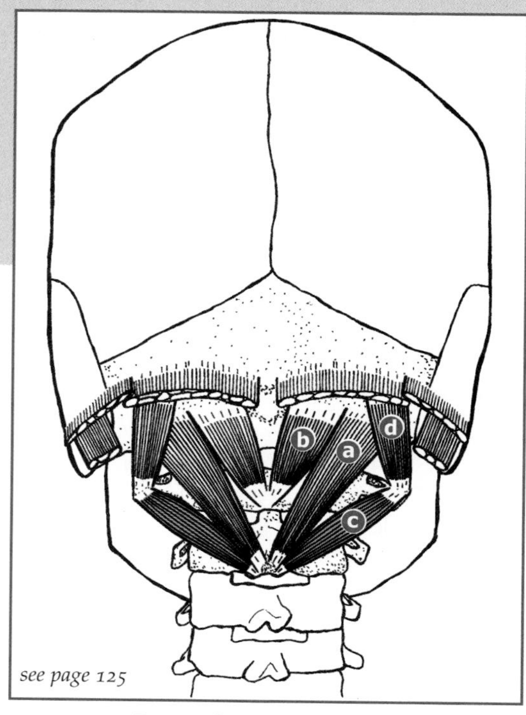

see page 125

Posterior View of the Suboccipital Muscle Group

a. Rectus Capitis Posterior Major
b. Rectus Capitis Posterior Minor
c. **Obliquus Capitis Inferior**
d. Obliquus Capitis Superior

RELATIONSHIP TO OTHER MUSCULOSKELETAL STRUCTURES

❑ 1. The obliquus capitis inferior, as with all of the suboccipital muscles, is very deep in the suboccipital region. The obliquus capitis inferior is deep to the trapezius and the semispinalis capitis.

❑ 2. Deep to the suboccipital muscle group are the occiput, the atlas (C1) and the axis (C2).

METHODOLOGY FOR LEARNING MUSCLE ACTIONS

❑ **Ipsilateral Rotation of the Atlas at the Atlantoaxial Joint:** The obliquus capitis inferior attaches from the S.P. of the axis (C2) to the T.P. of the atlas (C1, with its fibers running horizontally in the transverse plane). When the obliquus capitis inferior contracts, it pulls the T.P. of the atlas toward the S.P. of the axis, causing the anterior surface of the atlas to face the same side of the body that the obliquus capitis inferior is attached. Therefore, the obliquus capitis inferior ipsilaterally rotates the atlas upon the axis at the atlantoaxial joint. (Note: If the head is fixed to the atlas, the head will "go along for the ride" and the head and the atlas together will rotate upon the axis.)

MISCELLANEOUS

❑ 1. The obliquus capitis inferior is one of four muscles that are called the *suboccipital muscles*. They are the rectus capitis posterior major, rectus capitis posterior minor, obliquus capitis inferior and the obliquus capitis superior.

❑ 2. In addition to the four suboccipital muscles, there is a rectus capitis anterior and a rectus capitis lateralis.

❑ 3. The obliquus capitis inferior is the only one of the four suboccipital muscles that does not cross the atlanto-occipital joint to attach onto the head. Therefore, it cannot move the head, but rather moves the atlas (C1) at the atlantoaxial joint.

OBLIQUUS CAPITIS INFERIOR – continued

- ☐ 4. The suboccipital muscles are generally thought to be more important as postural muscles of the head/upper cervical region than as movers. However, of the four suboccipitals, the obliquus capitis inferior is the most important as a mover, due to the fact that its location affords it excellent leverage to rotate the atlas.
- ☐ 5. The obliquus capitis inferior and the obliquus capitis superior both attach to the T.P. of the atlas. Four other muscles also attach to the T.P. of the atlas: the levator scapulae, splenius cervicis, rectus capitis anterior and the rectus capitis lateralis.

❑ OBLIQUUS CAPITIS SUPERIOR
(OF THE SUBOCCIPITAL GROUP)

❑ **The name, obliquus capitis superior, tells us that the fibers of this muscle run obliquely (in comparison to the two rectus capitis posterior suboccipital muscles). It also tells us that this muscle attaches onto the head and is located superiorly (superior to the obliquus capitis inferior).**

DERIVATION ❑ obliquus: L. *oblique.*
capitis: L. *refers to the head.*
superior: L. *above.*

PRONUNCIATION ❑ ob-**lee**-kwus **kap**-i-tis sue-**pee**-ri-or

ATTACHMENTS

❑ **The Atlas (C1)**

- ❑ the T.P.

to the

❑ **Occiput**

- ❑ between the superior and inferior nuchal lines

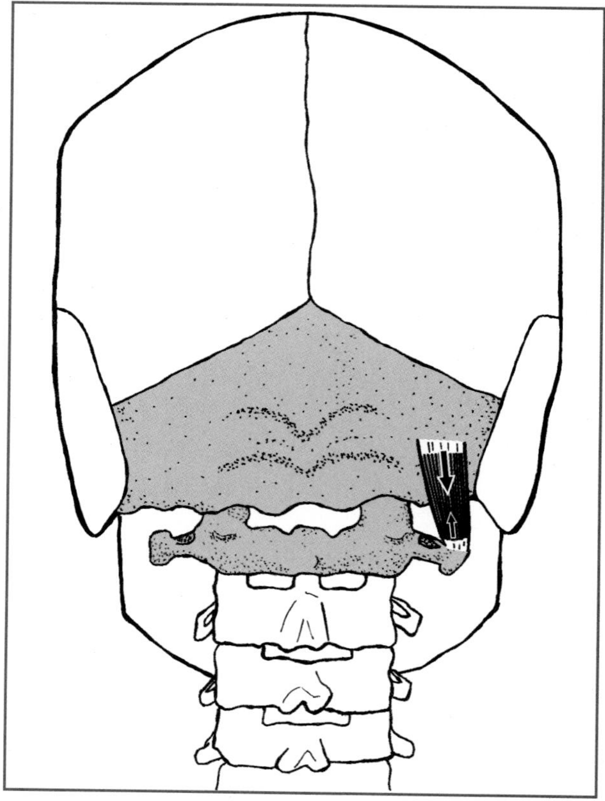

Posterior View of the Right Obliquus Capitis Superior

ACTIONS

❑ **1. Extension of the Head**

❑ **2.** Lateral Flexion of the Head

INNERVATION ❑ The Suboccipital Nerve ❑ dorsal ramus of C1

ARTERIAL SUPPLY ❑ The Occipital Artery (A Branch of the External Carotid Artery) and the Deep Cervical Artery (A Branch of the Costocervical Trunk)
❑ and the muscular branches of the vertebral artery (a branch of the subclavian artery)

PALPATION AND SUPPLEMENTARY TEXT

PALPATION

- ❑ As with all the suboccipital muscles, the obliquus capitis superior is very deep and difficult to palpate. However, if the superficial musculature is relaxed and the obliquus capitis superior is tight, it can be felt.
  - Have the client supine and as relaxed as possible.
  - Place palpating fingers lateral to the midline and just inferior to the occiput, between the T.P. of the atlas (C1) and the occiput and feel for the fibers of the obliquus capitis superior running superiorly and medially from the T.P. of the atlas toward the occiput.

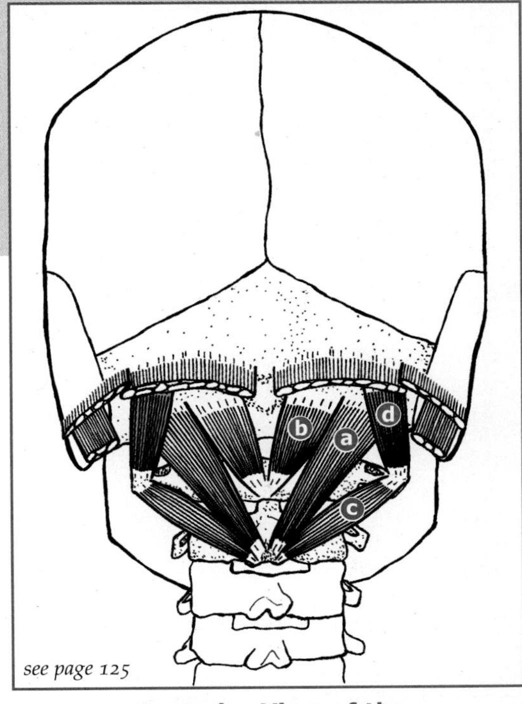

see page 125

Posterior View of the Suboccipital Muscle Group

a. Rectus Capitis Posterior Major
b. Rectus Capitis Posterior Minor
c. Obliquus Capitis Inferior
d. Obliquus Capitis Superior

RELATIONSHIP TO OTHER MUSCULOSKELETAL STRUCTURES

❑ 1. The obliquus capitis superior, as with all of the suboccipital muscles, is very deep in the suboccipital region. The obliquus capitis superior is deep to the trapezius and the semispinalis capitis.

❑ 2. Deep to the suboccipital muscle group are the occiput, the atlas (C1) and the axis (C2).

❑ 3. The occipital attachment of the obliquus capitis superior is superficial to the occipital attachment of the rectus capitis posterior major.

❑ 4. The occipital attachment of the obliquus capitis superior is slightly lateral (and partially deep) to the occipital attachment of the semispinalis capitis.

METHODOLOGY FOR LEARNING MUSCLE ACTIONS

❑ **1. Extension of the Head at the Atlanto-Occipital Joint:**
The obliquus capitis superior crosses the atlanto-occipital joint posteriorly (with its fibers running vertically in the sagittal plane); therefore, it extends the head upon the atlas (C1) at the atlanto-occipital joint.

❑ **2. Lateral Flexion of the Head at the Atlanto-Occipital Joint:**
The obliquus capitis superior crosses the atlanto-occipital joint laterally (with its fibers running vertically in the frontal plane); therefore, it laterally flexes the head upon the atlas (C1) at the atlanto-occipital joint.

MISCELLANEOUS

❑ 1. The obliquus capitis superior is one of four muscles that are called the *suboccipital muscles.* They are the rectus capitis posterior major, rectus capitis posterior minor, obliquus capitis inferior and the obliquus capitis superior.

OBLIQUUS CAPITIS SUPERIOR – continued

- ❑ 2. In addition to the four suboccipital muscles, there is a rectus capitis anterior and a rectus capitis lateralis.
- ❑ 3. The obliquus capitis superior and the obliquus capitis inferior both attach to the T.P. of the atlas (C1). Four other muscles also attach to the T.P. of the atlas: the levator scapulae, splenius cervicis, rectus capitis anterior and the rectus capitis lateralis.
- ❑ 4. The obliquus capitis superior also has the ability to contralaterally rotate the head upon the atlas (C1) at the atlanto-occipital joint.
- ❑ 5. The suboccipital muscles are generally thought to be more important as postural muscles, providing fine control of head posture, than as movers.

PLATYSMA

❑ The name, platysma, tells us that this muscle is broad and flat in shape.

DERIVATION ❑ platysma: Gr. *broad, plate.* **PRONUNCIATION** ❑ pla-**tiz**-ma

ATTACHMENTS

❑ **Subcutaneous Fascia of the Superior Chest**

- ❑ the pectoral and deltoid fascia

to the

❑ **Mandible and the Subcutaneous Fascia of the Lower Face**

ACTIONS

❑ **1. Draws Up the Skin of the Superior Chest and Neck, Creating Ridges of Skin in the Neck**

❑ **2.** Depresses and Draws the Lower Lip Laterally

❑ **3.** Depression of the Mandible

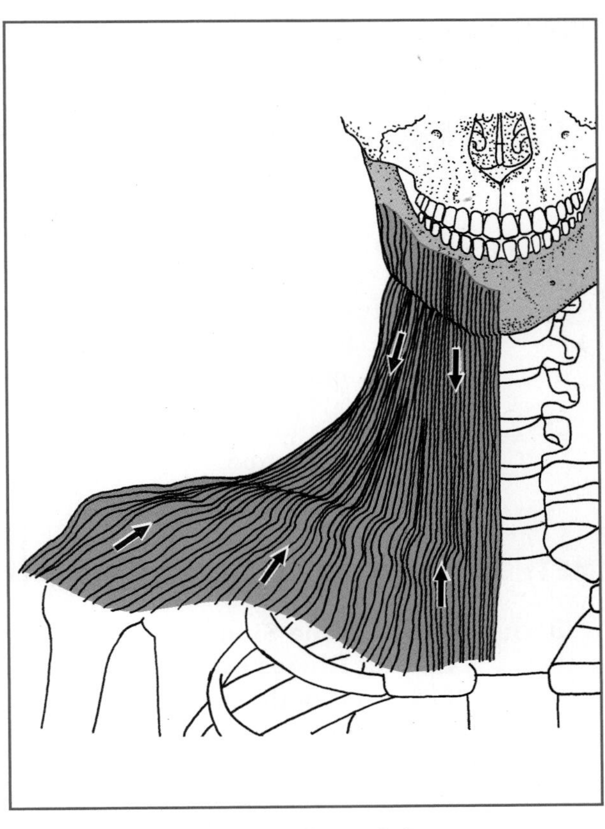

Anterior View of the Right Platysma

INNERVATION ❑ Facial Nerve (CN VII) ❑ cervical branch

ARTERIAL SUPPLY ❑ The Facial Artery (A Branch of the External Carotid Artery)
❑ and the transverse cervical artery (a branch of the thyrocervical trunk)

PLATYSMA – PALPATION AND SUPPLEMENTARY TEXT

PALPATION

- ❑ The ridges or wrinkling of the skin that are created in the neck by the contraction of the platysma are visible and easy to palpate.
    - Have the client seated or supine.
    - Place palpating hand on the anterolateral neck.
    - Ask the client to forcefully contract the platysma by depressing and drawing the lower lip laterally while keeping the mandible fixed in a position of slight depression. Observe and feel for the contraction of the platysma.

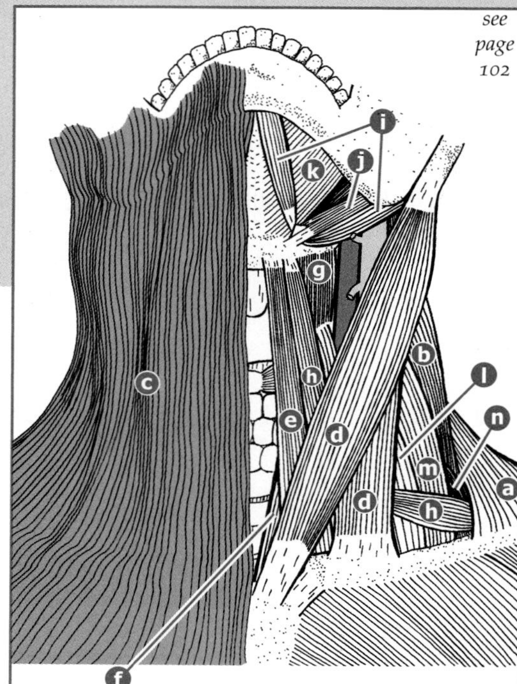

Anterior View of the Neck (Superficial)

a. Trapezius
b. Levator Scapulae
c. **Platysma** (removed on our right)
d. Sternocleidomastoid
e. Sternohyoid
f. Sternothyroid
g. Thyrohyoid
h. Omohyoid
i. Digastric
j. Stylohyoid
k. Mylohyoid
l. Anterior Scalene
m. Middle Scalene
n. Posterior Scalene

RELATIONSHIP TO OTHER MUSCULOSKELETAL STRUCTURES

❑ 1. The platysma is superficial in the chest and neck. In the face, it is deep to the depressor anguli oris, the depressor labii inferioris and the risorius.

❑ 2. The clavicle and parts of the deltoid, pectoralis major, sternocleidomastoid, infrahyoids and suprahyoids are all deep to the platysma.

METHODOLOGY FOR LEARNING MUSCLE ACTIONS

❑ **1. Draws Up the Skin of the Superior Chest and Neck, Creating Ridges of Skin in the Neck:** When both attachments of the platysma are fixed (i.e., the mandible is not allowed to move and the fascia of the chest can only move just so far) and the platysma is contracted forcefully, then the fibers of the platysma (attempting to move the attachments toward each other) tense and "ridges" of soft tissue will be seen standing out in the skin of the neck. (The lower lip will also be seen to move - see methodology #2.) Note: Some sources describe this as "wrinkling the skin of the neck."

❑ **2. Depresses and Draws the Lower Lip Laterally:** The platysma attaches to the fascia of the lower lip. From there, its fibers run primarily inferiorly, and a bit laterally, toward the fascia of the superior chest. When the superior attachment to the fascia of the inferior face moves, the lower lip is drawn inferiorly and the corner of the mouth is drawn laterally. This creates the facial expression of horror, surprise or disgust.

❑ **3. Depression of the Mandible at the Temporomandibular Joint:** Given the attachment directly into the mandible (as well as the attachment into the fascia overlying the mandible), and the fact that these fibers that attach into the mandible run vertically from the mandible down to the chest, the platysma can pull the mandible down toward the chest, thus depressing the mandible at the temporomandibular joint.

PLATYSMA – continued

MISCELLANEOUS

- ❑ 1. Although the platysma is placed in the neck chapter due to its location, by function it is primarily a muscle of facial expression. (Muscles of facial expression are found on page 22.)
- ❑ 2. The skeletal action of depression of the mandible by the platysma is extremely weak.
- ❑ 3. The platysma on one side blends with the contralateral platysma.
- ❑ 4. The platysma often blends with the other facial muscles in the lower face.
- ❑ 5. The platysma in humans is considered to be a remnant of a broader fascial muscle called the *panniculus carnosus* found in four-legged mammals. The panniculus carnosus is what enables a horse to shake off flies from its skin, and it is the same muscle that enables a cat to raise the hair on its back.
- ❑ 6. When the platysma contracts and the ridges or wrinkling of the skin of the neck occurs, it is reminiscent of the creature from the film, "The Creature From the Black Lagoon" (see illustration on page 33).

❑ STERNOCLEIDOMASTOID ("S.C.M.")

❑ **The name, sternocleidomastoid, tells us that this muscle attaches to the sternum, the clavicle and the mastoid process of the temporal bone.**

DERIVATION ❑ sterno: Gr. *refers to the sternum.*
cleido: Gr. *used for closing* (refers to the clavicle).
mastoid: Gr. *refers to the mastoid process.*

PRONUNCIATION ❑ **ster**-no-**kli**-do-**mas**-toyd

ATTACHMENTS

❑ **STERNAL HEAD: Manubrium of the Sternum**

- ❑ the anterior superior surface

❑ **CLAVICULAR HEAD: Medial Clavicle**

- ❑ the medial 1/3

to the

❑ **Mastoid Process of the Temporal Bone**

- ❑ and the lateral 1/2 of the superior nuchal line of the occipital bone

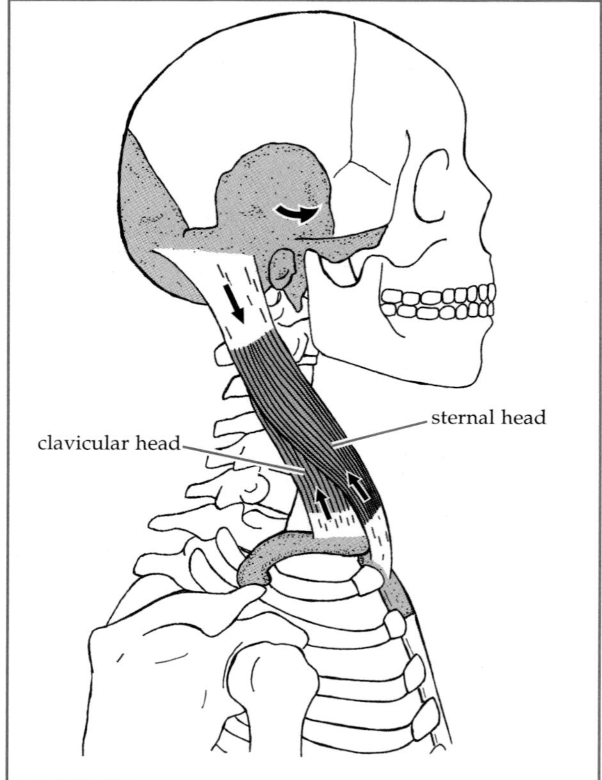

Lateral View of the Right Sternocleidomastoid

ACTIONS

❑ **1. Flexion of the Neck**

❑ **2. Lateral Flexion of the Neck and the Head**

❑ **3. Contralateral Rotation of the Neck and the Head**

❑ **4.** Extension of the Head

❑ **5.** Elevation of the Sternum and the Clavicle

INNERVATION ❑ Spinal Accessory Nerve (CN XI) ❑ and C2, 3

ARTERIAL SUPPLY ❑ The Occipital and Posterior Auricular Arteries (Branches of the External Carotid Artery)
❑ and the superior thyroid artery (a branch of the external carotid artery)

PALPATION AND SUPPLEMENTARY TEXT

PALPATION

- ❑ The sternocleidomastoid is superficial (except for the platysma), visible and easily palpable in the anterior/anterolateral neck.
  - Have the client seated with the neck and the head rotated to one side.
  - Stand on the other side of the client.
  - Place palpating hand on the anterolateral neck of the side where you are standing.
  - Now resist the client from laterally flexing the neck and the head toward the side where you are standing and feel for the contraction of the sternocleidomastoid.
  - Continue palpating the sternocleidomastoid from its inferior attachments toward its superior attachment.

see page 105

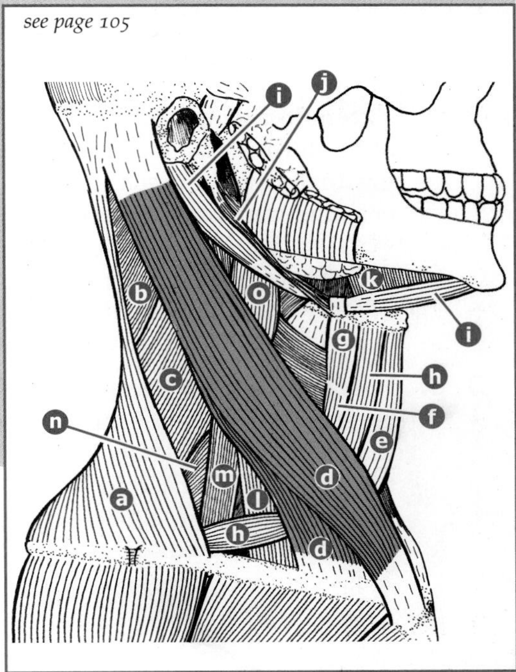

Lateral View of the Neck

a. Trapezius
b. Splenius Capitis
c. Levator Scapulae
d. **Sternocleidomastoid**
e. Sternohyoid
f. Sternothyroid
g. Thyrohyoid
h. Omohyoid
i. Digastric
j. Stylohyoid
k. Mylohyoid
l. Anterior Scalene
m. Middle Scalene
n. Posterior Scalene
o. Longus Capitis

RELATIONSHIP TO OTHER MUSCULOSKELETAL STRUCTURES

❑ 1. Except for the platysma, (which is superficial to all anterior neck muscles) the sternocleidomastoid is superficial throughout its entire course.

❑ 2. The following muscles are deep to the sternocleidomastoid (listed from inferior to superior): infrahyoids, scalenes, levator scapulae, digastric and the splenius capitis.

❑ 3. The attachment of the sternocleidomastoid onto the mastoid process of the temporal bone and the superior nuchal line of the occipital bone is superficial to the splenius capitis and lateral to the trapezius.

METHODOLOGY FOR LEARNING MUSCLE ACTIONS

❑ **1. Flexion of the Neck at the Spinal Joints:**
The sternocleidomastoid crosses the joints of the neck anteriorly (with its fibers running vertically in the sagittal plane); therefore, it flexes the neck at the cervical spinal joints. (Note: Although the sternocleidomastoid flexes the neck at the cervical spinal joints, it extends the head at the atlanto-occipital joint. See methodology #4.)

❑ **2. Lateral Flexion of the Neck and the Head at the Spinal Joints:** The sternocleidomastoid crosses the joints of the neck and the atlanto-occipital joint laterally (with its fibers running vertically in the frontal plane); therefore, it laterally flexes the neck at the cervical spinal joints and laterally flexes the head at the atlanto-occipital joint.

STERNOCLEIDOMASTOID – continued

- ❑ 3. **Contralateral Rotation of the Neck and the Head at the Spinal Joints:** The sternocleidomastoid wraps around the neck from the sternum/clavicle anteriorly to the cranium more posteriorly (with its fibers running somewhat horizontally in the transverse plane). When the sternocleidomastoid contracts, it pulls on the cranium, causing the anterior surface of the neck and/or the head to face the opposite side of the body from the side that the sternocleidomastoid is attached. Therefore, the sternocleidomastoid contralaterally rotates the neck at the cervical spinal joints and the head at the atlanto-occipital joint.

- ❑ 4. **Extension of the Head at the Atlanto-Occipital Joint:** The sternocleidomastoid begins anteriorly at its sternum/clavicle attachment. As it approaches its cranial attachment, the sternocleidomastoid gradually runs more and more posteriorly. By the time it crosses the atlanto-occipital joint, it is crossing that joint posteriorly (with its fibers running vertically in the sagittal plane). Therefore, since the sternocleidomastoid crosses the atlanto-occipital joint posteriorly, it extends the head at the atlanto-occipital joint. (Note: Although the sternocleidomastoid extends the head at the atlanto-occipital joint, it flexes the neck at the cervical spinal joints. See methodology #1.)

- ❑ 5. **Elevation of the Sternum and the Clavicle:** If the cranial attachment of the sternocleidomastoid is fixed, then the sternal/clavicular attachment must move. Since the sternocleidomastoid has its fibers running vertically from the sternum/clavicle, the sternum and the clavicle would be elevated toward the cranial attachment. (Note: This action is important for respiration.)

MISCELLANEOUS

- ❑ 1. The sternocleidomastoid attaches to the occipital bone as well as the mastoid process of the temporal bone superiorly. Because of this, some sources call this muscle the *sternocleidomastoidoccipitalis*.

- ❑ 2. The bulk of the superior attachment of the sternocleidomastoid is the mastoid attachment, which is a strong, thick rounded tendon. The occipital attachment is a thin aponeurosis.

- ❑ 3. Every muscle in the human body that crosses the cervical spinal joints and the atlanto-occipital joint (other than the sternocleidomastoid) has the same action at the neck that it has at the head. For example, the upper trapezius extends the neck and it extends the head; similarly, the longus capitis flexes the neck and it flexes the head. This is because these muscles cross the cervical joints of the neck in the same manner that that they cross the atlanto-occipital joint to attach onto the head. However, the sternocleidomastoid is unusual in that it crosses the cervical spinal joints anteriorly, yet crosses the atlanto-occipital joint posteriorly. Therefore, it flexes the neck at the cervical spinal joints, but it extends the head at the atlanto-occipital joint.

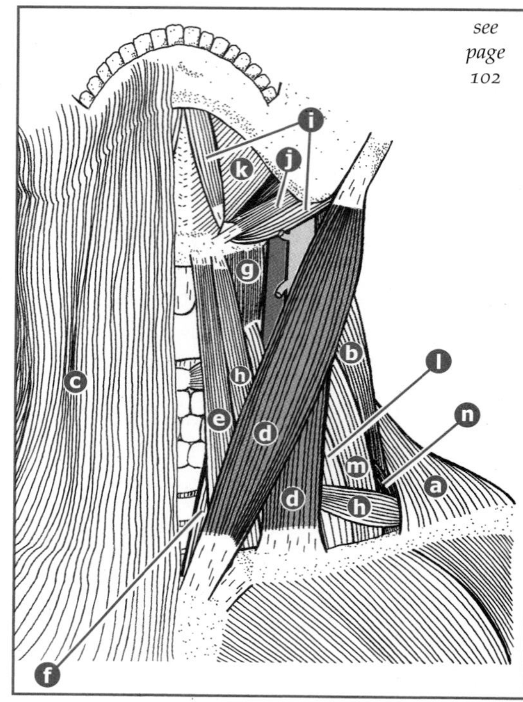

see page 102

Anterior View of the Neck (Superficial)

a. Trapezius
b. Levator Scapulae
c. Platysma (removed on our right)
d. Sternocleidomastoid
e. Sternohyoid
f. Sternothyroid
g. Thyrohyoid
h. Omohyoid
i. Digastric
j. Stylohyoid
k. Mylohyoid
l. Anterior Scalene
m. Middle Scalene
n. Posterior Scalene

STERNOCLEIDOMASTOID – continued

❑ 4. Some sources state that the action of the sternocleidomastoid upon the head at the atlanto-occipital joint can change from extension to flexion if the position of the head changes sufficiently, thus changing the line of pull of the sternocleidomastoid relative to the atlanto-occipital joint.

❑ 5. **Clavicular Actions:** Although the clavicle often moves passively by accompanying the scapula, the clavicle can be directly acted upon by musculature and therefore actively moved. The sternocleidomastoid attaches from the medial clavicle to the cranium. When the cranial attachment is fixed, the sternocleidomastoid can elevate the clavicle (along with the sternum, see methodology #5), and perhaps weakly upwardly rotate the clavicle (at the sternocostal joint).

❑ 6. By elevating the sternum, the sternocleidomastoid can help to elevate and expand the ribcage, which expands the thoracic cavity, creating more space for the lungs to expand for inspiration. Therefore, the sternocleidomastoid is an accessory muscle of respiration.

❑ 7. The carotid sinus of the common carotid artery lies directly medial to the sternocleidomastoid, midway up the neck. Given the neurological reflex that occurs to lower blood pressure when the carotid sinus is pressed, massage to this region must be done judiciously, especially with weak and/or elderly clients.

❑ 8. The sternocleidomastoid, as well as the scalenes, are often injured as a result of car accidents. This trauma is usually called *whiplash,* wherein the head and neck are forcefully thrown anteriorly and posteriorly (like a whip being lashed). When the head and the neck are thrown posteriorly, the anterior cervical musculature may be torn, or the muscle spindle reflex may occur, causing the anterior cervical musculature to spasm. When the head and the neck are thrown anteriorly, the same trauma may occur to the posterior musculature.

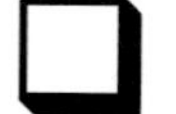

THE HYOIDS

The hyoids are a group of eight muscles that are superficial in the anterior neck.

THE HYOIDS ARE SUBDIVIDED INTO TWO GROUPS OF FOUR AS FOLLOWS:	
The Infrahyoids: Sternohyoid Sternothyroid Thyrohyoid Omohyoid	**The Suprahyoids:** Digastric Stylohyoid Mylohyoid Geniohyoid

Attachments:

- All the hyoid muscles (except the sternothyroid) attach into the hyoid bone.
- The infrahyoids are located inferior to the hyoid bone.
- The suprahyoids are located superior to the hyoid bone.

Actions:

- As a group, the infrahyoids depress the hyoid bone.
- As a group, the suprahyoids elevate the hyoid bone.
  - Therefore, the infrahyoids and the suprahyoids may be considered to be antagonistic to each other.
  - However, the infrahyoids and the suprahyoids may be contracted synergistically to fix the hyoid bone as a stable base of attachment for movements of the tongue.
- Movements of the hyoid bone are important in chewing, swallowing and speech.
- As a group, since the hyoids cross the cervical spinal joints anteriorly with their fibers running vertically, they can all assist with flexion of the neck at the spinal joints. For this to occur, the hyoid bone and the mandible must be fixed (stabilized).

Miscellaneous:

- The carotid sinus of the common carotid artery lies directly deep and lateral to the hyoid muscles midway up the neck. Given the neurological reflex that occurs to lower blood pressure when the carotid sinus is pressed, massage to this region must be done judiciously, especially with weak and/or elderly clients.

INNERVATION The hyoid muscles are innervated by the following nerves: the trigeminal nerve (CN V), the facial nerve (CN VII), the hypoglossal nerve (CN XII) and nerves from the cervical plexus.

ARTERIAL SUPPLY The infrahyoid muscles receive their arterial supply from the superior thyroid artery. Arterial supply to the suprahyoid muscles is varied.

ANTERIOR VIEW OF THE HYOIDS

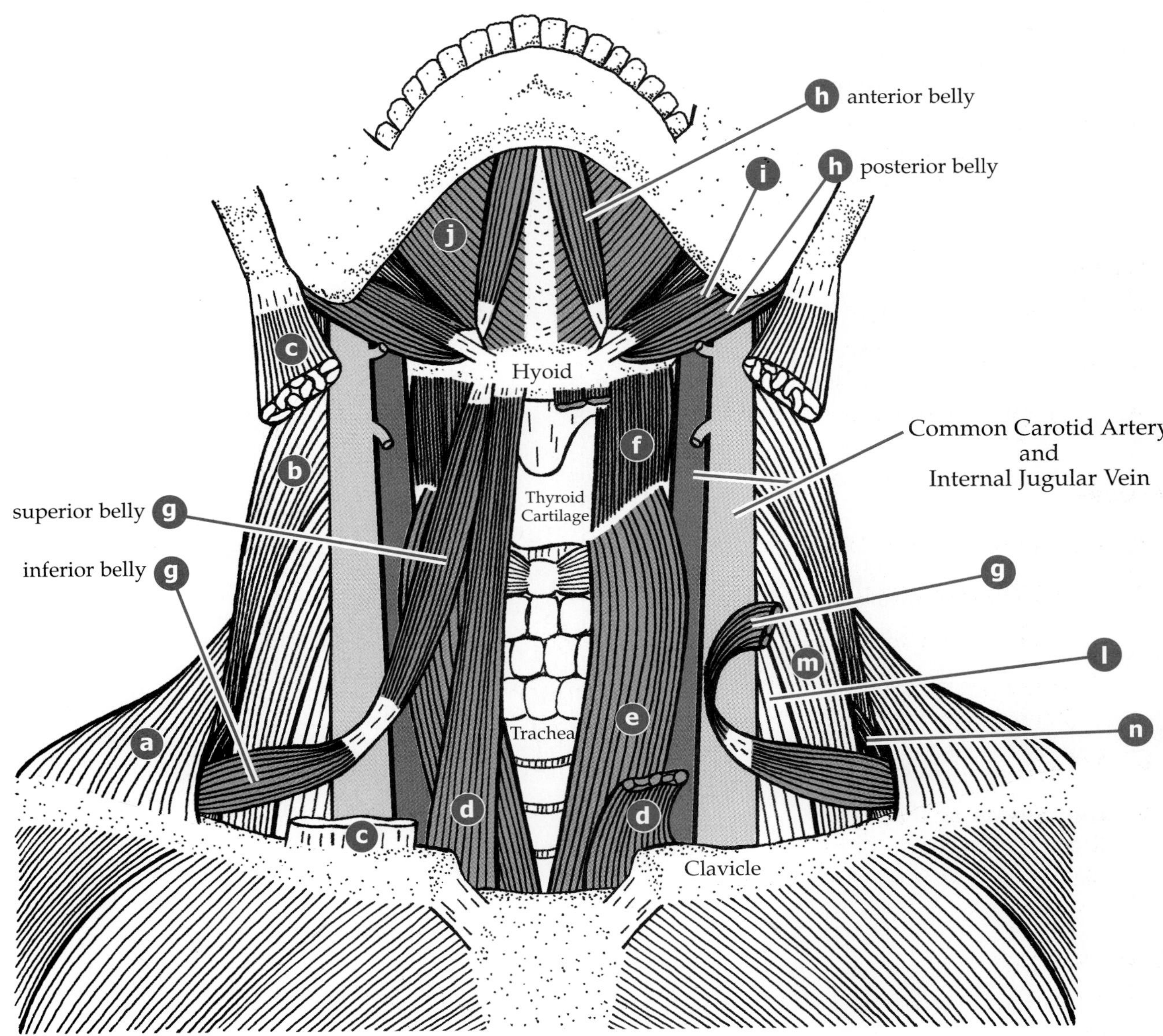

Note: The head is extended in this view.

a. **Trapezius**	h. **Digastric**
b. **Levator Scapulae**	i. **Stylohyoid**
c. **Sternocleidomastoid** (cut)	j. **Mylohyoid**
d. **Sternohyoid** (cut on our right)	k. **Geniohyoid** (not seen)
e. **Sternothyroid**	l. Anterior Scalene
f. **Thyrohyoid**	m. Middle Scalene
g. **Omohyoid** (cut and reflected on our right)	n. Posterior Scalene

❑ STERNOHYOID
(OF THE HYOID GROUP)

❑ **The name, sternohyoid, tells us that this muscle attaches from the sternum to the hyoid bone.**

DERIVATION ❑ sterno: L. *refers to the sternum.*
hyoid: Gr. *refers to the hyoid.*

PRONUNCIATION ❑ **ster**-no-**hi**-oyd

ATTACHMENTS

❑ **Sternum**

- ❑ the posterior surface of both the manubrium of the sternum and the medial clavicle

to the

❑ **Hyoid**

- ❑ the inferior surface of the body of the hyoid

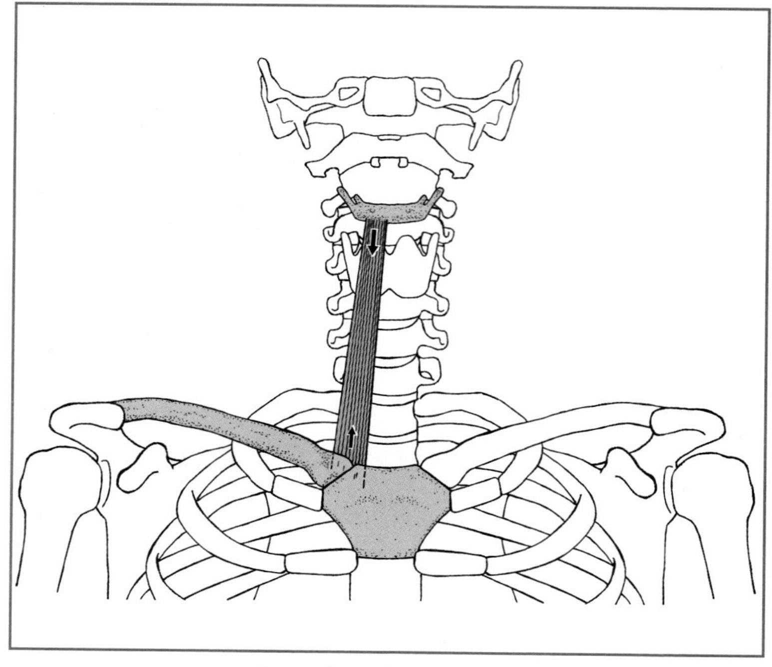

Anterior View of the Right Sternohyoid

ACTION

❑ **Depression of the Hyoid**

INNERVATION ❑ The Cervical Plexus ❑ ansa cervicalis (C1, 3)

ARTERIAL SUPPLY ❑ The Superior Thyroid Artery (A Branch of the External Carotid Artery)

PALPATION AND SUPPLEMENTARY TEXT

PALPATION

- ❑ The majority of the sternohyoid is superficial (except for the platysma) and easy to palpate, but it can be difficult to distinguish from the sternothyroid and thyrohyoid. Due to the presence of many delicate structures nearby (i.e., the trachea, thyroid gland and common carotid artery), care must be taken when palpating any structure in the anterior neck.
  - Have the client supine.
  - Locate the trachea, which may be found by palpating just inferior to the thyroid cartilage (the Adam's Apple) and the cricoid cartilage.
  - Place palpating fingers just lateral to the midline of the trachea and feel for the sternohyoid. Make sure that you stay medial to the sternocleidomastoid.
  - Continue palpating the sternohyoid superiorly toward the hyoid bone (using delicate pressure over the thyroid gland which is superficial to the thyroid cartilage).
  - To further bring out the sternohyoid, have the client swallow, which will momentarily make the sternohyoid contract; this is especially evident just inferior to the hyoid bone.

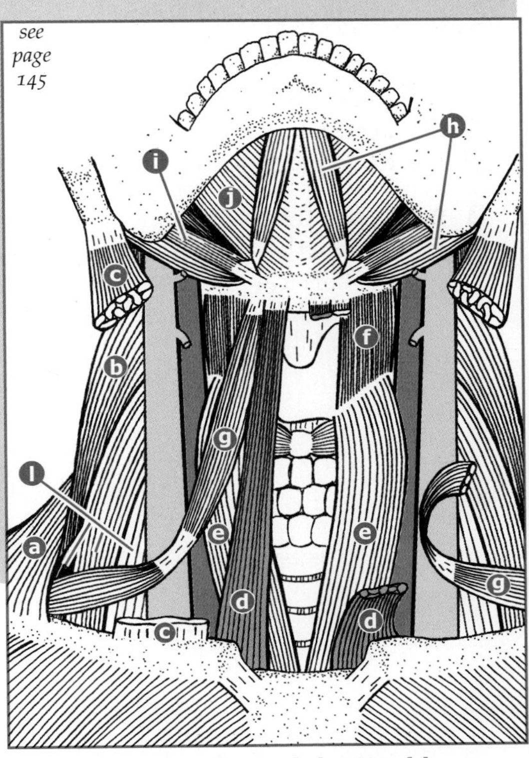

Anterior View of the Hyoids

a. Trapezius
b. Levator Scapulae
c. Sternocleidomastoid (cut)
d. **Sternohyoid** (cut on our right)
e. Sternothyroid
f. Thyrohyoid
g. Omohyoid (cut and reflected on our right)
h. Digastric
i. Stylohyoid
j. Mylohyoid
k. Geniohyoid (not seen)
l. Scalenes

RELATIONSHIP TO OTHER MUSCULOSKELETAL STRUCTURES

❑ 1. Nearly the entire sternohyoid is superficial in the anterior neck (except for the platysma, which is superficial to all anterior neck muscles). However, the inferior attachment of the sternohyoid is deep to the sternocleidomastoid.

❑ 2. The inferior portion of the sternohyoid lies directly medial to the sternocleidomastoid. The superior portion of the sternohyoid lies medial to the omohyoid.

❑ 3. The sternohyoid lies anterior to, and just lateral to, the midline of the trachea.

❑ 4. Deep to the sternohyoid are the sternothyroid and the thyrohyoid.

METHODOLOGY FOR LEARNING MUSCLE ACTIONS

❑ **Depression of the Hyoid:** The sternohyoid attaches from the hyoid bone superiorly, to the sternum inferiorly (with its fibers running vertically). When the sternohyoid contracts, it pulls the hyoid bone inferiorly toward the sternum. Therefore, the sternohyoid depresses the hyoid. (Note: Movements of the hyoid bone are important in chewing, swallowing and speech.)

STERNOHYOID – continued

MISCELLANEOUS

- ❑ 1. The sternohyoid is one of the four infrahyoid muscles. The four infrahyoid muscles are the sternohyoid, sternothyroid, thyrohyoid and the omohyoid. There are four suprahyoid muscles: the digastric, stylohyoid, mylohyoid and the geniohyoid. All the hyoid muscles are important in moving and/or fixating (stabilizing) the hyoid bone. These functions are necessary for chewing, swallowing and speech.
- ❑ 2. The carotid sinus of the common carotid artery lies slightly lateral to the sternohyoid (between the sternohyoid and the sternocleidomastoid, midway up the neck). Given the neurological reflex that occurs to lower blood pressure when the carotid sinus is pressed, massage to this region must be done judiciously, especially with weak and/or elderly clients.
- ❑ 3. When the hyoid bone and the mandible are fixed (stabilized), the hyoids as a group can be felt to contract with resisted neck flexion. Hence, the hyoids are all weak accessory flexors of the neck at the cervical spinal joints. This makes sense given their direction of fibers running vertically, anterior to the cervical vertebrae.

STERNOTHYROID

(OF THE HYOID GROUP)

❑ **The name, sternothyroid, tells us that this muscle attaches from the sternum to the thyroid cartilage.**

DERIVATION ❑ sterno: L. *refers to the sternum.*
thyroid: Gr. *refers to the thyroid cartilage.*

PRONUNCIATION ❑ **ster**-no-**thi**-royd

ATTACHMENTS

❑ **Sternum**

❑ the posterior surface of the manubrium of the sternum and the posterior surface of the cartilage of the 1st rib

to the

❑ **Thyroid Cartilage**

❑ the lamina of the thyroid cartilage

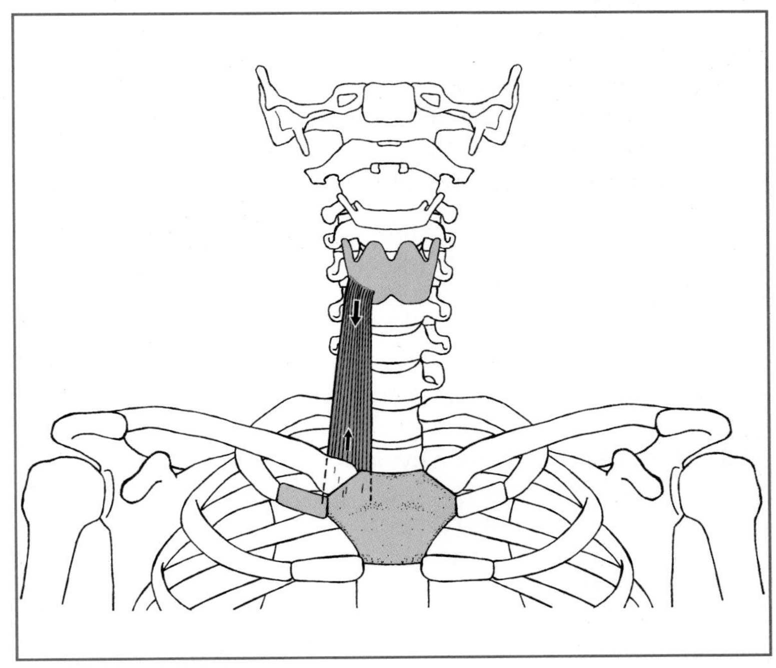

Anterior View of the Right Sternothyroid

ACTION

❑ **Depression of the Thyroid Cartilage**

INNERVATION ❑ The Cervical Plexus ❑ ansa cervicalis (C1, 3)

ARTERIAL SUPPLY ❑ The Superior Thyroid Artery (A Branch of the External Carotid Artery)

STERNOTHYROID – PALPATION AND SUPPLEMENTARY TEXT

PALPATION

- ❑ The sternothyroid is best palpated along with the sternohyoid (see the palpation section for this muscle on page 147). Keep in mind that the sternothyroid does not extend superiorly beyond the thyroid cartilage, as does the sternohyoid. Just superior to the manubrium, the sternothyroid is slightly medial to the sternohyoid; otherwise, these muscles are palpated together and distinguishing them from each other can be difficult.

RELATIONSHIP TO OTHER MUSCULOSKELETAL STRUCTURES

- ❑ 1. Most of the sternothyroid lies directly deep to the sternohyoid and the omohyoid. However, part of the sternothyroid is superficial (except for the platysma, which is superficial to all anterior neck muscles) just above the sternum.
- ❑ 2. The sternothyroid lies anterior to, and just lateral to, the midline of the trachea.
- ❑ 3. Deep to the sternothyroid is the trachea.

METHODOLOGY FOR LEARNING MUSCLE ACTIONS

- ❑ **Depression of the Thyroid Cartilage:** The sternothyroid attaches from the thyroid cartilage superiorly, to the sternum inferiorly (with its fibers running vertically). When the sternothyroid contracts, it pulls the thyroid cartilage inferiorly toward the sternum. Therefore, the sternothyroid depresses the thyroid cartilage. (Note: Movements of the thyroid cartilage are important in chewing, swallowing and speech.)

see page 145

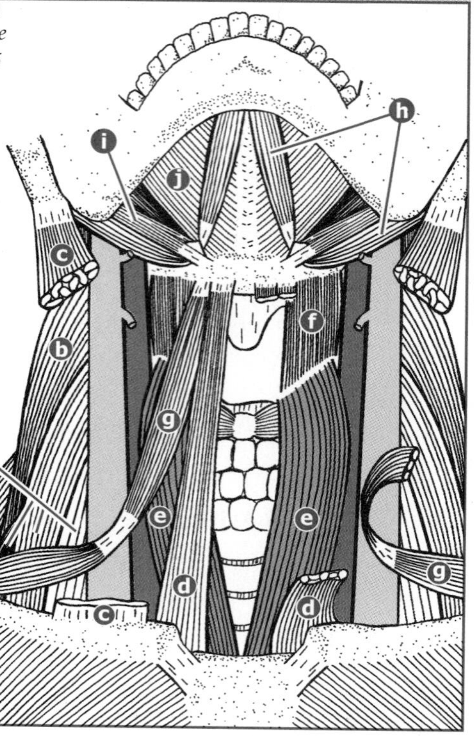

Anterior View of the Hyoids

a. Trapezius
b. Levator Scapulae
c. Sternocleidomastoid (cut)
d. Sternohyoid (cut on our right)
e. **Sternothyroid**
f. Thyrohyoid
g. Omohyoid (cut and reflected on our right)
h. Digastric
i. Stylohyoid
j. Mylohyoid
k. Geniohyoid (not seen)
l. Scalenes

MISCELLANEOUS

- ❑ 1. The sternothyroid is one of the four infrahyoid muscles. The four infrahyoid muscles are the sternohyoid, sternothyroid, thyrohyoid and the omohyoid. There are four suprahyoid muscles: the digastric, stylohyoid, mylohyoid and the geniohyoid. All the hyoid muscles are important in moving and/or fixating (stabilizing) the hyoid bone. These functions are necessary for chewing, swallowing and speech.
- ❑ 2. The carotid sinus of the common carotid artery lies slightly lateral to the sternothyroid (between the sternothyroid and the sternocleidomastoid, midway up the neck). Given the neurological reflex that occurs to lower blood pressure when the carotid sinus is pressed, massage to this region must be done judiciously, especially with weak and/or elderly clients.
- ❑ 3. When the hyoid bone and the mandible are fixed (stabilized), the hyoids as a group can be felt to contract with resisted neck flexion. Hence, the hyoids are all weak accessory flexors of the neck at the cervical spinal joints. This makes sense given their direction of fibers running vertically, anterior to the cervical vertebrae.

THYROHYOID

(OF THE HYOID GROUP)

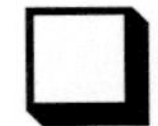

❑ **The name, thyrohyoid, tells us that this muscle attaches from the thyroid cartilage to the hyoid bone.**

DERIVATION ❑ thyro: Gr. *refers to the thyroid cartilage.*
hyoid: Gr. *refers to the hyoid bone.*

PRONUNCIATION ❑ **thi**-ro-**hi**-oyd

ATTACHMENTS

❑ **Thyroid Cartilage**

❑ the lamina of the thyroid cartilage

to the

❑ **Hyoid**

❑ the inferior surface of the greater cornu of the hyoid

ACTIONS

❑ **1. Depression of the Hyoid**

❑ **2. Elevation of the Thyroid Cartilage**

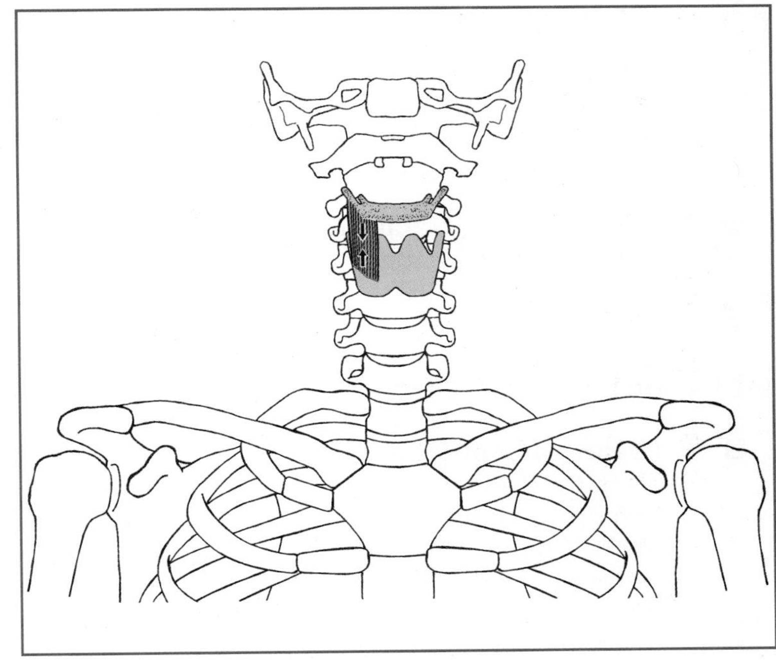

Anterior View of the Right Thyrohyoid

INNERVATION ❑ The Hypoglossal Nerve (CN XII)
❑ a branch of C1 through the hypoglossal nerve

ARTERIAL SUPPLY ❑ The Superior Thyroid Artery (A Branch of the External Carotid Artery)

THYROHYOID – PALPATION AND SUPPLEMENTARY TEXT

PALPATION

- ❑ The thyrohyoid is best palpated along with the sternohyoid (see the palpation section for this muscle on page 147). Keep in mind that the thyrohyoid does not extend inferiorly beyond the thyroid cartilage, as does the sternohyoid. The thyrohyoid is somewhat lateral to the sternohyoid (and the omohyoid), just superior to the larynx; otherwise, these muscles are palpated together and distinguishing them from each other can be difficult.

see page 145

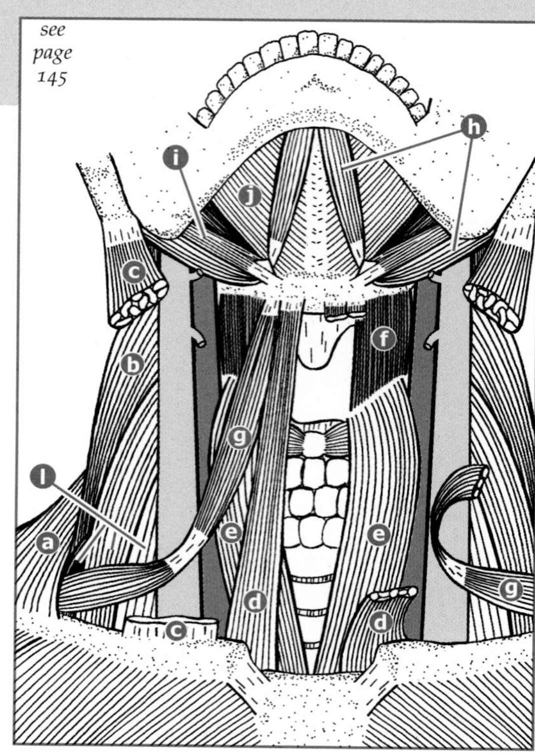

Anterior View of the Hyoids

a. Trapezius
b. Levator Scapulae
c. Sternocleidomastoid (cut)
d. Sternohyoid (cut on our right)
e. Sternothyroid
f. **Thyrohyoid**
g. Omohyoid (cut and reflected on our right)
h. Digastric
i. Stylohyoid
j. Mylohyoid
k. Geniohyoid (not seen)
l. Scalenes

RELATIONSHIP TO OTHER MUSCULOSKELETAL STRUCTURES

- ❑ 1. The inferior part of the thyrohyoid lies directly deep to the sternohyoid and omohyoid. However, its superior part is superficial (except for the platysma, which is superficial to all anterior neck muscles).
- ❑ 2. The thyrohyoid lies anterior to, and lateral to, the midline of the thyroid cartilage. It is inferior to the hyoid bone.
- ❑ 3. Deep to the thyrohyoid is the thyroid cartilage.

METHODOLOGY FOR LEARNING MUSCLE ACTIONS

- ❑ **1. Depression of the Hyoid:** The thyrohyoid attaches from the hyoid bone superiorly, to the thyroid cartilage inferiorly (with its fibers running vertically). When the thyroid cartilage is fixed (stabilized) and the thyrohyoid contracts, it pulls the hyoid bone inferiorly toward the thyroid cartilage. Therefore, the thyrohyoid depresses the hyoid. (Note: Movements of the hyoid bone are important in chewing, swallowing and speech.)
- ❑ **2. Elevation of the Thyroid Cartilage:** The thyrohyoid attaches from the thyroid cartilage inferiorly, to the hyoid bone superiorly (with its fibers running vertically). When the hyoid bone is fixed (stabilized) and the thyrohyoid contracts, it pulls the thyroid cartilage superiorly toward the hyoid bone. Therefore, the thyrohyoid elevates the thyroid cartilage. (Note: Movements of the thyroid cartilage are important in chewing, swallowing and speech.)

MISCELLANEOUS

- ❑ 1. The thyrohyoid is one of the four infrahyoid muscles. The four infrahyoid muscles are the sternohyoid, sternothyroid, thyrohyoid and the omohyoid. There are four suprahyoid muscles: the digastric, stylohyoid, mylohyoid and the geniohyoid. All the hyoid muscles are important in moving and/or fixating (stabilizing) the hyoid bone. These functions are necessary for chewing, swallowing and speech.

THYROHYOID – continued

- ❑ 2. The carotid sinus of the common carotid artery lies directly lateral to the thyrohyoid (between the thyrohyoid and the sternocleidomastoid, superior in the neck). Given the neurological reflex that occurs to lower blood pressure when the carotid sinus is pressed, massage to this region must be done judiciously, especially with weak and/or elderly clients.
- ❑ 3. The thyrohyoid can be considered to be an upward continuation of the sternothyroid muscle.
- ❑ 4. When the hyoid bone and the mandible are fixed (stabilized), the hyoids as a group can be felt to contract with resisted neck flexion. Hence, the hyoids are all weak accessory flexors of the neck at the cervical spinal joints. This makes sense given their direction of fibers running vertically, anterior to the cervical vertebrae.

OMOHYOID
(OF THE HYOID GROUP)

❑ **The name, omohyoid, tells us that this muscle attaches from the scapula ("omo" means shoulder, referring to the scapula) to the hyoid bone.**

DERIVATION ❑ omo: Gr. *shoulder.*
hyoid: Gr. *refers to the hyoid bone.*

PRONUNCIATION ❑ **o**-mo-**hi**-oyd

ATTACHMENTS

❑ **Scapula**

- ❑ the superior border

to the

❑ **INFERIOR BELLY: Clavicle**

- ❑ bound to the clavicle at its central tendon

❑ **SUPERIOR BELLY: Hyoid**

- ❑ the inferior surface of the body of the hyoid

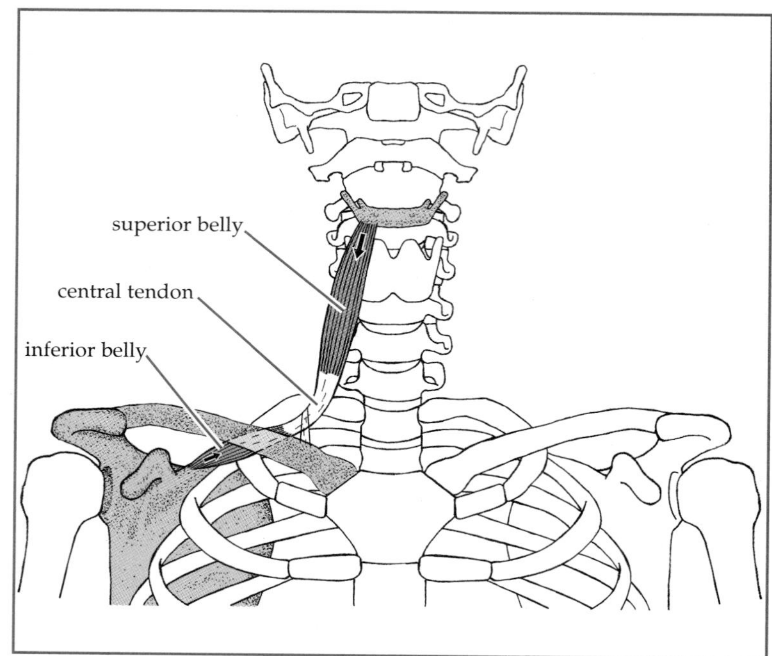

Anterior View of the Right Omohyoid

ACTION

❑ **Depression of the Hyoid**

INNERVATION ❑ The Cervical Plexus ❑ ansa cervicalis (C1-3)

ARTERIAL SUPPLY ❑ The Superior Thyroid Artery (A Branch of the External Carotid Artery) and the Transverse Cervical Artery (A Branch of the Thyrocervical Trunk)

PALPATION AND SUPPLEMENTARY TEXT

PALPATION

The omohyoid is superficial in the anterior neck (except for the platysma) and can be palpated between the sternocleidomastoid and the upper trapezius, just superior to the middle of the clavicle. The omohyoid can also be palpated lateral to the sternohyoid, superior to the medial border of the sternocleidomastoid. Differentiating the omohyoid from the sternohyoid is difficult.

- [ ] **To palpate from the lateral border of the sternocleidomastoid:**
  - Have the client supine.
  - Locate the lateral border of the sternocleidomastoid (see the palpation section for this muscle on page 141).
  - Place palpating hand lateral to the sternocleidomastoid, just superior to the clavicle, and feel for the fibers of the omohyoid running nearly horizontally. Make sure you are not palpating the scalenes, which are deep to the omohyoid (and have fibers running more vertically).
  - To further bring out the omohyoid, ask the client to swallow, which will cause the omohyoid to momentarily contract and help differentiate it from the scalenes.

- [ ] **To palpate from the lateral border of the sternohyoid:**
  - Have the client supine.
  - Locate the lateral border of the sternohyoid (see the palpation section for this muscle on page 147).
  - Place palpating hand lateral to the sternohyoid, and feel for the fibers of the omohyoid. Given the proximity of the common carotid artery, care must be taken with palpation.

To further bring out the omohyoid, ask the client to swallow, which will cause the omohyoid to momentarily contract (as well as the rest of the infrahyoids).

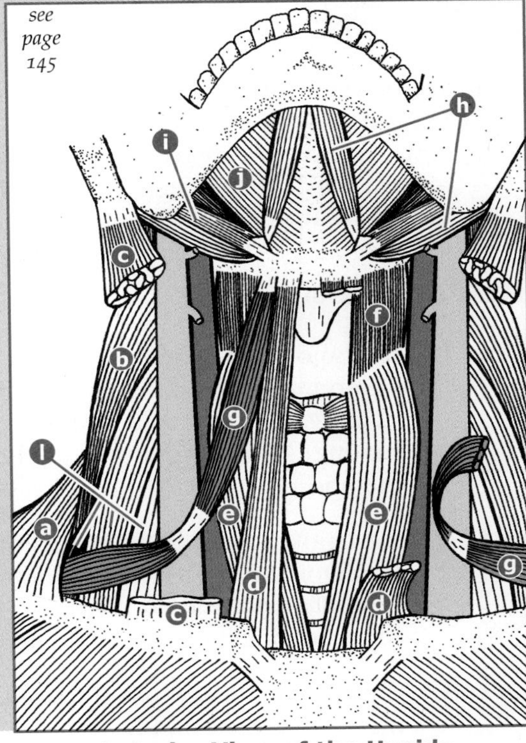

Anterior View of the Hyoids

a. Trapezius
b. Levator Scapulae
c. Sternocleidomastoid (cut)
d. Sternohyoid (cut on our right)
e. Sternothyroid
f. Thyrohyoid
g. **Omohyoid** (cut and reflected on our right)
h. Digastric
i. Stylohyoid
j. Mylohyoid
k. Geniohyoid (not seen)
l. Scalenes

OMOHYOID – continued

RELATIONSHIP TO OTHER MUSCULOSKELETAL STRUCTURES

❑ 1. The omohyoid runs an unusual course. The inferior belly of the omohyoid attaches onto the superior border of the scapula, just superior to the supraspinatus (near the scapular notch). From the scapula, the omohyoid runs anteriorly and slightly superiorly toward the clavicle, deep to the trapezius and superficial to the scalenes. Near the medial end of the clavicle, the omohyoid becomes tendinous (the central tendon). However, it does not attach directly to the clavicle, but rather its central tendon is attached to the clavicle by a fibrous sling of tissue. At this point, the omohyoid is deep to the sternocleidomastoid and superficial to the sternothyroid. Its superior belly then runs superiorly and attaches to the hyoid bone, just lateral to the sternohyoid.

❑ 2. Except for the platysma, the omohyoid is superficial in two locations: 1) slightly inferior to the hyoid bone and superior to the sternocleidomastoid in the anterior neck and 2) between the sternocleidomastoid and the trapezius in the inferolateral neck.

METHODOLOGY FOR LEARNING MUSCLE ACTIONS

❑ **Depression of the Hyoid:** The omohyoid attaches from the hyoid bone superiorly, to the clavicle inferiorly (with a continuation of its fibers to the scapula). Therefore, its fibers run vertically. When the scapula and the clavicle are fixed (stabilized) and the omohyoid contracts, it pulls the hyoid bone inferiorly toward the clavicle. Therefore, the omohyoid depresses the hyoid. (Note: Movements of the hyoid bone are important in chewing, swallowing and speech.)

MISCELLANEOUS

❑ 1. The omohyoid is one of the four infrahyoid muscles. The four infrahyoid muscles are the sternohyoid, sternothyroid, thyrohyoid and the omohyoid. There are four suprahyoid muscles: the digastric, stylohyoid, mylohyoid and the geniohyoid. All the hyoid muscles are important in moving and/or fixating (stabilizing) the hyoid bone. These functions are necessary for chewing, swallowing and speech.

❑ 2. The carotid sinus of the common carotid artery lies slightly lateral to the omohyoid (between the omohyoid and the sternocleidomastoid, midway up the neck). Given the neurological reflex that occurs to lower blood pressure when the carotid sinus is pressed, massage to this region must be done judiciously, especially with weak and/or elderly clients.

❑ 3. The omohyoid is unusual in that it has two bellies separated by its central tendon (also known as the *intermediate tendon*). Like the digastric (a suprahyoid muscle), the omohyoid's central tendon is tethered (attached) to bone by a fibrous sling of tissue.

❑ 4. When the hyoid bone and the mandible are fixed (stabilized), the hyoids as a group can be felt to contract with resisted neck flexion. Hence, the hyoids are all weak accessory flexors of the neck at the cervical spinal joints. This makes sense given their direction of fibers running vertically, anterior to the cervical vertebrae.

DIGASTRIC

(OF THE HYOID GROUP)

❑ **The name, digastric, tells us that this muscle has two bellies. ("Gaster" means belly.)**

DERIVATION ❑ di: Gr. *two.*
gastric: Gr. *belly.*

PRONUNCIATION ❑ di-**gas**-trik

ATTACHMENTS

❑ **POSTERIOR BELLY: Temporal Bone**

- ❑ the mastoid notch of the temporal bone

❑ **ANTERIOR BELLY: Mandible**

- ❑ the inner surface of the inferior border (the digastric fossa)

to the

❑ **Hyoid**

- ❑ the central tendon is bound to the hyoid bone at the body and the greater cornu

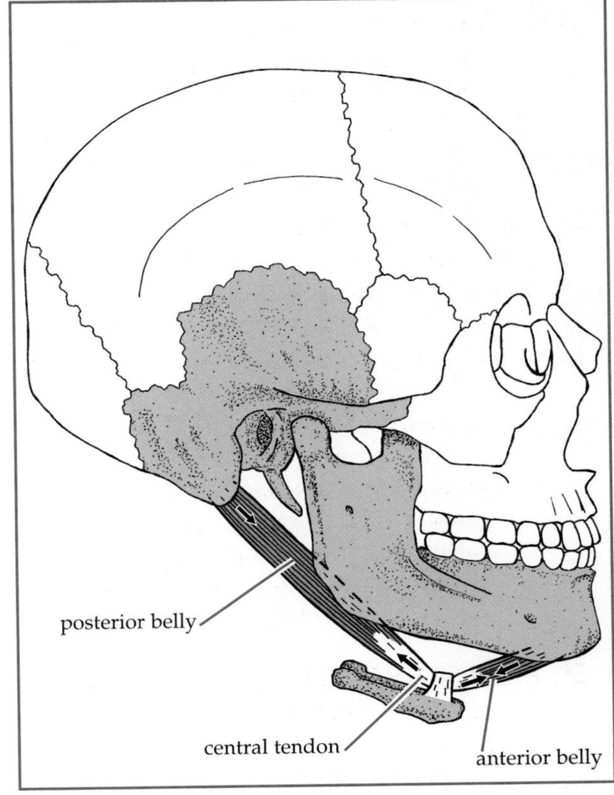

Lateral View of the Right Digastric

ACTIONS

❑ 1. **Elevation of the Hyoid**

❑ 2. Depression of the Mandible

❑ 3. Retraction of the Mandible

INNERVATION ❑ The Trigeminal (CN V) and the Facial Nerve (CN VII)
- ❑ anterior belly: mylohyoid branch of the inferior alveolar nerve of the posterior trunk of the mandibular division of the trigeminal nerve (CN V)
- ❑ posterior belly: facial nerve (CN VII)

ARTERIAL SUPPLY ❑ The Occipital, Posterior Auricular and Facial Arteries (Branches of the External Carotid Artery)

DIGASTRIC – PALPATION AND SUPPLEMENTARY TEXT

PALPATION

- ❑ The digastric is superficial for its entire course (except for the platysma) in the lateral and anterior neck until it dives deep to the sternocleidomastoid.
  - Have the client supine.
  - Place palpating hand just lateral to the hyoid bone and just inferior to the mandible.
  - Ask the client to actively but gently depress the mandible (open the mouth) and feel for the contraction of the digastric. It will be a pencil-thin muscle running horizontally.
  - Try to continue palpating the digastric posteriorly toward the mastoid process of the temporal bone until it dives deep to the sternocleidomastoid.

see page 145

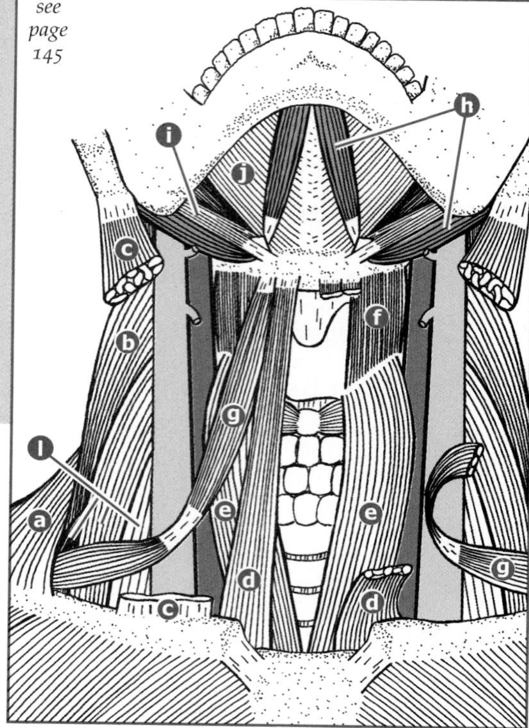

Anterior View of the Hyoids

a. Trapezius
b. Levator Scapulae
c. Sternocleidomastoid (cut)
d. Sternohyoid (cut on our right)
e. Sternothyroid
f. Thyrohyoid
g. Omohyoid (cut and reflected on our right)
h. **Digastric**
i. Stylohyoid
j. Mylohyoid
k. Geniohyoid (not seen)
l. Scalenes

RELATIONSHIP TO OTHER MUSCULOSKELETAL STRUCTURES

❑ 1. The digastric runs an unusual course. The posterior belly attaches to the mastoid notch of the temporal bone (deep to the sternocleidomastoid). It then runs anteriorly and slightly inferiorly toward the hyoid bone. Near the hyoid bone, the digastric becomes tendinous (the central tendon). However, the digastric does not attach directly to the hyoid bone, but rather its central tendon is attached to the hyoid by a fibrous sling of tissue. From there, the anterior belly runs superiorly and anteriorly to the inner surface of the mandible.

❑ 2. Except for the occipital attachment of the sternocleidomastoid and the platysma (which is superficial to all anterior neck muscles), the digastric is superficial for its entire course in the lateral and anterior neck. The submandibular salivary gland may also be superficial to the digastric.

❑ 3. The digastric runs inferior to, and parallel to, the stylohyoid.

❑ 4. Deep to the posterior belly of the digastric is the T.P. of the atlas (C1).

METHODOLOGY FOR LEARNING MUSCLE ACTIONS

❑ **1. Elevation of the Hyoid:** The anterior belly of the digastric attaches from the hyoid bone inferiorly, to the mandible superiorly (with its fibers running somewhat vertically). When the mandible is fixed (stabilized) and the digastric contracts, it pulls the hyoid bone superiorly toward the mandible. Therefore, the digastric elevates the hyoid. (Note: Movements of the hyoid bone are important in chewing, swallowing and speech.)

DIGASTRIC – continued

- ❑ 2. **Depression of the Mandible at the Temporomandibular Joint:** The anterior belly of the digastric attaches from the mandible inferiorly, to the hyoid bone superiorly (with its fibers running somewhat vertically). When the hyoid bone is fixed and the digastric contracts, it pulls the mandible inferiorly toward the hyoid bone. Therefore, the digastric depresses the mandible at the temporomandibular joint.

- ❑ 3. **Retraction of the Mandible at the Temporomandibular Joint:** The anterior belly of the digastric attaches from the hyoid bone posteriorly, to the mandible anteriorly (with its fibers running horizontally in the sagittal plane). When the hyoid bone is fixed (stabilized) and the digastric contracts, it pulls the mandible posteriorly toward the hyoid bone. Therefore, the digastric retracts the mandible at the temporomandibular joint.

MISCELLANEOUS

- ❑ 1. The digastric is one of the four suprahyoid muscles. The four suprahyoid muscles are the digastric, stylohyoid, mylohyoid and the geniohyoid. There are four infrahyoid muscles: the sternohyoid, sternothyroid, thyrohyoid and the omohyoid. All the hyoid muscles are important in moving and/or fixating (stabilizing) the hyoid bone. These functions are necessary for chewing, swallowing and speech.

- ❑ 2. The external carotid artery lies inferior and deep to the anterior belly of the digastric. Massage to this region must be done judiciously.

- ❑ 3. The digastric is unusual in that it has two bellies separated by its central tendon (also known as the *intermediate tendon*). Like the omohyoid (an infrahyoid muscle), the central tendon of the digastric is tethered (attached) to bone by a fibrous sling of tissue.

- ❑ 4. The attachment of the stylohyoid onto the hyoid bone is perforated by the central tendon of the digastric.

- ❑ 5. The digastric can also protract and retract the hyoid bone. The anterior belly of the digastric can protract the hyoid (draw the hyoid anteriorly), and the posterior belly of the digastric can retract the hyoid (draw the hyoid posteriorly).

- ❑ 6. When the hyoid bone and the mandible are fixed (stabilized), the hyoids as a group can be felt to contract with resisted neck flexion. Hence, they are weak accessory flexors of the neck at the cervical spinal joints. This makes sense given their direction of fibers running vertically, anterior to the cervical vertebrae.

❑

STYLOHYOID
(OF THE HYOID GROUP)

❑ **The name, stylohyoid, tells us that this muscle attaches from the styloid process (of the temporal bone) to the hyoid bone.**

DERIVATION ❑ stylo: Gr. *refers to the styloid process.*
hyoid: Gr. *refers to the hyoid bone.*

PRONUNCIATION ❑ **sti**-lo-**hi**-oyd

ATTACHMENTS

❑ **Styloid Process of the Temporal Bone**

- ❑ the posterior surface

to the

❑ **Hyoid**

- ❑ at the junction of the body and the greater cornu of the hyoid bone

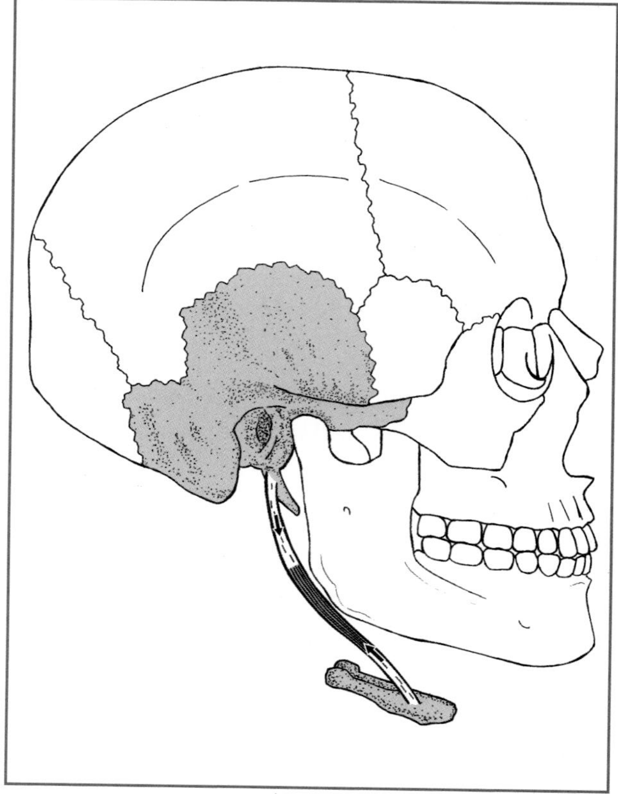

Lateral View of the Right Stylohyoid

ACTION

❑ **Elevation of the Hyoid**

INNERVATION ❑ The Facial Nerve (CN VII) ❑ the stylohyoid branch

ARTERIAL SUPPLY ❑ The Occipital, Posterior Auricular and Facial Arteries (Branches of the External Carotid Artery)

PALPATION AND SUPPLEMENTARY TEXT

PALPATION

The stylohyoid is best palpated at its styloid attachment. The belly is superficial (except for the platysma) and palpable, although it is difficult to distinguish from the posterior belly of the digastric, which lies inferior to it.

- Have the client supine.

❑ **To palpate the styloid attachment:**

- Place palpating fingers between the sternocleidomastoid and the posterior ramus of the mandible, i.e., over the styloid process of the temporal bone. Keep your pressure light to moderate since the styloid process of the temporal bone is a delicate structure.
- Ask the client to swallow and feel for the stylohyoid to contract.

❑ **To palpate the muscle belly:**

- Locate the digastric by palpating just lateral to the hyoid bone and asking the client to actively, but gently, depress the mandible (see page 158 for details).
- Palpate just superior to the posterior belly of the digastric and feel for the stylohyoid. It will be a thin muscle running parallel to the digastric.
- Ask the client to swallow, which will make the stylohyoid contract as well as the digastric. Keep in mind that the digastric contracts with depression of the mandible and the stylohyoid does not.

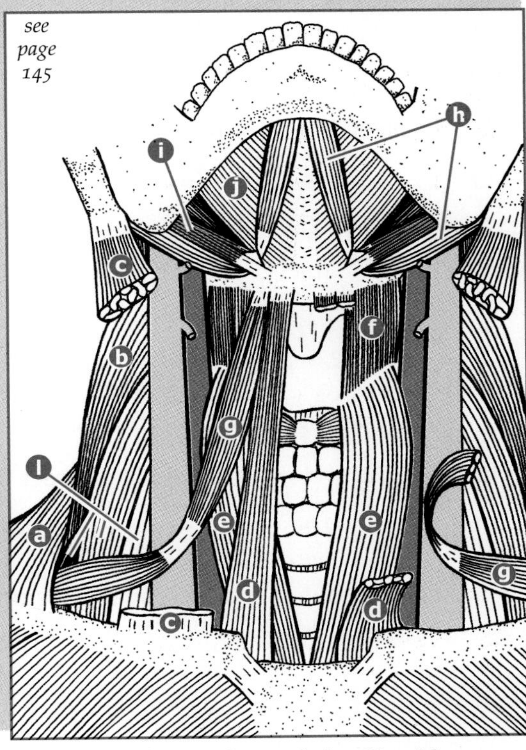

Anterior View of the Hyoids

a. Trapezius
b. Levator Scapulae
c. Sternocleidomastoid (cut)
d. Sternohyoid (cut on our right)
e. Sternothyroid
f. Thyrohyoid
g. Omohyoid (cut and reflected on our right)
h. Digastric
i. **Stylohyoid**
j. Mylohyoid
k. Geniohyoid (not seen)
l. Scalenes

RELATIONSHIP TO OTHER MUSCULOSKELETAL STRUCTURES

❑ 1. The stylohyoid is superior to, and runs parallel to, the posterior belly of the digastric.

❑ 2. Except for the platysma, which is superficial to all anterior neck muscles (and the submandibular salivary gland), the stylohyoid is superficial in the superolateral neck.

❑ 3. The attachment of the stylohyoid onto the hyoid bone is the same location where the digastric attaches (via its fibrous sling attachment that holds the central tendon of the digastric to the hyoid bone).

❑ 4. Deep to the stylohyoid is the T.P. of the Atlas (C1).

STYLOHYOID – continued

METHODOLOGY FOR LEARNING MUSCLE ACTIONS

- ❑ **Elevation of the Hyoid:** The stylohyoid attaches from the temporal bone superiorly, to the hyoid bone inferiorly (with its fibers running vertically). When the stylohyoid contracts, it pulls the hyoid bone superiorly toward the temporal bone. Therefore, the stylohyoid elevates the hyoid. (Note: Movements of the hyoid bone are important in chewing, swallowing and speech.)

MISCELLANEOUS

❑ 1. The stylohyoid is one of the four suprahyoid muscles. The four suprahyoid muscles are the digastric, stylohyoid, mylohyoid and the geniohyoid. There are four infrahyoid muscles: the sternohyoid, sternothyroid, thyrohyoid and the omohyoid. All the hyoid muscles are important in moving and/or fixating (stabilizing) the hyoid bone. These functions are necessary for chewing, swallowing and speech.

❑ 2. The external carotid artery lies inferior and deep to the stylohyoid. Massage to this region must be done judiciously.

❑ 3. The attachment of the stylohyoid onto the hyoid bone is perforated by the central tendon of the digastric.

❑ 4. There are two other small muscles that attach to the styloid process of the temporal bone. They are the styloglossus (a muscle that moves the tongue, see Appendix F, page 734) and the stylopharyngeus (a muscle that moves the pharynx, see Appendix F, page 738).

❑ 5. The stylohyoid can also retract the hyoid bone (draw the hyoid posteriorly).

❑ 6. When the hyoid bone and the mandible are fixed (stabilized), the hyoids as a group can be felt to contract with resisted neck flexion. Hence, the hyoids are all weak accessory flexors of the neck at the cervical spinal joints. This makes sense given their direction of fibers running vertically, anterior to the cervical vertebrae.

MYLOHYOID
(OF THE HYOID GROUP)

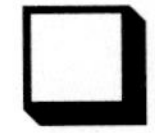

❑ **The name, mylohyoid, tells us that this muscle attaches to the hyoid bone. "Mylo," referring to the molar teeth, tells us that this muscle also attaches close to the molar teeth.**

DERIVATION ❑ mylo: Gr. *mill* (refers to the molar teeth).
hyoid: Gr. *refers to the hyoid bone.*

PRONUNCIATION ❑ **my**-lo-**hi**-oyd

ATTACHMENTS

❑ **Inner Surface of the Mandible**

❑ the mylohyoid line of the mandible (from the symphysis menti to the molars)

to the

❑ **Hyoid**

❑ the anterior surface of the body of the hyoid

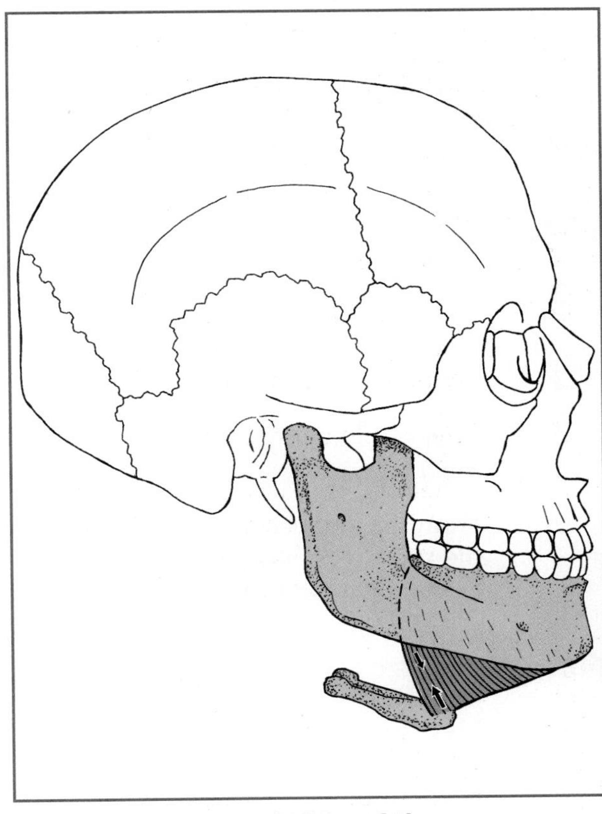

Lateral View of the Right Mylohyoid

ACTIONS

❑ **1. Elevation of the Hyoid**

❑ **2.** Depression of the Mandible

INNERVATION ❑ The Trigeminal Nerve (CN V)
❑ the mylohyoid branch of the inferior alveolar nerve of the posterior trunk of the mandibular division of the trigeminal nerve (CN V)

ARTERIAL SUPPLY ❑ The Inferior Alveolar Artery (A Branch of the Maxillary Artery)

MYLOHYOID – PALPATION AND SUPPLEMENTARY TEXT

PALPATION

- ❑ The mylohyoid is superficial (except for the platysma and the anterior belly of the digastric) and easy to palpate.
  - Have the client supine.
  - Place palpating fingers under the chin.
  - Ask the client to push the tip of the tongue against the roof of the mouth and feel for the contraction of the mylohyoid.
  - Asking the client to swallow or to depress the mandible against resistance will also cause the mylohyoid to palpably contract, as well as the anterior belly of the digastric and the geniohyoid.

see page 145

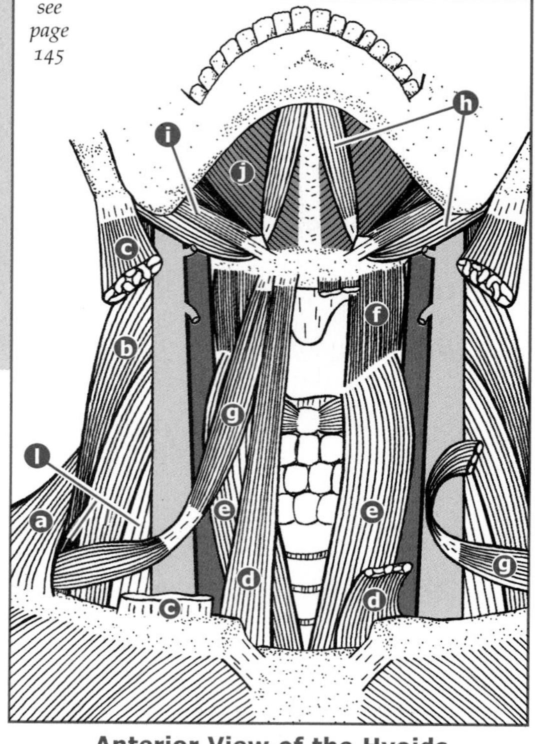

Anterior View of the Hyoids

a. Trapezius
b. Levator Scapulae
c. Sternocleidomastoid (cut)
d. Sternohyoid (cut on our right)
e. Sternothyroid
f. Thyrohyoid
g. Omohyoid (cut and reflected on our right)
h. Digastric
i. Stylohyoid
j. **Mylohyoid**
k. Geniohyoid (not seen)
l. Scalenes

RELATIONSHIP TO OTHER MUSCULOSKELETAL STRUCTURES

❑ 1. The mylohyoid is a broad, flat muscle that forms the muscular floor of the oral cavity.

❑ 2. Superior to the mylohyoid is the geniohyoid.

❑ 3. Inferior to the mylohyoid is the anterior belly of the digastric.

❑ 4. From the perspective of the underside of the mandible, the mylohyoid is superficial except for the anterior belly of the digastric and the platysma.

METHODOLOGY FOR LEARNING MUSCLE ACTIONS

❑ **1. Elevation of the Hyoid:** The mylohyoid attaches from the mandible superiorly, to the hyoid bone inferiorly (with its fibers running vertically). When the mandible is fixed and the mylohyoid contracts, it pulls the hyoid bone superiorly toward the mandible. Therefore, the mylohyoid elevates the hyoid. (Note: Movements of the hyoid bone are important in chewing, swallowing and speech.)

❑ **2. Depression of the Mandible at the Temporomandibular Joint:** The mylohyoid attaches from the mandible superiorly, to the hyoid bone inferiorly (with its fibers running somewhat vertically). When the hyoid bone is fixed and the mylohyoid contracts, it pulls the mandible inferiorly toward the hyoid bone. Therefore, the mylohyoid depresses the mandible.

MYLOHYOID – continued

MISCELLANEOUS

- ❑ 1. The mylohyoid is one of the four suprahyoid muscles. The four suprahyoid muscles are the digastric, stylohyoid, mylohyoid and the geniohyoid. There are four infrahyoid muscles: the sternohyoid, sternothyroid, thyrohyoid and the omohyoid. All the hyoid muscles are important in moving and/or fixating (stabilizing) the hyoid bone. These functions are necessary for chewing, swallowing and speech.
- ❑ 2. The fibers from the left and right mylohyoid muscles meet each other in the midline and form a median fibrous raphe. (A raphe is a seam of tissue formed by the union of the halves of a part.)
- ❑ 3. Another function of the mylohyoid is to elevate the floor of the mouth during the first stage of swallowing.
- ❑ 4. When the hyoid bone and the mandible are fixed (stabilized), the hyoids as a group can be felt to contract with resisted neck flexion. Hence, the hyoids are all weak accessory flexors of the neck at the cervical spinal joints. This makes sense given their direction of fibers running vertically, anterior to the cervical vertebrae.

GENIOHYOID
(OF THE HYOID GROUP)

❑ **The name, geniohyoid, tells us that this muscle attaches to the hyoid bone. "Genio," referring to the chin, tells us that this muscle also attaches to the mandible.**

DERIVATION ❑ genio: Gr. *chin.*
hyoid: Gr. *refers to the hyoid bone.*

PRONUNCIATION ❑ **jee**-nee-o-**hi**-oyd

ATTACHMENTS

❑ **Inner Surface of the Mandible**

- ❑ the inferior mental spine of the mandible

to the

❑ **Hyoid**

- ❑ the anterior surface of the body of the hyoid

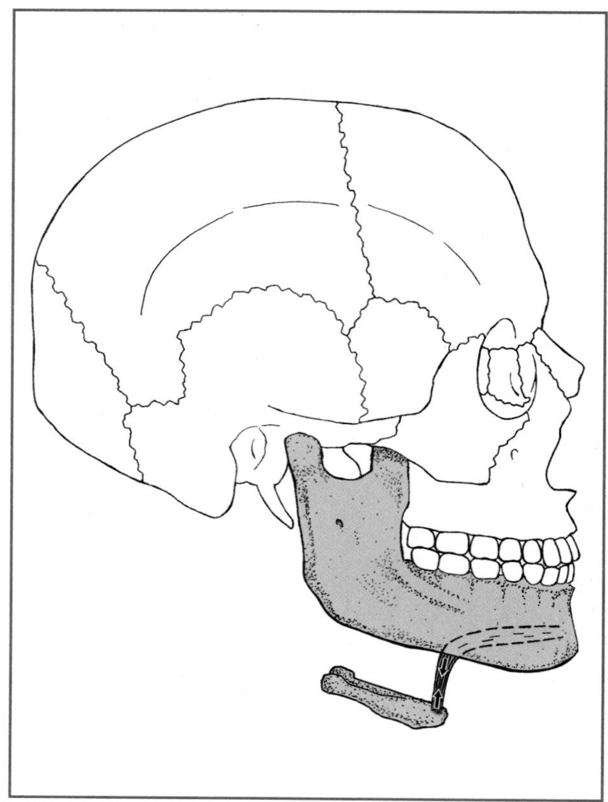

Lateral View of the Right Geniohyoid

ACTIONS

❑ 1. **Elevation of the Hyoid**

❑ 2. Depression of the Mandible

INNERVATION ❑ The Hypoglossal Nerve (CN XII)
❑ a branch of C1 through the hypoglossal nerve

ARTERIAL SUPPLY ❑ The Lingual Artery (A Branch of the External Carotid Artery)

PALPATION AND SUPPLEMENTARY TEXT

PALPATION

- [ ] The geniohyoid is a thin muscle located deep to the mylohyoid and the anterior belly of the digastric. It is difficult to distinguish the geniohyoid from these other two suprahyoid muscles, as actions that will cause the geniohyoid to contract will also cause the mylohyoid and/or anterior belly of the digastric to contract as well.
  - Have the client supine.
  - Place palpating fingers on the underside of the chin in the midline.
  - Ask the client to push the tip of the tongue against the roof of the mouth and feel for the contraction of the geniohyoid (as well as the mylohyoid).
  - Asking the client to swallow will also make the geniohyoid contract, as well as the mylohyoid and the anterior belly of the digastric.

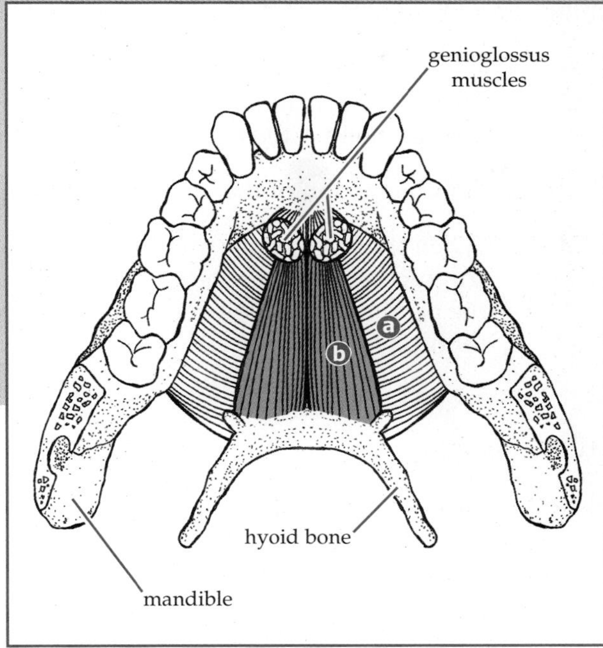

Superior View of the Floor of the Mouth

a. Mylohyoid
b. Geniohyoid

RELATIONSHIP TO OTHER MUSCULOSKELETAL STRUCTURES

- [ ] 1. The two geniohyoid muscles are two pencil-thin muscles that lie next to each other in the midline, sandwiched between the mylohyoid and the genioglossus muscles. The mylohyoids are inferior to the geniohyoids; the genioglossus muscles (muscles that move the tongue) are superior to the geniohyoids.
- [ ] 2. From the perspective of the underside of the mandible, the geniohyoid is deep to the mylohyoid, the anterior belly of the digastric and the platysma muscles.

METHODOLOGY FOR LEARNING MUSCLE ACTIONS

- [ ] **1. Elevation of the Hyoid:** The geniohyoid attaches from the hyoid bone inferiorly, to the mandible superiorly (with its fibers running somewhat vertically). When the mandible is fixed and the geniohyoid contracts, it pulls the hyoid bone superiorly toward the mandible. Therefore, the geniohyoid elevates the hyoid. (Note: Movements of the hyoid bone are important in chewing, swallowing and speech.)
- [ ] **2. Depression of the Mandible at the Temporomandibular Joint:** The geniohyoid attaches from the mandible superiorly, to the hyoid bone inferiorly (with its fibers running somewhat vertically). When the hyoid bone is fixed and the geniohyoid contracts, it pulls the mandible inferiorly toward the hyoid bone. Therefore, the geniohyoid depresses the mandible at the temporomandibular joint.

GENIOHYOID – continued

MISCELLANEOUS

- ❑ 1. The geniohyoid is one of the four suprahyoid muscles. The four suprahyoid muscles are the digastric, stylohyoid, mylohyoid and the geniohyoid. There are four infrahyoid muscles: the sternohyoid, sternothyroid, thyrohyoid and the omohyoid. All the hyoid muscles are important in moving and/or fixating (stabilizing) the hyoid bone. These functions are necessary for chewing, swallowing and speech.
- ❑ 2. The left and right geniohyoid muscles occasionally blend together.
- ❑ 3. The inferior mental spines are bony landmarks of the mandible that are on the posterior side, directly behind the symphysis menti, i.e., the midline of the mandible.
- ❑ 4. Another action of the geniohyoid is to protract the hyoid bone (draw the hyoid anteriorly).
- ❑ 5. When the hyoid bone and the mandible are fixed (stabilized), the hyoids as a group can be felt to contract with resisted neck flexion. Hence, the hyoids are all weak accessory flexors of the neck at the cervical spinal joints. This makes sense given their direction of fibers running vertically, anterior to the cervical vertebrae.

THE SCALENES

The scalenes are a group of muscles that are found in the anterolateral neck.

THERE ARE THREE SCALENE MUSCLES:		
Anterior Scalene	Middle Scalene	Posterior Scalene

Attachments:

- As a group, the scalenes attach from superiorly on the T.P.s of the cervical spine, to inferiorly on the 1st and 2nd ribs.
- The names of the scalenes refer to their relative location with respect to each other: the anterior scalene is the most anterior of the three; the posterior scalene is the most posterior of the three; the middle scalene is in the middle, sandwiched between the two.

Actions:

- As a group, the scalenes flex and laterally flex the cervical spine and/or elevate the 1st and 2nd ribs.
- The scalenes are considered to be the prime movers of lateral flexion of the neck.
- By elevating the 1st and 2nd ribs, the scalenes can help to elevate and expand the ribcage, which expands the thoracic cavity, thereby creating more space for the lungs to expand for inspiration. Therefore, the scalenes are accessory muscles of respiration.
- There is controversy regarding the role of the scalenes with respect to rotation of the neck. Some sources state that the scalenes perform contralateral rotation; other sources state that they perform ipsilateral rotation. Other sources state that the scalenes perform rotation without specifying whether it is contralateral or ipsilateral rotation. Still others are silent on this issue. Given the direction of fibers and the consequent line of pull, it seems likely that of all the scalenes, the anterior scalene is best suited for rotation, and that it would perform contralateral rotation of the neck at the cervical spinal joints.

Miscellaneous:

- Of the scalenes, the middle scalene is the longest and the largest and the posterior scalene is the shortest and the smallest.
- There is a fourth scalene muscle called the *scalenus minimus* that is present, on at least one side, in 50-75% of the population. When present, it is usually found posterior to the anterior scalene, attaching from the T.P. (anterior tubercle) of C7 to the 1st rib (inner border) and the pleural membrane of the lung.

INNERVATION The scalenes are innervated by cervical spinal nerves (ventral rami).

ARTERIAL SUPPLY Arterial supply to the scalenes is provided by either the ascending cervical artery or the transverse cervical artery.

Clinical Applications:

- The scalenes, as well as the sternocleidomastoid, are often injured as a result of car accidents. This trauma is usually called *whiplash,* wherein the head and neck are forcefully thrown anteriorly and posteriorly (like a whip being lashed). When the head and the neck are thrown posteriorly, the anterior cervical musculature may be torn, or the muscle spindle reflex may occur, causing the anterior cervical musculature to spasm. When the head and the neck are thrown anteriorly, the same trauma may occur to the posterior musculature.
- The brachial plexus of nerves and the subclavian artery run between the anterior and middle scalenes (see illustration on page 104). If these muscles are tight, then entrapment of these nerves and/or artery can occur. When this does happen, it is called *anterior scalene syndrome* (also known as *scalenus anticus syndrome*, one of the three types of *thoracic outlet syndrome*). This condition can cause sensory symptoms (e.g., tingling, pain or numbness) and/or motor symptoms (e.g., weakness and/or partial paralysis) in the upper extremity.

VIEWS OF THE SCALENES

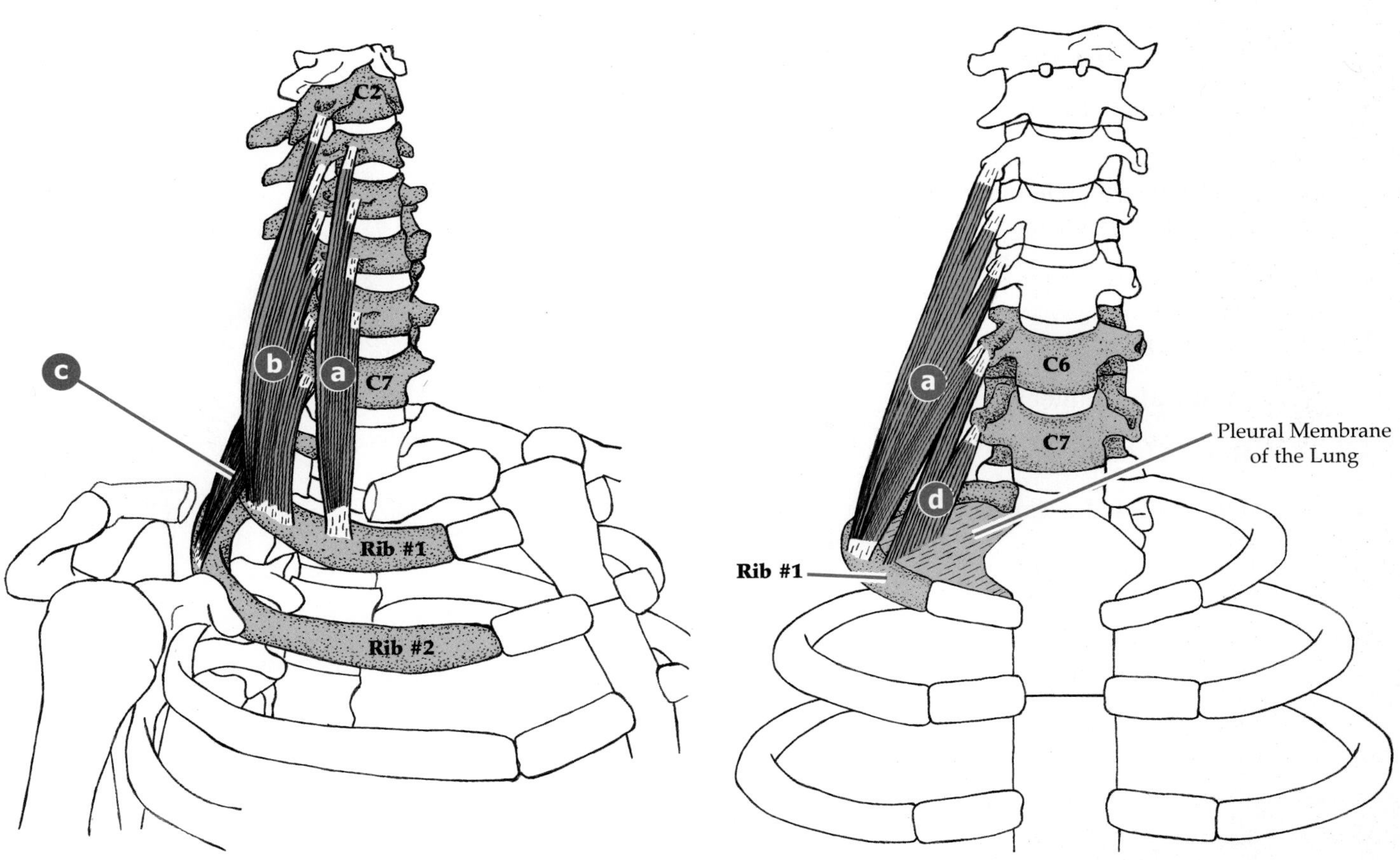

Anterolateral View of the Right Scalenes (the clavicle has been cut)

Anterior View of the Right Scalenus Minimus and Anterior Scalene

a. **Anterior Scalene**
b. **Middle Scalene**
c. **Posterior Scalene**
d. **Scalenus Minimus**

ANTERIOR SCALENE
(OF THE SCALENE GROUP)

❑ **The name, anterior scalene, tells us that this muscle has a step or ladder-like shape and is located anteriorly (anterior to the middle and posterior scalenes).**

DERIVATION ❑ anterior: L. *before, in front of.*
scalene: L. *uneven, ladder.*

PRONUNCIATION ❑ an-**tee**-ri-or **skay**-leen

ATTACHMENTS

❑ **T.P.s of the Cervical Spine**

- ❑ the anterior tubercles of C3-6

to the

❑ **1st Rib**

- ❑ the scalene tubercle on the inner border

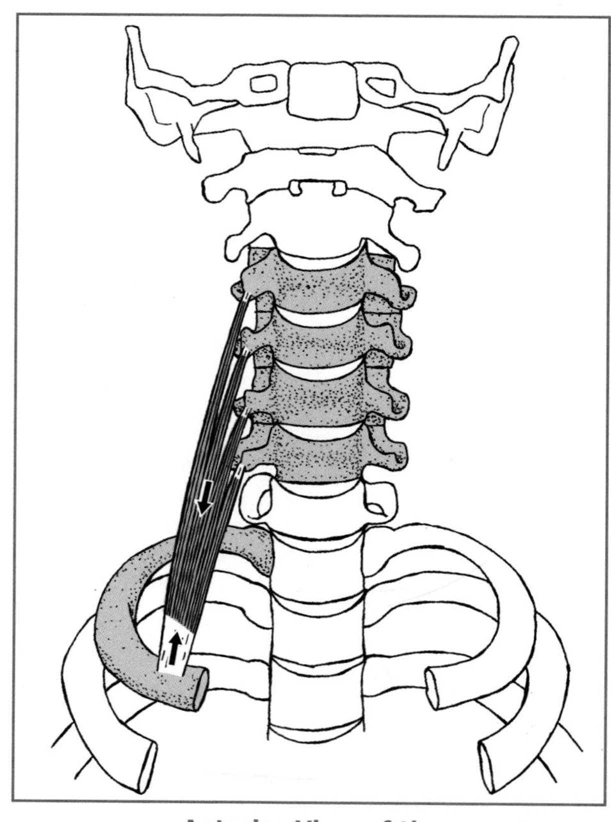

Anterior View of the Right Anterior Scalene

ACTIONS

❑ 1. **Flexion of the Neck**

❑ 2. **Lateral Flexion of the Neck**

❑ 3. **Elevation of the 1st Rib**

❑ 4. Contralateral Rotation of the Neck

INNERVATION ❑ Cervical Spinal Nerves ❑ ventral rami; C4-6

ARTERIAL SUPPLY ❑ The Ascending Cervical Artery (A Branch of the Inferior Thyroid Artery)

PALPATION AND SUPPLEMENTARY TEXT

PALPATION

- ❑ Part of the anterior scalene is superficial (except for the platysma) in the anterolateral neck.
  - Have the client seated.
  - Locate the lateral margin of the sternocleidomastoid (see the palpation section for this muscle on page 141).
  - Place palpating fingers slightly lateral to the lateral margin of the sternocleidomastoid and just superior to the clavicle.
  - Ask the client to take in a deep breath and feel for the contraction of the anterior and middle scalenes. Distinguishing the anterior scalene from the middle scalene can be difficult since they will both contract; palpate more medially for the anterior scalene, and slightly more laterally for the middle scalene.

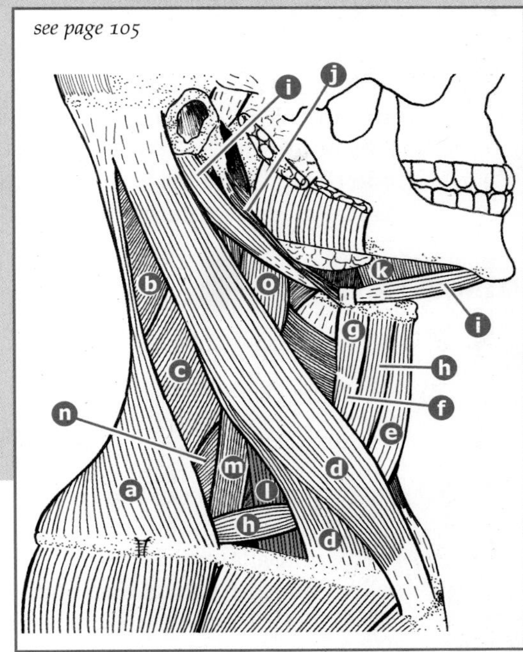

Lateral View of the Neck

a. Trapezius
b. Splenius Capitis
c. Levator Scapulae
d. Sternocleidomastoid
e. Sternohyoid
f. Sternothyroid
g. Thyrohyoid
h. Omohyoid
i. Digastric
j. Stylohyoid
k. Mylohyoid
l. **Anterior Scalene**
m. Middle Scalene
n. Posterior Scalene
o. Longus Capitis

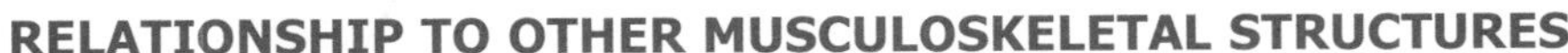

RELATIONSHIP TO OTHER MUSCULOSKELETAL STRUCTURES

❑ 1. The inferior portion of the anterior scalene is superficial, except where the clavicle and the omohyoid cross in front of it (and the platysma, which is superficial to all anterior neck muscles).

❑ 2. The superior portion of the anterior scalene is deep to the sternocleidomastoid.

❑ 3. Directly posterolateral to the anterior scalene is the middle scalene.

❑ 4. Deep to the anterior scalene are the brachial plexus of nerves, the subclavian artery and the pleural membrane of the lung.

❑ 5. If one looks at the relationship between the anterior scalene and the longus capitis, as well as the superior part of the longus colli, it can be seen that, except for the interruption of the attachment to the T.P.s of the cervical spine, there is a continuous line of pull from the 1st rib (the inferior most attachment of the anterior scalene) to the atlas (C1) and the head (the most superior attachment of the longus colli and capitis).

METHODOLOGY FOR LEARNING MUSCLE ACTIONS

❑ **1. Flexion of the Neck at the Spinal Joints:** The anterior scalene crosses the cervical spinal joints anteriorly (with its fibers running vertically in the sagittal plane); therefore, it flexes the neck at the cervical spinal joints.

❑ **2. Lateral Flexion of the Neck at the Spinal Joints:** The anterior scalene crosses the cervical spinal joints laterally (with its fibers running vertically in the frontal plane); therefore, it laterally flexes the neck at the cervical spinal joints.

ANTERIOR SCALENE – continued

❑ 3. **Elevation of the 1st Rib at the Sternocostal and Costovertebral Joints:** When the cervical attachment of the anterior scalene is fixed, the 1st rib must move. Given that the fiber direction of the anterior scalene is vertical from the 1st rib up to the cervical vertebrae, the anterior scalene elevates the 1st rib at the sternocostal and the costovertebral joints. (Note: This action is important for respiration.)

❑ 4. **Contralateral Rotation of the Neck at the Spinal Joints:** The attachment of the anterior scalene onto the 1st rib is more anterior than the transverse process attachments (therefore, the fibers are running slightly horizontally in the transverse plane). When the anterior scalene contracts, it pulls the T.P.s anteromedially toward the 1st rib, causing the anterior surface of the vertebrae to face the opposite side of the body from the side that the anterior scalene is attached. Therefore, the anterior scalene contralaterally rotates the neck at the cervical spinal joints.

MISCELLANEOUS

❑ 1. The anterior scalene is part of the scalene group, which is comprised of the anterior, middle, and posterior scalenes.

❑ 2. A fourth scalene, called the *scalenus minimus*, is often present.

❑ 3. There is controversy regarding the role of the scalene group with respect to rotation of the neck. Some sources state that the scalenes perform contralateral rotation; other sources state that they perform ipsilateral rotation. Other sources state rotation without specifying whether it is contralateral or ipsilateral rotation and still others are silent on this issue. Given the direction of fibers and the consequent line of pull, it seems likely that of all the scalenes, the anterior scalene is best suited for rotation, and it would perform contralateral rotation of the neck at the cervical spinal joints.

❑ 4. By elevating the 1st rib, the anterior scalene can help to elevate and expand the ribcage, which expands the thoracic cavity, thereby creating more space for the lungs to expand for inspiration. Therefore, the anterior scalene is an accessory muscle of respiration.

❑ 5. The brachial plexus of nerves and the subclavian artery run between the anterior and middle scalenes. If these muscles are tight, then entrapment of these nerves and/or artery can occur. When this happens, it is called *anterior scalene syndrome* (also known as *scalenus anticus syndrome)*, one of the three types of *thoracic outlet syndrome*. This condition can cause sensory symptoms (e.g., tingling, pain or numbness) and/or motor symptoms (e.g., weakness and/or partial paralysis) in the upper extremity.

❑ 6. Very close to the superior attachment of the anterior scalene is the common carotid artery. Given the neurological reflex that occurs to lower blood pressure when the carotid sinus of the common carotid artery is pressed, massage to this region must be done judiciously, especially with weak and/or elderly clients.

❑ 7. The scalenes, as well as the sternocleidomastoid, are often injured as a result of car accidents. This trauma is usually called *whiplash,* wherein the head and neck are forcefully thrown anteriorly and posteriorly (like a whip being lashed). When the head and neck are thrown posteriorly, the anterior cervical musculature may be torn, or the muscle spindle reflex may occur, causing the anterior cervical musculature to spasm. When the head and neck are thrown anteriorly, the same trauma may occur to the posterior musculature.

MIDDLE SCALENE
(OF THE SCALENE GROUP)

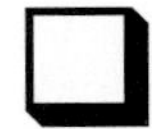

❑ **The name, middle scalene, tells us that this muscle has a step or ladder-like shape and is located in the middle of the scalene group (between the anterior and posterior scalenes).**

DERIVATION ❑ middle: L. *middle* (between).
scalene: L. *uneven, ladder.*

PRONUNCIATION ❑ **mi**-dil **skay**-leen

ATTACHMENTS

❑ **T.P.s of the Cervical Spine**

- ❑ the posterior tubercles of C2-7

to the

❑ **1st Rib**

- ❑ the superior surface

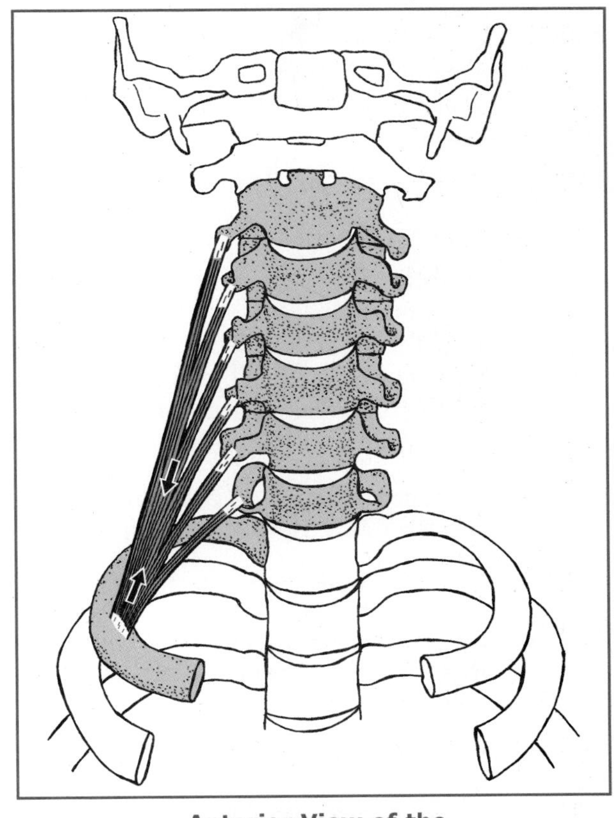

Anterior View of the Right Middle Scalene

ACTIONS

❑ 1. **Lateral Flexion of the Neck**

❑ 2. **Flexion of the Neck**

❑ 3. **Elevation of the 1st Rib**

INNERVATION ❑ Cervical Spinal Nerves ❑ ventral rami; C3-8

ARTERIAL SUPPLY ❑ The Transverse Cervical Artery (A Branch of the Thyrocervical Trunk)

MIDDLE SCALENE – PALPATION AND SUPPLEMENTARY TEXT

PALPATION

- ❑ Part of the middle scalene is superficial (except for the platysma) in the anterolateral neck.
  - Have the client seated.
  - Locate the lateral margin of the sternocleidomastoid (see the palpation section for this muscle on page 141).
  - Place palpating fingers slightly lateral to the lateral margin of the sternocleidomastoid and just superior to the clavicle.
  - Ask the client to take in a deep breath and feel for the contraction of the middle and anterior scalenes. Distinguishing the middle scalene from the anterior scalene can be difficult since they will both contract; palpate slightly more laterally for the middle scalene and more medially for the anterior scalene.

see page 105

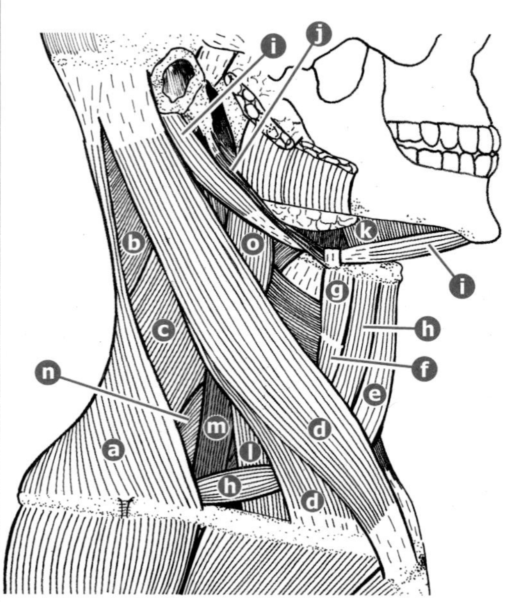

Lateral View of the Neck

a. Trapezius
b. Splenius Capitis
c. Levator Scapulae
d. Sternocleidomastoid
e. Sternohyoid
f. Sternothyroid
g. Thyrohyoid
h. Omohyoid
i. Digastric
j. Stylohyoid
k. Mylohyoid
l. Anterior Scalene
m. **Middle Scalene**
n. Posterior Scalene
o. Longus Capitis

RELATIONSHIP TO OTHER MUSCULOSKELETAL STRUCTURES

❑ 1. Like the anterior scalene, the inferior portion of the middle scalene is superficial, except where the clavicle and the omohyoid cross in front of it (and the platysma, which is superficial to all anterior neck muscles).

❑ 2. The superior portion of the middle scalene, like the anterior scalene, is deep to the sternocleidomastoid.

❑ 3. Directly anteromedial to the middle scalene is the anterior scalene.

❑ 4. The posterior scalene and the levator scapulae are posterolateral to the middle scalene.

METHODOLOGY FOR LEARNING MUSCLE ACTIONS

❑ **1. Lateral Flexion of the Neck at the Spinal Joints:** The middle scalene crosses the cervical spinal joints laterally (with its fibers running vertically in the frontal plane); therefore, it laterally flexes the neck at the cervical spinal joints.

❑ **2. Flexion of the Neck at the Spinal Joints:** The middle scalene crosses the cervical spinal joints anteriorly (with its fibers running vertically in the sagittal plane); therefore, it flexes the neck at the cervical spinal joints.

❑ **3. Elevation of the 1st Rib at the Sternocostal and Costovertebral Joints:** When the cervical attachment of the middle scalene is fixed, the 1st rib must move. Given that the fiber direction of the middle scalene is vertical from the 1st rib up to the cervical vertebrae, the middle scalene elevates the 1st rib at the sternocostal and costovertebral joints. (Note: This action is important for respiration.)

MIDDLE SCALENE – continued

MISCELLANEOUS

- ❑ 1. The middle scalene is part of the scalene group, which is comprised of the anterior, middle, and posterior scalenes.
- ❑ 2. A fourth scalene, called the *scalenus minimus*, is often present.
- ❑ 3. The middle scalene is the largest and the longest of the scalenes.
- ❑ 4. By elevating the 1st rib, the middle scalene can help to elevate and expand the ribcage, which expands the thoracic cavity, thereby creating more space for the lungs to expand for inspiration. Therefore, the middle scalene is an accessory muscle of respiration.
- ❑ 5. The nerve to the rhomboids (the dorsal scapula nerve) and some of the spinal nerve segments to the nerve to the serratus anterior (long thoracic nerve) pierce the middle scalene.
- ❑ 6. The brachial plexus of nerves and the subclavian artery run between the anterior and middle scalenes. If these muscles are tight, then entrapment of these nerves and/or artery can occur. When this happens, it is called *anterior scalene syndrome* (also known as *scalenus anticus syndrome)*, one of the three types of *thoracic outlet syndrome*. This condition can cause sensory symptoms (e.g., tingling, pain or numbness) and/or motor symptoms (e.g., weakness and/or partial paralysis) in the upper extremity.
- ❑ 7. The scalenes, as well as the sternocleidomastoid, are often injured as a result of car accidents. This trauma is usually called *whiplash,* wherein the head and neck are forcefully thrown anteriorly and posteriorly (like a whip being lashed). When the head and neck are thrown posteriorly, the anterior cervical musculature may be torn, or the muscle spindle reflex may occur, causing the anterior cervical musculature to spasm. When the head and neck are thrown anteriorly, the same trauma may occur to the posterior musculature.

❑

POSTERIOR SCALENE
(OF THE SCALENE GROUP)

❑ **The name, posterior scalene, tells us that this muscle has a step or ladder-like shape and is located posteriorly (posterior to the middle and anterior scalenes).**

DERIVATION ❑ posterior: L. *behind, toward the back.*
scalene: L. *uneven, ladder.*

PRONUNCIATION ❑ pos-**tee**-ri-or **skay**-leen

ATTACHMENTS

❑ **T.P.s of the Cervical Spine**

- ❑ the posterior tubercles of C5-7

to the

❑ **2nd Rib**

- ❑ the external surface

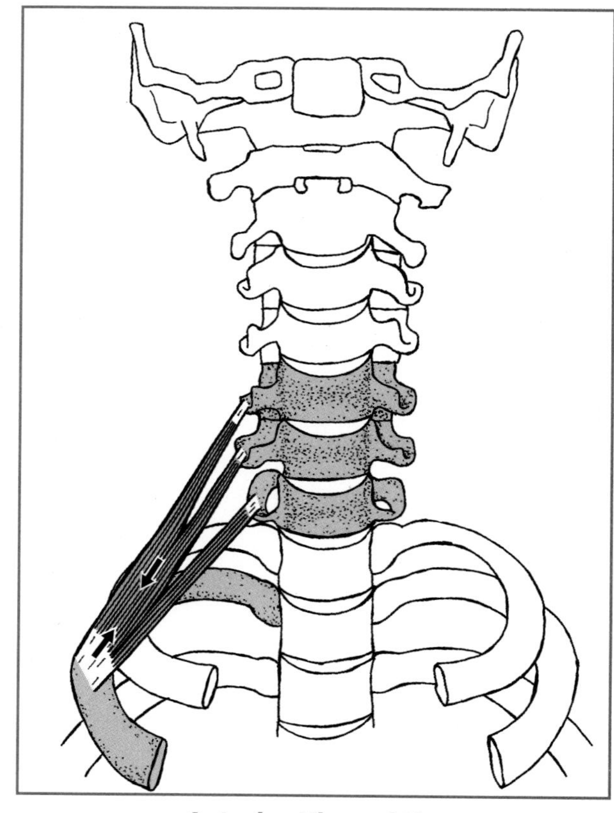

Anterior View of the Right Posterior Scalene

ACTIONS

❑ 1. **Lateral Flexion of the Neck**

❑ 2. **Elevation of the 2nd Rib**

INNERVATION ❑ Cervical Spinal Nerves ❑ ventral rami; C6-8

ARTERIAL SUPPLY ❑ The Transverse Cervical Artery (A Branch of the Thyrocervical Trunk)

PALPATION AND SUPPLEMENTARY TEXT

PALPATION

- ❑ Part of the posterior scalene is superficial (except for the platysma) in the lateral neck just anterior to the levator scapulae.
    - Have the client seated.
    - Locate the lateral margin of the sternocleidomastoid (see the palpation section for this muscle on page 141).
    - Place palpating fingers slightly lateral to the lateral margin of the sternocleidomastoid and just superior to the clavicle.
    - Ask the client to take in a deep breath and feel for the contractions of middle and anterior scalenes, then continue palpating more posteriorly for the posterior scalene. To distinguish the posterior scalene from the levator scapulae, which is directly posterior to it, have the client alternate between slightly elevating the scapula (which will cause the levator scapulae to contract) and taking in a deep breath (which will make the posterior scalene contract to elevate the 2nd rib).

see page 105

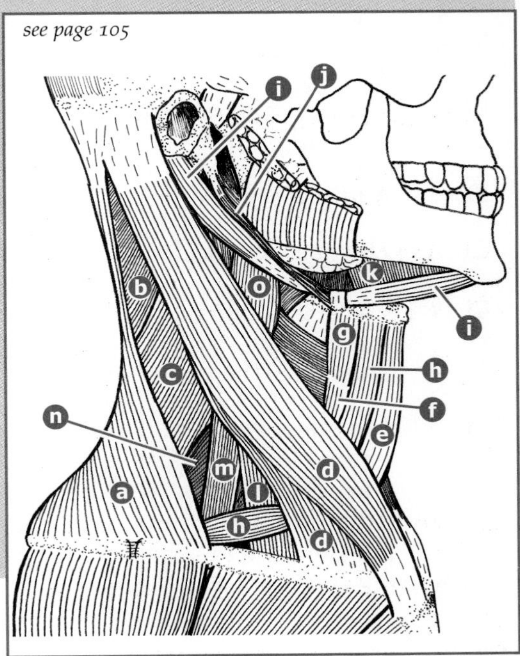

Lateral View of the Neck

a. Trapezius
b. Splenius Capitis
c. Levator Scapulae
d. Sternocleidomastoid
e. Sternohyoid
f. Sternothyroid
g. Thyrohyoid
h. Omohyoid
i. Digastric
j. Stylohyoid
k. Mylohyoid
l. Anterior Scalene
m. Middle Scalene
n. **Posterior Scalene**
o. Longus Capitis

RELATIONSHIP TO OTHER MUSCULOSKELETAL STRUCTURES

❑ 1. The posterior scalene is the most posterior of the three scalenes. Consequently, it is situated almost directly lateral in the inferior neck and is the most superficial from the lateral perspective.

❑ 2. There is a small area bounded by the trapezius and the levator scapulae (posteriorly), and the sternocleidomastoid (anteriorly), in which the posterior scalene is superficial. In this space, the posterior scalene is directly anterior to the levator scapulae and directly posterior to the middle scalene.

❑ 3. To attach onto the 2nd rib, the posterior scalene passes over (on the external side of) the 1st rib.

METHODOLOGY FOR LEARNING MUSCLE ACTIONS

❑ **1. Lateral Flexion of the Neck at the Spinal Joints:** The posterior scalene crosses the cervical spinal joints laterally (with its fibers running vertically in the frontal plane); therefore, it laterally flexes the neck at the cervical spinal joints. (Given that the posterior scalene only crosses the lower three cervical vertebrae, its action of lateral flexion would occur only at the lower neck.)

POSTERIOR SCALENE – continued

- ❑ 2. **Elevation of the 2nd Rib at the Sternocostal and Costovertebral Joints:** When the cervical attachment of the posterior scalene is fixed, the 2nd rib must move. Given that the fiber direction of the posterior scalene is vertical from the 2nd rib up to the cervical vertebrae, the posterior scalene elevates the 2nd rib at the sternocostal and costovertebral joints. (Note: This action is important for respiration.)

MISCELLANEOUS

- ❑ 1. The posterior scalene is part of the scalene group, which is comprised of the anterior, middle, and posterior scalenes.
- ❑ 2. A fourth scalene, called the *scalenus minimus*, is often present.
- ❑ 3. The posterior scalene is the smallest and the shortest of the three scalenes.
- ❑ 4. By elevating the 2nd rib, the posterior scalene can help to elevate and expand the ribcage, which expands the thoracic cavity, thereby creating more space for the lungs to expand for inspiration. Therefore, the posterior scalene is an accessory muscle of respiration.
- ❑ 5. The scalenes, as well as the sternocleidomastoid, are often injured as a result of car accidents. This trauma is usually called *whiplash,* wherein the head and neck are forcefully thrown anteriorly and posteriorly (like a whip being lashed). When the head and neck are thrown posteriorly, the anterior cervical musculature may be torn, or the muscle spindle reflex may occur, causing the anterior cervical musculature to spasm. When the head and neck are thrown anteriorly, the same trauma may occur to the posterior musculature.

LONGUS COLLI
(OF THE PREVERTEBRAL GROUP)

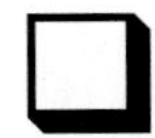

❑ **The name, longus colli, tells us that this muscle is long and found in the neck.**

DERIVATION ❑ longus: L. *long.* colli: L. *neck.*

PRONUNCIATION ❑ **long**-us **kol**-eye

ATTACHMENTS

❑ **ENTIRE MUSCLE: C3-T3 Vertebrae**

- ❑ the T.P.s and anterior bodies
  - ❑ SUPERIOR OBLIQUE PART: C3-5
    - ❑ the T.P.s of C3-5
  - ❑ INFERIOR OBLIQUE PART: T1-3
    - ❑ the anterior bodies of T1-3
  - ❑ VERTICAL PART: C5-T3
    - ❑ the anterior bodies of C5-T3

to the

❑ **ENTIRE MUSCLE: C1-C6 Vertebrae**

- ❑ the T.P.s and anterior bodies; and the anterior arch of the atlas
  - ❑ SUPERIOR OBLIQUE PART: C1
    - ❑ the anterior arch of the atlas
  - ❑ INFERIOR OBLIQUE PART: C5-6
    - ❑ the T.P.s of C5-6
  - ❑ VERTICAL PART: C2-4
    - ❑ the anterior bodies of C2-4

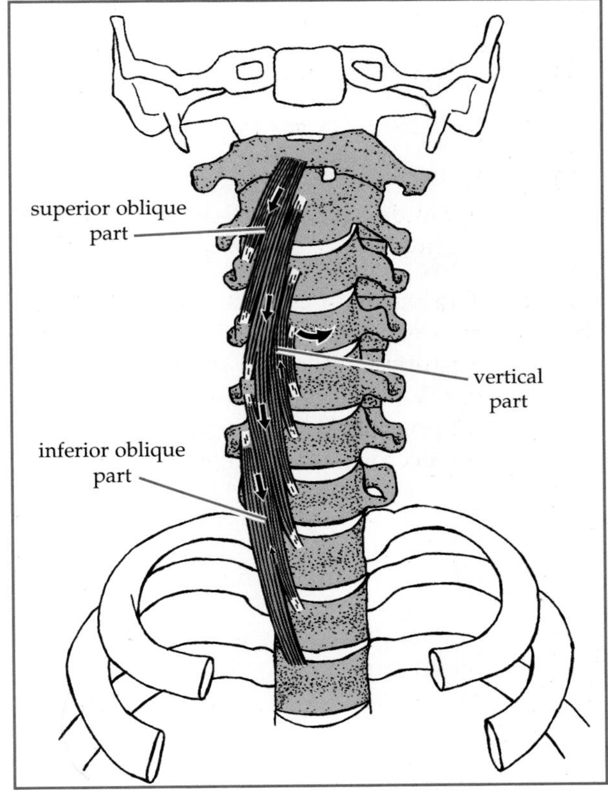

Anterior View of the Right Longus Colli

ACTIONS

❑ 1. **Flexion of the Neck**
❑ 2. Lateral Flexion of the Neck
❑ 3. Contralateral Rotation of the Neck

INNERVATION ❑ Cervical Spinal Nerves ❑ ventral rami; C2-6

ARTERIAL SUPPLY ❑ The Inferior Thyroid Artery (A Branch of the Thyrocervical Trunk) and the Vertebral Artery (A Branch of the Subclavian Artery)
❑ and the ascending pharyngeal artery (a branch of the external carotid artery)

LONGUS COLLI – PALPATION AND SUPPLEMENTARY TEXT

PALPATION

- ❑ Although the longus colli is located very deep in the anterior neck, it can be palpated.
  - Have the client seated or supine.
  - Stand to one side of the client.
  - Locate the sternocleidomastoid on the side where you are standing (see the palpation section for this muscle on page 141) and place palpating fingers just medial to the medial margin of it, pressing gently but firmly deep against the anterolateral cervical spine.
  - Ask the client to rotate the head to the side where you are standing (to relax the sternocleidomastoid).
  - Now resist the client from flexing the neck and feel for the contraction of the longus colli.

  Distinguishing the longus colli from the longus capitis will be difficult. The longus colli runs between T3 and C1 levels and the longus capitis runs between C6 and the occiput.

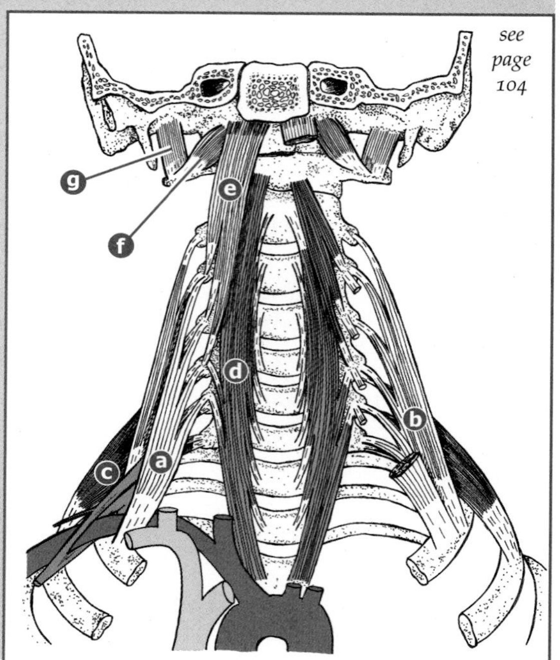

Anterior View of the Neck (Deep)

a. Anterior Scalene (cut on our right)
b. Middle Scalene
c. Posterior Scalene
d. Longus Colli
e. Longus Capitis (cut on our right)
f. Rectus Capitis Anterior
g. Rectus Capitis Lateralis

RELATIONSHIP TO OTHER MUSCULOSKELETAL STRUCTURES

❑ 1. The longus colli is very deep in the anterior neck (along with the longus capitis). The longus colli is deep to the hyoid bone, the suprahyoid and infrahyoid muscles, the trachea and the esophagus. The longus colli lies against the cervical and upper thoracic vertebral bodies.

❑ 2. The longus colli is generally inferior to the longus capitis. Where they overlap, the longus colli is deep to the longus capitis.

❑ 3. If one looks at the relationship between the longus colli (as well as the longus capitis) to the anterior scalene, it can be seen that, except for the interruption of the attachment to the T.P.s of the cervical spine, there is a continuous line of pull from the 1st rib (the inferior most attachment of the anterior scalene) to the atlas (C1) and the head (the most superior attachments of the longus colli and capitis).

❑ 4. The inferior part of the longus colli (the inferior part of the inferior oblique part) lies deep to the sternum.

METHODOLOGY FOR LEARNING MUSCLE ACTIONS

❑ **1. Flexion of the Neck at the Spinal Joints:** The longus colli crosses the joints of the neck anteriorly (with its fibers running vertically in the sagittal plane); therefore, it flexes the neck at the cervical spinal joints. (All parts of the longus colli perform this action.)

LONGUS COLLI – continued

- ❑ **2. Lateral Flexion of the Neck at the Spinal Joints:** The longus colli crosses the joints of the neck laterally (with its fibers running vertically in the frontal plane); therefore, it laterally flexes the neck at the cervical spinal joints. (Particularly the superior and inferior oblique parts of the longus colli perform this action.)

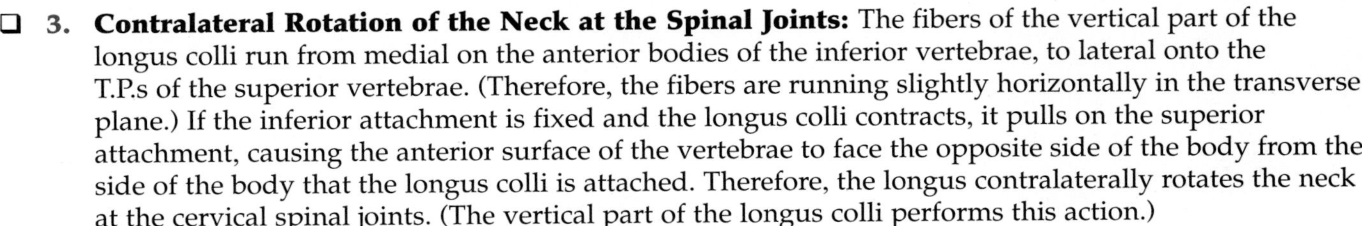

- ❑ **3. Contralateral Rotation of the Neck at the Spinal Joints:** The fibers of the vertical part of the longus colli run from medial on the anterior bodies of the inferior vertebrae, to lateral onto the T.P.s of the superior vertebrae. (Therefore, the fibers are running slightly horizontally in the transverse plane.) If the inferior attachment is fixed and the longus colli contracts, it pulls on the superior attachment, causing the anterior surface of the vertebrae to face the opposite side of the body from the side of the body that the longus colli is attached. Therefore, the longus contralaterally rotates the neck at the cervical spinal joints. (The vertical part of the longus colli performs this action.)

MISCELLANEOUS

- ❑ 1. The longus colli and the longus capitis along with the rectus capitis anterior and the rectus capitis lateralis are often grouped together and called the *prevertebral muscles.* (From an anterior perspective, they are just before, i.e., "pre," the vertebral column.)
- ❑ 2. The longus colli has three parts: the superior oblique part, the inferior oblique part and the vertical part.
- ❑ 3. There is a general pattern of attachments for the longus colli. The attachments of the vertical part are from anterior bodies to anterior bodies. The attachments of the inferior oblique part are from anterior bodies to T.P.s. The attachments of the superior oblique part are from T.P.s to the anterior arch of the atlas (C1). All T.P. attachments are to the anterior tubercles of the T.P.s.
- ❑ 4. The longus colli is considered to be a strong flexor of the neck at the cervical spinal joints.
- ❑ 5. The prevertebral muscles are important for fixating (stabilizing) the neck and the head while talking, swallowing, coughing and sneezing. The prevertebral muscles also fixate the neck during rapid arm movements.
- ❑ 6. All the activities listed in miscellaneous #5 can exacerbate deep anterior neck pain in people who have had a whiplash injury.

❑ LONGUS CAPITIS
(OF THE PREVERTEBRAL GROUP)

❑ **The name, longus capitis, tells us that this muscle is long and attaches to the head.**

DERIVATION ❑ longus: L. *long.*
capitis: L. *head.*

PRONUNCIATION ❑ **long**-us **kap**-i-tis

ATTACHMENTS

❑ **T.P.s of the Cervical Spine**

❑ the anterior tubercles of C3-5

to the

❑ **Occiput**

❑ the inferior surface of the basilar part of the occiput (just anterior to the foramen magnum)

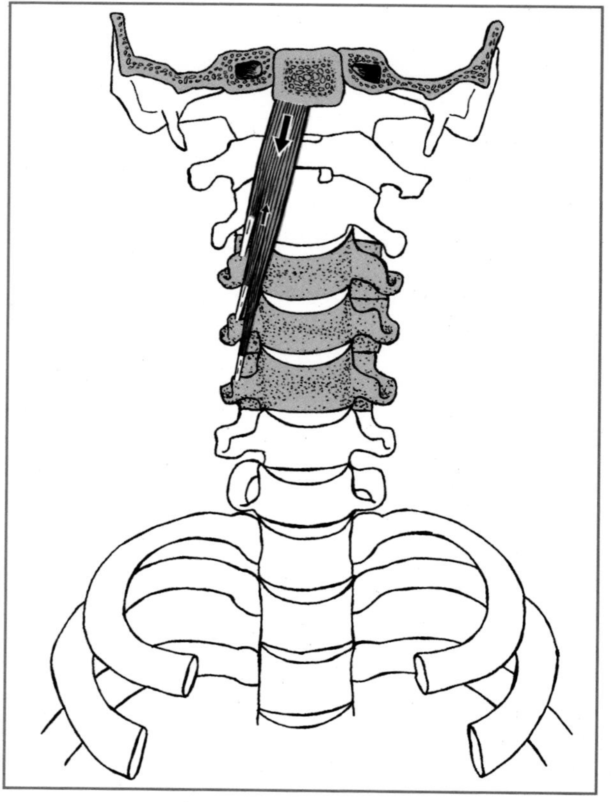

Anterior View of the Right Longus Capitis

ACTIONS

❑ 1. **Flexion of the Head and the Neck**

❑ 2. **Lateral Flexion of the Head and the Neck**

INNERVATION ❑ Cervical Spinal Nerves ❑ ventral rami; C1-3

ARTERIAL SUPPLY ❑ The Inferior Thyroid Artery (A Branch of the Thyrocervical Trunk) and the Vertebral Artery (A Branch of the Subclavian Artery)
❑ and the ascending pharyngeal artery (a branch of the external carotid artery)

PALPATION AND SUPPLEMENTARY TEXT

PALPATION

- ❑ Although the longus capitis is located very deep in the anterior neck, it can be palpated.
  - Have the client seated or supine.
  - Stand to one side of the client.
  - Locate the sternocleidomastoid on the side where you are standing (see the palpation section for this muscle on page 141) and place palpating fingers just medial to the medial margin of it, pressing gently but firmly deep against the anterolateral cervical spine.
  - Ask the client to rotate the head to the side where you are standing (to relax the sternocleidomastoid).
  - Now resist the client from flexing the neck and feel for the contraction of the longus capitis.

  Distinguishing the longus capitis from the longus colli will be difficult. The longus capitis runs between C6 and the occiput and the longus colli runs between T3 and C1 levels.

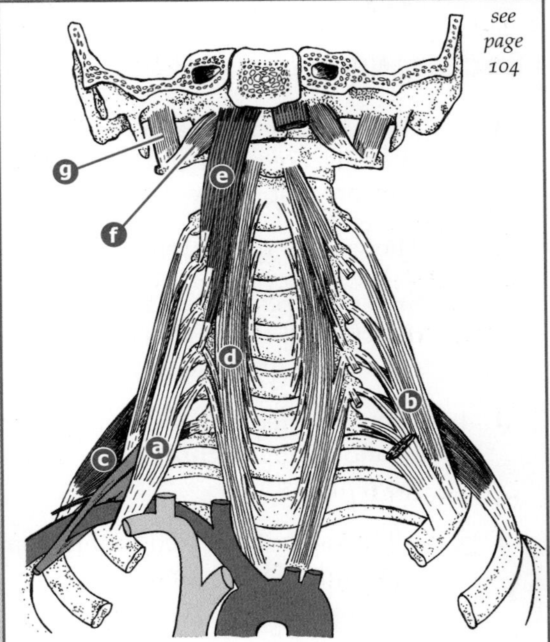

Anterior View of the Neck (Deep)

- **a.** Anterior Scalene (cut on our right)
- **b.** Middle Scalene
- **c.** Posterior Scalene
- **d.** Longus Colli
- **e.** **Longus Capitis** (cut on our right)
- **f.** Rectus Capitis Anterior
- **g.** Rectus Capitis Lateralis

RELATIONSHIP TO OTHER MUSCULOSKELETAL STRUCTURES

❑ 1. The longus capitis is very deep in the anterior neck (along with the longus colli). The longus capitis is deep to the hyoid bone, the suprahyoid muscles, the trachea and the esophagus.

❑ 2. The longus capitis is generally superior to the longus colli. Where they overlap, the longus colli is deep to the longus capitis. The rectus capitis anterior is also deep to the longus capitis.

❑ 3. If one looks at the relationship between the longus capitis (as well as the superior part of the longus colli) and the anterior scalene, it can be seen that, except for the interruption of the attachment to the T.P.s of the cervical spine, there is a continuous line of pull from the 1st rib (the inferior most attachment of the anterior scalene) to the atlas (C1) and the head (the most superior attachments of the longus colli and capitis).

METHODOLOGY FOR LEARNING MUSCLE ACTIONS

❑ **1. Flexion of the Head and the Neck at the Spinal Joints:** The longus capitis crosses the atlanto-occipital joint and the joints of the neck anteriorly (with its fibers running vertically in the sagittal plane); therefore, it flexes the head at the atlanto-occipital joint and the neck at the cervical spinal joints.

LONGUS CAPITIS – continued

- ❑ **2. Lateral Flexion of the Head and the Neck at the Spinal Joints:** The longus capitis crosses the atlanto-occipital joint and the joints of the neck laterally (with its fibers running vertically in the frontal plane); therefore, it laterally flexes the head at the atlanto-occipital joint and the neck at the cervical spinal joints.

MISCELLANEOUS

- ❑ 1. The longus capitis and the longus colli, along with the rectus capitis anterior and the rectus capitis lateralis, are often grouped together and called the *prevertebral muscles.* (From an anterior perspective, they are just before, i.e., "pre," the vertebral column.)
- ❑ 2. The vertebral attachments of the longus capitis are variable; the longus capitis often attaches to C6.
- ❑ 3. Some sources state that the longus capitis is capable of rotating the head and the neck. Given the fiber direction of the longus capitis, it would seem likely that the line of pull would cause contralateral rotation of the head and the neck.
- ❑ 4. The prevertebral muscles are important for fixating (stabilizing) the neck and the head while talking, swallowing, coughing and sneezing. The prevertebral muscles also fixate the neck during rapid arm movements.
- ❑ 5. All the activities listed in miscellaneous #4 can exacerbate deep anterior neck pain in people who have had a whiplash injury.

RECTUS CAPITIS ANTERIOR

(OF THE PREVERTEBRAL GROUP)

❑ **The name, rectus capitis anterior, tells us that the fibers of this muscle run straight and attach to the head anteriorly.**

DERIVATION ❑ rectus: L. *straight.*
capitis: L. *refers to the head.*
anterior: L. *before, in front of.*

PRONUNCIATION ❑ **rek**-tus **kap**-i-tis an-**tee**-ri-or

ATTACHMENTS

❑ **The Atlas (C1)**

❑ the anterior surface of the base of the T.P.

to the

❑ **Occiput**

❑ the inferior surface of the basilar part of the occiput (just anterior to the foramen magnum)

ACTION

❑ **Flexion of the Head**

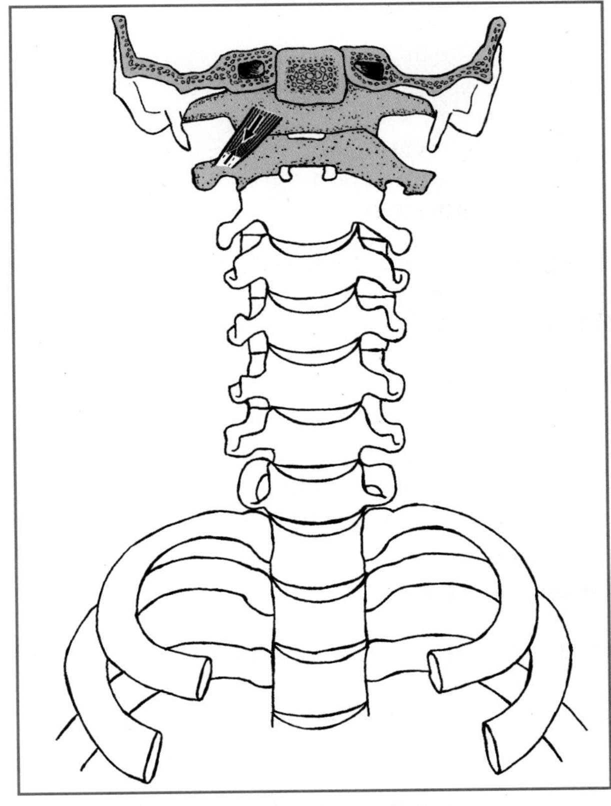

Anterior View of the Right Rectus Capitis Anterior

INNERVATION ❑ Cervical Spinal Nerves ❑ ventral rami; C1-2

ARTERIAL SUPPLY ❑ The Vertebral Artery (A Branch of the Subclavian Artery)

RECTUS CAPITIS ANTERIOR – PALPATION AND SUPPLEMENTARY TEXT

PALPATION

❑ The rectus capitis anterior is located very deep in the anterior neck between the atlas (C1) and the occiput and is not palpable.

RELATIONSHIP TO OTHER MUSCULOSKELETAL STRUCTURES

❑ 1. The rectus capitis anterior is very deep in the anterior neck.

❑ 2. Directly superficial to the rectus capitis anterior is the longus capitis.

❑ 3. The attachment of the rectus capitis anterior on the atlas (C1) is directly medial to the attachment of the rectus capitis lateralis on the atlas. From the atlas attachments, the rectus capitis anterior runs superiorly and medially to attach onto the occiput, whereas the rectus capitis lateralis runs superiorly and slightly laterally to attach onto the occiput.

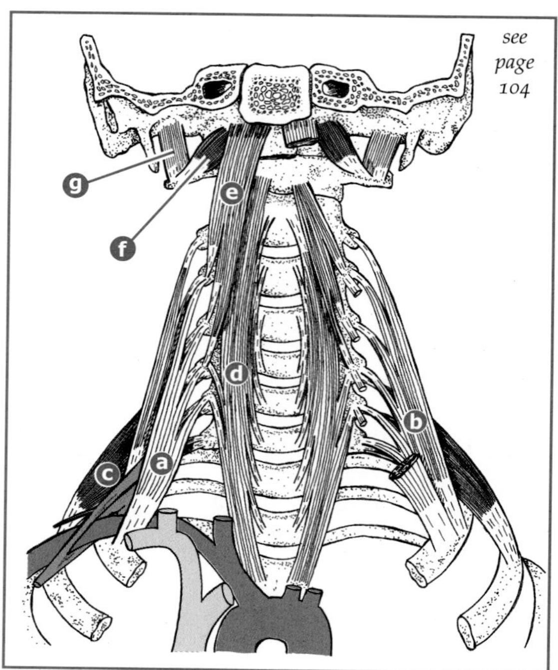

see page 104

Anterior View of the Neck (Deep)

a. Anterior Scalene (cut on our right)
b. Middle Scalene
c. Posterior Scalene
d. Longus Colli
e. Longus Capitis (cut on our right)
f. **Rectus Capitis Anterior**
g. Rectus Capitis Lateralis

METHODOLOGY FOR LEARNING MUSCLE ACTIONS

❑ **Flexion of the Head at the Atlanto-Occipital Joint:** The rectus capitis anterior crosses the joint between the atlas (C1) and the occiput anteriorly (with its fibers running vertically in the sagittal plane); therefore, it flexes the head upon the atlas at the atlanto-occipital joint.

MISCELLANEOUS

❑ 1. The rectus capitis anterior and the rectus capitis lateralis, along with the longus colli and the longus capitis, are often grouped together and called the *prevertebral muscles.* (From an anterior perspective, they are just before, i.e., "pre," the vertebral column.)

❑ 2. In addition to the rectus capitis anterior, there is also a rectus capitis lateralis, as well as a rectus capitis posterior major and a rectus capitis posterior minor. These four muscles attach onto the occiput (hence, capitis).

❑ 3. The prevertebral muscles are important for fixating (stabilizing) the neck and the head while talking, swallowing, coughing and sneezing.

❑ 4. All the activities listed in miscellaneous #3 can exacerbate deep anterior neck pain in people who have had a whiplash injury.

❑ 5. Some sources state that the rectus capitis anterior can also ipsilaterally rotate the head at the atlanto-occipital joint.

RECTUS CAPITIS LATERALIS ❑

(OF THE PREVERTEBRAL GROUP)

❑ **The name, rectus capitis lateralis, tells us that the fibers of this muscle run straight and attach to the head laterally.**

DERIVATION ❑ rectus: L. *straight.*
capitis: L. *refers to the head.*
lateralis: L. *refers to the side.*

PRONUNCIATION ❑ **rek**-tus **kap**-i-tis la-ter-**a**-lis

ATTACHMENTS

❑ **The Atlas (C1)**

❑ the superior surface of the T.P.

to the

❑ **Occiput**

❑ the inferior surface of the jugular process of the occiput

ACTION

❑ **Lateral Flexion of the Head**

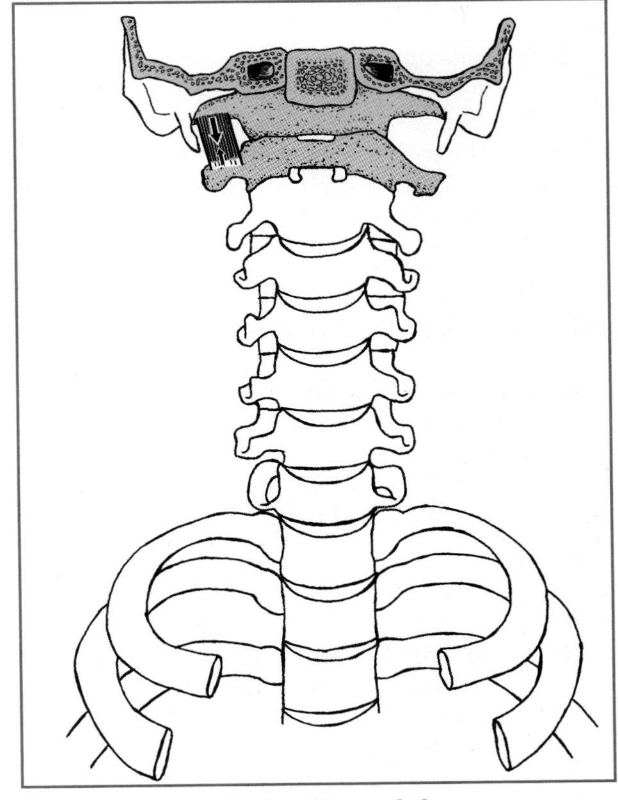

Anterior View of the Right Rectus Capitis Lateralis

INNERVATION ❑ Cervical Spinal Nerves ❑ ventral rami; C1-2

ARTERIAL SUPPLY ❑ The Vertebral Artery (A Branch of the Subclavian Artery) and the Occipital Artery (A Branch of the External Carotid Artery)

RECTUS CAPITIS LATERALIS PALPATION AND SUPPLEMENTARY TEXT

PALPATION

- ❑ The rectus capitis lateralis is located deep in the (antero)lateral neck between the atlas (C1) and the occiput and is difficult to palpate.
  - Have the client seated or supine.
  - Locate the T.P. of the atlas. To do this, first find the ramus of the mandible and palpate just posterior to it. (You should be anterior to the mastoid process of the temporal bone and inferior to the ear.)
  - Now feel for the T.P. of the atlas. (It is usually tender with pressure.)
  - Palpate superiorly to the T.P. of the atlas and a bit deeper and feel for the rectus capitis lateralis. Distinguishing its muscle belly from the adjacent musculature can be difficult.

    (Note: Very close to this region is the styloid process of the temporal bone. Care must be taken to not use too much pressure because the styloid process is a delicate structure.)

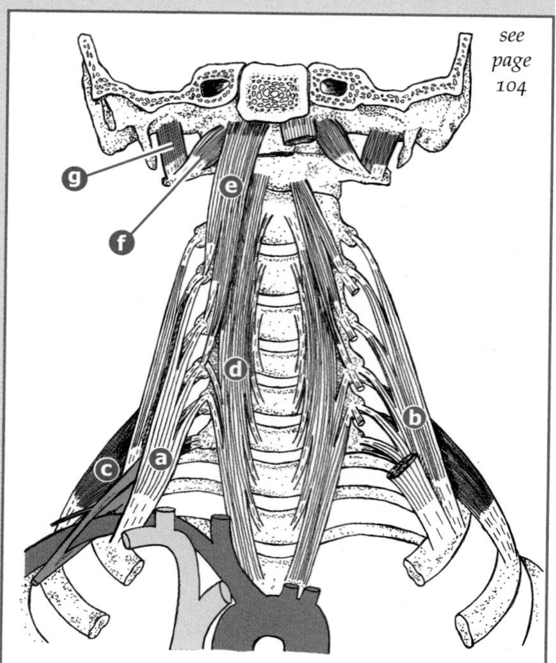

see page 104

Anterior View of the Neck (Deep)

a. Anterior Scalene (cut on our right)
b. Middle Scalene
c. Posterior Scalene
d. Longus Colli
e. Longus Capitis (cut on our right)
f. Rectus Capitis Anterior
g. **Rectus Capitis Lateralis**

RELATIONSHIP TO OTHER MUSCULOSKELETAL STRUCTURES

❑ 1. The rectus capitis lateralis is deep in the (antero)lateral neck.

❑ 2. The attachment of the rectus capitis lateralis on the atlas is directly lateral to the attachment of the rectus capitis anterior on the atlas. From the atlas attachments, the rectus capitis lateralis runs superiorly and slightly laterally to attach onto the occiput, whereas the rectus capitis anterior runs superiorly and medially to attach onto the occiput.

❑ 3. From a lateral perspective, the styloid process of the temporal bone is superficial to the rectus capitis lateralis.

METHODOLOGY FOR LEARNING MUSCLE ACTIONS

❑ **Lateral Flexion of the Head at the Atlanto-Occipital Joint:** The rectus capitis lateralis crosses the joint between the atlas (C1) and the occiput laterally (with its fibers running vertically in the frontal plane); therefore, it laterally flexes the head upon the atlas at the atlanto-occipital joint.

RECTUS CAPITIS LATERALIS – continued

MISCELLANEOUS

- ❑ 1. The rectus capitis lateralis and the rectus capitis anterior, along with the longus colli and the longus capitis, are often grouped together and called the *prevertebral muscles.* (From an anterior perspective, they are just before, i.e., "pre," the vertebral column.)
- ❑ 2. In addition to the rectus capitis lateralis, there is also a rectus capitis anterior, as well as a rectus capitis posterior major and a rectus capitis posterior minor. These four muscles attach onto the occiput (hence, capitis).
- ❑ 3. The prevertebral muscles are important for fixating (stabilizing) the neck and the head while talking, swallowing, coughing and sneezing.
- ❑ 4. All the activities listed in miscellaneous #3 can exacerbate deep anterior neck pain in people who have had a whiplash injury.
- ❑ 5. The rectus capitis lateralis muscles are considered to be homologous to the posterior intertransversarii muscles of the spine.

MUSCLES OF THE TRUNK

OVERVIEW OF THE MUSCLES OF THE TRUNK

ANATOMICALLY, THE MUSCLES OF THE TRUCK CAN BE DIVIDED INTO TWO MAJOR GROUPS:

The Posterior Trunk:

Superficial

- Latissimus Dorsi

Intermediate

- Rhomboids
- Serratus Anterior
- Serratus Posterior Superior
- Serratus Posterior Inferior

Deep

- Erector Spinae Group
- Transversospinalis Group
- Interspinales
- Intertransversarii
- Levatores Costarum
- Subcostales
- Quadratus Lumborum

The Anterior Trunk:

Muscles of the Chest

- Pectoralis Major
- Pectoralis Minor
- Subclavius
- External Intercostals
- Internal Intercostals
- Transversus Thoracis

Abdomen

Muscles of the Anterior Abdominal Wall

  - Rectus Abdominis
  - External Abdominal Oblique
  - Internal Abdominal Oblique
  - Transversus Abdominis
- Diaphragm

THE FOLLOWING MUSCLES ARE COVERED IN OTHER CHAPTERS OF THIS BOOK, BUT ARE ALSO PRESENT IN THE TRUNK:

Attaching from the trunk to the neck and/or head:

- Trapezius
- Splenius Capitis
- Splenius Cervicis
- Levator Scapulae
- Platysma

Attaching from the trunk to the pelvis and/or thigh:

- Psoas Major
- Psoas Minor

Attaching from the scapula to the arm and/or forearm:

- Supraspinatus
- Infraspinatus
- Teres Minor
- Subscapularis
- Teres Major
- Deltoid
- Coracobrachialis
- Biceps Brachii
- Triceps Brachii

Functionally, the muscles of the trunk cross spinal joints. Therefore, muscles of the trunk have their actions at these joints. The following general rules regarding actions can be stated for the muscles of the trunk:

► If a muscle crosses the trunk posteriorly, it can extend the trunk at the spinal joints.

- If a muscle crosses the trunk anteriorly, it can flex the trunk at the spinal joints.
- If a muscle crosses the trunk laterally on the right side, it can right laterally flex the trunk at the spinal joints.
- If a muscle crosses the trunk laterally on the left side, it can left laterally flex the trunk at the spinal joints.
- If a muscle wraps around the trunk, it can rotate the trunk at the spinal joints.
- Some of the muscles of the trunk considered here also cross the cervical spinal joints and/or the atlanto-occipital joint and can therefore move the neck and/or the head at these joints.

Some muscles of the trunk cross the lumbosacral joint to attach onto the pelvis. Therefore, these muscles can move the pelvis at the lumbosacral joint. The following general rules regarding actions can be stated for the muscles of the trunk that attach onto the pelvis:

- The spinal extensor muscles can anteriorly tilt the pelvis at the lumbosacral joint.
- The spinal flexor muscles can posteriorly tilt the pelvis at the lumbosacral joint.
- The spinal lateral flexor muscles can elevate the pelvis at the lumbosacral joint (on the side where they are located).
- The spinal rotator muscles can rotate the pelvis at the lumbosacral joint (in the direction opposite to how they rotate the trunk).
- All the muscles of the anterior abdominal wall can also compress the abdominal contents. Compression of the abdominal contents plays an important role in expiration and expulsion of abdominal contents (e.g., vomiting, expulsion of feces from the intestines and urine from the bladder).

Innervation and arterial supply of the trunk muscles are varied so it is difficult to state one generalization. The following should be noted:

INNERVATION

- Many of the deeper posterior trunk muscles are innervated by short unnamed branches of spinal nerves.

♥ ARTERIAL SUPPLY

- Many of the deeper posterior trunk muscles are supplied by branches directly off the aorta.

A NOTE REGARDING REVERSE ACTIONS

As a rule, this book does not employ the terms "origin" and "insertion." However, it is useful to utilize these terms to describe the concept of "reverse actions." The action section of this book describes the action of a muscle by stating the movement of a body part that is created by a muscle's contraction. The body part that usually moves when a muscle contracts is called the insertion. The methodology section further states at which joint the movement of the insertion occurs. However, the other body part that the muscle attaches to, the origin, can also move at that joint. *This movement can be called the reverse action of the muscle.* Keep in mind that the reverse action of a muscle is always possible. The likelihood that a reverse action will occur is based upon the ability of the insertion to be fixed so that the origin moves (instead of the insertion moving) when the muscle contracts. For more information and examples of reverse actions, see page 702.

❑ ANTERIOR VIEW OF THE BONES AND BONY LANDMARKS OF THE TRUNK

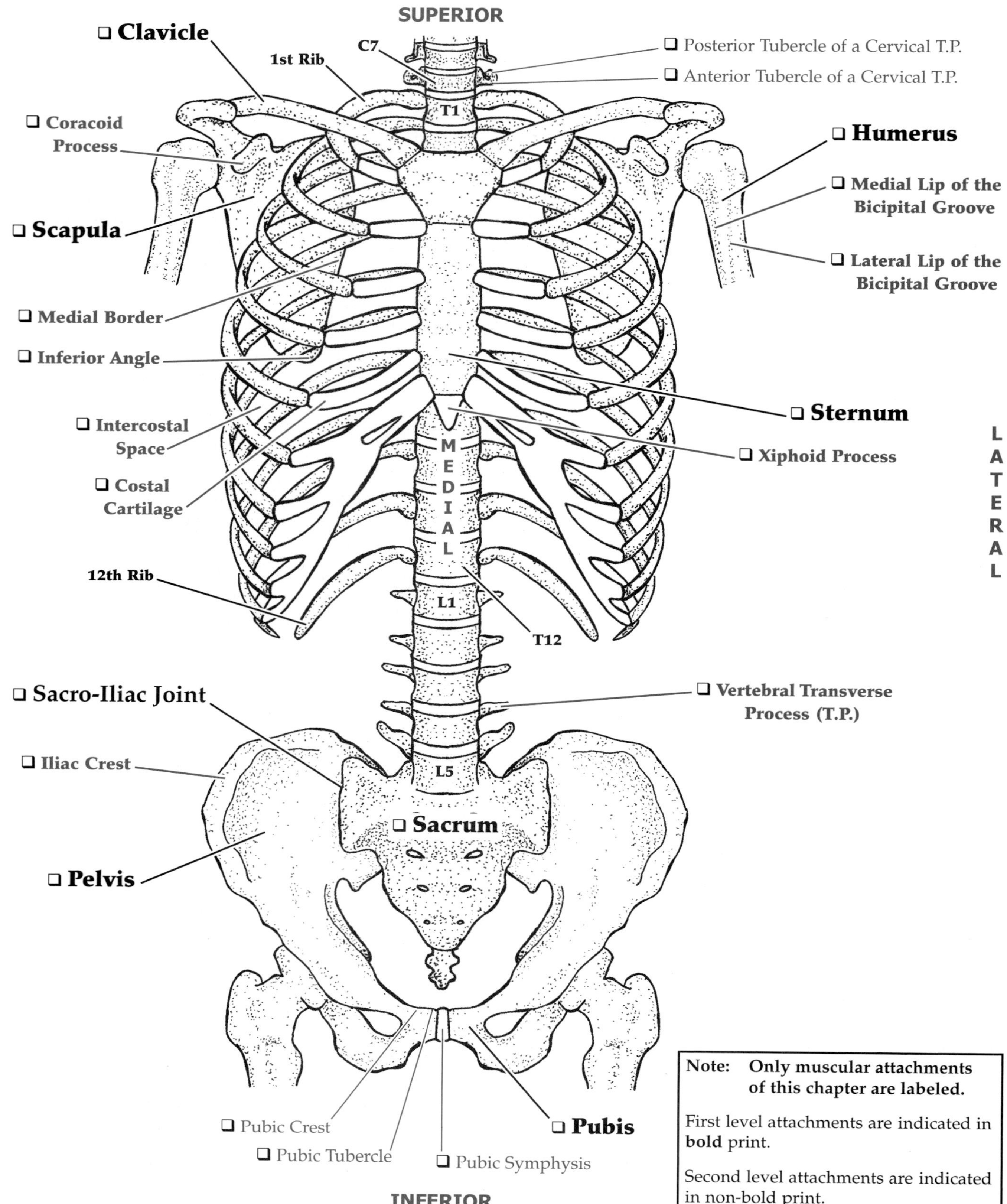

Note: **Only muscular attachments of this chapter are labeled.**

First level attachments are indicated in **bold** print.

Second level attachments are indicated in non-bold print.

ANTERIOR VIEW OF THE BONY ATTACHMENTS OF THE TRUNK

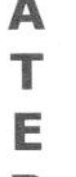

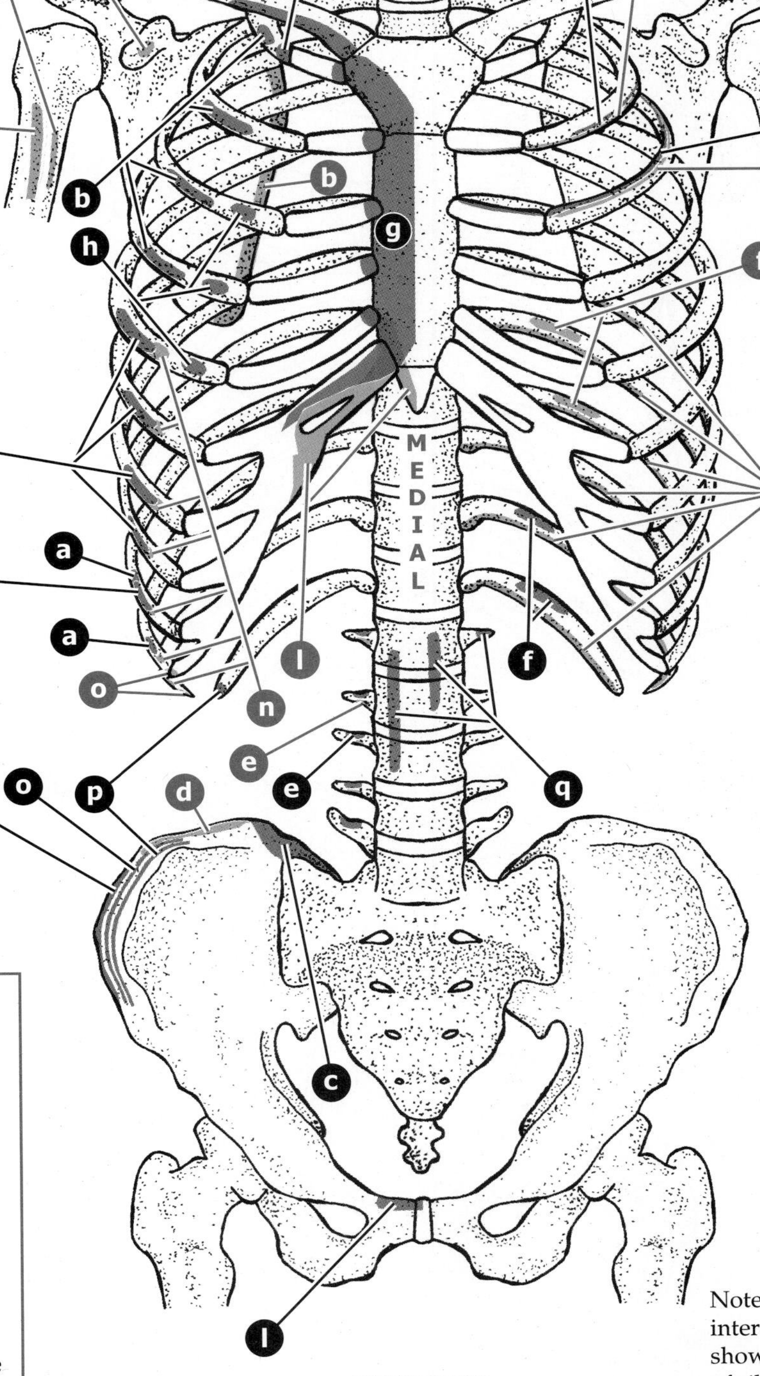

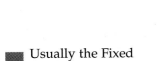

Usually the Fixed Attachment (Origin)

Usually the Mobile Attachment (Insertion)

- a. **Latissimus Dorsi**
- b. **Serratus Anterior**
- c. **Erector Spinae Group**
- d. **Quadratus Lumborum**
- e. **Intertransversarii**
- f. **Subcostales**
- g. **Pectoralis Major**
- h. **Pectoralis Minor**
- i. **Subclavius**
- j. **External Intercostals**
- k. **Internal Intercostals**
- l. **Rectus Abdominis**
- m. **Levatores Costarum**
- n. **External Abdominal Oblique**
- o. **Internal Abdominal Oblique**
- p. **Transversus Abdominis**
- q. **Diaphragm**

Note: The attachments of the intercostal muscles are only shown in the intercostal space of ribs 2-3 on our right. This pattern of attachments exists in all the intercostal spaces.

POSTERIOR VIEW OF THE BONES AND BONY LANDMARKS OF THE TRUNK

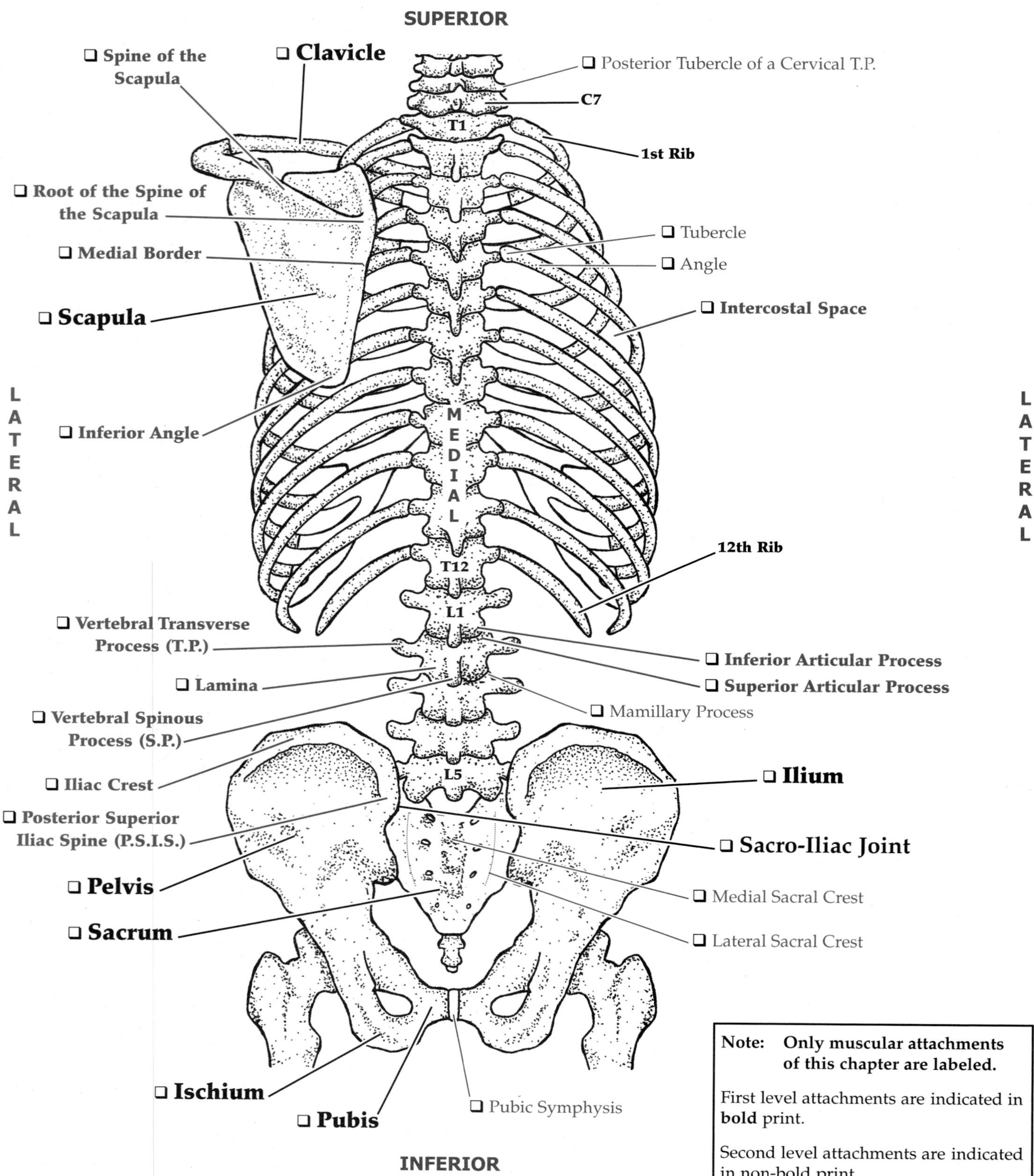

Note: **Only muscular attachments of this chapter are labeled.**

First level attachments are indicated in **bold** print.

Second level attachments are indicated in non-bold print.

POSTERIOR VIEW OF THE BONY ATTACHMENTS OF THE TRUNK

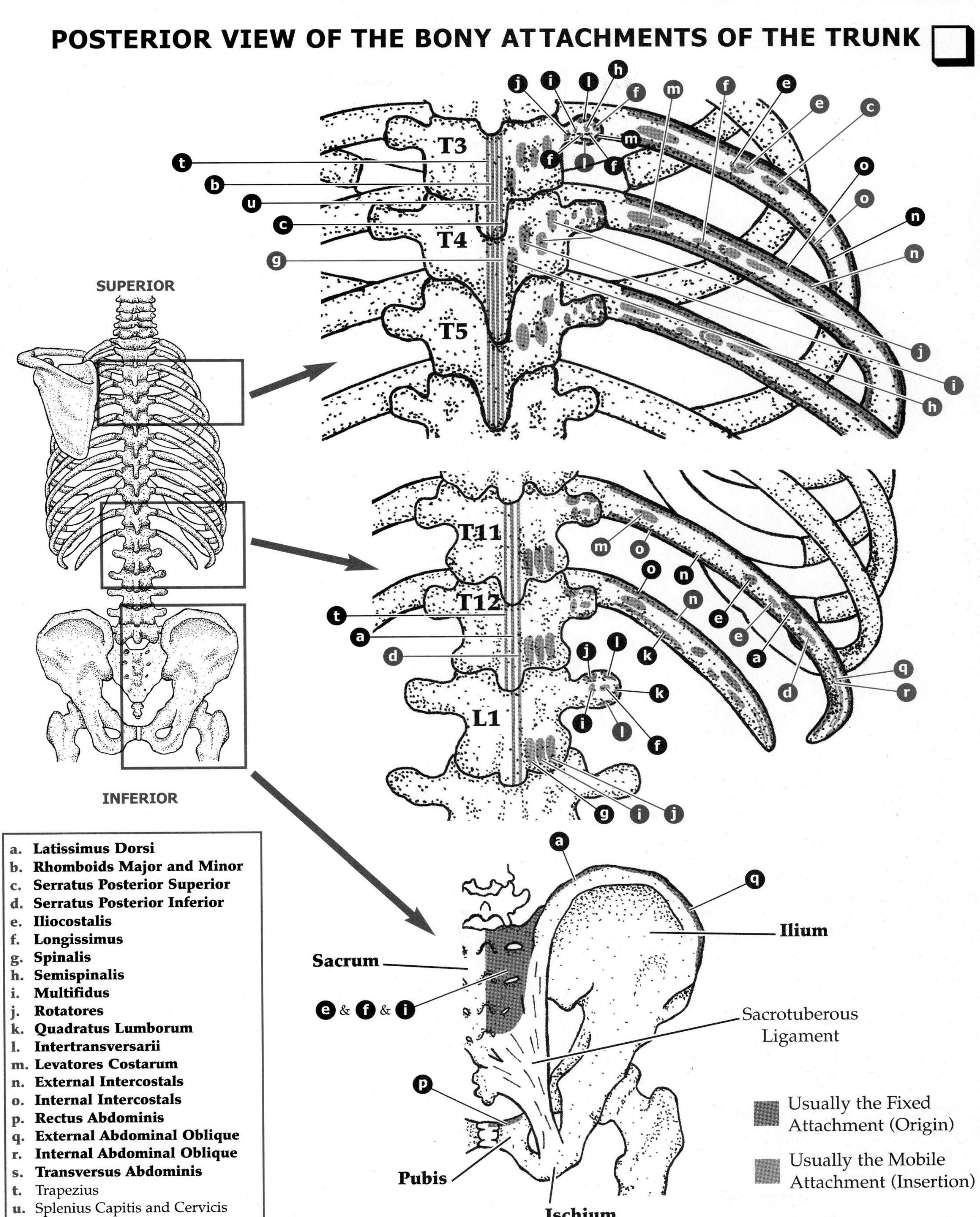

- a. **Latissimus Dorsi**
- b. **Rhomboids Major and Minor**
- c. **Serratus Posterior Superior**
- d. **Serratus Posterior Inferior**
- e. **Iliocostalis**
- f. **Longissimus**
- g. **Spinalis**
- h. **Semispinalis**
- i. **Multifidus**
- j. **Rotatores**
- k. **Quadratus Lumborum**
- l. **Intertransversarii**
- m. **Levatores Costarum**
- n. **External Intercostals**
- o. **Internal Intercostals**
- p. **Rectus Abdominis**
- q. **External Abdominal Oblique**
- r. **Internal Abdominal Oblique**
- s. **Transversus Abdominis**
- t. Trapezius
- u. Splenius Capitis and Cervicis

POSTERIOR VIEW OF THE TRUNK (SUPERFICIAL AND INTERMEDIATE)

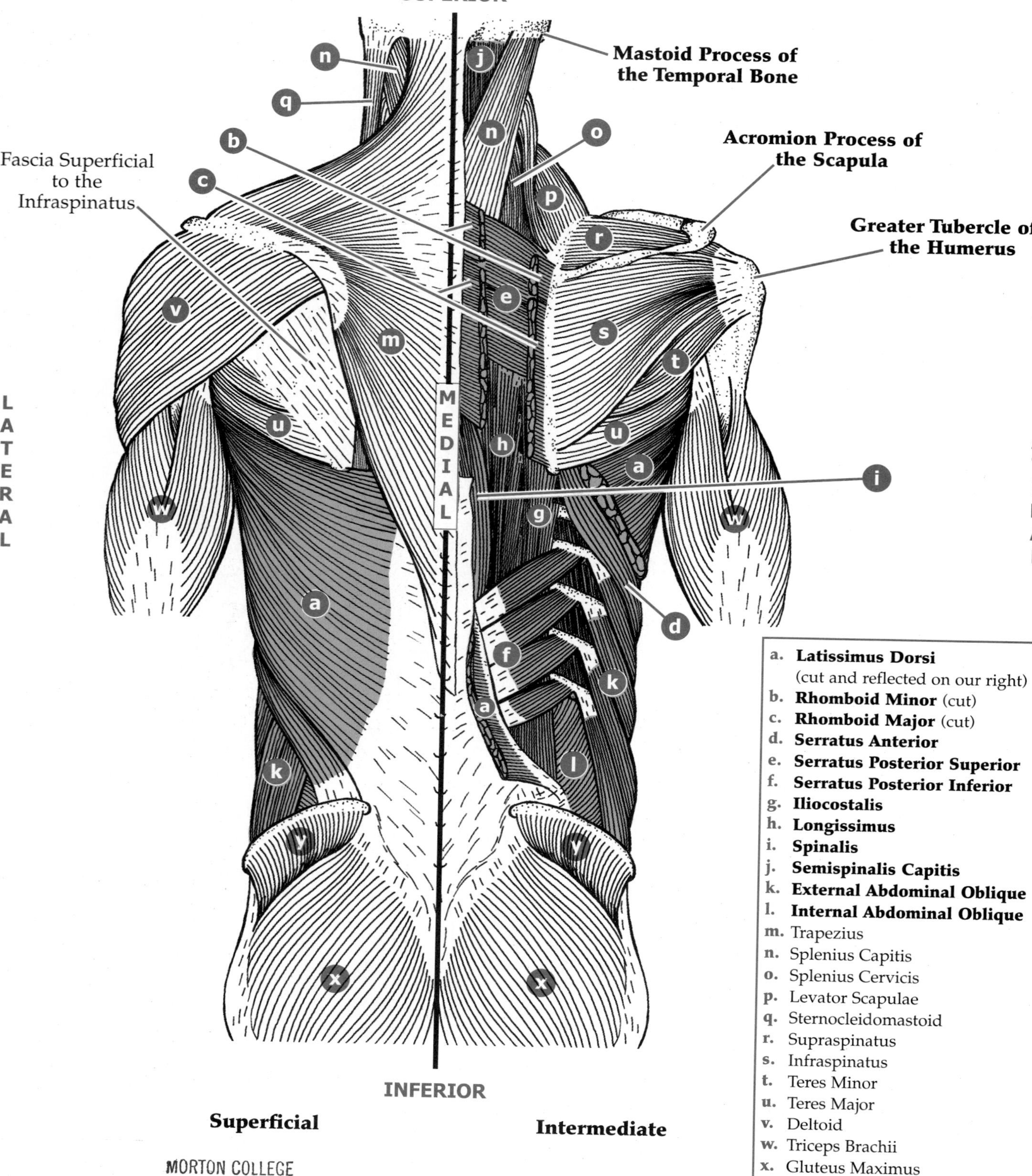
SUPERIOR
Mastoid Process of the Temporal Bone
Acromion Process of the Scapula
Greater Tubercle of the Humerus
Fascia Superficial to the Infraspinatus
LATERAL
MEDIAL
LATERAL
INFERIOR
Superficial
Intermediate
a. Latissimus Dorsi (cut and reflected on our right)
b. Rhomboid Minor (cut)
c. Rhomboid Major (cut)
d. Serratus Anterior
e. Serratus Posterior Superior
f. Serratus Posterior Inferior
g. Iliocostalis
h. Longissimus
i. Spinalis
j. Semispinalis Capitis
k. External Abdominal Oblique
l. Internal Abdominal Oblique
m. Trapezius
n. Splenius Capitis
o. Splenius Cervicis
p. Levator Scapulae
q. Sternocleidomastoid
r. Supraspinatus
s. Infraspinatus
t. Teres Minor
u. Teres Major
v. Deltoid
w. Triceps Brachii
x. Gluteus Maximus
y. Gluteus Medius

POSTERIOR VIEW OF THE TRUNK (DEEP LAYERS)

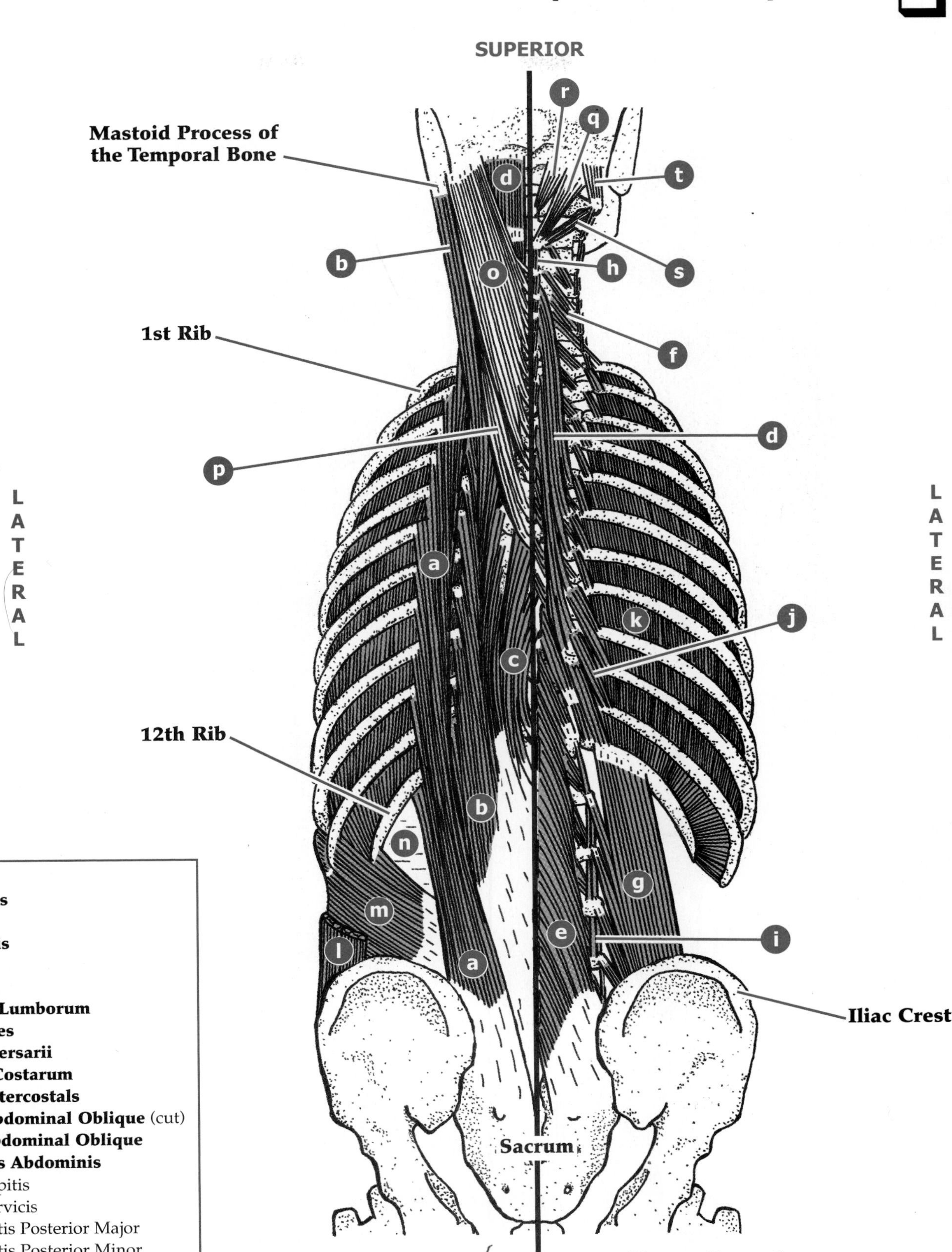

a. **Iliocostalis**
b. **Longissimus**
c. **Spinalis**
d. **Semispinalis**
e. **Multifidus**
f. **Rotatores**
g. **Quadratus Lumborum**
h. **Interspinales**
i. **Intertransversarii**
j. **Levatores Costarum**
k. **External Intercostals**
l. **External Abdominal Oblique** (cut)
m. **Internal Abdominal Oblique**
n. **Transversus Abdominis**
o. Splenius Capitis
p. Splenius Cervicis
q. Rectus Capitis Posterior Major
r. Rectus Capitis Posterior Minor
s. Obliquus Capitis Inferior
t. Obliquus Capitis Superior

ANTERIOR VIEW OF THE TRUNK (SUPERFICIAL AND INTERMEDIATE)

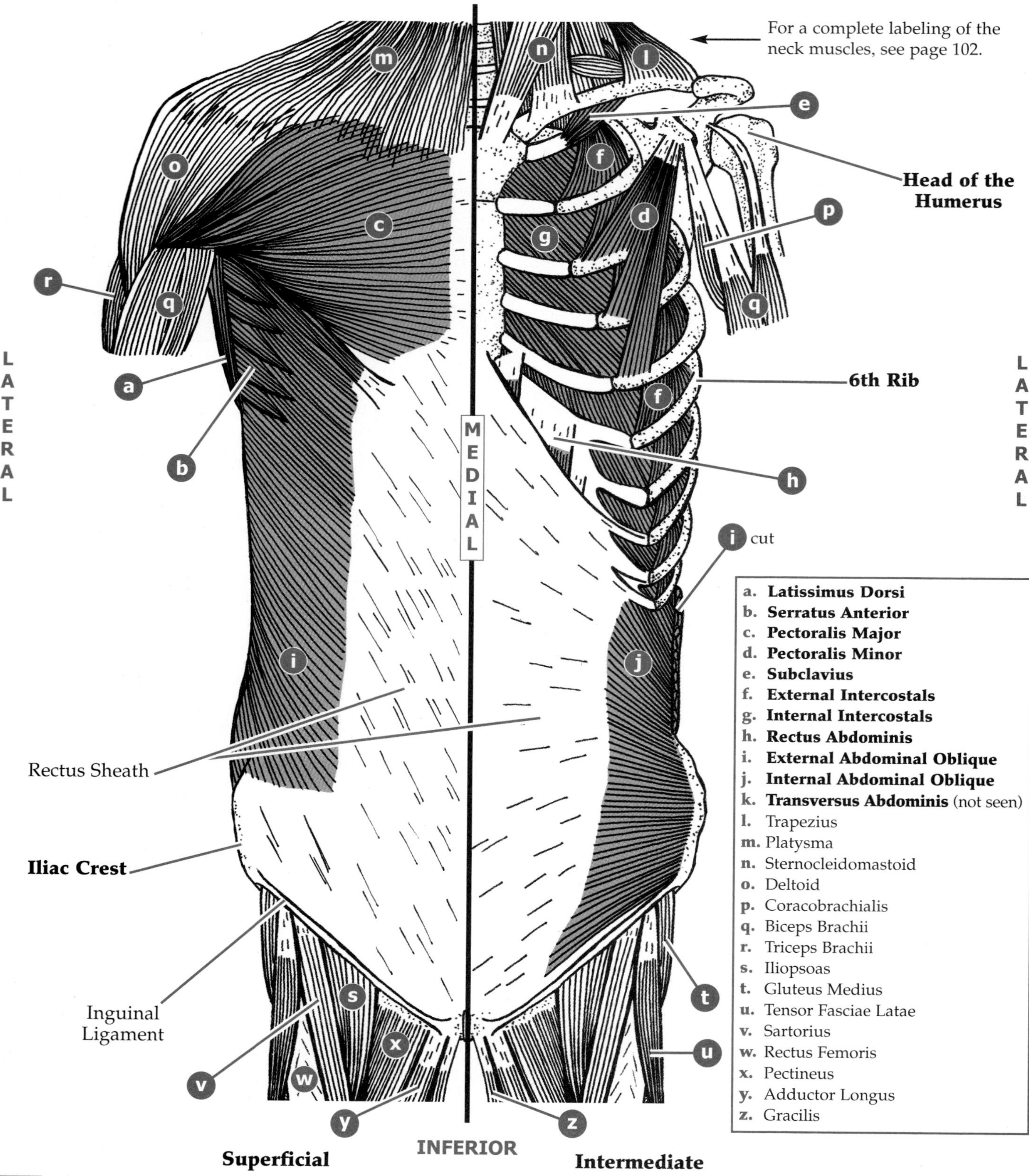

a. **Latissimus Dorsi**
b. **Serratus Anterior**
c. **Pectoralis Major**
d. **Pectoralis Minor**
e. **Subclavius**
f. **External Intercostals**
g. **Internal Intercostals**
h. **Rectus Abdominis**
i. **External Abdominal Oblique**
j. **Internal Abdominal Oblique**
k. **Transversus Abdominis** (not seen)
l. Trapezius
m. Platysma
n. Sternocleidomastoid
o. Deltoid
p. Coracobrachialis
q. Biceps Brachii
r. Triceps Brachii
s. Iliopsoas
t. Gluteus Medius
u. Tensor Fasciae Latae
v. Sartorius
w. Rectus Femoris
x. Pectineus
y. Adductor Longus
z. Gracilis

ANTERIOR VIEW OF THE TRUNK (INTERMEDIATE AND DEEP)

a. **Latissimus Dorsi** (not seen)
b. **Serratus Anterior** (not seen)
c. **Pectoralis Major** (not seen)
d. **Pectoralis Minor**
e. **Subclavius**
f. **External Intercostals**
g. **Internal Intercostals**
h. **Rectus Abdominis**
i. **External Abdominal Oblique**
j. **Internal Abdominal Oblique**
k. **Transversus Abdominis**
l. Trapezius
m. Platysma (not seen)
n. Sternocleidomastoid
o. Deltoid (not seen)
p. Coracobrachialis
q. Biceps Brachii
r. Triceps Brachii (not seen)
s. Iliopsoas
t. Gluteus Medius
u. Tensor Fasciae Latae
v. Sartorius
w. Rectus Femoris
x. Pectineus
y. Adductor Longus
z. Gracilis

LATERAL VIEW OF THE TRUNK

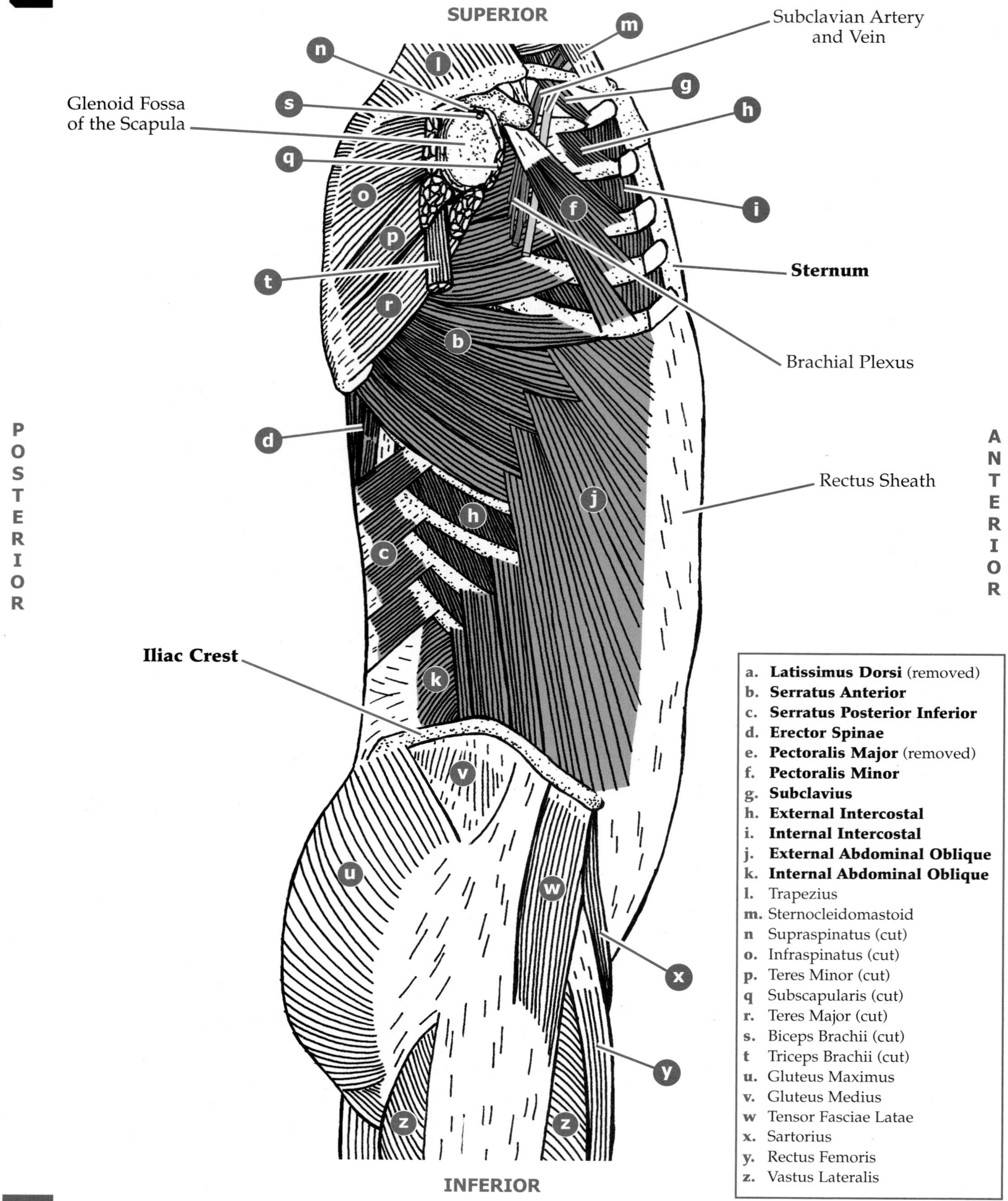

SUPERIOR

Subclavian Artery and Vein

Glenoid Fossa of the Scapula

Sternum

Brachial Plexus

POSTERIOR

ANTERIOR

Rectus Sheath

Iliac Crest

INFERIOR

- a. **Latissimus Dorsi** (removed)
- b. **Serratus Anterior**
- c. **Serratus Posterior Inferior**
- d. **Erector Spinae**
- e. **Pectoralis Major** (removed)
- f. **Pectoralis Minor**
- g. **Subclavius**
- h. **External Intercostal**
- i. **Internal Intercostal**
- j. **External Abdominal Oblique**
- k. **Internal Abdominal Oblique**
- l. Trapezius
- m. Sternocleidomastoid
- n Supraspinatus (cut)
- o. Infraspinatus (cut)
- p. Teres Minor (cut)
- q Subscapularis (cut)
- r. Teres Major (cut)
- s. Biceps Brachii (cut)
- t Triceps Brachii (cut)
- u. Gluteus Maximus
- v. Gluteus Medius
- w Tensor Fasciae Latae
- x. Sartorius
- y. Rectus Femoris
- z. Vastus Lateralis

CROSS SECTION VIEWS OF THE TRUNK

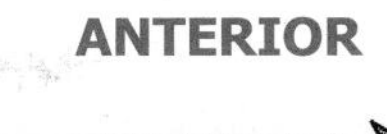

Thoracic Cross Section

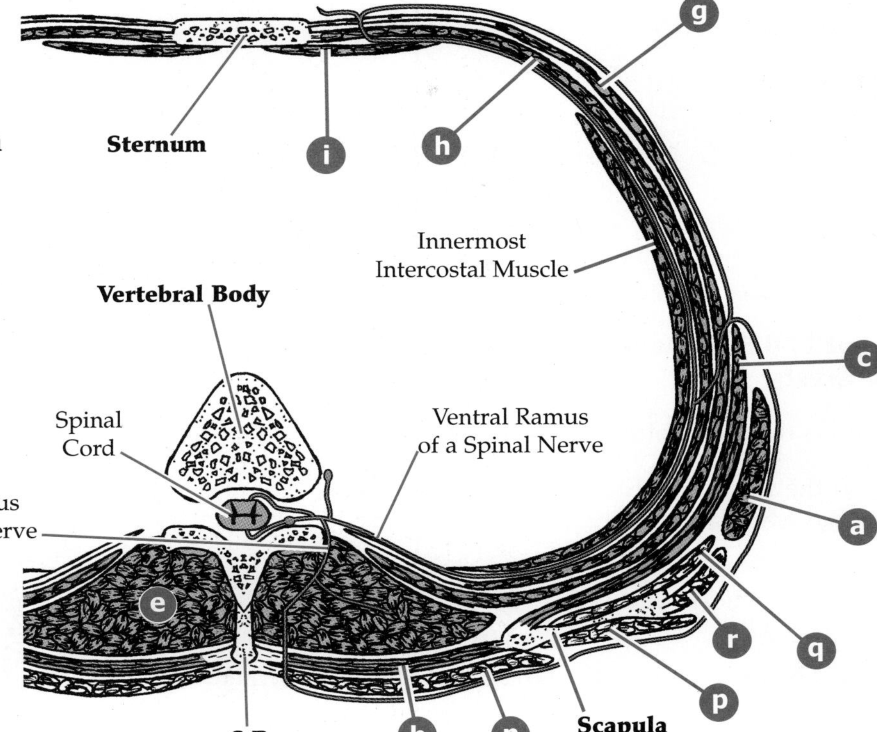

- **a. Latissimus Dorsi**
- **b. Rhomboid Major**
- **c. Serratus Anterior**
- **d. Serratus Posterior Inferior**
- **e. Erector Spinae Group**
- **f. Quadratus Lumborum**
- **g. External Intercostal**
- **h. Internal Intercostal**
- **i. Transversus Thoracis**
- **j. External Abdominal Oblique**
- **k. Internal Abdominal Oblique**
- **l. Transversus Abdominis**
- **m. Diaphragm (crura)**
- **n.** Trapezius
- **o.** Psoas Major
- **p.** Infraspinatus
- **q.** Subscapularis
- **r.** Teres Major

Lumbar Cross Section

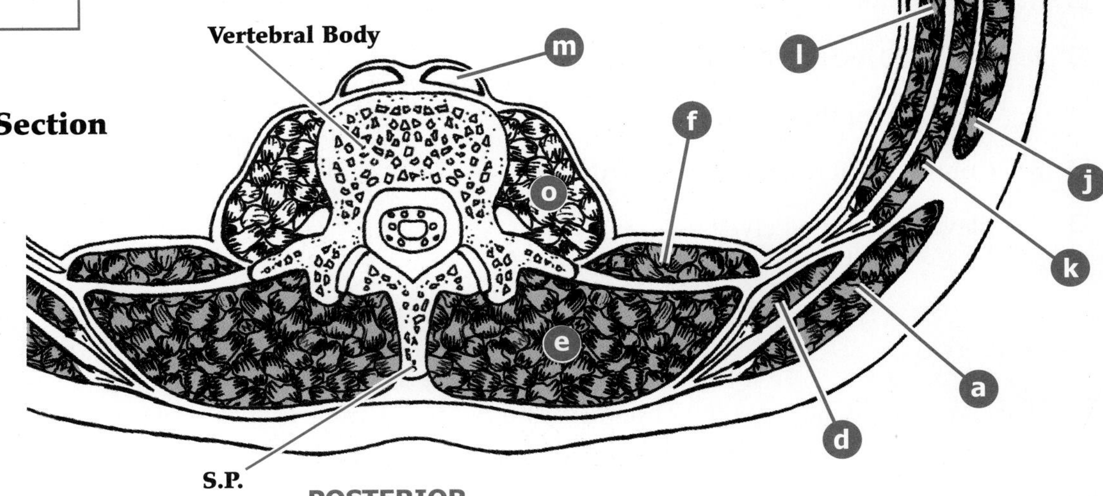

❑ LATISSIMUS DORSI (THE "LATS")

❑ **The name, latissimus dorsi, tells us that this muscle is a wide muscle of the back.**

DERIVATION ❑ latissimus: L. *wide.*
dorsi: L. *back.*

PRONUNCIATION ❑ la-**tis**-i-mus **door**-si

ATTACHMENTS

❑ **S.P.s of T7-L5, Posterior Sacrum, Posterior Iliac Crest**

- ❑ all via the thoracolumbar fascia
- ❑ and the lowest 3-4 ribs and the inferior angle of the scapula

to the

❑ **Medial Lip of the Bicipital Groove of the Humerus**

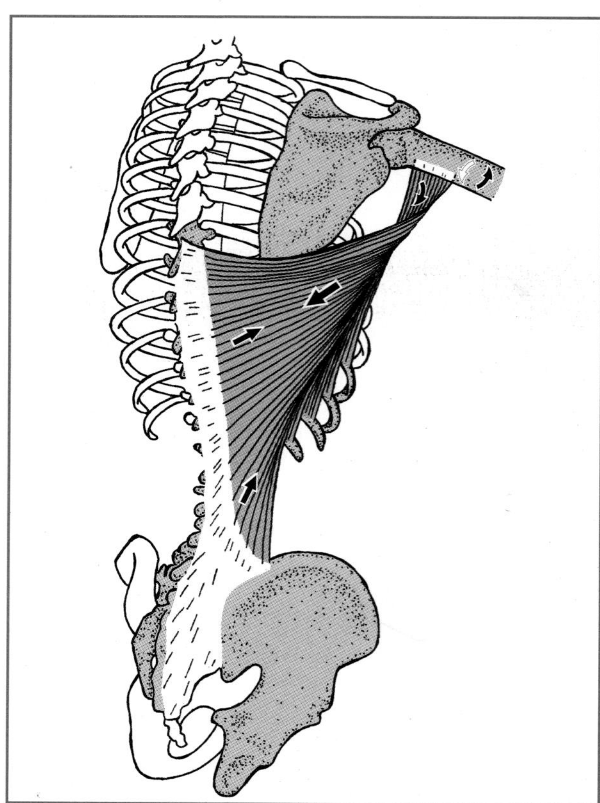

Posterolateral View of the Right Latissimus Dorsi

ACTIONS

❑ 1. **Medial Rotation of the Arm**

❑ 2. **Adduction of the Arm**

❑ 3. **Extension of the Arm**

❑ 4. **Anterior Tilt of the Pelvis**

❑ 5. Depression of the Scapula

❑ 6. Lateral Deviation of the Trunk

❑ 7. Elevation of the Trunk

❑ 8. Contralateral Rotation of the Trunk

❑ 9. Elevation of the Pelvis

INNERVATION ❑ The Thoracodorsal Nerve ❑ C6, **7**, 8

ARTERIAL SUPPLY ❑ The Thoracodorsal Artery (A Branch of the Subscapular Artery) and the Dorsal Branches of the Posterior Intercostal Arteries (Branches of the Aorta)

PALPATION AND SUPPLEMENTARY TEXT

PALPATION

The majority of the latissimus dorsi is thin and sheet-like and therefore, difficult to distinguish from adjacent musculature. However, the muscle becomes thicker and easier to palpate as it nears the axilla (the armpit) where it makes up the majority of the posterior axillary fold of tissue.

❑ **Standing:**

- Both the client and therapist should be standing and facing each other.
- Have the client place his/her arm (or forearm) on your shoulder.
- Place palpating hand on the client's posterior axillary fold.
- Ask the client to attempt to adduct and extend the arm at the shoulder joint (your body providing resistance to these actions) and feel for the contraction of the latissimus dorsi.
- Continue palpating the latissimus dorsi distally toward the humeral attachment. (Be careful with palpation in this region because the brachial plexus of nerves and brachial artery are superficial here.)
- It can be difficult to distinguish the tendon of the latissimus dorsi from the tendon of the teres major because they often blend together.

❑ **Seated:**

- Have the client seated with the hands at the sides.
- Place palpating hand on the client's posterior axillary fold.
- Ask the client to push down on the table with both hands, attempting to elevate the pelvis and trunk off the table, and feel for the contraction of the latissimus dorsi.
- Continue palpating the latissimus dorsi distally toward the humeral attachment. (Be careful with palpation in this region because the brachial plexus of nerves and brachial artery are superficial here.)
- It can be difficult to distinguish the tendon of the latissimus dorsi from the tendon of the teres major because they often blend together.

see page 200

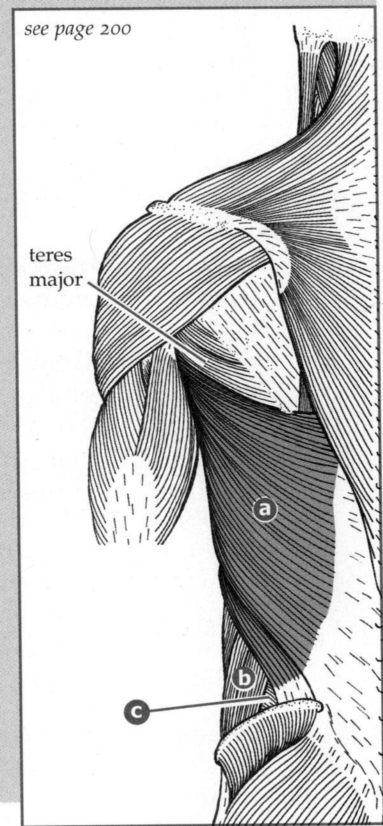

Posterior View of the Trunk

a. Latissimus Dorsi
b. External Abdominal Oblique
c. Internal Abdominal Oblique

RELATIONSHIP TO OTHER MUSCULOSKELETAL STRUCTURES

❑ 1. The latissimus dorsi is superficial except for a small portion that is deep to the lower trapezius.

❑ 2. The distal tendon of the latissimus dorsi runs parallel to the distal tendon of the teres major.

LATISSIMUS DORSI ("THE LATS") – continued

- ❑ 3. The teres major and the latissimus dorsi both attach onto the medial lip of the bicipital groove of the humerus. On the medial lip, the latissimus dorsi attaches more anteriorly, with the teres major attaching directly posterior to it.
- ❑ 4. The latissimus dorsi's attachments onto the ribs meet with and are approximately perpendicular to the external abdominal oblique's attachments onto the ribs (inferior to the interdigitation of the serratus anterior with the external abdominal oblique).
- ❑ 5. Deep to the latissimus dorsi in the lumbar region are the serratus posterior inferior, the most posterior attachments of the external and internal abdominal obliques, the erector spinae and the quadratus lumborum.
- ❑ 6. From the posterior perspective, the serratus anterior is deep to the latissimus dorsi in the axillary region.
- ❑ 7. From the anterior perspective, the humeral attachment of the latissimus dorsi is deep to the pectoralis major, the short head of the biceps brachii and the coracobrachialis.
- ❑ 8. The attachment of the distal tendon of the latissimus dorsi onto the humerus is between the teres major's humeral attachment (which is posterior to it) and the pectoralis major's humeral attachment (which is anterior to it). A saying to help one remember this is "The lady between two majors." The "Lady" (pronounce it like "Laty") refers to the latissimus dorsi; the two majors refer to the teres major and the pectoralis major.

METHODOLOGY FOR LEARNING MUSCLE ACTIONS

- ❑ **1. Medial Rotation of the Arm at the Shoulder Joint:** The latissimus dorsi crosses the shoulder joint from medial on the pelvis and trunk to lateral on the humerus (with its fibers oriented somewhat horizontally in the transverse plane). However, it does not attach onto the first aspect on the humerus that it reaches, but rather wraps around to the anterior side of the humerus to attach onto the medial lip of the bicipital groove of the humerus. When the latissimus dorsi contracts, it pulls the medial lip of the bicipital groove posteromedially, causing the anterior surface of the humerus to face medially. Therefore, the latissimus dorsi medially rotates the arm at the shoulder joint. (Note the similarity of the direction of fibers of the latissimus dorsi to the direction of fibers of the teres major.)
- ❑ **2. Adduction of the Arm at the Shoulder Joint:** The teres major crosses the shoulder joint posteriorly from medial on the trunk to lateral on the humerus (with fibers running horizontally in the frontal plane). Therefore, when the lateral attachment, the humerus, is pulled toward the medial attachment, the scapula, the humerus is pulled toward the midline. Therefore, the latissimus dorsi adducts the arm at the shoulder joint.
- ❑ **3. Extension of the Arm at the Shoulder Joint:** The latissimus dorsi crosses the shoulder joint posteriorly (with the fibers running vertically in the sagittal plane); therefore, it extends the arm at the shoulder joint.
- ❑ **4. Anterior Tilt of the Pelvis at the Lumbosacral Joint:** With the humeral attachment fixed, the latissimus dorsi, by pulling superiorly on the posterior pelvis, anteriorly tilts the pelvis at the lumbosacral joint.
- ❑ **5. Depression of the Scapula at the Scapulocostal Joint:** The latissimus dorsi attaches from inferiorly on the trunk to superiorly on the humerus (with its fibers running vertically). When the humerus is fixed to the scapula, and the latissimus dorsi contracts, it pulls the humerus and the scapula inferiorly. Therefore, when the humerus is fixed to the scapula, the latissimus dorsi depresses the scapula at the scapulocostal joint.

LATISSIMUS DORSI ("THE LATS") – continued

- ❑ **6. Lateral Deviation of the Trunk at the Shoulder Joint:** When the humeral attachment of the latissimus dorsi is fixed and the latissimus dorsi contracts, it pulls the trunk toward the humerus. This causes the trunk to move laterally toward the humerus (in the frontal plane since the fibers are running somewhat horizontally). Therefore, the latissimus dorsi laterally deviates the trunk at the shoulder joint. (Note: This movement of the trunk relative to the humerus at the shoulder joint requires the scapula to be fixed to the trunk.)
- ❑ **7. Elevation of the Trunk at the Shoulder Joint:** If the arm is first in an elevated position (whether it is flexed, extended, abducted or adducted) above the trunk and the humeral attachment of the latissimus dorsi is fixed, then, when the latissimus dorsi contracts, it pulls the trunk superiorly toward the humerus (since the fibers are running vertically). Therefore, the latissimus dorsi elevates the trunk at the shoulder joint. (Note: This movement of the trunk relative to the humerus at the shoulder joint requires the scapula to be fixed to the trunk.)
- ❑ **8. Contralateral Rotation of the Trunk at the Shoulder Joint:** When the humeral attachment of the latissimus dorsi is fixed and the latissimus dorsi contracts, it pulls the posterior trunk toward the humerus causing the anterior trunk to face the opposite side of the body from the side of the body that the latissimus dorsi is attached (since its fibers are running somewhat horizontally in the transverse plane). Therefore, the latissimus dorsi contralaterally rotates the trunk at the shoulder joint. (Note: This movement of the trunk relative to the humerus at the shoulder joint requires the scapula to be fixed to the trunk.)
- ❑ **9. Elevation of the Pelvis at the Lumbosacral Joint:** With the humeral attachment fixed, the latissimus dorsi, by pulling superiorly on the lateral pelvis (since the fibers are running vertically), elevates the pelvis at the lumbosacral joint.

MISCELLANEOUS

- ❑ 1. The fibers of the latissimus dorsi twist in such a way that the superior fibers attach distally on the humerus, and the inferior fibers attach proximally on the humerus.
- ❑ 2. The distal fibers of the pectoralis major also twist so that the superior fibers become most distal at the humeral attachment and the inferior fibers become most proximal at the humeral attachment.
- ❑ 3. The latissimus dorsi and the teres major make up the majority of the "posterior axillary fold" of tissue, which borders the axilla (armpit) posteriorly.
- ❑ 4. Sometimes the latissimus dorsi blends with the teres major.
- ❑ 5. The scapular attachment of the latissimus dorsi is often absent.
- ❑ 6. The spinal and pelvic attachments of the latissimus dorsi are all via the thoracolumbar fascia, a layer of fascia that covers the deeper muscles of the thoracic and lumbar regions. The thoracolumbar fascia is especially thick in the lumbar region, where it divides into three layers, investing and enveloping the deep muscles of the lumbar region and eventually attaching onto the posterior iliac crest and the S.P.s and T.P.s of the lumbar vertebrae.
- ❑ 7. Because the latissimus dorsi often has an attachment onto the inferior angle of the scapula, it can have the ability to act directly upon the scapula. When the trunk is fixed, the latissimus dorsi may depress, retract (adduct) and/or downwardly rotate the scapula at the scapulocostal joint. When the arm is fixed, the latissimus dorsi may elevate, protract (abduct) and/or upwardly rotate the scapula at the scapulocostal joint.

LATISSIMUS DORSI ("THE LATS") – continued

❑ 8. Scapular Tilt Actions: In addition to its other actions, the scapula can also tilt.

If the medial border of the scapula were to move away from the body wall, contraction of the latissimus dorsi would pull the medial border of the scapula back against the body wall. This movement of the medial border of the scapula moving toward the body wall is called medial tilt; therefore, the latissimus dorsi medially tilts the scapula at the scapulocostal joint.

If the inferior angle of the scapula were to move away from the body wall, contraction of the latissimus dorsi would pull the inferior angle of the scapula back against the body wall. This movement of the inferior angle of the scapula moving toward the body wall is called downward tilt; therefore, the latissimus dorsi downwardly tilts the scapula at the scapulocostal joint.

❑ 9. The latissimus dorsi does all three shoulder joint actions necessary to swim the "crawl" (freestyle stroke), namely, extension, adduction and medial rotation of the arm at the shoulder joint.

❑ 10. The teres major is sometimes called the *little brother* or the *little helper* of the latissimus dorsi because they run together between the scapula and the humerus, they attach together onto the medial lip of the bicipital groove of the humerus, and they have the same direction of muscle fibers and therefore, the same three actions of the arm at the shoulder joint (medial rotation, adduction and extension). However, perhaps a better name for the teres major would be the *fat little brother* or *fat little helper* because this muscle is extremely thick. ☺

❑ 11. To do a pull-up, elevation of the trunk must occur. The latissimus dorsi and the pectoralis major are particularly important for this action.

❑ 12. The latissimus dorsi is very important with respect to its function of elevating the pelvis and trunk superiorly toward the arm. For example, climbing utilizes this function. Also, a person in a wheelchair needs to use the latissimus dorsi by fixing the humeral attachment and contracting the latissimus dorsi to move the pelvis and trunk. Use of crutches similarly relies on the latissimus dorsi to move the pelvis and trunk. (Note: The pectoralis major also performs this action and assists with these movements.)

❑ 13. The latissimus dorsi and the pectoralis major are both large, powerful muscles that attach from the trunk to the arm. These two muscles are synergistic to each other with respect to their arm actions in that they both adduct and medially rotate the arm at the shoulder joint. However, they are antagonistic to each other with respect to their (sagittal plane) arm actions; the latissimus dorsi (being posterior) extends the arm at the shoulder joint, and the pectoralis major (being anterior) flexes the arm at the shoulder joint. (Note: Depending upon the position of the humerus, the pectoralis major can extend the arm at the shoulder joint, see methodology #4 of the pectoralis major on page 261.)

❑ 14. The latissimus dorsi and the pectoralis major are both large, powerful muscles that attach from the trunk to the arm. These two muscles are synergistic to each other with respect to their trunk actions in that they both elevate and laterally deviate the trunk at the shoulder joint. However, they are antagonistic to each other with respect to their trunk actions; the latissimus dorsi (being posterior) contralaterally rotates the trunk at the shoulder joint, and the pectoralis major (being anterior) ipsilaterally rotates the trunk at the shoulder joint.

RHOMBOIDS MAJOR AND MINOR

❑ **The name, rhomboids, tells us that these muscles have the geometric shape of a rhombus (a parallelogram or diamond shape). "Major" tells us that the rhomboid major is the larger muscle of the two; "minor" tells us that the rhomboid minor is smaller.**

DERIVATION ❑ rhomb: Gr. *rhombos* (the geometric shape).
oid: Gr. *shape, resemblance.*
major: L. *larger.*
minor: L. *smaller.*

PRONUNCIATION ❑ **rom**-boyd **may**-jor, **my**-nor

ATTACHMENTS

❑ **THE RHOMBOIDS: S.P.s of C7-T5**

- ❑ **MINOR:** S.P.s of C7-T1
  - ❑ and the inferior nuchal ligament
- ❑ **MAJOR:** S.P.s of T2-T5

to the

❑ **THE RHOMBOIDS: Medial Border of the Scapula from the Root of the Spine of the Scapula to the Inferior Angle of the Scapula**

- ❑ **MINOR:** at the Root of the Spine of the Scapula
- ❑ **MAJOR:** Between the Root of the Spine of the Scapula and the Inferior Angle of the Scapula

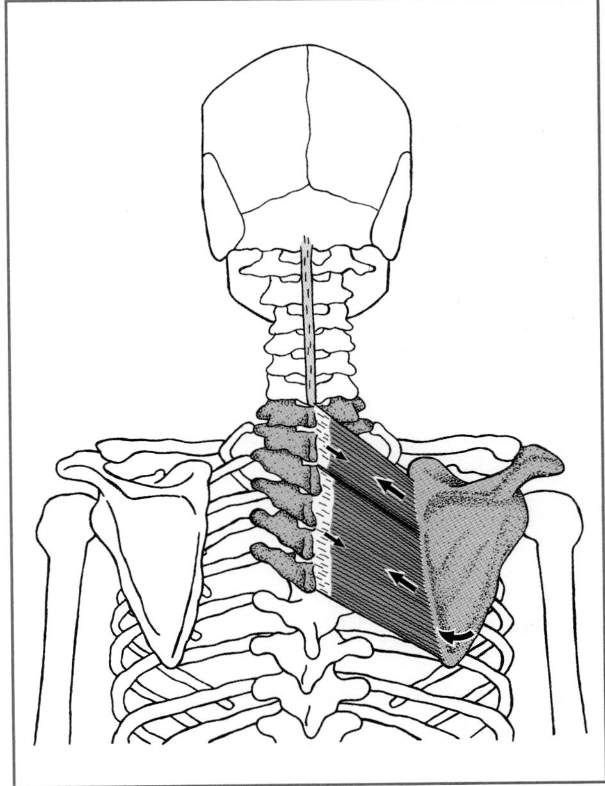

Posterior View of the Right Rhomboids Major and Minor

ACTIONS

❑ 1. **Retraction (Adduction) of the Scapula**

❑ 2. **Elevation of the Scapula**

❑ 3. Downward Rotation of the Scapula

❑ 4. Contralateral Rotation of the Trunk

INNERVATION ❑ The Dorsal Scapular Nerve ❑ C4, 5

ARTERIAL SUPPLY ❑ The Dorsal Scapular Artery (A Branch of the Subclavian Artery)

RHOMBOIDS MAJOR AND MINOR
PALPATION AND SUPPLEMENTARY TEXT

PALPATION

- ❑ The rhomboids are deep to the trapezius, but may be visible and are easily palpable if the trapezius is relaxed.
  - Have the client prone with a hand placed in the small of the back. (This action requires downward rotation of the scapula, an antagonistic action to the trapezius, which will cause it to relax.)
  - Place palpating hand between the scapula (at a level that is between the inferior angle and the root of the spine of the scapula) and the spine.
  - Ask the client to lift the hand away from the back and feel for the contraction of the rhomboids.

  Note the fiber direction running medially and superiorly from the scapula to the spine. Distinguishing the rhomboid minor from the rhomboid major can be very difficult.

see page 106

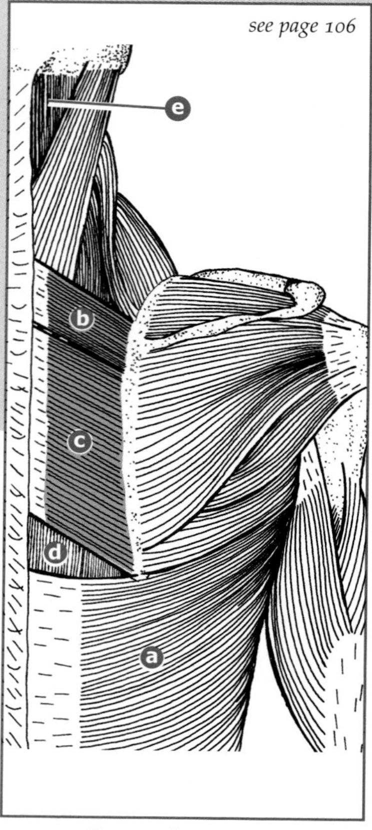

Posterior View of the Trunk

a. Latissimus Dorsi
b. **Rhomboid Minor**
c. **Rhomboid Major**
d. Erector Spinae
e. Semispinalis Capitis

RELATIONSHIP TO OTHER MUSCULOSKELETAL STRUCTURES

❑ 1. The rhomboids are deep to the trapezius.

❑ 2. The rhomboid minor is directly superior to the rhomboid major.

❑ 3. The rhomboid minor attaches onto the scapula, inferior to the levator scapulae's attachment onto the scapula.

❑ 4. Deep to the rhomboids are the splenius capitis, splenius cervicis, serratus posterior superior and the erector spinae.

METHODOLOGY FOR LEARNING MUSCLE ACTIONS

❑ 1. **Retraction (Adduction) of the Scapula at the Scapulocostal Joint:** The rhomboids attach from the spine medially, to the scapula laterally (with their fibers running somewhat horizontally in the frontal plane). When the rhomboids contract, they pull the scapula medially toward the spine; therefore, the rhomboids retract (adduct) the scapula at the scapulocostal joint.

❑ 2. **Elevation of the Scapula at the Scapulocostal Joint:** The rhomboids attach from the spine superiorly, to the scapula inferiorly (with their fibers running somewhat vertically). When the rhomboids contract, they pull the scapula superiorly toward the spine; therefore, the rhomboids elevate the scapula at the scapulocostal joint.

❑ 3. **Downward Rotation of the Scapula at the Scapulocostal Joint:** When the rhomboids contract, they pull on the scapula, causing the inferior angle of the scapula to swing up toward the spine. This will cause the glenoid fossa to orient downward; therefore, the rhomboids downwardly rotate the scapula at the scapulocostal joint.

RHOMBOIDS MAJOR AND MINOR – continued

❑ **4. Contralateral Rotation of the Trunk at the Spinal Joints:** When the scapula is fixed, and the rhomboids contract (with their fibers oriented somewhat horizontally in the transverse plane), they pull the spinous processes of the vertebrae toward the scapula, causing the anterior bodies of the vertebrae to face the opposite side of the body from the side of the body that the rhomboids are attached. Therefore, the rhomboids contralaterally rotate the trunk at the spinal joints.

MISCELLANEOUS

❑ 1. The rhomboids major and minor are considered together because they have identical fiber direction and, therefore, identical lines of pull and identical actions. (The rhomboid major is more powerful than the rhomboid minor at downward rotation of the scapula because its attachment on the scapula is more inferior. From there it has better leverage to rotate the scapula.)

❑ 2. There is usually a small interval of space between the two rhomboids, but sometimes there is not. These two muscles may even blend together.

❑ 3. **Scapular Tilt Actions:** In addition to its other actions, the scapula can also tilt. If the medial border of the scapula were to move away from the body wall, contraction of the rhomboids would pull the medial border of the scapula back against the body wall. This movement of the medial border of the scapula moving toward the body wall is called medial tilt and therefore, the rhomboids medially tilt the scapula at the scapulocostal joint.

❑ 4. The action of medial tilt of the scapula is particularly important when the scapula is protracted because the scapula tends to laterally tilt (wing out) when it protracts. Muscles that medially tilt the scapula keep the scapula from laterally tilting (winging out).

❑ 5. The rhomboid muscles are sometimes called the *Christmas Tree* muscles. When you look at the rhomboids bilaterally with the spinal column between them, they look like a Christmas tree in shape.

❑ 6. *Rounded Shoulders* is a common postural condition in which the scapulae are protracted (abducted) and depressed (at the scapulocostal joints) and the humeri are medially rotated (at the shoulder joints). Given the rhomboid's actions of both retraction and elevation of the scapula, when the rhomboid muscles are weak, they can contribute to this condition because they are unable to efficiently oppose protraction and depression of the scapulae. This is especially true if the protractors and/or depressors of the scapulae (often the pectoralis minor muscles) are tight.

❑ SERRATUS ANTERIOR

❑ **The name, serratus anterior, tells us that this muscle has a serrated appearance and is anterior (anterior to the serratus posterior superior and serratus posterior inferior).**

DERIVATION ❑ serratus: L. *a notching.*
anterior: L. *in front.*

PRONUNCIATION ❑ ser-**a**-tus an-**tee**-ri-or

ATTACHMENTS

❑ **Ribs #1-9**

- ❑ anterolaterally

to the

❑ **Anterior Surface of the Entire Medial Border of the Scapula**

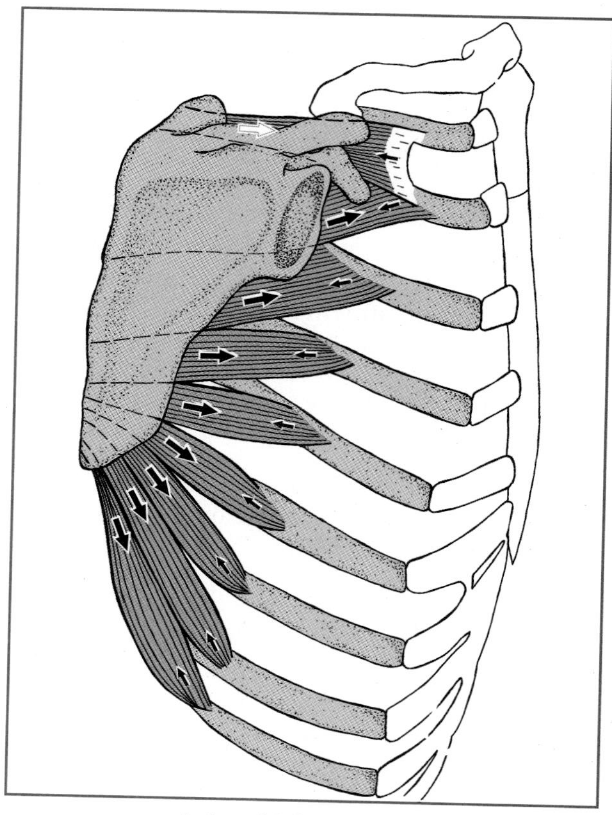

Lateral View of the Right Serratus Anterior

ACTIONS

❑ 1. **Protraction (Abduction) of the Scapula**

❑ 2. **Upward Rotation of the Scapula**

❑ 3. Elevation of the Scapula

❑ 4. Depression of the Scapula

INNERVATION ❑ The Long Thoracic Nerve ❑ **C5**, 6, 7

ARTERIAL SUPPLY ❑ The Dorsal Scapular Artery (A Branch of the Subclavian Artery) and the Lateral Thoracic Artery (A Branch of the Axillary Artery)
❑ and the superior thoracic artery (a branch of the axillary artery)

PALPATION AND SUPPLEMENTARY TEXT

PALPATION

- ❑ The serratus anterior is a large muscle found in the anterolateral trunk. Much of it is deep to the scapula.
  - Have the client supine with the arm flexed to 90° at the shoulder joint (hand pointed toward the ceiling).
  - Locate the lateral border of the pectoralis major (anterior axillary fold) and then locate the lateral border of the latissimus dorsi (posterior axillary fold).
  - Place palpating hand between these two borders in the axilla (the armpit) and feel for the ribs and the serratus anterior.
  - Now ask the client to actively protract the scapula at the scapulocostal joint by pushing the hand toward the ceiling and feel for the contraction of the serratus anterior. Resistance may be added.
  - Once located, try to follow the serratus anterior as far anterior as possible, (deep to the pectoralis major) and as far posterior as possible (deep to the latissimus dorsi and the scapula).

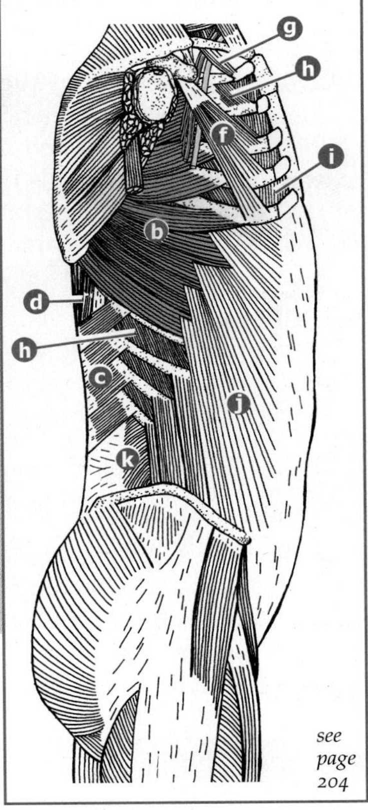

see page 204

Lateral View of the Trunk

a. Latissimus Dorsi (removed)
b. **Serratus Anterior**
c. Serratus Posterior Inferior
d. Erector Spinae
e. Pectoralis Major (removed)
f. Pectoralis Minor
g. Subclavius
h. External Intercostal
i. Internal Intercostal
j. External Abdominal Oblique
k. Internal Abdominal Oblique

RELATIONSHIP TO OTHER MUSCULOSKELETAL STRUCTURES

❑ 1. From the posterior perspective, the majority of the serratus anterior lies deep to the scapula and the latissimus dorsi. From the anterior perspective, its lies deep to the pectoralis major and minor.

❑ 2. The serratus anterior is superficial anterolaterally on the trunk where it meets the external abdominal oblique.

❑ 3. The lowest 4-5 slips of costal (rib) attachments of the serratus anterior interdigitate with the external abdominal oblique.

❑ 4. The serratus anterior lies next to (anterior to) the subscapularis muscle.

METHODOLOGY FOR LEARNING MUSCLE ACTIONS

❑ 1. **Protraction (Abduction) of the Scapula at the Scapulocostal Joint:** The costal (rib) attachment of the serratus anterior is more anterior than the scapular attachment. When the serratus anterior contracts, it pulls on the scapula anteriorly toward the ribs; therefore, the serratus anterior protracts (abducts) the scapula at the scapulocostal joint.

❑ 2. **Upward Rotation of the Scapula at the Scapulocostal Joint:** When the serratus anterior contracts, it pulls on the scapula (especially the fibers attaching to the inferior angle of the scapula), causing the inferior angle of the scapula to swing anteriorly and superiorly toward the rib attachment of the serratus anterior. This causes the glenoid fossa to orient upward; therefore, the serratus anterior upwardly rotates the scapula at the scapulocostal joint.

SERRATUS ANTERIOR – continued

- ❑ **3. Elevation of the Scapula at the Scapulocostal Joint:** The upper fibers of the serratus anterior attach from the scapula to ribs positioned more superiorly. When the serratus anterior contracts, it pulls the scapula superiorly toward these ribs; therefore, the serratus anterior elevates the scapula at the scapulocostal joint.

- ❑ **4. Depression of the Scapula at the Scapulocostal Joint:** The lower fibers of the serratus anterior attach from the scapula to ribs positioned more inferiorly. When the serratus anterior contracts, it pulls the scapula inferiorly toward these ribs; therefore, the serratus anterior depresses the scapula at the scapulocostal joint.

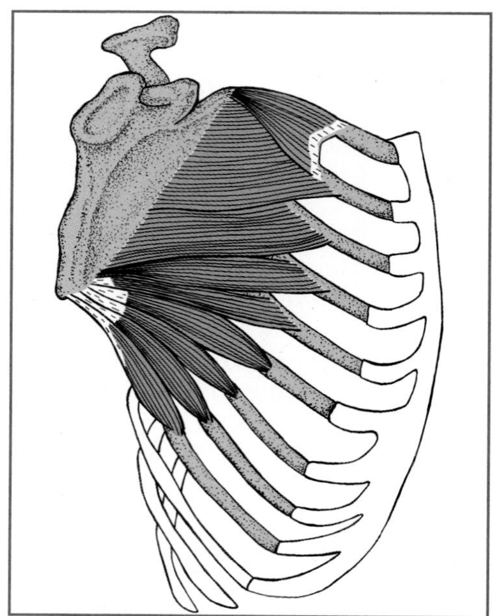

Lateral View of the Right Serratus Anterior (with the lateral border of the scapula pulled away from the trunk to view the scapular attachment of the serratus anterior)

MISCELLANEOUS

- ❑ 1. The serrated appearance comes from attaching onto separate ribs, which creates the notched look of a serrated knife.

- ❑ 2. In very well-developed individuals, the serratus anterior looks like ribs standing out in the anterolateral trunk.

- ❑ 3. The serratus anterior can be considered to have three parts: the first part attaching from ribs #1 and #2 to the superior angle of the scapula, the second part from ribs #2 and #3 to the length of the medial border of the scapula and the third part from ribs #4-9 to the inferior angle of the scapula.

- ❑ 4. The third part (most inferior part) of the serratus anterior is the strongest.

- ❑ 5. The serratus anterior is the prime mover of protraction, upward rotation and medial tilt of the scapula at the scapulocostal joint.

- ❑ 6. Scapular Tilt Actions: In addition to its other actions, the scapula can also tilt.

  If the medial border of the scapula were to move away from the body wall, contraction of the serratus anterior would pull the medial border of the scapula back against the body wall. This movement of the medial border of the scapula moving toward the body wall is called medial tilt; therefore, the serratus anterior medially tilts the scapula at the scapulocostal joint.

  If the inferior angle of the scapula were to move away from the body wall, contraction of the serratus anterior would pull the inferior angle of the scapula back against the body wall. This movement of the inferior angle of the scapula moving toward the body wall is called downward tilt; therefore, the serratus anterior downwardly tilts the scapula at the scapulocostal joint.

- ❑ 7. The action of medial tilt of the scapula at the scapulocostal joint is particularly important when the scapula is protracted because the scapula tends to laterally tilt (wing out) when it protracts. Muscles that medially tilt the scapula keep the scapula from laterally tilting (winging out) at the scapulocostal joint.

- ❑ 8. There is controversy as to the serratus anterior and its role with regard to medial/lateral tilt of the scapula. The serratus anterior has been listed here as a medial tilter of the scapula. However, some sources state that the upper fibers of the serratus anterior produce lateral tilt of the scapula at the scapulocostal joint.

SERRATUS ANTERIOR – continued

- ❑ 9. Some sources state that the uppermost fibers of the serratus anterior can downwardly rotate the scapula at the scapulocostal joint.
- ❑ 10. There is controversy regarding whether or not the serratus anterior is involved with respiration by moving the ribcage. Given its attachments onto the ribs, an accessory respiratory action seems likely.
- ❑ 11. The serratus anterior is important with motions that require forceful protraction of the scapula at the scapulocostal joint, such as reaching, pushing, punching and throwing.
- ❑ 12. Upward rotation of the scapula at the scapulocostal joint is a necessary coupled action that must accompany flexion and abduction (elevation) actions of the arm at the shoulder joint. Given its role as an upward rotator of the scapula, the serratus anterior is active during all elevation actions of flexion and/or abduction of the arm at the shoulder joint.
- ❑ 13. Flexion of the arm at the shoulder joint requires the coupled action of protraction of the scapula at the scapulocostal joint (in addition to the coupled action of upward rotation of the scapula at the scapulocostal joint, see miscellaneous #12). Given its ability to upwardly rotate and protract the scapula, the serratus anterior is ideally suited to be active during flexion movements that elevate the arm anteriorly. It is interesting to note that the trapezius, which is another upward rotator of the scapula, is active during abduction movements of the arm, but not during flexion movements of the arm. This is because the trapezius' action of retraction of the scapula at the scapulocostal joint is antagonistic to the necessary protraction of the scapula that must accompany flexion of the arm at the shoulder joint.

SERRATUS POSTERIOR SUPERIOR

❑ **The name, serratus posterior superior, tells us that this muscle has a serrated appearance and is posterior and superior in location (posterior to the serratus anterior and superior to the serratus posterior inferior).**

DERIVATION ❑ serratus: L. *a notching.*
superior: L. *above.*
posterior: L. *behind, toward the back.*

PRONUNCIATION ❑ ser-**a**-tus pos-**tee**-ri-or sue-**pee**-ri-or

ATTACHMENTS

❑ **S.P.s of C7-T3**

- ❑ and the lower nuchal ligament

to the

❑ **Ribs #2-5**

- ❑ the superior borders and the external surfaces

ACTION

❑ **Elevation of Ribs #2-5**

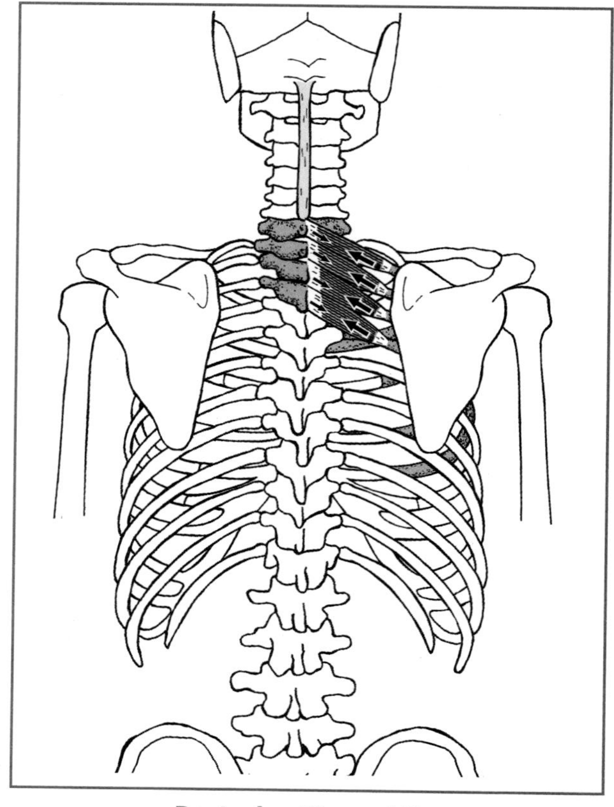

Posterior View of the
Right Serratus Posterior Superior

INNERVATION ❑ Intercostal Nerves ❑ intercostal nerves #2-5

ARTERIAL SUPPLY ❑ The Dorsal Branches of the Posterior Intercostal Arteries (Branches of the Aorta)

PALPATION AND SUPPLEMENTARY TEXT

PALPATION

- ❑ The serratus posterior superior is a thin muscle deep to the trapezius and the rhomboids and extremely difficult to palpate. If the rhomboids and the trapezius are relaxed, and the serratus posterior superior is tight, then it may be palpable.
  - Have the client prone.
  - Place palpating hand in the region of the upper rhomboids.
  - Ask the client to take in a moderately deep breath and feel for the contraction of the serratus posterior superior.

  Note: The fiber direction of the serratus posterior superior is identical to the overlying rhomboids.

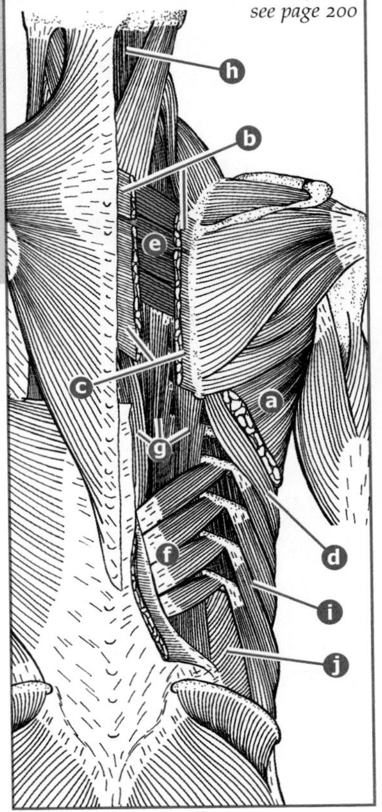

Posterior View of the Trunk

a. Latissimus Dorsi (cut)
b. Rhomboid Minor (cut)
c. Rhomboid Major (cut)
d. Serratus Anterior
e. **Serratus Posterior Superior**
f. Serratus Posterior Inferior
g. Erector Spinae
h. Semispinalis Capitis
i. External Abdominal Oblique
j. Internal Abdominal Oblique

RELATIONSHIP TO OTHER MUSCULOSKELETAL STRUCTURES

❑ 1. The serratus posterior superior is directly deep to the rhomboids.

❑ 2. The serratus posterior superior is directly superficial to the erector spinae musculature and the lower portions of the splenius capitis and the splenius cervicis.

METHODOLOGY FOR LEARNING MUSCLE ACTIONS

❑ **Elevation of Ribs #2-5 at the Sternocostal and Costovertebral Joints:** The serratus posterior superior attaches from ribs #2-5 inferiorly, to the vertebral column superiorly (with its fibers running somewhat vertically). When the serratus posterior superior contracts, it pulls the ribs superiorly toward the vertebral attachment. Therefore, the serratus posterior superior elevates ribs #2-5 at the sternocostal and costovertebral joints.

MISCELLANEOUS

❑ 1. The serrated appearance of the serratus posterior superior comes from attaching onto separate ribs, which creates the notched look of a serrated knife.

❑ 2. The serratus posterior superior is a thin, quadrilateral-shaped muscle.

❑ 3. The serratus posterior superior is variable with regard to its attachments. Its most common variation is that its spinal attachment is only C7-T2 instead of C7-T3.

❑ 4. The action of elevating ribs #2-5 at the sternocostal and costovertebral joints is considered to be important for respiration. More specifically, by elevating these upper ribs, the thoracic cavity expands, which creates more space for the lungs to expand. Therefore, the serratus posterior superior is a muscle of inspiration.

SERRATUS POSTERIOR INFERIOR

❑ **The name, serratus posterior inferior, tells us that this muscle has a serrated appearance and is posterior and inferior in location (posterior to the serratus anterior and inferior to the serratus posterior superior).**

DERIVATION ❑ serratus: L. *a notching*
inferior: L. *below.*
posterior: L. *behind, toward the back.*

PRONUNCIATION ❑ ser-**a**-tus pos**tee**-ri-or in-**fee**-ri-or

ATTACHMENTS

❑ **S.P.s of T11-L2**

to the

❑ **Ribs #9-12**

❑ the inferior borders and the external surfaces

ACTION

❑ **Depression of Ribs #9-12**

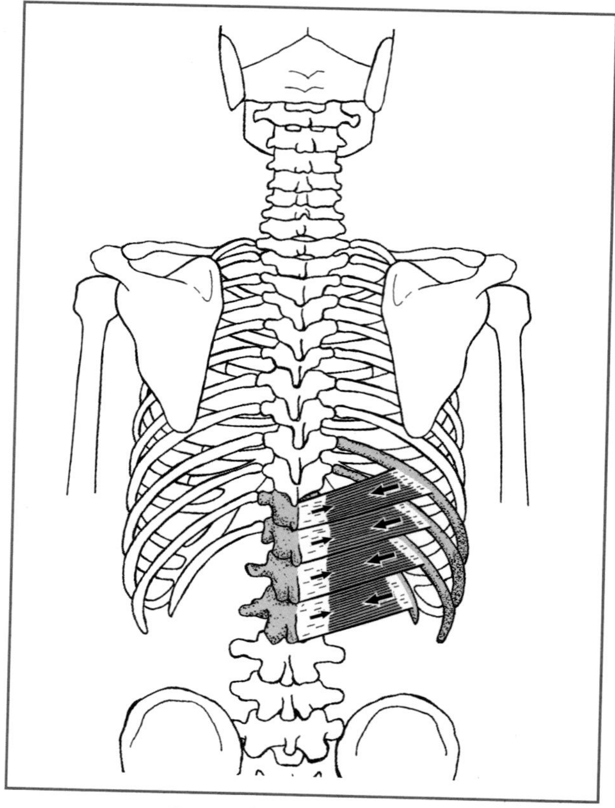

Posterior View of the Right Serratus Posterior Inferior

INNERVATION ❑ Subcostal Nerve and Intercostal Nerves
❑ intercostal nerves #9-11

ARTERIAL SUPPLY ❑ The Dorsal Branches of the Posterior Intercostal Arteries (Branches of the Aorta)

PALPATION AND SUPPLEMENTARY TEXT

PALPATION

- ❑ The serratus posterior inferior is a thin muscle deep to the latissimus dorsi and very difficult to palpate. If the latissimus dorsi is relaxed, and the serratus posterior inferior is tight, then it may be palpable.
  - Have the client prone.
  - Place palpating hands in the upper lumbar region.
  - Ask the client to take in a moderately deep breath and feel for the contraction of the serratus posterior inferior.

  Note: The fiber direction of the serratus posterior inferior is identical to the overlying latissimus dorsi.

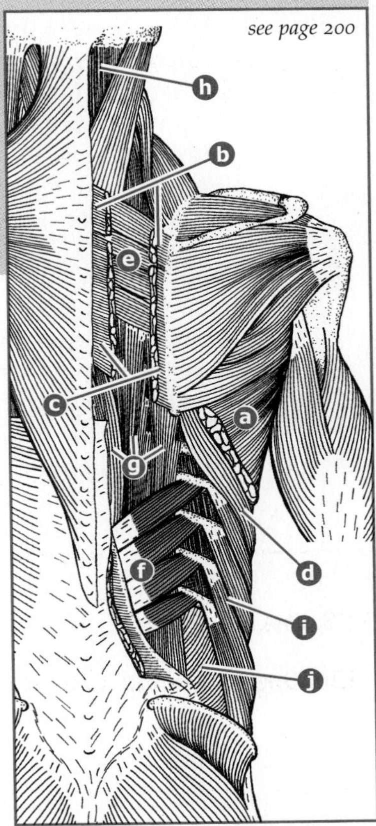

see page 200

Posterior View of the Trunk

a. Latissimus Dorsi (cut)
b. Rhomboid Minor (cut)
c. Rhomboid Major (cut)
d. Serratus Anterior
e. Serratus Posterior Superior
f. **Serratus Posterior Inferior**
g. Erector Spinae
h. Semispinalis Capitis
i. External Abdominal Oblique
j. Internal Abdominal Oblique

RELATIONSHIP TO OTHER MUSCULOSKELETAL STRUCTURES

❑ 1. The serratus posterior inferior is directly deep to the latissimus dorsi.

❑ 2. Directly deep to the serratus posterior inferior is the erector spinae group.

METHODOLOGY FOR LEARNING MUSCLE ACTIONS

❑ **Depression of Ribs #9-12 at the Sternocostal and Costovertebral Joints:** The serratus posterior inferior attaches from ribs #9-12 superiorly, to the vertebral column inferiorly (with its fibers running somewhat vertically). When the serratus posterior inferior contracts, it pulls the ribs inferiorly toward the vertebral attachment. Therefore, the serratus posterior inferior depresses ribs #9-12 at the sternocostal and costovertebral joints.

MISCELLANEOUS

❑ 1. The serrated appearance of the serratus posterior inferior comes from attaching onto separate ribs, which creates the notched look of a serrated knife.

❑ 2. The serratus posterior inferior is a thin, quadrilateral-shaped muscle.

❑ 3. The serratus posterior inferior is variable with regard to its spinal and costal (rib) attachments.

SERRATUS POSTERIOR INFERIOR – continued

❑ 4. The action of depressing ribs #9-12 is considered to be important for respiration. More specifically, by depressing these lower ribs, the thoracic cavity expands, which creates more space for the lungs to expand. However, its main function regarding the lower ribs is not to be a mover and actually move the lower ribs into depression, but rather to fix the lower ribs in place so that they do not elevate when the diaphragm contracts and exerts an upward pull upon them. In this manner, if the lower attachments of the diaphragm are fixed, the dome of the diaphragm contracts and drops down more efficiently, thus increasing the size of the thoracic cavity for the lungs to expand and fill with air. Therefore, the serratus posterior inferior is a muscle of inspiration (primarily as a fixator, i.e., stabilizer). It must be noted that there is some controversy regarding the role of the serratus posterior inferior with regard to respiration. Some sources state that it is not involved with respiration at all. Other sources list it as a muscle of expiration rather than inspiration. However, looking at its biomechanical role of fixating the lower ribs against the pull of the diaphragm clearly places the serratus posterior inferior as a muscle of inspiration.

❑ 5. Some sources state that the serratus posterior inferior should have a role in moving the trunk. Indeed, if the costal (rib) attachments are fixed and the vertebrae move, it seems likely that the serratus posterior inferior should be able to contralaterally rotate the trunk at the spinal joints. (Note the somewhat horizontal nature to the fiber direction in the transverse plane.) Further, given the fact that the spinal joints are crossed posteriorly (with the fibers running somewhat vertically in the sagittal plane), the serratus posterior inferior should be able to extend the trunk at the spinal joints.

THE ERECTOR SPINAE GROUP ❑

❑ **The name, erector spinae, tells us that this muscle makes the spine erect. (Given that the spine usually bends forward into flexion, to make it erect would be to perform extension of the spine.)**

DERIVATION ❑ erector: L. *to erect.*
spinae: L. *thorn* (refers to the spine).

PRONUNCIATION ❑ ee-**rek**-tor **spee**-nee

ATTACHMENTS

❑ **Pelvis**

to the

❑ **Spine, Ribcage and the Head**

ACTIONS

❑ 1. **Extension of the Trunk and the Neck and the Head**

❑ 2. **Lateral Flexion of the Trunk and the Neck and the Head**

❑ 3. **Ipsilateral Rotation of the Trunk and the Neck and the Head**

❑ 4. **Anterior Tilt of the Pelvis**

❑ 5. Elevation of the Pelvis

❑ 6. Contralateral Rotation of the Pelvis

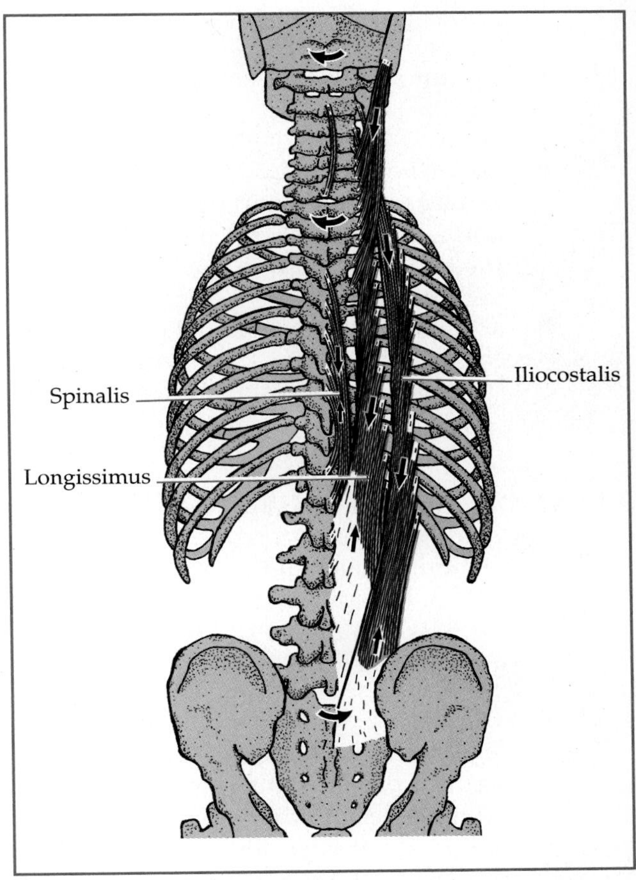

Posterior View of the Right Erector Spinae Group

INNERVATION ❑ Spinal Nerves
❑ dorsal rami of cervical, thoracic and lumbar spinal nerves

ARTERIAL SUPPLY ❑ The Dorsal Branches of the Posterior Intercostal and Lumbar Arteries (All Branches of the Aorta)
❑ and the thoracodorsal artery (a branch of the subclavian artery)

THE ERECTOR SPINAE GROUP PALPATION AND SUPPLEMENTARY TEXT

PALPATION

- ❑ The erector spinae is a deep, massive muscle group located lateral to the spine, running vertically from the pelvis to the head.
  - Have the client prone.
  - Place palpating hands lateral to the S.P.s of the vertebral column in the lumbar region and feel for the vertical orientation of the fibers of the erector spinae.
  - Continue palpating the erector spinae inferiorly and superiorly toward its attachments.
  - To further bring out the erector spinae group, ask the client to actively extend the upper part of the body (trunk, neck and head) off the table and feel for the contraction of the erector spinae group, particularly in the lumbar and lower thoracic regions.
  - To palpate the erector spinae of the neck, it is best to have the client supine. The erector spinae musculature in this region is deep and can be difficult to distinguish from other posterior cervical muscles.

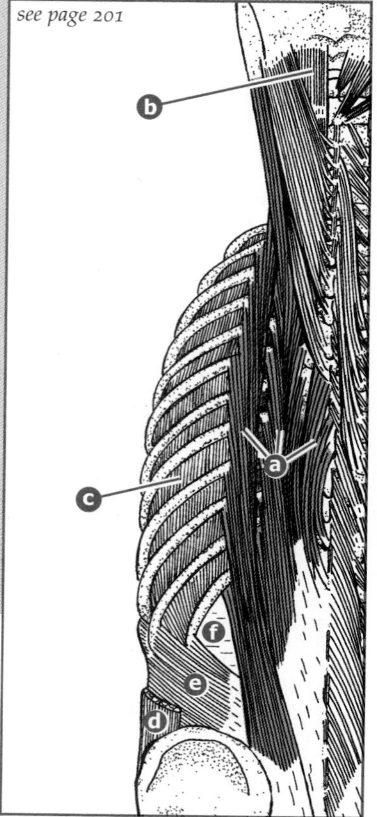

Posterior View of the Trunk

a. **Erector Spinae**
b. Transversospinalis
c. External Intercostals
d. External Abdominal Oblique (cut)
e. Internal Abdominal Oblique
f. Transversus Abdominis

RELATIONSHIP TO OTHER MUSCULOSKELETAL STRUCTURES

❑ 1. Although much of the erector spinae group lies on either side of the S.P.s of the spine in the laminar groove (over the laminae, between the S.P.s and the T.P.s), keep in mind that this group also attaches quite far laterally.

❑ 2. The erector spinae group is deep in the back and neck. In the lumbar region, the erector spinae group is deep to the latissimus dorsi and the serratus posterior inferior. In the thoracic region, the erector spinae group is deep to the trapezius, latissimus dorsi, rhomboids major and minor, serratus posterior superior, splenius capitis and the splenius cervicis. In the cervical region, the erector spinae group is deep to the trapezius, splenius capitis, splenius cervicis and the sternocleidomastoid.

❑ 3. In the trunk, the transversospinalis muscle group, quadratus lumborum and the ribcage are deep to the erector spinae group. In the neck, the suboccipital muscle group is deep to the erector spinae group.

METHODOLOGY FOR LEARNING MUSCLE ACTIONS

❑ 1. **Extension of the Trunk and the Neck and the Head at the Spinal Joints:** The erector spinae group crosses the spinal joints posteriorly from the pelvis all the way to the head (with its fibers running vertically in the sagittal plane). Therefore, the erector spinae group extends the trunk and the neck at the spinal joints, and extends the head at the atlanto-occipital joint.

THE ERECTOR SPINAE GROUP – continued

- ☐ 2. **Lateral Flexion of the Trunk and the Neck and the Head at the Spinal Joints:** The erector spinae group crosses the spinal joints laterally from the pelvis all the way to the head (with its fibers running vertically in the frontal plane). Therefore, the erector spinae group laterally flexes the trunk and the neck at the spinal joints, and laterally flexes the head at the atlanto-occipital joint.

- ☐ 3. **Ipsilateral Rotation of the Trunk and the Neck and the Head at the Spinal Joints:** The arrangement of the erector spinae group is generally such that its inferior attachment is medial and its fibers run up to the more superior attachment, which lies more laterally (with its fibers running somewhat horizontally in the transverse plane). When the erector spinae group contracts, it pulls this superolateral attachment posteromedially toward the midline, causing the anterior surface of the trunk and/or the neck and/or the head to face the same side of the body that the erector spinae group is attached. Therefore, the erector spinae group ipsilaterally rotates the trunk and the neck at the spinal joints, and ipsilaterally rotates the head at the atlanto-occipital joint.

- ☐ 4. **Anterior Tilt of the Pelvis at the Lumbosacral Joint:** With the superior attachments fixed, the erector spinae group, by pulling superiorly on the posterior pelvis, anteriorly tilts the pelvis at the lumbosacral joint.

- ☐ 5. **Elevation of the Pelvis at the Lumbosacral Joint:** With the superior attachments fixed, the erector spinae group, by pulling superiorly on the lateral pelvis (since the fibers are running vertically), elevates the pelvis at the lumbosacral joint.

- ☐ 6. **Contralateral Rotation of the Pelvis at the Lumbosacral Joint:** When the superior attachments of the erector spinae group are fixed and the erector spinae group contracts, it pulls on the inferior attachment, the pelvis. (Since the fibers of the erector spinae group have a slight horizontal orientation in the transverse plane, the pelvis will rotate.) When the erector spinae group contracts, it pulls the posterior pelvis posterolaterally toward the side of the body that the erector spinae group is attached, causing the anterior pelvis to face the opposite side of the body from the side of the body that the erector spinae group is attached. Therefore, the erector spinae group contralaterally rotates the pelvis at the lumbosacral joint.

MISCELLANEOUS

- ☐ 1. The erector spinae group can be divided into three subgroups. These three subgroups are, from lateral to medial, the iliocostalis, the longissimus and the spinalis.

- ☐ 2. Generally, the following statements can be made regarding the erector spinae subgroups:
  - The iliocostalis attaches from the ilium to the ribs.
  - The longissimus is the longest of the three subgroups.
  - The spinalis attaches from S.P.s to S.P.s.

- ☐ 3. Of the three subgroups of the erector spinae, only the iliocostalis and longissimus attach onto the pelvis, and only the longissimus attaches onto the head. (Occasionally, the spinalis capitis attaches to the head.)

- ☐ 4. Each of the three subgroups of the erector spinae can be further subdivided into three subgroups. They are the iliocostalis lumborum, thoracis and cervicis; the longissimus thoracis, cervicis and capitis; and the spinalis thoracis, cervicis and capitis. (Note: The spinalis capitis often blends with and therefore is considered to be a part of the semispinalis capitis of the transversospinalis group.)

- ☐ 5. The erector spinae is also known as the *sacrospinalis* group.

- ☐ 6. The term *paraspinal* musculature is also used to describe the erector spinae and the transversospinalis groups together.

ILIOCOSTALIS
(OF THE ERECTOR SPINAE GROUP)

❑ **The name, iliocostalis, tells us that this muscle attaches from the ilium to the ribs.**

DERIVATION ❑ ilio: L. *refers to the ilium.*
costalis: L. *refers to the ribs.*

PRONUNCIATION ❑ **il**-ee-o-kos-**ta**-lis

ATTACHMENTS

❑ **ENTIRE ILIOCOSTALIS: Sacrum, Iliac Crest and Ribs #3-12**

❑ ILIOCOSTALIS LUMBORUM: Medial Iliac Crest and the Medial and Lateral Sacral Crests

❑ ILIOCOSTALIS THORACIS: Angles of Ribs #7-12

❑ ILIOCOSTALIS CERVICIS: Angles of Ribs #3-6

to the

❑ **ENTIRE ILIOCOSTALIS: Ribs #1-12 and T.P.s of C4-7**

❑ ILIOCOSTALIS LUMBORUM: Angles of Ribs #7-12

❑ ILIOCOSTALIS THORACIS: Angles of Ribs #1-6 and the T.P. of C7

❑ ILIOCOSTALIS CERVICIS: T.P.s of C4-6

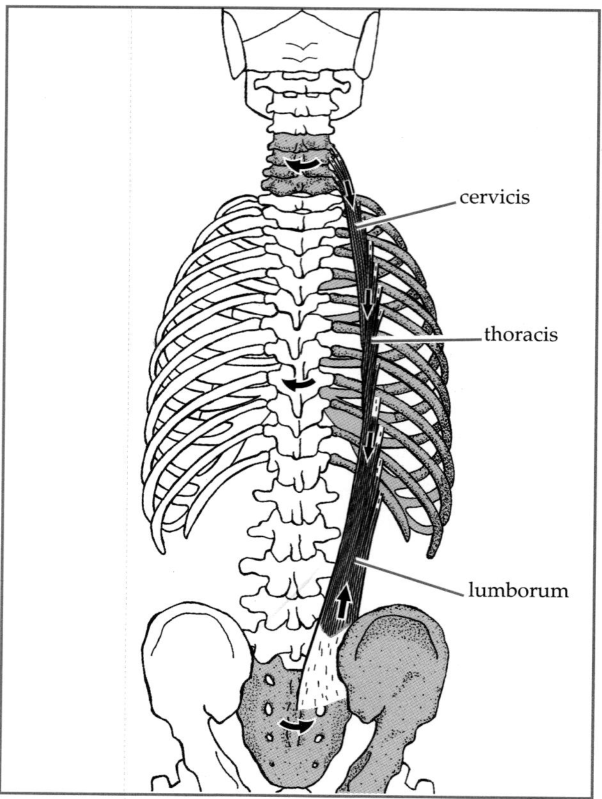

Posterior View of the Right Iliocostalis

ACTIONS

❑ 1. **Extension of the Trunk and the Neck**

❑ 2. **Lateral Flexion of the Trunk and the Neck**

❑ 3. **Ipsilateral Rotation of the Trunk and the Neck**

❑ 4. **Anterior Tilt of the Pelvis**

❑ 5. Elevation of the Pelvis

❑ 6. Contralateral Rotation of the Pelvis

INNERVATION ❑ Spinal Nerves
❑ dorsal rami of lower cervical, thoracic and upper lumbar spinal nerves

ARTERIAL SUPPLY ❑ The Dorsal Branches of the Posterior Intercostal Arteries (Branches of the Aorta)
❑ and the thoracodorsal artery (a branch of the subclavian artery)

PALPATION AND SUPPLEMENTARY TEXT

PALPATION

- ❑ The iliocostalis is the most lateral of the three erector spinae subgroups.
  - Have the client prone.
  - Locate the erector spinae group in the thoracic region (see the palpation section for this muscle group on page 224). Once located, the iliocostalis will be the most lateral fibers of the erector spinae group.
  - Palpate the iliocostalis' attachments onto the ribs.
  - Continue palpating the iliocostalis inferiorly (it may be possible to feel where the iliocostalis and the longissimus divide in the lumbar region) and superiorly toward its attachments.

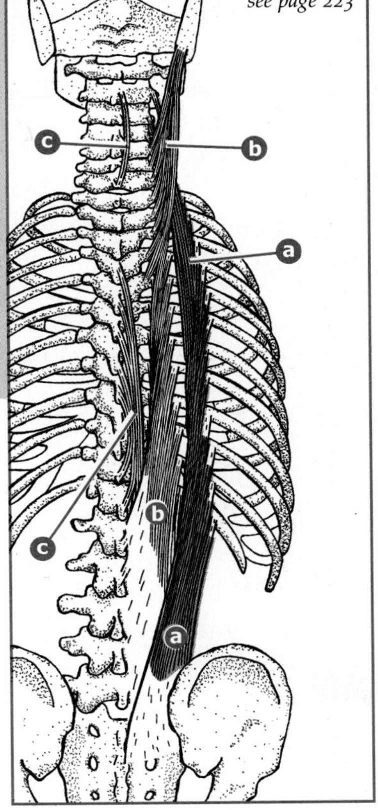

Posterior View of the Trunk

a. **Iliocostalis**
b. Longissimus
c. Spinalis

RELATIONSHIP TO OTHER MUSCULOSKELETAL STRUCTURES

❑ 1. The iliocostalis, as part of the erector spinae group, is fairly deep in the posterior trunk.

❑ 2. The iliocostalis is deep to the latissimus dorsi, serratus posterior inferior, trapezius, rhomboids major and minor, serratus posterior superior, splenius capitis and the splenius cervicis (as well as the longissimus and semispinalis capitis in the neck).

❑ 3. Deep to the iliocostalis are the multifidus, quadratus lumborum, the ribcage and the external and internal intercostal muscles.

❑ 4. The iliocostalis is the most lateral of the erector spinae muscles. It may run laterally enough to be deep to the scapula.

METHODOLOGY FOR LEARNING MUSCLE ACTIONS

❑ 1. **Extension of the Trunk and the Neck at the Spinal Joints:** The iliocostalis crosses the spinal joints posteriorly from the pelvis all the way to the lower neck (with its fibers running vertically in the sagittal plane); therefore, it extends the trunk and the neck at the spinal joints.

❑ 2. **Lateral Flexion of the Trunk and the Neck at the Spinal Joints:** The iliocostalis crosses the spinal joints laterally from the pelvis all the way to the lower neck (with its fibers running vertically in the frontal plane); therefore, it laterally flexes the trunk and the neck at the spinal joints.

❑ 3. **Ipsilateral Rotation of the Trunk and the Neck at the Spinal Joints:** The arrangement of the iliocostalis is generally such that its inferior attachment is medial and its fibers run up to the more superior attachment, which lies more laterally (with its fibers running somewhat horizontally in the transverse plane). When the iliocostalis contracts, it pulls this superolateral attachment posteromedially toward the midline, causing the anterior surface of the trunk and/or the neck to face the same side of the body that the iliocostalis is attached. Therefore, the iliocostalis ipsilaterally rotates the trunk and the neck at the spinal joints.

ILIOCOSTALIS – continued

- ❑ **4. Anterior Tilt of the Pelvis at the Lumbosacral Joint:** With the superior attachments fixed, the iliocostalis, by pulling superiorly on the posterior pelvis, anteriorly tilts the pelvis at the lumbosacral joint.

- ❑ **5. Elevation of the Pelvis:** With the superior attachments fixed, the iliocostalis, by pulling superiorly on the lateral pelvis (since the fibers are running vertically), elevates the pelvis at the lumbosacral joint.

- ❑ **6. Contralateral Rotation of the Pelvis:** When the superior attachments of the iliocostalis are fixed and the iliocostalis contracts, it pulls on the inferior attachment, the pelvis. (Since the fibers of the iliocostalis have a slight horizontal orientation in the transverse plane, the pelvis will rotate.) When the iliocostalis contracts, it pulls the posterior pelvis posterolaterally toward the side of the body that the iliocostalis is attached, causing the anterior pelvis to face the opposite side of the body from the side of the body that the iliocostalis is attached. Therefore, the iliocostalis contralaterally rotates the pelvis at the lumbosacral joint.

MISCELLANEOUS

- ❑ 1. The iliocostalis is also known as the *iliocostocervicalis*.

- ❑ 2. The iliocostalis can be subdivided into the iliocostalis lumborum, the iliocostalis thoracis and the iliocostalis cervicis.

- ❑ 3. Of the three subgroups of the erector spinae group, the iliocostalis has the most lateral attachment (onto the ribs). Keep this in mind when working on the erector spinae group. The iliocostalis often attaches lateral enough to be deep to the scapula!

LONGISSIMUS

(OF THE ERECTOR SPINAE GROUP)

❑ **The name, longissimus, tells us that this muscle is long. It is the longest of the erector spinae subgroups.**

DERIVATION ❑ longissimus: L. *very long.*

PRONUNCIATION ❑ lon-**jis**-i-mus

ATTACHMENTS

❑ **ENTIRE LONGISSIMUS: Sacrum, Iliac Crest and T.P.s of L1-5 and T1-5 and the Articular Processes of C5-7**

❑ LONGISSIMUS THORACIS: Medial Iliac Crest, Posterior Sacrum and the T.P.s of L1-5

❑ LONGISSIMUS CERVICIS: T.P.s of the Upper 5 Thoracic Vertebrae

❑ LONGISSIMUS CAPITIS: T.P.s of the Upper 5 Thoracic Vertebrae and the Articular Processes of the Lower 3 Cervical Vertebrae

to the

❑ **ENTIRE LONGISSIMUS: Ribs #4-12, T.P.s of T1-12 and C2-6 and the Mastoid Process of the Temporal Bone**

❑ LONGISSIMUS THORACIS: T.P.s of All the Thoracic Vertebrae and the Lower 9 Ribs (between the tubercles and the angles)

❑ LONGISSIMUS CERVICIS: T.P.s of C2-6 (posterior tubercles)

❑ LONGISSIMUS CAPITIS: Mastoid Process of the Temporal Bone

Posterior View of the Right Longissimus

ACTIONS

❑ 1. **Extension of the Trunk and the Neck and the Head**

❑ 2. **Lateral Flexion of the Trunk and the Neck and the Head**

❑ 3. **Ipsilateral Rotation of the Trunk and the Neck and the Head**

❑ 4. **Anterior Tilt of the Pelvis**

❑ 5. Elevation of the Pelvis

❑ 6. Contralateral Rotation of the Pelvis

INNERVATION ❑ Spinal Nerves
- ❑ dorsal rami of lower cervical, thoracic and lumbar spinal nerves

ARTERIAL SUPPLY ❑ The Dorsal Branches of the Posterior Intercostal and Lumbar Arteries (All Branches of the Aorta)

LONGISSIMUS – PALPATION AND SUPPLEMENTARY TEXT

PALPATION

❑ The longissimus makes up the bulk of the medial fibers of the erector spinae musculature.

- Have the client prone.
- Locate the erector spinae group in the thoracic region (see the palpation section for this muscle group on page 224).
- Once located, palpate the longissimus between the S.P.s and the iliocostalis (laterally). The longissimus will be clearly palpable as a mass of musculature running vertically alongside the S.P.s. It is extremely difficult to distinguish the medial margin of the longissimus from the spinalis.)
- Continue palpating the longissimus inferiorly (it may be possible to feel where the iliocostalis and the longissimus divide in the lumbar region) and superiorly toward its attachments.

see page 223

Posterior View of the Trunk

a. Iliocostalis
b. Longissimus
c. Spinalis

RELATIONSHIP TO OTHER MUSCULOSKELETAL STRUCTURES

❑ 1. The longissimus is located between the iliocostalis (which is directly lateral to it) and the spinalis (which is directly medial to it).

❑ 2. The longissimus is deep to the latissimus dorsi, serratus posterior inferior, trapezius, rhomboids major and minor, serratus posterior superior, splenius capitis and the splenius cervicis.

❑ 3. The longissimus attachment onto the mastoid process of the temporal bone is deep to the mastoid process attachment of the splenius capitis and the sternocleidomastoid.

❑ 4. Deep to the longissimus are the multifidus, rotatores, levatores costarum, intertransversarii, quadratus lumborum, the ribcage and the external and internal intercostal muscles.

❑ 5. The longissimus cervicis' inferior attachment is in the thoracic region, medial to the longissimus thoracis.

❑ 6. Most of the longissimus cervicis is deep to the longissimus capitis.

❑ 7. The longissimus capitis lies between the longissimus cervicis (which is directly lateral to it) and the splenius capitis (which is directly medial to it).

METHODOLOGY FOR LEARNING MUSCLE ACTIONS

❑ **1. Extension of the Trunk and the Neck and the Head at the Spinal Joints:** The longissimus crosses the spinal joints posteriorly from the pelvis all the way to the head (with its fibers running vertically in the sagittal plane). Therefore, the longissimus extends the trunk and the neck at the spinal joints, and extends the head at the atlanto-occipital joint.

LONGISSIMUS – continued

- ❑ **2. Lateral Flexion of the Trunk and the Neck and the Head at the Spinal Joints:** The longissimus crosses the spinal joints laterally from the pelvis all the way to the head (with its fibers running vertically in the frontal plane). Therefore, the longissimus laterally flexes the trunk and the neck at the spinal joints, and laterally flexes the head at the atlanto-occipital joint.
- ❑ **3. Ipsilateral Rotation of the Trunk and the Neck and the Head at the Spinal Joints:** The arrangement of the longissimus is generally such that its inferior attachment is medial and its fibers run up to the more superior attachment, which lies more laterally (with its fibers running somewhat horizontally in the transverse plane). When the longissimus contracts, it pulls this superolateral attachment posteromedially toward the midline, causing the anterior surface of the trunk and/or the neck and/or the head to face the same side of the body that the longissimus is attached. Therefore, the longissimus ipsilaterally rotates the trunk and the neck at the spinal joints, and ipsilaterally rotates the head at the atlanto-occipital joints.
- ❑ **4. Anterior Tilt of the Pelvis at the Lumbosacral Joint:** With the superior attachments fixed, the longissimus, by pulling superiorly on the posterior pelvis, anteriorly tilts the pelvis at the lumbosacral joint.
- ❑ **5. Elevation of the Pelvis at the Lumbosacral Joint:** With the superior attachments fixed, the longissimus, by pulling superiorly on the lateral pelvis (since the fibers are running vertically), elevates the pelvis at the lumbosacral joint.
- ❑ **6. Contralateral Rotation of the Pelvis at the Lumbosacral Joint:** When the superior attachments of the longissimus are fixed and the longissimus contracts, it pulls on the inferior attachment, the pelvis. (Since the fibers of the longissimus have a slight horizontal orientation in the transverse plane, the pelvis will rotate.) When the longissimus contracts, it pulls the posterior pelvis posterolaterally toward the side of the body that the longissimus is attached, causing the anterior pelvis to face the opposite side of the body from the side of the body that the longissimus is attached. Therefore, the longissimus contralaterally rotates the pelvis at the lumbosacral joint.

MISCELLANEOUS

- ❑ 1. The longissimus can be subdivided into the longissimus thoracis, the longissimus cervicis and the longissimus capitis.
- ❑ 2. The longissimus is the longest and the largest of the three subgroups of the erector spinae group.
- ❑ 3. Of the three subgroups of the erector spinae group, the longissimus has the most superior attachment (onto the mastoid process of the temporal bone).
- ❑ 4. In the lumbar region, the longissimus blends with the iliocostalis. In the thoracic region, the longissimus blends with the spinalis.
- ❑ 5. The longissimus thoracis also attaches into the thoracolumbar fascia.

SPINALIS
(OF THE ERECTOR SPINAE GROUP)

❑ **The name, spinalis, tells us that this muscle attaches from S.P.s to S.P.s.**

DERIVATION ❑ spinalis: L. *refers to spinous processes.*

PRONUNCIATION ❑ spy-**na**-lis

ATTACHMENTS

❑ **ENTIRE SPINALIS: S.P.s of T11-L2 and C7 and the Nuchal Ligament**

❑ SPINALIS THORACIS: S.P.s of T11-L2

❑ SPINALIS CERVICIS: Inferior Nuchal Ligament and the S.P. of C7

❑ SPINALIS CAPITIS: Usually Considered to be the Medial Part of the Semispinalis Capitis

to the

❑ **ENTIRE SPINALIS: S.P.s of T5-12 and C2**

❑ SPINALIS THORACIS: S.P.s of T4-8

❑ SPINALIS CERVICIS: S.P. of C2

❑ SPINALIS CAPITIS: Usually Considered to be the Medial Part of the Semispinalis Capitis

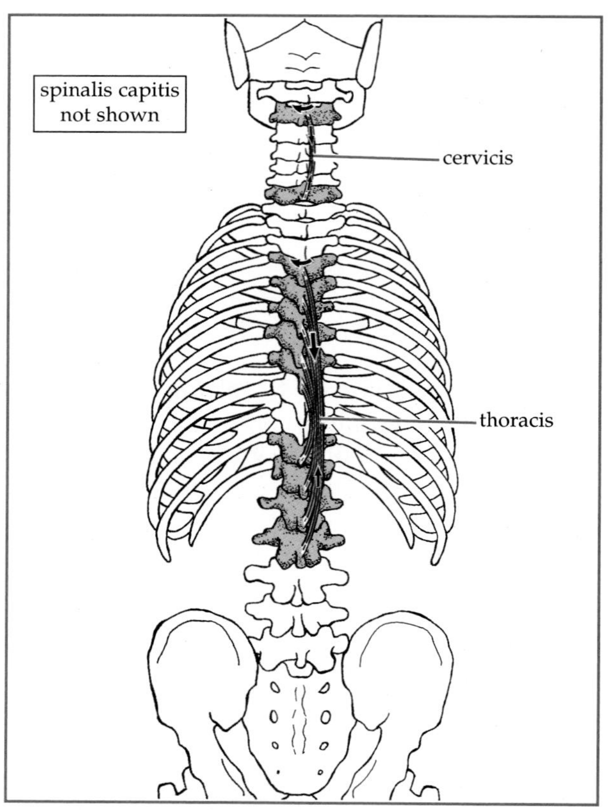

Posterior View of the Right Spinalis

ACTIONS

❑ 1. **Extension of the Trunk and the Neck and the Head**

❑ 2. **Lateral Flexion of the Trunk and the Neck and the Head**

❑ 3. **Ipsilateral Rotation of the Trunk and the Neck and the Head**

INNERVATION ❑ Spinal Nerves
❑ dorsal rami of the lower cervical and the thoracic spinal nerves

ARTERIAL SUPPLY ❑ The Dorsal Branches of the Posterior Intercostal and Lumbar Arteries (All Branches of the Aorta)

PALPATION AND SUPPLEMENTARY TEXT

PALPATION

- ❑ The spinalis is a small and deep muscle that blends with the longissimus and semispinalis. It is best palpated along with the longissimus (see the palpation section for this muscle on page 230). If palpable, the spinalis will be the deepest, most medial fibers of the erector spinae. It is effectively impossible to distinguish from the adjacent erector spinae and transversospinalis musculature.

RELATIONSHIP TO OTHER MUSCULOSKELETAL STRUCTURES

❑ 1 The spinalis fibers are the most medial of all the fibers of the erector spinae group.

❑ 2. The spinalis is deep to the latissimus dorsi, serratus posterior inferior, trapezius, rhomboids major and minor, serratus posterior superior, splenius capitis and the splenius cervicis.

❑ 3. Deep to the spinalis are the multifidus, rotatores and the vertebrae.

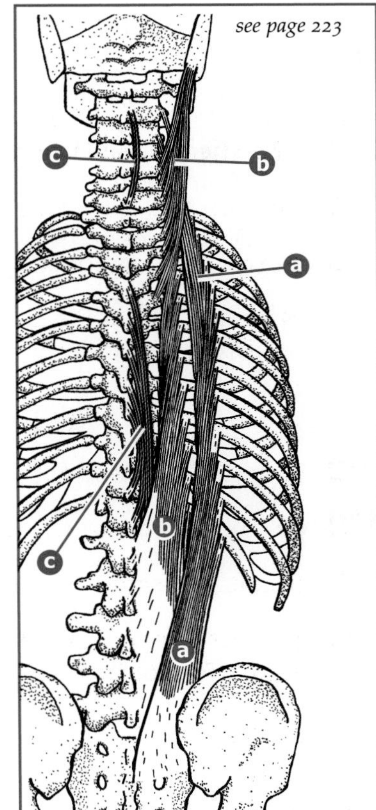

Posterior View of the Trunk

a. Iliocostalis
b. Longissimus
c. **Spinalis**

METHODOLOGY FOR LEARNING MUSCLE ACTIONS

❑ **1. Extension of the Trunk and the Neck and the Head at the Spinal Joints:** The spinalis crosses the spinal joints posteriorly from the upper lumbar region all the way to the head (with its fibers running vertically in the sagittal plane). Therefore, the spinalis extends the trunk and the neck at the spinal joints, and extends the head at the atlanto-occipital joint.

❑ **2. Lateral Flexion of the Trunk and the Neck and the Head at the Spinal Joints:** The spinalis crosses the spinal joints laterally from the upper lumbar region all the way to the head (with its fibers running vertically in the frontal plane). Therefore, the spinalis laterally flexes the trunk and the neck at the spinal joints, and laterally flexes the head at the atlanto-occipital joint.

❑ **3. Ipsilateral Rotation of the Trunk and the Neck and the Head at the Spinal Joints:** The arrangement of the spinalis is generally such that its inferior attachment is medial and its fibers run up to the more superior attachment, which lies more laterally (with its fibers running somewhat horizontally in the transverse plane). When the spinalis contracts, it pulls this superolateral attachment posteromedially toward the midline, causing the anterior surface of the trunk and/or the neck and/or the head to face the same side of the body that the spinalis is attached. Therefore, the spinalis ipsilaterally rotates the trunk and the neck at the spinal joints, and ipsilaterally rotates the head at the atlanto-occipital joints.

MISCELLANEOUS

❑ 1. The spinalis can be subdivided into the spinalis thoracis, the spinalis cervicis and the spinalis capitis.

❑ 2. Of the three subgroups of the erector spinae group, the spinalis is the smallest and located the most medial.

SPINALIS – continued

- ❑ 3. The spinalis is significant in the thoracic region only.
- ❑ 4. The spinalis thoracis usually blends intimately with the longissimus.
- ❑ 5. The spinalis capitis is also known as the *biventer cervicis* because a band of tendon cuts across it transversely, effectively dividing it into two bellies ("biventer" means two bellies).
- ❑ 6. Usually the spinalis capitis blends with the medial part of the semispinalis capitis (of the transversospinalis group) and is therefore usually considered to be a part of the semispinalis capitis. When the spinalis capitis is present as a distinct muscle, it is very small and deep to the semispinalis capitis.
- ❑ 7. The spinalis cervicis is often absent.
- ❑ 8. When present, the attachment levels of the spinalis cervicis are variable. Its inferior attachment often reaches to T1-2 and its superior attachment often reaches to C3-4.
- ❑ 9. Of its three possible actions, extension (of the trunk, neck and head at the spinal joints) is its strongest action. Lateral flexion and ipsilateral rotation (of the trunk, neck and head at the spinal joints) are weak.

THE TRANSVERSOSPINALIS GROUP

❑ **The name, transversospinalis, tells us that this muscle group attaches from T.P.s to S.P.s.**

DERIVATION ❑ transverso: L. *refers to transverse processes.*
spinalis: L. *refers to spinous processes.*

PRONUNCIATION ❑ trans-**ver**-so-spy-**na**-lis

ATTACHMENTS

❑ **Pelvis**

to the

❑ **Spine and the Head**

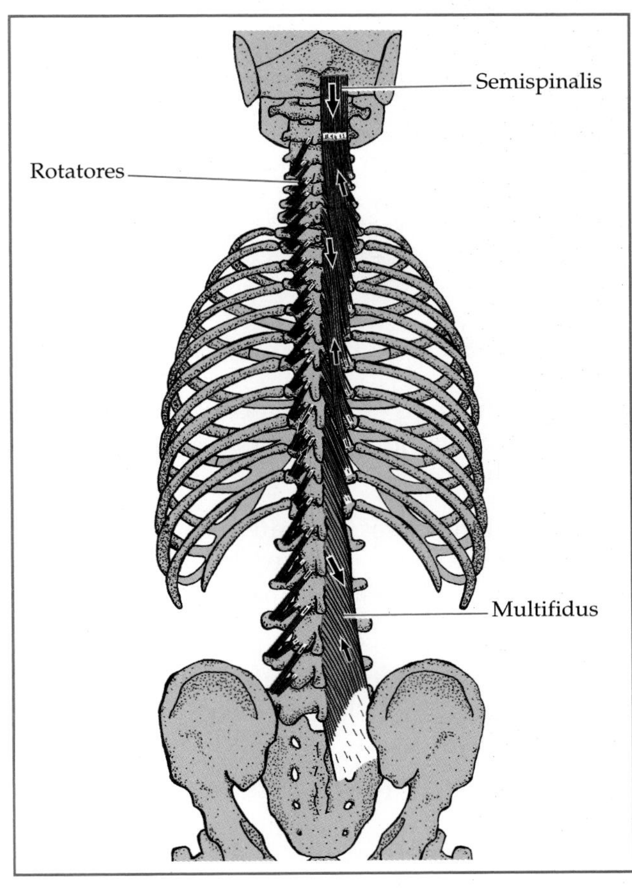

Posterior View of the Transversospinalis Group
(semispinalis and multifidus on the right)
(rotatores on the left)

ACTIONS

❑ **1. Extension of the Trunk and the Neck and the Head**

❑ **2. Lateral Flexion of the Trunk and the Neck and the Head**

❑ **3. Contralateral Rotation of the Trunk and the Neck**

❑ **4. Anterior Tilt of the Pelvis**

❑ **5.** Elevation of the Pelvis

❑ **6.** Ipsilateral Rotation of the Pelvis

INNERVATION ❑ Spinal Nerves
❑ dorsal rami of cervical, thoracic and lumbar spinal nerves

ARTERIAL SUPPLY ❑ The Occipital Artery (A Branch of the External Carotid Artery) and the Dorsal Branches of the Posterior Intercostal and Lumbar Arteries (All Branches of the Aorta)
❑ and the deep cervical artery (a branch of the thyrocervical trunk)

THE TRANSVERSOSPINALIS GROUP PALPATION AND SUPPLEMENTARY TEXT

PALPATION

- ❑ The transversospinalis is very deep and difficult to palpate. In the trunk, it may be sensed deep to the erector spinae musculature if the erector spinae musculature is relaxed. The multifidus in the sacral and lower lumbar regions and the semispinalis in the cervical region are bulky and may be palpated. Otherwise, distinguishing the transversospinalis from the more superficial musculature is extremely difficult.
    - To palpate the transversospinalis of the trunk, have the client prone and try to palpate deep to the erector spinae (see the palpation section for this group on page 224).
    - To palpate the transversospinalis of the neck, have the client supine and palpate deep to the upper trapezius between the spine and the splenius capitis (see the palpation sections for these muscles on pages 111 and 115, respectively).

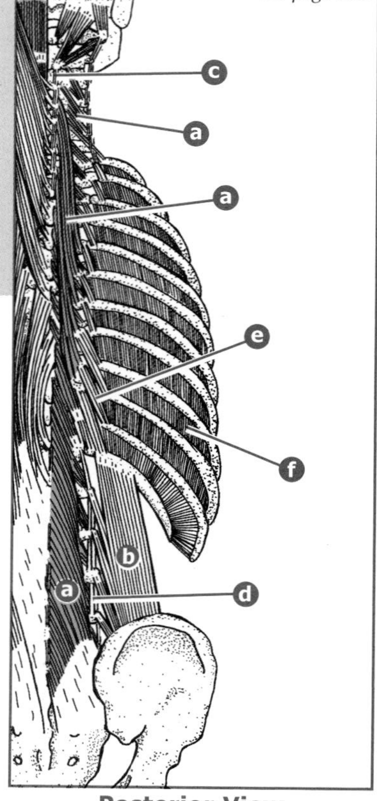

Posterior View of the Trunk

a. **Transversospinalis**
b. Quadratus Lumborum
c. Interspinales
d. Intertransversarii
e. Levatores Costarum
f. External Intercostals

RELATIONSHIP TO OTHER MUSCULOSKELETAL STRUCTURES

❑ 1. The transversospinalis group is very deep in the back and lies in the laminar groove (over the laminae, between the S.P.s and the T.P.s) of the spine.

❑ 2. In the trunk, the transversospinalis group is directly deep to the erector spinae group. In the neck, the transversospinalis group is deep to the trapezius, sternocleidomastoid and the splenius capitis.

❑ 3. In the trunk, the vertebrae are directly deep to the transversospinalis group. In the neck, the suboccipitals are directly deep to the transversospinalis group.

METHODOLOGY FOR LEARNING MUSCLE ACTIONS

❑ 1. **Extension of the Trunk and the Neck and the Head at the Spinal Joints:** The transversospinalis group crosses the spinal joints posteriorly from the pelvis all the way to the head (with its fibers running vertically in the sagittal plane). Therefore, the transversospinalis group extends the trunk and the neck at the spinal joints, and extends the head at the atlanto-occipital joint.

❑ 2. **Lateral Flexion of the Trunk and the Neck and the Head at the Spinal Joints:** The transversospinalis group crosses the spinal joints laterally from the pelvis all the way to the head (with its fibers running vertically in the frontal plane). Therefore, the transversospinalis group laterally flexes the trunk and the neck at the spinal joints, and laterally flexes the head at the atlanto-occipital joint.

THE TRANSVERSOSPINALIS GROUP – continued

- ❑ **3. Contralateral Rotation of the Trunk and the Neck at the Spinal Joints:** The arrangement of the transversospinalis group is generally from a T.P. inferolaterally to an S.P. superomedially (with its fibers running somewhat horizontally in the transverse plane). The inferior attachment is usually more fixed (since the inferior attachment on the trunk and/or pelvis is connected to the thighs, legs and feet, which are grounded); therefore, the superior attachment usually moves. When the transversospinalis group contracts, it pulls the superior attachment on the S.P. posterolaterally toward the more inferolateral T.P., causing the anterior surface of the body part that is moved to face the opposite side of the body from the side of the body that the transversospinalis group is attached. Therefore, the transversospinalis group contralaterally rotates the trunk and the neck at the spinal joints. (The transversospinalis group also crosses the atlanto-occipital joint to attach onto the head. However, the direction of fibers of the transversospinalis is nearly directly vertical at this point. Therefore, the transversospinalis has little or no ability to rotate the head at the atlanto-occipital joint.)
- ❑ **4. Anterior Tilt of the Pelvis at the Lumbosacral Joint:** With the superior attachments fixed, the transversospinalis group, by pulling superiorly on the posterior pelvis, anteriorly tilts the pelvis at the lumbosacral joint.
- ❑ **5. Elevation of the Pelvis at the Lumbosacral Joint:** With the superior attachments fixed, the transversospinalis group, by pulling superiorly on the lateral pelvis (since the fibers are running vertically), elevates the pelvis at the lumbosacral joint.
- ❑ **6. Ipsilateral Rotation of the Pelvis at the Lumbosacral Joint:** When the superior attachments of the transversospinalis group are fixed and the transversospinalis group contracts, it pulls on the inferior attachment, the pelvis. (Since the fibers of the transversospinalis group have a slight horizontal orientation in the transverse plane, the pelvis will rotate.) When the transversospinalis group contracts, it pulls the posterior pelvis posteromedially toward the spine, causing the anterior pelvis to face the same side of the body that the transversospinalis group is attached. Therefore, the transversospinalis group ipsilaterally rotates the pelvis at the lumbosacral joint.

MISCELLANEOUS

- ❑ 1. The name, transversospinalis, tells us that this muscle group attaches from a T.P. ("transverso") to an S.P. ("spinalis"). The transverse process attachment of the transversospinalis group is the inferior attachment; the spinous process attachment of the transversospinalis group is the superior attachment.
- ❑ 2. Actually, the inferior attachment of the transversospinalis group is not always precisely onto the transverse processes. Sometimes the inferior attachment is onto the mamillary or articular processes of the vertebrae.
- ❑ 3. The transversospinalis muscle group can be divided into three subgroups. These three subgroups are, from superficial to deep, the semispinalis, the multifidus and the rotatores.
- ❑ 4. The following statements can be made regarding the transversospinalis subgroups:
    - The semispinalis group attaches superiorly to vertebrae 5 or more levels above the inferior attachment.
    - The multifidus attaches superiorly to vertebrae 3-4 levels above the inferior attachment.
    - The rotatores attach superiorly to the vertebrae 1-2 levels above the inferior attachment.
- ❑ 5. Of the three subgroups of the transversospinalis, only the multifidus attaches onto the pelvis, and only the semispinalis attaches onto the head.

THE TRANSVERSOSPINALIS GROUP – continued

- ❑ 6. The direction of the fibers of the three subgroups of the transversospinalis varies. The semispinalis subgroup is the most vertical and the rotatores subgroup is the most horizontal and the multifidus subgroup is between the other two in orientation. Given these directions of fibers, it would make sense that the semispinalis is best suited for the extension/lateral flexion component of their spinal actions and the rotatores would be best suited for the contralateral rotation component of their spinal actions. (Hence the name "rotatores," since they are horizontal in the transverse plane to do "rotation.")
- ❑ 7. The term *paraspinal musculature* is also used to describe the erector spinae and the transversospinalis groups together.
- ❑ 8. The semispinalis of the transversospinalis can be further subdivided into three subgroups: the semispinalis thoracis, cervicis and capitis.
- ❑ 9. The spinalis capitis of the erector spinae group usually blends with the medial part of the semispinalis capitis and is usually considered to be a part of the semispinalis capitis.
- ❑ 10. The semispinalis is best developed and quite massive in the cervical region.
- ❑ 11. The multifidus is best developed and quite massive in the lumbar region.

SEMISPINALIS
(OF THE TRANSVERSOSPINALIS GROUP)

❑

❑ **The name, semispinalis, tells us that this muscle is associated with S.P.s.**

DERIVATION ❑ semi: L. *half.*
spinalis: L. *refers to spinous processes.*

PRONUNCIATION ❑ **sem**-ee-spy-**na**-lis

ATTACHMENTS

❑ **ENTIRE SEMISPINALIS: T.P.s of C7-T10 and the Articular Processes of C4-6**

❑ SEMISPINALIS THORACIS: T.P.s of T6-10

❑ SEMISPINALIS CERVICIS: T.P.s of T1-5

❑ SEMISPINALIS CAPITIS: T.P.s of C7-T6 and the Articular Processes of C4-6

to the

❑ **ENTIRE SEMISPINALIS: S.P.s of C2-T4 and the Occipital Bone**

❑ SEMISPINALIS THORACIS: S.P.s of C6-T4

❑ SEMISPINALIS CERVICIS: S.P.s of C2-5

❑ SEMISPINALIS CAPITIS: Occipital Bone Between the Superior and Inferior Nuchal Lines

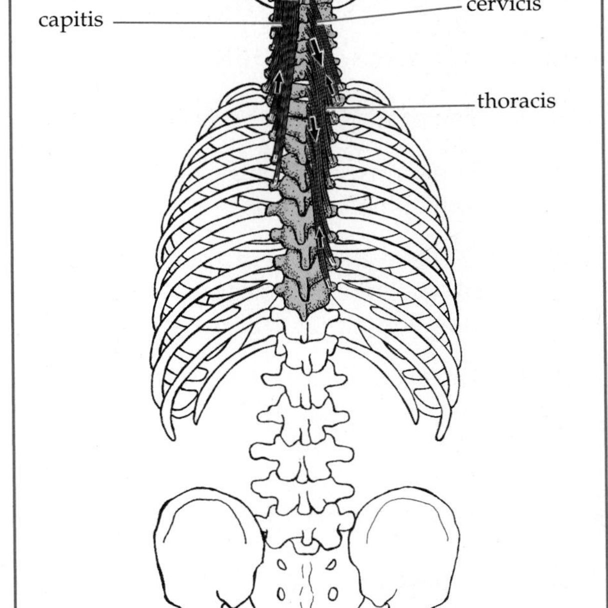

Posterior View of the Semispinalis
(semispinalis thoracis and cervicis on the right)
(semispinalis capitis on the left)

ACTIONS

❑ 1. **Extension of the Trunk and the Neck and the Head**

❑ 2. **Lateral Flexion of the Trunk and the Neck and the Head**

❑ 3. **Contralateral Rotation of the Trunk and the Neck**

INNERVATION ❑ Spinal Nerves
❑ dorsal rami of cervical and thoracic spinal nerves

ARTERIAL SUPPLY ❑ The Occipital Artery (A Branch of the External Carotid Artery) and the Dorsal Branches of the Posterior Intercostal Arteries (Branches of the Aorta)
❑ and the deep cervical artery (a branch of the costocervical trunk)

SEMISPINALIS – PALPATION AND SUPPLEMENTARY TEXT

PALPATION

- ❑ The semispinalis is best palpated in the cervical region where it is deep only to the trapezius between the spine and the splenius capitis. It can be best palpated if the trapezius is relaxed.
  - Have the client supine with the forearm in the small of the back (causing downward rotation of the scapula to relax the trapezius).
  - Place palpating hands in the posteromedial neck and feel for the semispinalis capitis.
  - Continue palpating the semispinalis superiorly toward the occipital attachment between the superior and inferior nuchal lines.

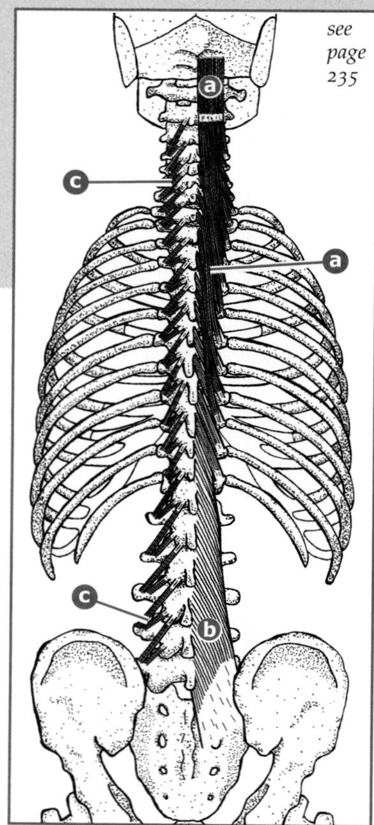

Posterior View of the Trunk

a. **Semispinales**
b. Multifidus
c. Rotatores

RELATIONSHIP TO OTHER MUSCULOSKELETAL STRUCTURES

❑ 1. The semispinalis thoracis is directly deep to the erector spinae.

❑ 2. The semispinalis cervicis is deep to the spinalis cervicis and the semispinalis capitis.

❑ 3. In the neck, the semispinalis capitis is superficial to the suboccipital muscles and deep to the upper trapezius, splenius capitis and the sternocleidomastoid.

❑ 4. The occipital attachment of the semispinalis capitis is sandwiched between the trapezius, sternocleidomastoid and splenius capitis more superficially, and the suboccipitals, deeper.

METHODOLOGY FOR LEARNING MUSCLE ACTIONS

❑ 1. **Extension of the Trunk and the Neck and the Head at the Spinal Joints:** The semispinalis crosses the spinal joints posteriorly from the thoracic region all the way to the head (with its fibers running vertically in the sagittal plane). Therefore, the semispinalis extends the trunk and the neck at the spinal joints, and extends the head at the atlanto-occipital joint.

❑ 2. **Lateral Flexion of the Trunk and the Neck and the Head at the Spinal Joints:** The semispinalis crosses the spinal joints laterally from the thoracic region all the way to the head (with its fibers running vertically in the frontal plane). Therefore, the semispinalis laterally flexes the trunk and the neck at the spinal joints, and laterally flexes the head at the atlanto-occipital joint.

SEMISPINALIS – continued

❑ 3. **Contralateral Rotation of the Trunk and the Neck at the Spinal Joints:** The arrangement of the semispinalis is generally from a T.P. inferolaterally to an S.P. superomedially (with its fibers running somewhat horizontally in the transverse plane). The inferior attachment is usually more fixed (since the inferior attachment on the trunk and/or pelvis is connected to the thighs, legs and feet, which are grounded); therefore, the superior attachment usually moves. When the semispinalis contracts, it pulls the superior attachment on the S.P. posterolaterally toward the more inferolateral T.P., causing the anterior surface of the body part that is moved to face the opposite side of the body from the side of the body that the semispinalis is attached. Therefore, the semispinalis contralaterally rotates the trunk and the neck at the spinal joints. (The semispinalis also crosses the atlanto-occipital joint to attach onto the head. However, the direction of fibers of the semispinalis is nearly directly vertical at this point. Therefore, the semispinalis has little or no ability to rotate the head at the atlanto-occipital joint.)

MISCELLANEOUS

❑ 1. A semispinalis muscle attaches to a T.P. inferiorly and runs superiorly to attach onto the S.P. of a vertebra, five or more levels above the inferior attachment. Most commonly, a semispinalis muscle attaches six levels superior to the inferior attachment.

❑ 2. The fiber direction of the semispinalis is the most vertical of the three transversospinalis groups; hence, its best action is extension of the spine in the sagittal plane.

❑ 3. The semispinalis can be subdivided into the semispinalis thoracis, the semispinalis cervicis and the semispinalis capitis.

❑ 4. The spinalis capitis (of the erector spinae group) usually blends with the medial part of the semispinalis capitis. Therefore, the spinalis capitis is usually considered to be a part of the semispinalis capitis. (Occasionally, the spinalis capitis is a distinct muscle.)

❑ 5. When the spinalis capitis does blend with the medial portion of the semispinalis capitis, this muscle may be known as the *biventer cervicis* because a band of tendon often cuts across it transversely effectively dividing it into two bellies ("biventer" means two bellies), and it is in the neck ("cervicis" means neck).

❑ 6. The semispinalis capitis is the largest of the three subdivisions of the semispinalis.

❑ 7. The inferior attachments of the semispinalis capitis are variable and often attach to the T.P. of T7 and/or to the S.P.s of C7-T1.

❑ 8. The inferior attachments of the semispinalis cervicis are variable and often attach to the T.P. of T6.

❑ 9. The greater occipital nerve, which innervates the posterior half of the scalp, pierces through the semispinalis capitis (as well as the upper trapezius). When the semispinalis capitis is tight, the greater occipital nerve can be compressed causing a *tension headache* that is felt in the posterior head. (This condition is also known as *greater occipital neuralgia*.)

MULTIFIDUS
(OF THE TRANSVERSOSPINALIS GROUP)

❑ **The name, multifidus, tells us that this muscle is made up of many separate muscles that split to go to separate attachments.**

DERIVATION ❑ multi: L. *many.*
fidus: L. *to split.*

PRONUNCIATION ❑ mul-**tif**-id-us

ATTACHMENTS

❑ **Posterior Sacrum, Posterior Superior Iliac Spine (P.S.I.S.), Posterior Sacro-iliac Ligament and L5-C4 Vertebrae**

- ❑ LUMBAR REGION: All Mamillary Processes (not T.P.s)
- ❑ THORACIC REGION: All T.P.s
- ❑ CERVICAL REGION: the Articular Processes of C4-7 (not T.P.s)

to the

❑ **S.P.s of Vertebrae 2-4 Segmental Levels Superior to the Inferior Attachment**

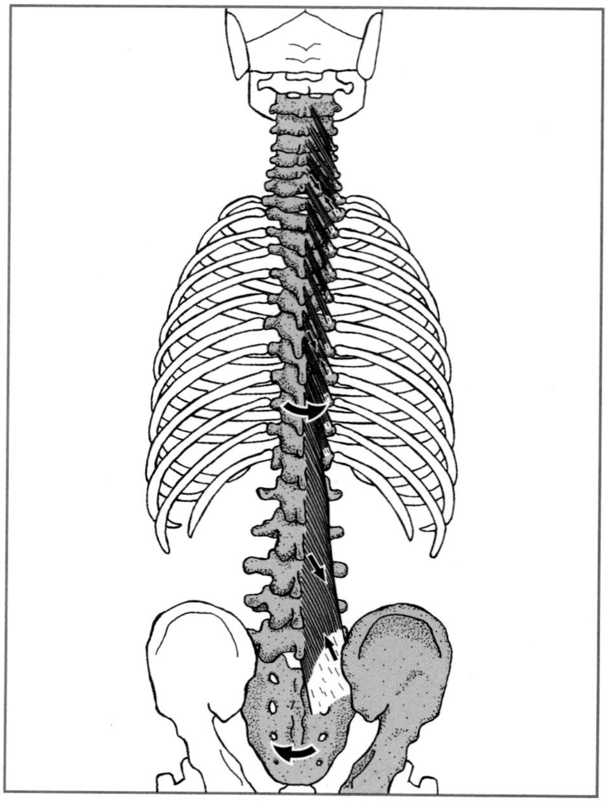

Posterior View of the Right Multifidus

ACTIONS

❑ **1. Extension of the Trunk and the Neck**

❑ **2. Lateral Flexion of the Trunk and the Neck**

❑ **3. Contralateral Rotation of the Trunk and the Neck**

❑ **4. Anterior Tilt of the Pelvis**

❑ **5.** Elevation of the Pelvis

❑ **6.** Ipsilateral Rotation of the Pelvis

INNERVATION ❑ Spinal Nerves ❑ dorsal rami

ARTERIAL SUPPLY ❑ The Dorsal Branches of the Posterior Intercostal and Lumbar Arteries (All Branches of the Aorta)

PALPATION AND SUPPLEMENTARY TEXT

PALPATION

- ❑ The multifidus is deep to the erector spinae group and best palpated in the lumbosacral region, where it is quite bulky. Its mass may be palpated although not precisely distinguished from adjacent musculature.
  - Have the client prone.
  - Place palpating hands on either side of the midline of the sacrum.
  - Ask the client to actively extend the upper part of the body (trunk, neck and head) off the table and feel for the contraction of the multifidus.
  - Continue palpating the multifidus on either side of the midline in the sacral and lumbar regions.

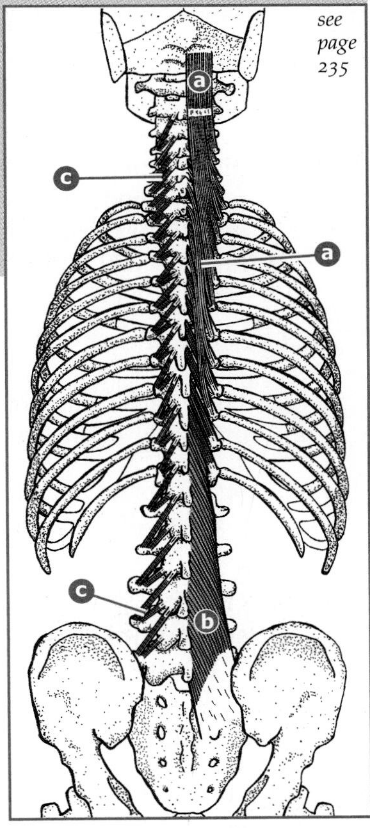

see page 235

Posterior View of the Trunk

a. Semispinales
b. Multifidus
c. Rotatores

RELATIONSHIP TO OTHER MUSCULOSKELETAL STRUCTURES

❑ 1. In the lumbar region, the multifidus group is directly deep to the erector spinae musculature. In the thoracic and cervical region, the multifidus group is directly deep to the semispinalis.

❑ 2. Where the rotatores are present, they are directly deep to the multifidus group. Where there are no rotatores, the vertebrae are directly deep to the multifidus group.

METHODOLOGY FOR LEARNING MUSCLE ACTIONS

❑ **1. Extension of the Trunk and the Neck at the Spinal Joints:** The multifidus group crosses the spinal joints posteriorly from the pelvis all the way to the cervical spine (with its fibers running vertically in the sagittal plane). Therefore, the multifidus group extends the trunk and the neck at the spinal joints.

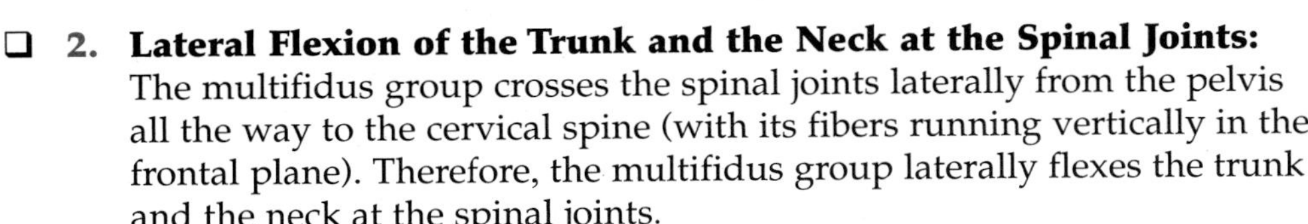

❑ **2. Lateral Flexion of the Trunk and the Neck at the Spinal Joints:** The multifidus group crosses the spinal joints laterally from the pelvis all the way to the cervical spine (with its fibers running vertically in the frontal plane). Therefore, the multifidus group laterally flexes the trunk and the neck at the spinal joints.

❑ **3. Contralateral Rotation of the Trunk and the Neck at the Spinal Joints:** The arrangement of the multifidus group is generally from a T.P. (or mamillary process or articular process) inferolaterally to an S.P. superomedially (with its fibers running somewhat horizontally in the transverse plane). The inferior attachment is usually more fixed (since the inferior attachment on the trunk and/or pelvis is connected to the thighs, legs and feet, which are grounded); therefore, the superior attachment usually moves. When the multifidus group contracts, it pulls the superior attachment on the S.P. posterolaterally toward the more inferolateral T.P., causing the anterior surface of the body part that is moved to face the opposite side of the body from the side of the body that the multifidus group is attached. Therefore, the multifidus group contralaterally rotates the trunk and the neck at the spinal joints.

MULTIFIDUS – continued

❑ **4. Anterior Tilt of the Pelvis at the Lumbosacral Joint:** With the superior attachments fixed, the multifidus group, by pulling superiorly on the posterior pelvis, anteriorly tilts the pelvis at the lumbosacral joint.

❑ **5. Elevation of the Pelvis at the Lumbosacral Joint:** With the superior attachments fixed, the multifidus group, by pulling superiorly on the lateral pelvis (since the fibers are running vertically), elevates the pelvis at the lumbosacral joint.

❑ **6. Ipsilateral Rotation of the Pelvis at the Lumbosacral Joint:** When the superior attachments of the multifidus group are fixed and the multifidus group contracts, it pulls on the inferior attachment, the pelvis. (Since the fibers of the multifidus group have a slight horizontal orientation in the transverse plane, the pelvis will rotate.) When the multifidus group contracts, it pulls the posterior pelvis posteromedially toward the spine, causing the anterior pelvis to face the same side of the body that the multifidus group is attached. Therefore, the multifidus group ipsilaterally rotates the pelvis at the lumbosacral joint.

MISCELLANEOUS

❑ 1. The attachments for the multifidus group are from a T.P. (or mamillary process or articular process) inferiorly to an S.P. superiorly.

❑ 2. By the usual definition, the multifidus group attaches to an S.P. 3-4 levels superior to its inferior attachment.

❑ 3. Some sources describe the multifidus group as having layers that span from 1- 4 vertebrae superior to the inferior attachment. More specifically, they describe three layers. The most superficial layer goes from a T.P. inferiorly, to an S.P. 3-4 levels superiorly. The next layer goes from the same T.P. to an S.P. 2-3 levels superior. Some sources state that the deepest layer goes from the same T.P. to the S.P. of the very next vertebra superiorly. (More conventional naming of the transversospinalis group would name these last fibers as rotatores.)

❑ 4. The multifidus group is bulkiest in the lumbosacral region.

❑ 5. There is actually very little erector spinae musculature that overlies the multifidus in the lumbar region. However, in this region, the tendinous fibers of the erector spinae are very thick and difficult to palpate through.

ROTATORES
(OF THE TRANSVERSOSPINALIS GROUP)

❑ **The name, rotatores, tells us that these muscles perform rotation.**

DERIVATION ❑ rotatores: L. *to turn, a muscle revolving a body part on its axis.*

PRONUNCIATION ❑ ro-ta-**to**-reez

ATTACHMENTS

❑ **T.P. (inferiorly)**

to the

❑ **Lamina (superiorly)**

- ❑ of the vertebrae 1-2 levels superior

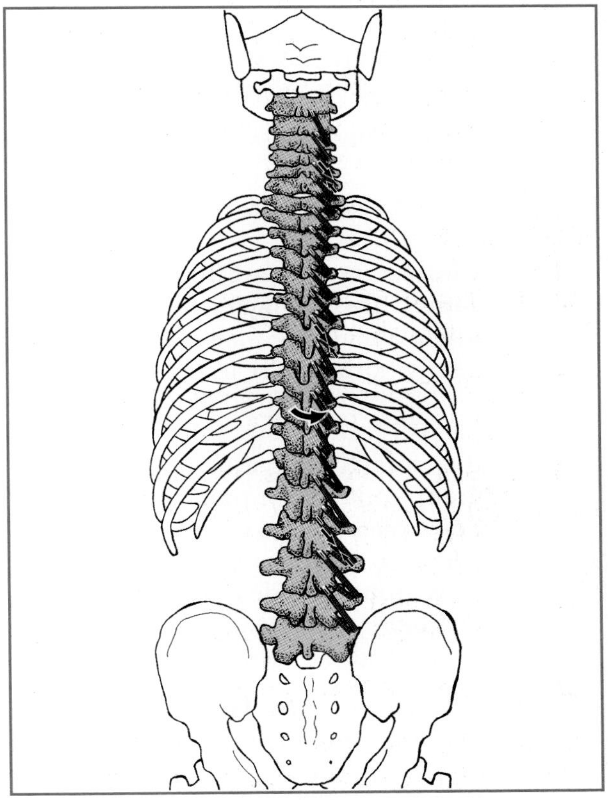

ACTIONS

❑ 1. **Contralateral Rotation of the Trunk and the Neck**

❑ 2. **Extension of the Trunk and the Neck**

Posterior View of the Right Rotatores

INNERVATION ❑ Spinal Nerves ❑ dorsal rami

ARTERIAL SUPPLY ❑ The Dorsal Branches of the Posterior Intercostal and Lumbar Arteries (All Branches of the Aorta)

ROTATORES – PALPATION AND SUPPLEMENTARY TEXT

PALPATION

❑ The rotatores are very small and extremely deep muscles that are virtually impossible to palpate. If palpation is to be attempted, have the client prone and place your palpating fingers in the client's laminar groove (over the laminae, between the S.P.s and the T.P.s) while asking the client to actively rotate the trunk away from you and feel for the contraction of the rotatores.

RELATIONSHIP TO OTHER MUSCULOSKELETAL STRUCTURES

❑ 1. The rotatores are extremely deep in the laminar groove. They are directly deep to the multifidus.

❑ 2. Deep to the rotatores are the vertebrae.

METHODOLOGY FOR LEARNING MUSCLE ACTIONS

❑ **1. Contralateral Rotation of the Trunk and the Neck at the Spinal Joints:** The arrangement of the rotatores group is generally from a T.P. inferolaterally to a lamina superomedially (with its fibers running nearly horizontally in the transverse plane). The inferior attachment is usually more fixed (since the inferior attachment on the trunk and/or pelvis is connected to the thighs, legs and feet, which are grounded); therefore, the superior attachment usually moves. When the rotatores group contracts, it pulls the superior attachment on the lamina posterolaterally toward the more inferolateral T.P., causing the anterior surface of the body part that is moved to face the opposite side of the body from the side of the body that the rotatores group is attached. Therefore, the rotatores group contralaterally rotates the trunk and the neck at the spinal joints.

❑ **2. Extension of the Trunk and the Neck at the Spinal Joints:** The rotatores group crosses the spinal joints posteriorly from a T.P. inferiorly, to a lamina superiorly (with their fibers running somewhat vertically in the sagittal plane). Therefore, the rotatores extend the trunk and the neck at the spinal joints.

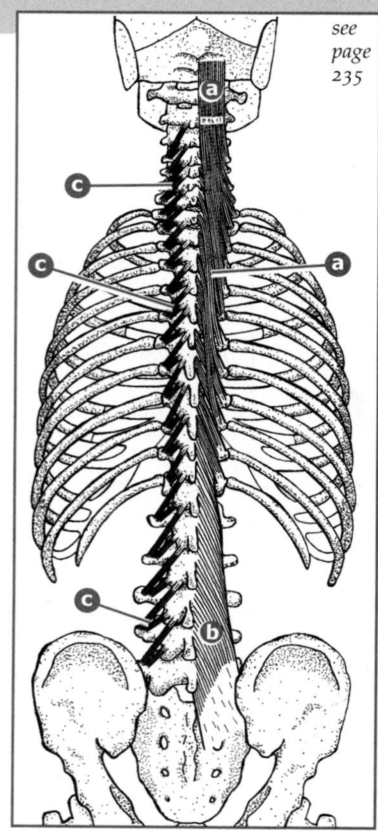

see page 235

Posterior View of the Trunk

a. Semispinales
b. Multifidus
c. **Rotatores**

MISCELLANEOUS

❑ 1. By the usual definition, the rotatores group attaches to an S.P. 1-2 levels superior to its inferior attachment.

❑ 2. The rotatores are usually divided into a brevis component that attaches to the vertebra immediately superior and a longus component that skips one vertebra to attach to the vertebra two above.

❑ 3. The fiber direction of the rotatores group is the most horizontal of the three transversospinalis groups. Being more horizontal gives it a line of pull in the transverse plane, creating the action of rotation, hence, its name "rotatores."

❑ 4. The rotatores are technically subdivided into three subgroups: the rotatores lumborum, rotatores thoracis and the rotatores cervicis.

❑ 5. Only the rotatores thoracis subgroup is well developed. The rotatores lumborum and rotatores cervicis are only represented by irregular muscle bundles that are similar in arrangement to the rotatores thoracis.

QUADRATUS LUMBORUM

❑ **The name, quadratus lumborum, tells us that this muscle is shaped somewhat like a square and is located in the lumbar, i.e., lower back, region.**

DERIVATION ❑ quadratus: L. *squared.*
lumborum: L. *loin* (low back).

PRONUNCIATION ❑ kwod-**ray**-tus lum-**bor**-um

ATTACHMENTS

❑ **12th Rib and the T.P.s of L1-4**

- ❑ the medial 1/2 of the inferior border of the 12th rib

to the

❑ **Posterior iliac Crest**

- ❑ the posteromedial iliac crest and the iliolumbar ligament

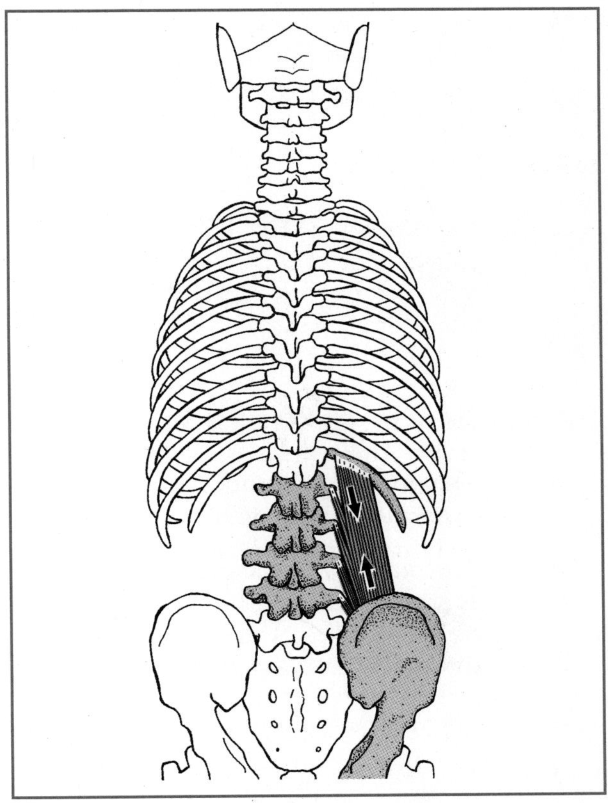

Posterior View of the Right Quadratus Lumborum

ACTIONS

❑ 1. **Elevation of the Pelvis**

❑ 2. **Anterior Tilt of the Pelvis** Tucks!

❑ 3. **Lateral Flexion of the Trunk**

❑ 4. **Extension of the Trunk**

❑ 5. Depression of the 12th Rib

INNERVATION ❑ Lumbar Plexus ❑ T12, L1, 2, 3

ARTERIAL SUPPLY ❑ Branches of the Subcostal and Lumbar Arteries (All Branches of the Aorta)
❑ and the iliolumbar artery (a branch of the internal iliac artery)

QUADRATUS LUMBORUM – PALPATION AND SUPPLEMENTARY TEXT

PALPATION

- ❑ The quadratus lumborum is a square-shaped muscle in the lumbar region. Given that it is deep to the erector spinae, the quadratus lumborum must be palpated from the side.
  - Have the client prone.
  - Place palpating hand superior to the iliac crest and just lateral to the erector spinae musculature.
  - Ask the client to elevate the pelvis (move the pelvis toward the head) on the side you are palpating and feel for the contraction of the quadratus lumborum.
  - It may be difficult to distinguish the quadratus lumborum from the adjacent musculature since elevation of the pelvis will also cause the erector spinae to contract, as well as the abdominal wall muscles and perhaps the latissimus dorsi.
  - Continue palpating the quadratus lumborum medially, attempting to feel it deep to the erector spinae.

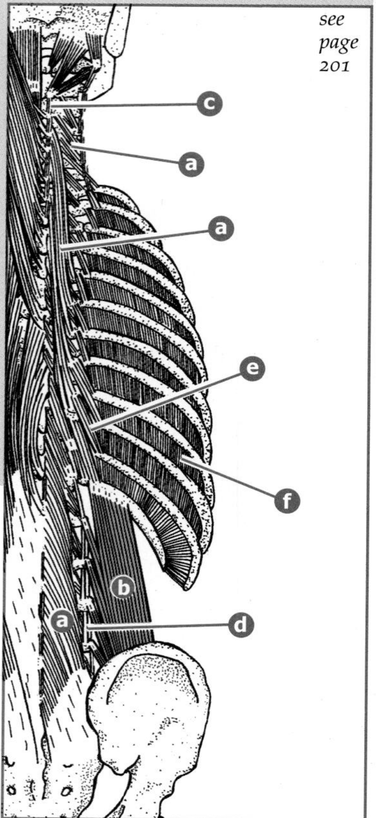

see page 201

Posterior View of the Trunk

a. Transversospinalis
b. Quadratus Lumborum
c. Interspinales
d. Intertransversarii
e. Levatores Costarum
f. External Intercostals

RELATIONSHIP TO OTHER MUSCULOSKELETAL STRUCTURES

❑ 1. The quadratus lumborum is very deep and forms part of the posterior abdominal body wall.

❑ 2. The majority of the quadratus lumborum is deep to the erector spinae. A small portion of the lateral part of the quadratus lumborum is deep to the muscles of the abdominal wall (external abdominal oblique, internal abdominal oblique and the transversus abdominis).

❑ 3. The abdominal viscera are deep (anterior) to the quadratus lumborum.

❑ 4. The psoas major lies slightly anterior and medial to the quadratus lumborum.

METHODOLOGY FOR LEARNING MUSCLE ACTIONS

❑ **1. Elevation of the Pelvis at the Lumbosacral Joint:** With the superior attachments fixed, the quadratus lumborum, by pulling superiorly on the lateral pelvis (since the fibers are running vertically), elevates the pelvis at the lumbosacral joint.

❑ **2. Anterior Tilt of the Pelvis at the Lumbosacral Joint:** With the superior attachments fixed, the quadratus lumborum, by pulling superiorly on the posterior pelvis, anteriorly tilts the pelvis at the lumbosacral joint.

❑ **3. Lateral Flexion of the Trunk at the Spinal Joints:** The quadratus lumborum crosses the spinal joints laterally (with its fibers running vertically in the frontal plane); therefore, it laterally flexes the trunk at the spinal joints.

QUADRATUS LUMBORUM – continued

- ❑ 4. **Extension of the Trunk at the Spinal Joints:** The quadratus lumborum crosses the spinal joints posteriorly (with its fibers running vertically in the sagittal plane); therefore, it extends the trunk at the spinal joints.
- ❑ 5. **Depression of the 12th Rib at the Costovertebral Joints:** When the pelvic attachment is fixed and the quadratus lumborum contracts, it pulls the 12th rib inferiorly toward the pelvis. Therefore, the quadratus lumborum depresses the 12th rib.

MISCELLANEOUS

- ❑ 1. A common variation of the quadratus lumborum is to also have an attachment onto the T.P. of L5.
- ❑ 2. The quadratus lumborum, by pulling inferiorly on the 12th rib, causes the thoracic cavity to expand, which creates more space for the lungs to expand. However, the main function of the quadratus lumborum regarding the 12th rib is not to be a mover and actually move the 12th rib into depression, but rather to fix the 12th rib in place so that it does not elevate when the diaphragm contracts and exerts an upward pull upon it. In this manner, if the lower attachments of the diaphragm are fixed, the diaphragm contracts and the dome of the diaphragm drops down more efficiently, thus increasing the size of the thoracic cavity for the lungs to expand and fill with air. Therefore, the quadratus lumborum is a muscle of inspiration primarily as a fixator (stabilizer).
- ❑ 3. When working on the quadratus lumborum, you can position the client either prone, supine or side lying. However, since it is so deep (to the massive erector spinae musculature), it must be accessed with palpatory pressure from lateral to medial (i.e., come in from the side).
- ❑ 4. Keep in mind that the quadratus lumborum is not the only muscle in the lateral lumbar region and should not be blamed for all pain in that area. The erector spinae is also present in the lateral lumbar region and is functionally active and just as likely or even more likely to develop tension and pain.
- ❑ 5. The quadratus lumborum can elevate the pelvis. Often the term "hiking up the hip" is used to describe this action. This term "hiking up the hip" can be very misleading and ambiguous. Generally, when the term "hip" is used (unless the context is otherwise made very clear) it is assumed that movement of the femur at the hip joint is meant, not movement of the pelvis at the lumbosacral joint.

INTERSPINALES

❑ **The name, interspinales, tells us that these muscles are located between spinous processes of the vertebrae.**

DERIVATION ❑ interspinales: L. *between spinous processes.*

PRONUNCIATION ❑ **in**-ter-spy-**na**-leez

ATTACHMENTS

❑ **From an S.P. to the S.P. directly superior**

- ❑ CERVICAL REGION: there are 6 pairs of interspinales located between T1-C2
- ❑ THORACIC REGION: there are 2 pairs of interspinales located between T2-T1 and T12-T11
- ❑ LUMBAR REGION: there are 4 pairs of interspinales located between L5-L1

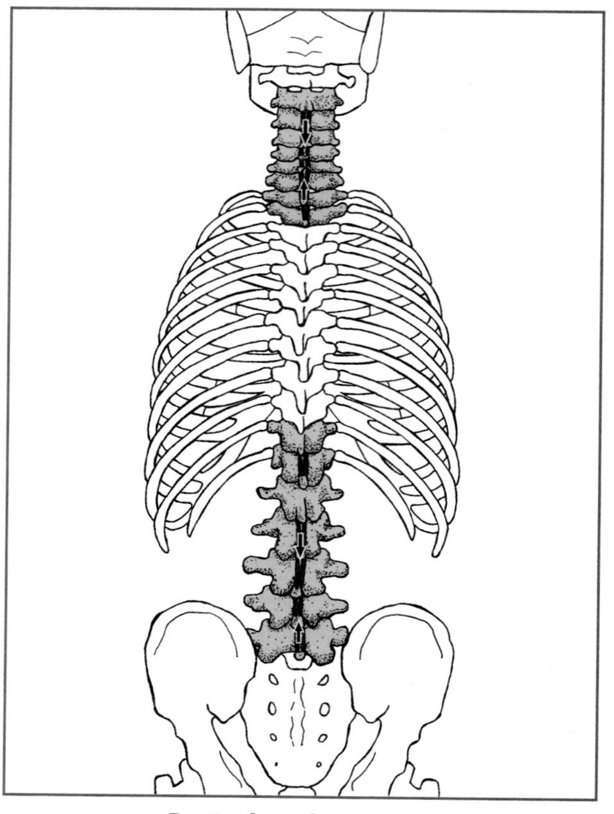

Posterior View of the Right and Left Interspinales

ACTION

❑ **Extension of the Neck and the Trunk**

INNERVATION ❑ Spinal Nerves ❑ dorsal rami

ARTERIAL SUPPLY ❑ The Dorsal Branches of the Posterior Intercostal Arteries (Branches of the Aorta)

PALPATION AND SUPPLEMENTARY TEXT

PALPATION

- ☐ The interspinales are small muscles located between the S.P.s of the spine, along with the interspinous ligaments and the supraspinous ligament. However, it is difficult to distinguish the interspinales muscles from these other tissues.
  - Have the client seated.
  - Place palpating fingers between the vertebral spinous processes.
  - Ask the client to flex the neck and/or trunk and feel for the interspinales.

    (Note: Flexion will increase the space between the S.P.s and make access to the interspinales easier. However, it will also cause the tissue to become stretched and taut.)

see page 201

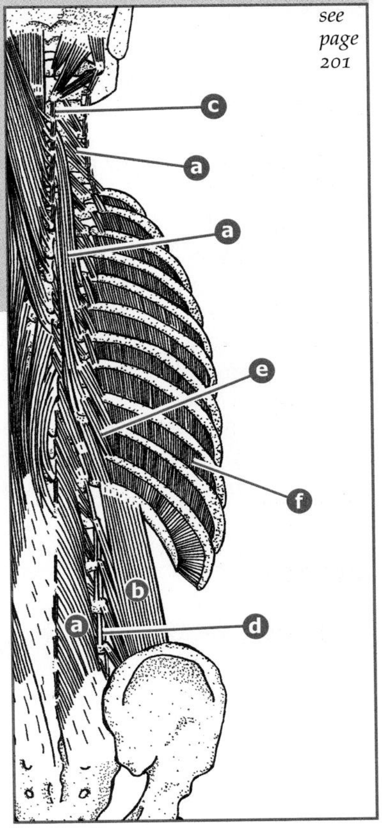

Posterior View of the Trunk

- **a.** Transversospinalis
- **b.** Quadratus Lumborum
- **c.** **Interspinales**
- **d.** Intertransversarii
- **e.** Levatores Costarum
- **f.** External Intercostals

RELATIONSHIP TO OTHER MUSCULOSKELETAL STRUCTURES

- ☐ 1. The interspinales are paired muscles that are located on either side of the interspinous ligaments, between the apices of S.P.s of adjacent vertebrae.
- ☐ 2. The interspinales are located deep to the supraspinous ligament (the nuchal ligament in the cervical region).

METHODOLOGY FOR LEARNING MUSCLE ACTIONS

- ☐ **Extension of the Neck and the Trunk at the Spinal Joints:** Each interspinalis muscle attaches from an S.P. of a vertebra inferiorly to the S.P. of the vertebra directly superior. Therefore, the interspinales cross the vertebral joints posteriorly (with their fibers running vertically in the sagittal plane). When an interspinalis muscle contracts, it pulls the more superior vertebra posteriorly and inferiorly toward the more inferior vertebra, which creates extension of that vertebra of the neck and/or trunk at the spinal joint between them.

MISCELLANEOUS

- ☐ 1. The interspinales are paired muscles on either side of the interspinous ligaments.
- ☐ 2. The interspinales are not located throughout the entire spine. They are primarily found in the cervical region (six pairs between C2 and T1) and the lumbar region (four pairs between L1 and L5). In the thoracic region, there are usually only two pairs found at T2-T1 and T12-11.
- ☐ 3. The interspinales vary in location and are occasionally also found at T3-2, L1-T12 and S1-L5.
- ☐ 4. Some sources believe that the interspinales do not have sufficient strength nor leverage to actually create movement of the spine, but may be important as fixating (stabilizing) muscles of the spine. Other sources believe that the interspinales are not even capable of fixating the vertebrae; instead, they conjecture that the interspinales are important for proprioception by providing precise monitoring of intervertebral positions.

INTERTRANSVERSARII

❑ **The name, intertransversarii, tells us that these muscles are located between transverse processes of the vertebrae.**

DERIVATION ❑ intertransversarii: L. *between transverse processes.*

PRONUNCIATION ❑ **in**-ter-trans-ver-**sa**-ri-eye

ATTACHMENTS

❑ **From a T.P. to the T.P. directly superior**

- ❑ CERVICAL REGION: There are 7 pairs of intertransversarii muscles (anterior and posterior sets) located between C1 and T1 on each side of the body.
- ❑ THORACIC REGION: There are 3 intertransversarii muscles between T10 and L1 on each side of the body.
- ❑ LUMBAR REGION: There are 4 pairs of intertransversarii muscles (medial and lateral sets) located between L1 and L5 on each side of the body.

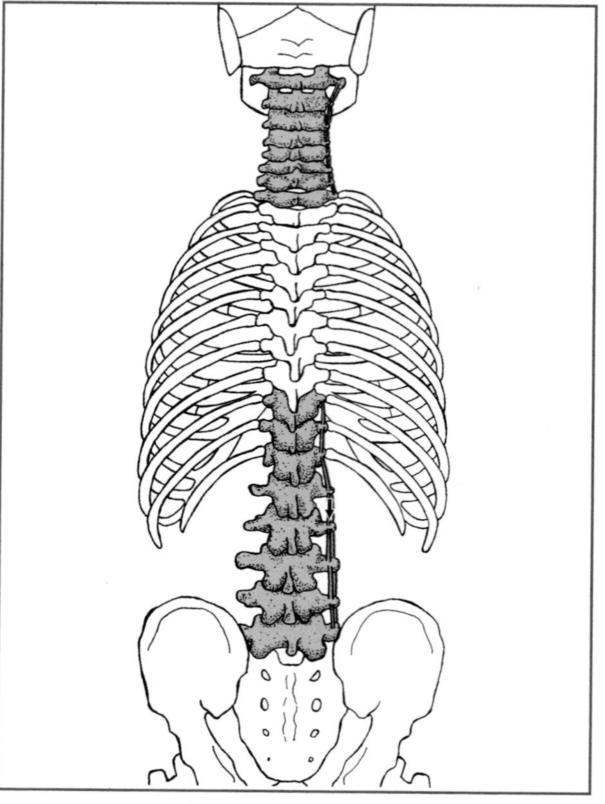

Posterior View of the Right Intertransversarii

ACTION

❑ **Lateral Flexion of the Neck and the Trunk**

INNERVATION ❑ Spinal Nerves ❑ dorsal and ventral rami

ARTERIAL SUPPLY ❑ The Dorsal Branches of the Posterior Intercostal Arteries (Branches of the Aorta)

PALPATION AND SUPPLEMENTARY TEXT

PALPATION

- ❑ The intertransversarii muscles are small and very deep muscles. Palpating and distinguishing them from adjacent musculature are nearly impossible.

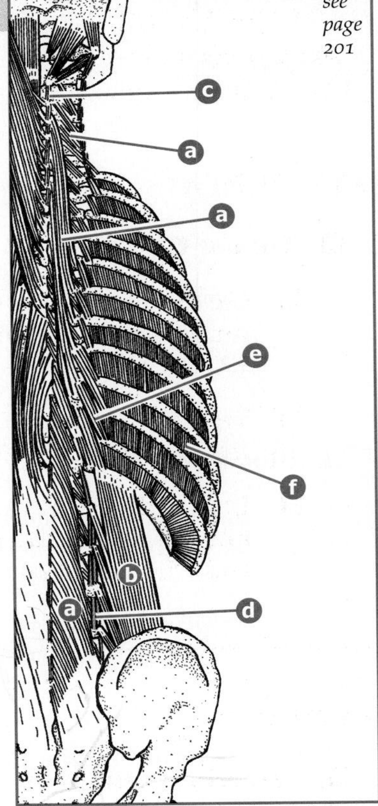

Posterior View of the Trunk

a. Transversospinalis
b. Quadratus Lumborum
c. Interspinales
d. Intertransversarii
e. Levatores Costarum
f. External Intercostals

RELATIONSHIP TO OTHER MUSCULOSKELETAL STRUCTURES

- ❑ 1. The thoracic and lumbar intertransversarii are located between T.P.s and are very deep. The latissimus dorsi, erector spinae and the serratus posterior inferior are all superficial to the thoracic and lumbar intertransversarii.
- ❑ 2. The cervical intertransversarii are located between the T.P.s and are very deep. The trapezius, splenius capitis, splenius cervicis and the semispinalis capitis are all superficial to the cervical intertransversarii.

METHODOLOGY FOR LEARNING MUSCLE ACTIONS

- ❑ **Lateral Flexion of the Neck and the Trunk at the Spinal Joints:** Each intertransversarii muscle attaches from a T.P. of one vertebra and runs superiorly to attach onto the T.P. of the vertebra directly superior. Therefore, they cross the vertebral joints laterally (with their fibers running vertically in the frontal plane). When an intertransversarii contracts, it pulls the more superior vertebra inferiorly and laterally toward the more inferior vertebra, which creates lateral flexion of that vertebra of the neck and/or trunk at the spinal joint between them.

MISCELLANEOUS

- ❑ 1. The anterior cervical intertransversarii attach onto the anterior tubercles of the T.P.s of the cervical spine and the posterior cervical intertransversarii attach onto the posterior tubercles of the T.P.s of the cervical spine. The lumbar medial intertransversarii attach to accessory and mamillary processes of the lumbar vertebrae and the lumbar lateral intertransversarii attach to T.P.s of the lumbar vertebrae.
- ❑ 2. The intertransversarii between C1 (atlas) and C2 (axis) are often absent.
- ❑ 3. Essentially, the intertransversarii do not exist in the thoracic region. The levatores costarum and the intercostals are considered to the homologous with the two sets of intertransversarii in the thoracic region.
- ❑ 4. Ventral and dorsal rami of spinal nerves run between and pierce through the intertransversarii, especially in the cervical region.
- ❑ 5. The intertransversarii are considered to be primarily important not as movers of the spine, but as fixating (stabilizing) postural muscles.

❑ LEVATORES COSTARUM

❑ **The name, levatores costarum, tells us that these muscles elevate the ribs.**

DERIVATION ❑ levator: L. *lifter.*
costarum: L. *refers to the ribs.*

PRONUNCIATION ❑ le-va-**to**-rez (singular: le-**vay**-tor) kos-**tar**-um

ATTACHMENTS

❑ **T.P.s of C7-T11**

- ❑ the tips of the T.P.s

to the

❑ **Ribs #1-12 (inferiorly)**

- ❑ the external surfaces of the ribs, between the tubercle and the angle

ACTIONS

❑ 1. **Elevation of the Ribs**

❑ 2. Extension of the Trunk

❑ 3. Lateral Flexion of the Trunk

❑ 4. Contralateral Rotation of the Trunk

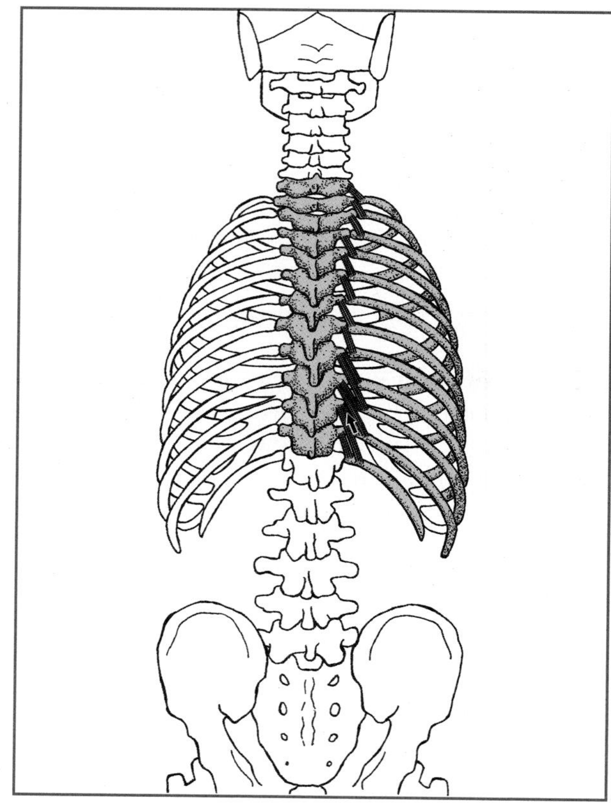

Posterior View of the Right Levatores Costarum

INNERVATION ❑ Spinal Nerves ❑ dorsal rami

ARTERIAL SUPPLY ❑ The Dorsal Branches of the Posterior Intercostal Arteries (Branches of the Aorta)

PALPATION AND SUPPLEMENTARY TEXT

PALPATION

- ❑ The levatores costarum are small and very deep muscles. Palpating and distinguishing the levatores costarum from the adjacent musculature are extremely difficult if not impossible. If palpation is to be attempted, have the client prone and place your palpating fingers between the mass of the erector spinae musculature and the angles of the ribs while asking the client to slowly and deeply breath in and out. Try to feel for the contraction of the levatores costarum.

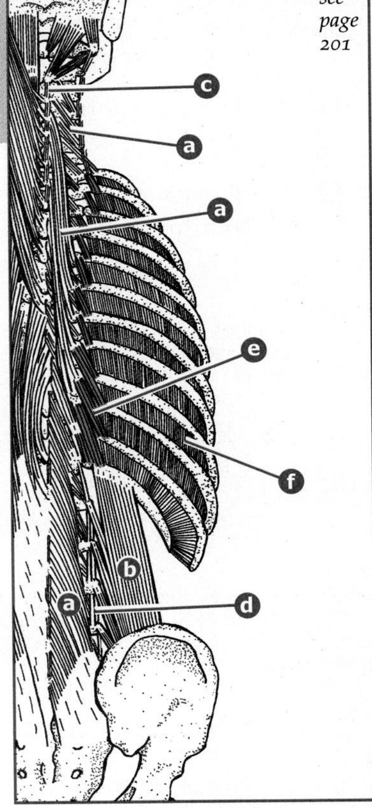

see page 201

Posterior View of the Trunk

a. Transversospinalis
b. Quadratus Lumborum
c. Interspinales
d. Intertransversarii
e. **Levatores Costarum**
f. External Intercostals

RELATIONSHIP TO OTHER MUSCULOSKELETAL STRUCTURES

- ❑ 1. The levatores costarum are deep to the trapezius, latissimus dorsi, serratus posterior superior, serratus posterior inferior and the erector spinae muscles.
- ❑ 2. Deep to the levatores costarum are the intercostal muscles.

METHODOLOGY FOR LEARNING MUSCLE ACTIONS

- ❑ 1. **Elevation of the Ribs at the Sternocostal and Costovertebral Joints:** The levatores costarum attach from superiorly on a vertebral T.P. to inferiorly onto a rib (with their fibers running vertically). When the vertebral attachment is fixed and the levatores costarum contract, they pull the costal attachments, i.e., the ribs, superiorly toward the vertebral attachment. Therefore, the levatores costarum elevate the ribs at the sternocostal and costovertebral joints.
- ❑ 2. **Extension of the Trunk at the Spinal Joints:** When the costal attachment of the levatores costarum is fixed and the levatores costarum contract, they pull the vertebral attachment toward the costal attachment. Since the levatores costarum cross the spinal joints posteriorly (with their fibers running vertically in the sagittal plane), they extend the trunk at the spinal joints.
- ❑ 3. **Lateral Flexion of the Trunk at the Spinal Joints:** When the costal attachment of the levatores costarum is fixed and the levatores costarum contract, they pull the vertebral attachment toward the costal attachment. Since the levatores costarum cross the spinal joints somewhat laterally (with their fibers running vertically in the frontal plane), they laterally flex the trunk at the spinal joints.
- ❑ 4. **Contralateral Rotation of the Trunk at the Spinal Joints:** When the costal attachment of the levatores costarum is fixed and the levatores costarum contract, they pull the vertebral attachment toward the costal attachment. When the levatores costarum contract, they pull the vertebral attachment posterolaterally (since the fibers are running somewhat horizontally in the transverse plane), causing the anterior surface of the trunk to face the opposite side of the body from the side of the body that the levatores costarum are attached. Therefore, the levatores costarum contralaterally rotate the trunk at the spinal joints.

LEVATORES COSTARUM – continued

MISCELLANEOUS

- ☐ 1. The levatores costarum attach from a T.P. of a vertebra and orient inferiorly and laterally to attach onto the rib directly inferior to the vertebral attachment. However, the levatores costarum that attach to vertebrae T8-10 have a second slip of tissue that also attaches to the second rib below that vertebral attachment (i.e., ribs #10-12). When this occurs, the two parts of the levatores costarum are called the *levatores costarum breves* and the *levatores costarum longi*.
- ☐ 2. There is controversy as to whether the primary role of the levatores costarum is as respiratory muscles that move the ribs or as muscles that move and/or fix (stabilize) the spinal joints.
- ☐ 3. The levatores costarum are considered to be homologous to the intertransversarii of the cervical and lumber regions.

SUBCOSTALES

❑ **The name, subcostales, tells us that these muscles are "under," i.e., deep, to the ribs.**

DERIVATION ❑ sub: L. *under.*
costales: L. *refers to the ribs.*

PRONUNCIATION ❑ sub-kos-**tal**-eez

ATTACHMENTS

❑ **Ribs #10-12**

❑ the internal surface of the ribs, near the angle

to the

❑ **Ribs #8-10**

❑ the internal surface of the ribs, near the angle

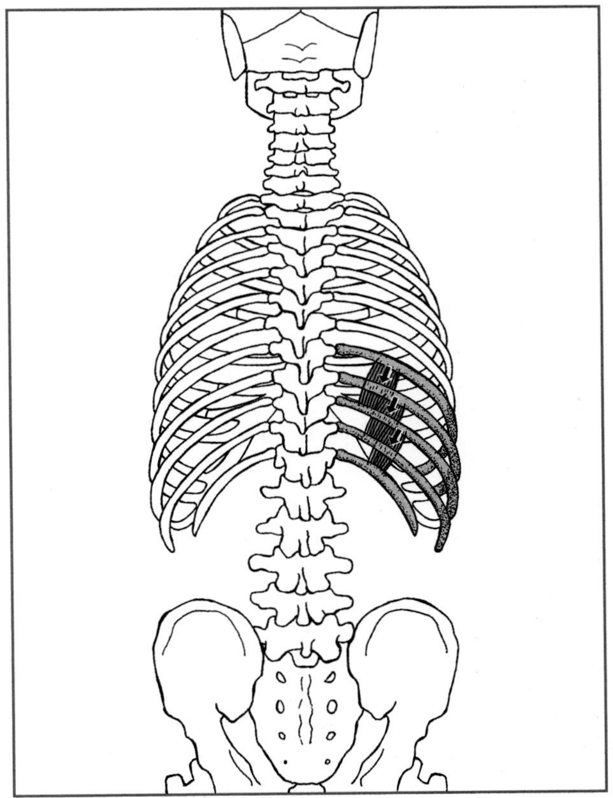

Posterior View of the Right Subcostales

ACTION

❑ **Depression of Ribs #8-10**

INNERVATION ❑ Intercostal Nerves

ARTERIAL SUPPLY ❑ The Dorsal Branches of the Posterior Intercostal Arteries (Branches of the Aorta)

SUBCOSTALES – PALPATION AND SUPPLEMENTARY TEXT

PALPATION

- ❑ The subcostales are deep to the ribcage itself and are essentially not palpable. If pressure were to translate through to them, it would have to be applied with your palpating fingers just lateral to the erector spinae's lateral border in the intercostal spaces between ribs #8-12.

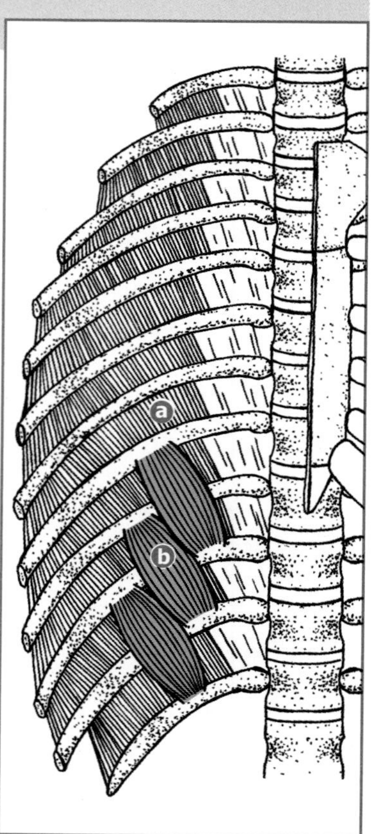

Anterior View of the Internal Wall of the Trunk

a. Internal Intercostals
b. Subcostales

RELATIONSHIP TO OTHER MUSCULOSKELETAL STRUCTURES

- ❑ 1. The subcostales are deep to the ribcage and all the musculature overlying the ribcage in the lower posterior thoracic region, as well as the external and internal intercostal muscles and the intercostal neurovascular bundle.
- ❑ 2. The subcostales are superficial to the pleural membrane of the lungs.

METHODOLOGY FOR LEARNING MUSCLE ACTIONS

- ❑ **Depression of Ribs #8-10 at the Sternocostal and Costovertebral Joints:** The subcostales attach from the internal surface of a rib and run superiorly (with their fibers running vertically), skipping one rib to attach onto the internal surface of a more superior rib. When the subcostales contract, they pull the more superior rib inferiorly toward the more inferior rib. Therefore, the subcostales depress ribs #8-10. This action assists forceful expiration by decreasing the size of the thoracic cavity; hence, the subcostales are respiratory muscles.

MISCELLANEOUS

- ❑ 1. The subcostales are variable in their presentation. They are usually well developed only in the lower thoracic region. Most often, there are three subcostales muscles running from rib #8 to rib #10, rib #9 to rib #11, and rib #10 to rib #12 (as presented earlier in the attachment section and shown in the individual illustration).
- ❑ 2. There is controversy as to the precise action(s) of the subcostales. It is supposed that they are respiratory muscles that depress the ribs for forced expiration. This action would be based upon their inferior attachment staying fixed, and the muscles pulling the superior attachment inferiorly. However, from their line of pull, if the superior attachment were to stay fixed, it is conceivable that they could also pull the lower attachment superiorly and elevate the lower ribs, i.e., ribs #10-12.

PECTORALIS MAJOR

❑ **The name, pectoralis major, tells us that this muscle is located in the pectoral (chest) region and is large (larger than the pectoralis minor).**

DERIVATION ❑ pectoralis: L. *refers to the chest.*
major: L. *larger.*

PRONUNCIATION ❑ **pek**-to-ra-lis **may**-jor

ATTACHMENTS

❑ **Medial Clavicle, Sternum and the Costal Cartilages of Ribs #1-7**

- ❑ the medial 1/2 of the clavicle and the aponeurosis of the external abdominal oblique

to the

❑ **Lateral Lip of the Bicipital Groove of the Humerus**

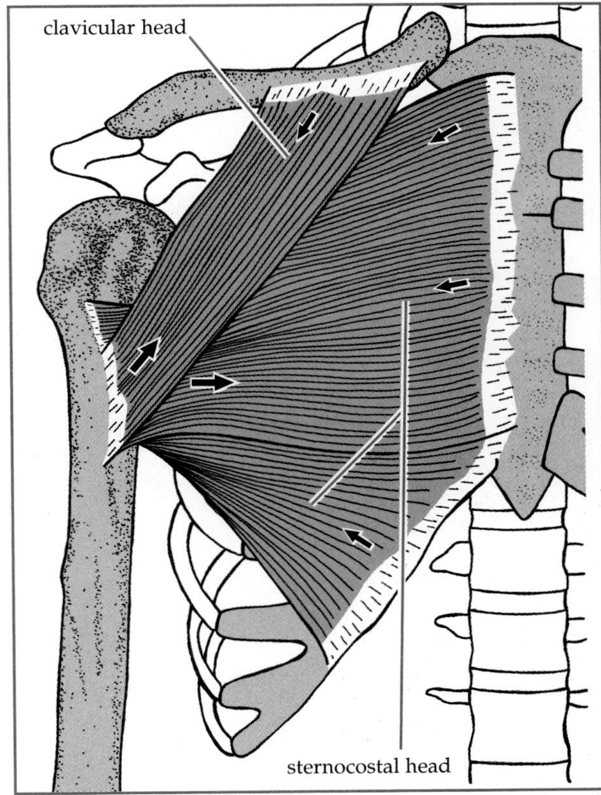

Anterior View of the Right Pectoralis Major

ACTIONS

❑ 1. **Adduction of the Arm**

❑ 2. **Medial Rotation of the Arm**

❑ 3. **Flexion of the Arm (clavicular head)**

❑ 4. Extension of the Arm (sternocostal head)

❑ 5. Abduction of the Arm (clavicular head, above 90°)

❑ 6. Depression of the Scapula

❑ 7. Elevation of the Trunk

❑ 8. Lateral Deviation of the Trunk

❑ 9. Ipsilateral Rotation of the Trunk

INNERVATION ❑ The Medial and Lateral Pectoral Nerves ❑ **C5**, 6, **7**, 8, T1

ARTERIAL SUPPLY ❑ The Pectoral Branches of the Thoracoacromial Trunk (A Branch of the Axillary Artery)

- ❑ and the posterior intercostal arteries (branches of the aorta) and the lateral thoracic artery (a branch of the axillary artery)

PECTORALIS MAJOR – PALPATION AND SUPPLEMENTARY TEXT

PALPATION

The pectoralis major is a large and superficial muscle in the chest that is both visible and palpable. It makes up the vast majority of the anterior axillary fold of tissue.

- Have the client seated.

❑ **To palpate the entire muscle:**

- Have the client raise the arm to 90° of abduction at the shoulder joint.
- Place palpating hand on the belly of the pectoralis major.
- Ask the client to actively horizontally flex the arm at the shoulder joint against resistance and feel for the contraction of the pectoralis major.
- Continue palpating the pectoralis major medially and superiorly toward its attachments on the trunk and distally toward its humeral attachment.

❑ **To palpate the clavicular head:**

- Place palpating hand inferior to the medial clavicle.
- Resist the client from moving the arm at the shoulder joint obliquely toward the head (i.e., flexion and adduction) and feel for the contraction of the pectoralis major.
- Continue palpating the pectoralis major distally toward its humeral attachment.

❑ **To palpate the sternocostal head:**

- Place palpating hand on the inferior aspect of the anterior axillary fold.
- Resist the client from adducting the arm at the shoulder joint and feel for the contraction of the sternocostal head of the pectoralis major.
- Continue palpating the sternocostal head of the pectoralis major medially toward its attachment on the trunk and distally toward its humeral attachment.

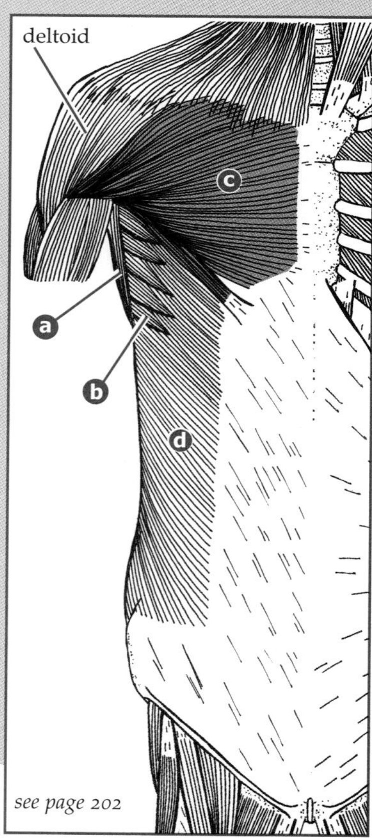

see page 202

Anterior View of the Trunk

a. Latissimus Dorsi
b. Serratus Anterior
c. **Pectoralis Major**
d. External Abdominal Oblique

RELATIONSHIP TO OTHER MUSCULOSKELETAL STRUCTURES

❑ 1. The pectoralis major is superficial in the chest.

❑ 2. Deep to the pectoralis major are the pectoralis minor and the subclavius, as well as the proximal attachments of the coracobrachialis and the short and long heads of the biceps brachii.

❑ 3. The anterior deltoid is lateral to the pectoralis major.

PECTORALIS MAJOR – continued

METHODOLOGY FOR LEARNING MUSCLE ACTIONS

- ☐ 1. **Adduction of the Arm at the Shoulder Joint:** The pectoralis major crosses the shoulder joint anteriorly, from medial on the trunk to lateral on the humerus (with the fibers running horizontally in the frontal plane and crossing below the center of the shoulder joint). When the pectoralis major contracts, it pulls the humerus medially toward the trunk; therefore, the pectoralis major adducts the humerus, i.e., the arm, at the shoulder joint.
- ☐ 2. **Medial Rotation of the Arm at the Shoulder Joint:** The pectoralis major crosses the shoulder joint anteriorly from the trunk to the humerus. However, the pectoralis major does not attach to the most medial aspect of the humerus, but rather wraps around the humerus to attach onto the lateral lip of the bicipital groove (with its fibers running horizontally in the transverse plane). When the pectoralis major contracts, it pulls the humeral attachment posteromedially, causing the anterior surface of the arm to face medially. Therefore, the pectoralis major medially rotates the arm at the shoulder joint.
- ☐ 3. **Flexion of the Arm at the Shoulder Joint (clavicular head):** The clavicular head of the pectoralis major crosses the shoulder joint anteriorly (with the fibers running vertically in the sagittal plane); therefore, it flexes the arm at the shoulder joint.
- ☐ 4. **Extension of the Arm at the Shoulder Joint (sternocostal head):** The sternocostal head of the pectoralis major crosses the shoulder joint in such a way (with its fibers running vertically in the sagittal plane) that if the arm is already in a position of flexion, these fibers can pull the arm, which is more anterior, posteriorly back toward the chest. Therefore, the pectoralis major can extend the arm at the shoulder joint. (Note: The pectoralis major cannot extend the arm at the shoulder joint beyond anatomical position.)
- ☐ 5. **Abduction of the Arm at the Shoulder Joint (clavicular head, above 90°):** If the arm is first in a position of approximately 90° or more of abduction at the shoulder joint, the clavicular fibers of the pectoralis major change their orientation with respect to the shoulder joint (running vertically in the frontal plane), and now cross above the center of the joint. (Note the similarity of how the deltoid or supraspinatus cross above the center of the shoulder joint.) Therefore, if the arm is already in a position of approximately 90° or more of abduction at the shoulder joint, the clavicular head of the pectoralis major can abduct the arm at the shoulder joint.
- ☐ 6. **Depression of the Scapula at the Scapulocostal Joint:** The sternocostal head of the pectoralis major attaches from inferiorly on the trunk to more superiorly on the humerus (with its fibers running somewhat vertically). When the humerus is fixed to the scapula and the sternocostal head of the pectoralis major contracts, it pulls inferiorly on the humerus, and the scapula is also pulled inferiorly. Therefore, when the humerus is fixed to the scapula, the pectoralis major depresses the scapula at the scapulocostal joint.
- ☐ 7. **Elevation of the Trunk at the Shoulder Joint:** If the arm is first in an elevated position (whether it is flexed, extended, abducted or adducted) above the trunk and the humeral attachment of the pectoralis major is fixed, then, when the pectoralis major contracts, it pulls the trunk superiorly toward the humerus (since the fibers are running somewhat vertically). Therefore, the pectoralis major elevates the trunk at the shoulder joint. (Note: This movement of the trunk relative to the humerus at the shoulder joint requires the scapula to be fixed to the trunk.)
- ☐ 8. **Lateral Deviation of the Trunk at the Shoulder Joint:** If the arm is first abducted away from the trunk and the humeral attachment of the pectoralis major is fixed, then, when the pectoralis major contracts, it pulls the trunk laterally toward the humerus. (This movement of the trunk will occur in the frontal plane since the fibers are running somewhat horizontally.) Therefore, the pectoralis major laterally deviates the trunk at the shoulder joint. (Note: This movement of the trunk relative to the humerus at the shoulder joint requires the scapula to be fixed to the trunk.)

PECTORALIS MAJOR – continued

- ❑ **9. Ipsilateral Rotation of the Trunk at the Shoulder Joint:** When the humeral attachment of the pectoralis major is fixed and the pectoralis major contracts, it pulls the trunk toward the humerus, causing the anterior trunk to face the same side of the body that the pectoralis major is attached (since the fibers are running somewhat horizontally in the transverse plane). Therefore, the pectoralis major ipsilaterally rotates the trunk at the shoulder joint. (Note: This movement of the trunk relative to the humerus at the shoulder joint requires the scapula to be fixed to the trunk.)

MISCELLANEOUS

- ❑ 1. Sources differ on how the pectoralis major is divided into parts. Some say that it has clavicular, sternal, costal and abdominal heads; others lump the sternal and costal heads into a sternocostal head; others omit the abdominal head altogether. Regardless of how it is divided, what is most important to realize is that the pectoralis major has upper fibers and lower fibers that cross the shoulder joint differently and therefore, have different actions at the shoulder joint.
- ❑ 2. The pectoralis major has layers: the clavicular fibers are the most superficial (anterior); the sternal fibers are deep to the clavicular fibers; and the costal and abdominal fibers are the deepest (most posterior).
- ❑ 3. The fibers of the pectoralis major twist so that the more superior clavicular fibers attach further distally on the humerus, and the more inferior sternal, costal and abdominal fibers attach more proximally on the humerus.
- ❑ 4. The distal fibers of the latissimus dorsi also twist so that the superior fibers become most distal at the humeral attachment and the inferior fibers become most proximal at the humeral attachment.
- ❑ 5. The pectoralis major makes up the vast majority of the "anterior axillary fold" of tissue, which borders the axilla (the armpit) anteriorly.
- ❑ 6. **Clavicular Actions:** Although the clavicle often moves passively by accompanying scapular movement, the clavicle can be directly acted upon by musculature and therefore actively moved. The clavicular section of the pectoralis major attaches from the medial clavicle to the humerus. When the humeral attachment is fixed, the pectoralis major depresses, downwardly rotates and/or protracts the clavicle at the sternocostal joint toward the humerus.
- ❑ 7. The pectoralis major (clavicular head) can only create flexion of the arm at the shoulder joint up to 60°.
- ❑ 8. The pectoralis major is a powerful horizontal flexor of the arm at the shoulder joint.
- ❑ 9. The pectoralis major is especially important and powerful in sagittal plane movements of the arm at the shoulder joint, such as pushing, pulling, throwing and punching.
- ❑ 10. To do a pull-up, elevation of the trunk must occur. The pectoralis major and the latissimus dorsi are particularly important for this action.
- ❑ 11. The pectoralis major and the latissimus dorsi are both large, powerful muscles that attach from the trunk to the arm. These two muscles are synergistic to each other with respect to their arm actions in that they both adduct and medially rotate the arm at the shoulder joint. However, they are antagonistic to each other with respect to their sagittal plane arm actions; the pectoralis major (being anterior) flexes the arm at the shoulder joint, and the latissimus dorsi (being posterior) extends the arm at the shoulder joint. (Note: Depending upon the position of the humerus, the pectoralis major can extend the arm at the shoulder joint, see methodology #4.)
- ❑ 12. The pectoralis major and the latissimus dorsi are both large, powerful muscles that attach from the trunk to the arm. These two muscles are synergistic to each other with respect to their trunk actions in that they both elevate and laterally deviate the trunk at the shoulder joint. However, they are antagonistic to each other with respect to their trunk actions; the pectoralis major (being anterior) ipsilaterally rotates the trunk at the shoulder joint, and the latissimus dorsi (being posterior) contralaterally rotates the trunk at the shoulder joint.

PECTORALIS MINOR

❑ **The name, pectoralis minor, tells us that this muscle is located in the pectoral (chest) region and is small (smaller than the pectoralis major).**

DERIVATION ❑ pectoralis: L. *refers to the chest.*
minor: L. *smaller.*

PRONUNCIATION ❑ pek-to-**ra**-lis **my**-nor

ATTACHMENTS

❑ **Ribs #3-5**

to the

❑ **Coracoid Process of the Scapula**

- ❑ the medial aspect

ACTIONS

❑ 1. **Protraction (Abduction) of the Scapula**

❑ 2. **Depression of the Scapula**

❑ 3. **Elevation of Ribs #3-5**

❑ 4. Downward Rotation of the Scapula

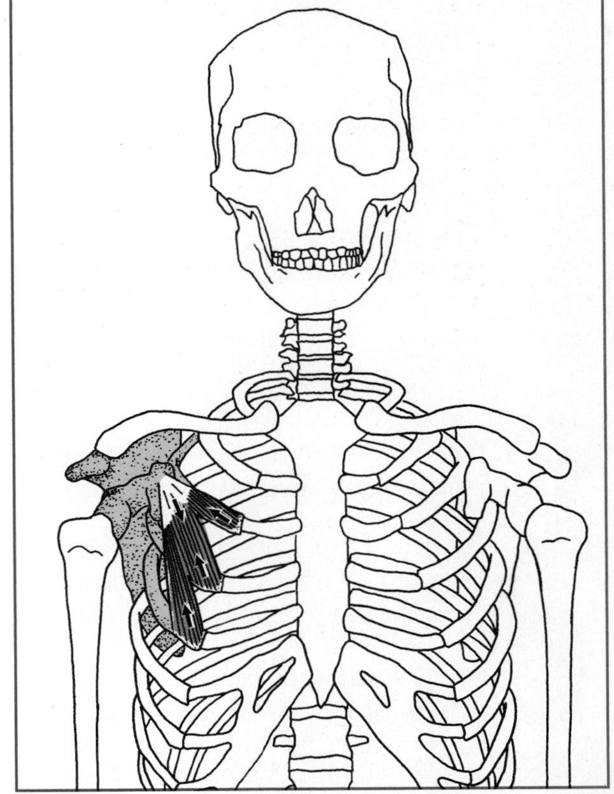

Anterior View of the Pectoralis Minor

INNERVATION ❑ The Medial and Lateral Pectoral Nerves ❑ C5, 6, **7**, **8**, T1

ARTERIAL SUPPLY ❑ The Pectoral Branches of the Thoracoacromial Trunk (A Branch of the Axillary Artery)
❑ and the posterior intercostal arteries (branches of the aorta) and the lateral thoracic artery (a branch of the axillary artery)

PECTORALIS MINOR – PALPATION AND SUPPLEMENTARY TEXT

PALPATION

The pectoralis minor is located in the chest deep to the pectoralis major. The lateral portion of the pectoralis minor can be directly palpated in the axilla (the armpit). However, if the pectoralis major is relaxed, contraction of the entire pectoralis minor is easily palpable through the pectoralis major.

❑ **Seated:**

- Have the client seated with the forearm relaxed in the small of the back.
- Place palpating fingers just inferior to the coracoid process of the scapula.
- Ask the client to lift the hand away from the back (causing extension of the arm at the shoulder joint, which requires downward rotation of the scapula at the scapulocostal joint, an action of the pectoralis minor) and feel for the contraction of the pectoralis minor.

❑ **Supine:**

- Have the client supine.
- Support the client's arm in abduction (passive abduction) at the shoulder joint and locate the lateral wall of the pectoralis major (i.e., the lateral wall of the anterior axillary fold).
- Place palpating fingers deep to the pectoralis major and the lateral portion of the pectoralis minor can be felt against the ribcage.
- To further bring out the pectoralis minor, ask the client to take in a deep breath which will cause the pectoralis minor to tighten (to elevate ribs #3-5) without tightening the nearby musculature.

  (Note: Asking the client to actively protract and depress the scapula at the scapulocostal joint will also bring out the pectoralis minor. However, the serratus anterior and pectoralis major will also contract, which will block palpation of the pectoralis minor through them.)

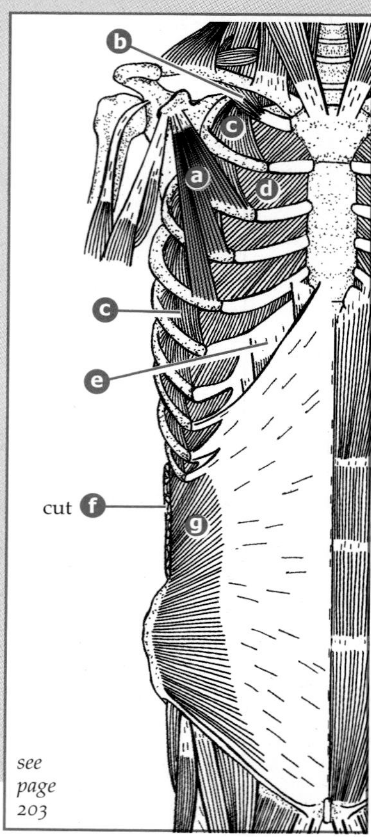

see page 203

Anterior View of the Trunk

a. **Pectoralis Minor**
b. Subclavius
c. External Intercostals
d. Internal Intercostals
e. Rectus Abdominis
f. External Abdominal Oblique
g. Internal Abdominal Oblique

RELATIONSHIP TO OTHER MUSCULOSKELETAL STRUCTURES

❑ 1. The pectoralis minor is deep to the pectoralis major.

❑ 2. Deep to the pectoralis minor are the serratus anterior and the ribcage.

❑ 3. The proximal attachment of the pectoralis minor is the coracoid process. The short head of the biceps brachii and the coracobrachialis also attach onto the coracoid process of the scapula.

PECTORALIS MINOR – continued

METHODOLOGY FOR LEARNING MUSCLE ACTIONS

- ❑ 1. **Protraction (Abduction) of the Scapula at the Scapulocostal Joint:** The pectoralis minor attaches from the scapula posteriorly, to the ribs anteriorly (with its fibers running horizontally). When the pectoralis minor contracts, it pulls the scapula anteriorly toward the ribs. Therefore, the pectoralis minor protracts (abducts) the scapula.
- ❑ 2. **Depression of the Scapula at the Scapulocostal Joint:** The pectoralis minor attaches from the scapula superiorly, to the ribs inferiorly (with its fibers running vertically). When the pectoralis minor contracts, it pulls the scapula inferiorly toward the ribs. Therefore, the pectoralis minor depresses the scapula.
- ❑ 3. **Elevation of Ribs #3-5 at the Sternocostal and Costovertebral Joints:** The pectoralis minor attaches from the scapula superiorly, to the ribs inferiorly (with its fibers running vertically). When the scapula is fixed and the pectoralis minor contracts, it pulls the ribs superiorly toward the scapula. Therefore, the pectoralis minor elevates ribs #3-5.
- ❑ 4. **Downward Rotation of the Scapula at the Scapulocostal Joint:** When the pectoralis minor contracts and pulls on the coracoid process of the scapula, it rotates the scapula in such a manner that the coracoid process (anteriorly) is pulled inferiorly and laterally, and the inferior angle of the scapula (posteriorly) elevates and moves medially. This rotation causes the glenoid fossa of the scapula to orient downward and therefore, the pectoralis minor downwardly rotates the scapula.

MISCELLANEOUS

- ❑ 1. Scapular Tilt Actions: In addition to its other actions, the scapula can also tilt.

  When the pectoralis minor contracts and pulls on the coracoid process, it pulls the scapula in such a manner that the lateral border of the scapula is pulled in toward the lateral body wall and the medial border of the scapula moves away from the posterior body wall. This movement of the medial border of the scapula coming away from the body wall is called lateral tilt; therefore, the pectoralis minor laterally tilts the scapula at the scapulocostal joint.

  When the pectoralis minor contracts and pulls on the coracoid process, it pulls the scapula in such a manner that the scapula is pulled inferiorly and toward the anterior body wall and the inferior angle of the scapula moves superiorly and away from the posterior body wall. This movement of the inferior angle of the scapula coming away from the body wall is called upward tilt; therefore, the pectoralis minor upwardly tilts the scapula at the scapulocostal joint.
- ❑ 2. The brachial plexus of nerves and the subclavian artery and vein are sandwiched between the pectoralis minor and the ribcage. Therefore, this is a common entrapment site for these nerves and blood vessels. If the pectoralis minor is tight, the vessels and nerves may be compressed and the condition is called *pectoralis minor syndrome* (one of three types of *thoracic outlet syndrome*).
- ❑ 3. *Rounded Shoulders* is a common postural condition in which the scapulae are protracted (abducted) and depressed (at the scapulocostal joints) and the humeri are medially rotated (at the shoulder joints). Given the pectoralis minor's actions of both protraction and depression of the scapula, when the pectoralis minor muscles are tight, they can significantly contribute to this condition.
- ❑ 4. By elevating ribs #3-5, the pectoralis minor can expand the ribcage, which expands the thoracic cavity, creating more space for the lungs to expand for inspiration. Therefore, the pectoralis minor is an accessory muscle of respiration.

❑ SUBCLAVIUS

❑ **The name, subclavius, tells us that this muscle is "under," i.e., inferior to the clavice.**

DERIVATION ❑ sub: L. *under.*
clavius: L. *key.*

PRONUNCIATION ❑ sub-**klay**-vee-us

ATTACHMENTS

❑ **1st Rib**

❑ at the junction with its costal cartilage

to the

❑ **Clavicle**

❑ the middle 1/3 of the inferior surface

ACTIONS

❑ 1. **Depression of the Clavicle**

❑ 2. **Elevation of the 1st Rib**

❑ 3. Protraction of the Clavicle

❑ 4. Downward Rotation of the Clavicle

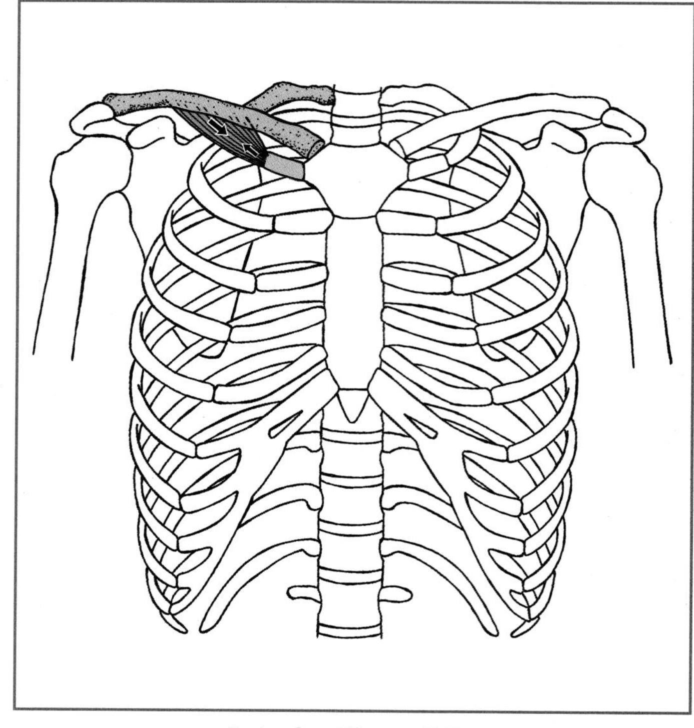

Anterior View of the Right Subclavius

INNERVATION ❑ A Nerve from the Brachial Plexus ❑ C5, 6

ARTERIAL SUPPLY ❑ The Clavicular Branch of the Thoracoacromial Trunk (A Branch of the Axillary Artery) and the Suprascapular Artery (A Branch of the Thyrocervical Trunk)

PALPATION AND SUPPLEMENTARY TEXT

PALPATION

- [ ] The subclavius, which is deep to the pectoralis major and located between the clavicle and the 1st rib, is very difficult to palpate and distinguish from the pectoralis major.
    - Have the client side-lying.
    - Support the client's arm in a position of partial flexion (passive flexion) to relax the pectoralis major.
    - Place palpating fingers slightly inferior to the middle 1/3 clavicle.
    - Now curl your fingers under the clavicle and feel for the subclavius against the inferior surface of the clavicle.

RELATIONSHIP TO OTHER MUSCULOSKELETAL STRUCTURES

- [ ] 1. The subclavius is located between the clavicle and the 1st rib.
- [ ] 2. The subclavius is deep to the pectoralis major.
- [ ] 3. Deep to the subclavius are the brachial plexus of nerves and the subclavian artery and vein.

METHODOLOGY FOR LEARNING MUSCLE ACTIONS

- [ ] **1. Depression of the Clavicle at the Sternoclavicular Joint:** The subclavius attaches to the clavicle superiorly, from the 1st rib inferiorly (with its fibers running somewhat vertically). When the subclavius contracts, it pulls the clavicle inferiorly toward the 1st rib. Therefore, the subclavius depresses the clavicle at the sternoclavicular joint.
- [ ] **2. Elevation of the First Rib at the Sternocostal and Costovertebral Joints:** The subclavius attaches to the 1st rib inferiorly, from the clavicle superiorly. When the subclavius contracts, it pulls the 1st rib superiorly toward the clavicle. Therefore, the subclavius elevates the 1st rib at the sternocostal and costovertebral joints.
- [ ] **3. Protraction of the Clavicle at the Sternoclavicular Joint:** The attachment of the subclavius onto the first rib is slightly more anterior than its clavicular attachment. When the subclavius pulls on the clavicle, the clavicle is pulled anteriorly toward the first rib; therefore, the subclavius protracts the clavicle at the sternoclavicular joint.

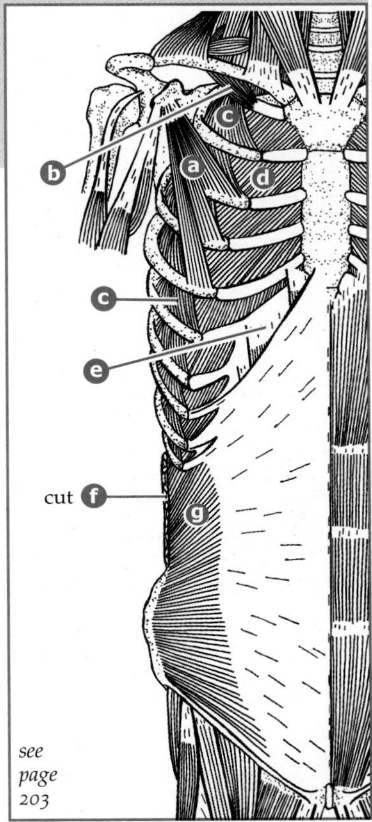

see page 203

Anterior View of the Trunk

a. Pectoralis Minor
b. **Subclavius**
c. External Intercostals
d. Internal Intercostals
e. Rectus Abdominis
f. External Abdominal Oblique
g. Internal Abdominal Oblique

SUBCLAVIUS – continued

❑ **4. Downward Rotation of the Clavicle at the Sternoclavicular Joint:** The subclavius attaches from the 1st rib to the inferior surface of the clavicle. When the subclavius contracts, it pulls the clavicle anteroinferiorly, causing the anterior surface of the clavicle to face inferiorly (since its pull is anterior to the axis about which the clavicle rotates). Therefore, the subclavius downwardly rotates the clavicle at the sternoclavicular joint. Note: The clavicle is fully downwardly rotated in anatomical position, so the subclavius must downwardly rotate a clavicle that is first upwardly rotated. (Since upward rotation of the clavicle causes the inferior surface of the clavicle to face anteriorly, the subclavius returns the inferior surface of the clavicle to face inferiorly again.)

MISCELLANEOUS

❑ 1. Given that the subclavius depresses the clavicle at the sternoclavicular joint, if the clavicle is fixed to the scapula (in fact, these two bones of the pectoral girdle often move together as a unit), then the subclavius can also depress the scapula at the scapulocostal joint.

❑ 2. The actions listed here for the subclavius are posited based upon the lines of pull of this muscle upon the bones to which it attaches. Electromyographic evidence as to when the subclavius is and is not recruited to contract is contradictory and unclear. Therefore, considerable controversy exists regarding exactly which actions this muscle performs and when it performs them.

❑ 3. Many sources believe that the main function of the subclavius is to act as a fixator of the clavicle during movements of the arm/shoulder girdle.

❑ 4. The brachial plexus of nerves and the subclavian artery and vein are located deep to the subclavius (between the clavicle and the 1st rib). This location is a fairly common entrapment site for these nerves and blood vessels. When entrapment of these nerves and/or vessels occurs in this location, it is called *costoclavicular syndrome* (one of three types of *thoracic outlet syndrome*).

EXTERNAL INTERCOSTALS

❑ **The name, external intercostals, tells us that these muscles are located between ribs and are external (superficial to the internal intercostals).**

DERIVATION ❑ external: L. *outside.*
inter: L. *between*
costals: L. *refers to the ribs.*

PRONUNCIATION ❑ **eks**-turn-al in-ter-**kos**-tal

ATTACHMENTS

❑ **In the Intercostal Spaces of Ribs #1-12**

- ❑ Each external intercostal attaches from the inferior border of one rib to the superior border of the rib directly inferior.

ACTIONS

❑ **1. Elevation of Ribs #2-12**

❑ 2. Depression of Ribs #1-11

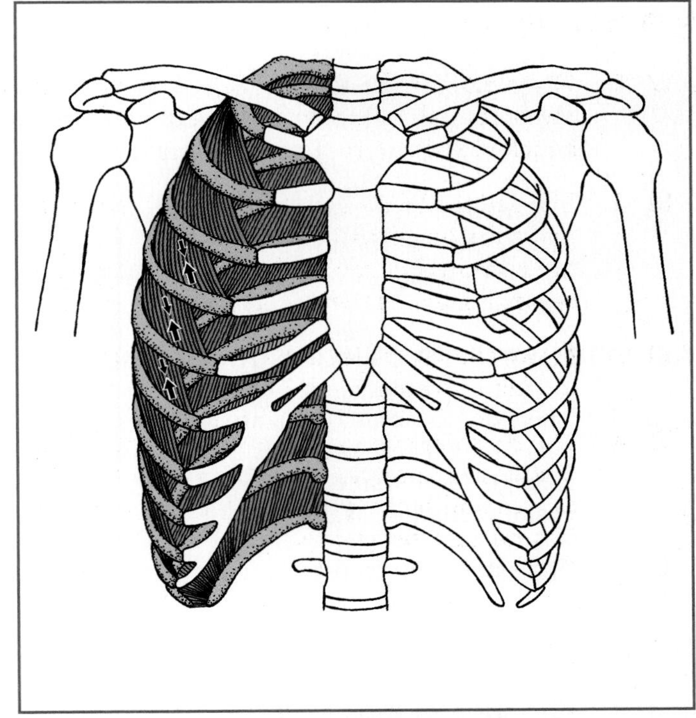

Anterior View of the Right External Intercostals

INNERVATION ❑ Intercostal Nerves

ARTERIAL SUPPLY ❑ Branches of the Costocervical Trunk (A Branch of the Subclavian Artery) and the Superior Thoracic Artery (A Branch of the Axillary Artery)

- ❑ and the anterior intercostal arteries (branches of the internal thoracic artery) and the posterior intercostal arteries (branches of the aorta)

EXTERNAL INTERCOSTALS PALPATION AND SUPPLEMENTARY TEXT

PALPATION

- ❑ The external intercostals (along with the internal intercostals) are located between the ribs (intercostal spaces) in the anterior, posterior and lateral trunk. In certain locations, these muscles are deep to many structures and difficult to palpate. In other locations, especially laterally on the body, the external intercostals may be superficial and easy to palpate.
  - Have the client supine.
  - Locate the hard surfaces of two adjacent ribs.
  - Place palpating fingers into the intercostal space between these two ribs and feel for the external intercostal muscle. Distinguishing between the external and internal intercostals can be very difficult.
  - To palpate the external intercostals in other regions of the ribcage, follow the above procedure.

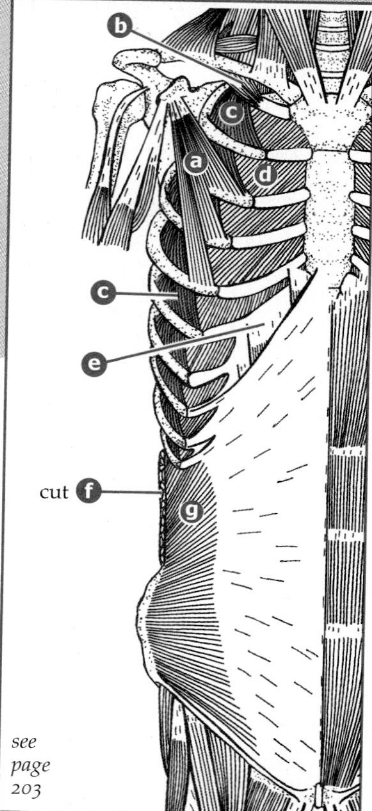

Anterior View of the Trunk

a. Pectoralis Minor
b. Subclavius
c. External Intercostals
d. Internal Intercostals
e. Rectus Abdominis
f. External Abdominal Oblique
g. Internal Abdominal Oblique

RELATIONSHIP TO OTHER MUSCULOSKELETAL STRUCTURES

❑ 1. The external intercostals are located in the intercostal spaces between ribs #1-12. Therefore, they are deep to all muscles that overlie the ribcage. Note that the external intercostals are not located between the costal cartilages of the ribs.

❑ 2. The external intercostals are directly superficial to the internal intercostals.

METHODOLOGY FOR LEARNING MUSCLE ACTIONS

❑ **1. Elevation of Ribs #2-12 at the Sternocostal and Costoclavicular Joints:** The external intercostals are located in the intercostal spaces and attach from the inferior margin of the more superior rib to the superior margin of the more inferior rib. When the superior rib is fixed and an external intercostal muscle contracts, it pulls superiorly on the inferior rib, thus, elevating it. Therefore, the external intercostals elevate ribs #2-12. Elevation of the ribs is necessary for inspiration; therefore, the external intercostals are respiratory muscles.

❑ **2. Depression of Ribs #1-11 at the Sternocostal and Costoclavicular Joints:** The external intercostals are located in the intercostal spaces and attach from the inferior margin of the more superior rib to the superior margin of the more inferior rib. If the lower rib is fixed and an external intercostal muscle contracts, it pulls inferiorly on the superior rib, thus depressing it. Therefore, the external intercostals depress ribs #1-11. Depression of the ribs is necessary for expiration; therefore, the external intercostals are respiratory muscles.

EXTERNAL INTERCOSTALS – continued

MISCELLANEOUS

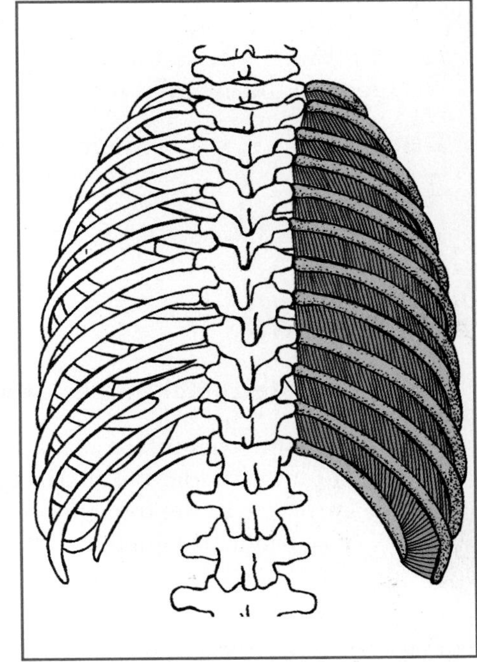

Posterior View of the Right External Intercostals

- ❑ 1 The fibers of the external intercostals are oriented in the same direction as the fibers of the external abdominal obliques. For this reason, the external intercostals between the ribs appear to be extensions of the external abdominal obliques of the abdomen.
- ❑ 2. The external intercostals are thicker than the internal intercostals.
- ❑ 3. Given the location of the external intercostals, it is clear that they are involved in respiration. However, there is controversy regarding whether the external intercostals elevate or depress the ribs during respiration. Generally, it is stated that they act during inspiration by elevating ribs, however, this is not known for certain. Given that the external intercostals are located in eleven intercostal spaces, and that these eleven intercostal spaces are located in the anterior, lateral and posterior trunk, it is likely that different parts of this muscle group are active in different parts of the respiratory cycle.
- ❑ 4. Regardless of the controversy over the exact actions of the external intercostals (see miscellaneous #3), it is clear that they are involved in respiration. Therefore, the external intercostals (and the internal intercostals) should be addressed in any client who has a respiratory condition. Further, athletes may also greatly benefit from having these muscles worked on due to the great demand for respiration during exercise.
- ❑ 5. The external intercostals (and the internal intercostals) are also involved in fixation (stabilization) of the ribcage during other movements of the body.
- ❑ 6. The intercostal muscles are the meat that is eaten when one eats ribs or spare ribs.

INTERNAL INTERCOSTALS

❑ **The name, internal intercostals, tells us that these muscles are located between ribs and are internal (deep to the external intercostals).**

DERIVATION ❑ internal: L. *inside.*
inter: L. *between.*
costals: L. *refers to the ribs.*

PRONUNCIATION ❑ **in**-turn-al in-ter-**kos**-tal

ATTACHMENTS

❑ **In the Intercostal Spaces of Ribs #1-12**

❑ Each internal intercostal attaches from the superior border of one rib and its costal cartilage, to the inferior border of the rib and its costal cartilage that is directly superior.

ACTIONS

❑ **1. Depression of Ribs #1-11**

❑ 2. Elevation of Ribs #2-12

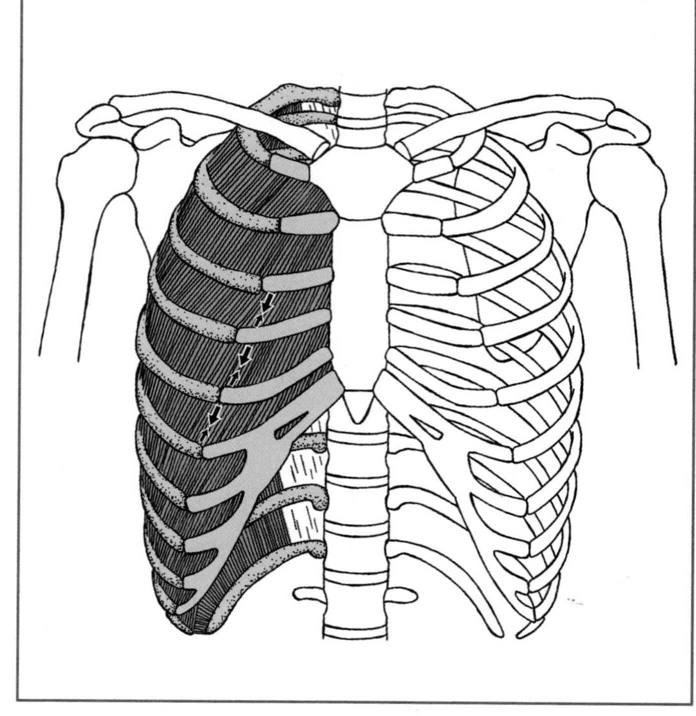

Anterior View of the Right Internal Intercostals

INNERVATION ❑ Intercostal Nerves

ARTERIAL SUPPLY ❑ Branches of the Costocervical Trunk (A Branch of the Subclavian Artery) and the Superior Thoracic Artery (A Branch of the Axillary Artery)

❑ and the anterior intercostal arteries (branches of the internal thoracic artery) and the posterior intercostal arteries (branches of the aorta)

PALPATION AND SUPPLEMENTARY TEXT

PALPATION

- ❑ The internal intercostals are deep to the external intercostals in the intercostal spaces and located in the anterior, posterior, and lateral trunk. (The exception to this is the intercostal spaces between the costal cartilages, where there are no external intercostals.) To palpate the internal intercostals, locate the external intercostals (see the palpation section for this muscle group on page 270). If the external intercostals are relaxed and the internal intercostals are tight, it may be possible to palpate and distinguish these two muscles.

RELATIONSHIP TO OTHER MUSCULOSKELETAL STRUCTURES

❑ 1. The internal intercostals are located in the intercostal spaces between ribs #1-12. Therefore, they are deep to all muscles that overlie the ribcage. They are directly deep to the external intercostals, except in the intercostal spaces between the costal cartilages where no external intercostals muscles are located.

❑ 2. The internal intercostals are superficial to the innermost intercostals, the subcostales and the pleural membrane of the lung.

METHODOLOGY FOR LEARNING MUSCLE ACTIONS

❑ 1. **Depression of Ribs #1-11 at the Sternocostal and Costoclavicular Joints:** The internal intercostals are located in the intercostal spaces and attach from the inferior margin of the more superior rib to the superior margin of the more inferior rib. If the lower rib is fixed and an internal intercostal muscle contracts, it pulls inferiorly on the superior rib, thus depressing it. Therefore, the internal intercostals depress ribs #1-11. Depression of the ribs is necessary for expiration; therefore, the internal intercostals are respiratory muscles.

❑ 2. **Elevation of Ribs #2-12 at the Sternocostal and Costoclavicular Joints:** The internal intercostals are located in the intercostal spaces and attach from the inferior margin of the more superior rib to the superior margin of the more inferior rib. When the superior rib is fixed and an internal intercostal muscle contracts, it pulls superiorly on the inferior rib, thus, elevating it. Therefore, the internal intercostals elevate ribs #2-12. Elevation of the ribs is necessary for inspiration; therefore, the internal intercostals are respiratory muscles.

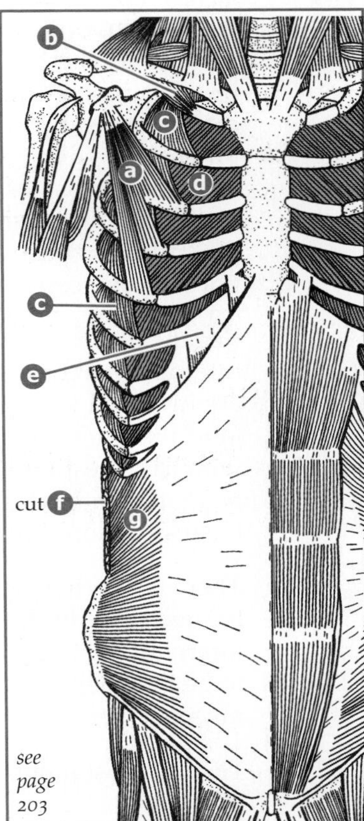

see page 203

Anterior View of the Trunk

- **a.** Pectoralis Minor
- **b.** Subclavius
- **c.** External Intercostals
- **d. Internal Intercostals**
- **e.** Rectus Abdominis
- **f.** External Abdominal Oblique
- **g.** Internal Abdominal Oblique

MISCELLANEOUS

❑ 1. Anteriorly, the internal intercostals are located in the spaces between the costal cartilages. (The external intercostals are not.)

❑ 2. Posteriorly, the fibers of the internal intercostals only reach as far as the angle of the ribs. However, the internal intercostals attach into the internal intercostal membrane, which reaches farther medially toward the spine.

INTERNAL INTERCOSTALS – continued

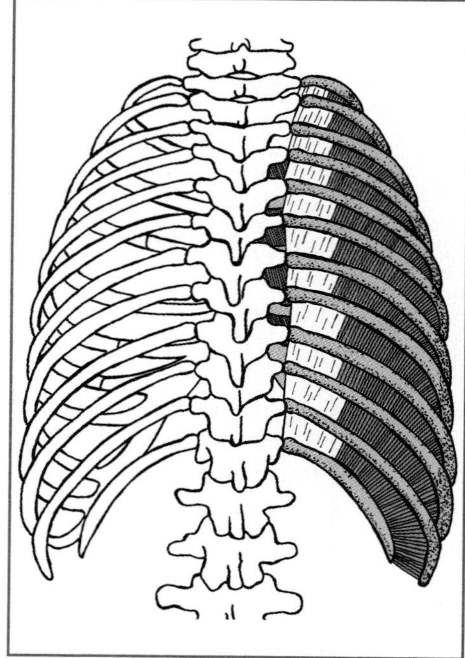

Posterior View of the Right Internal Intercostals

- ❑ 3. The fibers of the internal intercostals are oriented in the same direction as the fibers of the internal abdominal obliques. For this reason, the internal intercostals between the ribs appear to be extensions of the internal abdominal obliques of the abdomen.
- ❑ 4. The internal intercostals are generally thinner than the external intercostals. The thickest region of the internal intercostals is between the costal cartilages.
- ❑ 5. Given the location of the internal intercostals, it is clear that they are involved in respiration. However, there is controversy regarding whether the internal intercostals elevate or depress the ribs during respiration. Generally, it is stated that they act during expiration by depressing ribs; however, this is not known for certain. Given that the internal intercostals are located in eleven intercostal spaces, and that these eleven intercostal spaces are located in the anterior, lateral and posterior trunk, it is likely that different parts of this muscle group are active in different parts of the respiratory cycle.
- ❑ 6. Regardless of the controversy over the exact actions of the internal intercostals (see miscellaneous #5), it is clear that they are involved in respiration. Therefore, the internal intercostals (and the external intercostals) should be addressed in any client who has a respiratory condition. Further, athletes may also greatly benefit from having these muscles worked on due to the great demand for respiration during exercise.
- ❑ 7. There is another layer of muscles called the *innermost intercostals* or *intercostals intimi,* which are located directly deep to the internal intercostals and have an identical direction of fibers to the internal intercostals. This third layer of intercostal musculature, which has always been considered to be the deeper layer of the internal intercostals, is now considered by many sources to be a distinct muscle layer.
- ❑ 8. The intercostal muscles are the meat that is eaten when one eats ribs or spare ribs.

TRANSVERSUS THORACIS

❑ **The name, transversus thoracis, tells us that this muscle runs transversely across the thoracic region.**

DERIVATION ❑ transversus: L. *running transversely.*
thoracis: Gr. *refers to the thorax (chest).*

PRONUNCIATION ❑ trans-**ver**-sus thor-**as**-is

ATTACHMENTS

❑ **Internal Surfaces of the Sternum, Xiphoid Process and Adjacent Costal Cartilages**

❑ the inferior 1/3 of the sternum, and the costal cartilages of ribs #4-7

to the

❑ **Internal Surface of Costal Cartilages #2-6**

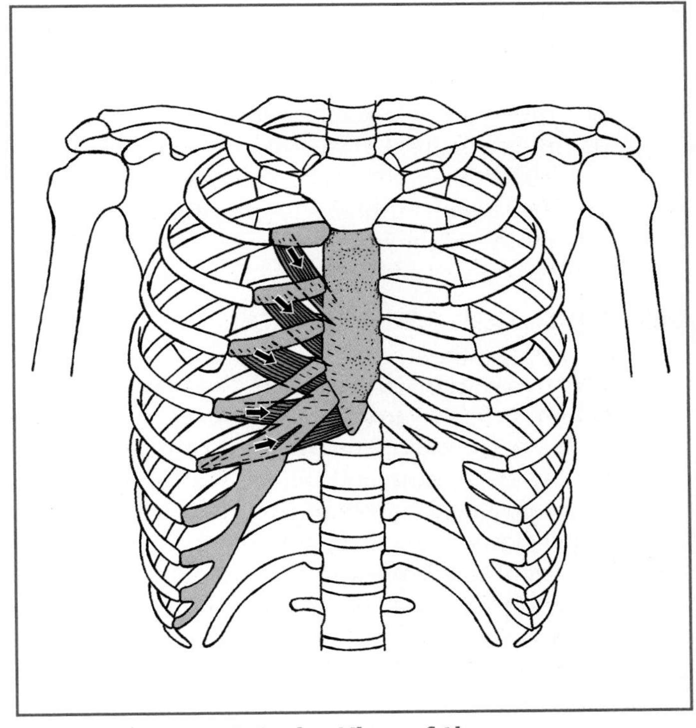

Anterior View of the Right Transversus Thoracis

ACTION

❑ **Depression of Ribs #2-6**

INNERVATION ❑ Intercostal Nerves

ARTERIAL SUPPLY ❑ The Anterior Intercostal Arteries (Branches of the Internal Thoracic Artery)

TRANSVERSUS THORACIS PALPATION AND SUPPLEMENTARY TEXT

PALPATION

- ❑ The transversus thoracis is deep to the ribcage itself and essentially not palpable. A small portion of it may be palpable just lateral to the xiphoid process of the sternum. Or, some pressure may translate through to it if applied with your palpating fingers in the medial intercostal spaces between ribs #2-6, just lateral to the sternum.

RELATIONSHIP TO OTHER MUSCULOSKELETAL STRUCTURES

- ❑ The transversus thoracis is deep to the ribcage and all the musculature that overlies the anterior thoracic region, as well as the external and internal intercostal muscles. The transversus thoracis is superficial to the pleural membrane of the lungs.

METHODOLOGY FOR LEARNING MUSCLE ACTIONS

- ❑ **Depression of Ribs #2-6 at the Sternocostal and Costovertebral Joints:** The transversus thoracis has its fibers running primarily vertically, attaching from the lower sternum and the xiphoid process inferiorly, to the costal cartilages of ribs #2-6 superiorly. When the transversus thoracis contracts, it pulls the 2nd through 6th costal cartilages inferiorly toward the sternum and xiphoid process. Therefore, the transversus thoracis depresses costal cartilages #2-6 and thereby depresses ribs #2-6 at the sternocostal and costovertebral joints. (Note: This action is necessary for inspiration.)

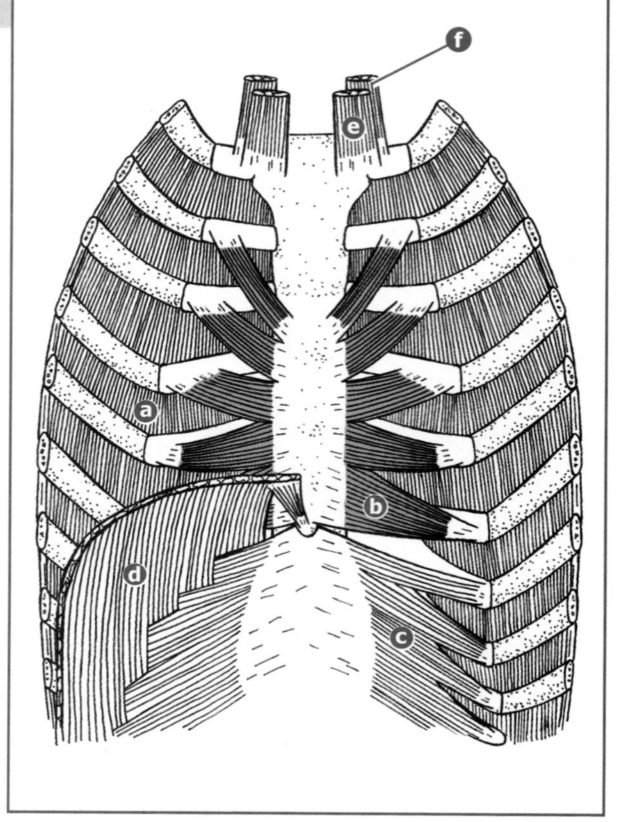

Posterior View of the Internal Wall of the Trunk

- **a.** Internal Intercostals
- **b. Transversus Thoracis**
- **c.** Transversus Abdominis
- **d.** Diaphragm
- **e.** Sternohyoid
- **f.** Sternothyroid

MISCELLANEOUS

- ❑ 1. The superior fibers of the transversus thoracis run primarily vertically, but the inferior fibers run horizontally, i.e., transversely.
- ❑ 2. The transversus thoracis is also known as the *sternocostalis* or as the *triangularis sternae*.
- ❑ 3. The transversus thoracis is internal, i.e., it is located within the thoracic cavity.
- ❑ 4. The inferior fibers of the transversus thoracis are contiguous with the superior fibers of the transversus abdominis, another deep trunk muscle that runs transversely.
- ❑ 5. The attachments of the transversus thoracis vary.
- ❑ 6. The primary role of the transversus thoracis is as a respiratory muscle. By depressing the costal cartilages, and therefore ribs #2-6, the volume of the ribcage expands for inspiration.

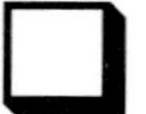

THE MUSCLES OF THE ANTERIOR ABDOMINAL WALL

The anterior abdominal wall consists of four muscles that attach from the trunk to the pelvis.

THERE ARE FOUR ANTERIOR ABDOMINAL WALL MUSCLES:	
Rectus Abdominis	External Abdominal Oblique Internal Abdominal Oblique Transversus Abdominis

Attachments:

- The rectus abdominis is located anteromedially.
- The external and internal abdominal obliques and the transversus abdominis are located anterolaterally.
  - The external abdominal oblique is the most superficial of the three anterolateral abdominal wall muscles.
  - The internal abdominal oblique is in the middle.
  - The transversus abdominis is the deepest of the three anterolateral abdominal wall muscles.
  - These three anterolateral abdominal muscles attach far posterior into the low back.
- The rectus abdominis is enclosed within the *rectus sheath* (a sheath of muscular fascia).
- The midline aponeuroses of the external abdominal oblique, internal abdominal oblique and the transversus abdominis muscles come together to form the rectus sheath (also known as the *abdominal aponeurosis*), which encloses the rectus abdominis.

Actions:

- ► All four muscles of the anterior abdominal wall can compress the abdominal contents, which plays an important role in expiration and expulsion of abdominal contents (e.g., vomiting, expulsion of feces from the intestines and expulsion of urine from the bladder).
- ► All the muscles of the anterior abdominal wall, except for the transversus abdominis, can flex the trunk at the spinal joints and/or posteriorly tilt the pelvis at the lumbosacral joint.
- ► The transversus abdominis cannot move the skeleton. Its primary action is compression of the abdominal contents.
- ► The external abdominal oblique of one side of the body is synergistic with the internal abdominal oblique on the opposite side of the body with respect to rotation of the trunk at the spinal joints. Note the similarity of the direction of fibers of these muscles.

Miscellaneous:

- ■ Two other muscles, the pyramidalis and the cremaster, are also located in the anterior abdominal wall. See Appendix F, page 730 for more details.

INNERVATION The anterior abdominal wall muscles are innervated by intercostal nerves.

♥ ARTERIAL SUPPLY The rectus abdominis receives the majority of its arterial supply from the superior and inferior epigastric arteries. The three lateral anterior abdominal wall muscles receive the majority of their arterial supply from the posterior intercostal and subcostal arteries.

VIEWS OF THE ANTERIOR ABDOMINAL WALL

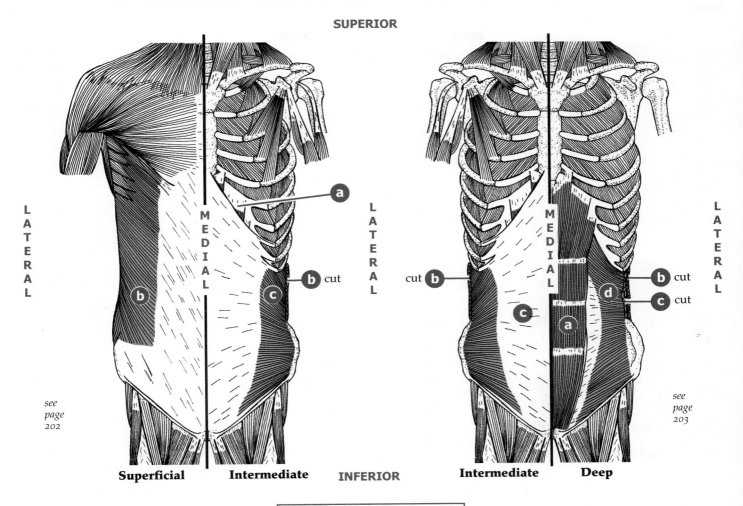

SUPERIOR

LATERAL

a

MEDIAL

b cut

c

b

LATERAL

cut b

c

MEDIAL

a

d

b cut

c cut

LATERAL

see page 202

see page 203

Superficial | Intermediate | INFERIOR | Intermediate | Deep

For a complete labeling of the trunk muscles, see page 202 and 203.

a. **Rectus Abdominis**
b. **External Abdominal Oblique**
c. **Internal Abdominal Oblique**
d. **Transversus Abdominis**

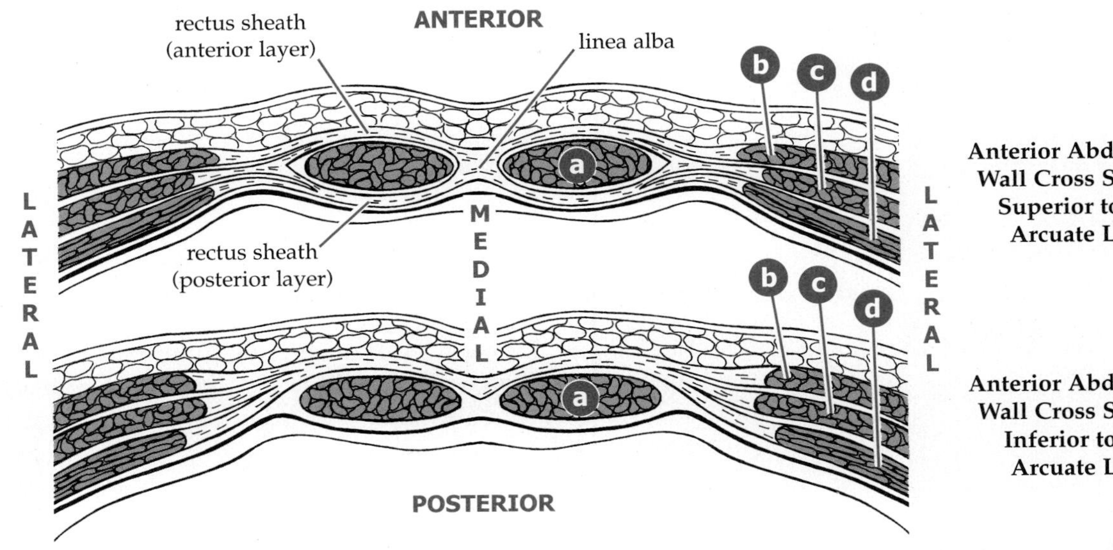

Anterior Abdominal Wall Cross Section Superior to the Arcuate Line

Anterior Abdominal Wall Cross Section Inferior to the Arcuate Line

❑ RECTUS ABDOMINIS

❑ **The name, rectus abdominis, tells us that this muscle runs straight up the abdomen.**

DERIVATION ❑ rectus: L. *straight.*
abdominis: L. *refers to the abdomen.*

PRONUNCIATION ❑ **rek**-tus ab-**dom**-i-nis

ATTACHMENTS

❑ **Pubis**

❑ the crest and symphysis of the pubis

to the

❑ **Xiphoid Process and the Cartilage of Ribs #5-7**

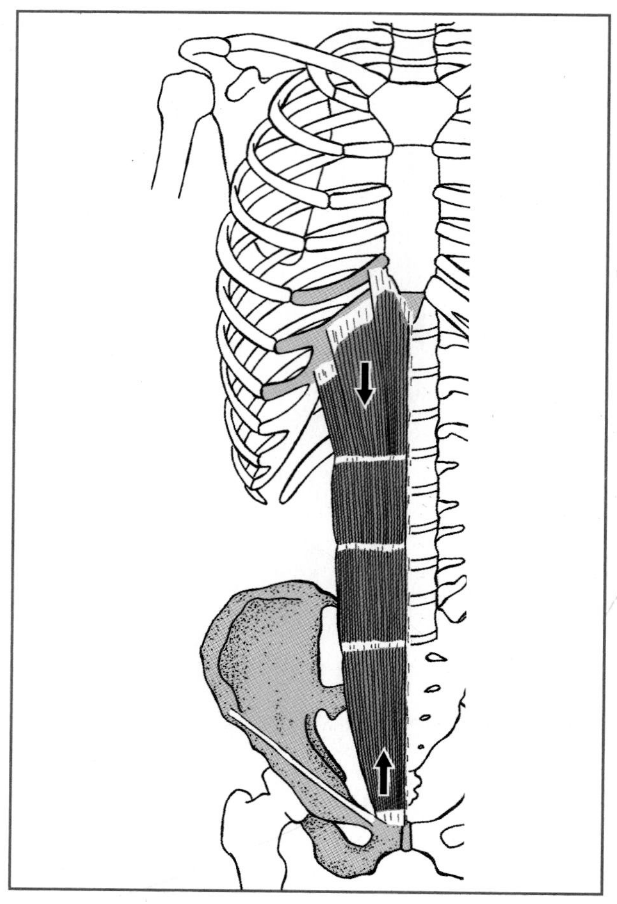

Anterior View of the Right Rectus Abdominis

ACTIONS

❑ 1. **Flexion of the Trunk**

❑ 2. **Posterior Tilt of the Pelvis**

❑ 3. Lateral Flexion of the Trunk

❑ 4. Compression of the Abdominal Contents

INNERVATION ❑ Intercostal Nerves ❑ ventral rami of T5-12

ARTERIAL SUPPLY ❑ The Superior Epigastric Artery (A Branch of the Internal Thoracic Artery) and the Inferior Epigastric Artery (A Branch of the External Iliac Artery)
❑ and the terminal branches of the subcostal and posterior intercostal arteries (all branches of the aorta)

PALPATION AND SUPPLEMENTARY TEXT

PALPATION

❑ The rectus abdominis is easily palpable and often visible.

- Have the client supine with a pillow placed under the knees to passively flex the thighs at the hip joints.
- Place palpating hands between the xiphoid process of the sternum and the adjacent ribs superiorly and the pubis inferiorly.
- Ask the client to alternately do mild flexion of the trunk (a small curl-up) and relax and feel for the contraction of the rectus abdominis.

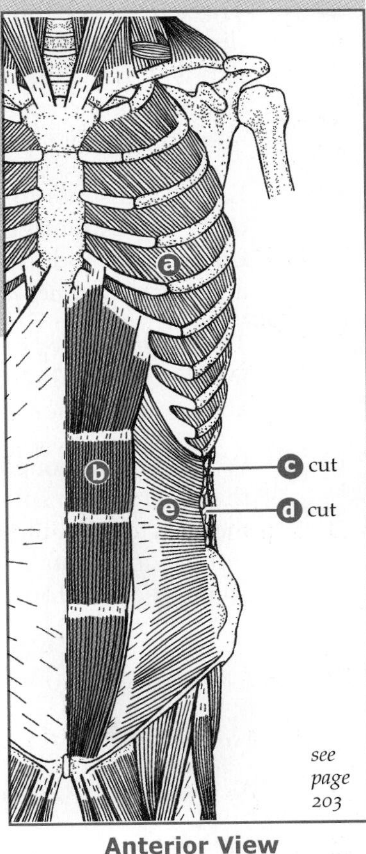
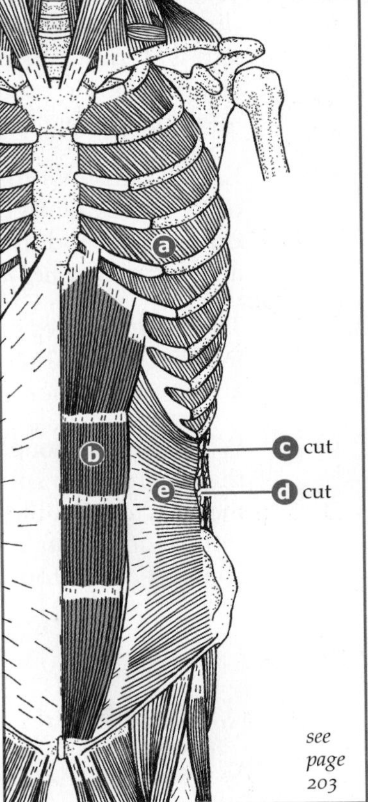

see page 203

Anterior View of the Trunk

a. Internal Intercostals
b. Rectus Abdominis
c. External Abdominal Oblique
d. Internal Abdominal Oblique
e. Transversus Abdominis

RELATIONSHIP TO OTHER MUSCULOSKELETAL STRUCTURES

❑ 1. The rectus abdominis is superficial in the anteromedial abdomen. It is encased in the rectus sheath, which is made up of the aponeuroses of the external and internal abdominal obliques as well as the transversus abdominis.

❑ 2. Deep to the rectus abdominis is the peritoneum of the abdominal cavity.

❑ 3. Lateral to the rectus abdominis are the other three muscles of the anterior abdominal wall: the external and internal abdominal obliques and the transversus abdominis.

❑ 4. Medial to the rectus abdominis is the linea alba (and then the contralateral rectus abdominis).

METHODOLOGY FOR LEARNING MUSCLE ACTIONS

❑ **1. Flexion of the Trunk at the Spinal Joints:** The rectus abdominis crosses the spinal joints anteriorly (with its fibers running vertically in the sagittal plane) and attaches onto the pelvis. When the pelvis is fixed and the rectus abdominis contracts, it pulls the trunk toward the pelvis anteriorly. Therefore, the rectus abdominis flexes the trunk at the spinal joints.

❑ **2. Posterior Tilt of the Pelvis at the Lumbosacral Joint:** The rectus abdominis crosses the spinal joints anteriorly (with its fibers running vertically in the sagittal plane) and attaches onto the pelvis. When the trunk is fixed and the rectus abdominis contracts, it pulls the pelvis toward the trunk anteriorly. This motion is called posterior tilt of the pelvis and occurs at the lumbosacral joint.

❑ **3. Lateral Flexion of the Trunk at the Spinal Joints:** The rectus abdominis crosses the spinal joints slightly on the lateral side (with its fibers running vertically in the frontal plane). When the pelvis is fixed and the rectus abdominis contracts, it pulls the trunk toward the pelvis laterally. Therefore, the rectus abdominis laterally flexes the trunk at the spinal joints.

❑ **4. Compression of the Abdominal Contents:** The rectus abdominis attaches from the trunk to the pelvis in the anterior abdominal wall (with its fibers running vertically). When both the trunk and the pelvis are fixed and the rectus abdominis contracts, it exerts a compressive force upon the abdomen. This plays an important role in expiration and expulsion of abdominal contents (e.g., vomiting, expulsion of feces from the intestines and urine from the bladder).

RECTUS ABDOMINIS – continued

MISCELLANEOUS

❑ 1. Three fibrous bands known as *tendinous inscriptions* transect the rectus abdominis muscles and divide each one of them into four sections or boxes. For this reason, the rectus abdominis muscles in a well-developed individual are often known as the *eight-pack (8-pack) muscle.* (Actually, it is more often incorrectly labeled the *six-pack (6-pack) muscle*, because six of the eight compartments are more visible.)

❑ 2. Each rectus abdominis is encased in the rectus sheath, which is made up of the aponeuroses of the other three anterior abdominal wall muscles (the external and internal abdominal obliques and the transversus abdominis). The two rectus sheaths (left and right) meet in the midline of the abdomen and form the *linea alba.*

❑ 3. The four muscles of the anterior abdominal wall are the rectus abdominis, external abdominal oblique, internal abdominal oblique and the transversus abdominis. All these muscles compress against the abdominal contents and help to create a flat abdomen.

❑ 4. When old-fashioned straight-legged sit-ups are done, the movement that occurs is not flexion of the trunk at the spinal joints, but rather is flexion of the hip joints with the pelvis (fixed to the trunk) moving toward the femurs. In this circumstance, the movers are not the abdominal wall muscles, but rather the flexors of the hip joints. The abdominal wall muscles do contract, but not as movers; they contract as fixators (stabilizers) of the pelvis, locking it to the trunk.

EXTERNAL ABDOMINAL OBLIQUE ❑

❑ **The name, external abdominal oblique, tells us that this muscle is located externally in the abdomen (superficial to the internal abdominal oblique) and its fibers are oriented obliquely.**

DERIVATION ❑ external: L. *outside.*
abdominal: L. *refers to the abdomen*
oblique: L. *slanting, diagonal.*

PRONUNCIATION ❑ **eks**-turn-al ab-**dom**-in-al o-**bleek**

ATTACHMENTS

❑ **Anterior Iliac Crest, Pubic Bone and the Abdominal Aponeurosis**

❑ the pubic crest and tubercle

to the

❑ **Lower 8 Ribs (Ribs #5-12)**

❑ the inferior border of the ribs

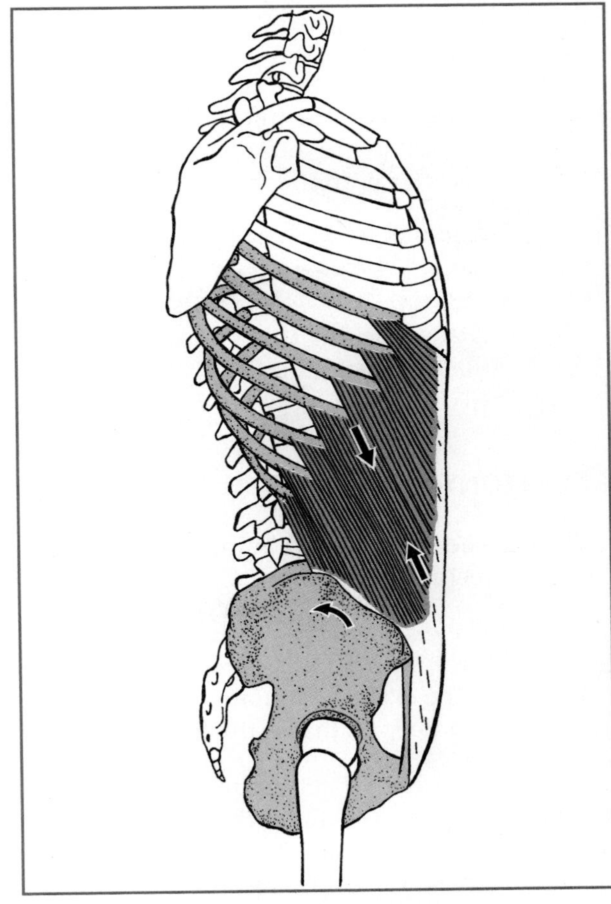

Lateral View of the
Right External Abdominal Oblique

ACTIONS

❑ 1. **Flexion of the Trunk**

❑ 2. **Lateral Flexion of the Trunk**

❑ 3. **Contralateral Rotation of the Trunk**

❑ 4. **Posterior Tilt of the Pelvis**

❑ 5. Ipsilateral Rotation of the Pelvis

❑ 6. Compression of the Abdominal Contents

INNERVATION ❑ Intercostal Nerves ❑ ventral rami of T7-12

ARTERIAL SUPPLY ❑ The Subcostal and Posterior Intercostal Arteries (All Branches of the Aorta) and the Deep Circumflex Iliac Artery (A Branch of the External Iliac Artery)
❑ and the inferior epigastric artery (a branch of the external iliac artery)

EXTERNAL ABDOMINAL OBLIQUE PALPATION AND SUPPLEMENTARY TEXT

PALPATION

- ❑ The external abdominal oblique is located lateral to the rectus abdominis and attaches all the way to the posterolateral trunk.
  - Have the client supine with a pillow placed under the knees to passively flex the thighs at the hip joints.
  - Place palpating hands on the anterolateral abdomen between the iliac crest and the lower ribs.
  - Ask the client to actively rotate the trunk at the spinal joints to the opposite side (along with slight flexion of the trunk) and feel for the contraction of the external abdominal oblique. (Keep in mind that the more flexion that is performed, the more the internal abdominal oblique will also contract.)
  - Continue palpating the external abdominal obliques superolaterally toward the rib attachments and inferomedially toward the iliac crest and the abdominal aponeurosis.
  - If possible, try to feel the oblique direction of the external abdominal oblique's fibers.

  Distinguishing the contraction of the external abdominal oblique from the contraction of the internal abdominal oblique may be difficult.

see page 202

Anterior View of the Trunk

a. Latissimus Dorsi
b. Serratus Anterior
c. Pectoralis Major
d. **External Abdominal Oblique**

RELATIONSHIP TO OTHER MUSCULOSKELETAL STRUCTURES

❑ 1. The external abdominal oblique is located lateral to the rectus abdominis.

❑ 2. The external abdominal oblique is the most superficial of the three layers of the anterolateral abdominal wall. Directly deep to the external abdominal oblique is the internal abdominal oblique, and deep to that is the transversus abdominis.

❑ 3. The external abdominal oblique interdigitates with the serratus anterior (at ribs #5-9) along the anterolateral body wall. The external abdominal oblique's fibers also meet fibers of the latissimus dorsi (at approximately a perpendicular angle at ribs #10-12) along the posterolateral body wall.

❑ 4. Keep in mind that the external abdominal oblique is not only located in the anterior abdominal region; it is also located in the lateral body wall and reaches all the way to the posterior body wall where it interdigitates with the latissimus dorsi at ribs #10-12.

METHODOLOGY FOR LEARNING MUSCLE ACTIONS

❑ **1. Flexion of the Trunk at the Spinal Joints:** The external abdominal oblique crosses the spinal joints anteriorly (with its fibers running vertically in the sagittal plane) and attaches onto the pelvis. When the pelvis is fixed, and the external abdominal oblique contracts, it pulls the trunk toward the pelvis anteriorly. Therefore, the external abdominal oblique flexes the trunk at the spinal joints.

EXTERNAL ABDOMINAL OBLIQUE – continued

❑ **2. Lateral Flexion of the Trunk at the Spinal Joints:** The external abdominal oblique crosses the spinal joints laterally (with its fibers running vertically in the frontal plane). When the pelvis is fixed, and the external abdominal oblique contracts, it pulls the trunk toward the pelvis laterally. Therefore, the external abdominal oblique laterally flexes the trunk at the spinal joints.

❑ **3. Contralateral Rotation of the Trunk at the Spinal Joints:** The external abdominal oblique wraps around the trunk (with its fibers running somewhat horizontally in the transverse plane). When the pelvis is fixed and the external abdominal oblique contracts, it pulls on the trunk, causing the anterior surface of the trunk to face the opposite side of the body from the side of the body that the external abdominal oblique is attached. Therefore, the external abdominal oblique contralaterally rotates the trunk at the spinal joints.

❑ **4. Posterior Tilt of the Pelvis at the Lumbosacral Joint:** The external abdominal oblique crosses the spinal joints anteriorly (with its fibers running vertically in the sagittal plane) and attaches onto the pelvis. When the trunk is fixed and the external abdominal oblique contracts, it pulls the pelvis toward the trunk anteriorly. This motion is called posterior tilt of the pelvis and occurs at the lumbosacral joint.

❑ **5. Ipsilateral Rotation of the Pelvis at the Lumbosacral Joint:** When the superior attachments of the external abdominal oblique are fixed and the external abdominal oblique contracts, it pulls on the inferior attachment, the pelvis, causing the anterior surface of the pelvis to face the same side of the body that the external abdominal oblique is attached (since the fibers of the external abdominal oblique have a horizontal orientation in the transverse plane). Therefore, the external abdominal oblique ipsilaterally rotates the pelvis at the lumbosacral joint.

❑ **6. Compression of the Abdominal Contents:** The external abdominal oblique attaches from the trunk to the pelvis in the anterior abdominal wall (with its fibers running vertically). When both the trunk and the pelvis are fixed and the external abdominal oblique contracts, it exerts a compressive force upon the abdomen. This plays an important role in expiration and expulsion of abdominal contents (e.g., vomiting, expulsion of feces from the intestines and urine from the bladder).

MISCELLANEOUS

❑ 1. If you were to put your hand into a coat pocket, your fingers would be pointing along the direction of the fibers of the external abdominal oblique on that side. For this reason, the external abdominal obliques are sometimes called the *pocket muscles*.

❑ 2. The aponeurosis of the external abdominal oblique, between the anterior superior iliac spine and the pubic tubercle, forms the inguinal ligament.

❑ 3. The abdominal aponeurosis is actually the midline aponeurosis of the external abdominal oblique. This external abdominal oblique aponeurosis, along with the aponeuroses of the internal abdominal oblique and the transversus abdominis, form the rectus sheath that envelops the rectus abdominis.

❑ 4. The external abdominal oblique is a contralateral rotator of the trunk at the spinal joints and the internal abdominal oblique is an ipsilateral rotator of the trunk at the spinal joints; hence with regard to trunk rotation (transverse plane actions), they are antagonistic to each other. However, the external abdominal oblique on one side of the body is synergistic with the internal abdominal oblique on the opposite side of the body during trunk rotation. Note the similarity of the direction of their fibers.

❑ 5. The external abdominal oblique is an ipsilateral rotator of the pelvis at the lumbosacral joint and the internal abdominal oblique is a contralateral rotator of the pelvis at the lumbosacral joint; hence with regard to pelvic rotation (transverse plane actions), they are antagonistic to each other. However, the external abdominal oblique on one side of the body is synergistic with the internal abdominal oblique on the opposite side of the body during pelvic rotation. Note the similarity of the direction of their fibers.

❑ 6. With regard to flexion and lateral flexion of the trunk at the spinal joints (sagittal and frontal plane actions), the external and internal abdominal obliques are synergistic to each other.

❑ INTERNAL ABDOMINAL OBLIQUE

❑ **The name, internal abdominal oblique, tells us that this muscle is located internally in the abdomen (deep to the external abdominal oblique) and its fibers are oriented obliquely.**

DERIVATION ❑ internal: L. *inside.*
abdominal: L. *refers to the abdomen.*
oblique: L. *slanting, diagonal.*

PRONUNCIATION ❑ in-**turn**-al ab-**dom**-in-al o-**bleek**

ATTACHMENTS

❑ **Inguinal Ligament, Iliac Crest and the Thoracolumbar Fascia**

❑ the lateral 2/3 of the inguinal ligament

to the

❑ **Lower 3 Ribs (#10-12) and the Abdominal Aponeurosis**

ACTIONS

❑ 1. **Flexion of the Trunk**

❑ 2. **Lateral Flexion of the Trunk**

❑ 3. **Ipsilateral Rotation of the Trunk**

❑ 4. **Posterior Tilt of the Pelvis**

❑ 5. Contralateral Rotation of the Pelvis

❑ 6. Compression of the Abdominal Contents

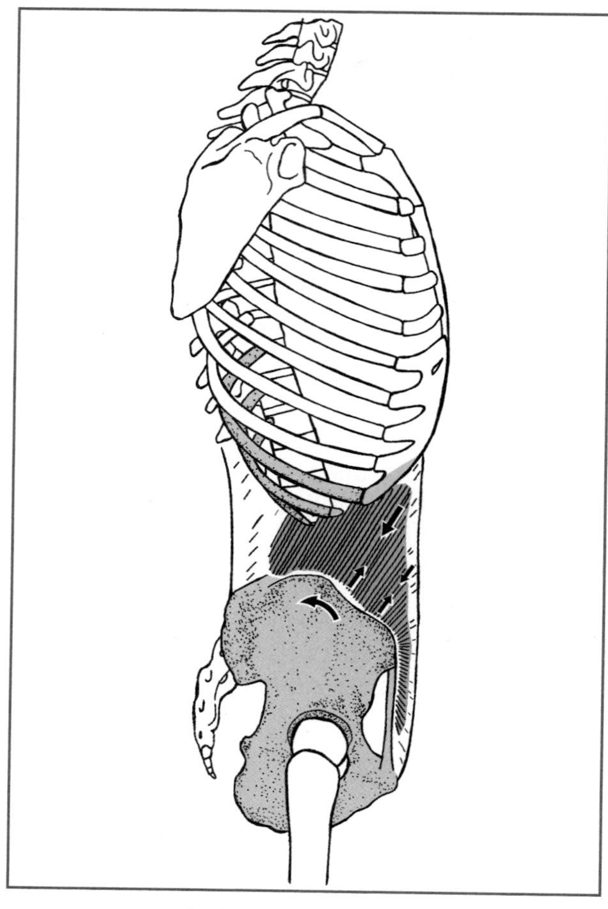

Lateral View of the Right Internal Abdominal Oblique

INNERVATION ❑ Intercostal Nerves ❑ ventral rami of T7-L1

ARTERIAL SUPPLY ❑ The Subcostal and Posterior Intercostal Arteries (All Branches of the Aorta) and the Deep Circumflex Iliac Artery (A Branch of the External Iliac Artery)
❑ and the inferior epigastric artery (a branch of the external iliac artery)

PALPATION AND SUPPLEMENTARY TEXT

PALPATION

- ❑ The internal abdominal oblique is deep to the external abdominal oblique. It is located lateral to the rectus abdominis and attaches all the way to the posterolateral trunk.
  - Have the client supine with a pillow placed under the knees to passively flex the thighs at the hip joints.
  - Place palpating hands on the anterolateral abdomen between the iliac crest and the lower ribs.
  - Ask the client to actively rotate the trunk at the spinal joints to the same side (along with slight flexion of the trunk) and feel for the contraction of the internal abdominal oblique. (Keep in mind that the more flexion that is performed, the more the external abdominal oblique will also contract.)

  Distinguishing the contraction of the internal abdominal oblique from the contraction of the external abdominal oblique will be difficult.

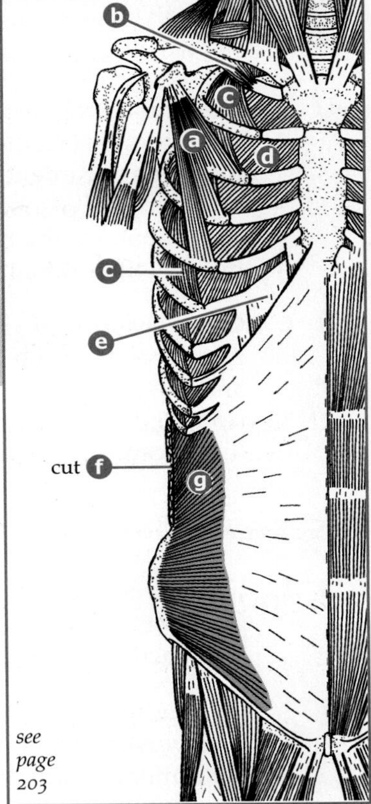

see page 203

Anterior View of the Trunk

a. Pectoralis Minor
b. Subclavius
c. External Intercostals
d. Internal Intercostals
e. Rectus Abdominis
f. External Abdominal Oblique
g. **Internal Abdominal Oblique**

RELATIONSHIP TO OTHER MUSCULOSKELETAL STRUCTURES

❑ 1. The internal abdominal oblique is located lateral to the rectus abdominis.

❑ 2. The internal abdominal oblique is the middle muscle of the three anterolateral abdominal wall muscles. It is deep to the external abdominal oblique and superficial to the transversus abdominis.

❑ 3. Keep in mind that the internal abdominal oblique is not only located in the anterior abdominal region; it is also located in the lateral body wall and reaches all the way to the posterior body wall where it attaches into the thoracolumbar fascia, just lateral to the erector spinae.

METHODOLOGY FOR LEARNING MUSCLE ACTIONS

❑ 1. **Flexion of the Trunk at the Spinal Joints:** The internal abdominal oblique crosses the spinal joints anteriorly (with its fibers running vertically in the sagittal plane) and attaches onto the pelvis. When the pelvis is fixed, and the internal abdominal oblique contracts, it pulls the trunk toward the pelvis anteriorly. Therefore, the internal abdominal oblique flexes the trunk at the spinal joints.

❑ 2. **Lateral Flexion of the Trunk at the Spinal Joints:** The internal abdominal oblique crosses the spinal joints laterally (with its fibers running vertically in the frontal plane). When the pelvis is fixed, and the internal abdominal oblique contracts, it pulls the trunk toward the pelvis laterally. Therefore, the internal abdominal oblique laterally flexes the trunk at the spinal joints.

INTERNAL ABDOMINAL OBLIQUE – continued

- ❑ 3. **Ipsilateral Rotation of the Trunk at the Spinal Joints:** The internal abdominal oblique wraps around the trunk (with its fibers running somewhat horizontally in the transverse plane). When the pelvis is fixed and the internal abdominal oblique contracts, it pulls on the trunk, causing the anterior surface of the trunk to face the same side of the body that the internal abdominal oblique is attached. Therefore, the internal abdominal oblique ipsilaterally rotates the trunk at the spinal joints.
- ❑ 4. **Posterior Tilt of the Pelvis at the Lumbosacral Joint:** The internal abdominal oblique crosses the spinal joints anteriorly (with its fibers running vertically in the sagittal plane) and attaches onto the pelvis. When the trunk is fixed and the internal abdominal oblique contracts, it pulls the pelvis toward the trunk anteriorly. This motion is called posterior tilt of the pelvis and occurs at the lumbosacral joint.
- ❑ 5. **Contralateral Rotation of the Pelvis at the Lumbosacral Joint:** When the superior attachments of the internal abdominal oblique are fixed and the internal abdominal oblique contracts, it pulls on the inferior attachment, the pelvis, causing the anterior surface of the pelvis to face the opposite side of the body from the side of the body that the internal abdominal oblique is attached (since the fibers of the internal abdominal oblique have a horizontal orientation in the transverse plane). Therefore, the internal abdominal oblique contralaterally rotates the pelvis at the lumbosacral joint.
- ❑ 6. **Compression of the Abdominal Contents:** The internal abdominal oblique attaches from the trunk to the pelvis in the anterior abdominal wall (with its fibers running vertically). When both the trunk and the pelvis are fixed and the internal abdominal oblique contracts, it exerts a compressive force upon the abdomen. This plays an important role in expiration and expulsion of abdominal contents (e.g., vomiting, expulsion of feces from the intestines and urine from the bladder).

MISCELLANEOUS

- ❑ 1. If you were to put your hand into a coat pocket, your fingers would be pointing along the direction of the fibers of the external abdominal oblique on that side. The fibers of the internal abdominal oblique are exactly 90° opposite (perpendicular) to those of the external abdominal oblique.
- ❑ 2. The midline aponeuroses of the external abdominal oblique, the internal abdominal oblique and the transversus abdominis form the rectus sheath that envelops the rectus abdominis. Part of the internal abdominal oblique's midline aponeurosis actually splits and wraps around the rectus abdominis both superficially and deep. (This occurs superior to the arcuate line, which is located approximately halfway between the umbilicus and the pubic bone. See cross section illustrations on page 279.)
- ❑ 3. The internal abdominal oblique is an ipsilateral rotator of the trunk at the spinal joints and the external abdominal oblique is a contralateral rotator of the trunk at the spinal joints; hence with regard to trunk rotation (transverse plane actions), they are antagonistic to each other. However, the internal abdominal oblique on one side of the body is synergistic with the external abdominal oblique on the opposite side of the body during trunk rotation. Note the similarity of the direction of their fibers.
- ❑ 4. The internal abdominal oblique is a contralateral rotator of the pelvis at the lumbosacral joint and the external abdominal oblique is an ipsilateral rotator of the pelvis at the lumbosacral joint; hence with regard to pelvic rotation (transverse plane actions), they are antagonistic to each other. However, the internal abdominal oblique on one side of the body is synergistic with the external abdominal oblique on the opposite side of the body during pelvic rotation. Note the similarity of the direction of their fibers.
- ❑ 5. With regard to flexion and lateral flexion of the trunk at the spinal joints (sagittal and frontal plane actions), the internal and external abdominal obliques are synergistic to each other

TRANSVERSUS ABDOMINIS ❑

❑ **The name, transversus abdominis, tells us that this muscle runs transversely across the abdomen.**

DERIVATION ❑ transversus: L. *running transversely.*
abdominis: L. *refers to the abdomen.*

PRONUNCIATION ❑ trans-**ver**-sus ab-**dom**-i-nis

ATTACHMENTS

❑ **Inguinal Ligament, Iliac Crest, Thoracolumbar Fascia and the Lower Costal Cartilages**

❑ the lateral 1/3 of the inguinal ligament;
the lower 6 costal cartilages (of ribs #7-12)

to the

❑ **Abdominal Aponeurosis**

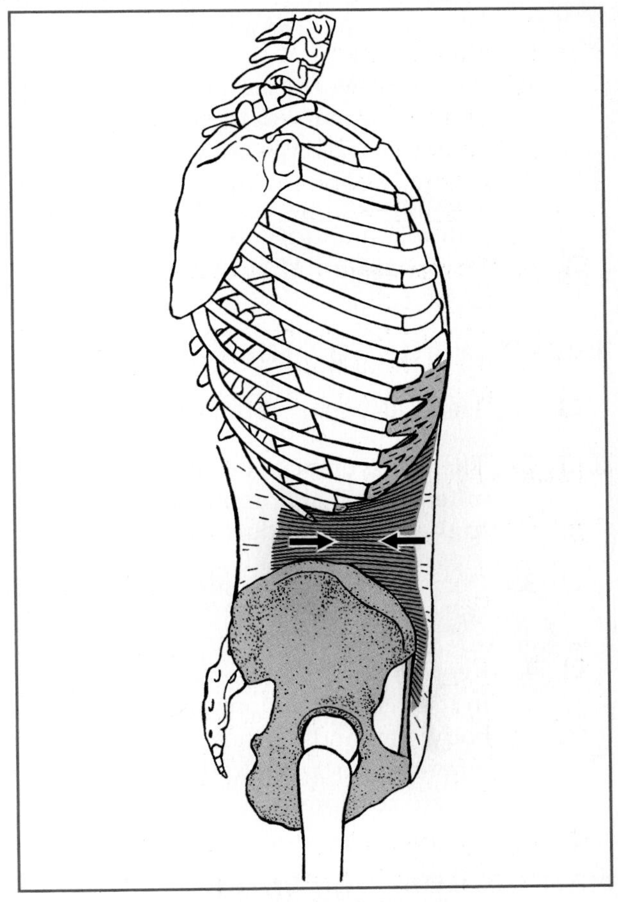

Lateral View of the Right Transversus Abdominis

ACTION

❑ **Compression of the Abdominal Contents**

INNERVATION ❑ Intercostal Nerves ❑ ventral rami of T7-L1

ARTERIAL SUPPLY ❑ The Subcostal and Posterior Intercostal Arteries (All Branches of the Aorta) and the Deep Circumflex Iliac Artery (A Branch of the External Iliac Artery)
❑ and the inferior epigastric artery (a branch of the external iliac artery)

TRANSVERSUS ABDOMINIS PALPATION AND SUPPLEMENTARY TEXT

PALPATION

- ❑ The transversus abdominis is deep to the external and internal abdominal obliques in the anterolateral abdominal wall.
    - Have the client supine with a pillow placed under the knees to passively flex the thighs at the hip joints.
    - Place palpating hands on the anterolateral abdomen between the iliac crest and the lower ribs.
    - Ask the client to forcefully exhale and feel for the contraction of the transversus abdominis (as well as the external and internal abdominal obliques).

    Distinguishing the contraction of the transversus abdominis from the contraction of the obliques will be extremely difficult, if not impossible.

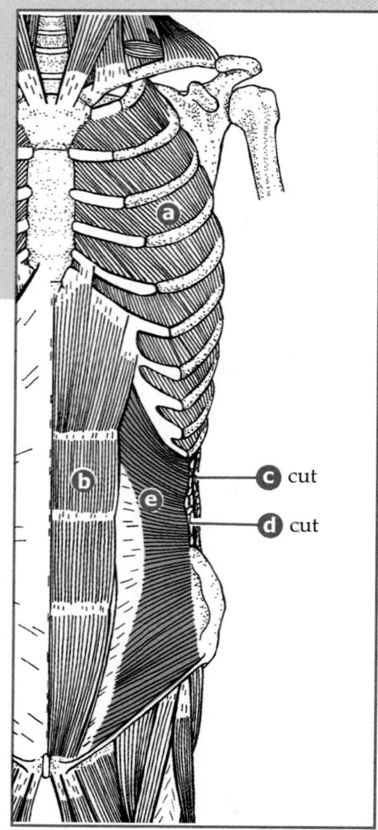

Anterior View of the Trunk

- **a.** Internal Intercostals
- **b.** Rectus Abdominis
- **c.** External Abdominal Oblique
- **d.** Internal Abdominal Oblique
- **e.** **Transversus Abdominis**

RELATIONSHIP TO OTHER MUSCULOSKELETAL STRUCTURES

- ❑ 1. The transversus abdominis is lateral to the rectus abdominis.
- ❑ 2. The transversus abdominis is the deepest of the three anterolateral abdominal wall muscles. It is directly deep to the internal abdominal oblique.
- ❑ 3. Deep to the transversus abdominis is the peritoneum of the abdominal cavity.
- ❑ 4. Keep in mind that the transversus abdominis is not only located in the anterior abdominal region; it is also located in the lateral body wall and reaches all the way to the posterior body wall where it attaches into the thoracolumbar fascia, just lateral to the erector spinae.

METHODOLOGY FOR LEARNING MUSCLE ACTIONS

- ❑ **Compression of the Abdominal Contents:** The transversus abdominis attaches from the thoracolumbar fascia posteriorly, to the linea alba anteriorly, and from the lower ribs superiorly, to the iliac crest inferiorly (with its fibers running horizontally). Given the direction of the fibers, contraction cannot cause skeletal movement. Instead, contraction of the transversus abdominis tightens the muscle against the abdomen, compressing the abdominal contents. This plays an important role in expiration and expulsion of abdominal contents (e.g., vomiting, expulsion of feces from the intestines and expulsion of urine from the bladder).

TRANSVERSUS ABDOMINIS – continued

MISCELLANEOUS

- ❑ 1. The transversus abdominis is the only anterior abdominal wall muscle that cannot act as a mover of a skeletal action. Its primary purpose is to compress the abdominal contents. It can also serve to pull on, and thereby fix, the linea alba. Fixing the linea alba creates a more stable base of attachment for other abdominal wall muscles.
- ❑ 2. The transversus abdominis contributes (along with the external and internal abdominal obliques) to the rectus sheath, which encloses the rectus abdominis.
- ❑ 3. The upper fibers of the transversus abdominis are contiguous with the diaphragm and the transversus thoracis (another muscle that runs transversely in the trunk).
- ❑ 4. The transversus abdominis is sometimes called the *corset* muscle because it wraps around the abdomen like a corset, and like a corset, it functions to hold in the abdomen.

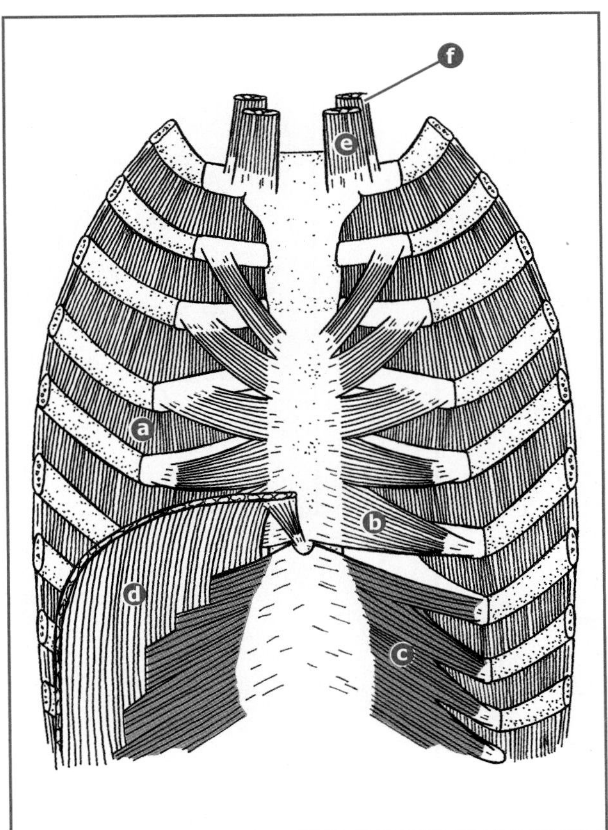

Posterior View of the Internal Wall of the Trunk

a. Internal Intercostals
b. Transversus Thoracis
c. **Transversus Abdominis**
d. Diaphragm
e. Sternohyoid
f. Sternothyroid

❑ DIAPHRAGM

❑ **The name, diaphragm, tells us that this muscle is a partition.**

DERIVATION ❑ diaphragm: Gr. *partition.*

PRONUNCIATION ❑ **di**-a-fram

ATTACHMENTS

❑ **ENTIRE MUSCLE: Internal Surfaces of the Ribcage and Sternum, and the Spine**

❑ STERNAL PART: Internal Surface of the Xiphoid Process of the Sternum

❑ COSTAL PART: Internal Surface of the Lower 6 Ribs (Ribs #7-12) and their Costal Cartilages

❑ LUMBAR PART: L1-L3

- ❑ The lumbar attachments consist of two aponeuroses called the medial and lateral arcuate ligaments and two tendons called the right and left crura.

to the

❑ **Central Tendon of the Diaphragm**

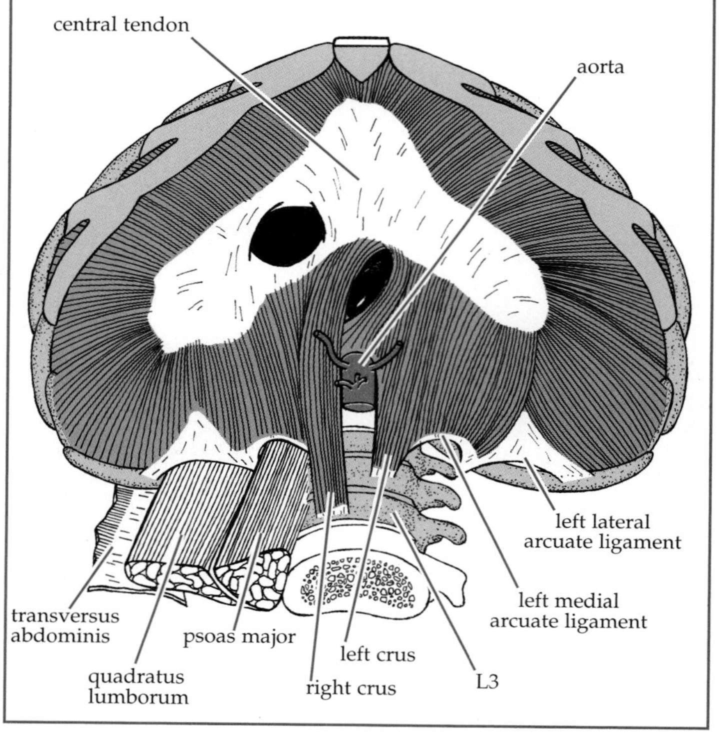

Inferior View of the Diaphragm
(the psoas major, quadratus lumborum and transversus abdominis are shown on our left)

ACTION

❑ **Increases the Volume of the Thoracic Cavity**

INNERVATION ❑ The Phrenic Nerve ❑ C3-5

ARTERIAL SUPPLY ❑ Branches of the Aorta and the Internal Thoracic Artery (A Branch of the Subclavian Artery)

- ❑ the superior and inferior phrenic arteries (both branches of the aorta), and the musculophrenic and pericardiacophrenic arteries (both branches of the internal thoracic artery)

PALPATION AND SUPPLEMENTARY TEXT

PALPATION

The diaphragm is a dome-shaped muscle, located internally, that separates the thoracic cavity from the abdominal cavity. Only part of the diaphragm is accessible for palpation. The client must be comfortable and relaxed.

❑ **Supine:**

- Have the client supine with a pillow placed under the knees to passively flex the thighs at the hip joints (This allows the pelvis to passively posterior tilt at the hip joints and the lumbosacral joint, which slackens the anterior abdominal wall allowing for better palpation of the diaphragm).
- Place palpating fingers on the inferior margin of the anterior ribcage.
- Ask the client to take in a deep breath and then slowly exhale.
- As the client slowly exhales, curl your fingertips under (inferior and then deep to) the ribcage and feel for the diaphragm, palpating gently, yet firmly, as deep as possible against the internal surface of the ribs.

❑ **Side-lying:**

- Have the client side-lying with the trunk slightly flexed. This position slackens the abdominal wall.
- Palpate the diaphragm that is on the upper side of the body by following the above procedure.

RELATIONSHIP TO OTHER MUSCULOSKELETAL STRUCTURES

❑ 1. The diaphragm separates the thoracic cavity from the abdominal cavity.

❑ 2. The medial and lateral arcuate ligaments of the lumbar part of the diaphragm actually attach across the quadratus lumborum and the psoas major muscles.

METHODOLOGY FOR LEARNING MUSCLE ACTIONS

❑ **Inspiration (Increases the Volume of the Thoracic Cavity):** The diaphragm is essentially shaped like a dome. This dome is somewhat asymmetrical with the anterior aspect of it being higher than the posterior aspect. Its attachments peripherally onto the posterior ribcage and the lumbar vertebrae are its lowest points. The attachments peripherally onto the anterior ribcage and the xiphoid process of the sternum are somewhat higher. From these peripheral attachments, the fibers essentially run vertically and toward the center of the body to converge together into the *central tendon* of the diaphragm. Thus the diaphragm attaches into itself centrally at the central tendon. When the diaphragm contracts, the volume of the thoracic cavity increases to allow the lungs to inflate and expand for inspiration. This process occurs in two steps. The mechanisms are as follows:

When the diaphragm contracts, the bony peripheral attachments are more fixed and the pull is on the central tendon, which causes the center (i.e., the top of the dome) to drop down (against the abdominal viscera). This raises the volume of the thoracic cavity to allow the lungs to inflate and expand for inspiration. This aspect of the diaphragm's contraction is usually called *abdominal breathing*.

DIAPHRAGM – continued

As the diaphragm continues to contract, the pressure caused by the resistance of the abdominal viscera prohibits the central dome from dropping any further and the dome now becomes less able to move (i.e., more fixed). The pull exerted by the contraction of the fibers of the diaphragm now pull peripherally on the ribcage, elevating the lower ribs and causing the anterior ribcage and sternum to push anteriorly. This further increases the volume of the thoracic cavity to allow the lungs to inflate and expand. This aspect of the diaphragm's contraction is usually called *thoracic breathing*.

MISCELLANEOUS

- ❑ 1. The diaphragm is a partition between the thoracic cavity and the abdominal (abdominopelvic) cavity.
- ❑ 2. The medial arcuate ligament of the diaphragm surrounds the psoas major and runs from the body of L2 to the T.P. of L2.
- ❑ 3. The lateral arcuate ligament of the diaphragm surrounds the quadratus lumborum and runs from the T.P. of L2 to the 12th rib.
- ❑ 4. The two crura (singular: crus) of the diaphragm are not symmetrical. The right crus is broader and attaches farther inferiorly than the left crus.
- ❑ 5. The central tendon of the diaphragm is a thin but strong aponeurosis located near the center of the muscle.
- ❑ 6. The costal fibers of the diaphragm interdigitate with the transversus abdominis.
- ❑ 7. There are a number of openings in the diaphragm to allow passage of structures between the thoracic and abdominal cavities. The largest openings are for the esophagus, the aorta and the inferior vena cava.
- ❑ 8. The diaphragm is the only muscle that must contract for quiet, relaxed inspiration. Many other muscles also contract to assist and create more forceful inspiration (such as during exercise). No contraction of any muscle is necessary for quiet relaxed expiration; elastic recoil of the diaphragm is sufficient to press against the lungs and push out the air. Many other muscles do contract when forceful expiration is needed (such as during exercise).
- ❑ 9. The diaphragm is unusual in that it is under both conscious control and unconscious control.
- ❑ 10. More specifically, contraction of the diaphragm is under constant unconscious regulation by the brainstem of the brain. However, we routinely override this brainstem control whenever we choose to sing, talk, sigh, hold our breath or otherwise consciously change our breathing pattern.
- ❑ 11. The innervation to the diaphragm is the phrenic nerve, composed of spinal nerves C3, 4, 5. ("C3, 4, 5 keeps the diaphragm alive!" ☺)
- ❑ 12. A *hiatal hernia* is when part of the stomach herniates (ruptures) through the diaphragm into the thoracic cavity.

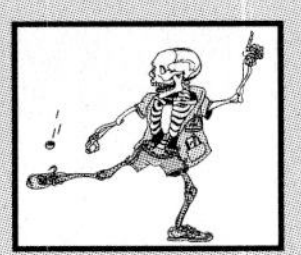

PART TWO – MUSCLES OF THE LOWER EXTREMITY

MUSCLES OF THE PELVIS

MUSCLES OF THE THIGH

MUSCLES OF THE LEG

INTRINSIC MUSCLES OF THE FOOT

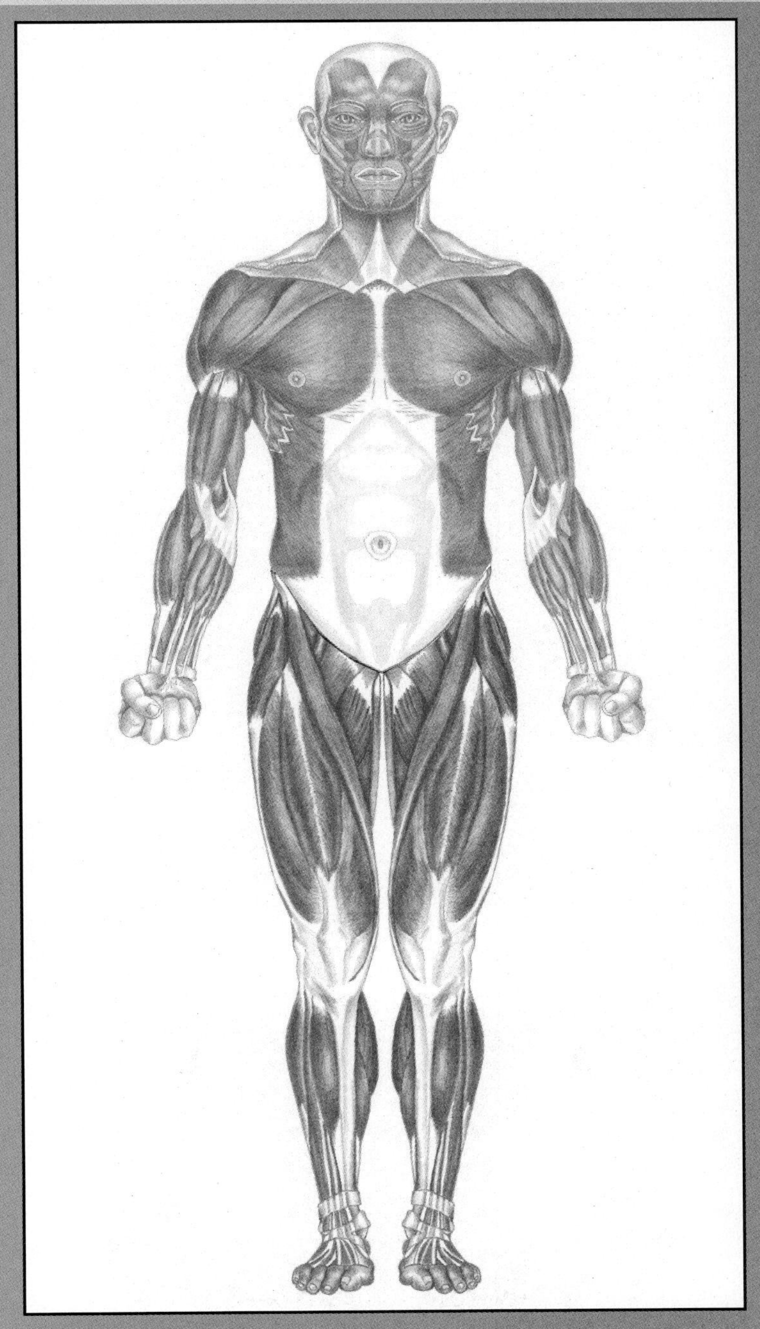

LOWER EXTREMITY

MUSCLES OF THE PELVIS

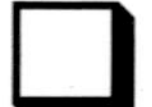

OVERVIEW OF THE MUSCLES OF THE PELVIS

ANATOMICALLY, THE MUSCLES OF THE PELVIS MAY BE DIVIDED INTO TWO GROUPS:	
The Anterior Group: ▪ Psoas Major ▪ Iliacus ▪ Psoas Minor	**The Posterior Group:** *Superficial* ▪ Gluteus Maximus *Intermediate* ▪ Gluteus Medius *Deep:* *The Deep Lateral Rotators of the Thigh* ▪ Piriformis ▪ Superior Gemellus ▪ Obturator Internus ▪ Inferior Gemellus ▪ Obturator Externus ▪ Quadratus Femoris ▪ Gluteus Minimus

THE FOLLOWING MUSCLES ARE COVERED IN OTHER CHAPTERS OF THIS BOOK, BUT ARE ALSO PRESENT IN THE PELVIS:

- The Erector Spinae Group
- The Transversospinalis Group
- Rectus Abdominis
- External Abdominal Oblique
- Internal Abdominal Oblique
- Transversus Abdominis
- Tensor Fasciae Latae
- Sartorius
- Rectus Femoris
- Pectineus
- Adductor Longus
- Gracilis
- Adductor Brevis
- Adductor Magnus
- Biceps Femoris
- Semitendinosus
- Semimembranosus

(Please see Appendix E for other muscles that attach to the pelvis.)

This is how the muscles of the pelvis are usually classified. However, like any classification it is overly simplistic and can be misleading. Please note the following:

- All the muscles of the posterior pelvis, while essentially posterior in location, also travel and attach fairly far laterally (onto or near to the greater trochanter of the femur). Some might even argue that the gluteus medius and the gluteus minimus are primarily lateral in location.

- The gluteus medius and the gluteus minimus have fibers that are not only posterior and lateral, but also somewhat anterior. (These anterior fibers are directly next to the tensor fasciae latae and are far enough anterior to be able to flex the thigh at the hip joint.)
- The gluteus maximus does not completely cover the gluteus medius; the middle portion of the gluteus medius is superficial.

Functionally, the muscles of the pelvis cross the hip joint. Therefore, muscles of the pelvis have their actions at the hip joint. The following general rules regarding actions can be stated for muscles of the pelvis:

- The muscles of the posterior pelvis, having a fiber direction that is primarily horizontal, can laterally rotate the thigh at the hip joint (or contralaterally rotate the pelvis at the hip joint).
- The gluteal muscles, having a vertical component to their fibers can also extend the thigh at the hip joint (or posteriorly tilt the pelvis at the hip joints) and abduct the thigh at the hip joint (or depress, i.e., laterally tilt, the pelvis at the hip joint).
- The gluteus medius and the gluteus minimus have anterior fibers that can flex the thigh at the hip joint (or anteriorly tilt the pelvis at the hip joint).
- Since the psoas major and the iliacus are anterior, they can flex the thigh at the hip joint (or anteriorly tilt the pelvis at the hip joint).
- Note that the psoas major is also a muscle of the trunk and can move the trunk at the spinal joints.

INNERVATION

- Generally, the anterior pelvis is innervated by the lumbar nerve segments L1, 2, and 3.
- Generally, the posterior pelvis is innervated by the inferior and superior gluteal nerves and branches of the lumbosacral plexus (except the obturator externus, which is innervated by the obturator nerve).

♥ ARTERIAL SUPPLY

- The anterior pelvis receives its arterial supply from branches of the descending aorta and branches of the internal iliac artery.
- The posterior pelvis receives its arterial supply from the superior and inferior gluteal arteries (except the obturator externus, which receives its arterial supply from the obturator artery).

A NOTE REGARDING REVERSE ACTIONS

As a rule, this book does not employ the terms "origin" and "insertion." However, it is useful to utilize these terms to describe the concept of "reverse actions." The action section of this book describes the action of a muscle by stating the movement of a body part that is created by a muscle's contraction. The body part that usually moves when a muscle contracts is called the insertion. The methodology section further states at which joint the movement of the insertion occurs. However, the other body part that the muscle attaches to, the origin, can also move at that joint. *This movement can be called the reverse action of the muscle.* Keep in mind that the reverse action of a muscle is always possible. The likelihood that a reverse action will occur is based upon the ability of the insertion to be fixed so that the origin moves (instead of the insertion moving) when the muscle contracts. For more information and examples of reverse actions, see page 702.

❑ ANTERIOR VIEW OF THE BONES AND BONY LANDMARKS OF THE RIGHT PELVIS

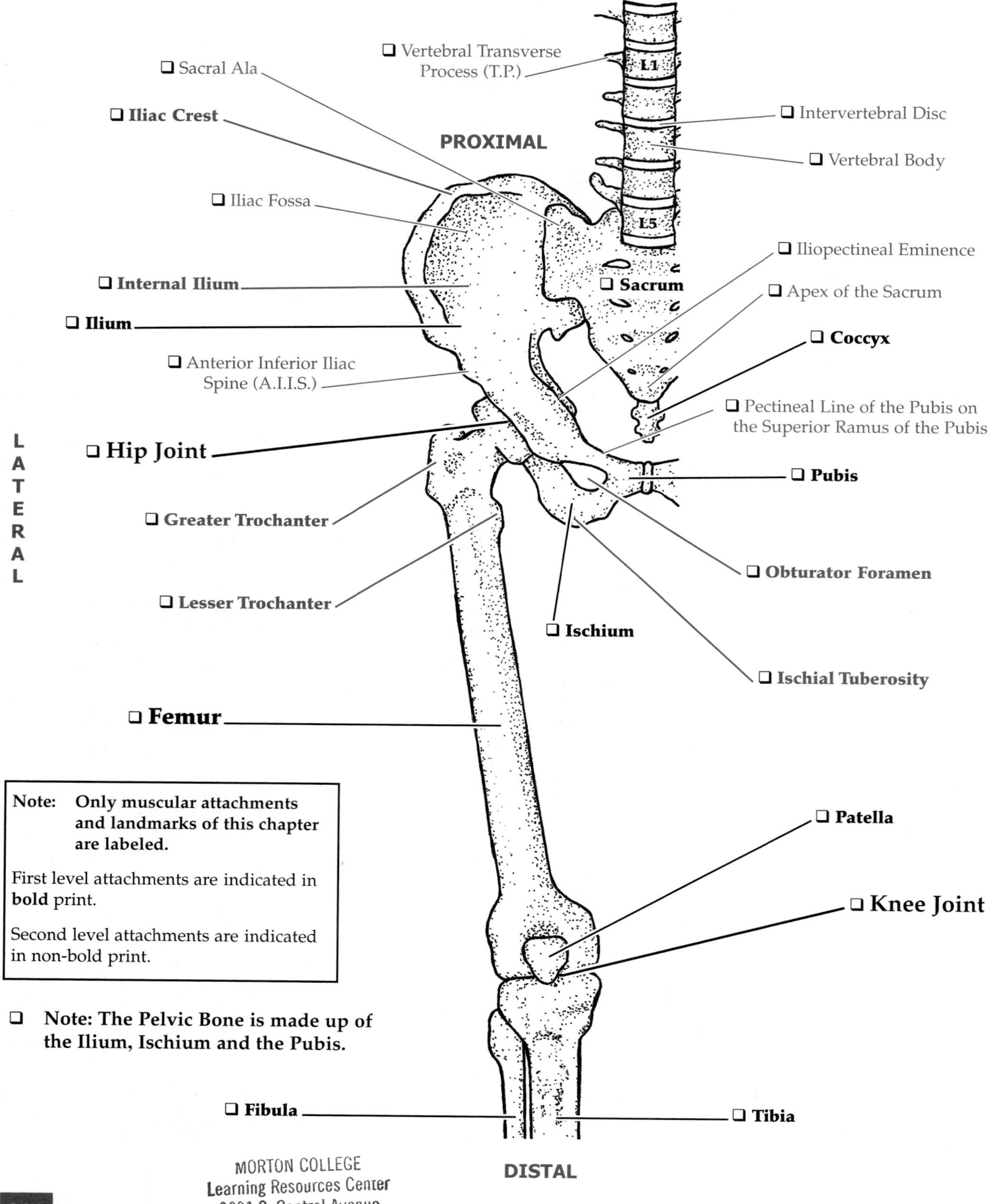

Note: Only muscular attachments and landmarks of this chapter are labeled.

First level attachments are indicated in **bold** print.

Second level attachments are indicated in non-bold print.

❑ **Note: The Pelvic Bone is made up of the Ilium, Ischium and the Pubis.**

ANTERIOR VIEW OF BONY ATTACHMENTS OF THE RIGHT PELVIS

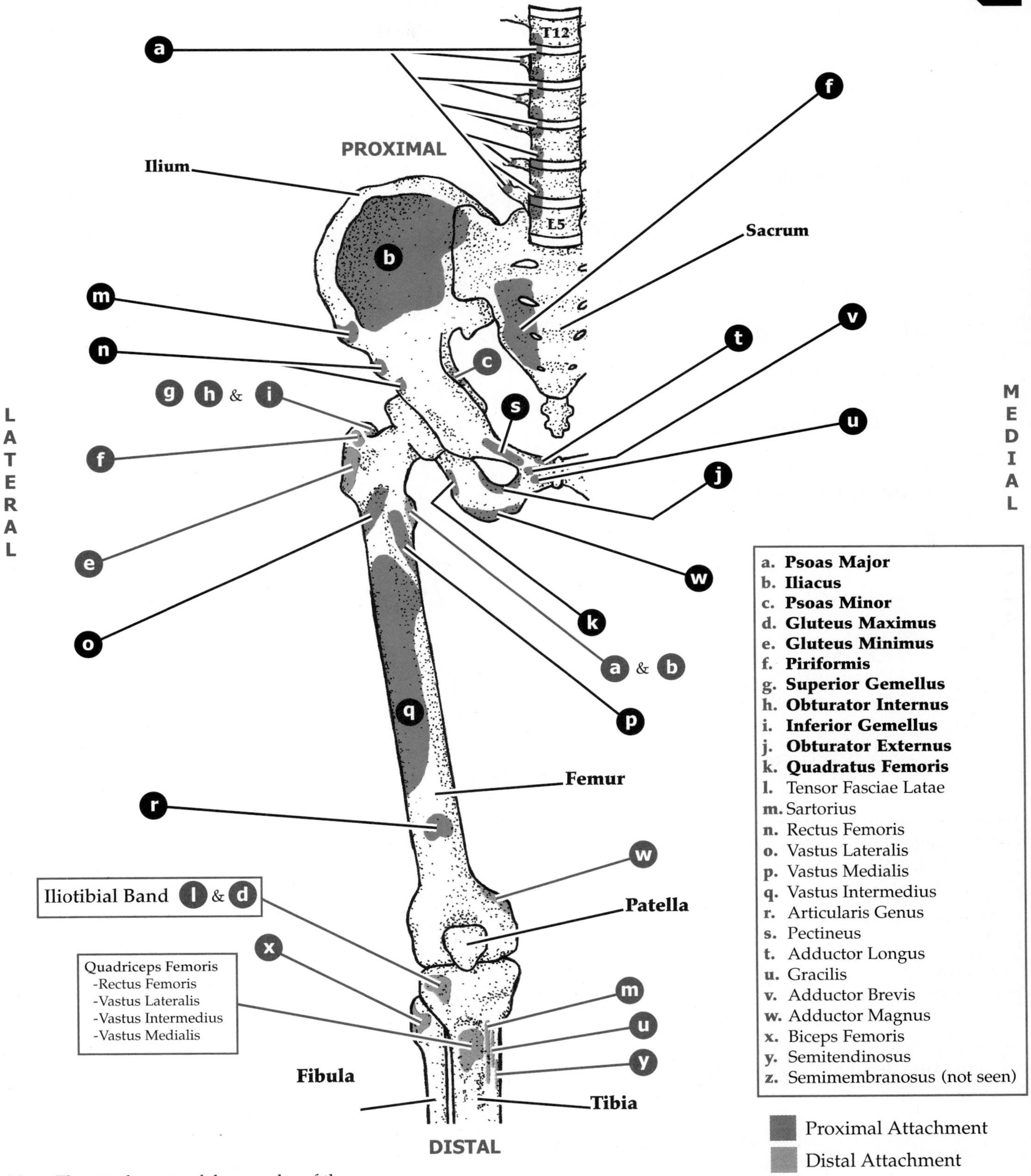

a. **Psoas Major**
b. **Iliacus**
c. **Psoas Minor**
d. **Gluteus Maximus**
e. **Gluteus Minimus**
f. **Piriformis**
g. **Superior Gemellus**
h. **Obturator Internus**
i. **Inferior Gemellus**
j. **Obturator Externus**
k. **Quadratus Femoris**
l. Tensor Fasciae Latae
m. Sartorius
n. Rectus Femoris
o. Vastus Lateralis
p. Vastus Medialis
q. Vastus Intermedius
r. Articularis Genus
s. Pectineus
t. Adductor Longus
u. Gracilis
v. Adductor Brevis
w. Adductor Magnus
x. Biceps Femoris
y. Semitendinosus
z. Semimembranosus (not seen)

Proximal Attachment
Distal Attachment

Note: The attachments of the muscles of the trunk chapter are not shown (see page 197).

❑ POSTERIOR VIEW OF THE BONES AND BONY LANDMARKS OF THE RIGHT PELVIS

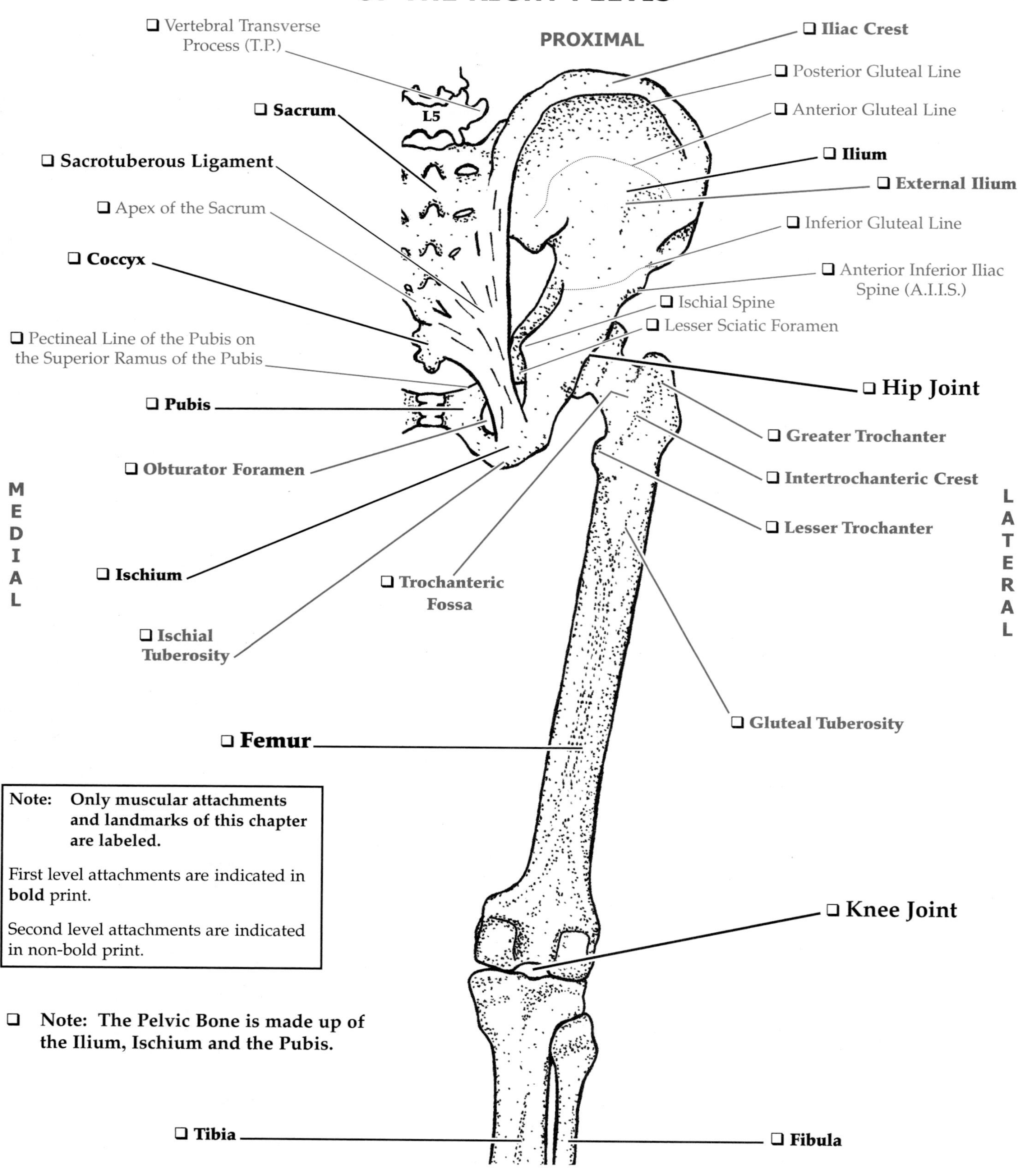

Note: **Only muscular attachments and landmarks of this chapter are labeled.**

First level attachments are indicated in **bold** print.

Second level attachments are indicated in non-bold print.

❑ **Note: The Pelvic Bone is made up of the Ilium, Ischium and the Pubis.**

POSTERIOR VIEW OF THE BONY ATTACHMENTS OF THE RIGHT PELVIS

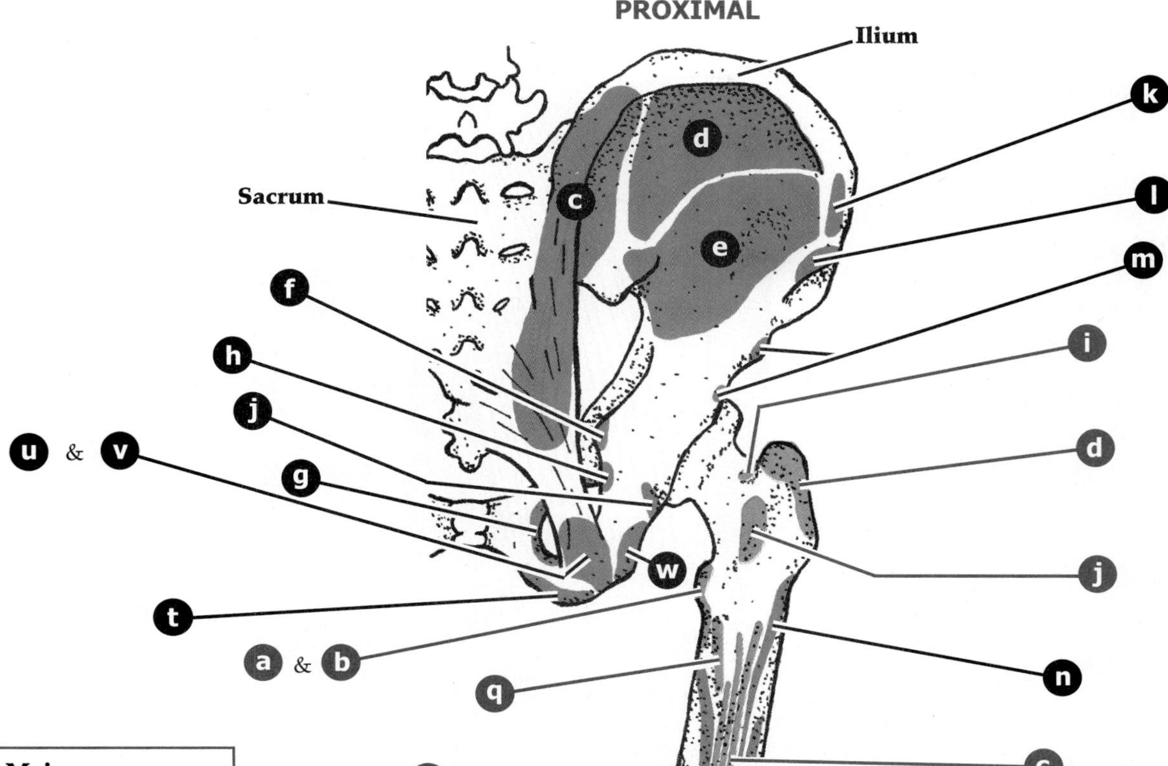

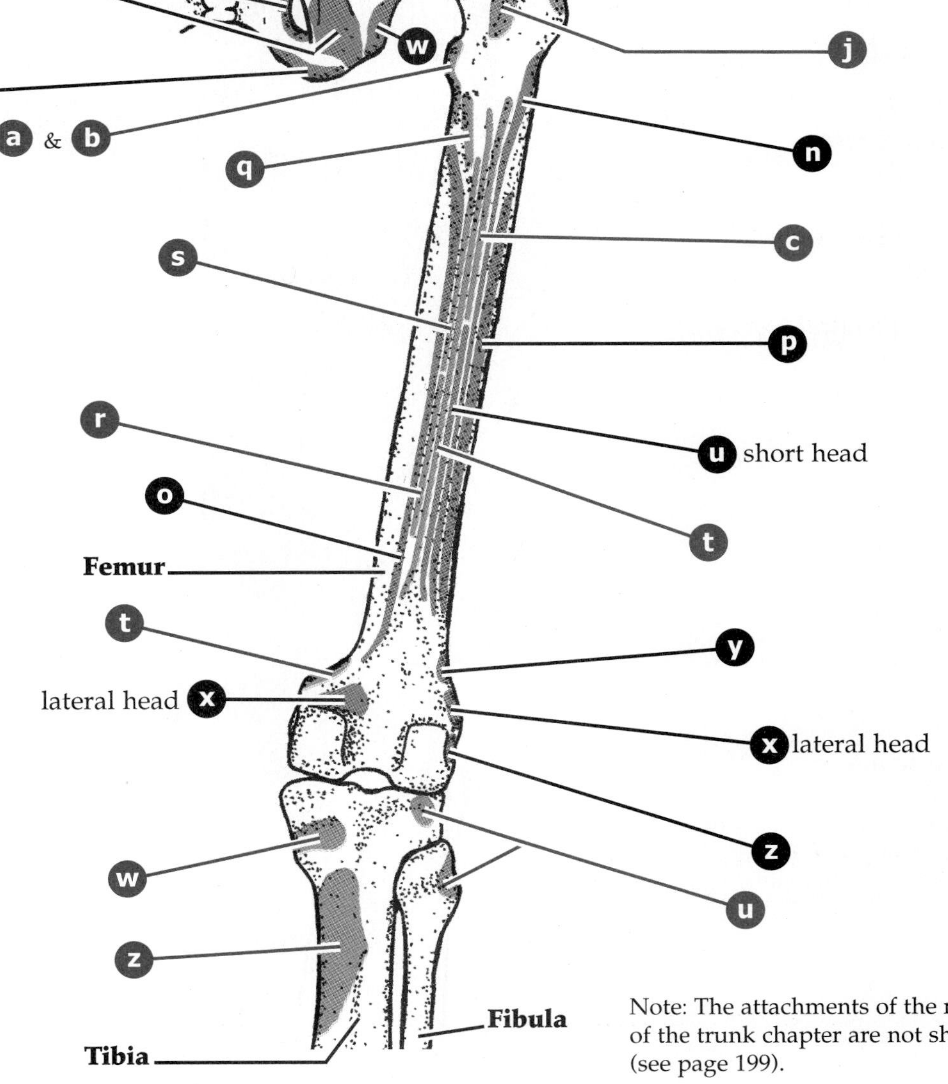

a. **Psoas Major**
b. **Iliacus**
c. **Gluteus Maximus**
d. **Gluteus Medius**
e. **Gluteus Minimus**
f. **Superior Gemellus**
g. **Obturator Internus**
h. **Inferior Gemellus**
i. **Obturator Externus**
j. **Quadratus Femoris**
k. Tensor Fasciae Latae
l. Sartorius
m. Rectus Femoris
n. Vastus Lateralis
o. Vastus Medialis
p. Vastus Intermedius
q. Pectineus
r. Adductor Longus
s. Adductor Brevis
t. Adductor Magnus
u. Biceps Femoris
v. Semitendinosus
w. Semimembranosus
x. Gastrocnemius
y. Plantaris
z. Popliteus

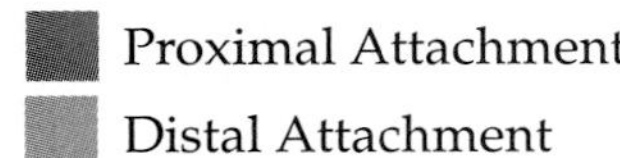

Note: The attachments of the muscles of the trunk chapter are not shown (see page 199).

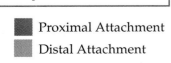

ANTERIOR VIEW OF THE RIGHT PELVIS

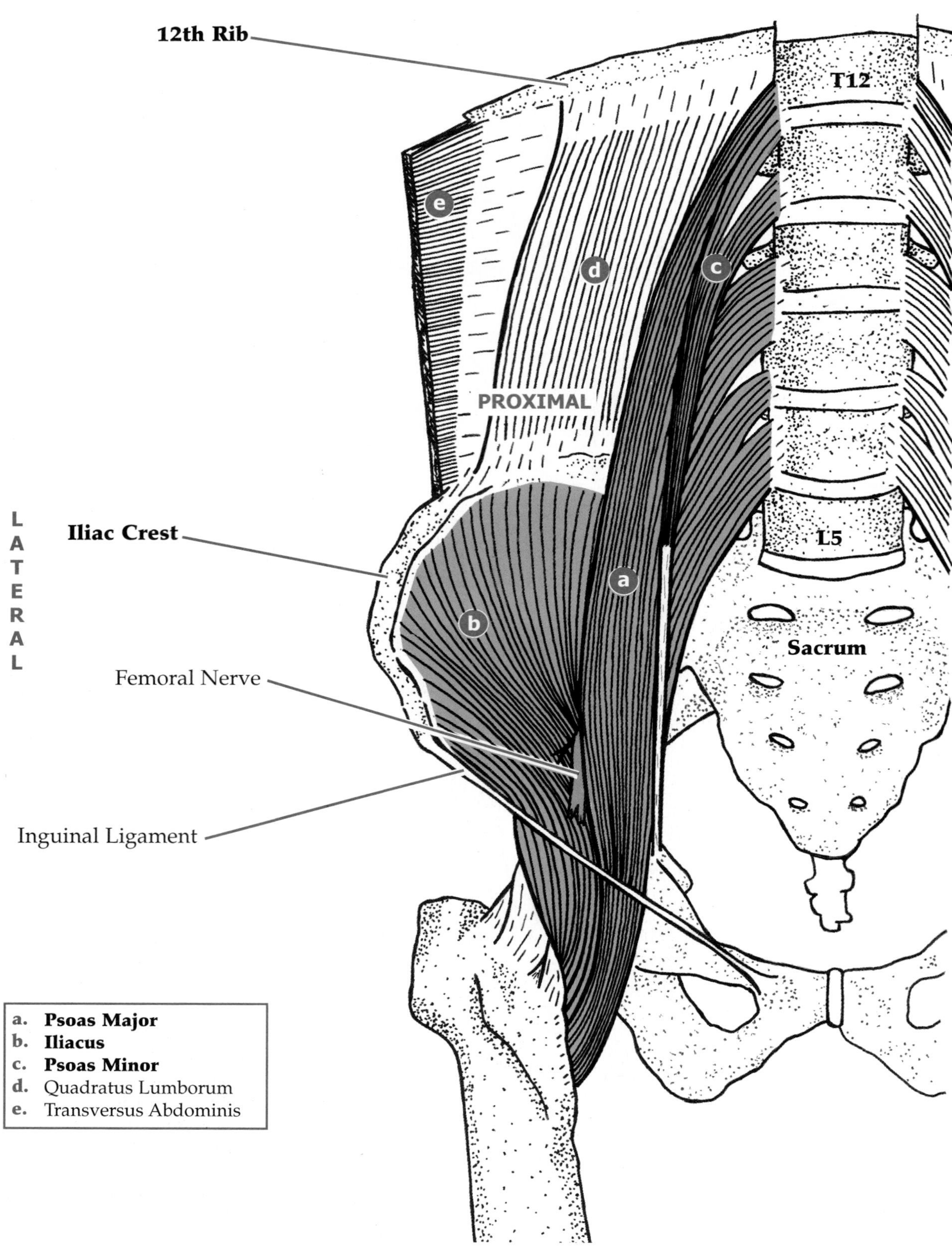

a. **Psoas Major**
b. **Iliacus**
c. **Psoas Minor**
d. Quadratus Lumborum
e. Transversus Abdominis

LATERAL VIEW OF THE RIGHT PELVIS

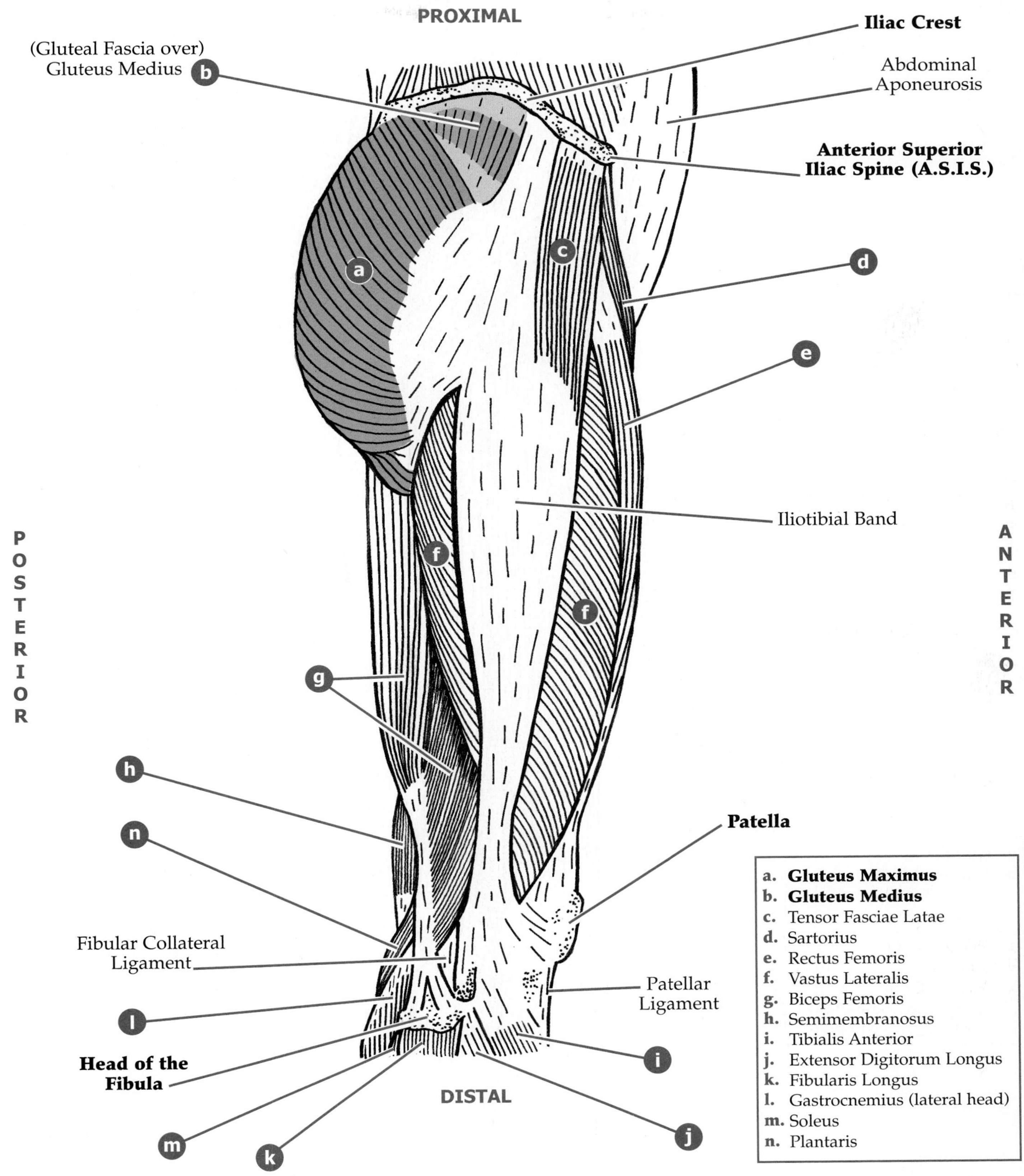

a. **Gluteus Maximus**
b. **Gluteus Medius**
c. Tensor Fasciae Latae
d. Sartorius
e. Rectus Femoris
f. Vastus Lateralis
g. Biceps Femoris
h. Semimembranosus
i. Tibialis Anterior
j. Extensor Digitorum Longus
k. Fibularis Longus
l. Gastrocnemius (lateral head)
m. Soleus
n. Plantaris

POSTERIOR VIEW OF THE RIGHT PELVIS (SUPERFICIAL)

PROXIMAL

Iliac Crest

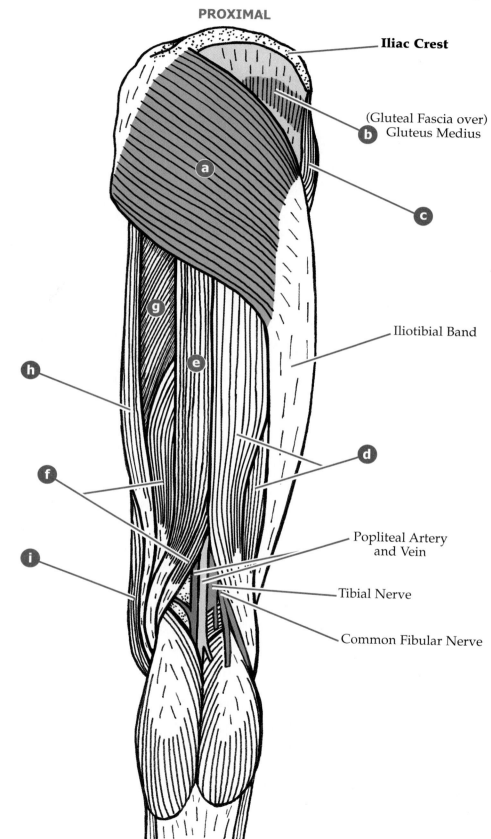

(Gluteal Fascia over)
b Gluteus Medius

a

c

g

Iliotibial Band

MEDIAL

LATERAL

h

e

d

f

Popliteal Artery
and Vein

i

Tibial Nerve

Common Fibular Nerve

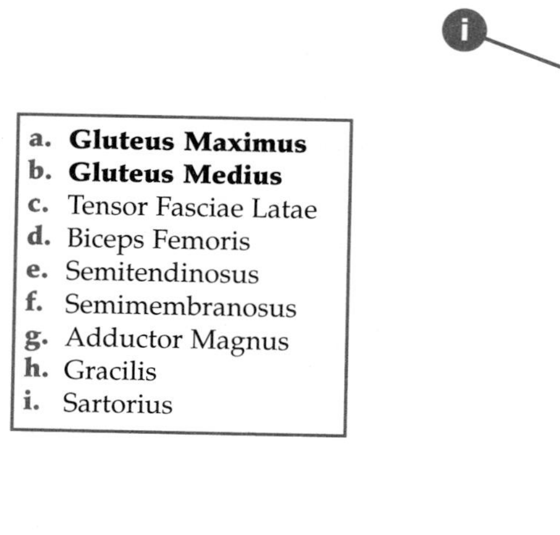

DISTAL

POSTERIOR VIEW OF THE RIGHT PELVIS (DEEP)

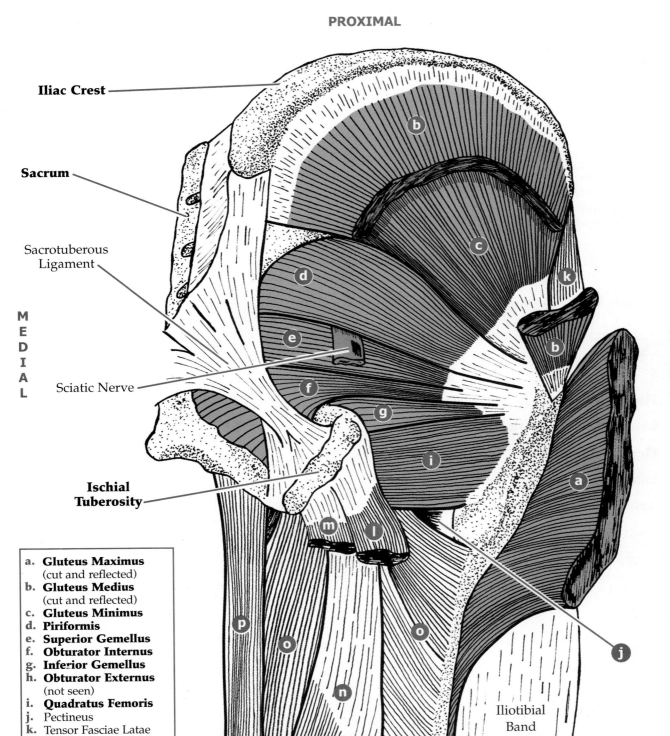

a. **Gluteus Maximus** (cut and reflected)
b. **Gluteus Medius** (cut and reflected)
c. **Gluteus Minimus**
d. **Piriformis**
e. **Superior Gemellus**
f. **Obturator Internus**
g. **Inferior Gemellus**
h. **Obturator Externus** (not seen)
i. **Quadratus Femoris**
j. Pectineus
k. Tensor Fasciae Latae
l. Biceps Femoris (cut)
m. Semitendinosus (cut)
n. Semimembranosus
o. Adductor Magnus
p. Gracilis

PSOAS MAJOR
(OF THE ILIOPSOAS)

❑ **The name, psoas major, tells us that this muscle is located in the loin (low back) area and is large (larger than the psoas minor).**

DERIVATION ❑ psoas: Gr. *loin.* major: L. *large.*

PRONUNCIATION ❑ **so**-as **may**-jor

ATTACHMENTS

❑ **Anterolateral Lumbar Spine**

❑ anterolaterally on the bodies of T12 - L5 and the intervertebral discs between, and anteriorly on the T.P.s of L1 - L5

to the

❑ **Lesser Trochanter of the Femur**

ACTIONS

❑ 1. **Flexion of the Thigh**

❑ 2. **Lateral Rotation of the Thigh**

❑ 3. **Flexion of the Trunk**

❑ 4. **Lateral Flexion of the Trunk**

❑ 5. **Anterior Tilt of the Pelvis**

❑ 6. Contralateral Rotation of the Trunk

❑ 7. Contralateral Rotation of the Pelvis

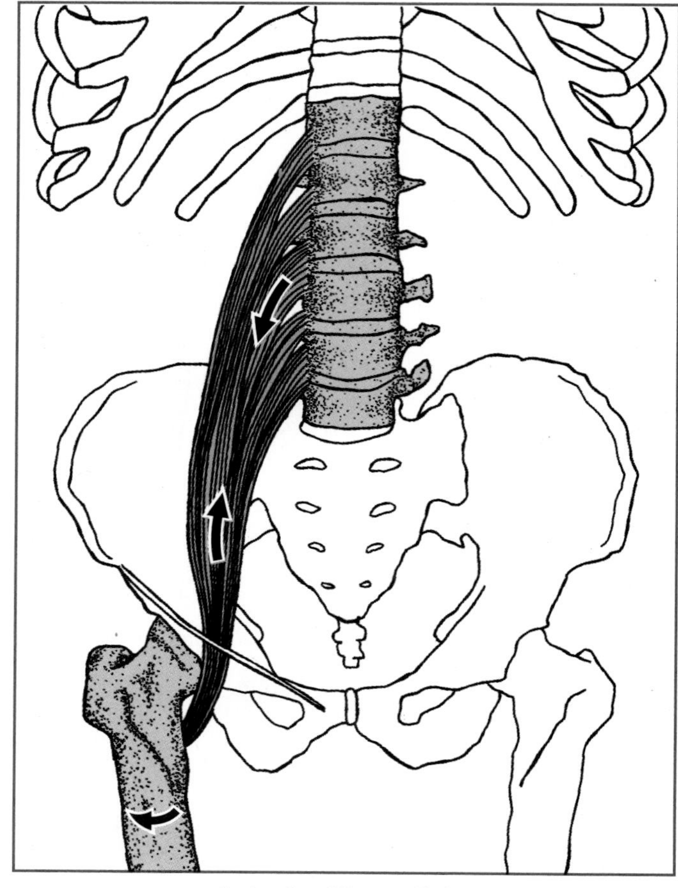

Anterior View of the Right Psoas Major

INNERVATION ❑ Lumbar Plexus ❑ **L1**, **2**, 3

ARTERIAL SUPPLY ❑ The Lumbar Arteries (Branches of the Aorta)
❑ and the iliolumbar artery (a branch of the internal iliac artery)

PALPATION AND SUPPLEMENTARY TEXT

PALPATION

- ❑ The psoas major is deep but palpable.
  - Have the client seated with the trunk slightly inclined forward (anterior tilt of the pelvis at the hip joint) to relax the anterior abdominal wall muscles.
  - Place palpating hand on the abdomen (between the iliac crest and the 12th rib) and palpate deeply with even pressure toward the psoas major.
  - Ask the client to flex the thigh at the hip joint (by lifting the foot off the floor) and feel for the contraction of the psoas major.

  The distal tendon of the psoas major is also palpable in the proximal anterior thigh between the pectineus and the sartorius. (Note: Be careful with palpation in this region because the femoral nerve, artery and vein lie over the iliopsoas and pectineus here. See illustration on page 352.)

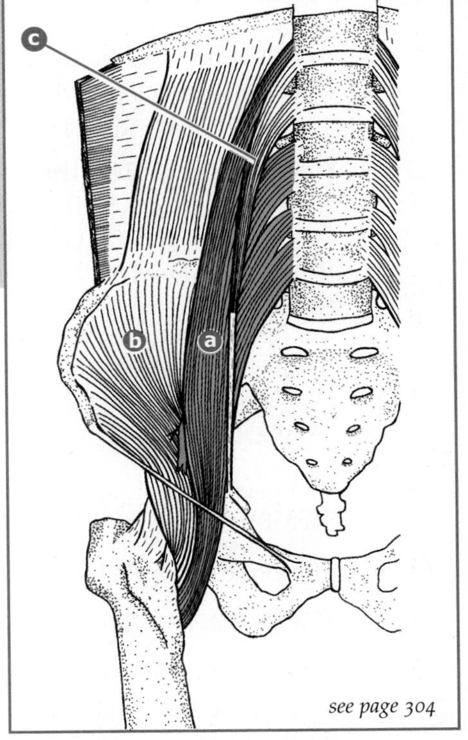

Anterior View of the Right Pelvis

a. **Psoas Major**
b. Iliacus
c. Psoas Minor

RELATIONSHIP TO OTHER MUSCULOSKELETAL STRUCTURES

❑ 1. The psoas major is deep in the abdomen and lies anteromedially to the quadratus lumborum.

❑ 2. Distally, the psoas major tendon is joined by the iliacus tendon to attach onto the lesser trochanter of the femur.

❑ 3. The psoas major lies deep to the inguinal ligament and directly anterior to the hip joint. The psoas minor lies directly anterior to the belly of the psoas major.

METHODOLOGY FOR LEARNING MUSCLE ACTIONS

❑ 1. **Flexion of the Thigh at the Hip Joint:** The psoas major crosses the hip joint anteriorly (with its fibers running vertically in the sagittal plane); therefore, it flexes the thigh at the hip joint.

❑ 2. **Lateral Rotation of the Thigh at the Hip Joint:** The psoas major crosses the hip joint anteriorly in such a way that it wraps around from the vertebral column to attach onto the lesser trochanter of the femur (with its fibers running somewhat horizontally in the transverse plane). When the psoas major contracts, it pulls the lesser trochanter anterolaterally and laterally rotates the femur, i.e., the thigh, at the hip joint.

❑ 3. **Flexion of the Trunk at the Spinal Joints:** The psoas major crosses the spinal joints anteriorly (with its fibers running vertically in the sagittal plane); therefore (with the femoral attachment fixed), the psoas major flexes the trunk at the spinal joints.

❑ 4. **Lateral Flexion of the Trunk at the Spinal Joints:** The psoas major crosses the spinal joints laterally (with its fibers running vertically in the frontal plane); therefore (with the femoral attachment fixed), the psoas major laterally flexes the trunk at the spinal joints.

PSOAS MAJOR – continued

❑ 5. **Anterior Tilt of the Pelvis at the Hip Joint:** When the trunk is fixed to the pelvis, and the psoas major contracts, the psoas major pulls the spinal attachment inferiorly toward the femurs, causing the pelvis to anteriorly tilt at the hip joint.

❑ 6. **Contralateral Rotation of the Trunk at the Spinal Joints:** The psoas major crosses the spinal joints, attaching from anterolaterally on the vertebral column to then attach further anteriorly onto the femur (with its fibers running somewhat horizontally in the transverse plane). When the femoral attachment is fixed and the psoas major contracts, it pulls the vertebrae, causing the anterior surface of the vertebrae to rotate toward the opposite side of the body from the side that the psoas major is attached. Therefore, the psoas major contralaterally rotates the trunk at the spinal joints.

❑ 7. **Contralateral Rotation of the Pelvis at the Hip Joint:** When the trunk is fixed to the pelvis, and the psoas major contracts, the psoas major pulls on the spinal attachment and rotates it in the transverse plane (see methodology #6). The trunk and the pelvis move as a unit and the pelvis rotates toward the opposite side of the body from the side that the psoas major is attached. Therefore, the psoas major contralaterally rotates the pelvis at the hip joint.

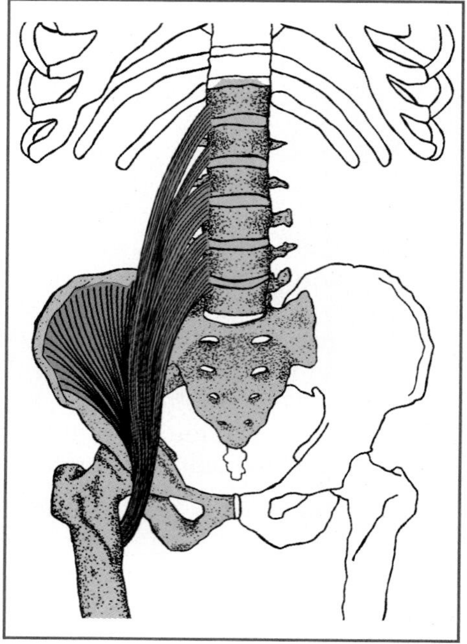

Anterior View of the Right Iliopsoas

MISCELLANEOUS

❑ 1. The psoas major, along with the iliacus muscle, is sometimes considered to be the *iliopsoas* muscle because of their common distal attachment onto the lesser trochanter of the femur.

❑ 2. The proximal attachment of the psoas major on the spine arises by five separate slips of tissue.

❑ 3. The iliopsoas is the prime mover of flexion of the thigh at the hip joint.

❑ 4. Lateral rotation of the thigh at the hip joint is a very weak action of the iliopsoas. In fact, the ability of the iliopsoas to do this action is dependent upon the amount of abduction and/or flexion of the thigh at the hip joint.

❑ 5. There is a great deal of controversy regarding the effect of the psoas major upon the lumbar spine. Generally, the psoas major is considered to be a flexor of the lumbar spine. However, when the lumbar spine is in an extended position, it is believed that the majority of the fibers of the psoas major cross posterior to the axis of movement and, therefore, extend the lumbar spine.

❑ 6. With regard to posture, a chronically tight psoas major anteriorly tilts the pelvis, causing the lumbar curve to increase (*hyperlordosis,* also known as *swayback*). Straight-legged sit-ups tend to disproportionately strengthen the psoas major in comparison to the anterior abdominal wall muscles. To avoid this, it is recommended to do curl ups, wherein the hip and knee joints are flexed and the trunk "curls" up (spinal flexion, not the pelvis anteriorly tilting at the hip joints) approximately 30°. With the hip joint flexed to 90°, the psoas major is slackened and will not be engaged if the curl up is restricted to approximately 30°.

❑ 7. The roots of the lumbar plexus of nerves enter the psoas major muscle directly; the lumbar plexus itself is located within the belly of the psoas major, and the branches of the lumbar plexus then emerge from the psoas major muscle. Therefore, a tight psoas major may entrap these nerves.

❑ 8. Tenderloin (also known as filet mignon) is the psoas major of a cow.

ILIACUS
(OF THE ILIOPSOAS)

❑ **The name, iliacus, tells us that this muscle attaches onto the ilium.**

DERIVATION ❑ iliacus: L. *refers to the ilium.*

PRONUNCIATION ❑ i-lee-**ak**-us

ATTACHMENTS

❑ **Internal Ilium**

❑ the upper 2/3 of the iliac fossa and the anterior inferior iliac spine (A.I.I.S.) and the sacral ala

to the

❑ **Lesser Trochanter of the Femur**

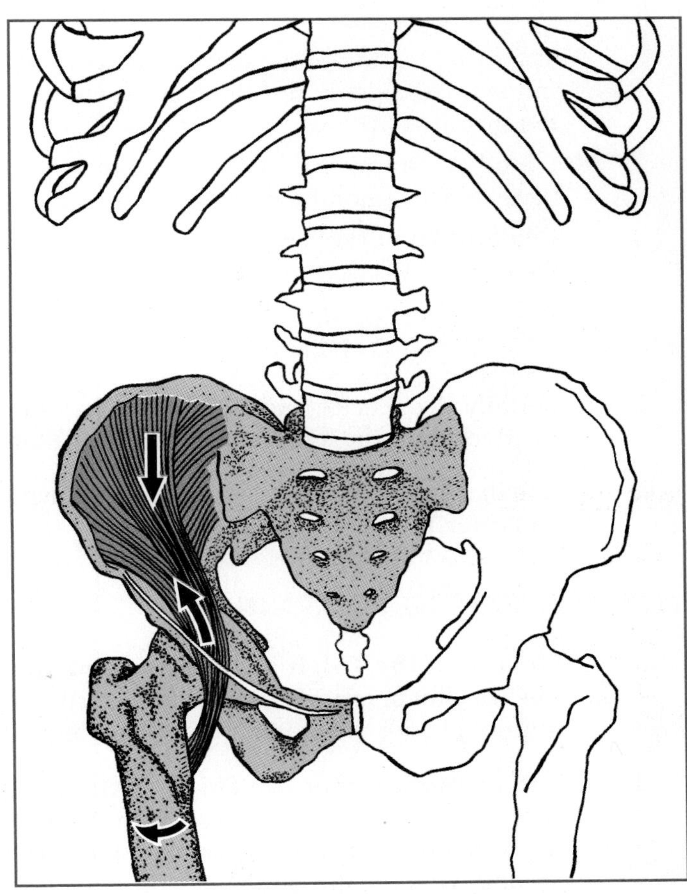

Anterior View of the Right Iliacus

ACTIONS

❑ 1. **Flexion of the Thigh**

❑ 2. **Lateral Rotation of the Thigh**

❑ 3. **Anterior Tilt of the Pelvis**

❑ 4. Contralateral Rotation of the Pelvis

INNERVATION ❑ The Femoral Nerve ❑ **L2**, 3

ARTERIAL SUPPLY ❑ The Iliolumbar Artery (A Branch of the Internal Iliac Artery)
❑ and the obturator artery (a branch of the internal iliac artery)

ILIACUS – PALPATION AND SUPPLEMENTARY TEXT

PALPATION

- [ ] Most of the iliacus is not palpable.
  - Have the client supine with the thighs slightly passively flexed and laterally rotated at the hip joints. This can be accomplished by placing a small pillow under the client's knees.
  - Place palpating hand on the anterior iliac crest and palpate into the iliac fossa with your fingertips.
  - Ask the client to actively flex the thigh at the hip joint and feel for the contraction of the iliacus.

  The distal tendon of the iliacus is also somewhat palpable in the proximal anterior thigh between the pectineus and the sartorius.

  (Note: Be careful with palpation in the anterior thigh region because the femoral nerve, artery and vein lie over the iliopsoas and pectineus here. See illustration on page 352.)

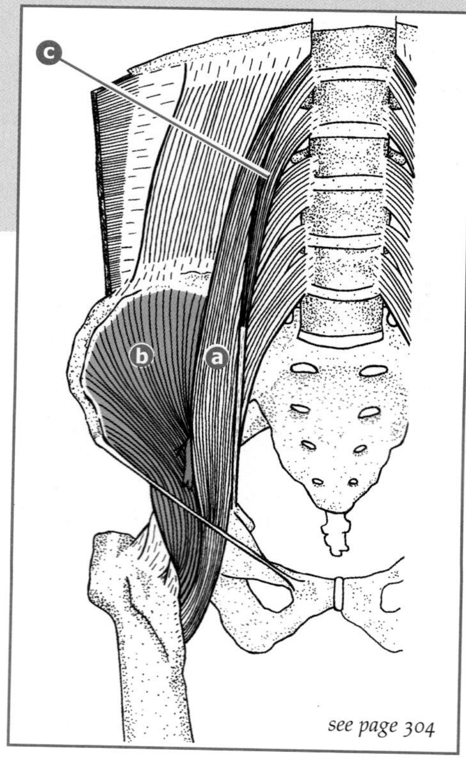

Anterior View of the Right Pelvis

a. Psoas Major
b. **Iliacus**
c. Psoas Minor

RELATIONSHIP TO OTHER MUSCULOSKELETAL STRUCTURES

- [ ] 1. Distally, the iliacus tendon joins the psoas major tendon to attach onto the lesser trochanter of the femur.
- [ ] 2. The iliacus lies deep to the inguinal ligament and directly anterior to the hip joint.

METHODOLOGY FOR LEARNING MUSCLE ACTIONS

- [ ] 1. **Flexion of the Thigh at the Hip Joint:** The iliacus crosses the hip joint anteriorly (with its fibers running vertically in the sagittal plane); therefore, it flexes the thigh at the hip joint.
- [ ] 2. **Lateral Rotation of the Thigh at the Hip Joint:** The iliacus crosses the hip joint anteriorly (with its fibers running somewhat horizontally in the transverse plane) in such a way that it wraps around from the ilium to attach onto the lesser trochanter of the femur. When the iliacus contracts, it pulls the lesser trochanter anterolaterally, and laterally rotates the femur, i.e., the thigh, at the hip joint.
- [ ] 3. **Anterior Tilt of the Pelvis at the Hip Joint:** When the thigh is fixed, the iliacus, by pulling inferiorly on the anterior pelvis, anteriorly tilts the pelvis at the hip joint.
- [ ] 4. **Contralateral Rotation of the Pelvis at the Hip Joint:** The iliacus crosses the hip joint anteriorly (with its fibers running somewhat horizontally in the transverse plane) in such a way that it wraps around from the femur to attach laterally onto the pelvis. When the femur is fixed, and the iliacus contracts, the iliacus rotates the pelvis (in the transverse plane) away from the side of the body that the iliacus is attached. Therefore, the iliacus contralaterally rotates the pelvis at the hip joint.

ILIACUS – continued

MISCELLANEOUS

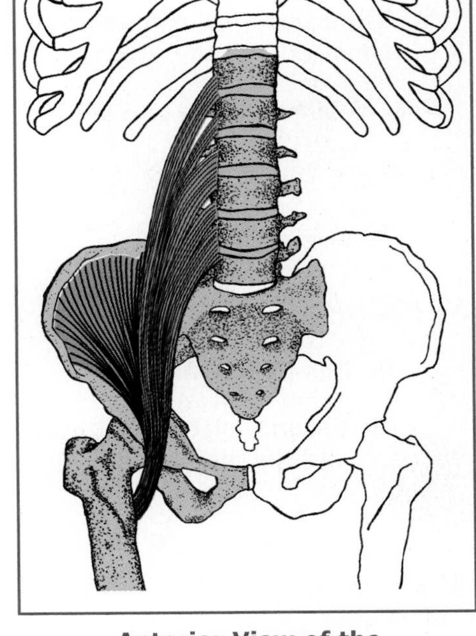

Anterior View of the Right Iliopsoas

- ❑ 1. The iliacus, along with the psoas major muscle, is sometimes considered, to be the *iliopsoas* muscle because of their common distal attachment onto the lesser trochanter of the femur.
- ❑ 2. The majority of the fibers of the distal iliacus actually attach into the psoas major's tendon (deep, on the posterior side) to then attach onto the lesser trochanter.
- ❑ 3. Some sources state that the iliacus can abduct the thigh at the hip joint. If this is true, then it would have to be the outermost (most lateral) fibers that would have the ability to do this (since their line of pull may fall just lateral to the mechanical axis of the femur).
- ❑ 4. The iliopsoas is the prime mover of thigh flexion.
- ❑ 5. Lateral rotation of the thigh at the hip joint is a very weak action of the iliopsoas. In fact, the ability of the iliopsoas to do this action is dependent upon the amount of abduction and/or flexion of the thigh at the hip joint.
- ❑ 6. With regard to posture, a chronically tight iliacus anteriorly tilts the pelvis, causing the lumbar curve to increase (*hyperlordosis*, also known as *swayback*). Straight-legged sit-ups tend to disproportionately strengthen the iliacus in comparison to the anterior abdominal wall muscles. To avoid this, it is recommended to do curl ups, wherein the hip and knee joints are flexed and the trunk "curls" up (spinal flexion, not the pelvis anteriorly tilting at the hip joints) approximately 30°. With the hip joint flexed to 90°, the iliacus is slackened and will not be engaged if the curl up is restricted to approximately 30°.

PSOAS MINOR

❑ **The name, psoas minor, tells us that this muscle is located in the loin (low back) area and is small (smaller than the psoas major).**

DERIVATION ❑ psoas: Gr. *loin.*
minor: L. *smaller.*

PRONUNCIATION ❑ **so**-as **my**-nor

ATTACHMENTS

❑ **Bodies of T12 and L1**

❑ the anterolateral bodies of T12-L1 and the disc between

to the

❑ **Pubis**

❑ the pectineal line of the pubis and the iliopectineal eminence (of the ilium and the pubis)

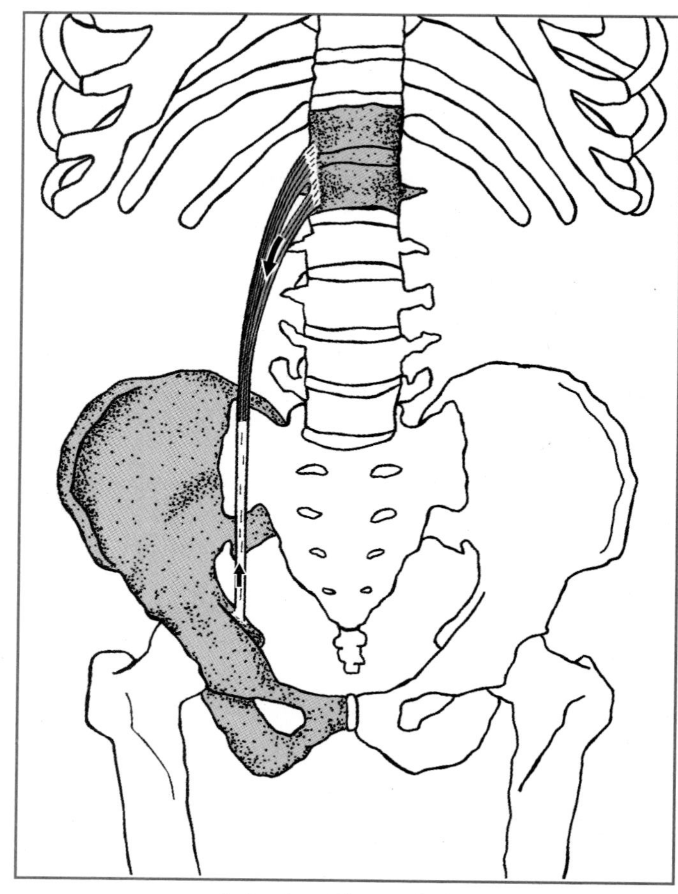

Anterior View of the Right Psoas Minor

ACTIONS

❑ 1. **Flexion of the Trunk**

❑ 2. **Posterior Tilt of the Pelvis**

INNERVATION ❑ L1 Spinal Nerve ❑ a branch from L1

ARTERIAL SUPPLY ❑ Lumbar Arteries (Branches of the Descending Aorta)

❑ and the arteria lumbalis ima of the median sacral artery (a branch of the aorta), the lumbar branch of the iliolumbar artery (a branch of the internal iliac artery) and the common iliac artery (a branch of the aorta)

PALPATION AND SUPPLEMENTARY TEXT

PALPATION

- ❑ Because the psoas minor is a fairly slender muscle that is deep in the abdomen (it lies directly on, i.e., anterior, to the psoas major), it is difficult to palpate. Given that the actions of the psoas minor are identical to the actions of the muscles of the anterior abdominal wall (through which one must try to palpate the psoas minor), it is not possible to palpate the psoas minor when it is contracting. In other words, when you have the client flex the trunk or posteriorly tilt the pelvis to contract the psoas minor, it also causes the rectus abdominis, external and internal abdominal obliques to contract, which will block you from palpating deeper into the abdomen. Therefore, the only way to palpate the psoas minor is to do so while it is relaxed.
  - First locate the psoas major (see the palpation section for this muscle on page 309).
  - Now palpate for the psoas minor. If the psoas major is relaxed and the psoas minor is tight, it may be possible to feel and distinguish the psoas minor.

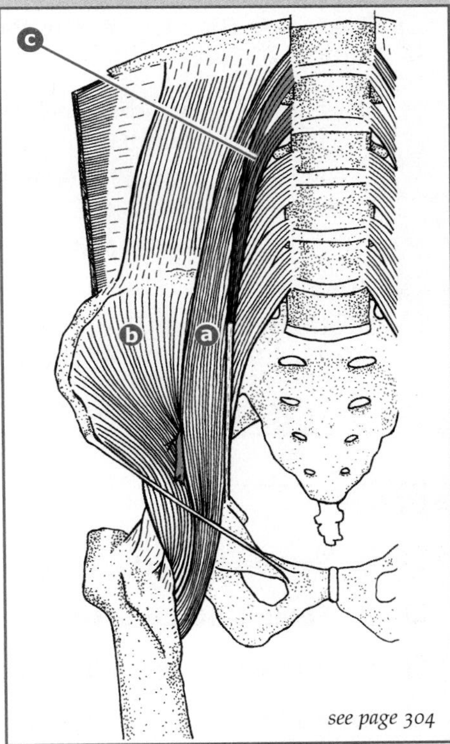

see page 304

Anterior View of the Right Pelvis

a. Psoas Major
b. Iliacus
c. **Psoas Minor**

RELATIONSHIP TO OTHER MUSCULOSKELETAL STRUCTURES

❑ 1. The psoas minor is deep in the abdomen and lies directly anterior to the psoas major.

❑ 2. Anterior (superficial) to the psoas minor are the abdominal viscera.

METHODOLOGY FOR LEARNING MUSCLE ACTIONS

❑ **1. Flexion of the Trunk at the Spinal Joints:** The psoas minor crosses the vertebral column anteriorly (with its fibers running vertically in the sagittal plane) and attaches onto the pelvis. When the psoas minor contracts, with the pelvis fixed, the trunk flexes at the spinal joints toward the pelvis.

❑ **2. Posterior Tilt of the Pelvis at the Lumbosacral Joint:** The psoas minor crosses the vertebral column anteriorly (with its fibers running vertically in the sagittal plane) and attaches onto the pelvis. When the trunk is fixed and the psoas minor contracts, it pulls the pelvis superiorly toward the spine. This motion is called posterior tilt of the pelvis and occurs at the lumbosacral joint.

MISCELLANEOUS

❑ 1. The psoas minor is absent in about 40% of the population.

❑ 2. The psoas minor is fairly weak and usually not considered to be a very important muscle.

❑ 3. The iliopectineal eminence (of the ilium and pubis) is also known as the *iliopubic eminence*.

❑ 4. A condition called *psoas minor syndrome* has been reported wherein the psoas minor in teenagers has not kept up with the growth of the trunk and pelvis and consequently is pulled taut and becomes painful.

GLUTEUS MAXIMUS

❑ **The name, gluteus maximus, tells us that this muscle is located in the gluteal (buttocks) region and is large (larger than the gluteus medius and the gluteus minimus).**

DERIVATION ❑ gluteus: Gr. *buttocks.*
maximus: L. *greatest.*

PRONUNCIATION ❑ **gloo**-tee-us **max**-i-mus

ATTACHMENTS

❑ **Posterior Iliac Crest, the Posterolateral Sacrum and the Coccyx**

❑ and the sacrotuberous ligament, the thoracolumbar fascia and the fascia over the gluteus medius

to the

❑ **Iliotibial Band (I.T.B.) and the Gluteal Tuberosity of the Femur**

ACTIONS

❑ 1. **Extension of the Thigh**

❑ 2. **Lateral Rotation of the Thigh**

❑ 3. **Abduction of the Thigh (upper 1/3)**

❑ 4. **Adduction of the Thigh (lower 2/3)**

❑ 5. **Posterior Tilt of the Pelvis**

❑ 6. Contralateral Rotation of the Pelvis

❑ 7. Extension of the Leg

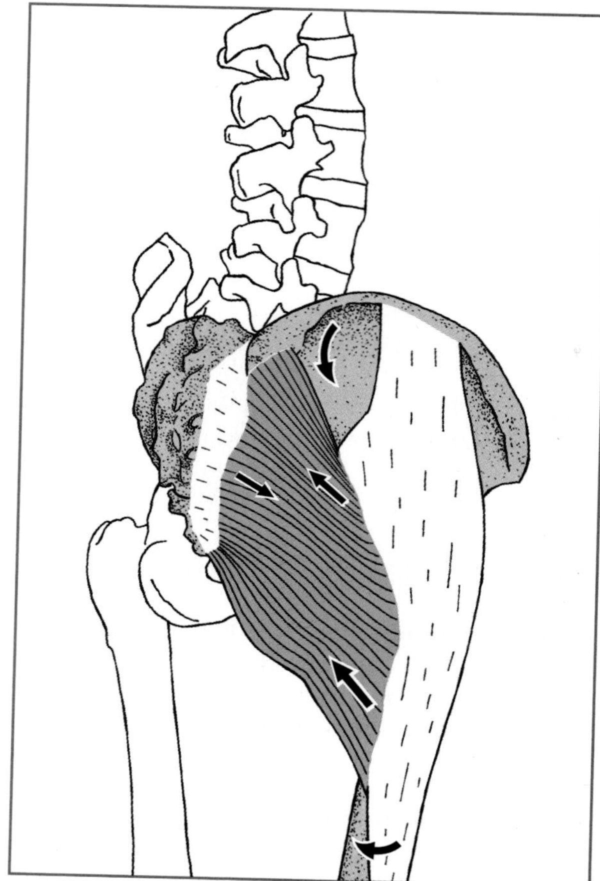

Posterolateral View of the Right Gluteus Maximus

INNERVATION ❑ The Inferior Gluteal Nerve ❑ **L5, S1,** 2

ARTERIAL SUPPLY ❑ The Superior Gluteal Artery and the Inferior Gluteal Artery (Branches of the Internal Iliac Artery)

PALPATION AND SUPPLEMENTARY TEXT

PALPATION

- ❑ The gluteus maximus is superficial and easy to palpate.
  - Have the client prone.
  - Place palpating hand on the lateral sacrum.
  - Palpate the gluteus maximus from its medial attachment (lateral sacrum) to its lateral attachment (I.T.B.).
  - To further bring out the gluteus maximus, have the client actively extend and laterally rotate the thigh at the hip joint.

    (Note: The gluteus maximus does not cover the entire buttocks; just inferior to the posterior iliac crest, the gluteus medius is superficial and directly palpable.)

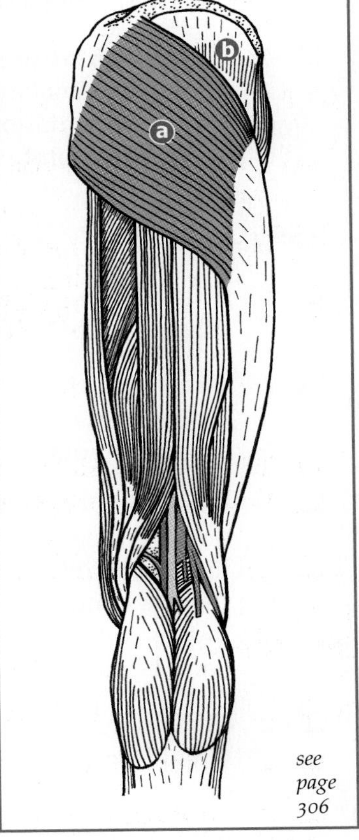

see page 306

Posterior View of the Right Pelvis (Superficial)

a. **Gluteus Maximus**
b. Gluteus Medius

RELATIONSHIP TO OTHER MUSCULOSKELETAL STRUCTURES

❑ 1. The gluteus maximus is superficial in the posterior pelvis and covers the posteroinferior portion of the gluteus medius. The gluteus maximus also covers the entire piriformis, superior gemellus, obturator internus, inferior gemellus, obturator externus, quadratus femoris and the ischial tuberosity.

❑ 2. The attachment of the gluteus maximus onto the gluteal tuberosity of the femur is between the vastus lateralis and adductor magnus attachments.

METHODOLOGY FOR LEARNING MUSCLE ACTIONS

❑ 1. **Extension of the Thigh at the Hip Joint:** The gluteus maximus crosses the hip joint posteriorly (with its fibers running vertically in the sagittal plane); therefore, it extends the thigh at the hip joint.

❑ 2. **Lateral Rotation of the Thigh at the Hip Joint:** The gluteus maximus wraps around the posterior pelvis to attach laterally onto the iliotibial band (with its fibers running somewhat horizontally in the transverse plane). When the gluteus maximus contracts, it pulls this lateral attachment posteromedially, causing the anterior surface of the thigh to face laterally. Therefore, the gluteus maximus laterally rotates the thigh at the hip joint.

❑ 3. **Abduction of the Thigh at the Hip Joint (upper 1/3):** The upper 1/3 of the gluteus maximus crosses the hip joint from medial to lateral above the center of the joint (with its fibers running vertically in the frontal plane). Therefore, this portion of the gluteus maximus abducts the thigh at the hip joint. (Note the similarity of the direction of fibers of the gluteus maximus to the direction of fibers of the gluteus medius.)

❑ 4. **Adduction of the Thigh at the Hip Joint (lower 2/3):** The lower 2/3 of the gluteus maximus crosses the hip joint from medial to lateral below the center of the joint (with its fibers running somewhat horizontally in the frontal plane). Therefore, this portion of the gluteus maximus adducts the thigh at the hip joint.

GLUTEUS MAXIMUS – continued

- ❑ **5. Posterior Tilt of the Pelvis at the Hip Joint:** When the thigh is fixed, the gluteus maximus, by pulling down on the posterior pelvis, posteriorly tilts the pelvis at the hip joint.
- ❑ **6. Contralateral Rotation of the Pelvis at the Hip Joint:** The gluteus maximus crosses the hip joint posteriorly (with its fibers running somewhat horizontally in the transverse plane). When the femoral attachment is fixed, and the gluteus maximus contracts, it pulls on the pelvis, causing the anterior pelvis to face the opposite side of the body from the side of the body that the gluteus maximus is attached. Therefore, the gluteus maximus contralaterally rotates the pelvis at the hip joint.
- ❑ **7. Extension of the Leg at the Knee Joint:** Due to its pull via the iliotibial band (which attaches to the proximal anterolateral tibia), the gluteus maximus crosses the knee joint anteriorly (with a vertical orientation to its pull in the sagittal plane). Therefore, the gluteus maximus extends the leg at the knee joint.

MISCELLANEOUS

- ❑ 1. There are two muscles that attach into the iliotibial band, the gluteus maximus and the tensor fasciae latae (T.F.L.).
- ❑ 2. Given that the gluteus maximus attaches into the iliotibial band from one direction and the tensor fasciae latae attaches into the iliotibial band from the opposite direction, they have opposite actions of rotation.
- ❑ 3. Given that both the gluteus maximus and the tensor fasciae latae attach into the iliotibial band, and the iliotibial band crosses the knee joint anteriorly, both of these muscles in effect cross the knee joint anteriorly and therefore, theoretically, can extend the leg at the knee joint. However, there is controversy over their ability to actually do this. Certainly, extension of the leg at the knee joint is not one of their major actions. It is likely that the role of these two muscles and the iliotibial band crossing the knee is primarily to help stabilize the knee joint.
- ❑ 4. The gluteus maximus, albeit the largest extensor and/or lateral rotator of the thigh, only contracts when forceful extension and/or lateral rotation of the thigh is required, such as running, jumping or climbing stairs.
- ❑ 5. It can be helpful to think of the gluteus maximus as the “speedskater’s muscle.” The gluteus maximus is powerful in extending, abducting and laterally rotating the thigh at the hip joint, which are all actions that are necessary when speedskating.
- ❑ 6. The action of posterior tilt of the pelvis at the hip joint by the gluteus maximus is important during walking, running and returning to an upright position from a stooped position.
- ❑ 7. If a person is standing and pinches the buttocks together, i.e., contracts the gluteus maximus muscles, an interesting postural effect occurs. The contraction of the gluteus maximus muscles should cause lateral rotation of the thighs at the hip joints. However, due to the friction between the bottom of the feet and the floor, the thighs cannot laterally rotate. Therefore, the rotatory force upon the thighs is translated all the way to the tarsal bones of the feet and the feet invert (supinate) instead, lifting up the arches of the feet. A conclusion from this might be that if a person’s gluteus maximus muscles are well developed and, therefore, have a stronger resting baseline tone, then the arches of their feet may gain extra support.
- ❑ 8. The gluteus maximus is the largest muscle in the human body.

GLUTEUS MEDIUS

❑ **The name, gluteus medius, tells us that this muscle is located in the gluteal (buttocks) region and is medium-sized (smaller than the gluteus maximus and larger than the gluteus minimus).**

DERIVATION ❑ gluteus: Gr. *buttocks.* medius: L. *middle.*

PRONUNCIATION ❑ **gloo**-tee-us **meed**- ee-us

ATTACHMENTS

❑ **External Ilium**

- ❑ inferior to the iliac crest and between the anterior and the posterior gluteal lines

to the

❑ **Greater Trochanter of the Femur**

- ❑ the lateral surface

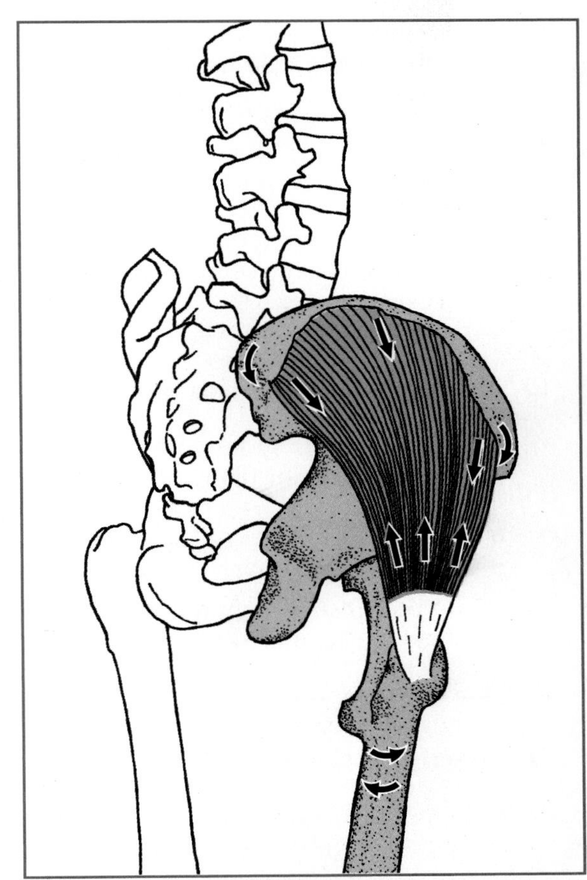

Posterolateral View of the Right Gluteus Medius

ACTIONS

❑ **1. Abduction of the Thigh (entire muscle)**

❑ **2. Flexion of the Thigh (anterior fibers)**

❑ **3. Medial Rotation of the Thigh (anterior fibers)**

❑ **4. Extension of the Thigh (posterior fibers)**

❑ **5. Lateral Rotation of the Thigh (posterior fibers)**

❑ **6. Posterior Tilt of the Pelvis (posterior fibers)**

❑ **7. Anterior Tilt of the Pelvis (anterior fibers)**

❑ 8. Depression (Lateral Tilt) of the Pelvis (entire muscle)

❑ 9. Ipsilateral Rotation of the Pelvis (anterior fibers)

❑ 10. Contralateral Rotation of the Pelvis (posterior fibers)

INNERVATION ❑ The Superior Gluteal Nerve ❑ **L4, 5,** S1

ARTERIAL SUPPLY ❑ The Superior Gluteal Artery (A Branch of the Internal Iliac Artery)

GLUTEUS MEDIUS – PALPATION AND SUPPLEMENTARY TEXT

PALPATION

The middle and anterior fibers of the gluteus medius are superficial and easy to palpate, while the posterior fibers are deep to the gluteus maximus.

- Have the client sidelying.

❑ **To palpate the middle portion:**

- Place palpating hand between the ilium (approximately halfway between the P.S.I.S. and the A.S.I.S.) and the greater trochanter of the femur and feel for the middle fibers of the gluteus medius. Remember that the middle portion of the gluteus medius is superficial and easily palpable.
- To further bring out the middle portion of the gluteus medius, ask the client to actively abduct the thigh at the hip joint.

❑ **To palpate the anterior portion:**

- Place palpating hand just posterior and inferior to the A.S.I.S. and feel for the anterior fibers of the gluteus medius.
- To further bring out the anterior section of the gluteus medius, ask the client to actively flex and medially rotate the thigh at the hip joint.

  (Note: Distinguishing the anterior fibers of the gluteus medius from the T.F.L. can be difficult.)

❑ **To palpate the posterior portion:**

- Palpate just deep to the (superolateral portion of the) gluteus maximus and feel for the posterior fibers of the gluteus medius deep to the gluteus maximus.
- Active extension and lateral rotation of the thigh at the hip joint will cause the posterior gluteus medius to contract. However, it will cause the gluteus maximus to contract as well.

  (Note: Distinguishing the posterior fibers of the gluteus medius from the gluteus maximus and the piriformis can be difficult.)

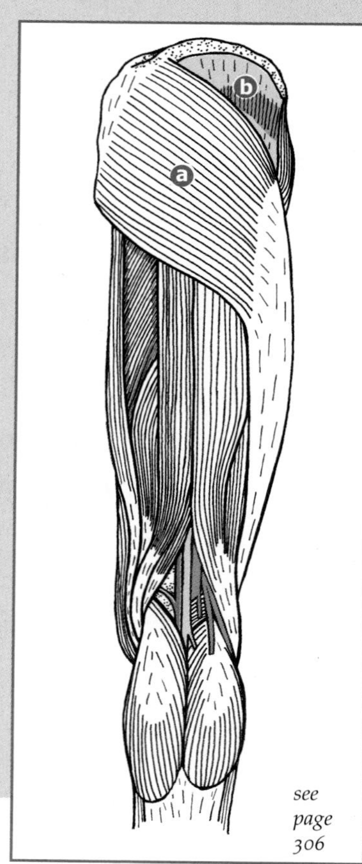

see page 306

Posterior View of the Right Pelvis (Superficial)

a. Gluteus Maximus
b. Gluteus Medius

RELATIONSHIP TO OTHER MUSCULOSKELETAL STRUCTURES

❑ 1. The posterior 1/3 of the gluteus medius is deep to the gluteus maximus. A small portion of the anterior gluteus medius is deep to the tensor fasciae latae.

❑ 2. The middle portion of the gluteus medius is superficial.

GLUTEUS MEDIUS – continued

- ❑ 3. The anterior fibers of the gluteus medius lie next to the tensor fasciae latae (with essentially an identical fiber direction) and the posterior fibers of the gluteus medius lie next to the piriformis (with essentially an identical fiber direction).
- ❑ 4. Deep to the gluteus medius is the gluteus minimus.

METHODOLOGY FOR LEARNING MUSCLE ACTIONS

- ❑ 1. **Abduction of the Thigh at the Hip Joint (entire muscle):** The gluteus medius crosses the hip joint laterally above the center of the joint (with its fibers running vertically in the frontal plane). Therefore, the gluteus medius abducts the thigh at the hip joint.
- ❑ 2. **Flexion of the Thigh at the Hip Joint (anterior fibers):** The anterior fibers of the gluteus medius cross the hip joint anteriorly (running vertically in the sagittal plane); therefore, they flex the thigh at the hip joint.
- ❑ 3. **Medial Rotation of the Thigh at the Hip Joint (anterior fibers):** The anterior fibers of the gluteus medius wrap around the anterior pelvis to attach laterally onto the greater trochanter (running somewhat horizontally in the transverse plane). When the gluteus medius contracts, it pulls the greater trochanter anteromedially, causing the anterior surface of the thigh to face medially. Therefore, the gluteus medius medially rotates the thigh at the hip joint. (Note the similarity of the direction of anterior fibers of the gluteus medius to the direction of fibers of the tensor fasciae latae.)
- ❑ 4. **Extension of the Thigh at the Hip Joint (posterior fibers):** The posterior fibers of the gluteus medius cross the hip joint posteriorly (running vertically in the sagittal plane); therefore, they extend the thigh at the hip joint.
- ❑ 5. **Lateral Rotation of the Thigh at the Hip Joint (posterior fibers):** The posterior fibers of the gluteus medius wrap around the posterior pelvis to attach laterally onto the greater trochanter (running somewhat horizontally in the transverse plane). When the gluteus medius contracts, it pulls the greater trochanter posteromedially, causing the anterior surface of the thigh to face laterally. Therefore, the gluteus medius laterally rotates the thigh at the hip joint. (Note the similarity of the direction of posterior fibers of the gluteus medius to the direction of fibers of the piriformis.)
- ❑ 6. **Posterior Tilt of the Pelvis at the Hip Joint (posterior fibers):** When the femoral attachment is fixed and the posterior fibers of the gluteus medius contract, they pull inferiorly on the posterior pelvis and posteriorly tilt the pelvis at the hip joint.
- ❑ 7. **Anterior Tilt of the Pelvis at the Hip Joint (anterior fibers):** When the femoral attachment is fixed and the anterior fibers of the gluteus medius contract, they pull inferiorly on the anterior pelvis and anteriorly tilt the pelvis at the hip joint.
- ❑ 8. **Depression (Lateral Tilt) of the Pelvis at the Hip Joint (entire muscle):** When the thigh is fixed, the gluteus medius, by pulling inferiorly on the pelvis laterally, depresses (laterally tilts) the pelvis on that side at the hip joint.
- ❑ 9. **Ipsilateral Rotation of the Pelvis at the Hip Joint (anterior fibers):** The anterior fibers of the gluteus medius cross the hip joint anteriorly (with their fibers running somewhat horizontally in the transverse plane). When the femoral attachment is fixed, and the anterior fibers of the gluteus medius contract, they pull on the pelvis, causing the anterior pelvis to face the same side of the body that the gluteus medius is attached. Therefore, the anterior fibers of the gluteus medius ipsilaterally rotate the pelvis at the hip joint. (Note the similarity of the direction of fibers of the anterior gluteus medius to the direction of fibers of the tensor fasciae latae.)

GLUTEUS MEDIUS – continued

❑ **10. Contralateral Rotation of the Pelvis at the Hip Joint (posterior fibers):** The posterior fibers of the gluteus medius cross the hip joint posteriorly (running somewhat horizontally in the transverse plane). When the femoral attachment is fixed, and the posterior fibers of the gluteus medius contract, they pull on the pelvis, causing the anterior pelvis to face the opposite side of the body from the side of the body that the gluteus medius is attached. Therefore, the posterior fibers of the gluteus medius contralaterally rotate the pelvis at the hip joint. (Note the similarity of the direction of fibers of the posterior gluteus medius to the direction of fibers of the piriformis.)

MISCELLANEOUS

❑ 1. Note how the gluteus medius fans around the hip joint. It crosses the hip joint anteriorly, laterally and posteriorly. Therefore, some sources consider the gluteus medius to have 3 sections: anterior, middle and posterior. This orientation is similar to the orientation of the deltoid to the shoulder joint. Therefore, both of these muscles can do the same actions at their respective joints. The gluteus medius can abduct, flex, extend, medially rotate, and laterally rotate the thigh at the hip joint. The deltoid can abduct, flex, extend, medially rotate, and laterally rotate the arm at the shoulder joint.

❑ 2. There is usually a thick layer of fascia overlying the gluteus medius muscle called the *gluteal fascia* or the *gluteal aponeurosis* (see posterior view of the pelvis on page 305).

❑ 3. Since the posterior portion of the gluteus medius is the thickest part, its actions are the strongest. Therefore, the strongest actions of the gluteus medius are abduction, extension and lateral rotation of the thigh at the hip joint.

❑ 4. Pelvic depression (lateral tilt) at the hip joint by the gluteus medius is actually its most important action. When one foot is lifted off the floor, the pelvis would fall to that side of the body because it is now unsupported; this is known as depression or lateral tilt of the pelvis to that side. If the pelvis did fall to the unsupported side, then the other side of the pelvis (on the support side) would have to lift up (elevate) away from the thigh on that side of the body. Simply put, the pelvis cannot depress on the unsupported side because the pelvis is not allowed to elevate on the support side. This is due to the contraction of the gluteus medius on the support side. For example, when the right foot lifts off the floor, the left-sided gluteus medius contracts, thereby depressing the left side of the pelvis and fixing it to the left thigh so that the pelvis cannot elevate on the left. If the left side of the pelvis cannot elevate, then the right side of the pelvis cannot depress; therefore, the pelvis remains level. With every step that a person takes when walking, contraction of the gluteus medius on the "support" side occurs. Therefore, the gluteus medius is important and necessary for proper gait.

❑ 5. The gluteus medius contracts to create a force of pelvic depression (lateral tilt) not only when a foot is lifted off the floor to walk (see miscellaneous #4), but also when weight is simply shifted to one foot. Therefore, the habitual practice of standing with all or most of the body weight on one side tends to cause the gluteus medius on that side to become overused and tight.

❑ 6. A chronically tight gluteus medius can create the postural conditions of a "functional" short lower extremity (usually called a "short leg") and a compensatory scoliosis. When the gluteus medius is tight, it pulls on and depresses (laterally tilts) the pelvis toward the thigh on that side. This results in a "functional short leg" (as opposed to a "structural short leg" wherein the femur and/or the tibia on one side is actually shorter than on the other side). Further, depressing the pelvis on one side creates an unlevel sacrum for the spine to sit on and a compensatory scoliosis must occur to return the head to a level position. (Note: The head must be level for proper proprioceptive balance in the inner ear and for the eyes to be level for visual proprioception.)

❑ 7. Understanding the role of the gluteus medius as a pelvis depressor whenever a person lifts a foot off the floor or simply shifts their weight to one side (see miscellaneous #4 and #5) gives us another easy way to palpate the gluteus medius. Stand and rock your weight back and forth from one foot to the other while palpating both gluteus medius muscles. The gluteus medius muscle on the support side (the side that you are bearing weight upon) will clearly be felt as it contracts.

GLUTEUS MINIMUS

❑ **The name, gluteus minimus, tells us that this muscle is located in the gluteal (buttocks) region and is small (smaller than the gluteus maximus and the gluteus medius).**

DERIVATION ❑ gluteus: Gr. *buttocks.* minimus: L. *least.*

PRONUNCIATION ❑ **gloo**-tee-us **min**-i-mus

ATTACHMENTS

❑ **External Ilium**

- ❑ between the anterior and inferior gluteal lines

to the

❑ **Greater Trochanter of the Femur**

- ❑ the anterior surface

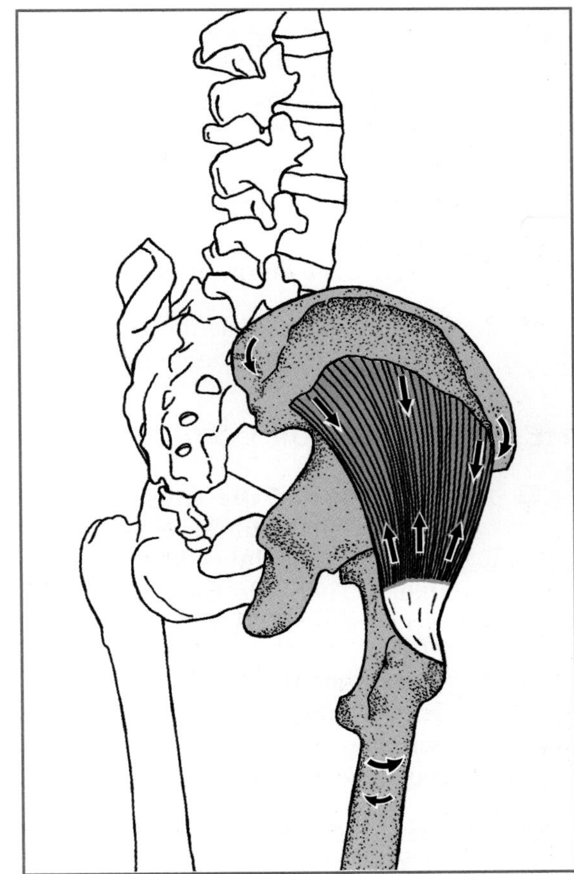

Posterolateral View of the Right Gluteus Minimus

ACTIONS

❑ 1. **Abduction of the Thigh (entire muscle)**
❑ 2. **Flexion of the Thigh (anterior fibers)**
❑ 3. **Medial Rotation of the Thigh (anterior fibers)**
❑ 4. **Extension of the Thigh (posterior fibers)**
❑ 5. **Lateral Rotation of the Thigh (posterior fibers)**
❑ 6. **Posterior Tilt of the Pelvis (posterior fibers)**
❑ 7. **Anterior Tilt of the Pelvis (anterior fibers)**
❑ 8. Depression (Lateral Tilt) of the Pelvis (entire muscle)
❑ 9. Ipsilateral Rotation of the Pelvis (anterior fibers)
❑ 10. Contralateral Rotation of the Pelvis (posterior fibers)

INNERVATION ❑ The Superior Gluteal Nerve ❑ **L4, 5,** S1

ARTERIAL SUPPLY ❑ The Superior Gluteal Artery (A Branch of the Internal Iliac Artery)

GLUTEUS MINIMUS – PALPATION AND SUPPLEMENTARY TEXT

PALPATION

- ❑ It is extremely difficult to differentiate the gluteus minimus from the gluteus medius since the gluteus medius entirely lies over the gluteus minimus and they have identical actions. The thickest part of the gluteus minimus is the anterior portion.
  - To palpate, follow the same procedure as for the gluteus medius (see the palpation section for this muscle on page 320) and try to palpate deeper for the gluteus minimus.

    If the superficial gluteus medius is relaxed and the gluteus minimus is very tight, it may be possible to feel and distinguish the gluteus minimus.

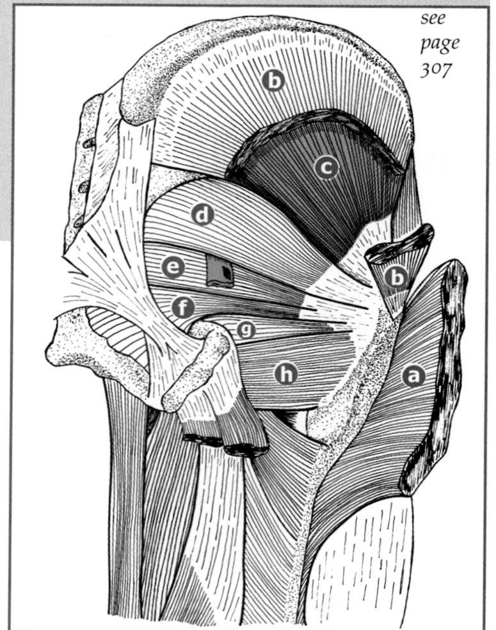

see page 307

Posterior View of the Right Pelvis (Deep)

- **a.** Gluteus Maximus (cut and reflected)
- **b.** Gluteus Medius (cut and reflected)
- **c. Gluteus Minimus**
- **d.** Piriformis
- **e.** Superior Gemellus
- **f.** Obturator Internus
- **g.** Inferior Gemellus
- **h.** Quadratus Femoris

RELATIONSHIP TO OTHER MUSCULOSKELETAL STRUCTURES

❑ 1. The gluteus minimus is deep to the gluteus medius.

❑ 2. Deep to the gluteus minimus are the joint capsule of the hip joint and the ilium.

METHODOLOGY FOR LEARNING MUSCLE ACTIONS

❑ **1. Abduction of the Thigh at the Hip Joint (entire muscle):** The gluteus minimus crosses the hip joint laterally above the center of the joint (with its fibers running vertically in the frontal plane). Therefore, the gluteus minimus abducts the thigh at the hip joint.

❑ **2. Flexion of the Thigh at the Hip Joint (anterior fibers):** The anterior fibers of the gluteus minimus cross the hip joint anteriorly (running vertically in the sagittal plane); therefore, they flex the thigh at the hip joint.

❑ **3. Medial Rotation of the Thigh at the Hip Joint (anterior fibers):** The anterior fibers of the gluteus minimus wrap around the anterior pelvis to attach laterally onto the greater trochanter (running somewhat horizontally in the transverse plane). When the gluteus minimus contracts, it pulls the greater trochanter anteromedially, causing the anterior surface of the thigh to face medially. Therefore, the gluteus minimus medially rotates the thigh at the hip joint. (Note the similarity of the direction of anterior fibers of the gluteus minimus to the direction of fibers of the tensor fasciae latae.)

❑ **4. Extension of the Thigh at the Hip Joint (posterior fibers):** The posterior fibers of the gluteus minimus cross the hip joint posteriorly (running vertically in the sagittal plane); therefore, they extend the thigh at the hip joint.

GLUTEUS MINIMUS – continued

❑ 5. **Lateral Rotation of the Thigh at the Hip Joint (posterior fibers):** The posterior fibers of the gluteus minimus wrap around the posterior pelvis to attach laterally onto the greater trochanter (running somewhat horizontally in the transverse plane). When the gluteus minimus contracts, it pulls the greater trochanter posteromedially, causing the anterior surface of the thigh to face laterally. Therefore, the gluteus minimus laterally rotates the thigh at the hip joint. (Note the similarity of the direction of posterior fibers of the gluteus minimus to the direction of fibers of the piriformis.)

❑ 6. **Posterior Tilt of the Pelvis at the Hip Joint (posterior fibers):** When the femoral attachment is fixed and the posterior fibers of the gluteus minimus contract, they pull inferiorly on the posterior pelvis and posteriorly tilt the pelvis at the hip joint.

❑ 7. **Anterior Tilt of the Pelvis at the Hip Joint (anterior fibers):** When the femoral attachment is fixed and the anterior fibers of the gluteus minimus contract, they pull inferiorly on the anterior pelvis and anteriorly tilt the pelvis at the hip joint.

❑ 8. **Depression (Lateral Tilt) of the Pelvis at the Hip Joint (entire muscle):** When the thigh is fixed, the gluteus minimus, by pulling inferiorly on the lateral pelvis, depresses (laterally tilts) the pelvis on that side at the hip joint.

❑ 9. **Ipsilateral Rotation of the Pelvis at the Hip Joint (anterior fibers):** The anterior fibers of the gluteus minimus cross the hip joint anteriorly (with their fibers running somewhat horizontally in the transverse plane). When the femoral attachment is fixed, and the anterior fibers of the gluteus minimus contract, they pull on the pelvis, causing the anterior pelvis to face the same side of the body that the gluteus minimus is attached. Therefore, the anterior fibers of the gluteus minimus ipsilaterally rotate the pelvis at the hip joint. (Note the similarity of the direction of fibers of the anterior gluteus minimus to the direction of fibers of the tensor fasciae latae.)

❑ 10. **Contralateral Rotation of the Pelvis at the Hip Joint (posterior fibers):** The posterior fibers of the gluteus minimus cross the hip joint posteriorly (with their fibers running somewhat horizontally in the transverse plane). When the femoral attachment is fixed, and the posterior fibers of the gluteus minimus contract, they pull on the pelvis, causing the anterior pelvis to face the opposite side of the body from the side of the body that the gluteus minimus is attached. Therefore, the posterior fibers of the gluteus minimus contralaterally rotate the pelvis at the hip joint. (Note the similarity of the direction of fibers of the posterior gluteus minimus to the direction of fibers of the piriformis.)

MISCELLANEOUS

❑ 1. The direction of fibers of the gluteus minimus is essentially identical to that of the gluteus medius; therefore, the actions are identical. The only difference is that the gluteus medius fans out more anteriorly and posteriorly around the hip joint. The gluteus medius is much more powerful than the gluteus minimus because of its greater size and greater coverage around the hip joint.

❑ 2. Since the anterior portion of the gluteus minimus is the thickest part, its actions are the strongest. Therefore, the strongest actions of the gluteus minimus are abduction, flexion and medial rotation of the thigh at the hip joint.

❑ 3. As with the gluteus medius, pelvic depression (lateral tilt) at the hip joint by the gluteus minimus is actually its most important action. (See miscellaneous #4, 5 and 7 of the gluteus medius on page 322.)

❑ 4. A chronically tight gluteus minimus can contribute to the related biomechanical postural conditions of a functional "short lower extremity" (usually called a "short leg") with a compensatory scoliosis. (See miscellaneous #6 of the gluteus medius on page 322.)

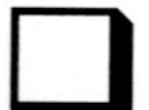

THE DEEP LATERAL ROTATORS OF THE THIGH

Deep to the gluteus maximus, there is a second layer of muscles that laterally rotates the thigh at the hip joint. These muscles are usually grouped together as the "Deep Lateral Rotators of the Thigh" or the "Deep Six."

THE DEEP LATERAL ROTATOR MUSCLES ARE (FROM SUPERIOR TO INFERIOR):	
Piriformis Superior Gemellus Obturator Internus	Inferior Gemellus Obturator Externus Quadratus Femoris

Attachments:

- Upon observation, it is clear that all the deep lateral rotators of the thigh have a nearly identical direction of fibers. They lie approximately horizontal in the transverse plane, and they attach laterally onto or near the greater trochanter of the femur.
- From a posterior perspective, all these muscles are at the same depth (except for the obturator externus, which lies deep to the quadratus femoris and is either entirely covered or nearly entirely covered by it).
- The piriformis and obturator internus both arise from the internal surface of the pelvic bone. All the other muscles of the posterior pelvis arise from the external surface of the pelvic bone.

Actions:

- When the deep lateral rotators of the thigh pull the femur toward their more medial attachment in the posterior buttocks region, they cause lateral rotation of the thigh at the hip joint.
- When the femoral attachment of the deep lateral rotators of the thigh is fixed, the pelvis rotates instead of the femur. This rotation causes the pelvis to rotate away from the side of the body that these muscles are attached. Therefore, these muscles contralaterally rotate the pelvis at the hip joint. (Note: All muscles that laterally rotate the thigh at the hip joint can also contralaterally rotate the pelvis at the hip joint.)

Miscellaneous:

- The gluteus maximus can also laterally rotate the thigh at the hip joint, but it is superficial to this group.
- Although it is at the same depth, the gluteus medius is usually not included in this group. The posterior fibers of the gluteus medius have the same direction as the piriformis, which lies directly inferior to it, and these fibers laterally rotate the thigh at the hip joint.
- The posterior fibers of the gluteus minimus can also laterally rotate the thigh at the hip joint, but the gluteus minimus is considered to be at a third deeper layer of musculature in the posterior pelvis.

INNERVATION	The deep lateral rotators of the thigh are innervated by branches of the sacral plexus, except the obturator externus, which is innervated by the obturator nerve.
♥ **ARTERIAL SUPPLY**	The deep lateral rotators of the thigh receive their arterial supply from the superior and inferior gluteal arteries and the obturator artery.

POSTERIOR VIEWS OF THE DEEP LATERAL ROTATORS OF THE RIGHT THIGH

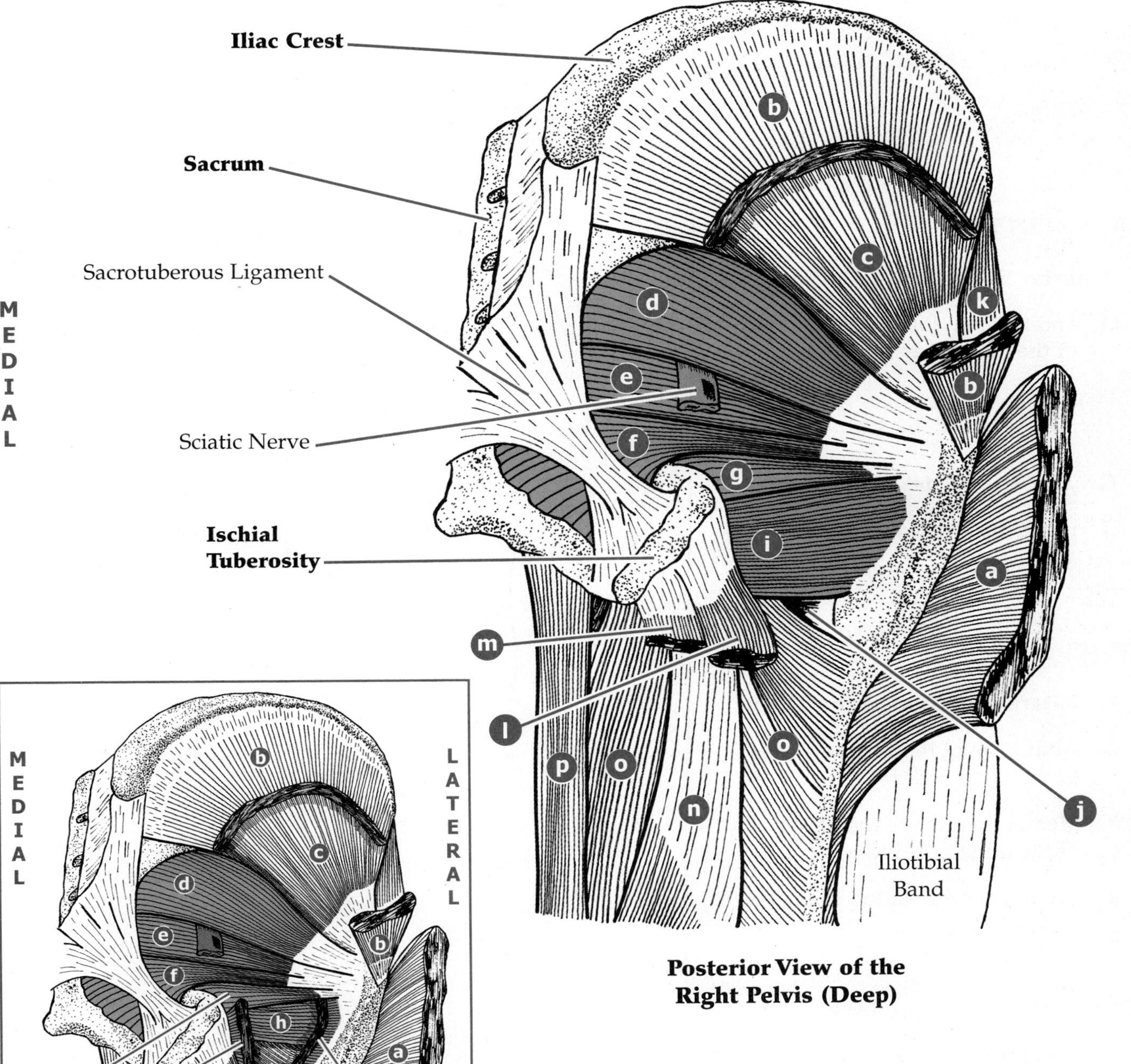

Posterior View of the Right Pelvis (Deep)

Quadratus Femoris Cut and Reflected to Show Obturator Externus

- **a.** Gluteus Maximus (cut and reflected)
- **b.** Gluteus Medius (cut and reflected)
- **c.** Gluteus Minimus
- **d. Piriformis**
- **e. Superior Gemellus**
- **f. Obturator Internus**
- **g. Inferior Gemellus**
- **h. Obturator Externus**
- **i. Quadratus Femoris**
- **j.** Pectineus
- **k.** Tensor Fasciae Latae
- **l.** Biceps Femoris (cut)
- **m.** Semitendinosus (cut)
- **n.** Semimembranosus
- **o.** Adductor Magnus
- **p.** Gracilis

❑

PIRIFORMIS

(OF THE DEEP LATERAL ROTATORS OF THE THIGH)

❑ **The name, piriformis, tells us that this muscle is shaped like a pear.**

DERIVATION ❑ piriformis: L. *pear shaped.* **PRONUNCIATION** ❑ pi-ri-**for**-mis

ATTACHMENTS

❑ **Anterior Sacrum**

- ❑ and the anterior surface of the sacrotuberous ligament

to the

❑ **Greater Trochanter of the Femur**

- ❑ the superomedial surface

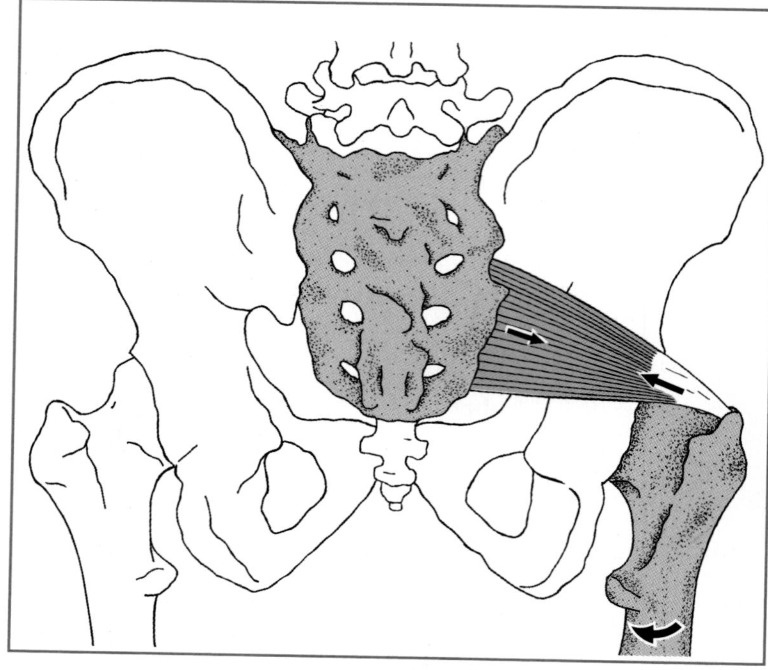

Posterior View of the Right Piriformis
(sacrotuberous ligament not shown)

ACTIONS

❑ **1. Lateral Rotation of the Thigh**

❑ **2.** Abduction of the Thigh (if the thigh is flexed)

❑ **3.** Medial Rotation of the Thigh (if the thigh is flexed)

❑ **4.** Contralateral Rotation of the Pelvis

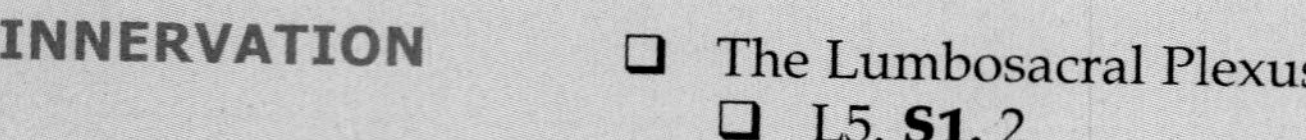

INNERVATION ❑ The Lumbosacral Plexus
- ❑ L5, **S1**, 2

ARTERIAL SUPPLY ❑ The Superior and Inferior Gluteal Arteries (Branches of the Internal Iliac Artery)

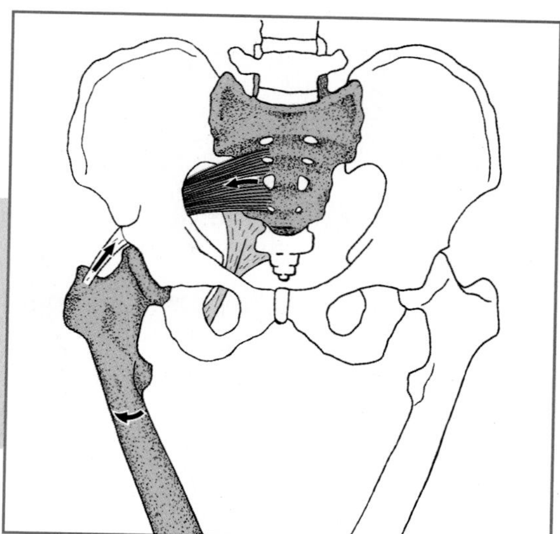

Anterior View of the Right Piriformis
(sacrotuberous ligament shown)

PALPATION AND SUPPLEMENTARY TEXT

PALPATION

- ❑ The piriformis can be palpated as part of the deep lateral rotator group of the thigh, but it is difficult to distinguish from the others.
  - Have the client prone.
  - Place palpating hand just lateral to the sacrum, at a point halfway between the P.S.I.S. and the apex of the sacrum.
  - Ask the client to flex the leg at the knee joint to 90°.
  - Ask the client to laterally rotate the thigh at the hip joint against resistance and feel for the contraction of the piriformis.

    (Note: In this position, lateral rotation of the thigh at the hip joint on the client's part will involve attempting to move the foot toward the opposite side of the body.)
  - Continue palpating the piriformis laterally toward the greater trochanter of the femur.

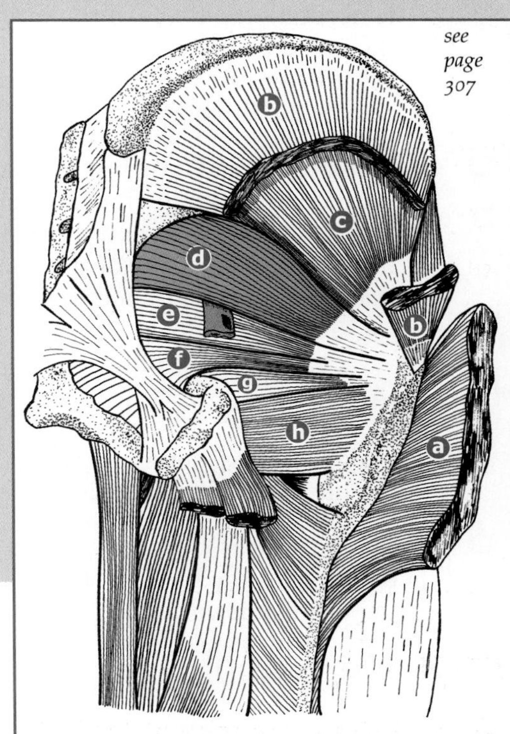

Posterior View of the Right Pelvis (Deep)

a. Gluteus Maximus (cut and reflected)
b. Gluteus Medius (cut and reflected)
c. Gluteus Minimus
d. **Piriformis**
e. Superior Gemellus
f. Obturator Internus
g. Inferior Gemellus
h. Quadratus Femoris

RELATIONSHIP TO OTHER MUSCULOSKELETAL STRUCTURES

❑ 1. The piriformis is deep to the gluteus maximus.

❑ 2. The piriformis is located between the gluteus medius (which is superior to it) and the superior gemellus (which is inferior to it).

METHODOLOGY FOR LEARNING MUSCLE ACTIONS

❑ 1. **Lateral Rotation of the Thigh at the Hip Joint:** The piriformis attaches from the sacrum medially and wraps around to the greater trochanter of the femur laterally (with its fibers running horizontally in the transverse plane). When the piriformis contracts, it pulls the greater trochanter posteromedially, causing the anterior surface of the thigh to face laterally. Therefore, the piriformis laterally rotates the thigh at the hip joint.

❑ 2. **Abduction of the Thigh at the Hip Joint (if the thigh is flexed):** When the thigh is already flexed, the orientation of the line of pull of the piriformis relative to the hip joint changes. The fibers (running horizontally) can now pull the femur away from the midline in the frontal plane. Therefore, the femur, i.e., the thigh, abducts at the hip joint.

PIRIFORMIS – continued

❑ 3. **Medial Rotation of the Thigh at the Hip Joint (if the thigh is flexed):** When the thigh is already flexed, the orientation of the line of pull of the piriformis relative to the hip joint changes. When the thigh is not in flexion, the fibers of the piriformis wrap around the posterior side of the femur to attach onto the greater trochanter. However, if the thigh is sufficiently flexed (sources state a minimum of 60° is needed), the fibers of the piriformis now wrap around the anterior side of the femur to attach onto the greater trochanter. Given this direction of fibers relative to the hip joint, the piriformis now pulls the greater trochanter anteromedially instead of posteromedially. Therefore, the piriformis medially rotates the thigh at the hip joint instead of laterally rotating the thigh at the hip joint.

❑ 4. **Contralateral Rotation of the Pelvis at the Hip Joint:** The piriformis crosses the hip joint posteriorly (with its fibers running somewhat horizontally in the transverse plane). When the femoral attachment is fixed, and the piriformis contracts, it pulls on the pelvis, causing the anterior pelvis to face the opposite side of the body from the side of the body that the piriformis is attached. Therefore, the piriformis contralaterally rotates the pelvis at the hip joint.

MISCELLANEOUS

❑ 1. The piriformis, superior gemellus, obturator internus and inferior gemellus can all abduct the thigh at the hip joint if the thigh is flexed.

❑ 2. The piriformis can change from being a lateral rotator of the thigh at the hip joint to a medial rotator of the thigh at the hip joint (if the thigh is first flexed at the hip joint); therefore, the method of stretching the piriformis varies with the position of the client's thigh. If the client's thigh is flexed, lateral rotation must be used to stretch the piriformis. If the client's thigh is not flexed, then medial rotation would be used. The thigh must be flexed to at least 60° for the piriformis to become a medial rotator of the thigh.

❑ 3. The piriformis sometimes blends with the gluteus medius.

❑ 4. The relationship of the sciatic nerve to the piriformis varies. Although it normally exits from the pelvis between the piriformis and the superior gemellus, in approximately 10-20% of individuals, the common fibular portion of the sciatic nerve (occasionally even the entire sciatic nerve) may pierce the piriformis muscle, exiting through the middle of it. This makes the sciatic nerve more susceptible to being compressed by the piriformis if the piriformis is tight. When the piriformis does compress the sciatic nerve, regardless of the relationship between the piriformis and the sciatic nerve, this condition is called *piriformis syndrome* and can result in symptoms of *sciatica*.

SUPERIOR GEMELLUS

(OF THE DEEP LATERAL ROTATORS OF THE THIGH)

❑ **The name, superior gemellus, tells us that this muscle is the more superior muscle of a pair of similar muscles.**

DERIVATION ❑ superior: L. *upper.*
gemellus: L. *twin.*

PRONUNCIATION ❑ su-**pee**-ree-or jee-**mel**-us

ATTACHMENTS

❑ **Ischial Spine**

to the

❑ **Greater Trochanter of the Femur**

- ❑ the medial surface

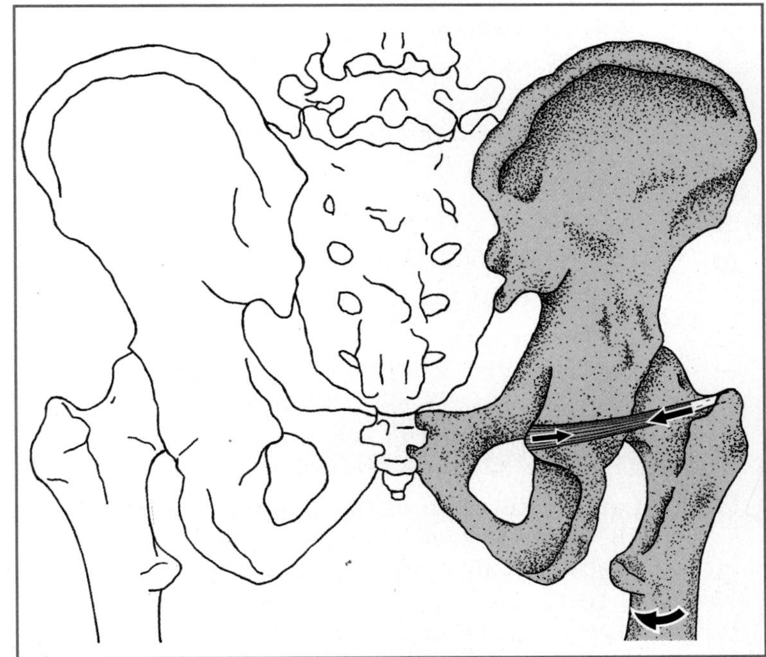

Posterior View of the Right Superior Gemellus

ACTIONS

❑ **1. Lateral Rotation of the Thigh**

❑ 2. Abduction of the Thigh (if the thigh is flexed)

❑ 3. Contralateral Rotation of the Pelvis

INNERVATION ❑ The Lumbosacral Plexus ❑ L5, S1

ARTERIAL SUPPLY ❑ The Inferior Gluteal Artery (A Branch of the Internal Iliac Artery)

SUPERIOR GEMELLUS – PALPATION AND SUPPLEMENTARY TEXT

PALPATION

- ❑ The superior gemellus can be palpated as part of the deep lateral rotator group of the thigh, but it is difficult to distinguish from the others.
  - Have the client prone.
  - Place palpating hand just inferior to the piriformis (see the palpation section for this muscle on page 329).
  - Ask the client to flex the leg at the knee joint to 90°.
  - Ask the client to laterally rotate the thigh at the hip joint against resistance and feel for the contraction of the superior gemellus.

  (Note: In this position, lateral rotation of the thigh at the hip joint on the client's part will involve attempting to move the foot toward the opposite side of the body.)

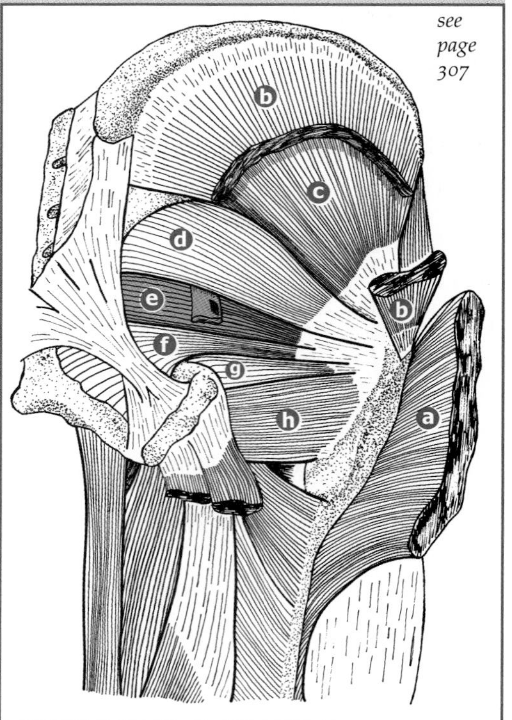

Posterior View of the Right Pelvis (Deep)

a. Gluteus Maximus (cut and reflected)
b. Gluteus Medius (cut and reflected)
c. Gluteus Minimus
d. Piriformis
e. **Superior Gemellus**
f. Obturator Internus
g. Inferior Gemellus
h. Quadratus Femoris

RELATIONSHIP TO OTHER MUSCULOSKELETAL STRUCTURES

❑ 1. The superior gemellus lies between the piriformis (which is superior to it) and the obturator internus (which is inferior to it).

❑ 2. The sciatic nerve normally exits the pelvis between the piriformis and the superior gemellus.

METHODOLOGY FOR LEARNING MUSCLE ACTIONS

❑ 1. **Lateral Rotation of the Thigh at the Hip Joint:** The superior gemellus wraps around the posterior pelvis to attach laterally onto the greater trochanter of the femur (with its fibers running horizontally in the transverse plane). When the superior gemellus contracts, it pulls the greater trochanter posteromedially, causing the anterior surface of the thigh to face laterally. Therefore, the superior gemellus laterally rotates the thigh at the hip joint. (Note the similarity of the direction of fibers of the superior gemellus to the direction of fibers of the piriformis.)

❑ 2. **Abduction of the Thigh at the Hip Joint (if the thigh is flexed):** As with the piriformis, if the thigh is already flexed, the orientation of the line of pull of the superior gemellus to the femur changes. The fibers (running horizontally) can now pull the femur away from the midline in the frontal plane. Therefore, the femur, i.e., the thigh, abducts at the hip joint.

❑ 3. **Contralateral Rotation of the Pelvis at the Hip Joint:** The superior gemellus crosses the hip joint posteriorly (with its fibers running somewhat horizontally in the transverse plane). When the femoral attachment is fixed, and the superior gemellus contracts, it pulls on the pelvis, causing the anterior pelvis to face the opposite side of the body from the side of the body that the superior gemellus is attached. Therefore, the superior gemellus contralaterally rotates the pelvis at the hip joint. (Note the similarity of the direction of fibers of the superior gemellus to the direction of fibers of the piriformis.)

MISCELLANEOUS

❑ 1. The lateral tendons of the superior gemellus, obturator internus and inferior gemellus usually blend together.

❑ 2. The piriformis, superior gemellus, obturator internus and inferior gemellus can all abduct the thigh at the hip joint if the thigh is flexed.

OBTURATOR INTERNUS
(OF THE DEEP LATERAL ROTATORS OF THE THIGH)

❑ **The name, obturator internus, tells us that this muscle attaches to the internal surface of the obturator foramen.**

DERIVATION ❑ obturator: L. *to stop up, obstruct.*
internus: L. *inner.*

PRONUNCIATION ❑ ob-too-**ray**-tor in-**ter**-nus

ATTACHMENTS

❑ **Internal Surface of the Pelvic Bone Surrounding the Obturator Foramen**

❑ the internal surfaces of:
the margin of the obturator foramen,
the obturator membrane,
the ischium, the pubis and the ilium

to the

❑ **Greater Trochanter of the Femur**

❑ the medial surface

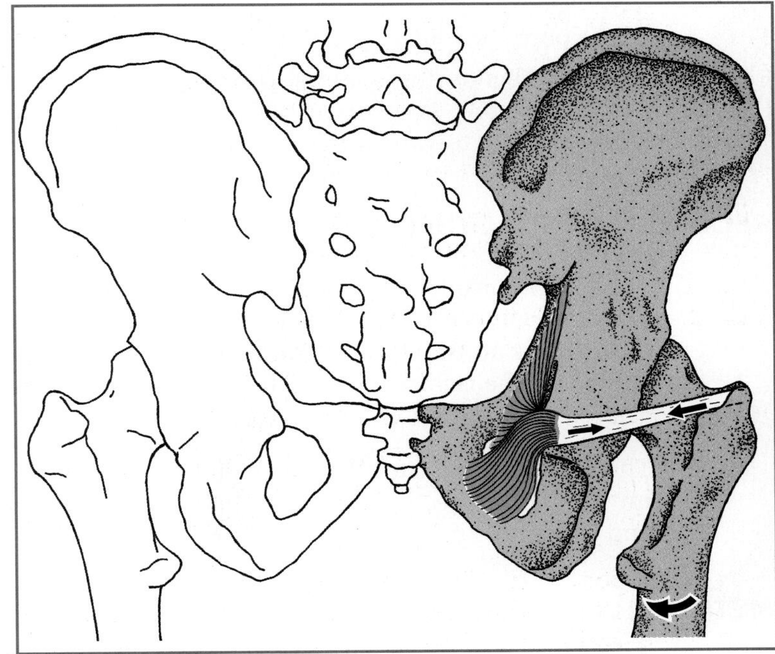

Posterior View of the Right Obturator Internus

ACTIONS

❑ 1. **Lateral Rotation of the Thigh**

❑ 2. Abduction of the Thigh
(if the thigh is flexed)

❑ 3. Contralateral Rotation of the Pelvis

INNERVATION ❑ The Lumbosacral Plexus ❑ L5, **S1**

ARTERIAL SUPPLY ❑ The Superior and Inferior Gluteal Arteries
(Branches of the Internal Iliac Artery)
❑ and the obturator artery (a branch of the internal iliac artery)

OBTURATOR INTERNUS – PALPATION AND SUPPLEMENTARY TEXT

PALPATION

- ❑ The obturator internus can be palpated as part of the deep lateral rotator group of the thigh, but it is difficult to distinguish from the others.
    - Have the client prone.
    - Place palpating hand inferior to the piriformis and the superior gemellus (see the palpation sections for these muscles on pages 329 and 332).
    - Ask the client to flex the leg at the knee joint to 90°.
    - Ask the client to laterally rotate the thigh at the hip joint against resistance and feel for the contraction of the obturator internus.

      (Note: In this position, lateral rotation of the thigh at the hip joint on the client's part will involve attempting to move the foot toward the opposite side of the body.)

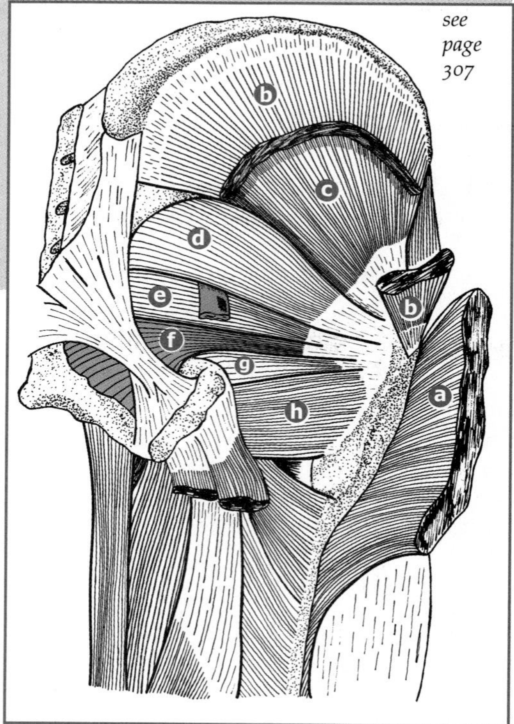

Posterior View of the Right Pelvis (Deep)

a. Gluteus Maximus (cut and reflected)
b. Gluteus Medius (cut and reflected)
c. Gluteus Minimus
d. Piriformis
e. Superior Gemellus
f. **Obturator Internus**
g. Inferior Gemellus
h. Quadratus Femoris

RELATIONSHIP TO OTHER MUSCULOSKELETAL STRUCTURES

❑ 1. The obturator internus begins inside the pelvis and exits the pelvis through the lesser sciatic foramen. It then wraps around the ischium between the ischial spine and the ischial tuberosity to join the other lateral rotators of the thigh.

❑ 2. The obturator internus lies between the two gemelli muscles. It is directly inferior to the superior gemellus and directly superior to the inferior gemellus.

METHODOLOGY FOR LEARNING MUSCLE ACTIONS

❑ 1. **Lateral Rotation of the Thigh at the Hip Joint:** The obturator internus wraps around the posterior pelvis to attach laterally onto the greater trochanter of the femur (with its fibers running horizontally in the transverse plane). When the obturator internus contracts, it pulls the greater trochanter posteromedially, causing the anterior surface of the thigh to face laterally. Therefore, the obturator internus laterally rotates the thigh at the hip joint. (Note the similarity of the direction of fibers of the obturator internus to the direction of fibers of the piriformis and superior gemellus.)

❑ 2. **Abduction of the Thigh at the Hip Joint (if the thigh is flexed):** As with the piriformis and the superior gemellus, if the thigh is already flexed, the orientation of the line of pull of the obturator internus to the femur changes. The fibers (running horizontally) can now pull the femur away from the midline in the frontal plane. Therefore, the femur, i.e., the thigh, abducts at the hip joint.

OBTURATOR INTERNUS – continued

- ❑ **3. Contralateral Rotation of the Pelvis at the Hip Joint:** The obturator internus crosses the hip joint posteriorly (with its fibers running somewhat horizontally in the transverse plane). When the femoral attachment is fixed, and the obturator internus contracts, it pulls on the pelvis, causing the anterior pelvis to face the opposite side of the body from the side of the body that the obturator internus is attached. Therefore, the obturator internus contralaterally rotates the pelvis at the hip joint. (Note the similarity of the direction of fibers of the obturator internus to the direction of fibers of the piriformis and superior gemellus.)

MISCELLANEOUS

- ❑ 1. "Obturator" means to stop up or obstruct. The obturator foramen is obstructed by the obturator membrane, as well as the obturator internus and obturator externus.
- ❑ 2. The lateral tendons of the superior gemellus, obturator internus and inferior gemellus usually blend together.
- ❑ 3. The obturator internus has a much larger pelvic attachment than the obturator externus.
- ❑ 4. The obturator internus is one of only a few muscles in the body that has a tendon that makes an abrupt turn of 90° or more. (Other muscles that do this are the fibularis longus, tibialis posterior, flexor digitorum longus, flexor hallucis longus, tensor palati and the superior oblique.)
- ❑ 5. The piriformis, superior gemellus, obturator internus and inferior gemellus can all abduct the thigh at the hip joint if the thigh is flexed.

❑

INFERIOR GEMELLUS

(OF THE DEEP LATERAL ROTATORS OF THE THIGH)

❑ **The name, inferior gemellus, tells us that this muscle is the more inferior muscle of a pair of similar muscles.**

DERIVATION ❑ inferior: L. *lower*.
gemellus: L. *twin*.

PRONUNCIATION ❑ in-**fee**-ree-or jee-**mel**-us

ATTACHMENTS

❑ **Ischial Tuberosity**

❑ the superior aspect

to the

❑ **Greater Trochanter of the Femur**

❑ the medial surface

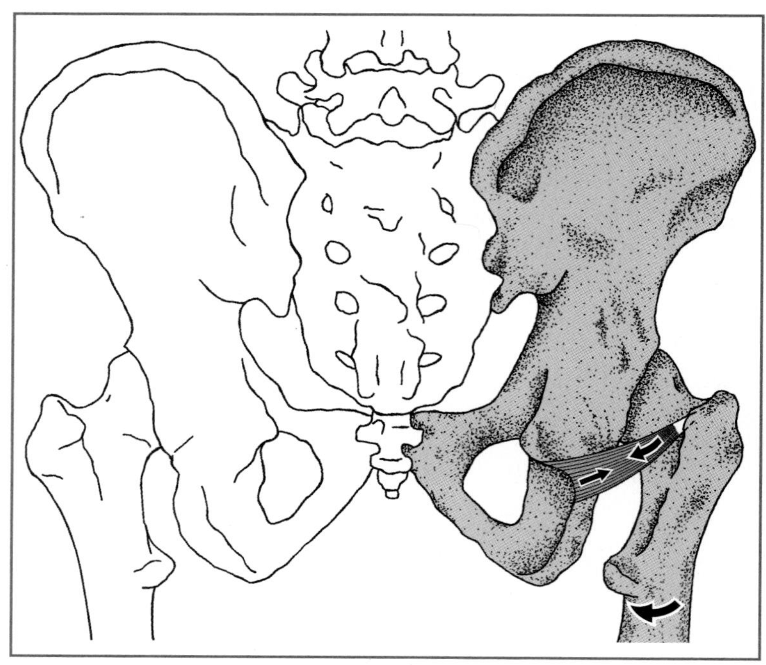

Posterior View of the Right Inferior Gemellus

ACTIONS

❑ **1. Lateral Rotation of the Thigh**

❑ **2.** Abduction of the Thigh (if the thigh is flexed)

❑ **3.** Contralateral Rotation of the Pelvis

INNERVATION ❑ The Lumbosacral Plexus ❑ L5, S1

ARTERIAL SUPPLY ❑ The Inferior Gluteal Artery (A Branch of the Internal Iliac Artery)
❑ and the obturator artery (a branch of the internal iliac artery)

PALPATION AND SUPPLEMENTARY TEXT

PALPATION

- ❑ The inferior gemellus can be palpated as part of the deep lateral rotator group of the thigh, but it is difficult to distinguish from the others.
  - Have the client prone.
  - Place palpating hand just lateral and slightly superior to the superior margin of the ischial tuberosity.
  - Ask the client to flex the leg at the knee joint to 90°.
  - Ask the client to laterally rotate the thigh at the hip joint against resistance and feel for the contraction of the inferior gemellus.

    (Note: In this position, lateral rotation of the thigh at the hip joint on the client's part will involve attempting to move the foot toward the opposite side of the body.)

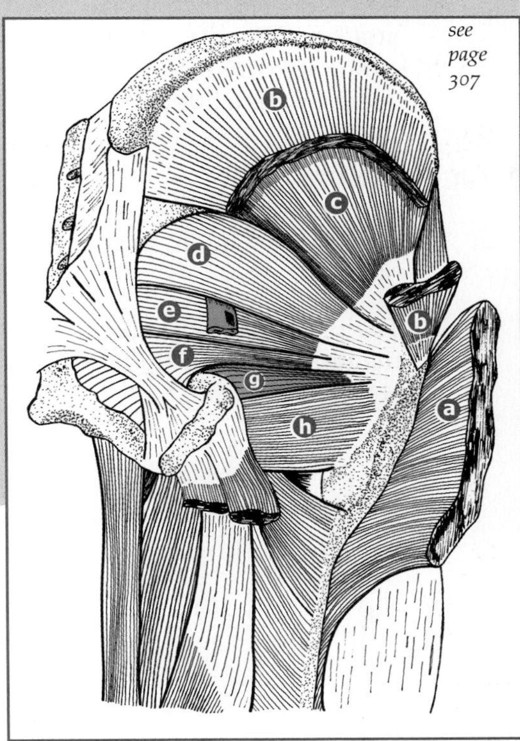

see page 307

Posterior View of the Right Pelvis (Deep)

a. Gluteus Maximus (cut and reflected)
b. Gluteus Medius (cut and reflected)
c. Gluteus Minimus
d. Piriformis
e. Superior Gemellus
f. Obturator Internus
g. Inferior Gemellus
h. Quadratus Femoris

RELATIONSHIP TO OTHER MUSCULOSKELETAL STRUCTURES

❑ 1. The inferior gemellus is inferior to the obturator internus.

❑ 2. The inferior gemellus is superior to the obturator externus and the quadratus femoris.

METHODOLOGY FOR LEARNING MUSCLE ACTIONS

❑ **1. Lateral Rotation of the Thigh at the Hip Joint:** The inferior gemellus wraps around the posterior pelvis to attach laterally onto the greater trochanter (with its fibers running horizontally in the transverse plane). When the inferior gemellus contracts, it pulls the greater trochanter posteromedially, causing the anterior surface of the thigh to face laterally. Therefore, the inferior gemellus laterally rotates the thigh at the hip joint. (Note the similarity of the direction of fibers of the inferior gemellus to the direction of fibers of the piriformis, superior gemellus and obturator internus.)

❑ **2. Abduction of the Thigh at the Hip Joint (if the thigh is flexed):** As with the piriformis, superior gemellus and obturator internus, if the thigh is already flexed, the orientation of the line of pull of the inferior gemellus to the femur changes. The fibers (running horizontally) can now pull the femur away from the midline in the frontal plane. Therefore, the femur, i.e., the thigh, abducts at the hip joint.

INFERIOR GEMELLUS – continued

❑ **3. Contralateral Rotation of the Pelvis at the Hip Joint:** The inferior gemellus crosses the hip joint posteriorly (with its fibers running somewhat horizontally in the transverse plane). When the femoral attachment is fixed, and the inferior gemellus contracts, it pulls on the pelvis, causing the anterior pelvis to face the opposite side of the body from the side of the body that the inferior gemellus is attached. Therefore, the inferior gemellus contralaterally rotates the pelvis at the hip joint. (Note the similarity of the direction of fibers of the inferior gemellus to the direction of fibers of the piriformis, superior gemellus and obturator internus.)

MISCELLANEOUS

❑ 1. The lateral tendons of the superior gemellus, obturator internus and inferior gemellus usually blend together.

❑ 2. The piriformis, superior gemellus, obturator internus and inferior gemellus can all abduct the thigh at the hip joint if the thigh is flexed.

OBTURATOR EXTERNUS

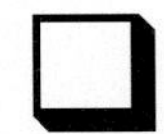

(OF THE DEEP LATERAL ROTATORS OF THE THIGH)

❑ **The name, obturator externus, tells us that this muscle attaches to the external surface of the obturator foramen.**

DERIVATION ❑ obturator: L. *to stop up, obstruct.*
externus: L. *outer.*

PRONUNCIATION ❑ ob-too-**ray**-tor ex-**ter**-nus

ATTACHMENTS

❑ **External Surface of the Pelvic Bone Surrounding the Obturator Foramen**

- ❑ the external surfaces of:
  the margin of the obturator foramen on the ischium and the pubis,
  and the obturator membrane

to the

❑ **Trochanteric Fossa of the Femur**

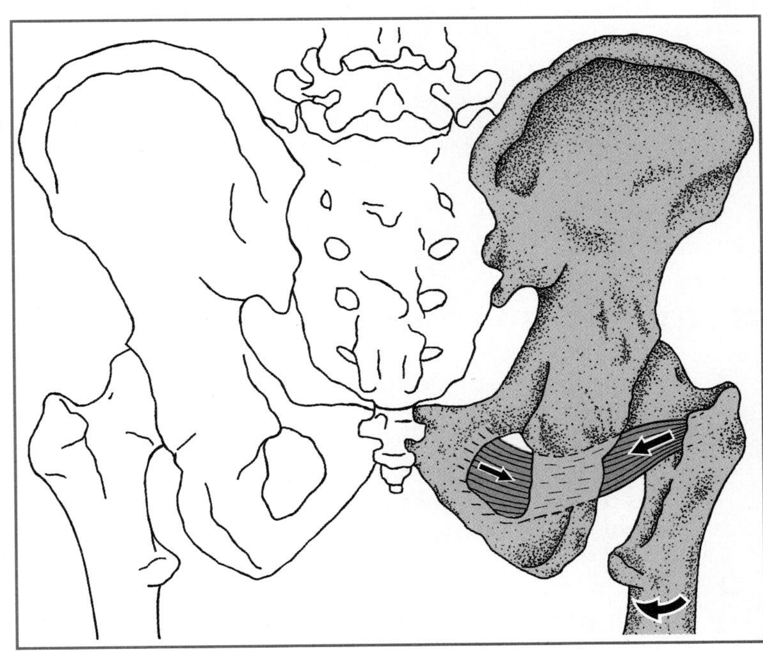

Posterior View of the Right Obturator Externus

ACTIONS

❑ 1. **Lateral Rotation of the Thigh**

❑ 2. Contralateral Rotation of the Pelvis

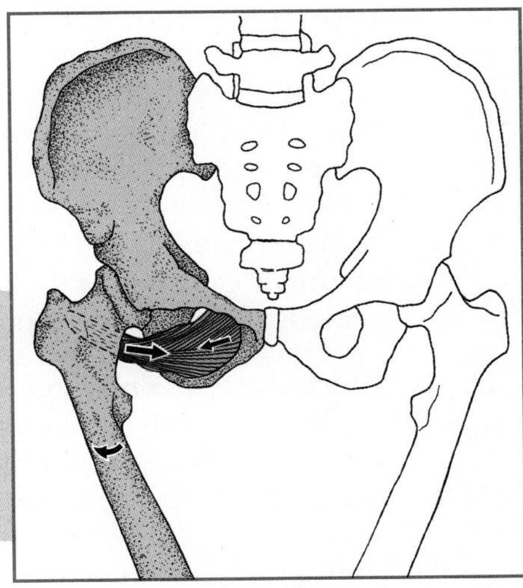

Anterior View of the Right Obturator Externus

INNERVATION ❑ The Obturator Nerve
❑ L3, **4**

ARTERIAL SUPPLY ❑ The Obturator Artery
(A Branch of the Internal Iliac Artery)

OBTURATOR EXTERNUS – PALPATION AND SUPPLEMENTARY TEXT

PALPATION

- ❑ The obturator externus can be palpated as part of the deep lateral rotator group of the thigh. Given how deep it is, it is extremely difficult to distinguish from the others.
  - Have the client prone.
  - Place palpating hand slightly lateral to the superior margin of the ischial tuberosity.
  - Ask the client to flex the leg at the knee joint to 90°.
  - Ask the client to laterally rotate the thigh at the hip joint against resistance and feel for the contraction of the obturator externus.

    (Note: In this position, lateral rotation of the thigh at the hip joint on the client's part will involve attempting to move the foot toward the opposite side of the body.)

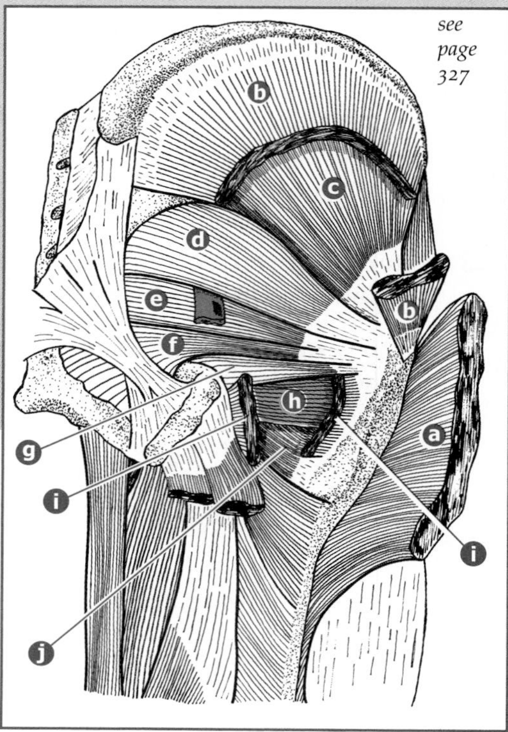

see page 327

Posterior View of the Right Pelvis (Deep)

a. Gluteus Maximus (cut and reflected)
b. Gluteus Medius (cut and reflected)
c. Gluteus Minimus
d. Piriformis
e. Superior Gemellus
f. Obturator Internus
g. Inferior Gemellus
h. **Obturator Externus**
i. Quadratus Femoris (cut and reflected)
j. Pectineus

RELATIONSHIP TO OTHER MUSCULOSKELETAL STRUCTURES

❑ 1. The obturator externus is directly inferior to the inferior gemellus.

❑ 2. From the posterior perspective, the obturator externus is deep to the quadratus femoris and is either entirely covered or nearly entirely covered by it.

❑ 3. From the anterior perspective, the obturator externus is directly deep to the pectineus.

METHODOLOGY FOR LEARNING MUSCLE ACTIONS

❑ 1. **Lateral Rotation of the Thigh at the Hip Joint:** The obturator externus wraps around the posterior pelvis to attach laterally onto the femur (with its fibers running horizontally in the transverse plane). When the obturator externus contracts, it pulls the greater trochanter posteromedially, causing the anterior surface of the thigh to face laterally. Therefore, the obturator externus laterally rotates the thigh at the hip joint. (Note the similarity of the direction of fibers of the obturator externus to the direction of fibers of the piriformis, superior gemellus, obturator internus and the inferior gemellus.)

❑ 2. **Contralateral Rotation of the Pelvis at the Hip Joint:** The obturator externus crosses the hip joint posteriorly (with its fibers running somewhat horizontally in the transverse plane). When the femoral attachment is fixed, and the obturator externus contracts, it pulls on the pelvis, causing the anterior pelvis to face the opposite side of the body from the side of the body that the obturator externus is attached. Therefore, the obturator externus contralaterally rotates the pelvis at the hip joint. (Note the similarity of the direction of fibers of the obturator externus to the direction of fibers of the piriformis, superior gemellus, obturator internus and inferior gemellus.)

OBTURATOR EXTERNUS – continued

MISCELLANEOUS

❑ 1. "Obturator" means to stop up or obstruct. The obturator foramen is obstructed by the obturator membrane, as well as the obturator internus and obturator externus.

❑ 2. The obturator externus is the only muscle of the deep lateral rotator group of the thigh that is not visible in the second layer of the posterior pelvic muscles. It is either entirely covered or nearly entirely covered by the quadratus femoris. When the obturator externus is visible in this layer, it is located between the inferior gemellus and the quadratus femoris.

❑ 3. As with the quadratus femoris, some sources state that the obturator externus can adduct the thigh at the hip joint because it crosses the hip joint low enough to be below the center of the joint.

❑ 4. The obturator externus is the only deep lateral rotator of the thigh that is not innervated by the lumbosacral plexus. It is innervated by the obturator nerve.

❑ QUADRATUS FEMORIS
(OF THE DEEP LATERAL ROTATORS OF THE THIGH)

❑ **The name, quadratus femoris, tells us that this muscle is square in shape and attaches to the femur.**

DERIVATION ❑ quadratus: L. *squared.*
femoris: L. *refers to the femur.*

PRONUNCIATION ❑ kwod-**rate**-us **fem**-o-ris

ATTACHMENTS

❑ **Ischial Tuberosity**

❑ the lateral border

to the

❑ **Intertrochanteric Crest of the Femur**

❑ and inferior to the intertrochanteric crest of the femur

ACTIONS

❑ 1. **Lateral Rotation of the Thigh**

❑ 2. Adduction of the Thigh

❑ 3. Contralateral Rotation of the Pelvis

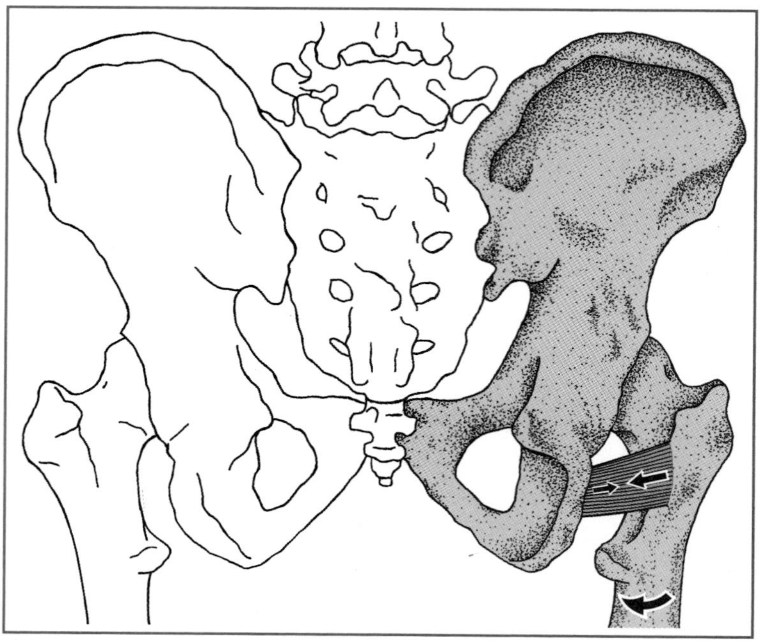

Posterior View of the Right Quadratus Femoris

INNERVATION ❑ The Lumbosacral Plexus ❑ L5, S1

ARTERIAL SUPPLY ❑ The Inferior Gluteal Artery (A Branch of the Internal Iliac Artery)
❑ and the obturator artery (a branch of the internal iliac artery)

QUADRATUS FEMORIS – PALPATION AND SUPPLEMENTARY TEXT

PALPATION

- ❑ The quadratus femoris can be palpated as part of the deep lateral rotator group of the thigh, but it is difficult to distinguish from the others.
  - Have the client prone.
  - Place palpating hand slightly lateral to the ischial tuberosity.
  - Ask the client to flex the leg at the knee joint to 90°.
  - Ask the client to laterally rotate the thigh at the hip joint against resistance and feel for the contraction of the quadratus femoris.

    (Note: In this position, lateral rotation of the thigh at the hip joint on the client's part will involve attempting to move the foot toward the opposite side of the body.)

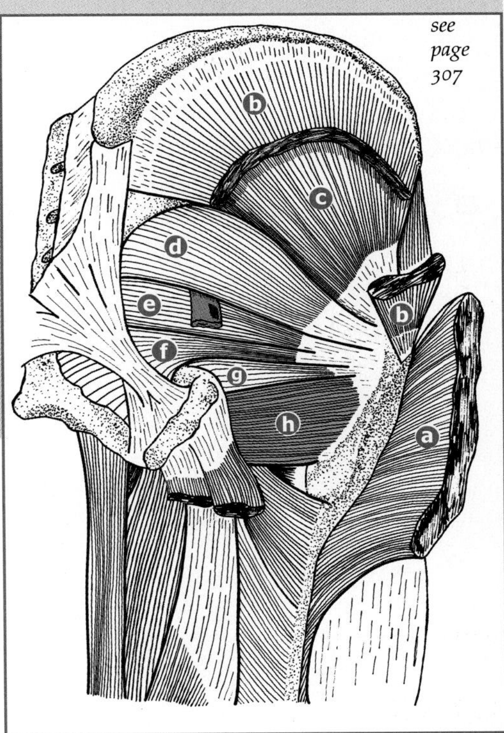

see page 307

Posterior View of the Right Pelvis (Deep)

a. Gluteus Maximus (cut and reflected)
b. Gluteus Medius (cut and reflected)
c. Gluteus Minimus
d. Piriformis
e. Superior Gemellus
f. Obturator Internus
g. Inferior Gemellus
h. **Quadratus Femoris**

RELATIONSHIP TO OTHER MUSCULOSKELETAL STRUCTURES

❑ 1. The quadratus femoris is directly inferior to the inferior gemellus and directly superior to the adductor magnus.

❑ 2. From the posterior perspective, the quadratus femoris is superficial to and either entirely covers or nearly entirely covers the obturator externus.

METHODOLOGY FOR LEARNING MUSCLE ACTIONS

❑ 1. **Lateral Rotation of the Thigh at the Hip Joint:** The quadratus femoris wraps around the posterior pelvis to attach laterally onto the femur (with its fibers running horizontally in the transverse plane). When the quadratus femoris contracts, it pulls the greater trochanter posteromedially, causing the anterior surface of the thigh to face laterally. Therefore, the quadratus femoris laterally rotates the thigh at the hip joint. (Note the similarity of the direction of fibers of the quadratus femoris to the direction of fibers of the piriformis, superior gemellus, obturator internus, inferior gemellus and obturator externus.)

❑ 2. **Adduction of the Thigh at the Hip Joint:** The quadratus femoris attaches sufficiently inferior on the pelvis and distal on the femur to cross the hip joint medially below the center of the joint (with its fibers running horizontally in the frontal plane). When the quadratus femoris contracts, it pulls the lateral attachment, i.e., the thigh, medially in the frontal plane. Therefore, the quadratus femoris adducts the thigh at the hip joint.

QUADRATUS FEMORIS – continued

- ❑ 3. **Contralateral Rotation of the Pelvis at the Hip Joint:** The quadratus femoris crosses the hip joint posteriorly (with its fibers running somewhat horizontally in the transverse plane). When the femoral attachment is fixed, and the quadratus femoris contracts, it pulls on the pelvis, causing the anterior pelvis to face the opposite side of the body from the side of the body that the quadratus femoris is attached. Therefore, the quadratus femoris contralaterally rotates the pelvis at the hip joint. (Note the similarity of the direction of fibers of the quadratus femoris to the direction of fibers of the piriformis, superior gemellus, obturator internus, inferior gemellus and obturator externus.)

MISCELLANEOUS

- ❑ As with the obturator externus, some sources state that the quadratus femoris can adduct the thigh at the hip joint because it crosses the hip joint low enough to be below the center of the joint.

MUSCLES OF THE THIGH

OVERVIEW OF THE MUSCLES OF THE THIGH

ANATOMICALLY, THE MUSCLES OF THE THIGH ARE USUALLY DIVIDED INTO THREE GROUPS:		
The Anterior Group: ▪ Tensor Fasciae Latae ▪ Sartorius *The Quadriceps Femoris:* ▪ Rectus Femoris ▪ Vastus Lateralis ▪ Vastus Medialis ▪ Vastus Intermedius ▪ Articularis Genus	**The Medial Group:** *The Adductor Group:* ▪ Pectineus ▪ Adductor Longus ▪ Gracilis ▪ Adductor Brevis ▪ Adductor Magnus	**The Posterior Group:** *The Hamstring Group:* ▪ Biceps Femoris ▪ Semitendinosus ▪ Semimembranosus

THE FOLLOWING MUSCLES ARE COVERED IN OTHER CHAPTERS OF THIS BOOK, BUT ARE ALSO PRESENT IN THE THIGH:	
▪ Psoas Major	▪ Obturator Internus
▪ Iliacus	▪ Inferior Gemellus
▪ Gluteus Maximus	▪ Obturator Externus
▪ Gluteus Medius	▪ Quadratus Femoris
▪ Gluteus Minimus	▪ Gastrocnemius
▪ Piriformis	▪ Plantaris
▪ Superior Gemellus	▪ Popliteus

This is the usual classification of the muscles of the thigh. However, like any classification, it is overly simplistic and can be misleading. Please note the following:

- Although no lateral group is listed, it does not mean that there is no musculature in the lateral thigh. Superficially, the lateral thigh contains the iliotibial band. However, deep to the iliotibial band are the vastus lateralis and the vastus intermedius. Also, the tensor fasciae latae is quite lateral as are the attachments of the sartorius and some of the posterior pelvic musculature; all of these muscles have a presence in the lateral thigh.
- The quadriceps muscles, although superficial in the anterior thigh, wrap around nearly the entire thigh to attach to the linea aspera on the posterior side of the femur. As noted above, the quadriceps can be found deeper in the lateral thigh, as well as the medial and posterior thigh.
- The adductor musculature, primarily medial as a group, can also be considered to be anterior or posterior in location. The pectineus, adductor longus, gracilis and the adductor brevis can be considered to be anterior as well as medial. The adductor magnus is quite posterior and can be considered to be posterior as well as medial.

Functionally, the muscles of the thigh either cross the hip joint and/or the knee joint. Therefore, muscles of the thigh have their actions at one or both of these joints. The following general rules regarding actions can be stated for muscles of the thigh:

- ► If a muscle crosses the hip joint anteriorly, it can flex the thigh at the hip joint and/or anteriorly tilt the pelvis at the hip joint.
- ► If a muscle crosses the hip joint posteriorly, it can extend the thigh at the hip joint and/or posteriorly tilt the pelvis at the hip joint.
- ► If a muscle crosses the hip joint laterally, it can abduct the thigh at the hip joint and/or depress (laterally tilt) the pelvis at the hip joint.
- ► If a muscle crosses the hip joint medially, it can adduct the thigh at the hip joint and/or elevate the pelvis at the hip joint.
- ► If a muscle crosses the knee joint anteriorly, it can extend the leg at the knee joint.
- ► If a muscle crosses the knee joint posteriorly, it can flex the leg at the knee joint.
- ► Actions of rotation can occur when the muscle's fiber direction has a horizontal component that wraps around the bone to which it attaches.

INNERVATION

- The anterior thigh is innervated by the femoral nerve (except the tensor fasciae latae).
- The medial thigh is innervated by the obturator nerve (except the pectineus and part of the adductor magnus).
- The posterior thigh is innervated by the sciatic nerve.

♥ ARTERIAL SUPPLY

- The anterior thigh receives its arterial supply from the femoral artery or the deep femoral artery (except the tensor fasciae latae).
- The medial thigh receives its arterial supply from the deep femoral artery.
- The posterior thigh receives its arterial supply from the inferior gluteal artery, the obturator artery, perforating branches of the deep femoral artery and the popliteal artery.

A NOTE REGARDING REVERSE ACTIONS

As a rule, this book does not employ the terms "origin" and "insertion." However, it is useful to utilize these terms to describe the concept of "reverse actions." The action section of this book describes the action of a muscle by stating the movement of a body part that is created by a muscle's contraction. The body part that usually moves when a muscle contracts is called the insertion. The methodology section further states at which joint the movement of the insertion occurs. However, the other body part that the muscle attaches to, the origin, can also move at that joint. *This movement can be called the reverse action of the muscle.* Keep in mind that the reverse action of a muscle is always possible. The likelihood that a reverse action will occur is based upon the ability of the insertion to be fixed so that the origin moves (instead of the insertion moving) when the muscle contracts. For more information and examples of reverse actions, see page 702.

❑ ANTERIOR VIEW OF THE BONES AND BONY LANDMARKS OF THE RIGHT THIGH

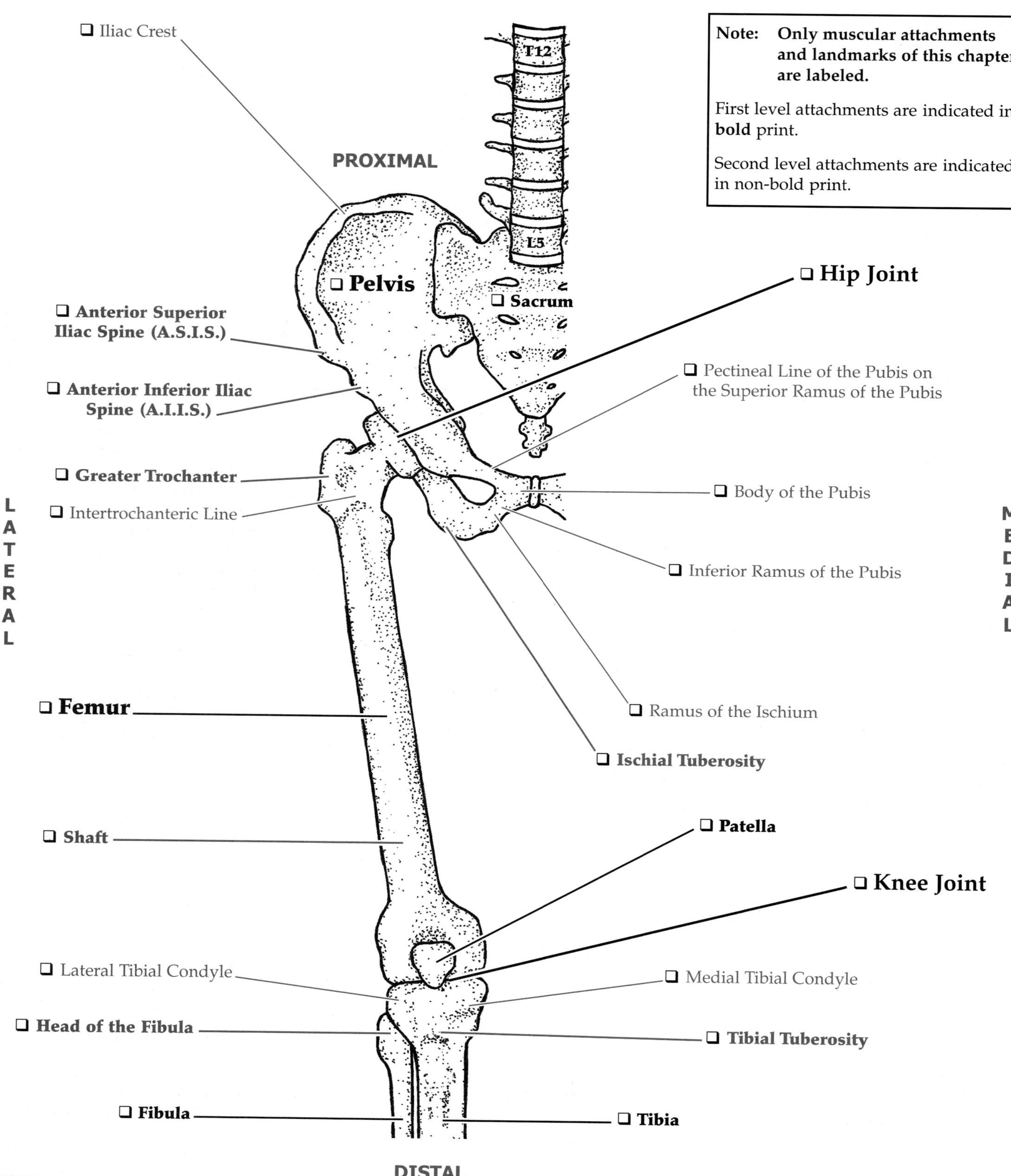

Note: **Only muscular attachments and landmarks of this chapter are labeled.**

First level attachments are indicated in **bold** print.

Second level attachments are indicated in non-bold print.

ANTERIOR VIEW OF THE BONY ATTACHMENTS OF THE RIGHT THIGH

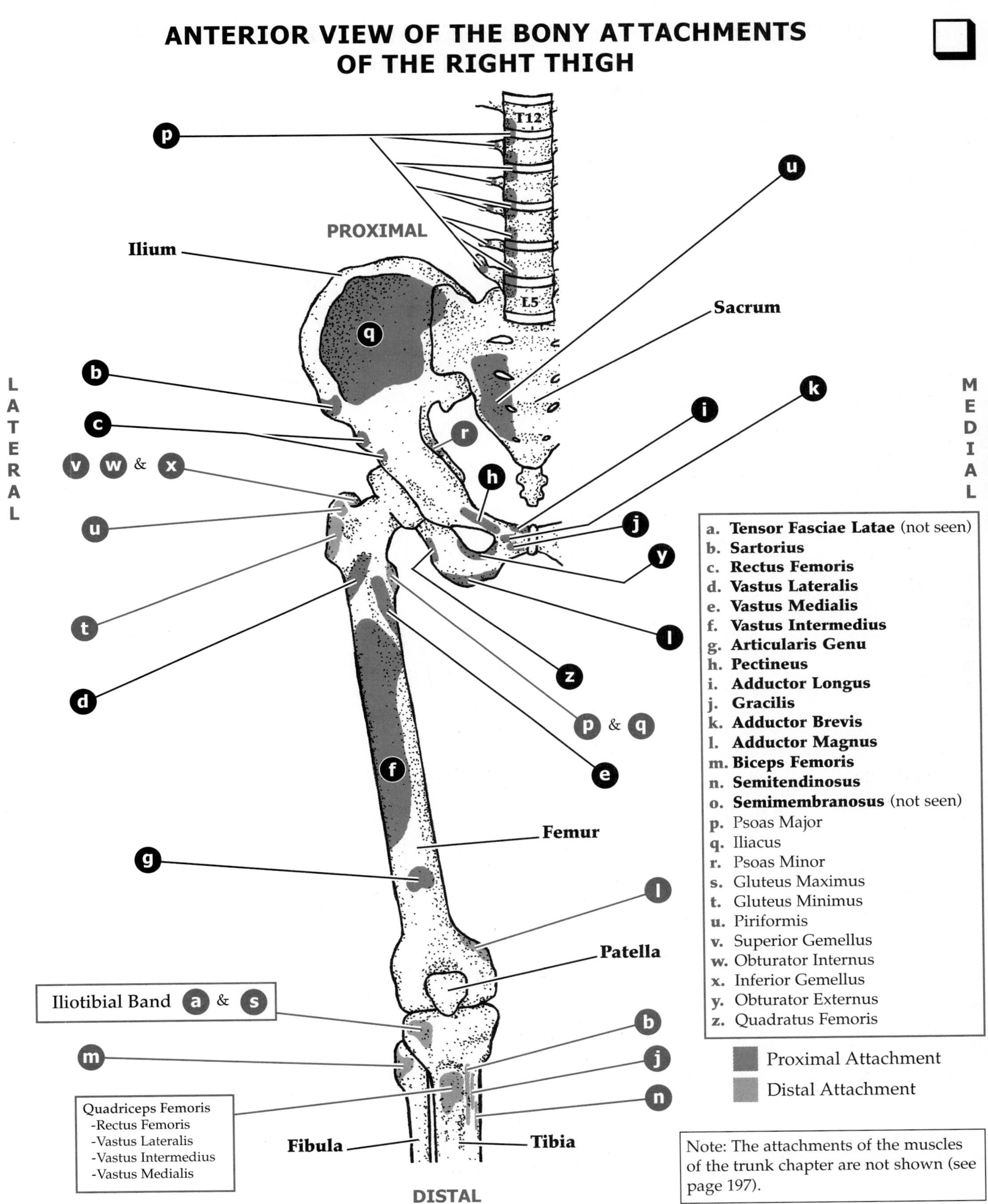

T12
L5
p
PROXIMAL
Ilium
q
u
Sacrum
b
c
v w & x
u
t
d
r
h
i
k
j
y
l
z
p & q
e
f
Femur
g
l
Patella
Iliotibial Band a & s
m
b
j
n
Quadriceps Femoris
-Rectus Femoris
-Vastus Lateralis
-Vastus Intermedius
-Vastus Medialis
Fibula
Tibia
DISTAL
LATERAL
MEDIAL
a. Tensor Fasciae Latae (not seen)
b. Sartorius
c. Rectus Femoris
d. Vastus Lateralis
e. Vastus Medialis
f. Vastus Intermedius
g. Articularis Genu
h. Pectineus
i. Adductor Longus
j. Gracilis
k. Adductor Brevis
l. Adductor Magnus
m. Biceps Femoris
n. Semitendinosus
o. Semimembranosus (not seen)
p. Psoas Major
q. Iliacus
r. Psoas Minor
s. Gluteus Maximus
t. Gluteus Minimus
u. Piriformis
v. Superior Gemellus
w. Obturator Internus
x. Inferior Gemellus
y. Obturator Externus
z. Quadratus Femoris
Proximal Attachment
Distal Attachment
Note: The attachments of the muscles of the trunk chapter are not shown (see page 197).

❑ POSTERIOR VIEW OF THE BONES AND BONY LANDMARKS OF THE RIGHT THIGH

Note: Only muscular attachments and landmarks of this chapter are labeled.

First level attachments are indicated in **bold** print.

Second level attachments are indicated in non-bold print.

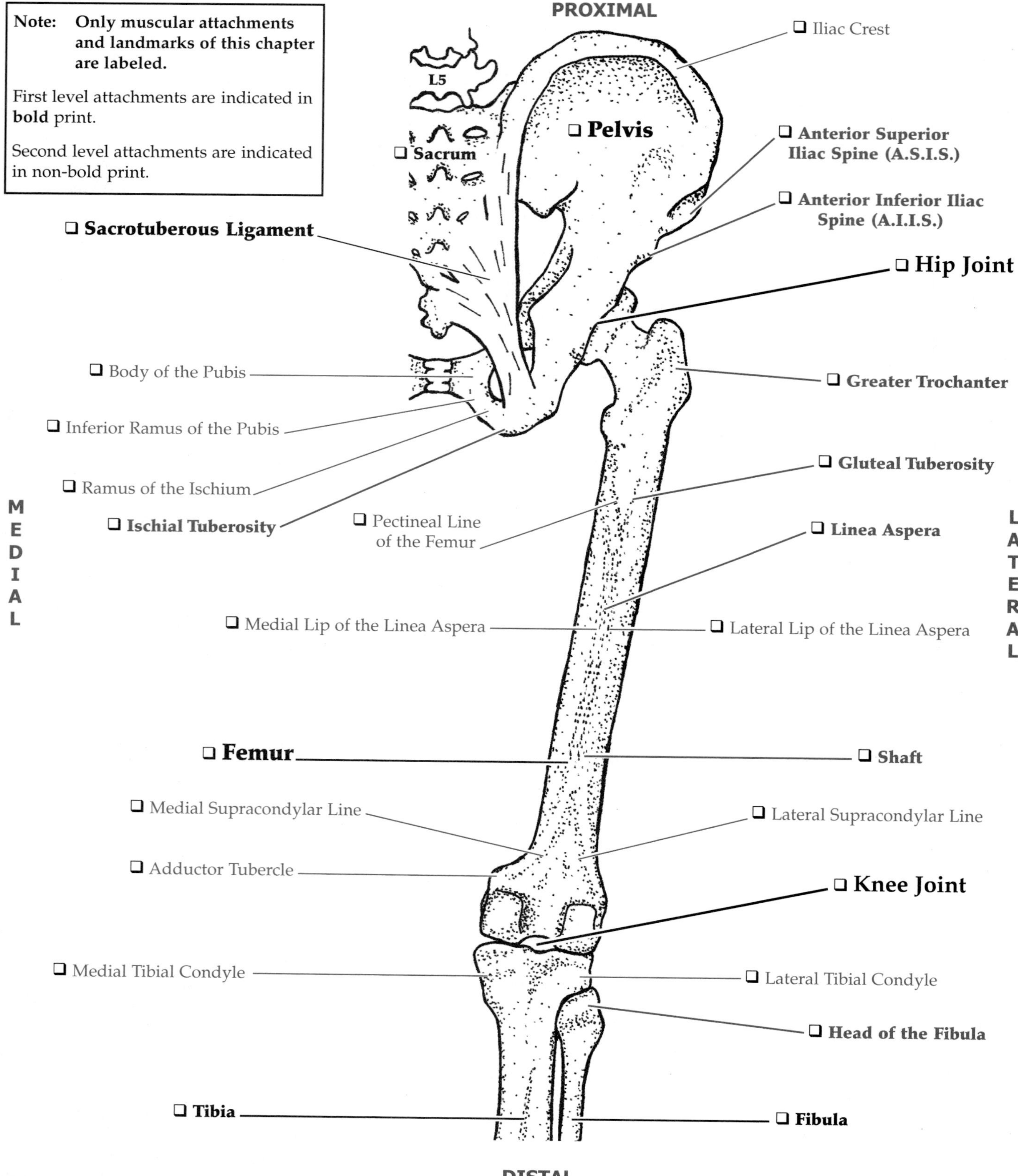

POSTERIOR VIEW OF THE BONY ATTACHMENTS OF THE RIGHT THIGH

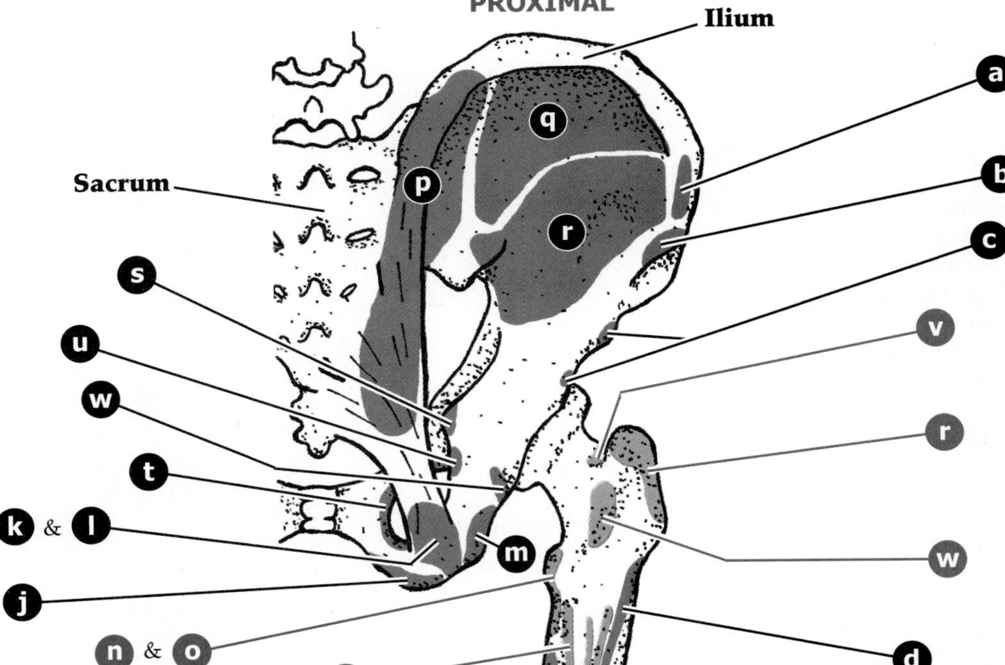

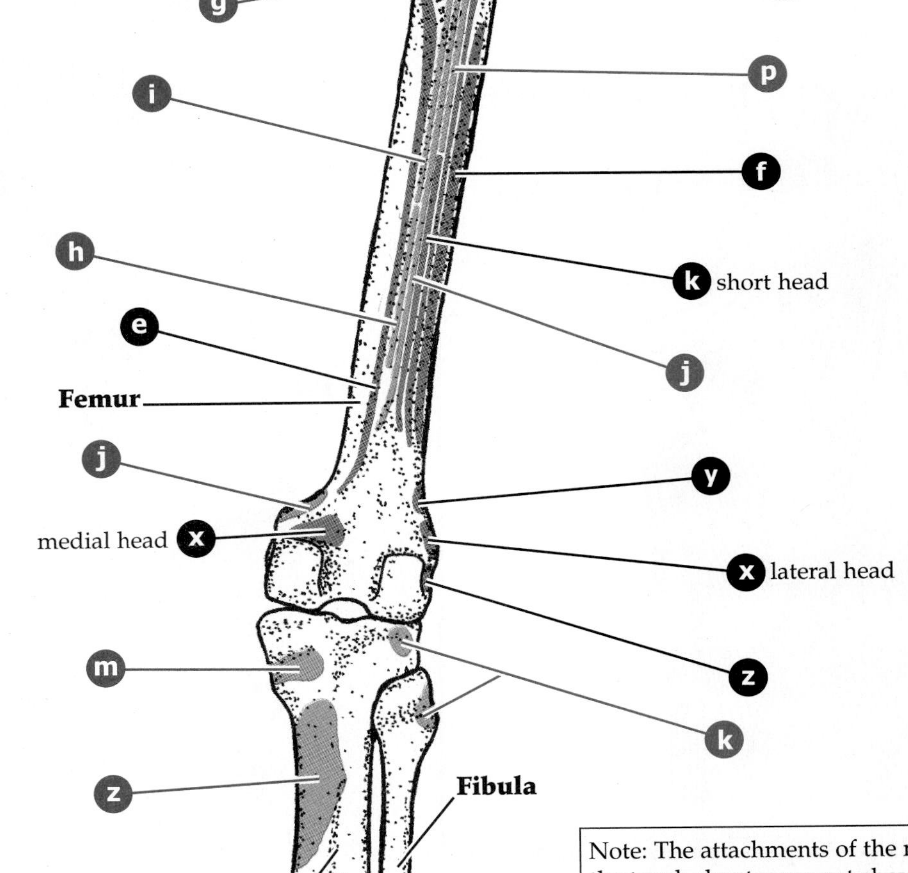

a. **Tensor Fasciae Latae**
b. **Sartorius**
c. **Rectus Femoris**
d. **Vastus Lateralis**
e. **Vastus Medialis**
f. **Vastus Intermedius**
g. **Pectineus**
h. **Adductor Longus**
i. **Adductor Brevis**
j. **Adductor Magnus**
k. **Biceps Femoris**
l. **Semitendinosus**
m. **Semimembranosus**
n. Psoas Major
o. Iliacus
p. Gluteus Maximus
q. Gluteus Medius
r. Gluteus Minimus
s. Superior Gemellus
t. Obturator Internus
u. Inferior Gemellus
v. Obturator Externus
w. Quadratus Femoris
x. Gastrocnemius
y. Plantaris
z. Popliteus

Proximal Attachment
Distal Attachment

Note: The attachments of the muscles of the trunk chapter are not shown (see page 199).

☐ ANTERIOR VIEW OF THE RIGHT THIGH (SUPERFICIAL)

PROXIMAL

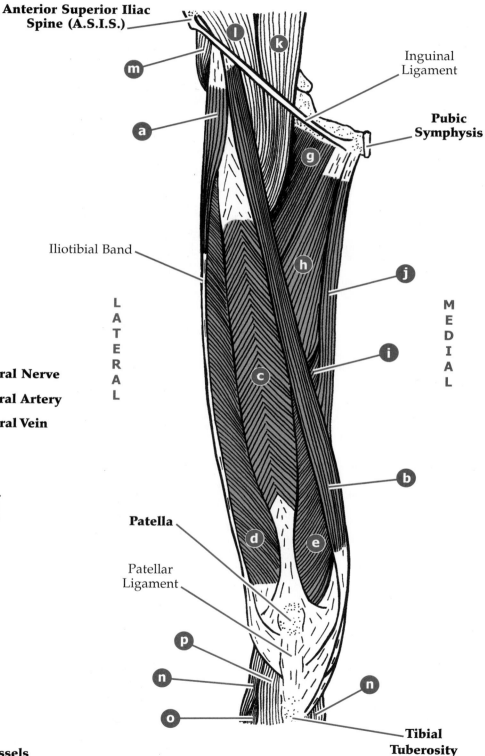

Anterior Superior Iliac Spine (A.S.I.S.)

l
k
m
Inguinal Ligament
a
Pubic Symphysis
g
Iliotibial Band
h
j
LATERAL
MEDIAL
i
c
b
Patella
d
e
Patellar Ligament
p
n
n
o
Tibial Tuberosity

DISTAL

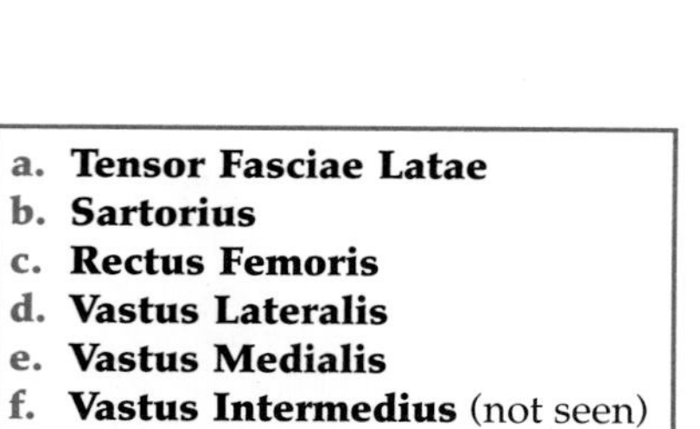
a. **Tensor Fasciae Latae**
b. **Sartorius**
c. **Rectus Femoris**
d. **Vastus Lateralis**
e. **Vastus Medialis**
f. **Vastus Intermedius** (not seen)
g. **Pectineus**
h. **Adductor Longus**
i. **Adductor Magnus**
j. **Gracilis**
k. Psoas Major
l. Iliacus
m. Gluteus Medius
n. Gastrocnemius
o. Fibularis Longus
p. Tibialis Anterior

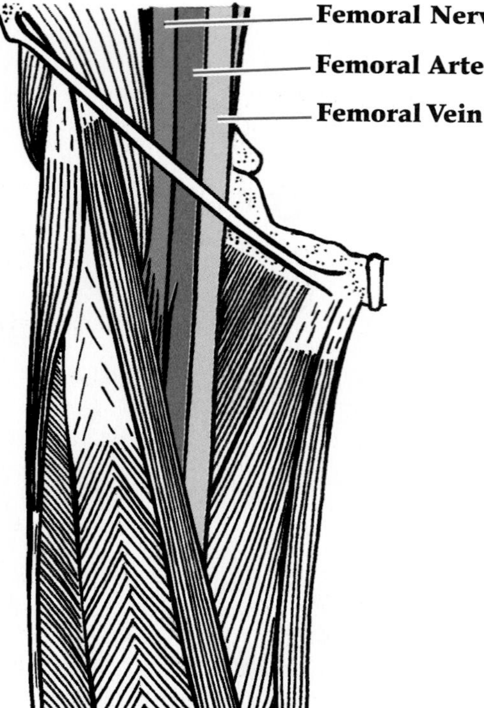

Relationship of Femoral Vessels to Anterior Thigh

ANTERIOR VIEW OF THE RIGHT THIGH (DEEP)

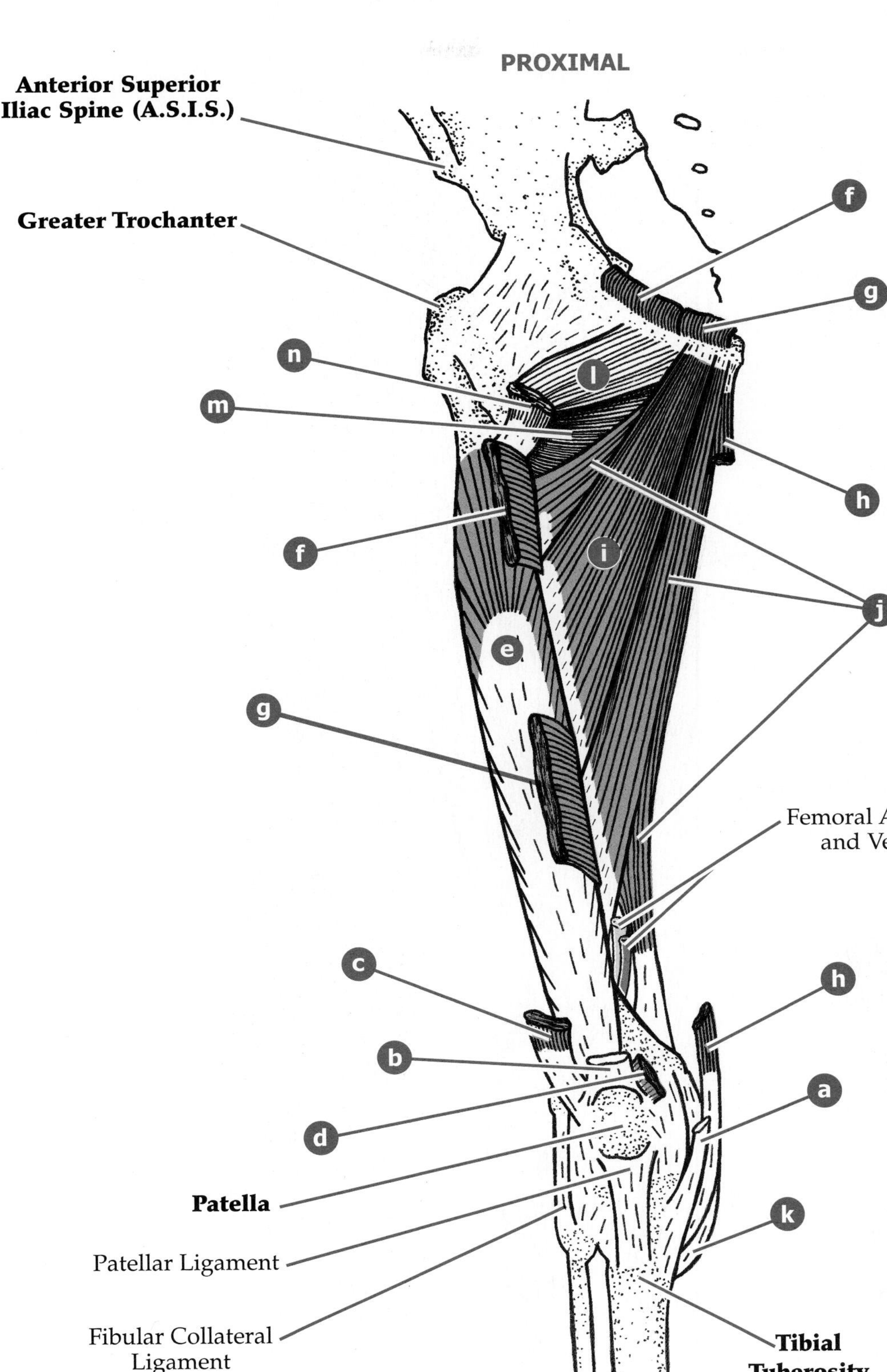

- a. **Sartorius** (cut)
- b. **Rectus Femoris** (cut)
- c. **Vastus Lateralis** (cut)
- d. **Vastus Medialis** (cut)
- e. **Vastus Intermedius**
- f. **Pectineus** (cut and reflected)
- g. **Adductor Longus** (cut and reflected)
- h. **Gracilis** (cut)
- i. **Adductor Brevis**
- j. **Adductor Magnus**
- k. **Semitendinosus**
- l. Obturator Externus
- m. Quadratus Femoris
- n. Iliopsoas (cut)

☐ POSTERIOR VIEW OF THE RIGHT THIGH (SUPERFICIAL)

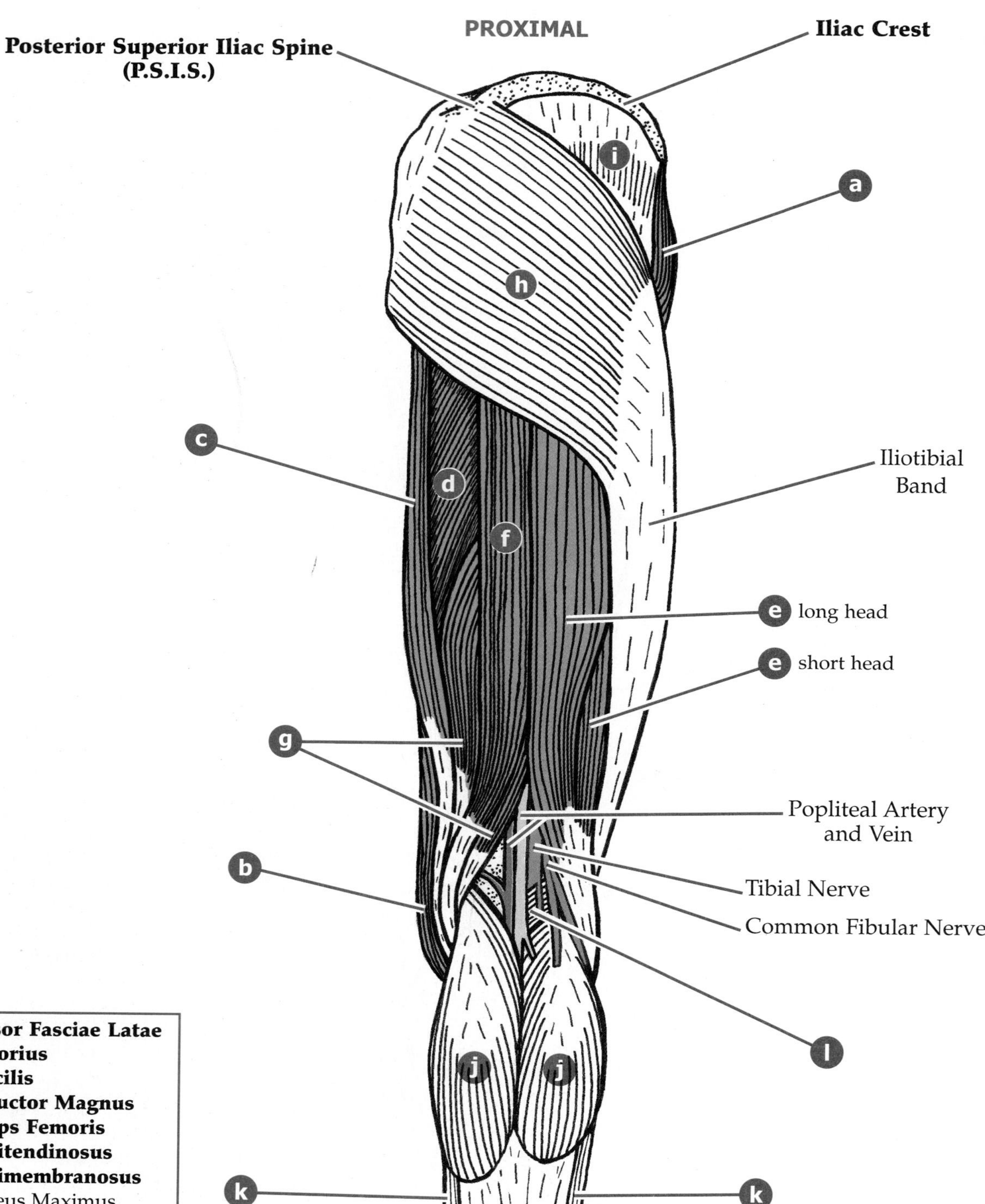

a. **Tensor Fasciae Latae**
b. **Sartorius**
c. **Gracilis**
d. **Adductor Magnus**
e. **Biceps Femoris**
f. **Semitendinosus**
g. **Semimembranosus**
h. Gluteus Maximus
i. Gluteus Medius
j. Gastrocnemius
k. Soleus
l. Plantaris

POSTERIOR VIEW OF THE RIGHT THIGH (DEEP)

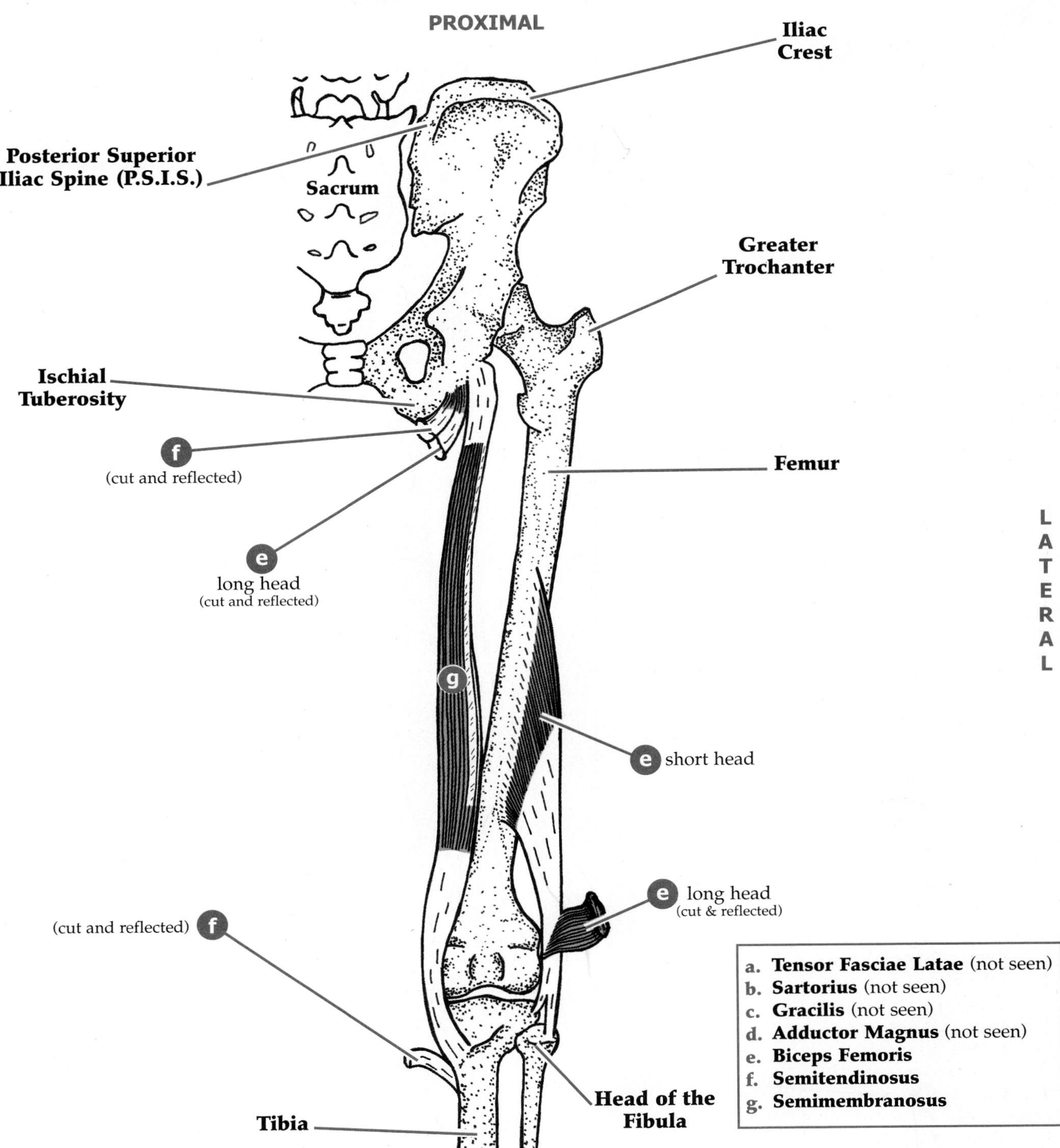

a. **Tensor Fasciae Latae** (not seen)
b. **Sartorius** (not seen)
c. **Gracilis** (not seen)
d. **Adductor Magnus** (not seen)
e. **Biceps Femoris**
f. **Semitendinosus**
g. **Semimembranosus**

LATERAL VIEW OF THE RIGHT THIGH

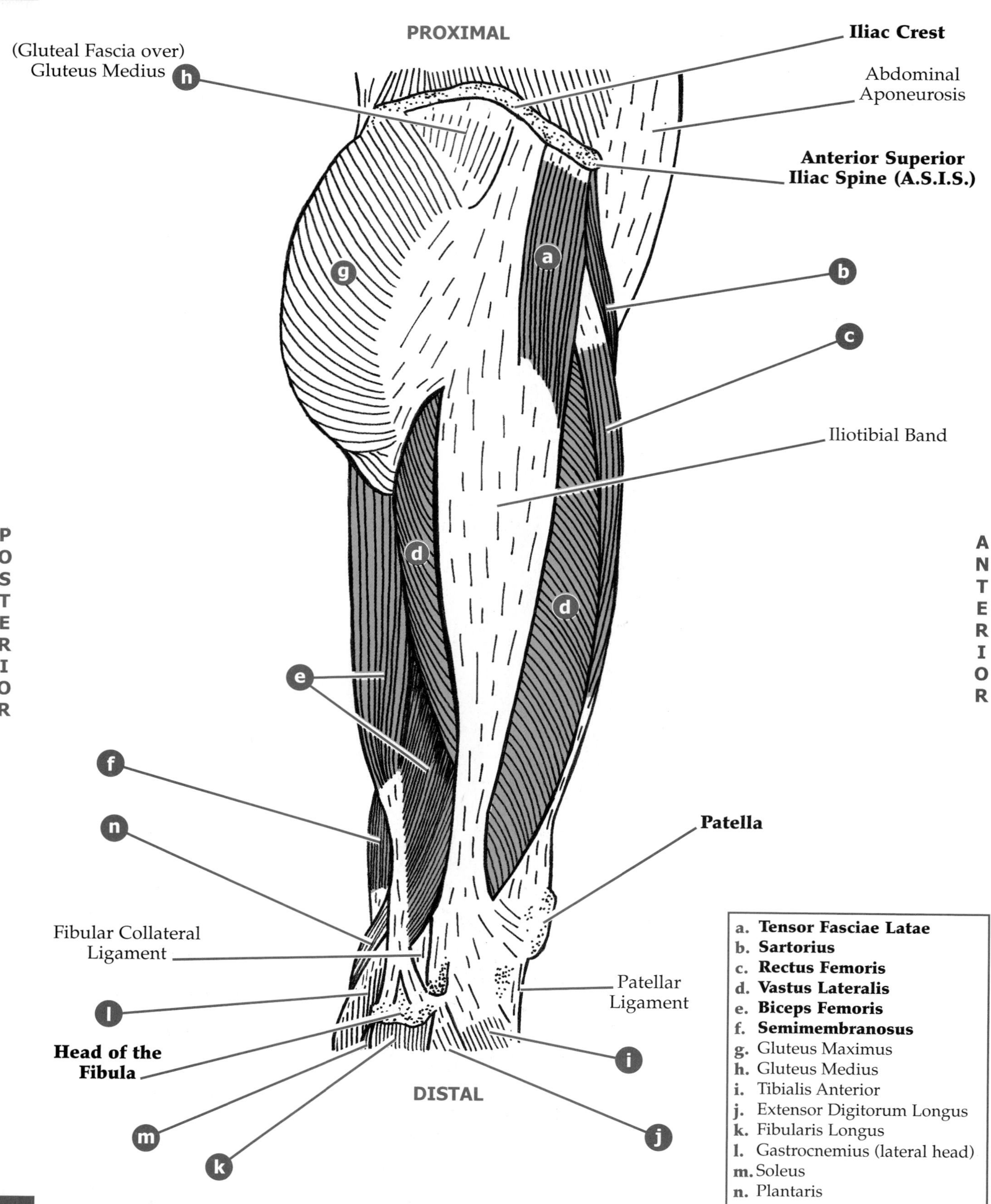

a. **Tensor Fasciae Latae**
b. **Sartorius**
c. **Rectus Femoris**
d. **Vastus Lateralis**
e. **Biceps Femoris**
f. **Semimembranosus**
g. Gluteus Maximus
h. Gluteus Medius
i. Tibialis Anterior
j. Extensor Digitorum Longus
k. Fibularis Longus
l. Gastrocnemius (lateral head)
m. Soleus
n. Plantaris

MEDIAL VIEW OF THE RIGHT THIGH

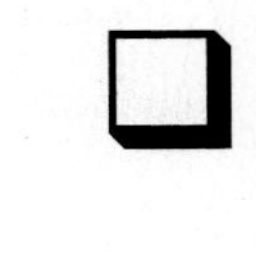

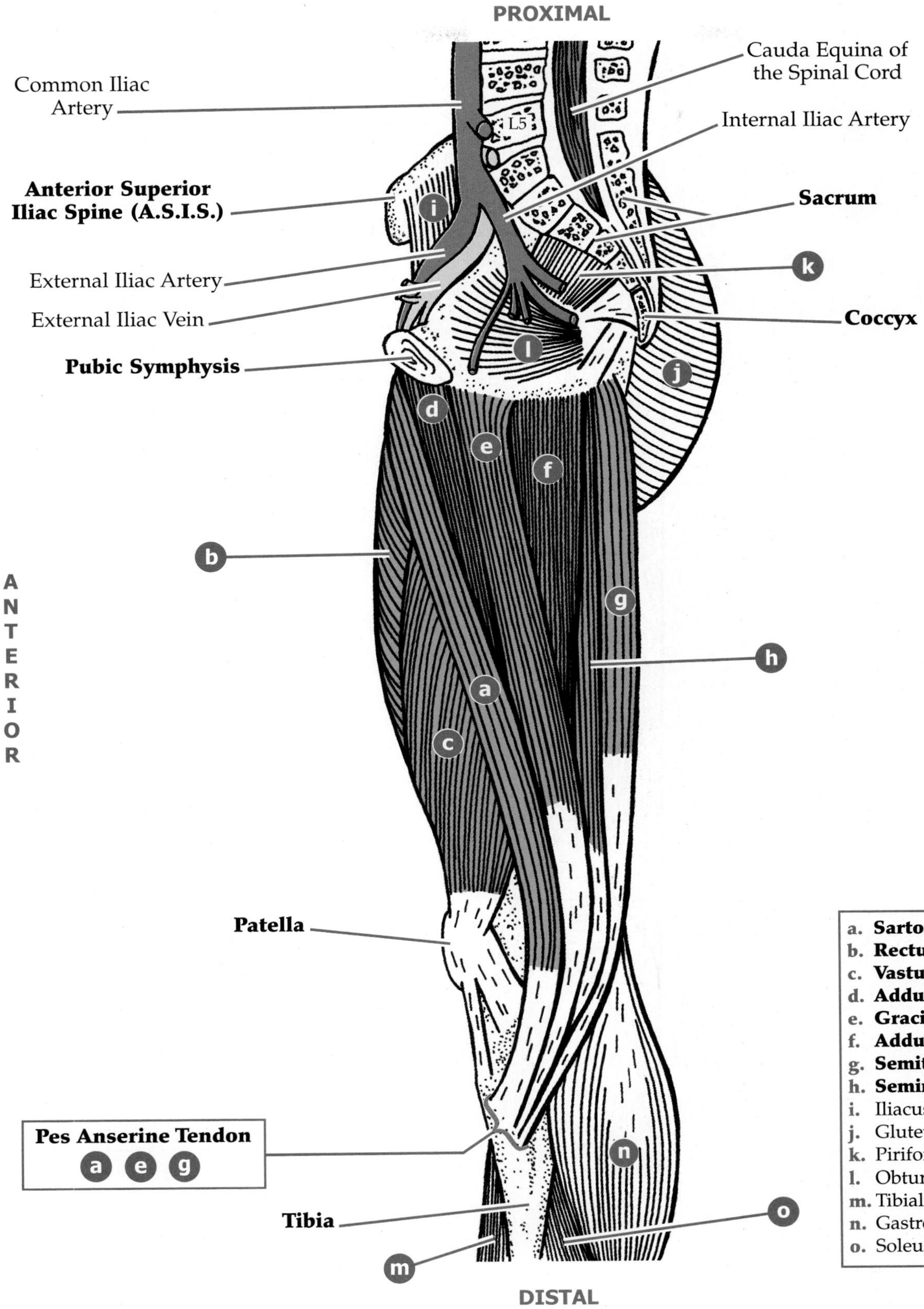

a. **Sartorius**
b. **Rectus Femoris**
c. **Vastus Medialis**
d. **Adductor Longus**
e. **Gracilis**
f. **Adductor Magnus**
g. **Semitendinosus**
h. **Semimembranosus**
i. Iliacus
j. Gluteus Maximus
k. Piriformis
l. Obturator Internus
m. Tibialis Anterior
n. Gastrocnemius (medial head)
o. Soleus

CROSS SECTION VIEWS OF THE RIGHT THIGH

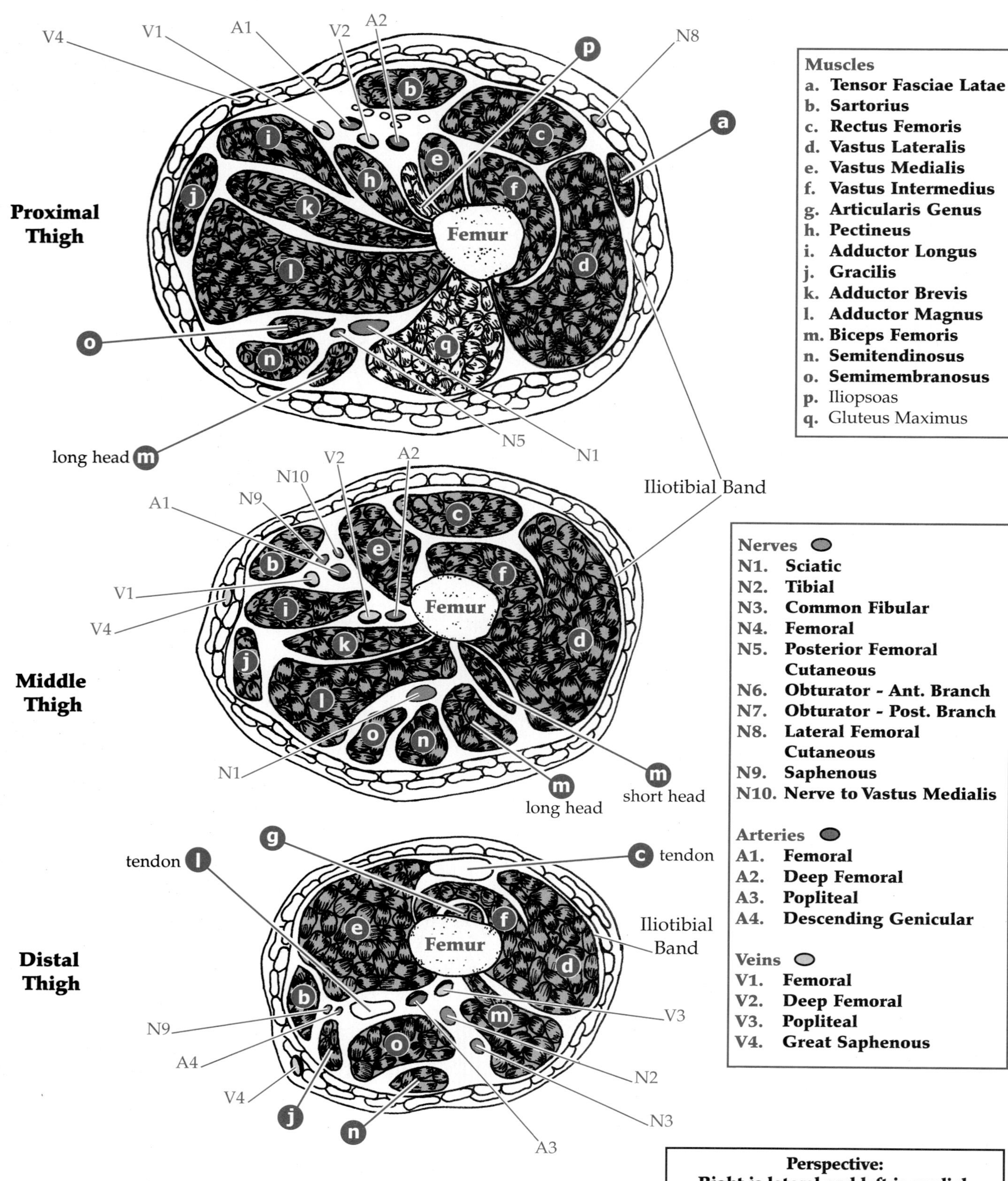
Proximal Thigh
V4
V1
A1
V2
A2
N8
Femur
long head m
N5
N1
Iliotibial Band
Middle Thigh
N10
N9
A1
V1
V4
N1
long head
short head
Distal Thigh
tendon l
tendon c
Iliotibial Band
N9
A4
V4
V3
N2
N3
A3
Muscles
a. Tensor Fasciae Latae
b. Sartorius
c. Rectus Femoris
d. Vastus Lateralis
e. Vastus Medialis
f. Vastus Intermedius
g. Articularis Genus
h. Pectineus
i. Adductor Longus
j. Gracilis
k. Adductor Brevis
l. Adductor Magnus
m. Biceps Femoris
n. Semitendinosus
o. Semimembranosus
p. Iliopsoas
q. Gluteus Maximus
Nerves
N1. Sciatic
N2. Tibial
N3. Common Fibular
N4. Femoral
N5. Posterior Femoral Cutaneous
N6. Obturator - Ant. Branch
N7. Obturator - Post. Branch
N8. Lateral Femoral Cutaneous
N9. Saphenous
N10. Nerve to Vastus Medialis
Arteries
A1. Femoral
A2. Deep Femoral
A3. Popliteal
A4. Descending Genicular
Veins
V1. Femoral
V2. Deep Femoral
V3. Popliteal
V4. Great Saphenous
Perspective:
Right is lateral and left is medial.
Top is anterior and bottom is posterior.

❑ TENSOR FASCIAE LATAE ("T.F.L.")

❑ **The name, tensor fasciae latae, tells us that this muscle "tenses" the "fascia latae." The fascia latae is the broad covering of fascia that lies over the muscles of the thigh.**

DERIVATION ❑ tensor: L. *stretcher.*
fasciae: L. *band/bandage.*
latae: L. *broad, refers to the side.*

PRONUNCIATION ❑ **ten**-sor **fash**-ee-a **la**-tee

ATTACHMENTS

❑ **Anterior Superior Iliac Spine (A.S.I.S.)**

- ❑ and the anterior iliac crest

to the

❑ **Iliotibial Band (I.T.B.)**

- ❑ 1/3 of the way down the thigh

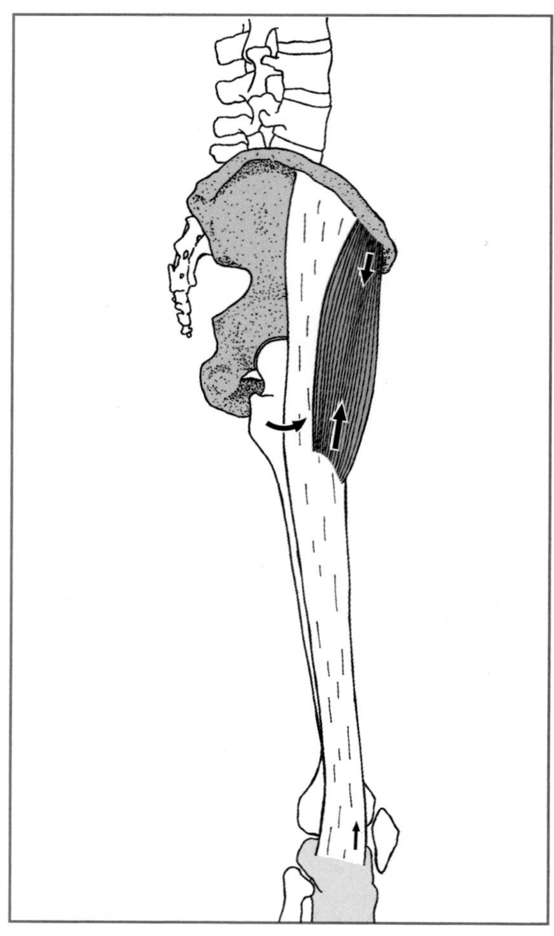

Lateral View of the
Right Tensor Fasciae Latae

ACTIONS

❑ 1. **Flexion of the Thigh**

❑ 2. **Abduction of the Thigh**

❑ 3. **Medial Rotation of the Thigh**

❑ 4. **Anterior Tilt of the Pelvis**

❑ 5. Depression (Lateral Tilt) of the Pelvis

❑ 6. Ipsilateral Rotation of the Pelvis

❑ 7. Extension of the Leg

INNERVATION ❑ The Superior Gluteal Nerve ❑ **L4, 5,** S1

ARTERIAL SUPPLY ❑ The Superior Gluteal Artery (A Branch of the Internal Iliac Artery)
❑ and the deep femoral artery (a major branch of the femoral artery)

PALPATION AND SUPPLEMENTARY TEXT

PALPATION

- ☐ The tensor fasciae latae is superficial and easy to palpate.
  - Have the client supine.
  - Place palpating hand just distal to the A.S.I.S.
  - Have the client actively hold the thigh in a position of flexion and medial rotation at the hip.
  - Resist the client from further flexion of the thigh at the hip joint and feel for the contraction of the T.F.L.
  - Continue palpating the T.F.L. distally and slightly posteriorly toward the I.T.B. attachment.

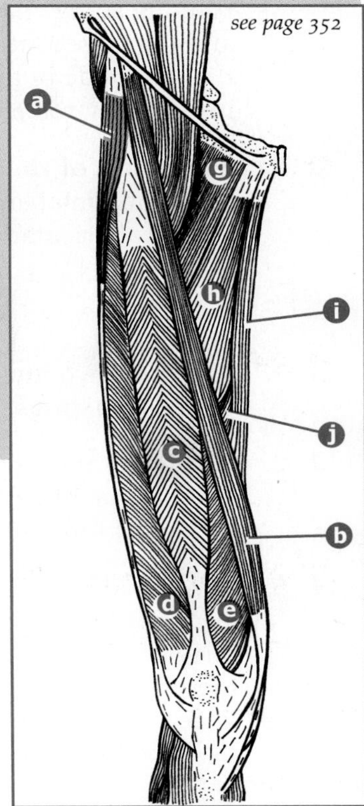

Anterior View of the Right Thigh (Superficial)

a. **Tensor Fasciae Latae**
b. Sartorius
c. Rectus Femoris
d. Vastus Lateralis
e. Vastus Medialis
f. Vastus Intermedius (not seen)
g. Pectineus
h. Adductor Longus
i. Gracilis
j. Adductor Magnus

RELATIONSHIP TO OTHER MUSCULOSKELETAL STRUCTURES

☐ 1. The tensor fasciae latae is anterior to the gluteus medius and posterior to the sartorius.

☐ 2. The tensor fasciae latae is superficial to the vastus lateralis. At its proximal attachment, the tensor fasciae latae is superficial to the proximal attachment of the rectus femoris.

METHODOLOGY FOR LEARNING MUSCLE ACTIONS

☐ 1. **Flexion of the Thigh at the Hip Joint:** The tensor fasciae latae crosses the hip joint anteriorly (with its fibers running vertically in the sagittal plane); therefore, it flexes the thigh at the hip joint.

☐ 2. **Abduction of the Thigh at the Hip Joint:** The tensor fasciae latae crosses the hip joint laterally (with its fibers running vertically in the frontal plane); therefore, it abducts the thigh at the hip joint.

☐ 3. **Medial Rotation of the Thigh at the Hip Joint:** The tensor fasciae latae crosses the hip joint laterally in such a way that it wraps from anteriorly on the pelvis to posteriorly into the iliotibial band (with its fibers running somewhat horizontally in the transverse plane). When the tensor fasciae pulls on the iliotibial band, it pulls this lateral attachment anteromedially, causing the anterior thigh to face medially. Therefore, the tensor fasciae latae medially rotates the thigh at the hip joint.

☐ 4. **Anterior Tilt of the Pelvis at the Hip Joint:** With the distal attachment fixed, the tensor fasciae latae, by pulling inferiorly on the anterior pelvis, anteriorly tilts the pelvis at the hip joint.

☐ 5. **Depression (Lateral Tilt) of the Pelvis at the Hip Joint:** With the distal attachment fixed, the tensor fasciae latae, by pulling inferiorly on the pelvis laterally, depresses (laterally tilts) the pelvis on that side at the hip joint.

TENSOR FASCIAE LATAE – continued

- ❑ 6. **Ipsilateral Rotation of the Pelvis at the Hip Joint:** The tensor fasciae latae crosses the hip joint in such a way that it wraps from medially on the pelvis to laterally into the iliotibial band (with its fibers running somewhat horizontally in the transverse plane). When the iliotibial band attachment is fixed and the tensor fasciae latae contracts, it pulls on the pelvis, causing the anterior pelvis to face toward the same side of the body that the tensor fasciae latae is attached. Therefore, the tensor fasciae latae ipsilaterally rotates the pelvis at the hip joint.
- ❑ 7. **Extension of the Leg at the Knee Joint:** Due to its pull via the iliotibial band (which attaches to the proximal anterolateral tibia), the tensor fasciae latae crosses the knee joint anteriorly (with a vertical orientation to its pull in the sagittal plane); therefore, it extends the leg at the knee joint.

MISCELLANEOUS

- ❑ 1. There are two muscles that attach into the iliotibial band, the tensor fasciae latae and the gluteus maximus.
- ❑ 2. Given that the tensor fasciae latae attaches into the iliotibial band from one direction and the gluteus maximus attaches into the iliotibial band from the opposite direction, they have opposite actions of rotation.
- ❑ 3. Given that both the tensor fasciae latae and the gluteus maximus attach into the iliotibial band, and the iliotibial band crosses the knee joint anteriorly, both of these muscles in effect cross the knee joint anteriorly and therefore, theoretically, can extend the leg at the knee joint. However, there is controversy over their ability to actually do this. Certainly, extension of the leg at the knee joint is not one of their major actions. It is likely that the role of these two muscles and the iliotibial band crossing the knee is primarily to help stabilize the knee joint.
- ❑ 4. A chronically tight tensor fasciae latae can create the postural conditions of a "functional" short lower extremity (usually called a "short leg") and a compensatory scoliosis. When the tensor fasciae latae is tight, it pulls on and depresses (laterally tilts) the pelvis toward the thigh on that side. This results in a "functional short leg" (as opposed to a "structural short leg" wherein the femur and/or the tibia on one side is actually shorter than on the other side). Further, depressing the pelvis on one side creates an unlevel sacrum for the spine to sit on and a compensatory scoliosis must occur to return the head to a level position. (Note: The head must be level for proper proprioceptive balance in the inner ear and for the eyes to be level for visual proprioception.)
- ❑ 5. The iliotibial band is a thickening of the fascia lata in the lateral thigh.

VIEWS OF THE QUADRICEPS

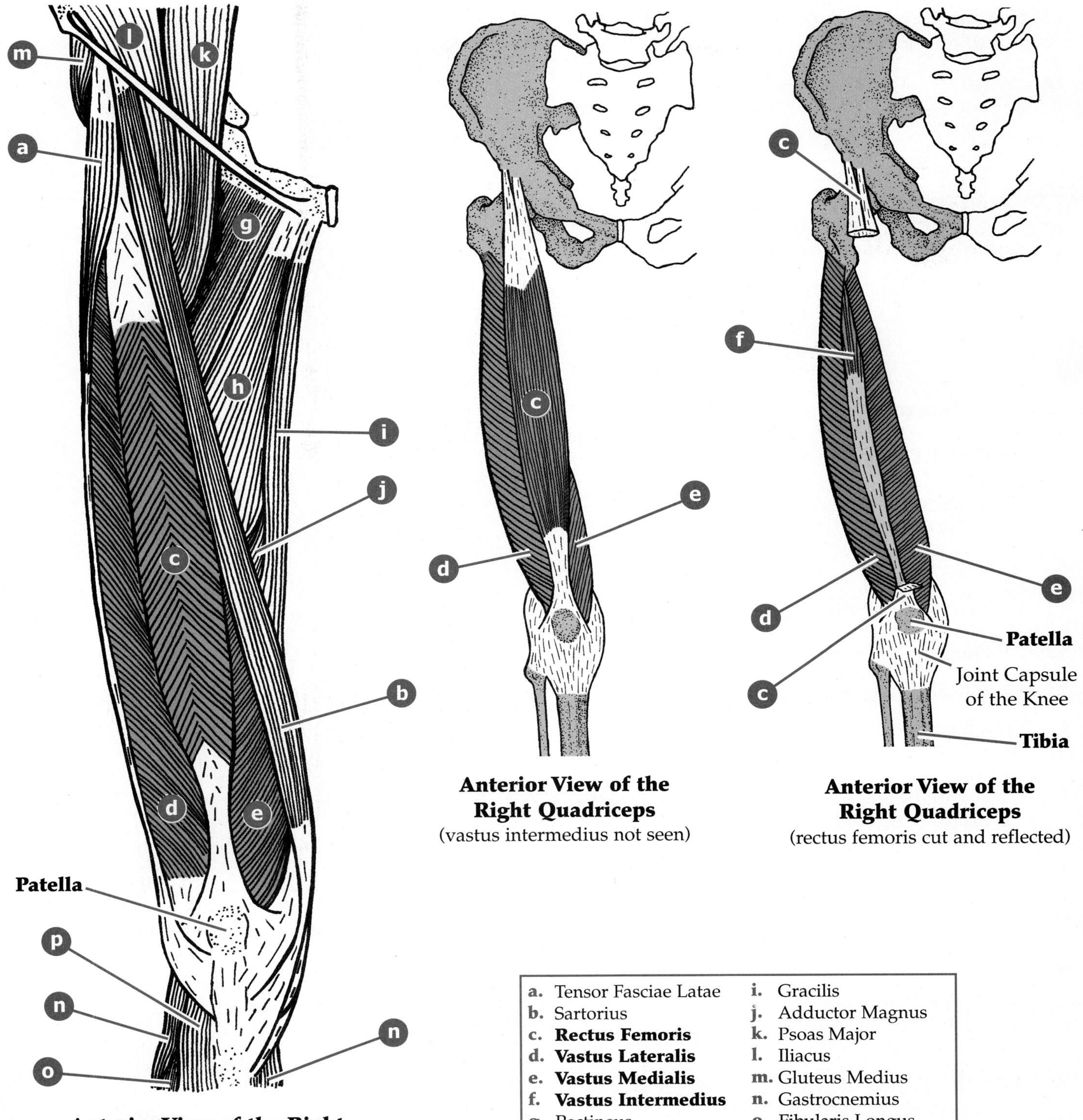

Anterior View of the Right Thigh (Superficial)

Anterior View of the Right Quadriceps
(vastus intermedius not seen)

Anterior View of the Right Quadriceps
(rectus femoris cut and reflected)

a. Tensor Fasciae Latae	**i.** Gracilis
b. Sartorius	**j.** Adductor Magnus
c. **Rectus Femoris**	**k.** Psoas Major
d. **Vastus Lateralis**	**l.** Iliacus
e. **Vastus Medialis**	**m.** Gluteus Medius
f. **Vastus Intermedius**	**n.** Gastrocnemius
g. Pectineus	**o.** Fibularis Longus
h. Adductor Longus	**p.** Tibialis Anterior

❑ RECTUS FEMORIS
(OF THE QUADRICEPS)

❑ **The name, rectus femoris, tells us that the fibers of this muscle run straight up and down (proximal to distal) on the femur.**

DERIVATION ❑ rectus: L. *straight.*
femoris: L. *refers to the femur.*

PRONUNCIATION ❑ **rek**-tus **fem**-o-ris

ATTACHMENTS

❑ **Anterior Inferior Iliac Spine (A.I.I.S.)**

- ❑ and just superior to the brim of the acetabulum

to the

❑ **Tibial Tuberosity**

- ❑ via the patella and the patellar ligament

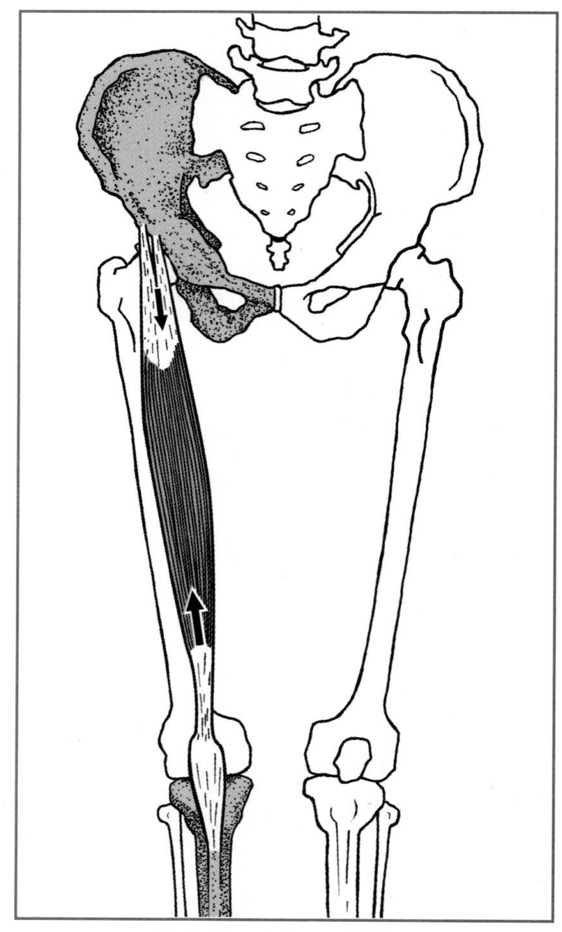

Anterior View of the Right Rectus Femoris

ACTIONS

❑ 1. **Extension of the Leg**

❑ 2. **Flexion of the Thigh**

❑ 3. **Anterior Tilt of the Pelvis**

INNERVATION ❑ The Femoral Nerve ❑ L2, **3, 4**

ARTERIAL SUPPLY ❑ The Femoral Artery (The Continuation of the External Iliac Artery) and the Deep Femoral Artery (A Major Branch of the Femoral Artery)

PALPATION AND SUPPLEMENTARY TEXT

PALPATION

- ❑ The rectus femoris is superficial and easy to palpate.
  - Have the client supine with a pillow under the knees.
  - Place palpating hand just proximal to the patella.
  - Resist the client from actively extending the leg at the knee joint and feel for the contraction of the rectus femoris.
  - Continue palpating the rectus femoris toward the A.I.I.S.
  - To palpate the proximal tendon of the rectus femoris, passively flex the thigh at the hip joint and palpate slightly distal to the A.I.I.S.

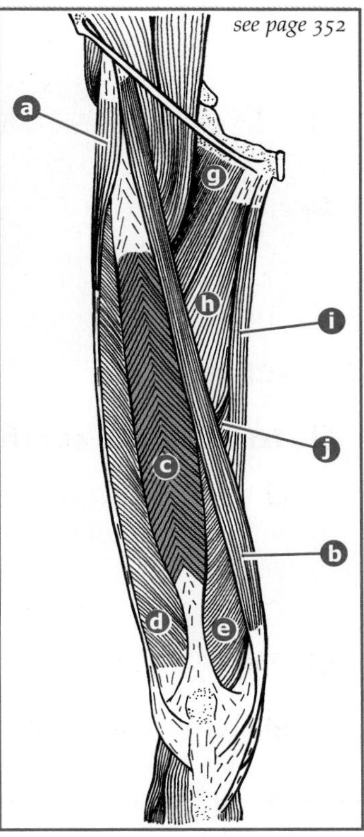

see page 352

Anterior View of the Right Thigh (Superficial)

- **a.** Tensor Fasciae Latae
- **b.** Sartorius
- **c.** **Rectus Femoris**
- **d.** Vastus Lateralis
- **e.** Vastus Medialis
- **f.** Vastus Intermedius (not seen)
- **g.** Pectineus
- **h.** Adductor Longus
- **i.** Gracilis
- **j.** Adductor Magnus

RELATIONSHIP TO OTHER MUSCULOSKELETAL STRUCTURES

❑ 1. The rectus femoris is superficial for its entire course except proximally, where its proximal attachment is deep to the sartorius and the tensor fasciae latae.

❑ 2. Deep to the rectus femoris is the vastus intermedius.

❑ 3. The rectus femoris is primarily located between the vastus lateralis (laterally) and the vastus medialis (medially) but it slightly overlies the two.

METHODOLOGY FOR LEARNING MUSCLE ACTIONS

❑ **1. Extension of the Leg at the Knee Joint:** The rectus femoris crosses the knee joint anteriorly (with its fibers running vertically in the sagittal plane); therefore, it extends the leg at the knee joint.

❑ **2. Flexion of the Thigh at the Hip Joint:** The rectus femoris crosses the hip joint anteriorly (with its fibers running vertically in the sagittal plane); therefore, it flexes the thigh at the hip joint.

❑ **3. Anterior Tilt of the Pelvis at the Hip Joint:** With the distal attachment fixed, the rectus femoris, by pulling inferiorly on the anterior pelvis, anteriorly tilts the pelvis at the hip joint.

MISCELLANEOUS

❑ 1. The proximal attachment of the rectus femoris onto the anterior inferior iliac spine (A.I.I.S.) is known as the *straight tendon*.

❑ 2. The proximal attachment of the rectus femoris, which attaches just superior to the brim of the acetabulum, is known as the *reflected tendon*.

❑ 3. Since it is the only quadriceps muscle that crosses the hip joint, the rectus femoris is the only quadriceps muscle that can move the thigh at the hip joint.

❑ 4. The reason that the quadriceps are so large and strong is not just to move the leg into extension at the knee joint, but rather to do the reverse action, i.e., move the thigh into extension at the knee joint (see page 702). This happens every time a person stands up from a seated position. To move the thigh at the knee joint requires moving the entire body along with the thigh; hence, the quadriceps need to be very large and strong.

❑ VASTUS LATERALIS

(OF THE QUADRICEPS)

❑ **The name, vastus lateralis, tells us that this muscle is vast in size and located laterally.**

DERIVATION ❑ vastus: L. *vast.*
lateralis: L. *lateral.*

PRONUNCIATION ❑ **vas**-tus lat-er-**a**-lis

ATTACHMENTS

❑ **Linea Aspera of the Femur**

❑ the lateral lip of the linea aspera of the femur and the anterior aspect of the greater trochanter and the gluteal tuberosity

to the

❑ **Tibial Tuberosity**

❑ via the patella and the patellar ligament

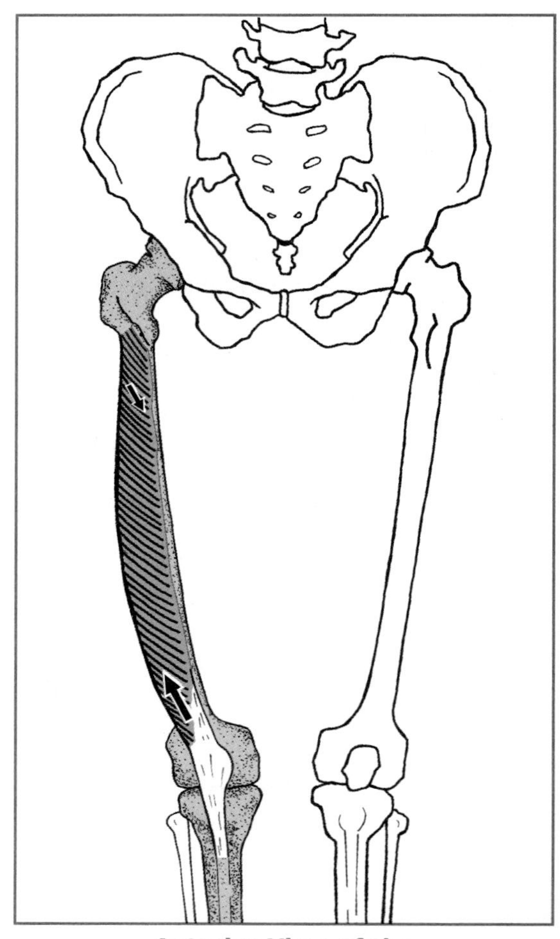

Anterior View of the Right Vastus Lateralis

ACTION

❑ **Extension of the Leg**

INNERVATION ❑ The Femoral Nerve ❑ L2, **3**, **4**

ARTERIAL SUPPLY ❑ The Femoral Artery (The Continuation of the External Iliac Artery) and the Deep Femoral Artery (A Major Branch of the Femoral Artery)
❑ and branches of the popliteal artery (the continuation of the femoral artery)

PALPATION AND SUPPLEMENTARY TEXT

PALPATION

- ❑ The vastus lateralis is visible and palpable from slightly distal to the greater trochanter all the way to its distal attachment on the patella.
  - Have the client supine.
  - Place palpating hand just distal to the greater trochanter.
  - Ask the client to contract the quadriceps and feel for the contraction of the vastus lateralis.
  - Continue palpating the vastus lateralis distally toward the patella.

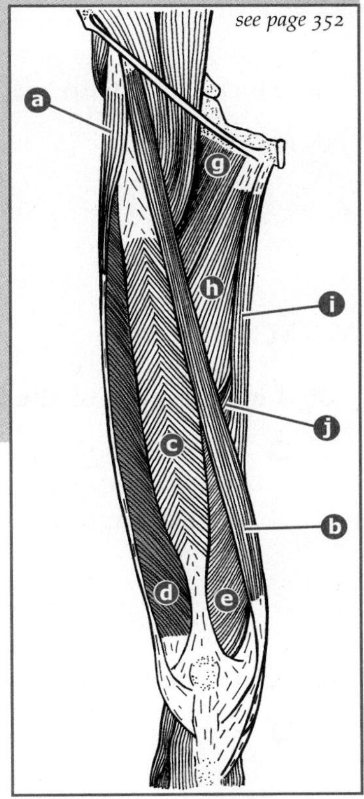

Anterior View of the Right Thigh (Superficial)

- **a.** Tensor Fasciae Latae
- **b.** Sartorius
- **c.** Rectus Femoris
- **d. Vastus Lateralis**
- **e.** Vastus Medialis
- **f.** Vastus Intermedius (not seen)
- **g.** Pectineus
- **h.** Adductor Longus
- **i.** Gracilis
- **j.** Adductor Magnus

RELATIONSHIP TO OTHER MUSCULOSKELETAL STRUCTURES

❑ 1. Anteriorly, the vastus lateralis is lateral and partially deep to the rectus femoris.

❑ 2. In the lateral thigh, the vastus lateralis is deep to the tensor fasciae latae and the iliotibial band.

❑ 3. Posteriorly, the vastus lateralis is superficial between the iliotibial band and the biceps femoris.

❑ 4. Deep to the vastus lateralis are the vastus intermedius and the femur.

METHODOLOGY FOR LEARNING MUSCLE ACTIONS

❑ **Extension of the Leg at the Knee Joint:** The vastus lateralis crosses the knee joint anteriorly (with its fibers running vertically in the sagittal plane); therefore, it extends the leg at the knee joint.

MISCELLANEOUS

❑ 1. The vastus lateralis is the largest of the four quadriceps femoris muscles.

❑ 2. The fibers of the vastus lateralis are oriented somewhat horizontally, which creates a line of pull on the patella that can pull it slightly laterally, in addition to proximally, when the quadriceps contract to extend the leg at the knee joint. Similarly, the vastus medialis can pull the patella slightly medially as the leg extends at the knee joint. The counterbalancing forces of the vastus lateralis and the vastus medialis help to assure that the patella tracks correctly on the femur as the leg extends at the knee joint.

❑ 3. The reason that the quadriceps are so large and strong is not just to move the leg into extension at the knee joint, but rather to do the reverse action, i.e., move the thigh into extension at the knee joint (see page 702). This happens every time a person stands up from a seated position. To move the thigh at the knee joint requires moving the entire body along with the thigh; hence, the quadriceps need to be very large and strong.

❑ 4. Pain attributed to the iliotibial band is often due to tightness of the vastus lateralis, which is deep to the iliotibial band.

❑

VASTUS MEDIALIS
(OF THE QUADRICEPS)

❑ **The name, vastus medialis, tells us that this muscle is vast in size and located medially.**

DERIVATION ❑ vastus: L. *vast.*
medialis: L. *medial.*

PRONUNCIATION ❑ **vas**-tus mee-dee-**a**-lis

ATTACHMENTS

❑ **Linea Aspera of the Femur**

❑ the medial lip of the linea aspera and the intertrochanteric line and the medial supracondylar line of the femur

to the

❑ **Tibial Tuberosity**

❑ via the patella and the patellar ligament

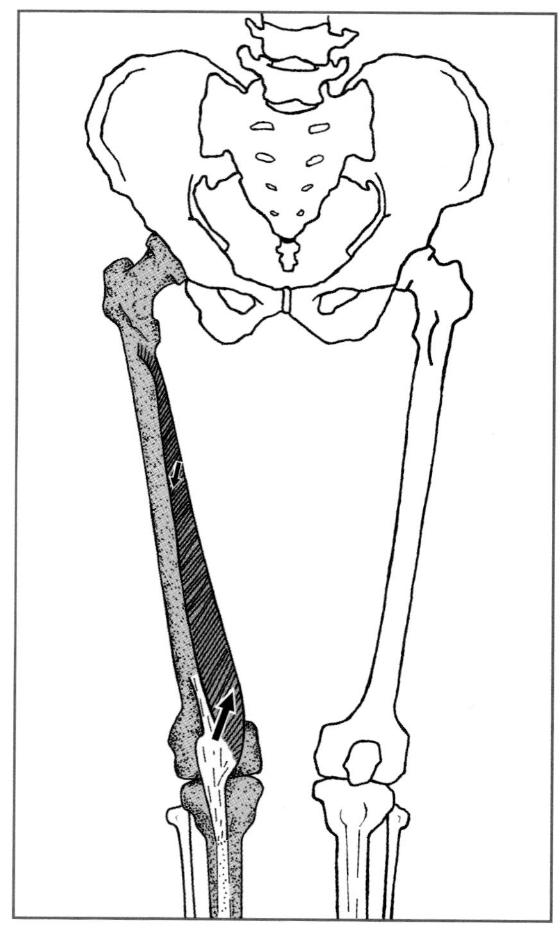

Anterior View of the Right Vastus Medialis

ACTION

❑ **Extension of the Leg**

INNERVATION ❑ The Femoral Nerve ❑ L2, **3, 4**

ARTERIAL SUPPLY ❑ The Femoral Artery (The Continuation of the External Iliac Artery)

PALPATION AND SUPPLEMENTARY TEXT

PALPATION

- ❑ The vastus medialis is best palpated medially in the distal 1/3 of the thigh.
  - Have the client supine.
  - Place palpating hand just proximal and medial to the patella.
  - Ask the client to contract the quadriceps and feel for the contraction of the vastus medialis.
  - Continue palpating the vastus medialis proximally as far as possible. (Note: The vastus medialis is deep to the sartorius and other muscles in the proximal 2/3 of the thigh.)

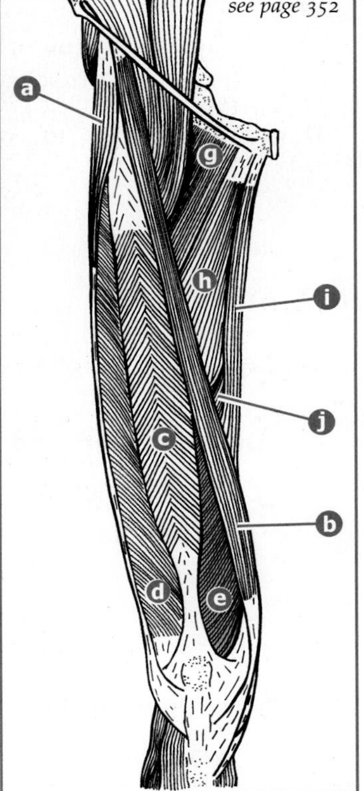

Anterior View of the Right Thigh (Superficial)

- **a.** Tensor Fasciae Latae
- **b.** Sartorius
- **c.** Rectus Femoris
- **d.** Vastus Lateralis
- **e. Vastus Medialis**
- **f.** Vastus Intermedius (not seen)
- **g.** Pectineus
- **h.** Adductor Longus
- **i.** Gracilis
- **j.** Adductor Magnus

RELATIONSHIP TO OTHER MUSCULOSKELETAL STRUCTURES

❑ 1. Anteriorly, the vastus medialis is medial and slightly deep to the rectus femoris. It is also deep to the sartorius.

❑ 2. The vastus medialis is anterior to the adductor group.

❑ 3. Deep to the vastus medialis is the femur.

METHODOLOGY FOR LEARNING MUSCLE ACTIONS

❑ **Extension of the Leg at the Knee Joint:** The vastus medialis crosses the knee joint anteriorly (with its fibers running vertically in the sagittal plane); therefore, it extends the leg at the knee joint.

MISCELLANEOUS

❑ 1. The most distal aspect of the vastus medialis is the bulkiest and may form a bulge in well-toned individuals.

❑ 2. The fibers of the vastus medialis are oriented somewhat horizontally, which creates a line of pull on the patella that can pull it slightly medially, in addition to proximally, when the quadriceps contract to extend the leg at the knee joint. Similarly, the vastus lateralis can pull the patella slightly laterally as the leg extends at the knee joint. The counterbalancing forces of the vastus medialis and the vastus lateralis help to assure that the patella tracks correctly on the femur as the leg extends at the knee joint.

❑ 3. Some sources refer to the upper fibers of the vastus medialis as the *vastus medialis longus* (V.M.L.) and the lower fibers as the *vastus medialis oblique* (V.M.O.) because of the drastic difference in the direction of the upper fibers compared to the lower fibers.

❑ 4. The reason that the quadriceps are so large and strong is not just to move the leg into extension at the knee joint, but rather to do the reverse action, i.e., move the thigh into extension at the knee joint (see page 702). This happens every time a person stands up from a seated position. To move the thigh at the knee joint requires moving the entire body along with the thigh; hence, the quadriceps need to be very large and strong.

❑

VASTUS INTERMEDIUS
(OF THE QUADRICEPS)

❑ **The name, vastus intermedius, tells us that this muscle is vast in size and located between the two other vastus muscles.**

DERIVATION ❑ vastus: L. *vast.*
inter: L. *between.*
medius: L. *middle.*

PRONUNCIATION ❑ **vas**-tus in-ter-**mee**-dee-us

ATTACHMENTS

❑ **Anterior Shaft and Linea Aspera of the Femur**

- ❑ the anterior and lateral surfaces of the femur and the lateral lip of the linea aspera

to the

❑ **Tibial Tuberosity**

- ❑ via the patella and the patellar ligament

ACTION

❑ **Extension of the Leg**

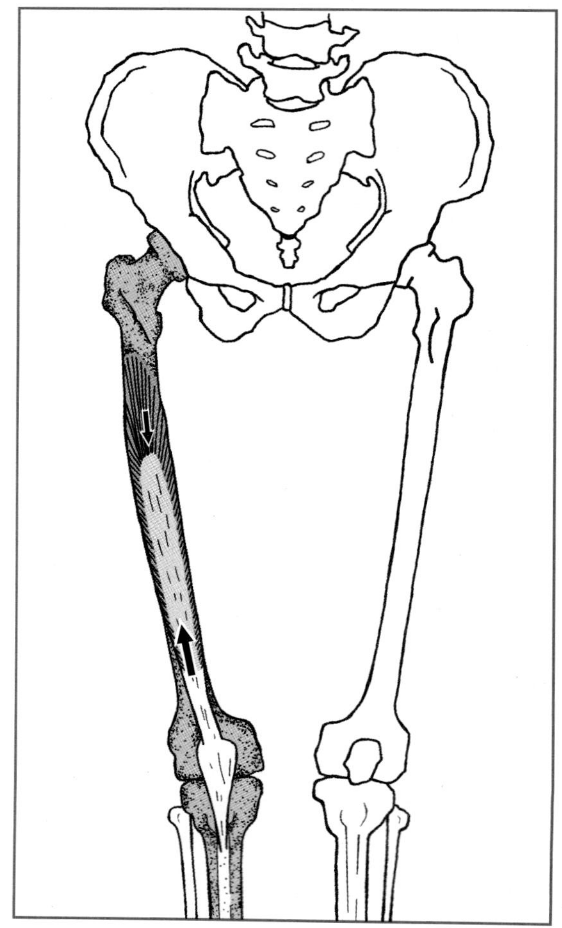

Anterior View of the
Right Vastus Intermedius

INNERVATION ❑ The Femoral Nerve ❑ L2, **3, 4**

ARTERIAL SUPPLY ❑ The Deep Femoral Artery (A Major Branch of the Femoral Artery)

PALPATION AND SUPPLEMENTARY TEXT

PALPATION

- ❑ The vastus intermedius is deep and difficult to palpate. The quadriceps must be relaxed in order to attempt to palpate the vastus intermedius.
  - Have the client supine.
  - Place palpating hand just proximal to the patella.
  - If the rectus femoris can be lifted and/or moved aside, the distal vastus intermedius may be palpated deep to the rectus femoris when approached from either the medial or the lateral side.
  - Use your palpating hand to palpate into the vastus intermedius from the medial and/or lateral side of the rectus femoris.

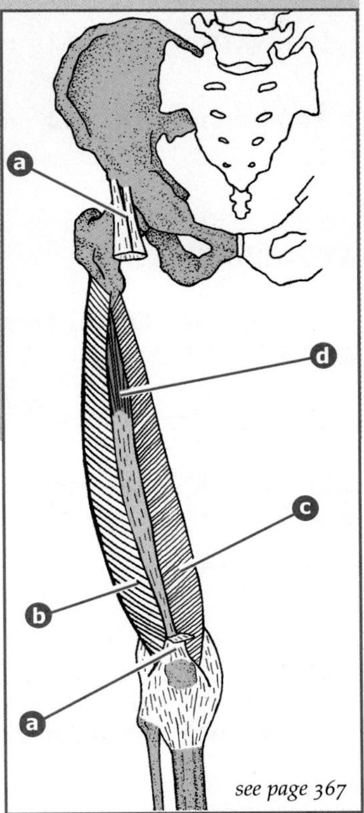

Anterior View of the Right Quadriceps
(rectus femoris cut and reflected)

a. Rectus Femoris (cut and reflected)
b. Vastus Lateralis
c. Vastus Medialis
d. **Vastus Intermedius**

RELATIONSHIP TO OTHER MUSCULOSKELETAL STRUCTURES

❑ 1. The vastus intermedius is deep to the rectus femoris and the vastus lateralis.

❑ 2. Deep to the vastus intermedius is a small muscle called the articularis genus and the femur.

METHODOLOGY FOR LEARNING MUSCLE ACTIONS

❑ **Extension of the Leg at the Knee Joint:** The vastus intermedius crosses the knee joint anteriorly (with its fibers running vertically in the sagittal plane); therefore, it extends the leg at the knee joint.

MISCELLANEOUS

❑ 1. The vastus intermedius somewhat blends into the vastus lateralis and the vastus medialis.

❑ 2. The vastus intermedius sometimes blends with the articularis genus.

❑ 3. The reason that the quadriceps are so large and strong is not just to move the leg into extension at the knee joint, but rather to do the reverse action, i.e., move the thigh into extension at the knee joint (see page 702). This happens every time a person stands up from a seated position. To move the thigh at the knee joint requires moving the entire body along with the thigh; hence, the quadriceps need to be very large and strong.

❑ ARTICULARIS GENUS

❑ **The name, articularis genus, tells us that this muscle is involved with the knee joint.**

DERIVATION ❑ articularis: L. *refers to a joint.*
genu: L. *knee.*

PRONUNCIATION ❑ ar-**tik**-you-**la**-ris **je**-new

ATTACHMENTS

❑ **Anterior Distal Femoral Shaft**

to the

❑ **Joint Capsule of the Knee Joint**

ACTION

❑ **Tenses and Pulls the Joint Capsule of the Knee Joint Proximally**

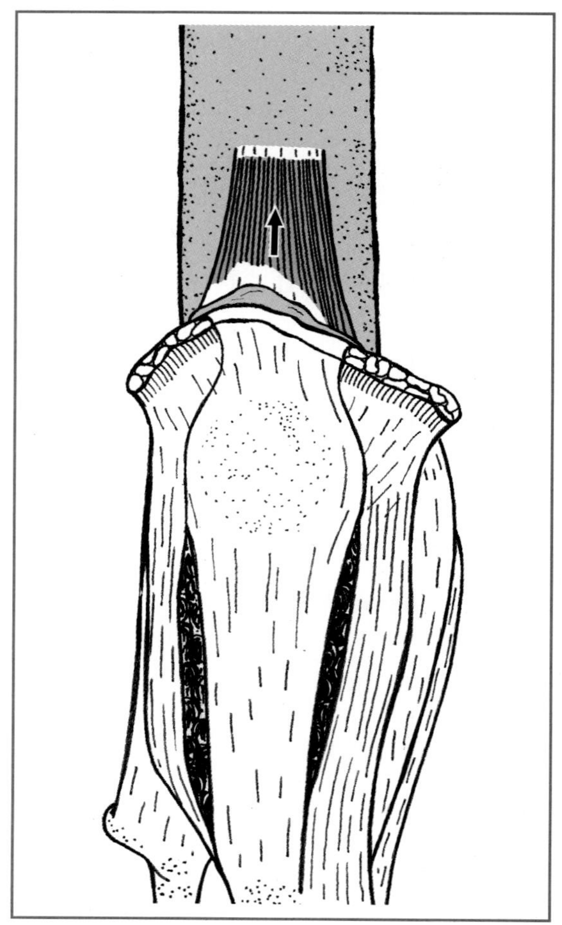

Anterior View of the Right Articularis Genus

INNERVATION ❑ The Femoral Nerve ❑ L2, **3, 4**

ARTERIAL SUPPLY ❑ The Deep Femoral Artery (A Major Branch of the Femoral Artery)

PALPATION AND SUPPLEMENTARY TEXT

PALPATION

- ❑ The articularis genus is a small muscle deep to the rectus femoris and vastus intermedius and is extremely difficult, if not impossible, to palpate.

RELATIONSHIP TO OTHER MUSCULOSKELETAL STRUCTURES

- ❑ 1. The articularis genus is deep to the vastus intermedius.
- ❑ 2. Deep to the articularis genus is the femur.

METHODOLOGY FOR LEARNING MUSCLE ACTIONS

- ❑ **Tenses and Pulls the Joint Capsule of the Knee Joint Proximally:** The articularis genus (with its fibers oriented vertically) pulls its distal attachment, the joint capsule of the knee joint, toward its proximal attachment (the anterior distal shaft of the femur).

MISCELLANEOUS

- ❑ 1. When the knee joint extends, the patella tracks up and down along the femur. The purpose of lifting the joint capsule of the knee joint proximally is to prevent the joint capsule from getting pinched between the patella and the femur during extension of the knee joint.
- ❑ 2. The articularis genus is sometimes a distinct muscle and sometimes it blends with the vastus intermedius.

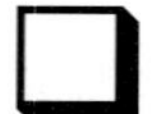

THE ADDUCTORS OF THE THIGH

These muscles are grouped together because they all adduct the thigh at the hip joint, as they all cross the hip joint medially with their fibers running from proximal and medial on the pelvic bone, to distal and lateral on the femur.

THERE ARE FIVE ADDUCTOR MUSCLES OF THE THIGH:	
Pectineus Adductor Longus Gracilis	Adductor Brevis Adductor Magnus

Attachments:

- Anatomically, the adductor muscle group of the thigh makes up the majority of the musculature of the medial thigh. Their relative anatomical relationships from the anterior perspective are as follows:
  - Superficially, from lateral to medial, one will see the pectineus, then the adductor longus, then the gracilis.
  - The adductor brevis is deep to the adductor longus.
  - The adductor magnus is the deepest of the entire group.
- All three "adductor" muscles attach onto the linea aspera of the femur.

Actions:

- All five adductors can also flex the thigh at the hip joint because they are all anterior to the hip joint (except the adductor magnus, which extends the thigh at the hip joint because it is posterior to the hip joint).
- There is some controversy about the role of all three "adductors" (adductor longus, adductor brevis, and adductor magnus) regarding rotation of the thigh at the hip joint. Some sources state these three adductor muscles medially rotate the thigh at the hip joint; other sources state that they laterally rotate the thigh at the hip joint. Although the evidence is not yet conclusive, much of the confusion arises due to the difference between the shaft of the femur and the mechanical axis of the femur. Usually, the mechanical axis of a long bone runs through its shaft. However, due to the change in angulation between the neck and the shaft of the femur, the mechanical axis of the femur lies posterior to its shaft. (The mechanical axis can be determined by drawing a line from the center of the femoral head to the midpoint between the femoral condyles.)

  When one first looks at the attachment of these three adductors onto the linea aspera of the femur, it seems that their attachment site is posterior to the axis of the femur, and therefore, they should laterally rotate the femur. However, considering that the mechanical axis is posterior to the shaft of the femur, the attachment of the adductors onto the linea aspera is actually anterior to the mechanical axis of the femur. For this reason, the weight of the evidence seems to favor the adductors' role as medial rotators of the thigh at the hip joint. (However, if the position of the femur changes, the relationship between the attachment site of the adductors and the mechanical axis of the femur changes, and therefore, the role of the three adductors can change to that of lateral rotation of the thigh at the hip joint.)

Miscellaneous:

- When the adductor muscles are strained and pain is felt at their proximal attachment, it is usually called a *groin pull* in lay terms.
- Although the obturator externus, quadratus femoris and the lower fibers of the gluteus maximus can also adduct the thigh, they are not considered to be part of the adductor group, proper.
- The gracilis muscle is also known as the *adductor gracilis*.

INNERVATION	The adductors are innervated by the obturator nerve except the pectineus, which is innervated by the femoral nerve. (The adductor magnus is innervated by the obturator nerve and the sciatic nerve.)
ARTERIAL SUPPLY	The adductors receive the majority of their blood supply from the deep femoral artery.

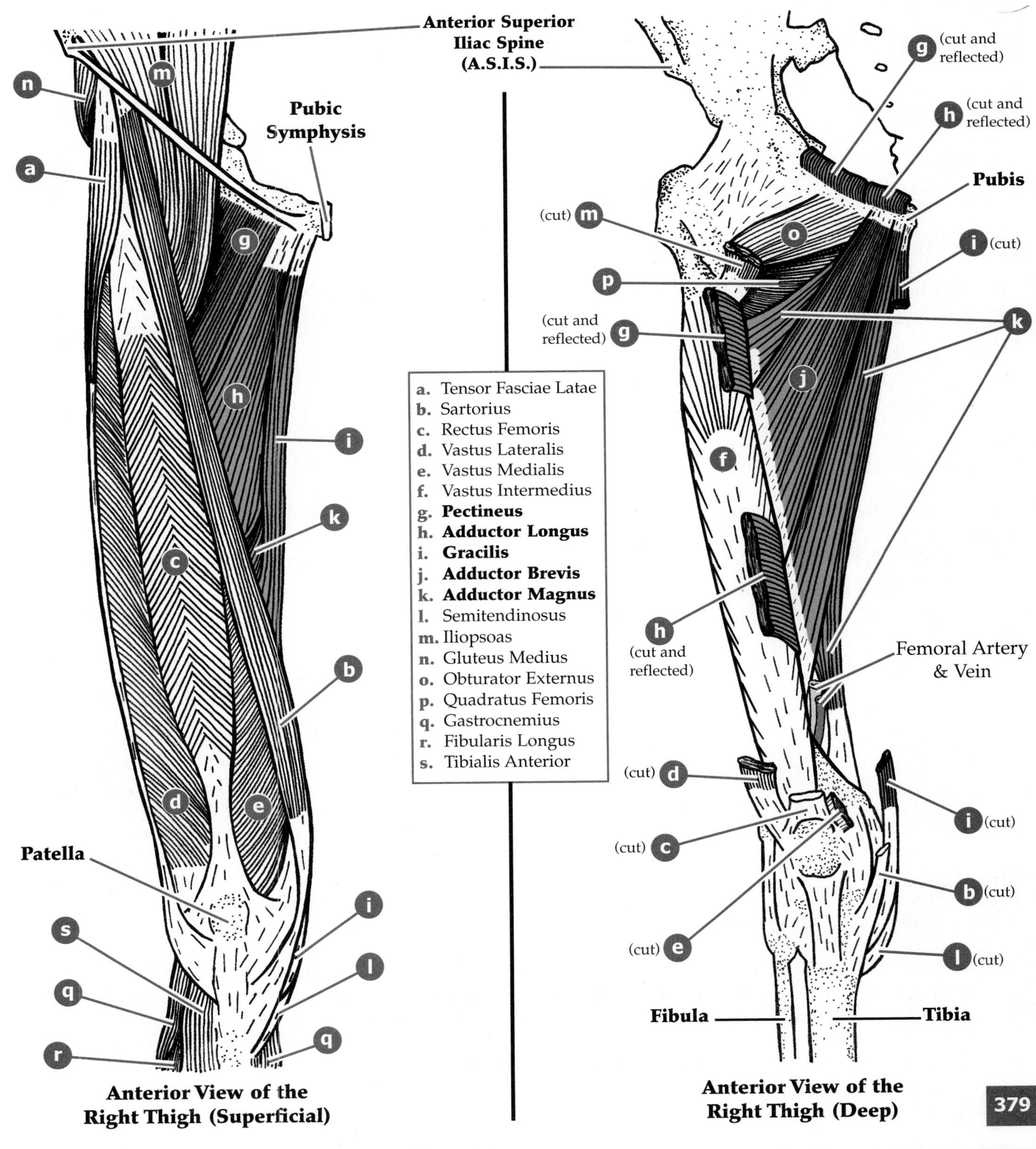

Anterior View of the Right Thigh (Superficial)

Anterior View of the Right Thigh (Deep)

❑

PECTINEUS

(OF THE ADDUCTOR GROUP)

❑ **The name, pectineus, means comb. This muscle has a comb-like appearance because the flat bands of its muscle fibers form a flat surface as they leave the pubic bone.**

DERIVATION ❑ pectineus: L. *comb.* **PRONUNCIATION** ❑ pek-**tin**-ee-us

ATTACHMENTS

❑ **Pubis**

❑ the pectineal line on the superior pubic ramus

to the

❑ **Proximal Posterior Shaft of the Femur**

❑ the pectineal line of the femur

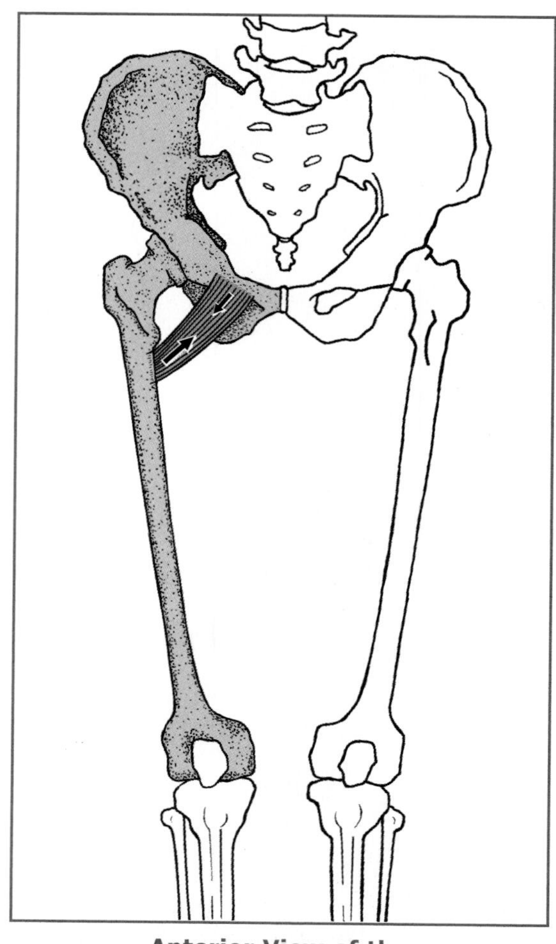

Anterior View of the Right Pectineus

ACTIONS

❑ 1. **Adduction of the Thigh**

❑ 2. **Flexion of the Thigh**

❑ 3. **Anterior Tilt of the Pelvis**

INNERVATION ❑ The Femoral Nerve ❑ **L2**, 3

ARTERIAL SUPPLY ❑ The Femoral Artery (The Continuation of the External Iliac Artery) and the Deep Femoral Artery (A Major Branch of the Femoral Artery)
❑ and the obturator artery (a branch of the internal iliac artery)

PALPATION AND SUPPLEMENTARY TEXT

PALPATION

❑ Although much of the pectineus is superficial, it can be a bit difficult to distinguish from the other adductors of the thigh.

- Have the client supine.
- Place palpating hand just lateral to the pubic tubercle (the most prominent aspect of the pubis anteriorly) and feel for the pectineus.
- Continue palpating just lateral and slightly proximal to the adductor longus (see the palpation section for this muscle on page 383).

  (Note: The adductor longus' tendon is the most prominent tendon in the groin region.)
- To further bring out the pectineus, ask the client to actively adduct the thigh at the hip joint. Keep in mind that active thigh adduction will cause all the thigh adductors to contract.

  (Note: Be careful with palpation in the proximal anterior thigh because the femoral nerve, artery and vein lie over the iliopsoas and pectineus here. See illustration on page 352.)

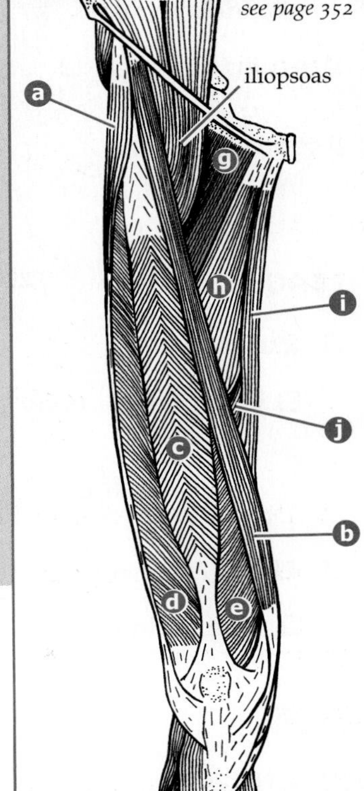

Anterior View of the Right Thigh (Superficial)

a. Tensor Fasciae Latae
b. Sartorius
c. Rectus Femoris
d. Vastus Lateralis
e. Vastus Medialis
f. Vastus Intermedius (not seen)
g. **Pectineus**
h. Adductor Longus
i. Gracilis
j. Adductor Magnus

RELATIONSHIP TO OTHER MUSCULOSKELETAL STRUCTURES

❑ 1. In the proximal anteromedial thigh, part of the pectineus is superficial and lies medial to the iliopsoas and lateral to the adductor longus.

❑ 2. The lateral part of the pectineus lies deep to the iliopsoas.

❑ 3. From the anterior perspective, the obturator externus and the quadratus femoris are directly deep to the pectineus.

METHODOLOGY FOR LEARNING MUSCLE ACTIONS

❑ 1. **Adduction of the Thigh at the Hip Joint:** The pectineus crosses the hip joint medially (with its fibers running somewhat horizontally in the frontal plane); therefore, it adducts the thigh at the hip joint.

❑ 2. **Flexion of the Thigh at the Hip Joint:** The pectineus crosses the hip joint anteriorly (with its fibers running vertically in the sagittal plane); therefore, it flexes the thigh at the hip joint.

❑ 3. **Anterior Tilt of the Pelvis at the Hip Joint:** With the distal attachment fixed, the pectineus, by pulling inferiorly on the anterior pelvis, anteriorly tilts the pelvis at the hip joint.

MISCELLANEOUS

❑ 1. Although some sources do not include it, the pectineus belongs in the adductor group of muscles (adductor longus, brevis, magnus and gracilis). Note the similarity of the direction of fibers of the pectineus to the direction of fibers of the adductor longus.

❑ 2. Do not confuse the pectineal line of the pubis (which is along the superior pubic ramus and is also known as the pecten of the pubis) with the pectineal line of the femur (which runs on the posterior femur between the lesser trochanter and the linea aspera of the femur).

❑ ADDUCTOR LONGUS

(OF THE ADDUCTOR GROUP)

❑ **The name, adductor longus, tells us that this muscle is an adductor and is long (longer than the adductor brevis).**

DERIVATION ❑ adductor: L. *a muscle that adducts a body part.*
longus: L. *long.*

PRONUNCIATION ❑ ad-**duk**-tor **long**-us

ATTACHMENTS

❑ **Pubis**

- ❑ the anterior body

to the

❑ **Linea Aspera of the Femur**

- ❑ the middle 1/3 at the medial lip

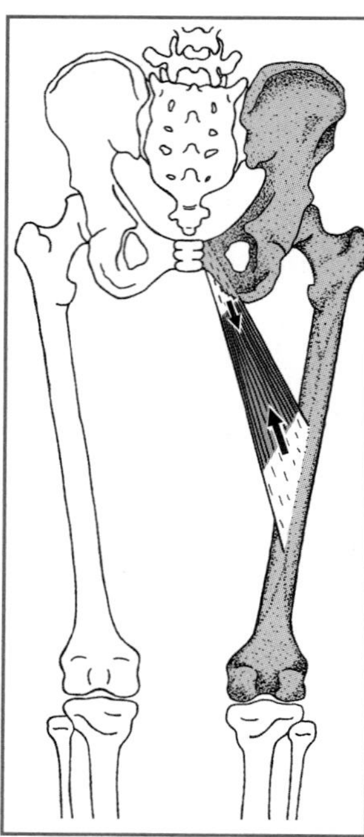

Posterior View of the Right Adductor Longus

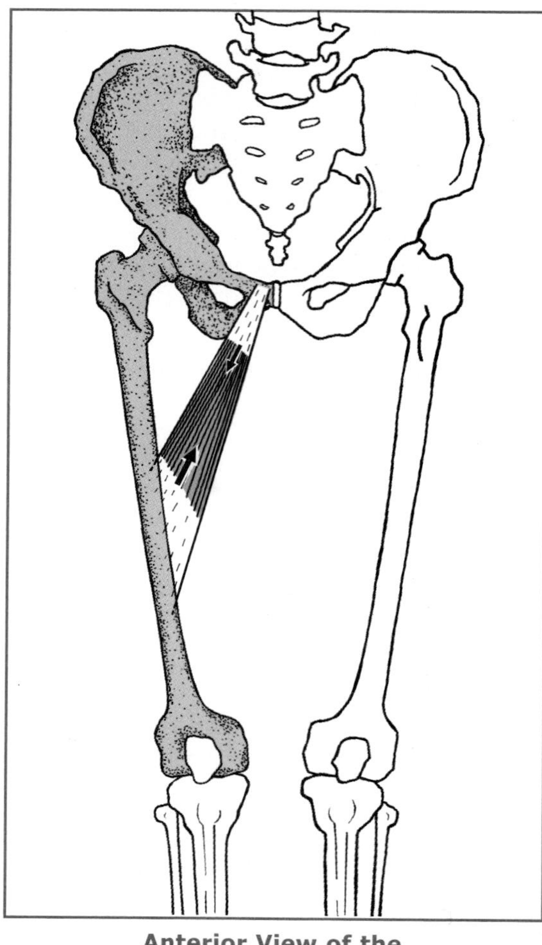

Anterior View of the Right Adductor Longus

ACTIONS

❑ 1. **Adduction of the Thigh**

❑ 2. **Flexion of the Thigh**

❑ 3. **Anterior Tilt of the Pelvis**

INNERVATION ❑ The Obturator Nerve ❑ **L2, 3,** 4

ARTERIAL SUPPLY ❑ The Femoral Artery (The Continuation of the External Iliac Artery) and the Deep Femoral Artery (A Major Branch of the Femoral Artery)
❑ and the obturator artery (a branch of the internal iliac artery)

PALPATION AND SUPPLEMENTARY TEXT

PALPATION

- ❑ The adductor longus has the most prominent tendon in the groin region.
  - Have the client supine.
  - Place palpating hand on the proximal anteromedial thigh.
  - Ask the client to actively adduct the thigh at the hip joint and feel for the proximal tendon of the adductor longus. It will be the most prominent tendon in the proximal anteromedial thigh.
  - Once located, follow the adductor longus' tendon proximally toward the pubis.
  - Next, try to follow the adductor longus distally as far as possible. At a certain point, the adductor longus will be posterior (deep) to the sartorius.

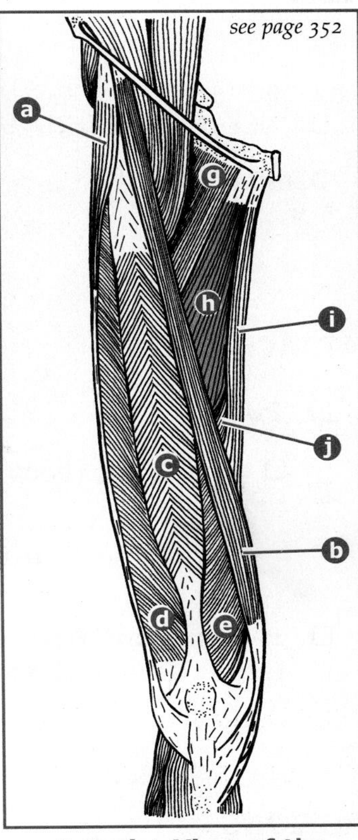

Anterior View of the Right Thigh (Superficial)

a. Tensor Fasciae Latae
b. Sartorius
c. Rectus Femoris
d. Vastus Lateralis
e. Vastus Medialis
f. Vastus Intermedius (not seen)
g. Pectineus
h. Adductor Longus
i. Gracilis
j. Adductor Magnus

RELATIONSHIP TO OTHER MUSCULOSKELETAL STRUCTURES

❑ 1. Much of the adductor longus is superficial in the proximal anteromedial thigh.

❑ 2. The adductor longus is medial to the pectineus and lateral to the gracilis.

❑ 3. From the anterior perspective, the adductor brevis is directly deep to the adductor longus. (The adductor magnus is directly deep to the adductor brevis.)

❑ 4. All three "adductors" attach distally onto the linea aspera. The attachment of the adductor longus on the linea aspera is the most medial of the three adductor muscles.

❑ 5. The vastus medialis attaches onto the medial lip of the linea aspera, medial to the adductor longus.

METHODOLOGY FOR LEARNING MUSCLE ACTIONS

❑ **1. Adduction of the Thigh at the Hip Joint:** The adductor longus crosses the hip joint medially (with its fibers running somewhat horizontally in the frontal plane); therefore, it adducts the thigh at the hip joint.

❑ **2. Flexion of the Thigh at the Hip Joint:** The adductor longus crosses the hip joint anteriorly (with its fibers running vertically in the sagittal plane); therefore, it flexes the thigh at the hip joint.

❑ **3. Anterior Tilt of the Pelvis at the Hip Joint:** With the distal attachment fixed, the adductor longus, by pulling inferiorly on the anterior pelvis, anteriorly tilts the pelvis at the hip joint.

MISCELLANEOUS

❑ 1. The adductor longus has the most prominent proximal tendon in the groin region.

❑ 2. The attachment of the adductor longus at the linea aspera often blends with the attachment of the vastus medialis.

❑

GRACILIS
(OF THE ADDUCTOR GROUP)

❑ **The name, gracilis, tells us that the shape of this muscle is slender and graceful.**

DERIVATION ❑ gracilis: L. *slender, graceful.* **PRONUNCIATION** ❑ gra-**sil**-is

ATTACHMENTS

❑ **Pubis**

- ❑ the anterior body and the inferior ramus

to the

❑ **Pes Anserine Tendon (at the Proximal Anteromedial Tibia)**

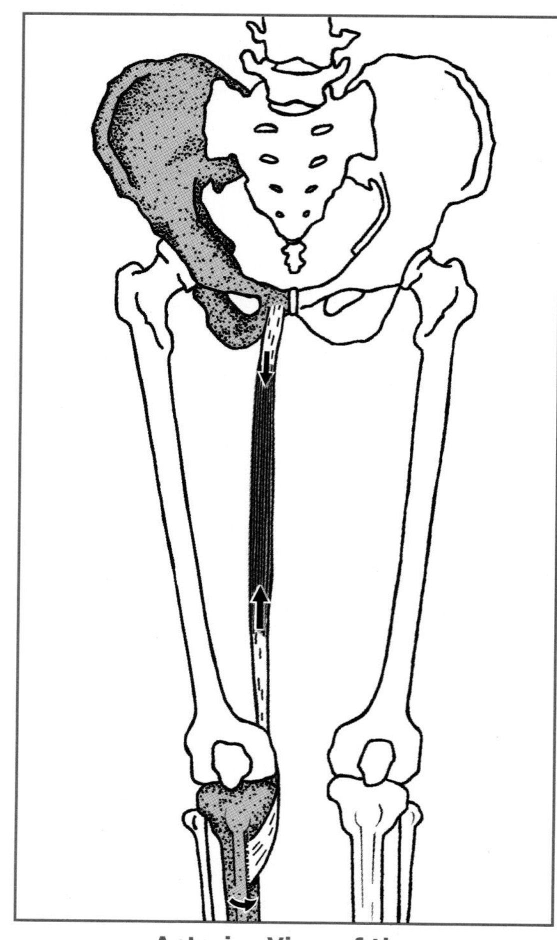

Anterior View of the Right Gracilis

ACTIONS

❑ 1. **Adduction of the Thigh**

❑ 2. **Flexion of the Thigh**

❑ 3. **Flexion of the Leg**

❑ 4. **Anterior Tilt of the Pelvis**

❑ 5. Medial Rotation of the Leg

INNERVATION ❑ The Obturator Nerve ❑ L2, 3

ARTERIAL SUPPLY ❑ The Deep Femoral Artery (A Major Branch of the Femoral Artery)
❑ and the obturator artery (a branch of the internal iliac artery)

PALPATION AND SUPPLEMENTARY TEXT

PALPATION

- ❑ The gracilis is located in the medial thigh and is superficial for its entire course.
  - Have the client seated.
  - Place palpating hand on the distal posteromedial thigh.
  - Ask the client to actively flex the leg at the knee joint. The gracilis and semitendinosus tendons will clearly be palpable. The gracilis will be the smaller and slightly more medial one of the two.
  - Once located, continue palpating the gracilis proximally toward the pubic bone.
  - To further bring out the gracilis, resistance can be added.

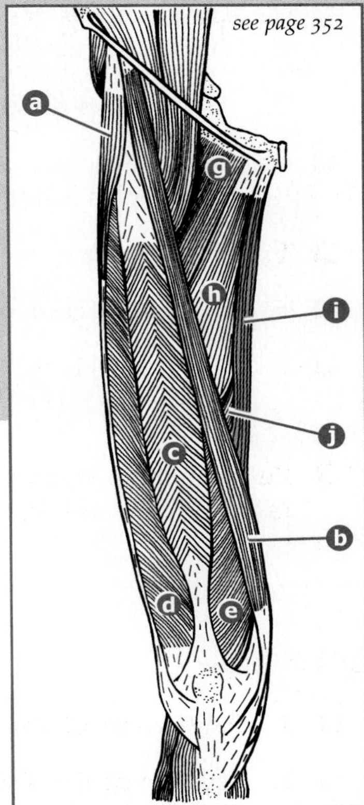

Anterior View of the Right Thigh (Superficial)

- **a.** Tensor Fasciae Latae
- **b.** Sartorius
- **c.** Rectus Femoris
- **d.** Vastus Lateralis
- **e.** Vastus Medialis
- **f.** Vastus Intermedius (not seen)
- **g.** Pectineus
- **h.** Adductor Longus
- **i.** **Gracilis**
- **j.** Adductor Magnus

RELATIONSHIP TO OTHER MUSCULOSKELETAL STRUCTURES

❑ 1. The gracilis is located in the medial thigh and is superficial for its entire course.

❑ 2. Proximally, the adductor longus is anterior and lateral to the gracilis. More distally, the sartorius is anterior to the gracilis.

❑ 3. Proximally, the adductor magnus is posterior to the gracilis. More distally, the semimembranosus and the semitendinosus are posterior to the gracilis.

❑ 4. The gracilis is one of three muscles that attach into the pes anserine tendon, and it attaches between the sartorius and the semitendinosus.

METHODOLOGY FOR LEARNING MUSCLE ACTIONS

❑ 1. **Adduction of the Thigh at the Hip Joint:** The gracilis crosses the hip joint medially (with its fibers running somewhat horizontally in the frontal plane); therefore, it adducts the thigh at the hip joint.

❑ 2. **Flexion of the Thigh at the Hip Joint:** The gracilis crosses the hip joint anteriorly (with its fibers running vertically in the sagittal plane); therefore, it flexes the thigh at the hip joint.

❑ 3. **Flexion of the Leg at the Knee Joint:** The gracilis crosses the knee joint posteriorly (with its fibers running vertically in the sagittal plane); therefore, it flexes the leg at the knee joint.

❑ 4. **Anterior Tilt of the Pelvis at the Hip Joint:** With the distal attachment fixed, the gracilis, by pulling inferiorly on the anterior pelvis, anteriorly tilts the pelvis at the hip joint.

❑ 5. **Medial Rotation of the Leg at the Knee Joint:** The gracilis crosses the knee joint medially from posterior to anterior (with its fibers running somewhat horizontally in the transverse plane) to attach into the pes anserine tendon at the medial tibia. When the gracilis pulls at the tibial attachment, the tibial attachment rotates posteromedially, causing the anterior tibia to face somewhat medially. Therefore, the gracilis medially rotates the leg at the knee joint.

GRACILIS – continued

MISCELLANEOUS

- ❑ 1. The gracilis is also known as the *adductor gracilis*.
- ❑ 2. The gracilis is one of three muscles that attach into the pes anserine tendon. The other two muscles that attach here are the sartorius and the semitendinosus.
- ❑ 3. All three pes anserine muscles flex and medially rotate the leg at the knee joint.
- ❑ 4. Of the muscles that attach into the pes anserine, the **S**artorius attaches the most anterior of the three, the **G**racilis is in the middle, and the **S**emitendinosus attaches the most posterior. (Think **SGS**. ☺)
- ❑ 5. "Pes Anserine" means goose foot.
- ❑ 6. The major action of the gracilis is adduction of the thigh.
- ❑ 7. The gracilis is the second longest muscle in the human body. (The sartorius is the longest.)

ADDUCTOR BREVIS

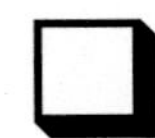

(OF THE ADDUCTOR GROUP)

❑ **The name, adductor brevis, tells us that this muscle is an adductor and is short (shorter than the adductor longus).**

DERIVATION ❑ adductor: L. *a muscle that adducts a body part.*
brevis: L. *short.*

PRONUNCIATION ❑ ad-**duk**-tor **bre**-vis

ATTACHMENTS

❑ **Pubis**

- ❑ the inferior ramus

to the

❑ **Linea Aspera of the Femur**

- ❑ the proximal 1/3

ACTIONS

❑ **1. Adduction of the Thigh**

❑ **2. Flexion of the Thigh**

❑ **3. Anterior Tilt of the Pelvis**

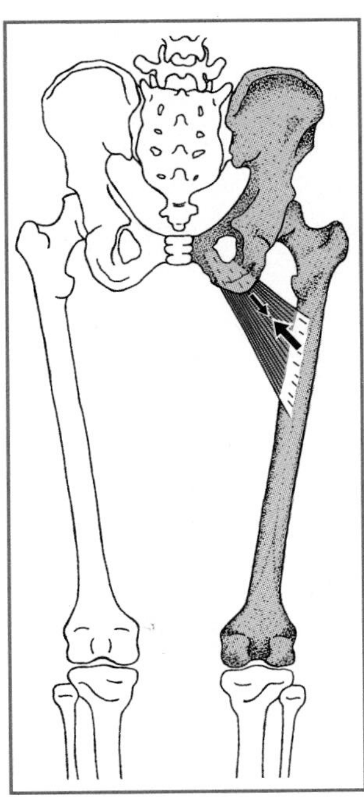

Posterior View of the Right Adductor Brevis

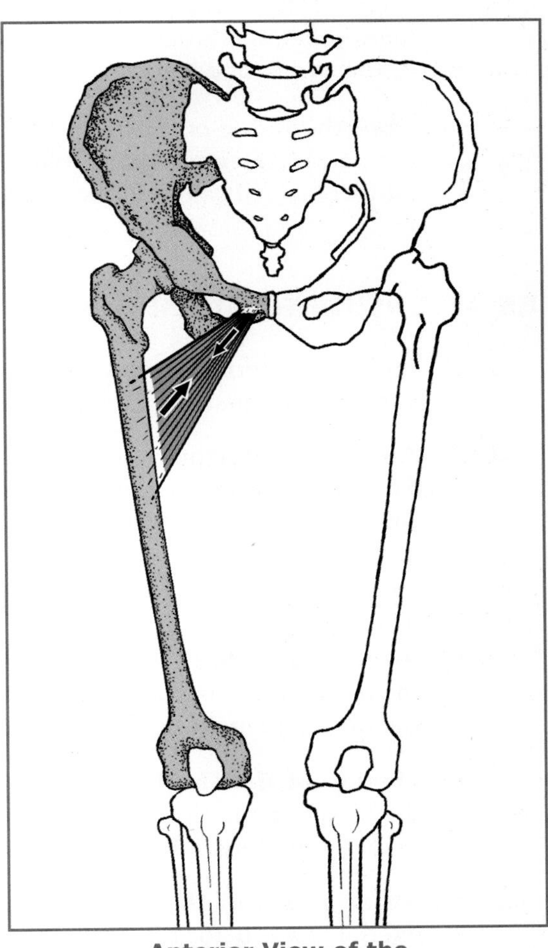

Anterior View of the Right Adductor Brevis

INNERVATION ❑ The Obturator Nerve ❑ L2, 3

ARTERIAL SUPPLY ❑ The Femoral Artery (The Continuation of the External Iliac Artery) and the Deep Femoral Artery (A Major Branch of the Femoral Artery)
❑ and the obturator artery (a branch of the internal iliac artery)

ADDUCTOR BREVIS – PALPATION AND SUPPLEMENTARY TEXT

PALPATION

- ❑ The adductor brevis is difficult to distinguish from the other adductors.
  - Have the client supine.
  - Place palpating hand on the proximal tendon of the adductor longus (see the palpation section for this muscle on page 383). The proximal tendon of the adductor longus is the most prominent tendon in the groin region.
  - Once the proximal tendon of the adductor longus is located, palpate for the adductor brevis deep to the adductor longus. The proximal tendon of the adductor brevis is slightly lateral to the proximal tendon of the adductor longus.
  - To further bring out the adductor brevis, ask the client to actively adduct the thigh at the hip joint. Keep in mind that active thigh adduction will cause all the thigh adductors to contract.

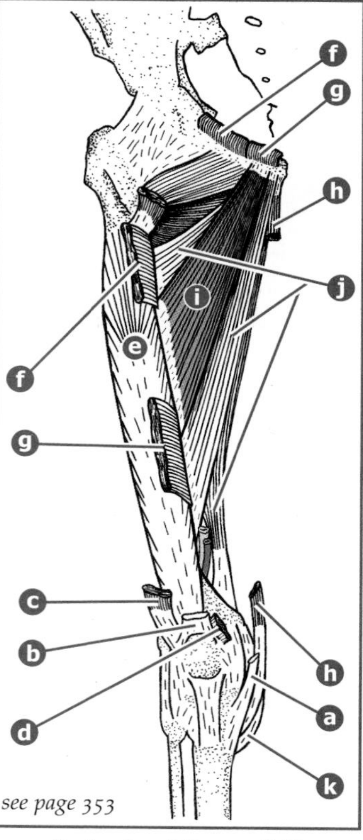

see page 353

Anterior View of the Right Thigh (Deep)

a. Sartorius (cut)
b. Rectus Femoris (cut)
c. Vastus Lateralis (cut)
d. Vastus Medialis (cut)
e. Vastus Intermedius
f. Pectineus (cut and reflected)
g. Adductor Longus (cut and reflected)
h. Gracilis (cut)
i. **Adductor Brevis**
j. Adductor Magnus
k. Semitendinosus

RELATIONSHIP TO OTHER MUSCULOSKELETAL STRUCTURES

❑ 1. From the anterior perspective, the adductor brevis is deep to the adductor longus and superficial to the adductor magnus.

❑ 2. All three "adductors" attach distally onto the linea aspera. The adductor brevis attaches onto the linea aspera between the attachments of the adductor longus and adductor magnus.

METHODOLOGY FOR LEARNING MUSCLE ACTIONS

❑ 1. **Adduction of the Thigh at the Hip Joint:** The adductor brevis crosses the hip joint medially (with its fibers running somewhat horizontally in the frontal plane); therefore, it adducts the thigh at the hip joint.

❑ 2. **Flexion of the Thigh at the Hip Joint:** The adductor brevis crosses the hip joint anteriorly (with its fibers running vertically in the sagittal plane); therefore, it flexes the thigh at the hip joint.

❑ 3. **Anterior Tilt of the Pelvis at the Hip Joint:** With the distal attachment fixed, the adductor brevis, by pulling inferiorly on the anterior pelvis, anteriorly tilts the pelvis at the hip joint.

MISCELLANEOUS

❑ The adductor brevis is located between the adductor longus and the adductor magnus.

ADDUCTOR MAGNUS

(OF THE ADDUCTOR GROUP)

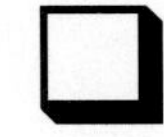

❑ **The name, adductor magnus, tells us that this muscle is an adductor and is large (larger than the adductor longus and the adductor brevis).**

DERIVATION ❑ adductor: L. *a muscle that adducts a body part.*
magnus: L. *great, large.*

PRONUNCIATION ❑ ad-**duk**-tor **mag**-nus

ATTACHMENTS

❑ **Pubis and Ischial Tuberosity**

❑ the inferior ramus of the pubis and the ramus of the ischium

to the

❑ **Linea Aspera of the Femur**

❑ and the gluteal tuberosity, medial supracondylar line and adductor tubercle of the femur

ACTIONS

❑ 1. **Adduction of the Thigh**

❑ 2. **Extension of the Thigh**

❑ 3. **Posterior Tilt of the Pelvis**

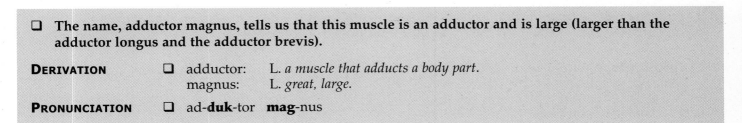

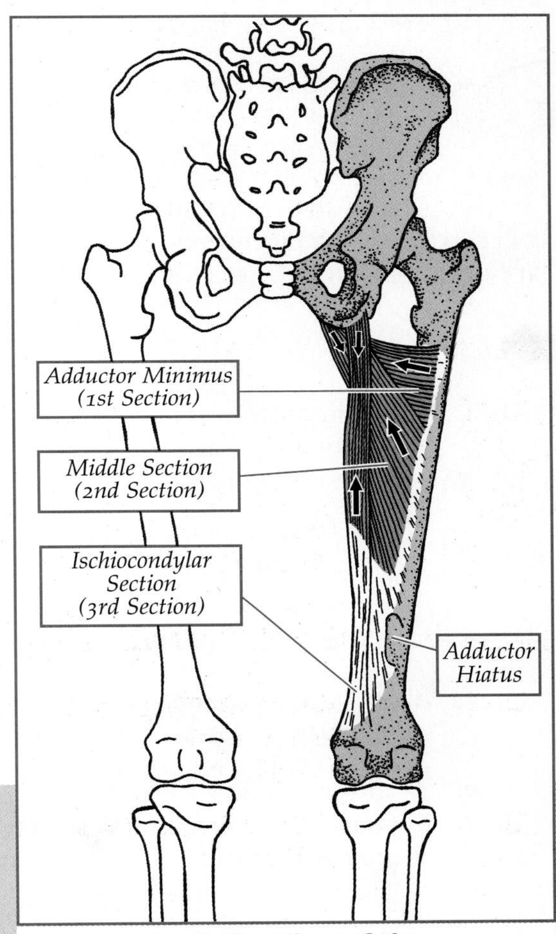

Posterior View of the Right Adductor Magnus

INNERVATION ❑ The Obturator Nerve and the Sciatic Nerve
- ❑ the obturator branch innervates the first two sections
- ❑ the tibial branch of the sciatic nerve innervates the third section
- ❑ **L2, 3,** 4

ARTERIAL SUPPLY

Pubic and Ischial Ramus Fibers:

❑ The Femoral Artery (The Continuation of the External Iliac Artery) and the Deep Femoral Artery (A Major Branch of the Femoral Artery)
- ❑ and the obturator artery (a branch of the internal iliac artery)

Ischial Tuberosity Fibers:

❑ The Deep Femoral Artery (A Major Branch of the Femoral Artery) and the Inferior Gluteal Artery (A Branch of the Internal Iliac Artery)
- ❑ and the obturator artery (a branch of the internal iliac artery) and branches of the popliteal artery (the continuation of the femoral artery)

ADDUCTOR MAGNUS – PALPATION AND SUPPLEMENTARY TEXT

PALPATION

The adductor magnus is difficult to palpate in its entirety since it is a deep muscle from most every perspective. However, portions of it are superficial and can be easily palpated.

❑ **Posteriorly:** A portion of the adductor magnus is superficial in the proximal 1/2 of the posteromedial thigh (see illustration on page 357).

- Have the client prone.
- Place palpating hand on the proximal posteromedial thigh.
- Palpate distal to the gluteus maximus, posterior to the gracilis, and anterior to the semitendinosus and semimembranosus (see the palpation sections for these muscles on pages 317, 385, 398, and 401 respectively).
- The adductor magnus may also be palpated posteriorly at the adductor tubercle on the medial condyle of the femur.
- To further bring out the adductor magnus, ask the client to actively adduct the thigh at the hip joint. Resistance may also be added. Keep in mind that active thigh adduction will cause all the thigh adductors to contract.

❑ **Anteriorly:** A portion of the adductor magnus is superficial in the proximal 1/2 of the posteromedial thigh (posterior to the gracilis and anterior to the semitendinosus and semimembranosus, see the palpation sections for these muscles on pages 385, 398, and 401 respectively).

- Have the client supine.
- Place palpating hand posterior to the gracilis and anterior to the semitendinosus and semimembranosus and feel for the adductor magnus.
- To further bring out the adductor magnus, ask the client to actively adduct the thigh at the hip joint. Resistance may also be added. Keep in mind that active thigh adduction will cause all the thigh adductors to contract.

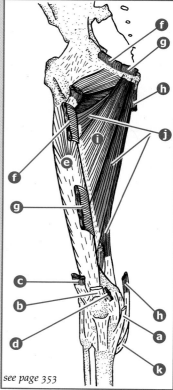

see page 353

Anterior View of the Right Thigh (Deep)

a. Sartorius (cut)
b. Rectus Femoris (cut)
c. Vastus Lateralis (cut)
d. Vastus Medialis (cut)
e. Vastus Intermedius
f. Pectineus (cut and reflected)
g. Adductor Longus (cut and reflected)
h. Gracilis (cut)
i. Adductor Brevis
j. **Adductor Magnus**
k. Semitendinosus

RELATIONSHIP TO OTHER MUSCULOSKELETAL STRUCTURES

❑ 1. From the anterior perspective, the adductor magnus is deep to the pectineus, the adductor longus and the adductor brevis. (There is a small portion of the adductor magnus that is superficial from the anterior perspective between the sartorius, adductor longus and the gracilis, see illustration on page 352.)

ADDUCTOR MAGNUS – continued

- ❑ 2. From the posterior perspective, the adductor magnus is deep to all three hamstring muscles. (There is a portion of the adductor magnus that is superficial from the posterior perspective between the gluteus maximus, gracilis, semitendinosus and the semimembranosus, see illustration on page 354.)
- ❑ 3. All three "adductors" attach distally onto the linea aspera. The adductor longus and adductor brevis attach directly medial to the adductor magnus on the linea aspera of the femur.
- ❑ 4. The gluteus maximus and the short head of the biceps femoris attach directly lateral to the adductor magnus onto the femur. (They attach onto the gluteal tuberosity and the linea aspera of the femur.)
- ❑ 5. The obturator externus and the quadratus femoris lie directly proximal to the adductor magnus.

METHODOLOGY FOR LEARNING MUSCLE ACTIONS

- ❑ **1. Adduction of the Thigh at the Hip Joint:** The adductor magnus crosses the hip joint medially (with its fibers running somewhat horizontally in the frontal plane); therefore, it adducts the thigh at the hip joint.
- ❑ **2. Extension of the Thigh at the Hip Joint:** The adductor magnus crosses the hip joint posteriorly (with its fibers running vertically in the sagittal plane); therefore, it extends the thigh at the hip joint.
- ❑ **3. Posterior Tilt of the Pelvis at the Hip Joint:** With the distal attachment fixed, the adductor magnus, by pulling inferiorly on the posterior pelvis, posteriorly tilts the pelvis at the hip joint.

MISCELLANEOUS

- ❑ 1. The adductor magnus has three sections.
- ❑ 2. The first section of the adductor magnus is sometimes referred to as the *adductor minimus*.
- ❑ 3. The second and third sections (the middle section and the ischiocondylar section) are separated by a hiatus called the *adductor hiatus*.
- ❑ 4. The femoral artery and vein pass through the adductor hiatus becoming the popliteal artery and vein.
- ❑ 5. The third section of the adductor magnus is called the *ischiocondylar section* because it attaches from the ischial tuberosity to the adductor tubercle, which is on the medial condyle of the femur.
- ❑ 6. Some sources state that the most anterior fibers of the adductor magnus can flex the thigh at the hip joint.

THE HAMSTRINGS

The hamstrings are a group of muscles in the posterior thigh.

THERE ARE THREE HAMSTRING MUSCLES:		
Biceps Femoris	Semitendinosus	Semimembranosus

Attachments:

- These muscles are grouped together as the hamstrings because they all attach proximally onto the ischial tuberosity.
- The semitendinosus and the semimembranosus are located medially in the posterior thigh and are sometimes referred to as the *medial hamstrings*.
- The biceps femoris is located laterally in the posterior thigh and is sometimes referred to as the *lateral hamstrings*. (Hamstrings is plural because the biceps femoris has two heads.)
- The biceps femoris and the semitendinosus are more superficial and the semimembranosus is deeper.

Actions:

- As a group, all three hamstrings flex the leg at the knee joint.
- As a group, all three hamstrings (except the short head of the biceps femoris) extend the thigh at the hip joint and/or posteriorly tilt the pelvis at the hip joint.

Miscellaneous:

- The hamstrings, as a group, were given this name because butchers used to hang the carcass of a pig by the hamstring tendons.

INNERVATION The three hamstrings are innervated by the sciatic nerve.

ARTERIAL SUPPLY The upper 1/3 of the hamstrings receives its arterial supply from the inferior gluteal artery and the obturator artery.

The middle 1/3 of the hamstrings receives its arterial supply from perforating branches of the deep femoral artery.

The distal 1/3 of the hamstrings receives its arterial supply from the popliteal artery.

VIEWS OF THE HAMSTRINGS

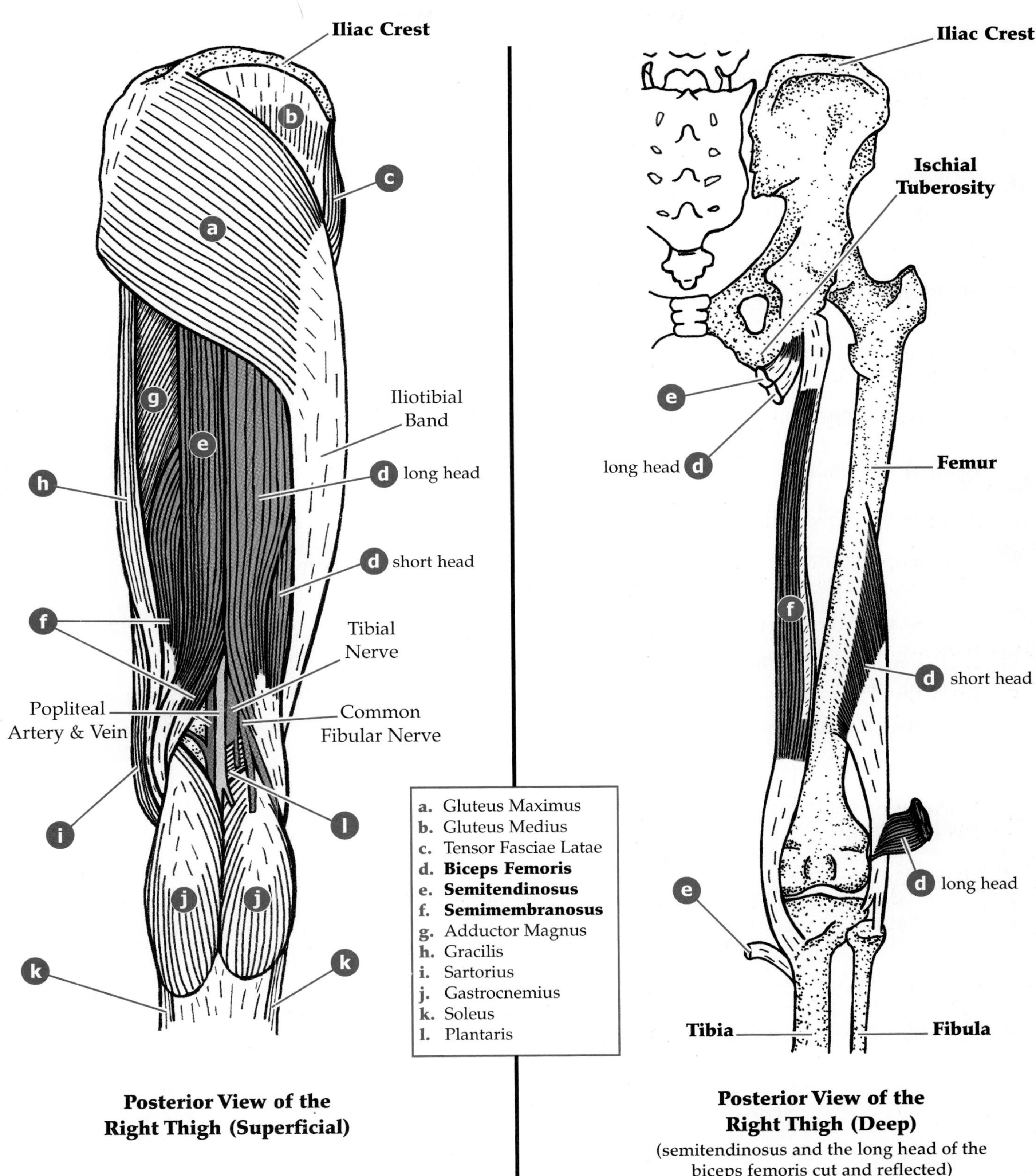

Posterior View of the Right Thigh (Superficial)

Posterior View of the Right Thigh (Deep)
(semitendinosus and the long head of the biceps femoris cut and reflected)

❑

BICEPS FEMORIS
(OF THE HAMSTRING GROUP)

❑ **The name, biceps femoris, tells us that this muscle has two heads and lies over the femur.**

DERIVATION ❑ biceps: L. *two heads.*
femoris: L. *refers to the femur.*

PRONUNCIATION ❑ **by**-seps **fem**-o-ris

ATTACHMENTS

❑ **Long Head: Ischial Tuberosity**

❑ and the sacrotuberous ligament

❑ **Short Head: Linea Aspera**

❑ and the lateral supracondylar line of the femur

to the

❑ **Head of the Fibula**

❑ and the lateral tibial condyle

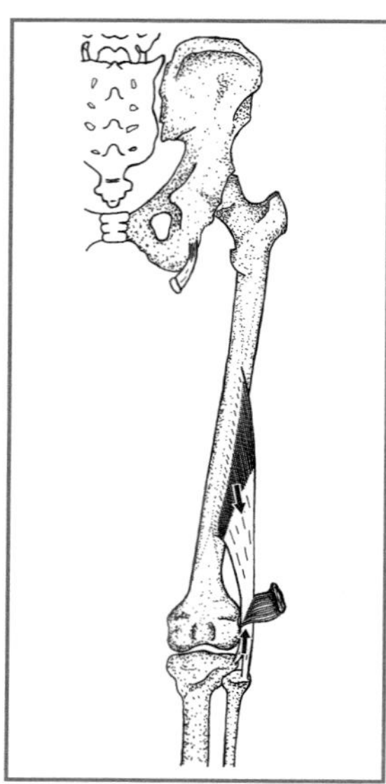

Posterior View of the Right Biceps Femoris Short Head
(biceps femoris long head cut and reflected)

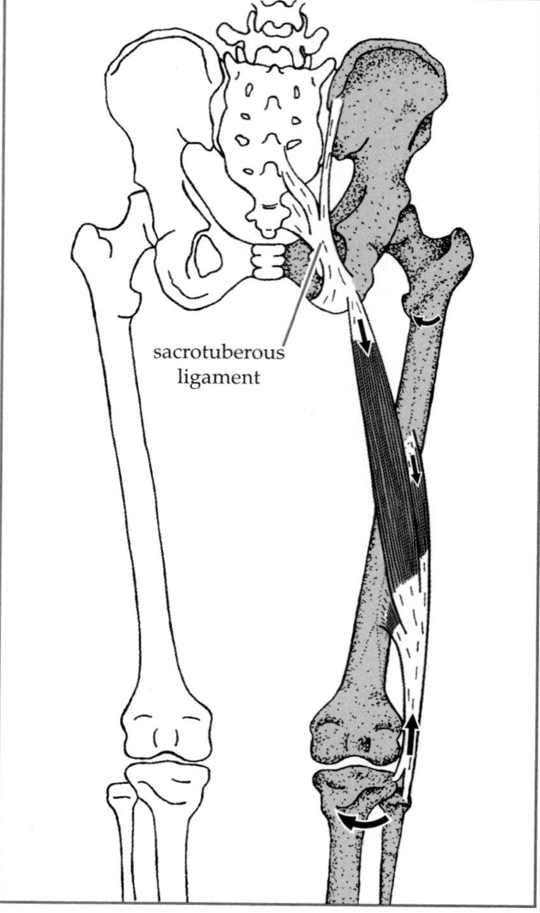

Posterior View of the Right Biceps Femoris

ACTIONS

❑ 1. **Flexion of the Leg (entire muscle)**

❑ 2. **Extension of the Thigh (long head)**

❑ 3. **Posterior Tilt of the Pelvis (long head)**

❑ 4. Lateral Rotation of the Leg (entire muscle)

❑ 5. Adduction of the Thigh (long head)

❑ 6. Lateral Rotation of the Thigh (long head)

INNERVATION

❑ The Sciatic Nerve
❑ the tibial nerve and the common fibular nerve; L5, **S1**, 2

ARTERIAL SUPPLY

Long Head:
❑ The Inferior Gluteal Artery (A Branch of the Internal Iliac Artery) and Perforating Branches of the Deep Femoral Artery (A Major Branch of the Femoral Artery)
❑ and the obturator artery (a branch of the internal iliac artery) and branches of the popliteal artery (the continuation of the femoral artery)

Short Head:
❑ Perforating Branches of the Deep Femoral Artery (A Major Branch of the Femoral Artery)
❑ and branches of the popliteal artery (the continuation of the femoral artery)

PALPATION AND SUPPLEMENTARY TEXT

PALPATION

The biceps femoris is superficial for most of its course in the posterolateral thigh and easy to palpate.

❑ **Seated:**

- Have the client seated.
- Place palpating hand on the distal posterolateral thigh.
- Ask the client to actively laterally rotate the leg at the knee joint and feel for the distal tendon of the biceps femoris. It will be the most prominent tendon in the distal posterolateral thigh.
- Continue palpating the biceps femoris proximally toward the ischial tuberosity.

❑ **Prone:**

- Have the client prone with the leg partially flexed at the knee joint.
- Place palpating hand on the distal posterolateral thigh.
- Resist the client from performing further flexion of the leg at the knee joint and feel for the distal tendon of the biceps femoris.
- Continue palpating the biceps femoris proximally toward the ischial tuberosity.

❑ **Proximal attachment:** To more easily palpate the proximal attachment of the biceps femoris (which is deep to the gluteus maximus) at the ischial tuberosity:

- Have the client prone with the leg partially flexed at the knee joint.
- Place palpating hand just distal to the ischial tuberosity.
- Ask the client to medially rotate the thigh at the hip joint. (Medial rotation will cause the gluteus maximus to relax.)
- Now have the client actively extend the thigh at the hip joint and feel for the tensing of the proximal tendon of the biceps femoris.

Note: The short head of the biceps femoris is deep to the long head and therefore is difficult to distinguish except distally near the knee, where some of its fibers are superficial and palpable lateral to the long head of the biceps femoris.

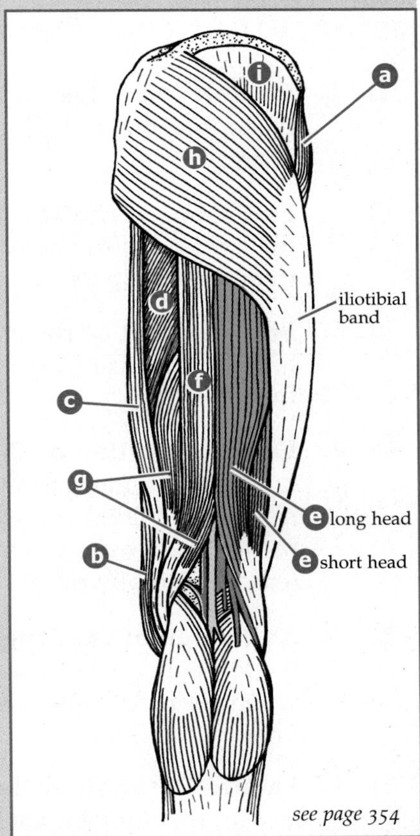

see page 354

Posterior View of the Right Thigh (Superficial)

a. Tensor Fasciae Latae
b. Sartorius
c. Gracilis
d. Adductor Magnus
e. **Biceps Femoris**
f. Semitendinosus
g. Semimembranosus
h. Gluteus Maximus
i. Gluteus Medius

BICEPS FEMORIS – continued

RELATIONSHIP TO OTHER MUSCULOSKELETAL STRUCTURES

- ❑ 1. The biceps femoris is a lateral hamstring muscle.
- ❑ 2. The biceps femoris is superficial in the posterolateral thigh, except proximally where it is deep to the gluteus maximus.
- ❑ 3. All the fibers of the short head of the biceps femoris are deep to the long head except distally near the knee, where some of the fibers of the short head are superficial, lateral to the long head of the biceps femoris.
- ❑ 4. The biceps femoris is just lateral to the semitendinosus and just medial (and also superficial) to the vastus lateralis.

METHODOLOGY FOR LEARNING MUSCLE ACTIONS

- ❑ **1. Flexion of the Leg at the Knee Joint (entire muscle):** The biceps femoris crosses the knee joint posteriorly (with its fibers running vertically in the sagittal plane); therefore, it flexes the leg at the knee joint.
- ❑ **2. Extension of the Thigh at the Hip Joint (long head):** The long head of the biceps femoris crosses the hip joint posteriorly (with its fibers running vertically in the sagittal plane); therefore, it extends the thigh at the hip joint.
- ❑ **3. Posterior Tilt of the Pelvis at the Hip Joint (long head):** With the distal attachment fixed, the long head of the biceps femoris, by pulling inferiorly on the posterior pelvis, posteriorly tilts the pelvis at the hip joint.
- ❑ **4. Lateral Rotation of the Leg at the Knee Joint (entire muscle):** The biceps femoris crosses the knee joint laterally from posterior to anterior (with its fibers running somewhat horizontally in the transverse plane) and attaches to the lateral leg. When the biceps femoris pulls at the leg attachment, the leg rotates posterolaterally, causing the anterior leg to face somewhat laterally. Therefore, the biceps femoris laterally rotates the leg at the knee joint.
- ❑ **5. Adduction of the Thigh at the Hip Joint (long head):** The long head of the biceps femoris crosses the hip joint posteriorly (with its fibers running somewhat horizontally in the frontal plane). Therefore, when the biceps femoris pulls its lateral attachment (the leg) medially, it adducts the thigh at the hip joint.
- ❑ **6. Lateral Rotation of the Thigh at the Hip Joint (long head):** The long head of the biceps femoris crosses the hip joint laterally, wrapping around the thigh from posteriorly on the pelvis to more anteriorly onto the leg (with its fibers running somewhat horizontally in the transverse plane). If the leg is fixed to the thigh, and the long head of the biceps femoris pulls on the leg, the leg and thigh rotates posterolaterally, causing the anterior thigh to face laterally. Therefore, the biceps femoris laterally rotates the thigh at the hip joint.

MISCELLANEOUS

- ❑ The proximal attachment of the biceps femoris' long head blends with the proximal attachment of the semitendinosus.

SEMITENDINOSUS
(OF THE HAMSTRING GROUP)

❑

❑ **The name, semitendinosus, tells us that this muscle has a long, slender (distal) tendon.**

DERIVATION ❑ semitendinosus: L. *refers to its long tendon.*

PRONUNCIATION ❑ **sem**-i-**ten**-di-**no**-sus

ATTACHMENTS

❑ **Ischial Tuberosity**

to the

❑ **Pes Anserine Tendon (at the Proximal Anteromedial Tibia)**

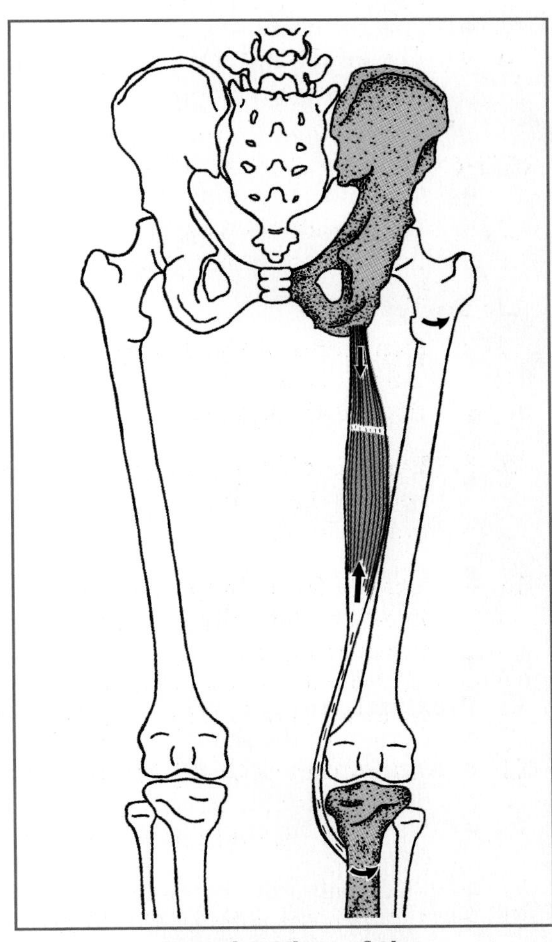

Posterior View of the Right Semitendinosus

ACTIONS

❑ 1. **Flexion of the Leg**

❑ 2. **Extension of the Thigh**

❑ 3. **Posterior Tilt of the Pelvis**

❑ 4. Medial Rotation of the Leg

❑ 5. Medial Rotation of the Thigh

INNERVATION ❑ The Sciatic Nerve ❑ the tibial nerve; L5, **S1**, 2

ARTERIAL SUPPLY ❑ The Inferior Gluteal Artery (A Branch of the Internal Iliac Artery) and Perforating Branches of the Deep Femoral Artery (A Major Branch of the Femoral Artery)
❑ and the obturator artery (a branch of the internal iliac artery) and branches of the popliteal artery (the continuation of the femoral artery)

SEMITENDINOSUS – PALPATION AND SUPPLEMENTARY TEXT

PALPATION

The semitendinosus is superficial for most of its course in the posteromedial thigh and easy to palpate.

❑ **Seated:**

- Have the client seated.
- Place palpating hand in the distal posteromedial thigh.
- Ask the client to actively contract the hamstrings without moving the knee joint and feel for the distal tendon of the semitendinosus.
  (Note: The semitendinosus and gracilis tendons will be clearly palpable. The semitendinosus will be the larger and more lateral one of the two muscles.)
- Continue palpating the semitendinosus proximally toward the ischial tuberosity.

❑ **Prone:**

- Have the client prone with the leg partially flexed at the knee joint.
- Place palpating hand on the distal posteromedial thigh.
- Resist further flexion of the leg at the knee joint and feel for the distal tendon of the semitendinosus.
- Continue palpating the semitendinosus proximally toward the ischial tuberosity.

❑ **Proximal attachment:** To more easily palpate the proximal attachment of the semitendinosus (which is deep to the gluteus maximus) at the ischial tuberosity:

- Have the client prone with the leg partially flexed at the knee joint.
- Place palpating hand just distal to the ischial tuberosity.
- Ask the client to medially rotate the thigh at the hip joint. (Medial rotation will cause the gluteus maximus to relax.)
- Now have the client actively extend the thigh and feel for the tensing of the proximal tendon of the semitendinosus.

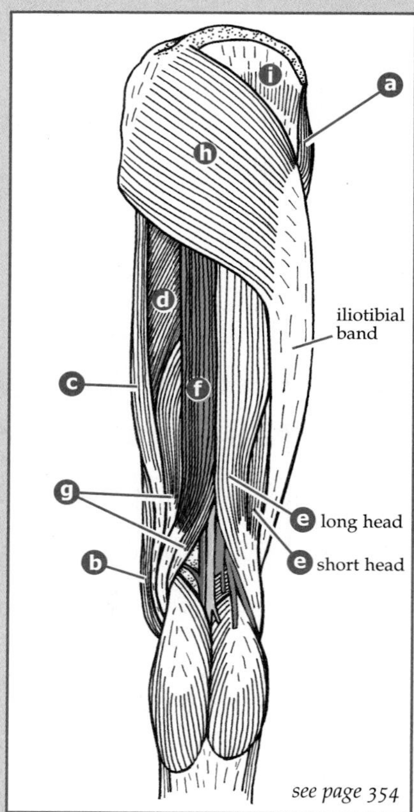

see page 354

Posterior View of the Right Thigh (Superficial)

a. Tensor Fasciae Latae
b. Sartorius
c. Gracilis
d. Adductor Magnus
e. Biceps Femoris
f. **Semitendinosus**
g. Semimembranosus
h. Gluteus Maximus
i. Gluteus Medius

SEMITENDINOSUS – continued

RELATIONSHIP TO OTHER MUSCULOSKELETAL STRUCTURES

- ❑ 1. The semitendinosus is a medial hamstring muscle.
- ❑ 2. The semitendinosus is superficial in the posteromedial thigh.
- ❑ 3. The proximal attachment of the semitendinosus is deep to the gluteus maximus.
- ❑ 4. The biceps femoris is lateral to the semitendinosus. More distally, a portion of the semimembranosus is distal to the semitendinosus.
- ❑ 5. Medial to the semitendinosus is the adductor magnus and a portion of the semimembranosus.
- ❑ 6. The majority of the semimembranosus is deep to the semitendinosus.
- ❑ 7. Of the three muscles that attach into the pes anserine tendon, the semitendinosus attaches the most posteriorly.

METHODOLOGY FOR LEARNING MUSCLE ACTIONS

- ❑ **1. Flexion of the Leg at the Knee Joint:** The semitendinosus crosses the knee joint posteriorly (with its fibers running vertically in the sagittal plane); therefore, it flexes the leg at the knee joint.
- ❑ **2. Extension of the Thigh at the Hip Joint:** The semitendinosus crosses the hip joint posteriorly (with its fibers running vertically in the sagittal plane); therefore, it extends the thigh at the hip joint.
- ❑ **3. Posterior Tilt of the Pelvis at the Hip Joint:** With the distal attachment fixed, the semitendinosus, by pulling inferiorly on the posterior pelvis, posteriorly tilts the pelvis at the hip joint.
- ❑ **4. Medial Rotation of the Leg at the Knee Joint:** The semitendinosus crosses the knee joint medially from posterior to anterior (with its fibers running somewhat horizontally in the transverse plane) to attach into the pes anserine tendon at the medial tibia. When the semitendinosus pulls at the leg attachment, the leg rotates posteromedially, causing the anterior tibia to face somewhat medially. Therefore, the semitendinosus medially rotates the leg at the knee joint.
- ❑ **5. Medial Rotation of the Thigh at the Hip Joint:** The semitendinosus crosses the hip joint medially, wrapping around the thigh from posteriorly on the pelvis to more anteriorly onto the leg (with its fibers running somewhat horizontally in the transverse plane). If the leg is fixed to the thigh, and the semitendinosus pulls on the leg, the leg and thigh rotate posteromedially, causing the anterior thigh to face medially. Therefore, the semitendinosus medially rotates the thigh at the hip joint.

MISCELLANEOUS

- ❑ 1. The semitendinosus is one of three muscles that attach into the pes anserine tendon. The other two muscles that attach here are the sartorius and the gracilis.
- ❑ 2. Of the muscles that attach into the pes anserine, the **S**artorius attaches the most anterior of the three, the **G**racilis is in the middle, and the **S**emitendinosus attaches the most posterior. (Think **SGS**. ☺)
- ❑ 3. All three pes anserine muscles flex and medially rotate the leg at the knee joint.
- ❑ 4. "Pes Anserine" means goose foot.
- ❑ 5. The proximal tendon of the semitendinosus blends with the proximal tendon of the biceps femoris.
- ❑ 6. The semitendinosus has a fibrous septum that divides it into distinct proximal and distal portions.

❑ SEMIMEMBRANOSUS
(OF THE HAMSTRING GROUP)

❑ **The name, semimembranosus, tells us that this muscle has a flattened, membranous (proximal) attachment.**

DERIVATION ❑ semimembranosus: L. *refers to its flattened, membranous tendon.*

PRONUNCIATION ❑ **sem**-i-**mem**-bra-**no**-sus

ATTACHMENTS

❑ **Ischial Tuberosity**

to the

❑ **Medial Condyle of the Tibia**

- ❑ the posterior surface

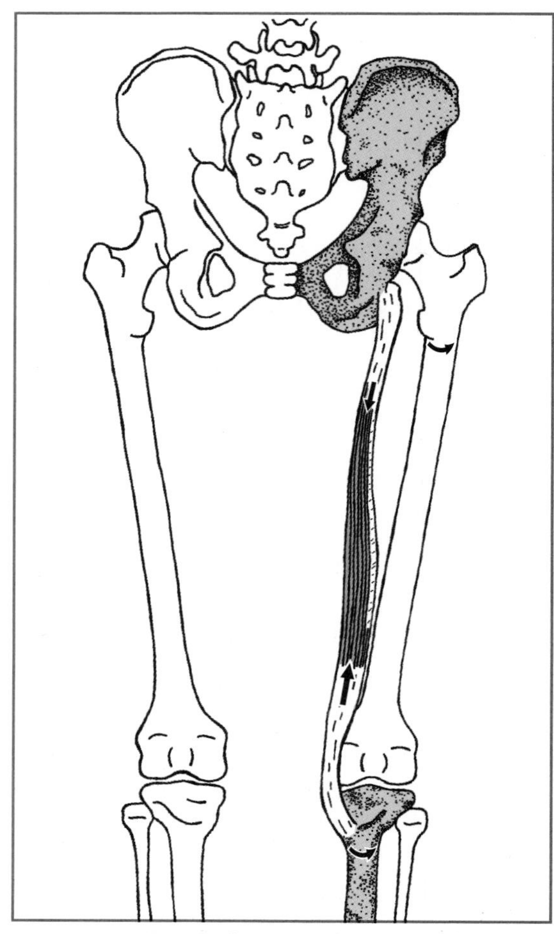

Posterior View of the Right Semimembranosus

ACTIONS

❑ 1. **Flexion of the Leg**

❑ 2. **Extension of the Thigh**

❑ 3. **Posterior Tilt of the Pelvis**

❑ 4. Medial Rotation of the Leg

❑ 5. Medial Rotation of the Thigh

INNERVATION ❑ The Sciatic Nerve ❑ the tibial nerve; L5, **S1**, 2

ARTERIAL SUPPLY ❑ The Inferior Gluteal Artery (A Branch of the Internal Iliac Artery) and Perforating Branches of the Deep Femoral Artery (A Major Branch of the Femoral Artery)

- ❑ and the obturator artery (a branch of the internal iliac artery) and branches of the popliteal artery (the continuation of the femoral artery)

PALPATION AND SUPPLEMENTARY TEXT

PALPATION

The semimembranosus can be best palpated distally in the posterior thigh, medial to the belly of the semitendinosus, and on either side of the distal tendon of the semitendinosus (see the palpation section for this muscle on page 398).

❑ **Prone:**

- Have the client prone with the leg partially flexed at the knee joint.
- Place palpating hand on the distal posteromedial thigh.
- Resist the client from performing further flexion of the leg at the knee joint and feel for the contraction of the semimembranosus. It will be medial to the semitendinosus and on either side of the distal tendon of the semitendinosus. Keep in mind that this will also make the semitendinosus and the biceps femoris contract.

❑ **Proximal attachment:** To more easily palpate the proximal attachment of the semimembranosus (which is deep to the gluteus maximus) at the ischial tuberosity:

- Place palpating hand just distal to the ischial tuberosity.
- Ask the client to medially rotate the thigh at the hip joint. (Medial rotation will cause the gluteus maximus to relax.)
- Now have the client actively extend the thigh and feel for the tensing of the proximal tendon of the semimembranosus.

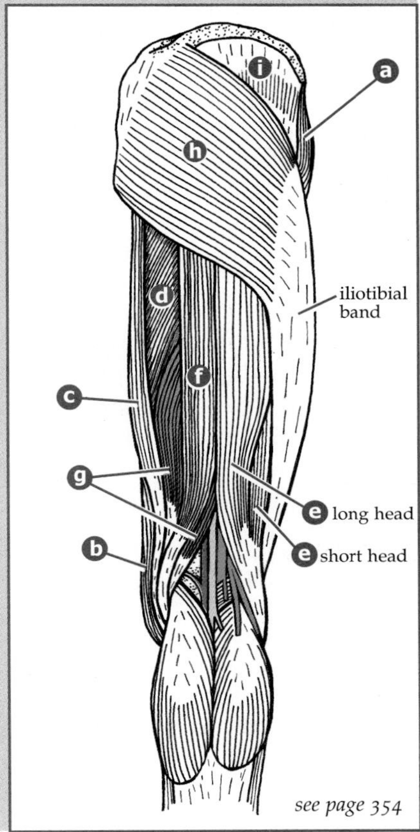

see page 354

Posterior View of the Right Thigh (Superficial)

a. Tensor Fasciae Latae
b. Sartorius
c. Gracilis
d. Adductor Magnus
e. Biceps Femoris
f. Semitendinosus
g. Semimembranosus
h. Gluteus Maximus
i. Gluteus Medius

RELATIONSHIP TO OTHER MUSCULOSKELETAL STRUCTURES

❑ 1. The semimembranosus is a medial hamstring muscle.

❑ 2. The semimembranosus is generally deep to the semitendinosus. However, part of it is superficial and found medial to the semitendinosus. More distally, the muscle belly of the semimembranosus is superficial on both sides of the distal tendon of the semitendinosus.

❑ 3. The proximal attachment of the semimembranosus is deep to the gluteus maximus.

❑ 4. The proximal attachment of the semimembranosus is located more laterally on the ischial tuberosity than the proximal attachments of the semitendinosus and biceps femoris.

❑ 5. Deep to the semimembranosus is the adductor magnus.

SEMIMEMBRANOSUS – continued

METHODOLOGY FOR LEARNING MUSCLE ACTIONS

- ❑ **1. Flexion of the Leg at the Knee Joint:** The semimembranosus crosses the knee joint posteriorly (with its fibers running vertically in the sagittal plane); therefore, it flexes the leg at the knee joint.
- ❑ **2. Extension of the Thigh at the Hip Joint:** The semimembranosus crosses the hip joint posteriorly (with its fibers running vertically in the sagittal plane); therefore, it extends the thigh at the hip joint.
- ❑ **3. Posterior Tilt of the Pelvis at the Hip Joint:** With the distal attachment fixed, the semimembranosus, by pulling inferiorly on the posterior pelvis, posteriorly tilts the pelvis at the hip joint.
- ❑ **4. Medial Rotation of the Leg at the Knee Joint:** The semimembranosus crosses the knee joint medially from posterior to anterior (with its fibers running somewhat horizontally in the transverse plane) and attaches to the medial leg. When the semimembranosus pulls at the leg attachment, the leg rotates posteromedially, causing the anterior tibia to face somewhat medially. Therefore, the semimembranosus medially rotates the leg at the knee joint.
- ❑ **5. Medial Rotation of the Thigh at the Hip Joint:** The semimembranosus crosses the hip joint medially, wrapping around the thigh from posteriorly on the pelvis to more anteriorly onto the leg (with its fibers running somewhat horizontally in the transverse plane). If the leg is fixed to the thigh, and the semimembranosus pulls on the leg, the leg and thigh rotate posteromedially, causing the anterior thigh to face medially. Therefore, the semimembranosus medially rotates the thigh at the hip joint.

MISCELLANEOUS

- ❑ 1. The semimembranosus is the largest of the three hamstring muscles.
- ❑ 2. The semimembranosus also attaches into the medial meniscus of the knee joint. This attachment facilitates the posterior movement of the medial meniscus during knee flexion. Posterior movement of the medial meniscus helps to prevent impingement of the medial meniscus between the femur and tibia during flexion of the knee joint. (Note: The popliteus has the same action with regard to the lateral meniscus.)

MUSCLES OF THE LEG

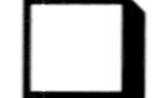

OVERVIEW OF THE MUSCLES OF THE LEG

ANATOMICALLY, THE MUSCLES OF THE LEG CAN BE DIVIDED INTO THREE MAJOR GROUPS:

The Anterior Compartment:

- Tibialis Anterior
- Extensor Digitorum Longus
- Extensor Hallucis Longus
- Fibularis Tertius

The Lateral Compartment:

- Fibularis Longus
- Fibularis Brevis

The Posterior Compartment:

Superficial:

- Gastrocnemius
- Soleus
- Plantaris

Deep:

- Popliteus
- Tibialis Posterior
- Flexor Digitorum Longus
- Flexor Hallucis Longus

THE FOLLOWING MUSCLES ARE COVERED IN OTHER CHAPTERS OF THIS BOOK, BUT ARE ALSO PRESENT IN THE LEG:

- The Quadriceps Femoris Group:
  - Rectus Femoris
  - Vastus Lateralis
  - Vastus Medialis
  - Vastus Intermedius
- The Hamstring Group:
  - Biceps Femoris
  - Semitendinosus
  - Semimembranosus
- Gracilis

The leg is a body part that has clearly divisible compartments. Therefore, the above classification is consistently used.

Functionally, since the muscles of the leg have their bellies in the leg and their distal tendons cross the ankle joint to attach into the foot, these muscles move the foot at the ankle or tarsal joints (except for the popliteus, which does not cross the ankle joint at all). The following general rules regarding actions can be stated for muscles of the leg:

- Any muscle that crosses the ankle joint must either cross it anteriorly or posteriorly (either anterior or posterior to the malleoli).
  - All the muscles of the anterior compartment cross the ankle joint anteriorly and can dorsiflex the foot at the ankle joint.
  - All the muscles of the lateral and posterior compartments cross the ankle joint posteriorly and can plantarflex the foot at the ankle joint (except the popliteus, which does not cross the ankle joint).

- Any muscle that crosses into the foot on the medial side crosses the tarsals medially and can invert the foot at the tarsal joints. The following muscles all invert the foot at the tarsal joints:
  - All the deep muscles of the posterior leg (except the popliteus).
  - The medial anterior compartment leg muscles, i.e., the tibialis anterior and the extensor hallucis longus.
- Any muscle that crosses into the foot on the lateral side crosses the tarsals laterally and can evert the foot at the tarsal joints. The following muscles all evert the foot at the tarsal joints:
  - All the muscles of the lateral compartment.
  - The lateral muscles of the anterior compartment, i.e., the extensor digitorum longus and the fibularis tertius.
- The gastrocnemius, plantaris and the popliteus cross the knee joint and can, therefore, move the knee joint. (They cross the knee joint posteriorly, so they can all flex the leg at the knee joint.)
- Some muscles of the leg also cross joints in the foot and can move the toes (at the metatarsophalangeal and interphalangeal joints.)

INNERVATION

- The anterior compartment of the leg is innervated by the deep fibular nerve.
- The lateral compartment of the leg is innervated by the superficial fibular nerve.
- The posterior compartment of the leg is innervated by the tibial nerve.

♥ ARTERIAL SUPPLY

- The anterior compartment of the leg receives its arterial supply from the anterior tibial artery.
- The lateral compartment of the leg receives its arterial supply from the fibular artery.
- The superficial posterior compartment of the leg receives its arterial supply from branches of the popliteal artery.
- The deep posterior compartment of the leg receives its arterial supply from the posterior tibial artery.

A NOTE REGARDING REVERSE ACTIONS

As a rule, this book does not employ the terms "origin" and "insertion." However, it is useful to utilize these terms to describe the concept of "reverse actions." The action section of this book describes the action of a muscle by stating the movement of a body part that is created by a muscle's contraction. The body part that usually moves when a muscle contracts is called the insertion. The methodology section further states at which joint the movement of the insertion occurs. However, the other body part that the muscle attaches to, the origin, can also move at that joint. *This movement can be called the reverse action of the muscle.* Keep in mind that the reverse action of a muscle is always possible. The likelihood that a reverse action will occur is based upon the ability of the insertion to be fixed so that the origin moves (instead of the insertion moving) when the muscle contracts. For more information and examples of reverse actions, see page 702.

❑ ANTERIOR VIEW OF THE BONES AND BONY LANDMARKS OF THE RIGHT LEG

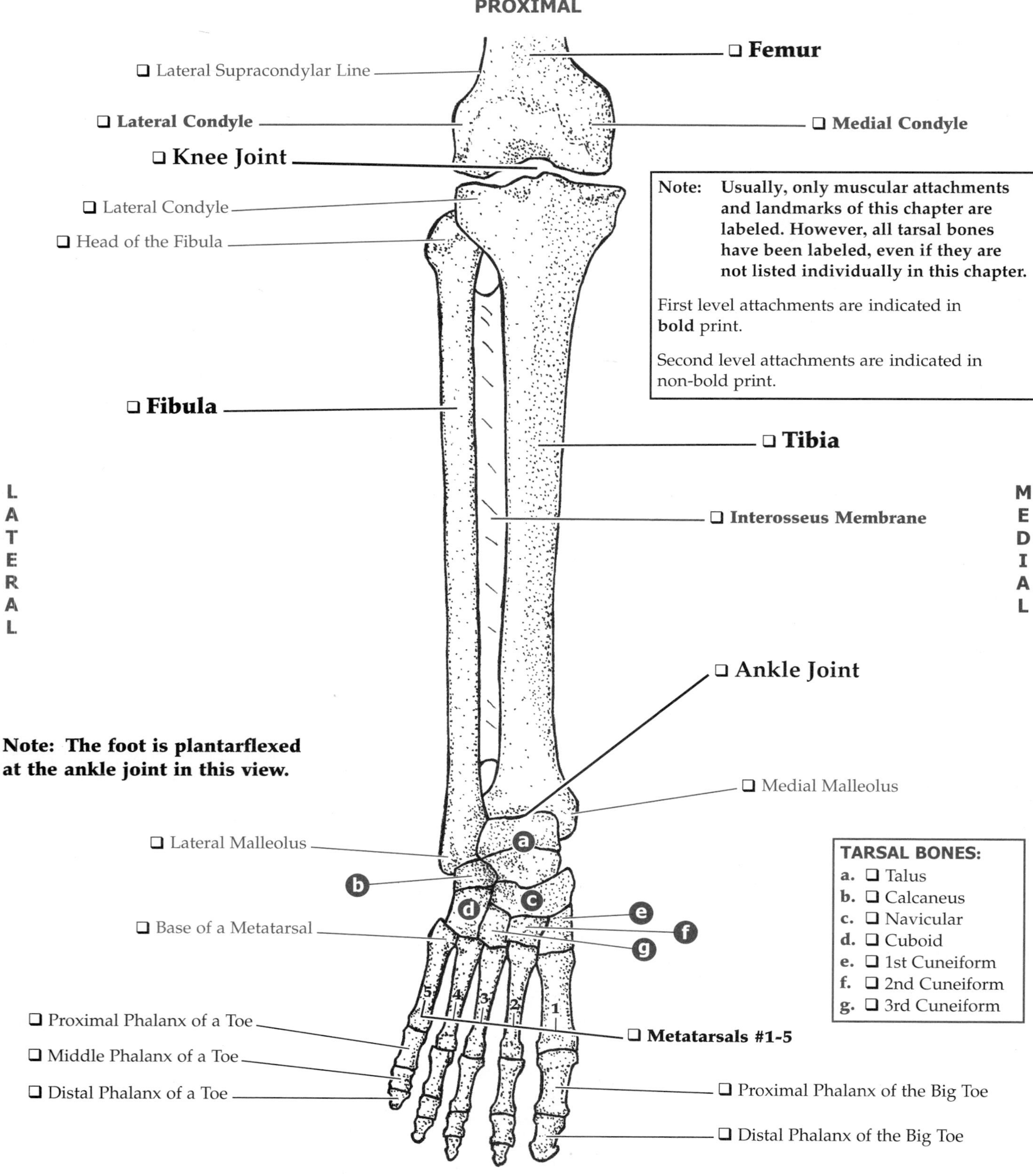

Note: **Usually, only muscular attachments and landmarks of this chapter are labeled. However, all tarsal bones have been labeled, even if they are not listed individually in this chapter.**

First level attachments are indicated in **bold** print.

Second level attachments are indicated in non-bold print.

Note: The foot is plantarflexed at the ankle joint in this view.

TARSAL BONES:
- **a.** ❑ Talus
- **b.** ❑ Calcaneus
- **c.** ❑ Navicular
- **d.** ❑ Cuboid
- **e.** ❑ 1st Cuneiform
- **f.** ❑ 2nd Cuneiform
- **g.** ❑ 3rd Cuneiform

ANTERIOR VIEW OF THE BONY ATTACHMENTS OF THE RIGHT LEG

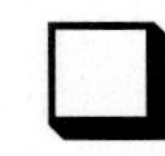

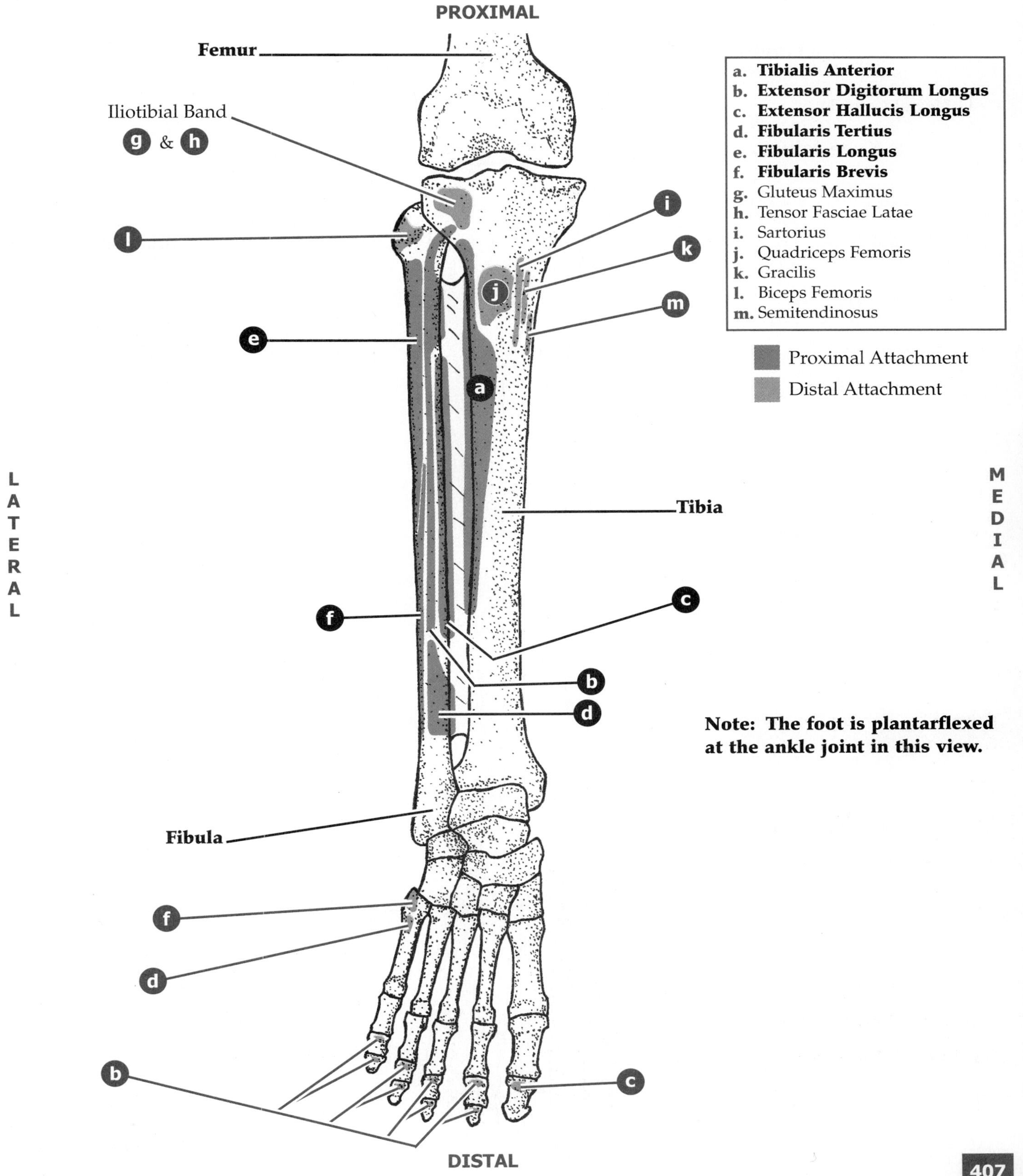

PROXIMAL

Femur

Iliotibial Band
g & h

l

e

a

j

i

k

m

Tibia

f

c

b

d

Fibula

f

d

b

c

DISTAL

LATERAL

MEDIAL

a. **Tibialis Anterior**
b. **Extensor Digitorum Longus**
c. **Extensor Hallucis Longus**
d. **Fibularis Tertius**
e. **Fibularis Longus**
f. **Fibularis Brevis**
g. Gluteus Maximus
h. Tensor Fasciae Latae
i. Sartorius
j. Quadriceps Femoris
k. Gracilis
l. Biceps Femoris
m. Semitendinosus

Proximal Attachment

Distal Attachment

Note: The foot is plantarflexed at the ankle joint in this view.

❑ POSTERIOR VIEW OF THE BONES AND BONY LANDMARKS OF THE RIGHT LEG

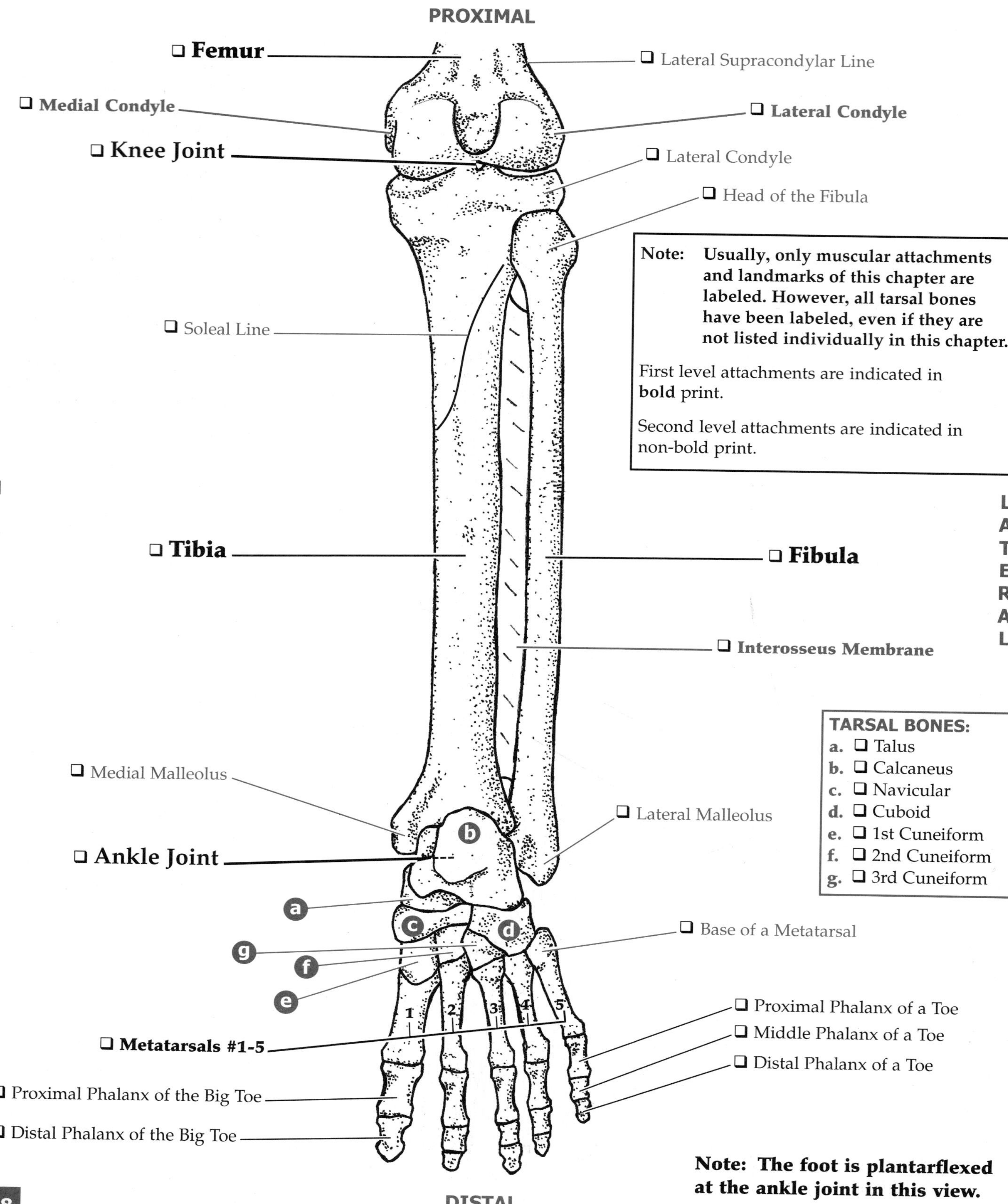

Note: Usually, only muscular attachments and landmarks of this chapter are labeled. However, all tarsal bones have been labeled, even if they are not listed individually in this chapter.

First level attachments are indicated in **bold** print.

Second level attachments are indicated in non-bold print.

TARSAL BONES:
- **a.** ❑ Talus
- **b.** ❑ Calcaneus
- **c.** ❑ Navicular
- **d.** ❑ Cuboid
- **e.** ❑ 1st Cuneiform
- **f.** ❑ 2nd Cuneiform
- **g.** ❑ 3rd Cuneiform

Note: The foot is plantarflexed at the ankle joint in this view.

POSTERIOR VIEW OF THE BONY ATTACHMENTS OF THE RIGHT LEG

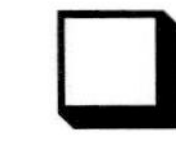

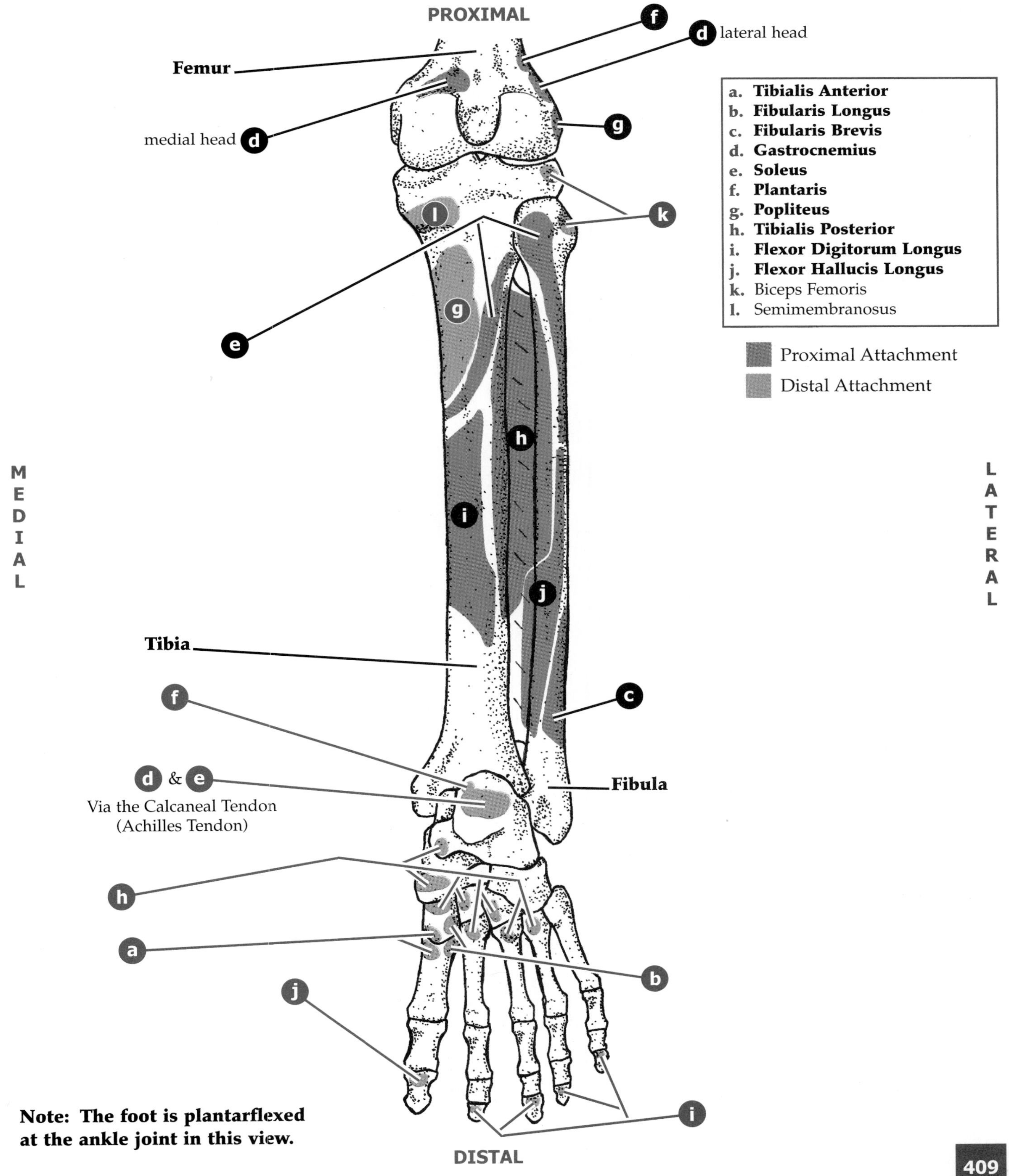

PROXIMAL
Femur
f
d lateral head
medial head d
g
k
l
e
g
h
i
j
MEDIAL
LATERAL
Tibia
c
f
d & e
Via the Calcaneal Tendon
(Achilles Tendon)
Fibula
h
a
b
j
i
DISTAL
a. Tibialis Anterior
b. Fibularis Longus
c. Fibularis Brevis
d. Gastrocnemius
e. Soleus
f. Plantaris
g. Popliteus
h. Tibialis Posterior
i. Flexor Digitorum Longus
j. Flexor Hallucis Longus
k. Biceps Femoris
l. Semimembranosus
Proximal Attachment
Distal Attachment

Note: The foot is plantarflexed at the ankle joint in this view.

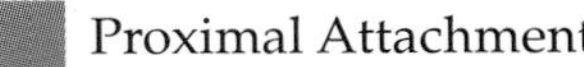

ANTERIOR VIEW OF THE RIGHT LEG

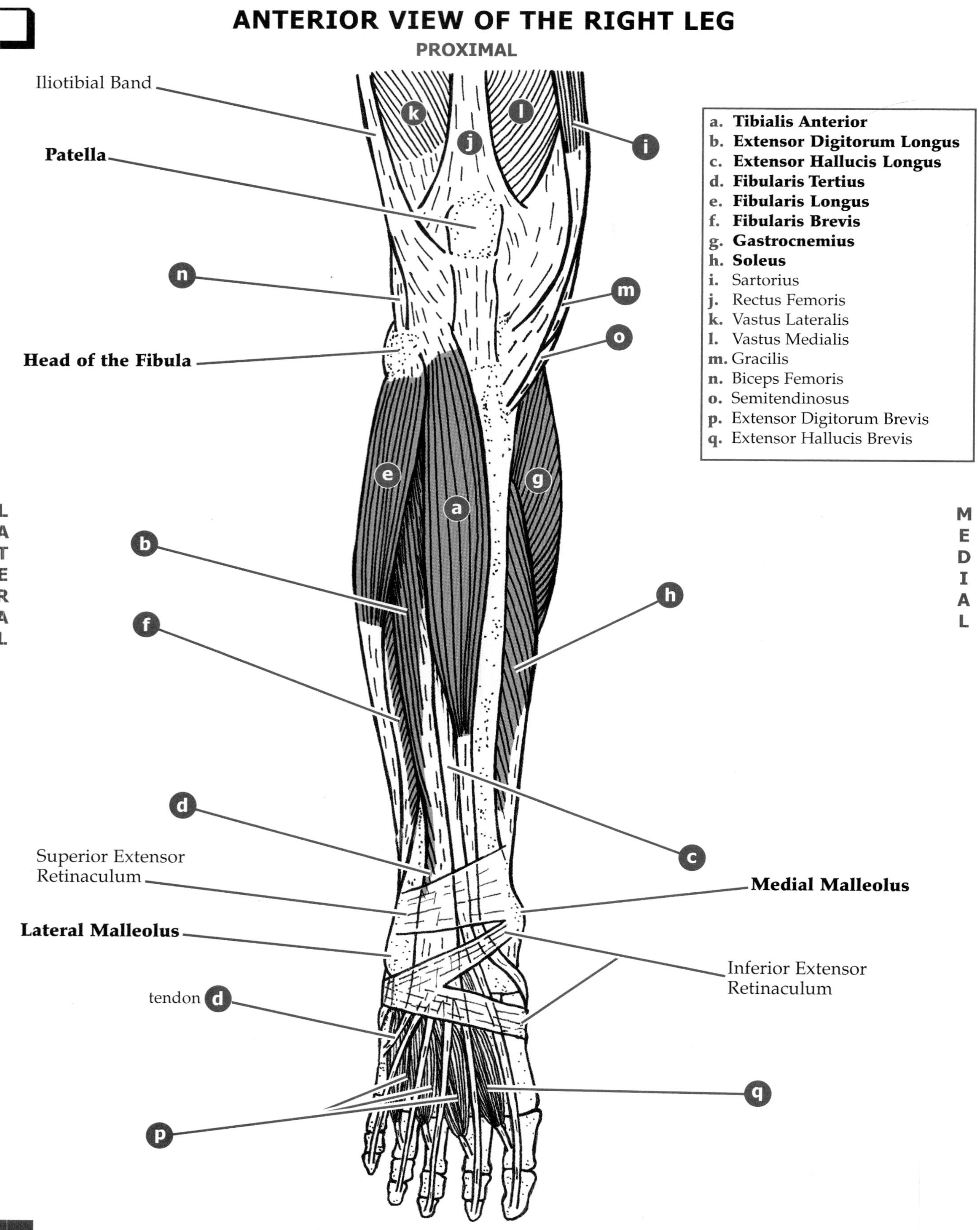
PROXIMAL
Iliotibial Band
Patella
Head of the Fibula
Superior Extensor Retinaculum
Lateral Malleolus
tendon d
Medial Malleolus
Inferior Extensor Retinaculum
LATERAL
MEDIAL
DISTAL
a. Tibialis Anterior
b. Extensor Digitorum Longus
c. Extensor Hallucis Longus
d. Fibularis Tertius
e. Fibularis Longus
f. Fibularis Brevis
g. Gastrocnemius
h. Soleus
i. Sartorius
j. Rectus Femoris
k. Vastus Lateralis
l. Vastus Medialis
m. Gracilis
n. Biceps Femoris
o. Semitendinosus
p. Extensor Digitorum Brevis
q. Extensor Hallucis Brevis

POSTERIOR VIEW OF THE RIGHT LEG (SUPERFICIAL)

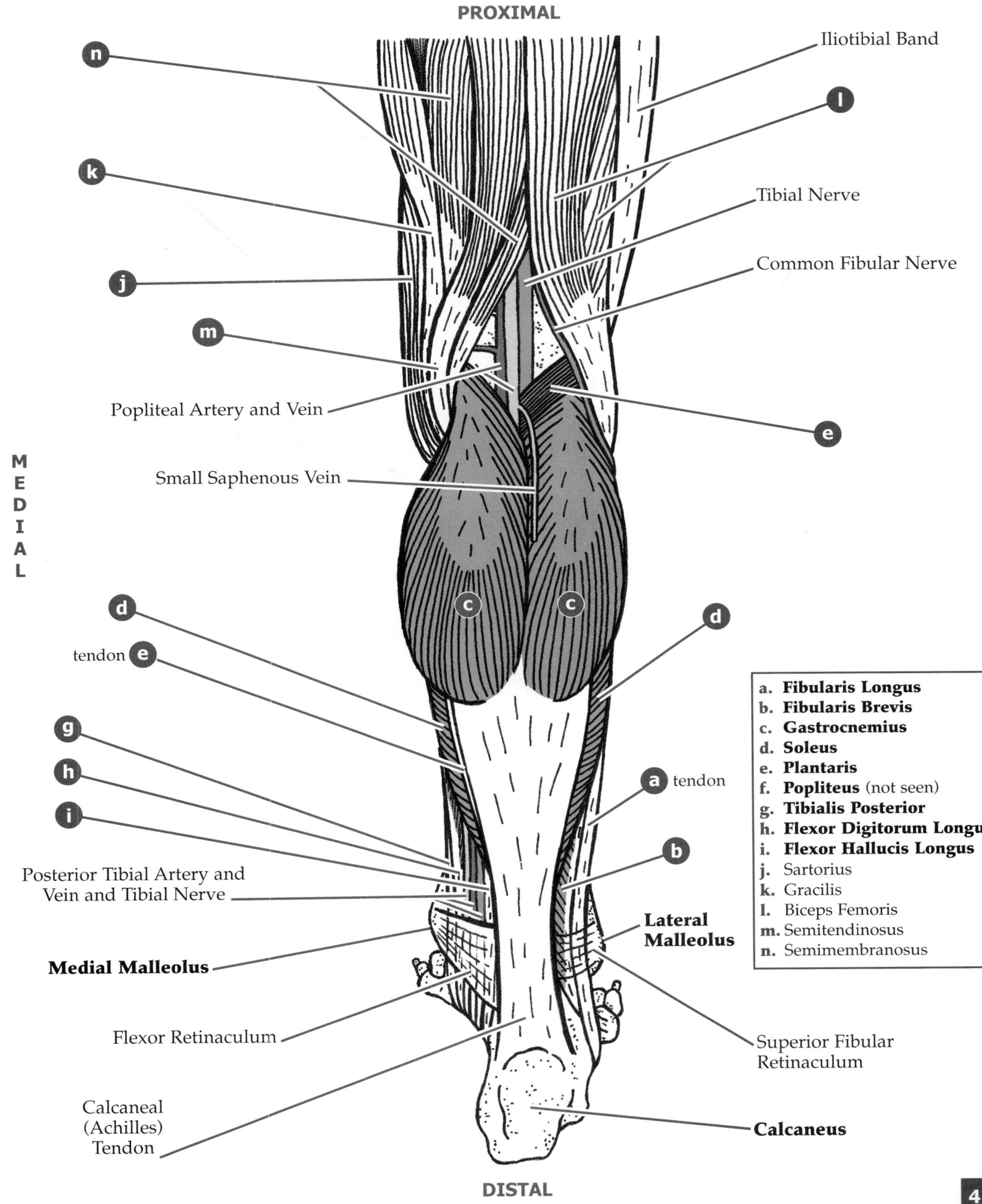

- a. **Fibularis Longus**
- b. **Fibularis Brevis**
- c. **Gastrocnemius**
- d. **Soleus**
- e. **Plantaris**
- f. **Popliteus** (not seen)
- g. **Tibialis Posterior**
- h. **Flexor Digitorum Longus**
- i. **Flexor Hallucis Longus**
- j. Sartorius
- k. Gracilis
- l. Biceps Femoris
- m. Semitendinosus
- n. Semimembranosus

POSTERIOR VIEW OF THE RIGHT LEG (INTERMEDIATE)

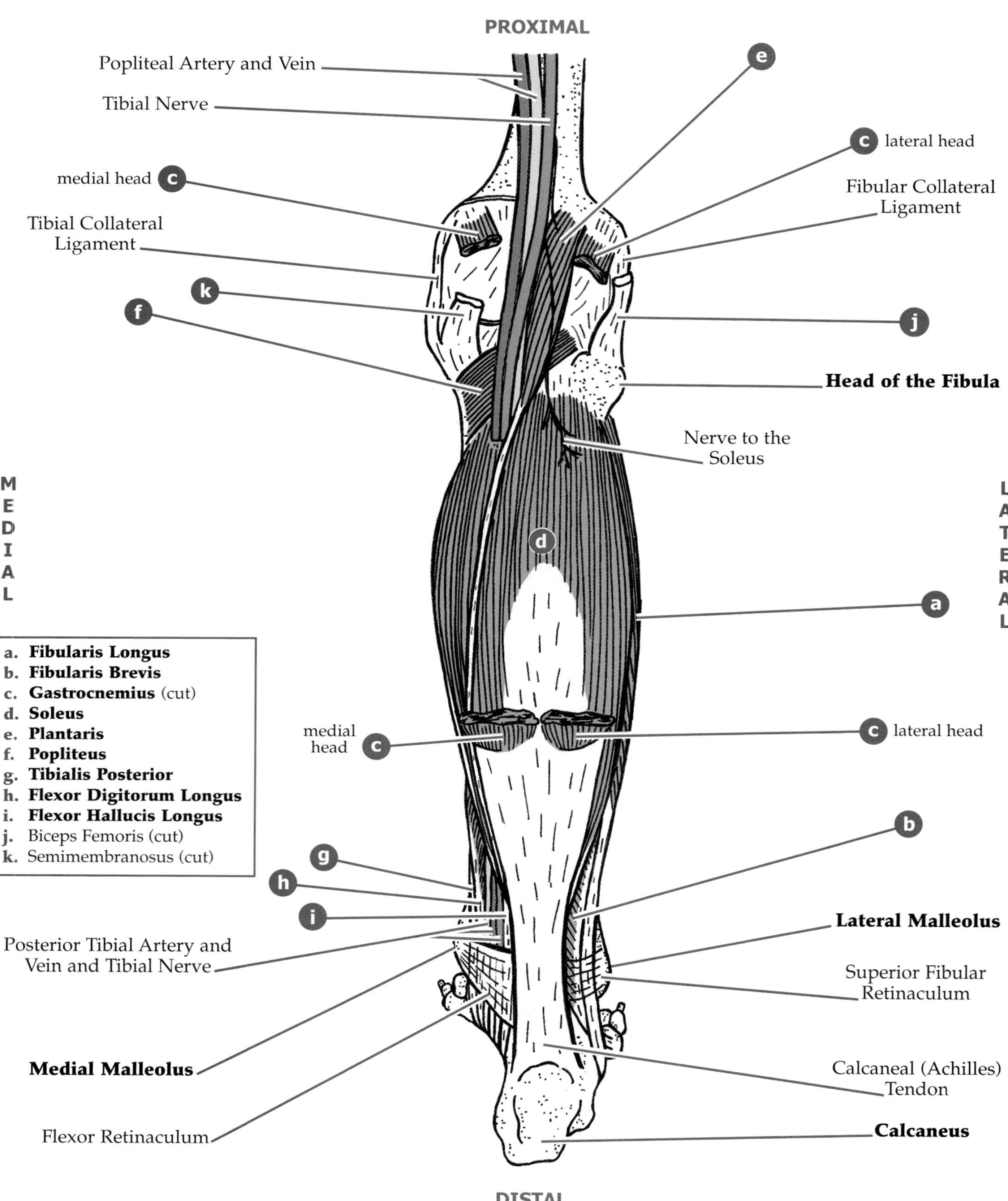

a. **Fibularis Longus**
b. **Fibularis Brevis**
c. **Gastrocnemius** (cut)
d. **Soleus**
e. **Plantaris**
f. **Popliteus**
g. **Tibialis Posterior**
h. **Flexor Digitorum Longus**
i. **Flexor Hallucis Longus**
j. Biceps Femoris (cut)
k. Semimembranosus (cut)

POSTERIOR VIEW OF THE RIGHT LEG (DEEP)

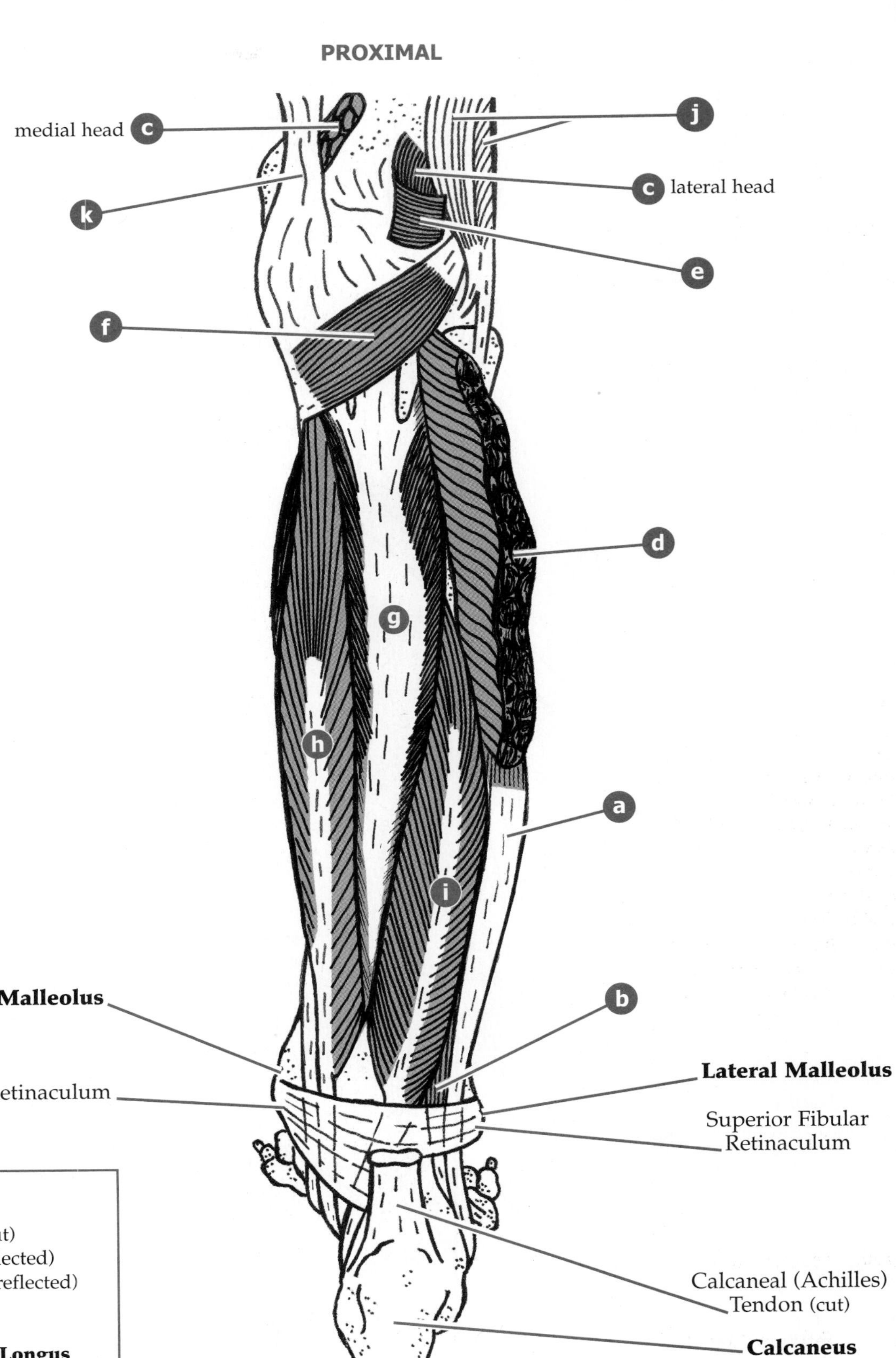

a. **Fibularis Longus**
b. **Fibularis Brevis**
c. **Gastrocnemius** (cut)
d. **Soleus** (cut and reflected)
e. **Plantaris** (cut and reflected)
f. **Popliteus**
g. **Tibialis Posterior**
h. **Flexor Digitorum Longus**
i. **Flexor Hallucis Longus**
j. Biceps Femoris
k. Semimembranosus

LATERAL VIEW OF THE RIGHT LEG

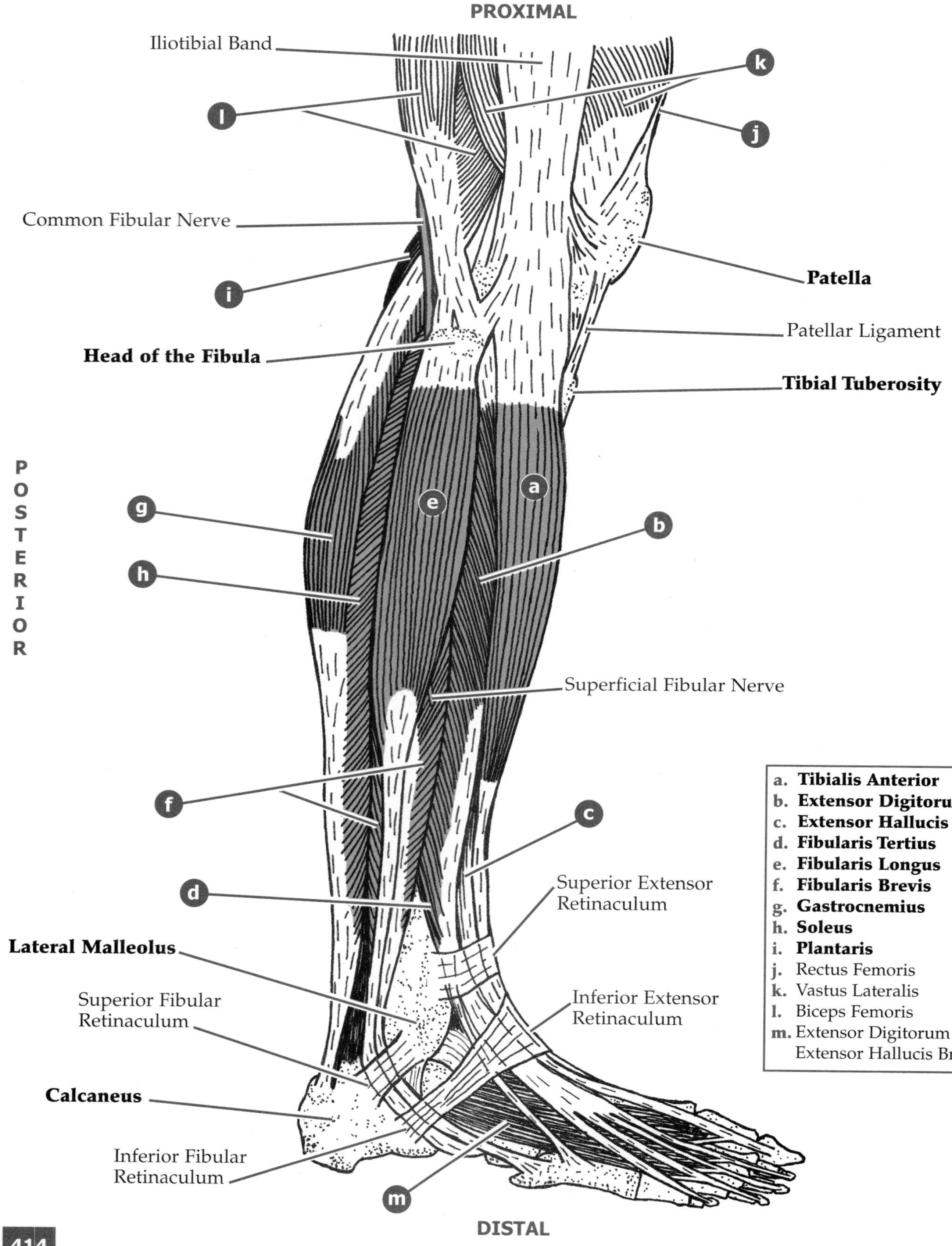

a. **Tibialis Anterior**
b. **Extensor Digitorum Longus**
c. **Extensor Hallucis Longus**
d. **Fibularis Tertius**
e. **Fibularis Longus**
f. **Fibularis Brevis**
g. **Gastrocnemius**
h. **Soleus**
i. **Plantaris**
j. Rectus Femoris
k. Vastus Lateralis
l. Biceps Femoris
m. Extensor Digitorum Brevis & Extensor Hallucis Brevis

MEDIAL VIEW OF THE RIGHT LEG

- a. **Tibialis Anterior**
- b. **Extensor Digitorum Longus**
- c. **Extensor Hallucis Longus**
- d. **Gastrocnemius**
- e. **Soleus**
- f. **Plantaris**
- g. **Tibialis Posterior**
- h. **Flexor Digitorum Longus**
- i. **Flexor Hallucis Longus**
- j. Sartorius
- k. Rectus Femoris
- l. Vastus Medialis
- m. Gracilis
- n. Adductor Magnus
- o. Semitendinosus
- p. Semimembranosus

COMPARTMENTS OF THE RIGHT LEG

ANTERIOR

MEDIAL

LATERAL

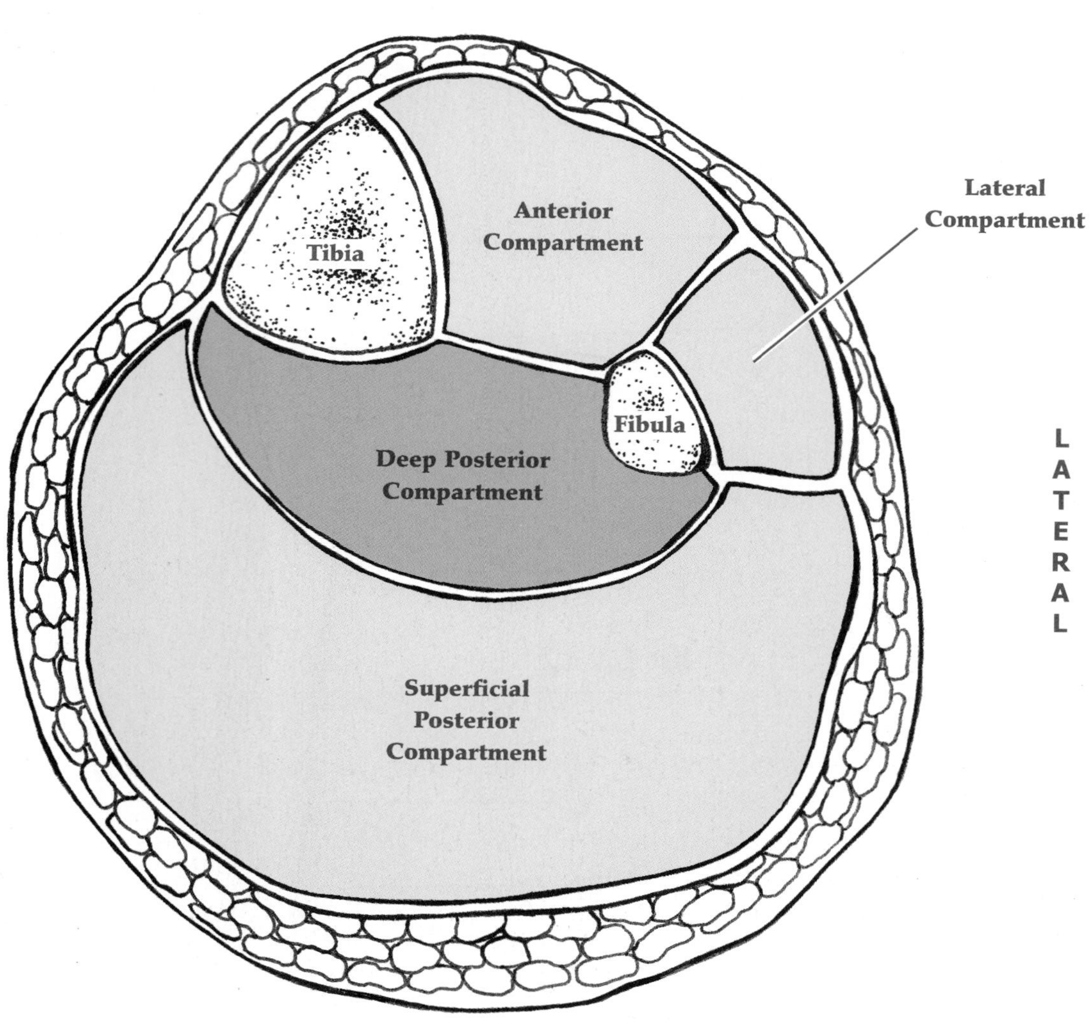

POSTERIOR

Anterior Compartment:	Tibialis Anterior Extensor Digitorum Longus Extensor Hallucis Longus Fibularis Tertius	**Superficial Posterior Compartment:**	Gastrocnemius Soleus Plantaris
Lateral Compartment:	Fibularis Longus Fibularis Brevis	**Deep Posterior Compartment:**	Popliteus Tibialis Posterior Flexor Digitorum Longus Flexor Hallucis Longus

CROSS SECTION VIEW OF THE RIGHT LEG

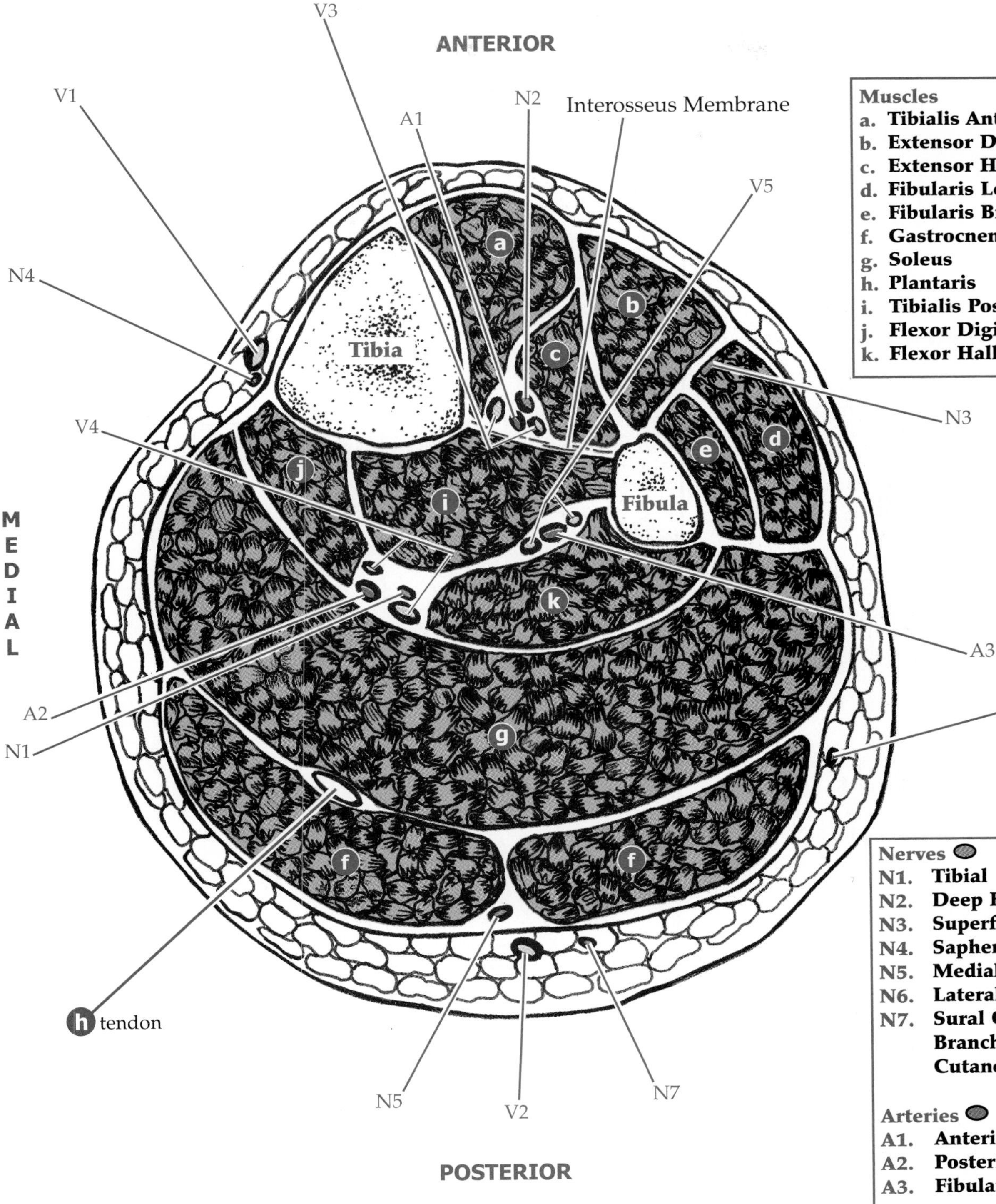

Muscles
- a. **Tibialis Anterior**
- b. **Extensor Digitorum Longus**
- c. **Extensor Hallucis Longus**
- d. **Fibularis Longus**
- e. **Fibularis Brevis**
- f. **Gastrocnemius**
- g. **Soleus**
- h. **Plantaris**
- i. **Tibialis Posterior**
- j. **Flexor Digitorum Longus**
- k. **Flexor Hallucis Longus**

Nerves
- N1. **Tibial**
- N2. **Deep Fibular**
- N3. **Superficial Fibular**
- N4. **Saphenous**
- N5. **Medial Sural Cutaneous**
- N6. **Lateral Sural Cutaneous**
- N7. **Sural Communicating Branch of Lateral Sural Cutaneous**

Arteries
- A1. **Anterior Tibial**
- A2. **Posterior Tibial**
- A3. **Fibular**

Veins
- V1. **Great Saphenous**
- V2. **Small Saphenous**
- V3. **Anterior Tibial**
- V4. **Posterior Tibial**
- V5. **Fibular**

Note: View is 1/3 of the way down the right leg.

❑ TIBIALIS ANTERIOR
(IN THE ANTERIOR COMPARTMENT)

❑ **The name, tibialis anterior, tells us that this muscle attaches to the tibia and is located anteriorly.**

DERIVATION ❑ tibialis: L. *refers to the tibia.*
anterior: L. *before, in front of.*

PRONUNCIATION ❑ tib-ee-**a**-lis an-**tee**-ri-or

ATTACHMENTS

❑ **Proximal Anterior Tibia**

❑ the lateral tibial condyle,
the proximal 2/3 of the anterior tibia
and the proximal 2/3 of the interosseus membrane

to the

❑ **Medial Foot**

❑ the 1st cuneiform and 1st metatarsal

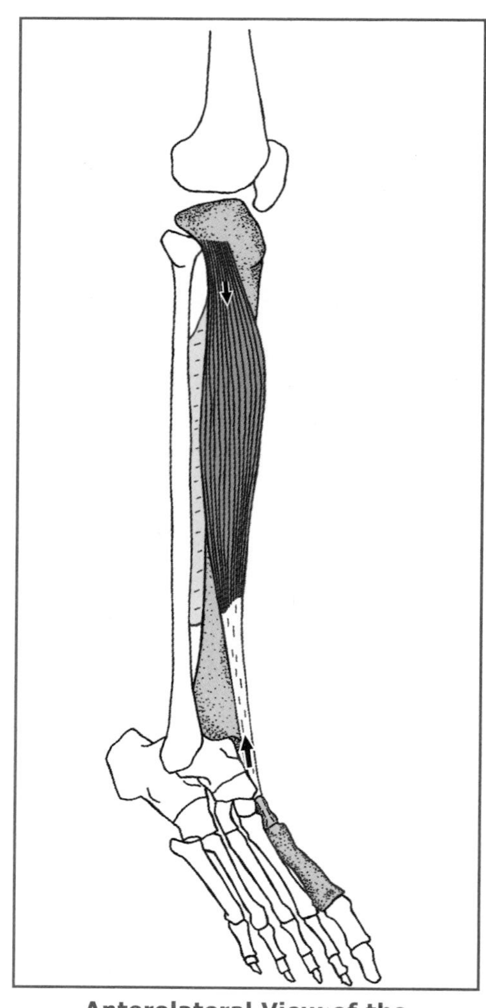

Anterolateral View of the Right Tibialis Anterior

ACTIONS

❑ 1. **Dorsiflexion of the Foot**

❑ 2. **Inversion of the Foot**

INNERVATION ❑ The Deep Fibular Nerve ❑ **L4**, 5

ARTERIAL SUPPLY ❑ The Anterior Tibial Artery (A Terminal Branch of the Popliteal Artery)

PALPATION AND SUPPLEMENTARY TEXT

PALPATION

The belly of the tibialis anterior is superficial and easy to palpate just lateral to the tibia in the anterolateral leg. Its distal tendon is superficial, visible and easy to palpate as it crosses the ankle joint anteriorly.

❑ **To visualize and palpate the distal tendon:**

- Have the client seated or supine.
- Ask the client to actively dorsiflex the foot (at the ankle joint) and invert the foot (at the tarsal joints). The distal tendon of the tibialis anterior will stand out crossing the ankle joint anteriorly.
  (Note: The extensor hallucis longus tendon will be directly lateral to the tibialis anterior tendon; if necessary, have the client flex the big toe to help eliminate the extensor hallucis longus from contracting.)

❑ **To palpate the belly:**

- Place palpating hand just lateral to the shaft of the tibia.
- Ask the client to actively dorsiflex and invert the foot and feel for the contraction of the tibialis anterior.
- Continue palpating the tibialis anterior proximally and distally toward its attachments.

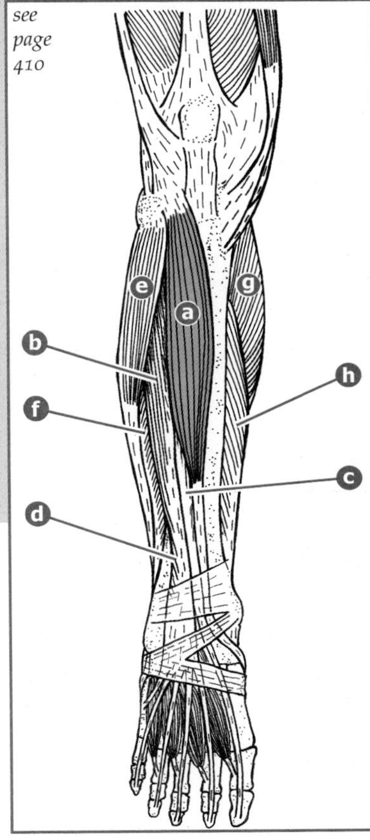

Anterior View of the Right Leg

a. **Tibialis Anterior**
b. Extensor Digitorum Longus
c. Extensor Hallucis Longus
d. Fibularis Tertius
e. Fibularis Longus
f. Fibularis Brevis
g. Gastrocnemius
h. Soleus

RELATIONSHIP TO OTHER MUSCULOSKELETAL STRUCTURES

❑ 1. The tibialis anterior is superficial in the anterolateral leg.

❑ 2. The tibialis anterior lies just lateral to the tibia.

❑ 3. The fibularis longus is lateral to the proximal attachment of the tibialis anterior. Slightly more distal, the extensor digitorum longus is lateral to the tibialis anterior, and more distally, the extensor hallucis longus is lateral to the tibialis anterior.

❑ 4. Deep to the belly of the tibialis anterior are the extensor digitorum longus and the extensor hallucis longus.

METHODOLOGY FOR LEARNING MUSCLE ACTIONS

❑ **1. Dorsiflexion of the Foot at the Ankle Joint:** The tibialis anterior crosses the ankle joint anteriorly (with its fibers running vertically in the sagittal plane); therefore, it dorsiflexes the foot at the ankle joint.

❑ **2. Inversion of the Foot at the Tarsal Joints:** The tibialis anterior crosses the foot medially (with its fibers running vertically in the frontal plane); therefore, it inverts the foot at the tarsal joints.

TIBIALIS ANTERIOR – continued

MISCELLANEOUS

- ❑ 1. The tibialis anterior is located in the anterior compartment of the leg.
- ❑ 2. The tibialis anterior has a very prominent distal tendon.
- ❑ 3. The tibialis anterior and the fibularis longus are known as the *stirrup muscles*. These two muscles both attach at the same location on the foot (1st cuneiform and 1st metatarsal) and may be viewed as a stirrup to support the arch (medial longitudinal arch) of the foot.
- ❑ 4. The tibialis anterior and the tibialis posterior both invert the foot (at the tarsal joints). However, since the tibialis anterior is anterior, it can also dorsiflex the foot at the ankle joint, whereas the tibialis posterior, being posterior, can plantarflex the foot.
- ❑ 5. When the tibialis anterior is tight and painful, especially along its tibial attachment, this condition is usually called *shin splints*. (Note: Shin splints is a general term that is applied to most any painful condition that occurs in the leg, i.e., between the knee and the ankle. Shin splints due to a painful tibialis anterior is probably the most common form of shin splints.)

EXTENSOR DIGITORUM LONGUS
(IN THE ANTERIOR COMPARTMENT)

❑ **The name, extensor digitorum longus, tells us that this muscle extends the digits, i.e., toes #2-5, and is long (longer than the extensor digitorum brevis).**

DERIVATION ❑ extensor: L. *a muscle that extends a body part.*
digitorum: L. *refers to a digit* (toe).
longus: L. *long.*

PRONUNCIATION ❑ eks-**ten**-sor dij-i-**toe**-rum **long**-us

ATTACHMENTS

❑ **Proximal Anterior Fibula**

❑ the proximal 2/3 of the fibula, the proximal 1/3 of the interosseus membrane, and the lateral tibial condyle

to the

❑ **Dorsal Surface of Toes #2-5**

❑ via its dorsal digital expansion onto the dorsal surface of the middle and distal phalanges

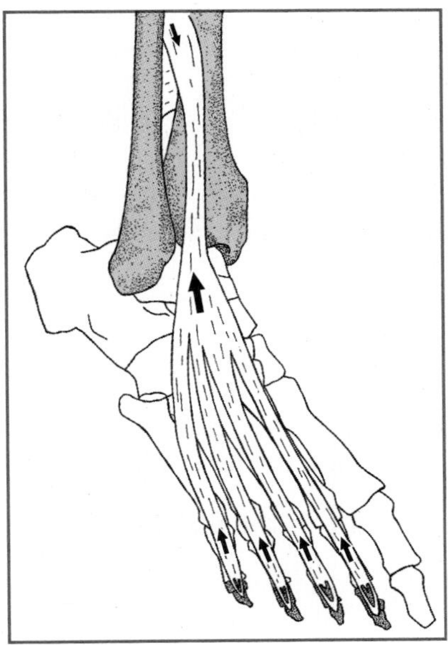

Anterolateral View of the Distal Tendons of the Right Extensor Digitorum Longus

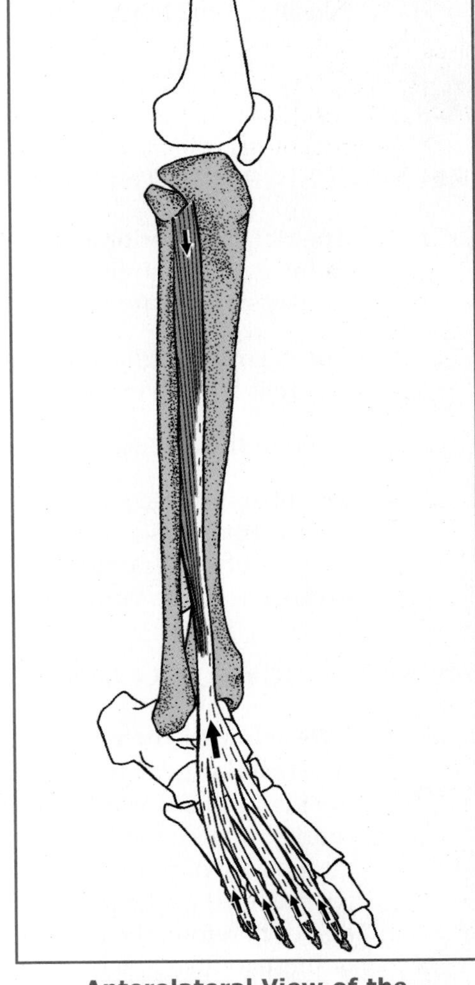

Anterolateral View of the Right Extensor Digitorum Longus

ACTIONS

❑ 1. **Extension of Toes #2-5**

❑ 2. **Dorsiflexion of the Foot**

❑ 3. Eversion of the Foot

INNERVATION ❑ The Deep Fibular Nerve ❑ L5, S1

ARTERIAL SUPPLY ❑ The Anterior Tibial Artery (A Terminal Branch of the Popliteal Artery)

EXTENSOR DIGITORUM LONGUS PALPATION AND SUPPLEMENTARY TEXT

PALPATION

- ❑ The distal tendons of the extensor digitorum longus are clearly visible on the dorsum of the foot, especially if the toes are extended. The majority of the belly of the extensor digitorum longus is palpable between the tibialis anterior and the fibularis longus.
  - Have the client seated or spine.
  - Place palpating hand on the dorsum of the foot.
  - Ask the client to actively extend toes #2-5 and feel for the tensing of the tendons of the extensor digitorum longus.
  - Follow the extensor digitorum longus proximally as far as possible.

see page 410

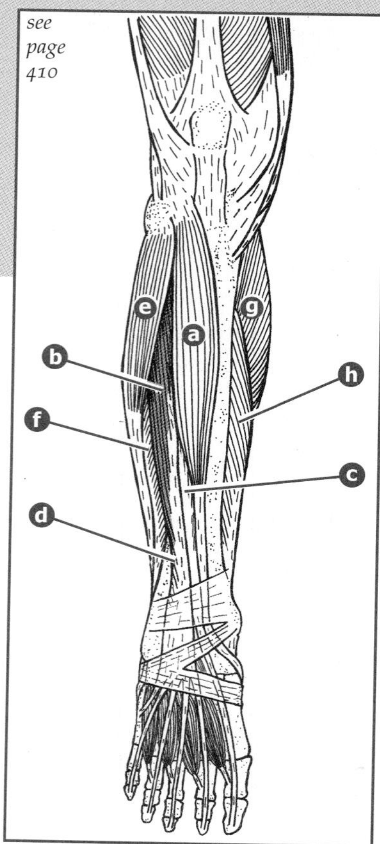

Anterior View of the Right Leg

a. Tibialis Anterior
b. Extensor Digitorum Longus
c. Extensor Hallucis Longus
d. Fibularis Tertius
e. Fibularis Longus
f. Fibularis Brevis
g. Gastrocnemius
h. Soleus

RELATIONSHIP TO OTHER MUSCULOSKELETAL STRUCTURES

❑ 1. The tibialis anterior and the extensor hallucis longus are medial to the extensor digitorum longus. The fibularis longus and the fibularis brevis are lateral to the extensor digitorum longus.

❑ 2. The extensor digitorum longus is superficial, except proximally, where it is deep to the tibialis anterior and the fibularis longus.

❑ 3. Deep to the extensor digitorum longus is the fibula.

❑ 4. The fibers of the most distal and lateral part of the extensor digitorum longus (that arise from the distal 1/3 of the fibula) do not attach onto digits, but rather onto the 5th metatarsal. This portion of the muscle is given a separate name, the fibularis tertius.

METHODOLOGY FOR LEARNING MUSCLE ACTIONS

❑ **1. Extension of Toes #2-5 at the Metatarsophalangeal Joint and the Interphalangeal Joints:** The extensor digitorum longus crosses toe joints #2-5 dorsally (with its fibers running horizontally in the sagittal plane); therefore, it extends toes #2-5. Given that it attaches all the way onto the distal phalanx, it crosses the metatarsophalangeal joint as well as the proximal and distal interphalangeal joints of toes #2-5. Therefore, the extensor digitorum longus extends toes #2-5 at all of these joints.

❑ **2. Dorsiflexion of the Foot at the Ankle Joint:** The extensor digitorum longus crosses the ankle joint anteriorly (with its fibers running vertically in the sagittal plane); therefore, it dorsiflexes the foot at the ankle joint.

❑ **3. Eversion of the Foot at the Tarsal Joints:** Much of the extensor digitorum longus crosses over the lateral side of the foot (with its fibers running vertically in the frontal plane); therefore, it everts the foot at the tarsal joints.

EXTENSOR DIGITORUM LONGUS – continued

MISCELLANEOUS

- ❑ 1. The extensor digitorum longus is located in the anterior compartment of the leg.
- ❑ 2. The distal attachment of the extensor digitorum longus spreads out to become a fibrous aponeurotic expansion that covers the dorsal, medial and lateral sides of the proximal phalanx. It then continues distally to attach onto the dorsal sides of the middle and distal phalanges. This structure is called the *dorsal digital expansion* (see page 457). The dorsal digital expansion also serves as an attachment site for the lumbricals pedis, dorsal interossei pedis and plantar interossei muscles.
- ❑ 3. The most distal and lateral part of the extensor digitorum longus (that arises from the distal 1/3 of the fibula) does not attach onto the digits; therefore, it is given a separate name, the fibularis tertius (see pages 426-7).

❑ EXTENSOR HALLUCIS LONGUS
(IN THE ANTERIOR COMPARTMENT)

❑ **The name, extensor hallucis longus, tells us that this muscle extends the big toe and is long (longer than the extensor hallucis brevis).**

DERIVATION ❑ extensor: L. *a muscle that extends a body part.*
hallucis: L. *refers to the big toe.*
longus: L. *long.*

PRONUNCIATION ❑ eks-**ten**-sor hal-**oo**-sis **long**-us

ATTACHMENTS

❑ **Middle Anterior Fibula**

❑ the middle 1/3 of the anterior fibula and the middle 1/3 of the interosseus membrane

to the

❑ **Dorsal Surface of the Big Toe (Toe #1)**

❑ the distal phalanx

ACTIONS

❑ 1. **Extension of the Big Toe (Toe #1)**

❑ 2. **Dorsiflexion of the Foot**

❑ 3. Inversion of the Foot

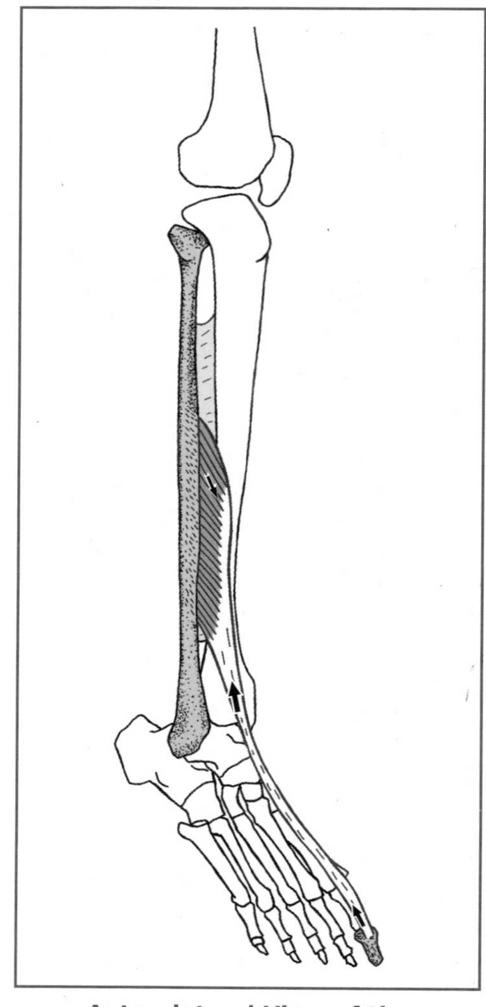

Anterolateral View of the Right Extensor Hallucis Longus

INNERVATION ❑ The Deep Fibular Nerve ❑ **L5**, S1

ARTERIAL SUPPLY ❑ The Anterior Tibial Artery (A Terminal Branch of the Popliteal Artery)

PALPATION AND SUPPLEMENTARY TEXT

PALPATION

❑ The distal tendon of the extensor hallucis longus is clearly visible on the dorsum of the foot (directly lateral to the tendon of the tibialis anterior), especially if the big toe is extended. Only a small portion of the belly of the extensor hallucis longus is easily palpable in the leg.

- Have the client either sitting or supine.
- Place palpating hand on the dorsum of the foot.
- Ask the client to actively extend the big toe and feel for the tensing of the tendon of the extensor hallucis longus.
- Follow the extensor hallucis longus proximally. It may be palpated in the distal half of the leg between the tibialis anterior tendon and the extensor digitorum longus.

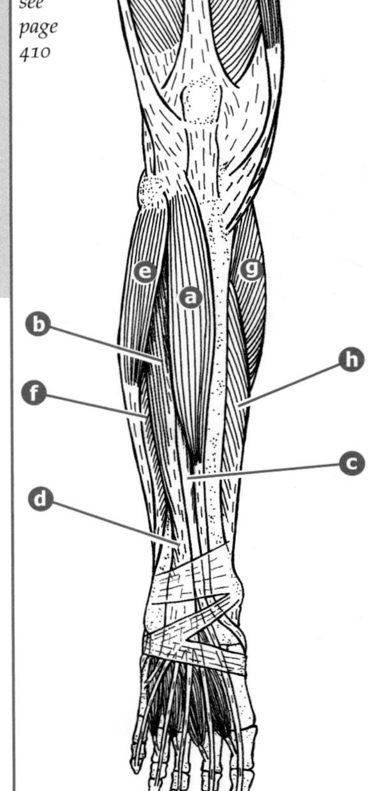

see page 410

Anterior View of the Right Leg

a. Tibialis Anterior
b. Extensor Digitorum Longus
c. **Extensor Hallucis Longus**
d. Fibularis Tertius
e. Fibularis Longus
f. Fibularis Brevis
g. Gastrocnemius
h. Soleus

RELATIONSHIP TO OTHER MUSCULOSKELETAL STRUCTURES

❑ 1. The extensor hallucis longus arises between the tibialis anterior and the extensor digitorum longus, and is deep to these muscles proximally.

❑ 2. A small portion of the belly of the extensor hallucis longus is superficial in the distal half of the leg between the tendons of the tibialis anterior and the extensor digitorum longus.

❑ 3. The distal tendon of the extensor hallucis longus becomes superficial and lies just lateral to the distal tendon of the tibialis anterior.

❑ 4. Deep to the extensor hallucis longus is the fibula.

METHODOLOGY FOR LEARNING MUSCLE ACTIONS

❑ **1. Extension of the Big Toe (Toe #1) at the Metatarsophalangeal Joint and the Interphalangeal Joint:** The extensor hallucis longus crosses the big toe dorsally (with its fibers running horizontally in the sagittal plane); therefore, it extends the big toe. Since it attaches onto the distal phalanx, it crosses both the metatarsophalangeal and the interphalangeal joints of the big toe. Therefore, the extensor hallucis longus extends the big toe at both of these joints.

❑ **2. Dorsiflexion of the Foot at the Ankle Joint:** The extensor hallucis longus crosses the ankle joint anteriorly (with its fibers running vertically in the sagittal plane); therefore, it dorsiflexes the foot at the ankle joint.

❑ **3. Inversion of the Foot at the Tarsal Joints:** The extensor hallucis longus crosses over the medial side of the foot (with its fibers running vertically in the frontal plane); therefore, it inverts the foot at the tarsal joints.

MISCELLANEOUS

❑ The extensor hallucis longus is located in the anterior compartment of the leg.

FIBULARIS TERTIUS
(IN THE ANTERIOR COMPARTMENT)

❑ **The name, fibularis tertius, tells us that this muscle attaches to the fibula and is the third "fibularis" muscle. The first two fibularis muscles are the fibularis longus and fibularis brevis.**

DERIVATION ❑ fibularis: L. *refers to the fibula.*
tertius: L. *third.*

PRONUNCIATION ❑ fib-you **la**-ris **ter**-she-us

ATTACHMENTS

❑ **Distal Anterior Fibula**

❑ the distal 1/3 of the anterior fibula and the distal 1/3 of the interosseus membrane

to the

❑ **5th Metatarsal**

❑ the dorsal surface of the base of the 5th metatarsal

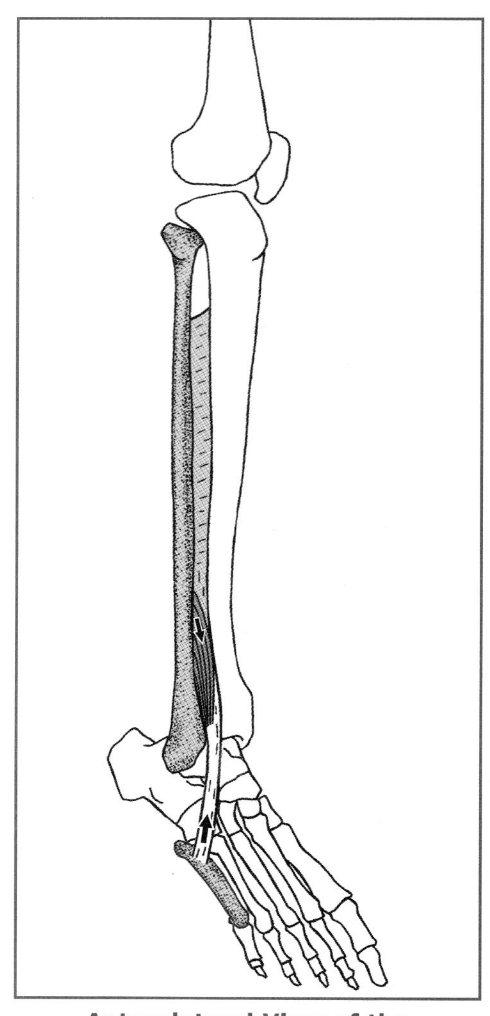

Anterolateral View of the Right Fibularis Tertius

ACTIONS

❑ 1. **Dorsiflexion of the Foot**

❑ 2. **Eversion of the Foot**

INNERVATION ❑ The Deep Fibular Nerve ❑ L5, S1

ARTERIAL SUPPLY ❑ The Anterior Tibial Artery (A Terminal Branch of the Popliteal Artery)

PALPATION AND SUPPLEMENTARY TEXT

PALPATION

The belly of the fibularis tertius, or one could say the portion of the extensor digitorum longus that makes up the fibularis tertius (which is the most distal and lateral part), is superficial and palpable. The distal tendon may also be palpated.

- ❑ **To palpate the belly:**
  - Have the client supine.
  - Place palpating hand on the distal shaft and the lateral malleolus of the fibula.
  - Palpate just medial to the distal shaft and lateral malleolus and you will be on the belly of the fibularis tertius.
  - To further bring out the fibularis tertius, ask the client to actively evert the foot (at the tarsal joints).

- ❑ **To palpate the distal tendon:**
  - Place palpating hand just lateral to the tendon of the extensor digitorum longus going to the 5th toe (see the palpation section for this muscle on page 422).
  - Ask the client to actively evert and dorsiflex the foot to make the tendon of the fibularis tertius visible as well as palpable.

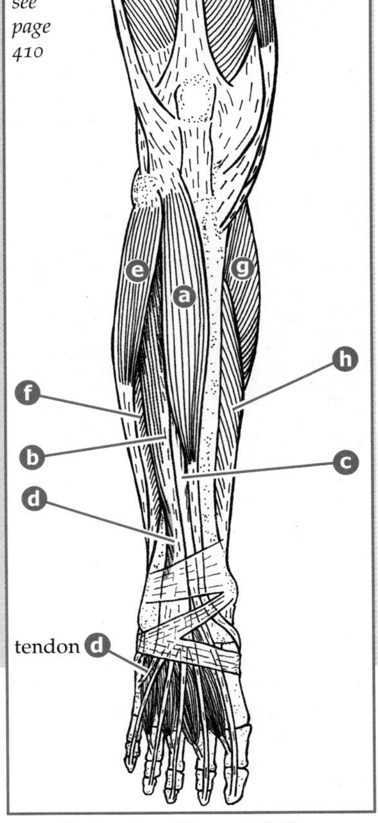

Anterior View of the Right Leg

a. Tibialis Anterior
b. Extensor Digitorum Longus
c. Extensor Hallucis Longus
d. Fibularis Tertius
e. Fibularis Longus
f. Fibularis Brevis
g. Gastrocnemius
h. Soleus

RELATIONSHIP TO OTHER MUSCULOSKELETAL STRUCTURES

❑ 1. The fibularis tertius is actually part of the extensor digitorum longus. It comprises the most distal part of the belly of the extensor digitorum longus, which becomes the most lateral tendon (and attaches to the 5th metatarsal).

❑ 2. Deep to the fibularis tertius is the fibula.

METHODOLOGY FOR LEARNING MUSCLE ACTIONS

❑ **1. Dorsiflexion of the Foot at the Ankle Joint:** The fibularis tertius crosses the ankle joint anteriorly (with its fibers running vertically in the sagittal plane); therefore, it dorsiflexes the foot at the ankle joint.

❑ **2. Eversion of the Foot at the Tarsal Joints:** The fibularis tertius crosses onto the foot laterally (with its fibers running vertically in the frontal plane); therefore, it everts the foot at the tarsal joints.

MISCELLANEOUS

❑ 1. The fibularis tertius is located in the anterior compartment of the leg.

❑ 2. The three "fibularis" muscles are grouped together because they all evert the foot at the tarsal joints.

❑ 3. The fibularis tertius was formerly named the *peroneus tertius*.

❑ 4. The fibularis tertius is actually the most distal and lateral part of the extensor digitorum longus. Its fibers do not attach onto a digit (a phalanx) and for this reason, the fibularis tertius is given a separate name and is not called part of the extensor digitorum longus.

FIBULARIS LONGUS
(IN THE LATERAL COMPARTMENT)

❑ **The name, fibularis longus, tells us that this muscle attaches to the fibula and is long (longer than the fibularis brevis).**

DERIVATION ❑ fibularis: L. *refers to the fibula.*
longus: L. *long.*

PRONUNCIATION ❑ fib-you-**la**-ris **long**-us

ATTACHMENTS

❑ **Proximal Lateral Fibula**

❑ the head of the fibula and the proximal 1/2 of the lateral fibula

to the

❑ **Medial Foot**

❑ the 1st cuneiform and 1st metatarsal

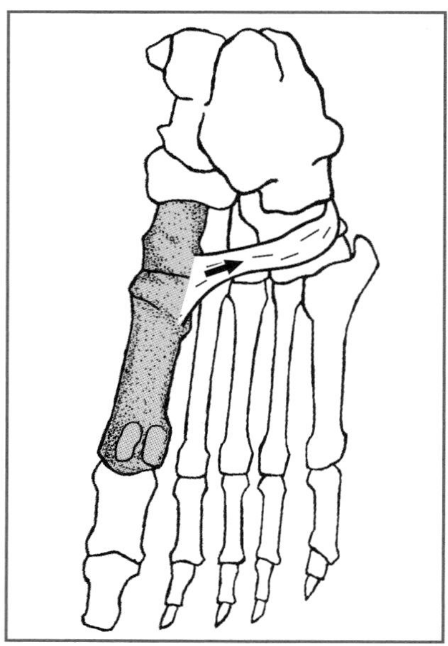

Plantar Surface of the Right Foot
(to view the distal tendon of the fibularis longus)

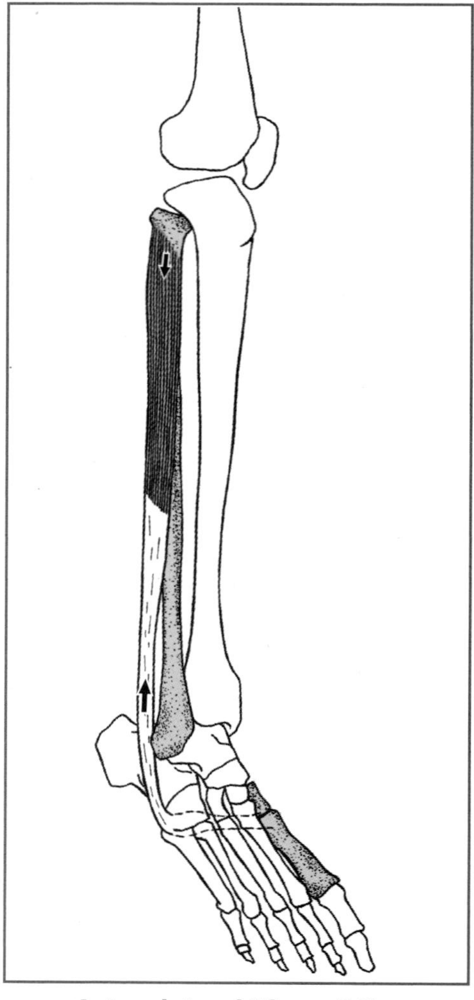

Anterolateral View of the Right Fibularis Longus

ACTIONS

❑ 1. **Eversion of the Foot**

❑ 2. **Plantarflexion of the Foot**

INNERVATION ❑ The Superficial Fibular Nerve ❑ L5, S1

ARTERIAL SUPPLY ❑ The Fibular Artery (A Branch of the Posterior Tibial Artery)

PALPATION AND SUPPLEMENTARY TEXT

PALPATION

- ❑ The belly of the fibularis longus is superficial and can be palpated for its entire length from the head of the fibula to the point where it becomes tendon halfway down the leg.
  - Have the client prone, supine, or side-lying.
  - Place palpating hand on the proximal lateral leg.
  - Ask the client to actively evert the foot (at the tarsal joints) and feel for the contraction of the belly of the fibularis longus from the head of the fibula to the point where it becomes tendon halfway down the leg.
  - Continue palpating distally to palpate the distal tendon of the fibularis longus. The distal tendon of the fibularis longus is superficial to the fibularis brevis muscle belly and care must be taken to distinguish the two.
  - The tendon of the fibularis longus is usually visible, as well as palpable, from posterior to the lateral malleolus all the way until it dives into the plantar side of the foot, inferior to the cuboid bone.
  - At the lateral malleolus, the tendon of the fibularis longus will be directly posterior to the tendon of the fibularis brevis (which will be closer to the lateral malleolus and more prominent).
  - Again, active eversion of the foot (at the tarsal joints) will make the distal tendon of the fibularis longus (as well as the distal tendon of the fibularis brevis) stand out.

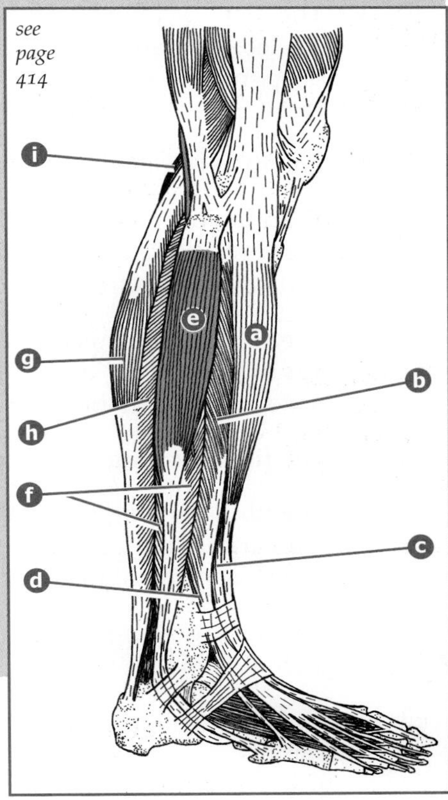

Lateral View of the Right Leg

a. Tibialis Anterior
b. Extensor Digitorum Longus
c. Extensor Hallucis Longus
d. Fibularis Tertius
e. **Fibularis Longus**
f. Fibularis Brevis
g. Gastrocnemius
h. Soleus
i. Plantaris

RELATIONSHIP TO OTHER MUSCULOSKELETAL STRUCTURES

❑ 1. Proximally, the fibularis longus is lateral to the tibialis anterior and the extensor digitorum longus.

❑ 2. Proximally, the fibularis longus is superficial to the extensor digitorum longus. Distally, the fibularis longus is superficial to the fibularis brevis.

❑ 3. The fibularis longus is anterior to the soleus.

❑ 4. The distal tendon of the fibularis longus is very deep and found in the fourth layer of muscles of the plantar surface of the foot.

METHODOLOGY FOR LEARNING MUSCLE ACTIONS

❑ **1. Eversion of the Foot at the Tarsal Joints:** The fibularis longus crosses onto the foot laterally (with its fibers running vertically in the frontal plane); therefore, it everts the foot at the tarsal joints.

FIBULARIS LONGUS – continued

- ❑ **2. Plantarflexion of the Foot at the Ankle Joint:** The fibularis longus crosses the ankle joint posteriorly (with its fibers running vertically in the sagittal plane); therefore, it plantarflexes the foot at the ankle joint.

MISCELLANEOUS

- ❑ 1. The fibularis longus is located in the lateral compartment of the leg.
- ❑ 2. The fibularis longus becomes tendon halfway down the leg.
- ❑ 3. The distal tendon of the fibularis longus follows an unusual path; it crosses posterior to the lateral malleolus to enter the lateral side of the foot, where it crosses posterior to the cuboid and then dives deep into the plantar side of the foot. It finally attaches onto the medial side of the foot at the same location as the attachment of the tibialis anterior (1st cuneiform and 1st metatarsal).
- ❑ 4. The three "fibularis" muscles are grouped together because they all evert the foot at the tarsal joints.
- ❑ 5. The fibularis longus and the fibularis brevis both cross posterior to the lateral malleolus; therefore, they both plantarflex the foot at the ankle joint. The fibularis tertius crosses anterior to the lateral malleolus; therefore, it dorsiflexes the foot at the ankle joint.
- ❑ 6. The fibularis longus is one of only a few muscles in the body that has a tendon that makes an abrupt turn of 90° or more. (Other muscles that do this are the obturator internus, tibialis posterior, flexor digitorum longus, flexor hallucis longus, tensor palati and the superior oblique.)
- ❑ 7. The fibularis longus was formerly named the *peroneus longus*.
- ❑ 8. The fibularis longus and the tibialis anterior are known as the *stirrup muscles*. These two muscles both attach at the same location on the foot (1st cuneiform and 1st metatarsal) and may be viewed to act as a stirrup to support the arch (medial longitudinal arch) of the foot.
- ❑ 9. The fibularis longus is also credited with supporting the transverse arch and the lateral longitudinal arch of the foot.
- ❑ 10. The fibularis longus and the fibularis brevis should be strengthened in people who have had inversion sprains of the ankle.

FIBULARIS BREVIS
(IN THE LATERAL COMPARTMENT)

❑ **The name, fibularis brevis, tells us that this muscle attaches onto the fibula and is short (shorter than the fibularis longus).**

DERIVATION ❑ fibularis: L. *refers to the fibula.*
brevis: L. *short.*

PRONUNCIATION ❑ fib-you-**la**-ris **bre**-vis

ATTACHMENTS

❑ **Distal Lateral Fibula**

❑ the distal 1/2 of the lateral fibula

to the

❑ **Lateral Foot**

❑ the lateral side of the base of the 5th metatarsal

ACTIONS

❑ **1. Eversion of the Foot**

❑ **2. Plantarflexion of the Foot**

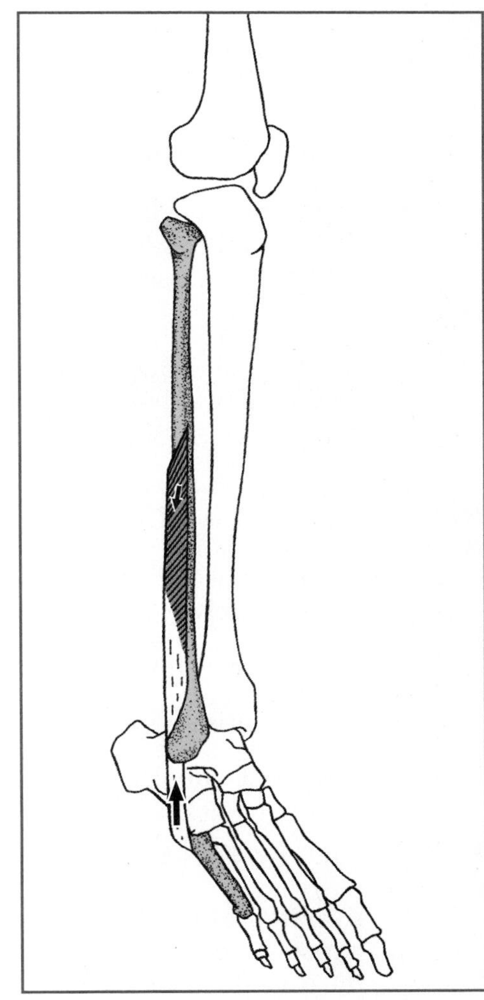

Anterolateral View of the Right Fibularis Brevis

INNERVATION ❑ The Superficial Fibular Nerve ❑ L5, S1

ARTERIAL SUPPLY ❑ The Fibular Artery (A Branch of the Posterior Tibial Artery)

FIBULARIS BREVIS – PALPATION AND SUPPLEMENTARY TEXT

PALPATION

- ❑ Much of the belly of the fibularis brevis is deep to the fibularis longus and difficult to palpate and distinguish from the fibularis longus.
  - Have the client either prone, supine or side lying.
  - Place palpating hand on the distal lateral leg.
  - Ask the client to actively evert the foot (at the tarsal joints) and feel for the belly of the fibularis brevis on either side of the fibularis longus' distal tendon. Keep in mind that this will make both the fibularis longus and the fibularis brevis stand out.
  - The distal tendon of the fibularis brevis is visible and palpable from the lateral malleolus to the base of the 5th metatarsal.
  - At the lateral malleolus, the tendon of the fibularis brevis is the one that is directly anterior to the tendon of the fibularis longus (and will be closer to the lateral malleolus and more prominent).
  - Again, active eversion of the foot (at the tarsal joints) will make the distal tendon of the fibularis brevis (as well as the distal tendon of the fibularis longus) stand out.

RELATIONSHIP TO OTHER MUSCULOSKELETAL STRUCTURES

- ❑ 1. The fibularis brevis is deep to the fibularis longus, but it is not entirely covered by the fibularis longus.
- ❑ 2. The fibularis brevis is posterior to the extensor digitorum longus.
- ❑ 3. The fibularis brevis is anterior to the soleus.
- ❑ 4. Deep to the fibularis brevis is the fibula.

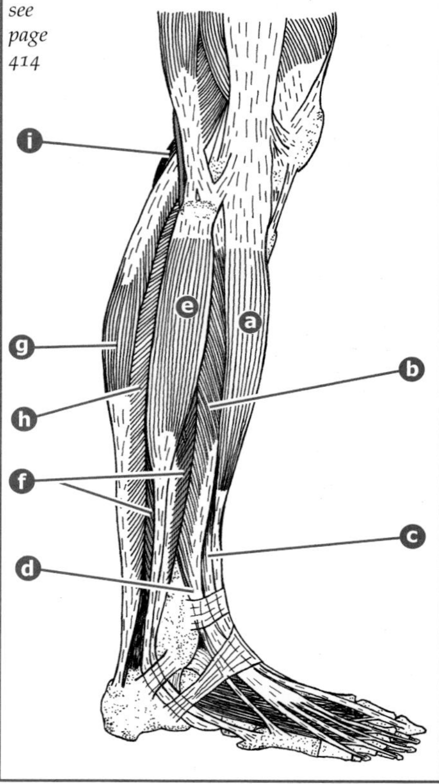

Lateral View of the Right Leg

a. Tibialis Anterior
b. Extensor Digitorum Longus
c. Extensor Hallucis Longus
d. Fibularis Tertius
e. Fibularis Longus
f. **Fibularis Brevis**
g. Gastrocnemius
h. Soleus
i. Plantaris

METHODOLOGY FOR LEARNING MUSCLE ACTIONS

- ❑ **1. Eversion of the Foot at the Tarsal Joints:** The fibularis brevis crosses onto the foot laterally (with its fibers running vertically in the frontal plane); therefore, it everts the foot at the tarsal joints.
- ❑ **2. Plantarflexion of the Foot at the Ankle Joint:** The fibularis brevis crosses the ankle joint posteriorly (with its fibers running vertically in the sagittal plane); therefore, it plantarflexes the foot at the ankle joint.

FIBULARIS BREVIS – continued

MISCELLANEOUS

- ❑ 1. The fibularis brevis is located in the lateral compartment of the leg.
- ❑ 2. The three "fibularis" muscles are grouped together because they all evert the foot at the tarsal joints.
- ❑ 3. The distal tendon of the fibularis brevis travels with the distal tendon of the fibularis longus. Together, they both cross posterior to the lateral malleolus. Therefore, they both plantarflex the foot at the ankle joint.
- ❑ 4. The fibularis brevis was formerly named the *peroneus brevis*.
- ❑ 5. The fibularis longus and the fibularis brevis should be strengthened in people who have had inversion sprains of the ankle.

❑ GASTROCNEMIUS ("GASTROCS")

(OF THE TRICEPS SURAE AND IN THE SUPERFICIAL POSTERIOR COMPARTMENT)

❑ **The name, gastrocnemius, tells us that this muscle gives the posterior leg its belly shape. (The contour of the posterior leg is due to the two bellies of the gastrocnemius.)**

DERIVATION ❑ gastro: Gr. *stomach.*
nemius: Gr. *leg.*

PRONUNCIATION ❑ **gas**-trok-**nee**-me-us

ATTACHMENTS

❑ **Medial and Lateral Femoral Condyles**

❑ and the distal posteromedial femur
and the distal posterolateral femur

to the

❑ **Calcaneus via the Calcaneal Tendon**

❑ the posterior surface

ACTIONS

❑ 1. **Plantarflexion of the Foot**

❑ 2. **Flexion of the Leg**

❑ 3. Inversion of the Foot

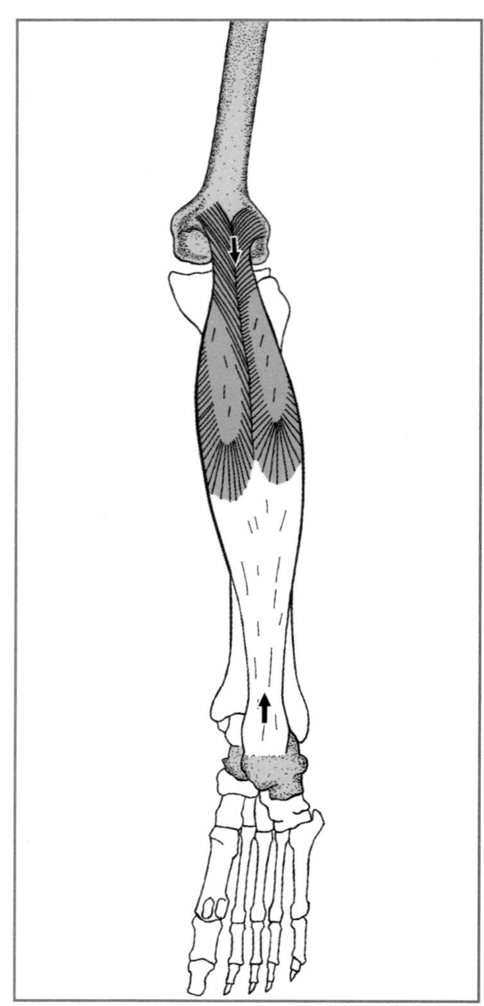

Posterior View of the Right Gastrocnemius
(with the foot plantarflexed)

INNERVATION ❑ The Tibial Nerve ❑ S1, 2

ARTERIAL SUPPLY ❑ Sural Branches of the Popliteal Artery (The Continuation of the Femoral Artery)

PALPATION AND SUPPLEMENTARY TEXT

PALPATION

- ❑ The gastrocnemius is superficial, visible and easy to palpate.
  - Have the client prone with the leg extended at the knee joint.
  - Place palpating hand on the proximal posterior leg.
  - To visualize and better palpate, ask the client to actively plantarflex the foot at the ankle joint against resistance and feel for the contraction of the gastrocnemius. It can be palpated from its proximal attachments to its distal attachment.

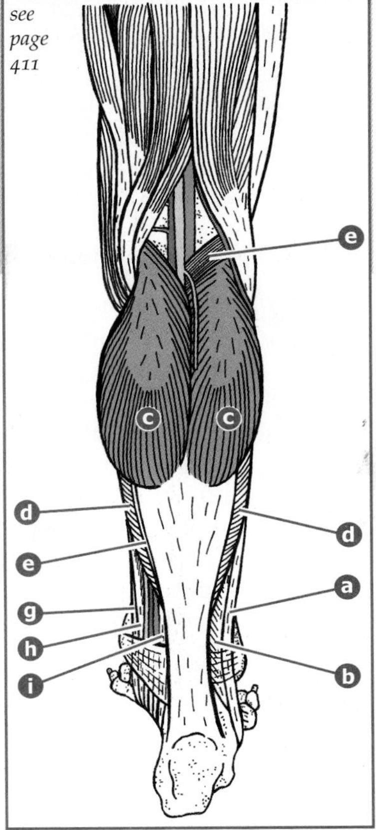

Posterior View of the Right Leg (Superficial)

a. Fibularis Longus
b. Fibularis Brevis
c. **Gastrocnemius**
d. Soleus
e. Plantaris
f. Popliteus (not seen)
g. Tibialis Posterior
h. Flexor Digitorum Longus
i. Flexor Hallucis Longus

RELATIONSHIP TO OTHER MUSCULOSKELETAL STRUCTURES

❑ 1. The gastrocnemius is superficial in the posterior leg.

❑ 2. The soleus is deep to the gastrocnemius and is largely, but not entirely, covered by it.

❑ 3. The distal belly and tendon of the biceps femoris is superficial to the proximal attachment of the lateral gastrocnemius.

METHODOLOGY FOR LEARNING MUSCLE ACTIONS

❑ 1. **Plantarflexion of the Foot at the Ankle Joint:** The gastrocnemius crosses the ankle joint posteriorly (with its fibers running vertically in the sagittal plane); therefore, it plantarflexes the foot at the ankle joint.

❑ 2. **Flexion of the Leg at the Knee Joint:** The gastrocnemius crosses the knee joint posteriorly (with its fibers running vertically in the sagittal plane); therefore, it flexes the leg at the knee joint.

❑ 3. **Inversion of the Foot at the Tarsal Joints:** The gastrocnemius crosses into the foot to attach onto the calcaneus medial to the axis of the tarsal joints where inversion occurs. Therefore, the gastrocnemius inverts the foot at the tarsal joints.

MISCELLANEOUS

❑ 1. The gastrocnemius is located in the superficial posterior compartment of the leg.

❑ 2. The gastrocnemius and the soleus together are sometimes called the *triceps surae*. Triceps refers to having three heads (medial gastrocnemius, lateral gastrocnemius and the soleus) and surae (**sur**-eye) refers to the calf of the leg. They are grouped together as the triceps surae because they all attach to the calcaneus via the calcaneal (Achilles) tendon.

❑ 3. Given that the distal tendon of the plantaris is directly next to (and often melds with) the calcaneal (Achilles) tendon, the plantaris is often grouped with the gastrocnemius and the soleus. This group is sometimes called the *quadriceps surae*.

GASTROCNEMIUS – continued

- ❑ 4. The gastrocnemius attaches to the calcaneus via the calcaneal tendon, which is also known as the *Achilles tendon*.
- ❑ 5. The Achilles tendon derives its name from the Greek mythological story in which Achilles was to go into battle to rescue Helen of Troy. When he was young, to make him invulnerable to poison arrows, his mother dipped him into the River Styx. However, she held him by his posterior ankle (i.e., heel). Therefore, he was vulnerable in that one spot, hence, the expression "Achilles heel" denoting a person's weakness. Unfortunately, Paris hit him with a poison arrow in his heel and he died. The relevance to anatomy is that the muscles of the triceps surae are the prime movers of foot plantarflexion, which is needed to push the foot off the ground when walking and/or running. If the Achilles tendon ruptures, one loses the ability to walk and/or run, which makes one vulnerable and weak.
- ❑ 6. The gastrocnemius becomes tendon approximately halfway down the leg.
- ❑ 7. Even though plantarflexion of the foot at the ankle joint is a very important action during walking, there is very little gastrocnemius activity in walking. The gastrocnemius is not appreciably recruited unless one walks uphill or up stairs, runs, jumps or tip-toes.
- ❑ 8. In most situations, since the gastrocnemius crosses the knee joint posteriorly, it will contribute to flexion of the knee joint. However, when a person is standing, it is extremely difficult for the knee joints to flex unless the ankle joints simultaneously dorsiflex. Therefore, if a person is standing and dorsiflexion of the ankle joints is prevented, then the gastrocnemius action at the knee joint changes. Unable to create flexion at the knee, the gastrocnemius pulls the femoral condyles posteriorly and inferiorly, contributing to extension at the knee joint. Therefore, in a typical standing posture, the gastrocnemius muscles can help to maintain knee extension.

SOLEUS

(OF THE TRICEPS SURAE AND IN THE SUPERFICIAL POSTERIOR COMPARTMENT) ❑

❑ **The name, soleus, tells us that this muscle attaches onto the sole of the foot (the calcaneus).**

DERIVATION ❑ soleus: L. *sole of the foot.*

PRONUNCIATION ❑ **so**-lee-us

ATTACHMENTS

❑ **Posterior Tibia and Fibula**

- ❑ the soleal line of the tibia and the head and proximal 1/3 of the fibula

to the

❑ **Calcaneus via the Calcaneal Tendon**

- ❑ the posterior surface

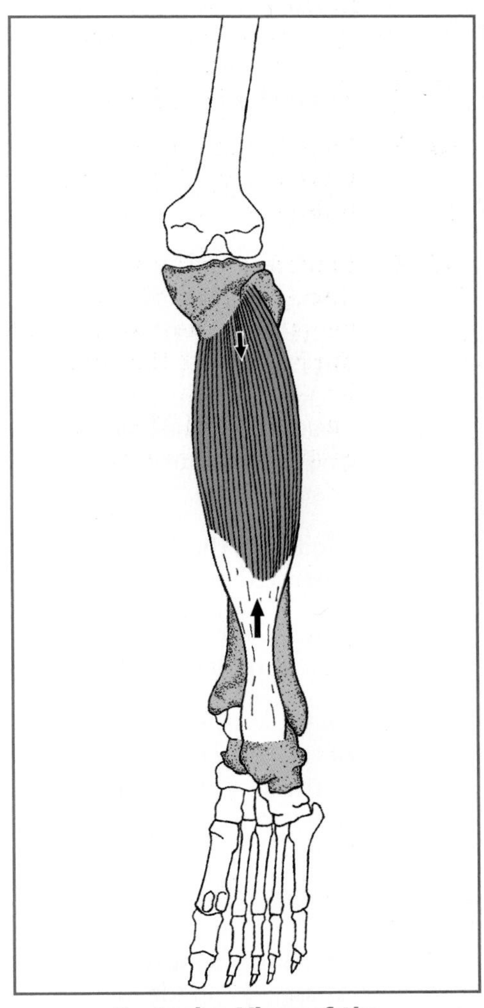

Posterior View of the Right Soleus
(with the foot plantarflexed)

ACTIONS

❑ 1. **Plantarflexion of the Foot**

❑ 2. Inversion of the Foot

INNERVATION ❑ The Tibial Nerve ❑ S1, 2

ARTERIAL SUPPLY ❑ Sural Branches of the Popliteal Artery (The Continuation of the Femoral Artery)

SOLEUS – PALPATION AND SUPPLEMENTARY TEXT

PALPATION

- ❑ The soleus may be visualized and/or palpated on either side of the gastrocnemius.
  - Have the client prone with the leg flexed at the knee joint. (Having the leg flexed slackens the gastrocnemius and lessens its contraction with plantarflexion of the foot.)
  - Place palpating hand on the proximal posterior leg.
  - Ask the client to actively plantarflex the foot at the ankle joint against mild resistance and feel for the contraction of the soleus.
  - The soleus is superficial on either side of the belly of the gastrocnemius or you may palpate it deep to the gastrocnemius in the posterior leg.

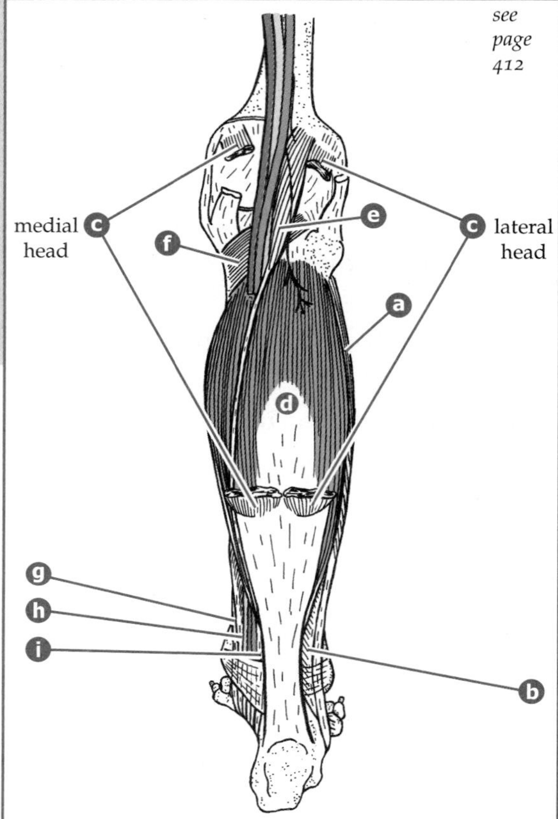

Posterior View of the Right Leg (Intermediate)

- **a.** Fibularis Longus
- **b.** Fibularis Brevis
- **c.** Gastrocnemius (cut)
- **d.** **Soleus**
- **e.** Plantaris
- **f.** Popliteus
- **g.** Tibialis Posterior
- **h.** Flexor Digitorum Longus
- **i.** Flexor Hallucis Longus

RELATIONSHIP TO OTHER MUSCULOSKELETAL STRUCTURES

❑ 1. Posteriorly, the soleus is deep to the gastrocnemius and the plantaris, but medially and laterally, the soleus is superficial.

❑ 2. Medially, the soleus is located between the gastrocnemius and the tibia.

❑ 3. Laterally, the soleus is located between the gastrocnemius and the fibularis longus.

❑ 4. The soleus is superficial to the three deep muscles of the posterior leg: the tibialis posterior, the flexor digitorum longus and the flexor hallucis longus (the "Tom, Dick and Harry" muscles).

METHODOLOGY FOR LEARNING MUSCLE ACTIONS

❑ **1. Plantarflexion of the Foot at the Ankle Joint:** The soleus crosses the ankle joint posteriorly (with its fibers running vertically in the sagittal plane); therefore, it plantarflexes the foot at the ankle joint.

❑ **2. Inversion of the Foot at the Tarsal Joints:** The soleus crosses into the foot to attach onto the calcaneus medial to the axis of the tarsal joints where inversion occurs. Therefore, the soleus inverts the foot at the tarsal joints.

SOLEUS – continued

MISCELLANEOUS

- ❑ 1. The soleus is located in the superficial posterior compartment of the leg.
- ❑ 2. The soleus and the gastrocnemius together are sometimes called the *triceps surae*. Triceps refers to having three heads (the medial gastrocnemius, the lateral gastrocnemius and the soleus) and surae (**sur**-eye) refers to the calf of the leg. They are grouped together as the triceps surae because they all attach to the calcaneus via the calcaneal tendon.
- ❑ 3. Given that the distal tendon of the plantaris is directly next to (and often melds with) the calcaneal (Achilles) tendon, the plantaris is often grouped with the gastrocnemius and the soleus. This group is sometimes called the *quadriceps surae*.
- ❑ 4. The soleus attaches to the calcaneus via the calcaneal tendon, which is also known as the *Achilles tendon*.
- ❑ 5. The Achilles tendon derives its name from the Greek mythological story in which Achilles was to go into battle to rescue Helen of Troy. When he was young, to make him invulnerable to poison arrows, his mother dipped him into the River Styx. However, she held him by his posterior ankle (i.e., heel). Therefore, he was vulnerable in that one spot, hence, the expression *Achilles heel* denoting a person's weakness. Unfortunately, Paris hit him with a poison arrow in his heel and he died. The relevance to anatomy is that the triceps surae are the prime movers of foot plantarflexion, which is needed to push the foot off the ground when walking and/or running. If the Achilles tendon ruptures, one loses the ability to walk and/or run, which makes one vulnerable and weak.
- ❑ 6. The soleus becomes tendon much further distally in the leg than the gastrocnemius.
- ❑ 7. The soleus is a thick muscle, largely accounting for the contours of the gastrocnemius being so visible. ("Behind every great gastrocnemius is a great soleus." ☺)

❑ PLANTARIS

(IN THE SUPERFICIAL POSTERIOR COMPARTMENT)

❑ **The name, plantaris, tells us that this muscle attaches onto the calcaneus, a bone of the plantar surface of the foot (see miscellaneous #7).**

DERIVATION ❑ plantaris: L. *refers to the plantar side of the foot.*

PRONUNCIATION ❑ plan-**ta**-ris

ATTACHMENTS

❑ **Distal Posterolateral Femur**

- ❑ the lateral condyle and the distal lateral supracondylar line of the femur

to the

❑ **Calcaneus**

- ❑ the posterior surface

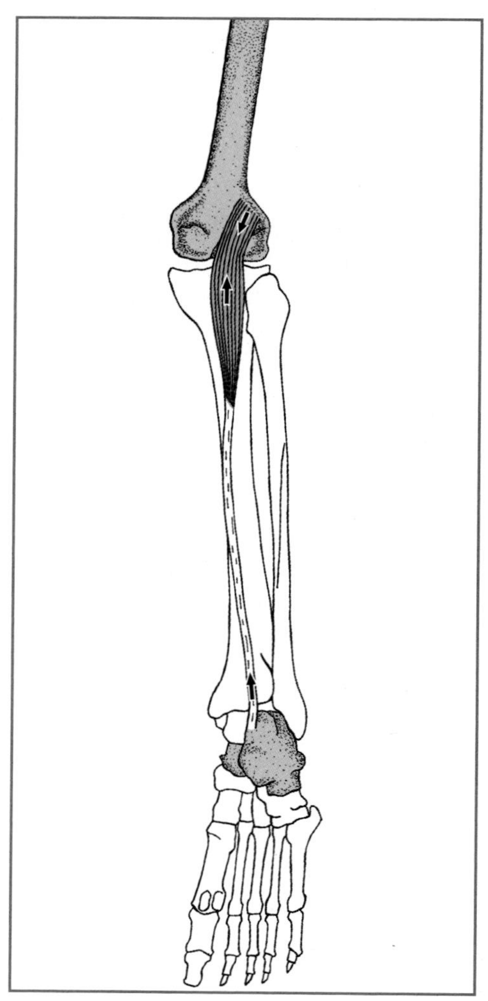

Posterior View of the Right Plantaris
(with the foot plantarflexed)

ACTIONS

❑ 1. **Plantarflexion of the Foot**

❑ 2. **Flexion of the Leg**

INNERVATION ❑ The Tibial Nerve ❑ S1, 2

ARTERIAL SUPPLY ❑ Sural Branches of the Popliteal Artery (The Continuation of the Femoral Artery)

PALPATION AND SUPPLEMENTARY TEXT

PALPATION

- ❑ The small muscle belly of the plantaris is superficial and palpable just medial to the distal attachment of the biceps femoris and the proximal attachment of the lateral head of the gastrocnemius.
  - Have the client prone with the leg extended at the knee joint.
  - Place palpating hand on the proximal posterior leg.
  - Ask the client to actively flex the leg at the knee joint and plantarflex the foot at the ankle joint and feel for the contraction of the plantaris.

    Distinguishing the plantaris from the lateral head of the gastrocnemius will be difficult given that the gastrocnemius will also contract with these two actions.

    (Note: The long distal tendon of the plantaris is so slender that it is not palpable even where it is superficial.)

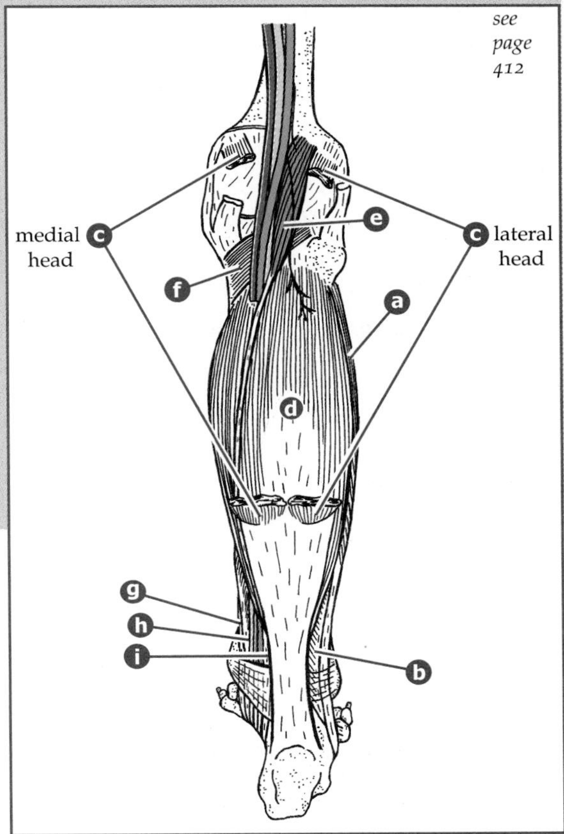

Posterior View of the Right Leg (Intermediate)

a. Fibularis Longus
b. Fibularis Brevis
c. Gastrocnemius (cut)
d. Soleus
e. Plantaris
f. Popliteus
g. Tibialis Posterior
h. Flexor Digitorum Longus
i. Flexor Hallucis Longus

RELATIONSHIP TO OTHER MUSCULOSKELETAL STRUCTURES

❑ 1. The plantaris attaches just medial to the lateral head of the gastrocnemius and the distal tendon of the biceps femoris.

❑ 2. Much of the belly of the plantaris is superficial in the posterior knee just medial to the lateral head of the gastrocnemius. Here, the plantaris is superficial to the popliteus.

❑ 3. The rest of the belly and the proximal 1/2 of the long distal tendon of the plantaris are sandwiched between the gastrocnemius and the soleus. (The tendon is deep to the gastrocnemius and superficial to the soleus.) The distal 1/2 of the long distal tendon is superficial just medial to the medial margin of the distal tendon of the gastrocnemius.

METHODOLOGY FOR LEARNING MUSCLE ACTIONS

❑ **1. Plantarflexion of the Foot at the Ankle Joint:** The plantaris crosses the ankle joint posteriorly (with its fibers running vertically in the sagittal plane); therefore, it plantarflexes the foot at the ankle joint.

❑ **2. Flexion of the Leg at the Knee Joint:** The plantaris crosses the knee joint posteriorly (with its fibers running vertically in the sagittal plane); therefore, it flexes the leg at the knee joint.

PLANTARIS – continued

MISCELLANEOUS

- ❑ 1. The plantaris is located in the superficial posterior compartment of the leg.
- ❑ 2. After crossing the knee joint, the plantaris becomes a very long, thin tendon that runs between the gastrocnemius and the soleus.
- ❑ 3. The distal tendon of the plantaris often joins with the calcaneal (Achilles) tendon of the gastrocnemius and soleus.
- ❑ 4. Given that the distal tendon of the plantaris is directly next to (and often melds with) the calcaneal (Achilles) tendon, the plantaris is often grouped with the gastrocnemius and the soleus. This group is sometimes called the *quadriceps surae*.
- ❑ 5. The plantaris muscle is so weak that many sources consider its function to be negligible.
- ❑ 6. The plantaris of the leg is considered to be analogous to the palmaris longus of the forearm.
- ❑ 7. The name plantaris is misleading because this muscle does not attach onto the plantar surface of the foot in humans (although it does attach onto the posterior calcaneus, which is near the plantar surface). In other primates, the plantaris curves around the calcaneus to attach into the plantar fascia, thereby actually attaching onto the plantar surface of the foot.

POPLITEUS
(IN THE DEEP POSTERIOR COMPARTMENT)

❑ **The name, popliteus, tells us that this muscle is located in the posterior knee.**

DERIVATION ❑ popliteus: L. *ham of the knee* (refers to the posterior knee).

PRONUNCIATION ❑ pop-**lit**-ee-us

ATTACHMENTS

❑ **Distal Posterolateral Femur**

- ❑ the lateral surface of the lateral condyle of the femur

to the

❑ **Proximal Posterior Tibia**

- ❑ the medial side

ACTIONS

❑ 1. **Medial Rotation of the Leg**

❑ 2. **Flexion of the Leg**

❑ 3. Lateral Rotation of the Thigh

Posterior View of the Right Popliteus
(with the foot plantarflexed)

INNERVATION ❑ The Tibial Nerve ❑ L4, 5, S1

ARTERIAL SUPPLY ❑ Branches of the Popliteal Artery (The Continuation of the Femoral Artery)

POPLITEUS – PALPATION AND SUPPLEMENTARY TEXT

PALPATION

❑ The popliteus is deep and difficult to palpate. However, the tibial attachment can be palpated.

- Have the client seated.
- Place palpating hand on the tibial tuberosity and slide around medially until you are on the posterior shaft of the tibia.
- Palpate deep to the gastrocnemius in that location.
- Ask the client to actively medially rotate the leg at the knee joint and feel for the contraction of the popliteus. (The tibial attachment of the popliteus will be distal to the tibial attachment of the semimembranosus.)

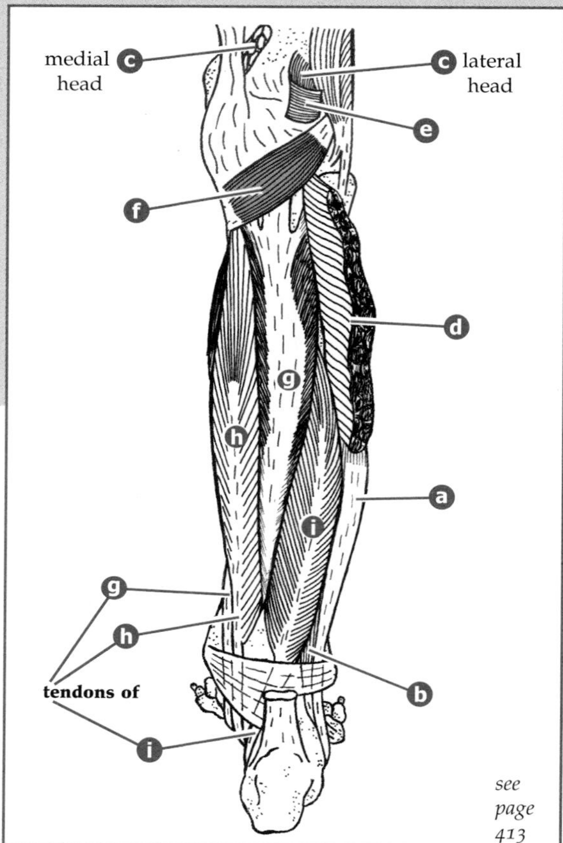

Posterior View of the Right Leg (Deep)

a. Fibularis Longus
b. Fibularis Brevis
c. Gastrocnemius (cut)
d. Soleus (cut and reflected)
e. Plantaris (cut and reflected)
f. Popliteus
g. Tibialis Posterior
h. Flexor Digitorum Longus
i. Flexor Hallucis Longus

RELATIONSHIP TO OTHER MUSCULOSKELETAL STRUCTURES

❑ 1. The popliteus is deep to the lateral head of the gastrocnemius and the plantaris.

❑ 2. The popliteus is proximal to the soleus.

❑ 3. Deep to the popliteus are the femur and the tibia.

METHODOLOGY FOR LEARNING MUSCLE ACTIONS

❑ **1. Medial Rotation of the Leg at the Knee Joint:** At the posterior knee, the popliteus wraps around the knee joint from the lateral femur to the medial tibia (with its fibers running horizontally in the transverse plane). When the popliteus contracts, it pulls the tibial attachment posterolaterally toward the femoral attachment. This causes the anterior leg to face somewhat medially. Therefore, the popliteus medially rotates the leg at the knee joint.

❑ **2. Flexion of the Leg at the Knee Joint:** The popliteus crosses the knee joint posteriorly (with its fibers running somewhat vertically in the sagittal plane); therefore, it flexes the leg at the knee joint.

❑ **3. Lateral Rotation of the Thigh at the Knee Joint:** Given that the popliteus wraps around the posterior knee joint from the medial tibia to the lateral femur (with its fibers running horizontally in the transverse plane), the popliteus can rotate the knee joint. When the attachment of the popliteus onto the leg is fixed (as is often the case with the foot planted on the ground), then instead of rotating the leg medially (see methodology #1), the reverse action occurs; i.e., the thigh is rotated laterally. When the popliteus contracts, it pulls the femur, causing the anterior surface of the thigh to face laterally. Therefore, the popliteus laterally rotates the thigh at the knee joint. (See note regarding reverse actions on page 405.)

POPLITEUS – continued

MISCELLANEOUS

- ❑ 1. The popliteus is located in the deep posterior compartment of the leg.
- ❑ 2. To flex a fully extended knee joint, medial rotation of the leg at the knee joint is required. Of all the medial rotators of the leg at the knee joint, the popliteus is thought to perform this initial medial rotation of the leg at the knee joint. When this occurs, it is often said that the popliteus "unlocks" the extended knee.
- ❑ 3. The popliteus also attaches into the lateral meniscus of the knee joint. This attachment facilitates the posterior movement of the lateral meniscus during knee flexion. Posterior movement of the lateral meniscus helps prevent impingement of the lateral meniscus between the femur and tibia during flexion of the knee joint. (Note: The semimembranosus has the same action with regard to the medial meniscus.)

❑ TIBIALIS POSTERIOR

("TOM" OF THE "TOM, DICK AND HARRY" MUSCLES AND IN THE DEEP POSTERIOR COMPARTMENT)

❑ **The name, tibialis posterior, tells us that this muscle attaches to the tibia and is located in the posterior leg.**

DERIVATION ❑ tibialis: L. *refers to the tibia.*
posterior: L. *behind, toward the back.*

PRONUNCIATION ❑ tib-ee-**a**-lis pos-**tee**-ri-or

ATTACHMENTS

❑ **Proximal Posterior Tibia and Fibula**

❑ the proximal 2/3 of:
the posterior tibia, fibula and interosseus membrane

to the

❑ **Plantar Surface of the Foot**

❑ metatarsals #2-4 and all the tarsal bones except the talus

ACTIONS

❑ **1. Plantarflexion of the Foot**

❑ **2 Inversion of the Foot**

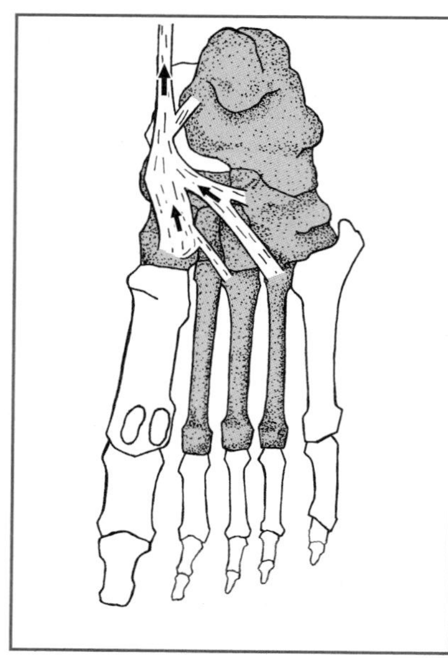

Plantar Surface of the Right Foot
(to view the distal tendon of the tibialis posterior)

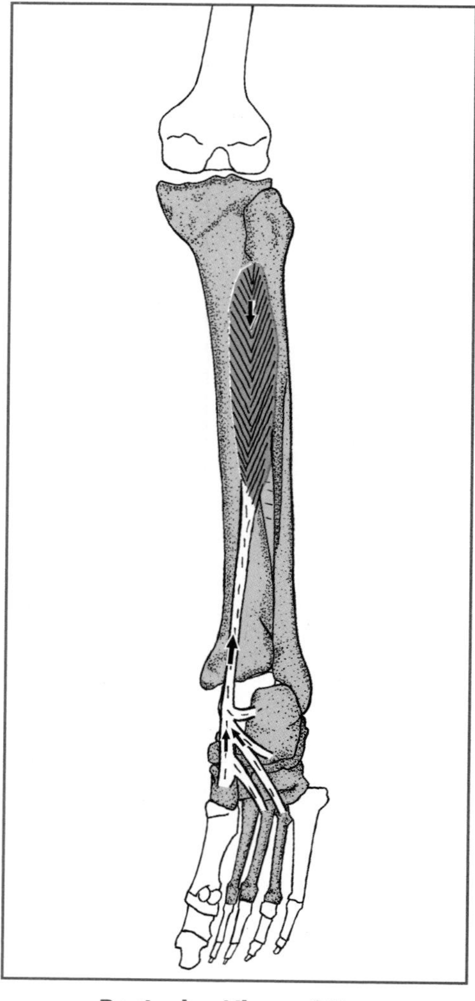

Posterior View of the Right Tibialis Posterior
(with the foot plantarflexed)

INNERVATION ❑ The Tibial Nerve ❑ L4, 5

ARTERIAL SUPPLY ❑ The Posterior Tibial Artery (A Terminal Branch of the Popliteal Artery)

PALPATION AND SUPPLEMENTARY TEXT

PALPATION

❑ The distal tendon of the tibialis posterior is visible and easily palpable proximal, posterior and distal to the medial malleolus. The belly of the tibialis posterior is very deep in the posterior leg and extremely difficult to palpate.

- Have the client seated or supine.
- To visualize and palpate the distal tendon of the tibialis posterior, have the client actively invert the foot (at the tarsal joints) and plantarflex the foot (at the ankle joint). Of the three tendons (tibialis posterior, flexor digitorum longus and flexor hallucis longus, i.e., the "Tom, Dick and Harry" muscles) that cross posterior to the medial malleolus, the distal tendon of the tibialis posterior is the closest to the medial malleolus.

  (Note: Asking the client to extend all five toes will help to eliminate contraction of the flexor digitorum longus and the flexor hallucis longus.)

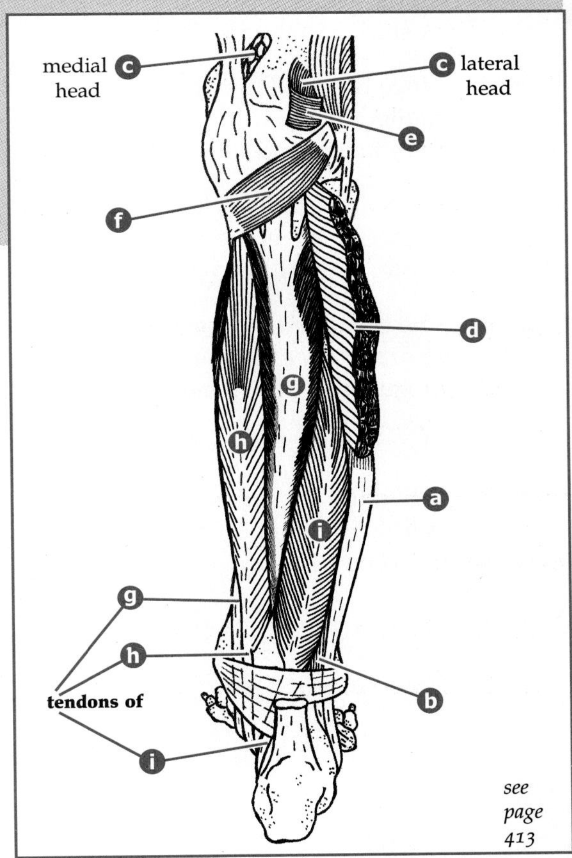

Posterior View of the Right Leg (Deep)

a. Fibularis Longus
b. Fibularis Brevis
c. Gastrocnemius (cut)
d. Soleus (cut and reflected)
e. Plantaris (cut and reflected)
f. Popliteus
g. **Tibialis Posterior**
h. Flexor Digitorum Longus
i. Flexor Hallucis Longus

RELATIONSHIP TO OTHER MUSCULOSKELETAL STRUCTURES

❑ 1. The tibialis posterior, flexor digitorum longus and flexor hallucis longus are the deepest muscles in the posterior leg. Where these muscles overlap, the tibialis posterior is the deepest of the three.

❑ 2. The tibialis posterior is deep to the soleus.

❑ 3. Deep to the tibialis posterior are the tibia, the fibula and the interosseus membrane.

❑ 4. Lateral to the tibialis posterior is the flexor digitorum longus and medial to the tibialis posterior is the flexor hallucis longus.

❑ 5. The distal tendon of the tibialis posterior crosses posterior to the medial malleolus along with the distal tendons of the flexor digitorum longus and the flexor hallucis longus.

❑ 6. The distal tendon of the tibialis posterior is very deep and found in the fourth layer of muscles of the plantar surface of the foot.

METHODOLOGY FOR LEARNING MUSCLE ACTIONS

❑ 1. **Plantarflexion of the Foot at the Ankle Joint:**
The tibialis posterior crosses the ankle joint posteriorly with its fibers running vertically in the sagittal plane); therefore, it plantarflexes the foot at the ankle joint.

TIBIALIS POSTERIOR – continued

❑ **2. Inversion of the Foot at the Tarsal Joints:** The tibialis posterior crosses the foot medially (with its fibers running vertically in the frontal plane); therefore, it inverts the foot at the tarsal joints.

MISCELLANEOUS

❑ 1. The tibialis posterior is located in the deep posterior compartment of the leg.

❑ 2. The tibialis posterior is the prime mover of inversion of the foot at the tarsal joints.

❑ 3. The **T**ibialis posterior is "**T**om" of the "**T**om, Dick and Harry" muscles. The Tom, Dick and Harry muscles are the tibialis posterior, flexor digitorum longus and flexor hallucis longus. Tom, Dick and Harry are grouped together because they are all deep in the posterior leg and their distal tendons cross posterior to the medial malleolus of the tibia (in order from anterior to posterior, Tom, Dick and Harry).

❑ 4. Since the tendons of the Tom, Dick and Harry group cross into the foot posterior to the medial malleolus, their line of pull is posteromedial. Therefore, all three Tom, Dick and Harry muscles plantarflex and invert the foot (at the ankle and tarsal joints respectively).

❑ 5. It is worth noting that the location of the muscle bellies of the Tom, Dick and Harry muscles in the posterior leg is, from medial to lateral, Dick, Tom and Harry (i.e., flexor digitorum longus, tibialis posterior and flexor hallucis longus).

❑ 6. The tibialis posterior is one of only a few muscles in the body that has a tendon that makes an abrupt turn of 90° or more. (Other muscles that do this are the obturator internus, fibularis longus, flexor digitorum longus, flexor hallucis longus, tensor palati and the superior oblique.)

❑ 7. The tibialis posterior helps to support the arch (medial longitudinal arch) of the foot.

❑ 8. When the tibialis posterior is tight and painful, this condition is often called *shin splints*. (Note: Shin splints is a general term that is applied to most any painful condition that occurs in the leg, i.e., between the knee and the ankle.)

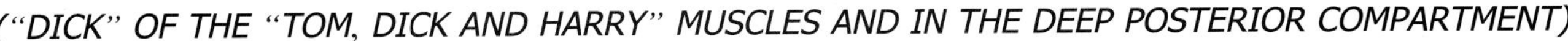

FLEXOR DIGITORUM LONGUS

("DICK" OF THE "TOM, DICK AND HARRY" MUSCLES AND IN THE DEEP POSTERIOR COMPARTMENT)

❑ **The name, flexor digitorum longus, tells us that this muscle flexes the digits, i.e., toes, and is long (longer than the flexor digitorum brevis).**

DERIVATION ❑ flexor: L. *a muscle that flexes a body part.*
digitorum: L. *refers to a digit* (toe).
longus: L. *long.*

PRONUNCIATION ❑ **fleks**-or dij-i-**toe**-rum **long**-us

ATTACHMENTS

❑ **Middle Posterior Tibia**

❑ the middle 1/3 of the posterior tibia

to the

❑ **Plantar Surface of Toes #2-5**

❑ the distal phalanges

ACTIONS

❑ 1. **Flexion of Toes #2-5**

❑ 2. **Plantarflexion of the Foot**

❑ 3. **Inversion of the Foot**

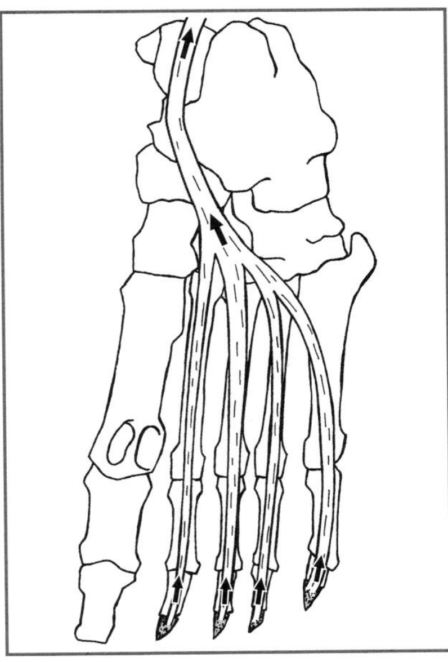

Plantar Surface of the Right Foot
(to view the distal tendons of the flexor digitorum longus)

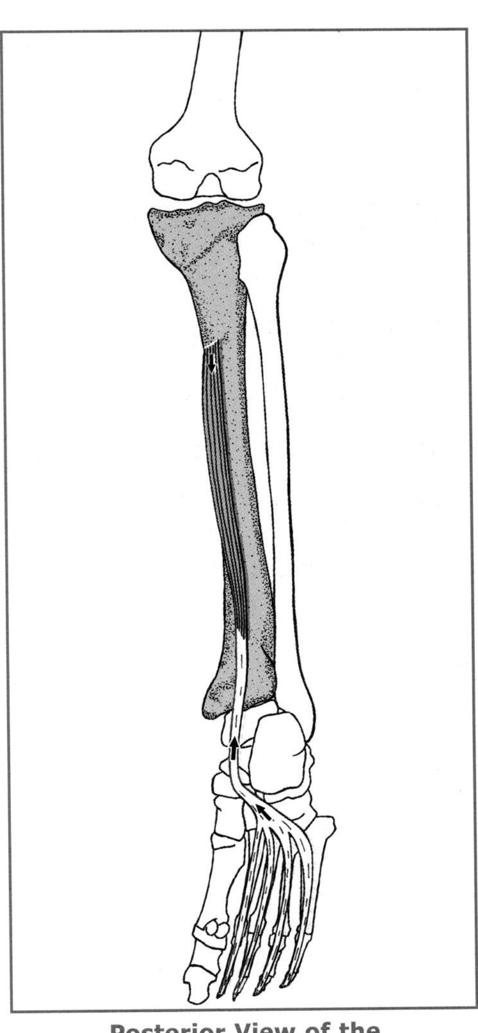

Posterior View of the Right Flexor Digitorum Longus
(with the foot plantarflexed)

INNERVATION ❑ The Tibial Nerve L5, **S1, 2**

ARTERIAL SUPPLY ❑ The Posterior Tibial Artery (A Terminal Branch of the Popliteal Artery)

FLEXOR DIGITORUM LONGUS – PALPATION AND SUPPLEMENTARY TEXT

PALPATION

The distal tendon of the flexor digitorum longus is one of three tendons that are palpable posterior to the medial malleolus. The majority of the belly of the flexor digitorum longus is very deep in the posterior leg and is extremely difficult to palpate. However, a small part of it is superficial and easily palpable in the distal medial leg, between the tibia and the soleus (see illustration on page 415).

❑ **To palpate the distal tendon:**

- Have the client seated or supine.
- Place palpating hand posterior to the medial malleolus.
- Have the client actively flex the toes and feel for the tensing of the distal tendon of the flexor digitorum longus.

  (Note: The tendons of the tibialis posterior and the flexor hallucis longus might also be palpable. To lessen their tendons from tensing, make sure that the client is not flexing the big toe and not inverting nor plantarflexing the foot.)

❑ **To palpate the belly in the posterior leg:**

- Locate the soleus (see the palpation section for this muscle on page 438) and palpate between the soleus and the shaft of the tibia in the medial leg.
- To further bring out the flexor digitorum longus, resistance may be added as the client actively flexes the toes.

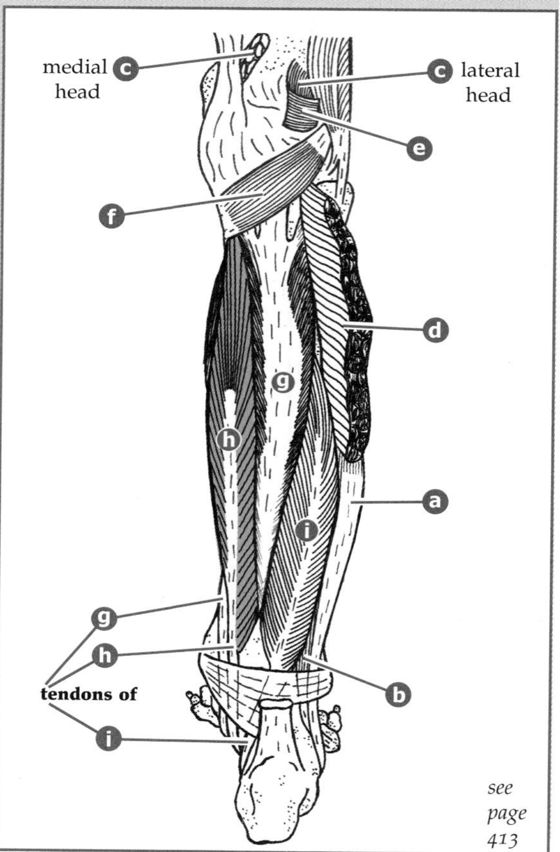

Posterior View of the Right Leg (Deep)

a. Fibularis Longus
b. Fibularis Brevis
c. Gastrocnemius (cut)
d. Soleus (cut and reflected)
e. Plantaris (cut and reflected)
f. Popliteus
g. Tibialis Posterior
h. **Flexor Digitorum Longus**
i. Flexor Hallucis Longus

RELATIONSHIP TO OTHER MUSCULOSKELETAL STRUCTURES

❑ 1. The flexor digitorum longus, tibialis posterior and flexor hallucis longus are the deepest muscles in the posterior leg. Where these muscles overlap, the tibialis posterior is the deepest of the three.

❑ 2. The flexor digitorum longus is deep to the soleus.

❑ 3. Deep to the flexor digitorum longus is the tibia.

❑ 4. The flexor digitorum longus is medial to the tibialis posterior and the flexor hallucis longus.

❑ 5. The distal tendon of the flexor digitorum longus crosses posterior to the medial malleolus along with the distal tendons of the tibialis posterior and the flexor hallucis longus.

FLEXOR DIGITORUM LONGUS – continued

METHODOLOGY FOR LEARNING MUSCLE ACTIONS

❑ **1. Flexion of Toes #2-5 at the Metatarsophalangeal Joint and the Interphalangeal Joints:** The flexor digitorum longus crosses the toe joints on the plantar side (with its fibers running horizontally in the sagittal plane); therefore, it flexes toes #2-5. Given that the flexor digitorum longus attaches onto the distal phalanx, it crosses the metatarsophalangeal joint and the proximal and distal interphalangeal joints of toes #2-5. Therefore, the flexor digitorum longus flexes the toes at all of these joints.

❑ **2. Plantarflexion of the Foot at the Ankle Joint:** The flexor digitorum longus crosses the ankle joint posteriorly (with its fibers running vertically in the sagittal plane); therefore, it plantarflexes the foot at the ankle joint.

❑ **3. Inversion of the Foot at the Tarsal Joints:** The flexor digitorum longus crosses the foot medially (with its fibers running vertically in the frontal plane); therefore, it inverts the foot at the tarsal joints.

MISCELLANEOUS

❑ 1. The flexor digitorum longus is located in the deep posterior compartment of the leg.

❑ 2. The flexor **D**igitorum longus is "**D**ick" of the "Tom, **D**ick and Harry" muscles. The Tom, Dick and Harry muscles are the tibialis posterior, flexor digitorum longus and flexor hallucis longus. Tom, Dick and Harry are grouped together because they are all deep in the posterior leg and all of their distal tendons cross posterior to the medial malleolus of the tibia (in order from anterior to posterior, Tom, Dick and Harry).

❑ 3. Since the tendons of the Tom, Dick and Harry group cross into the foot posterior to the medial malleolus, their line of pull is posteromedial. Therefore, all three Tom, Dick and Harry muscles plantarflex and invert the foot (at the ankle and tarsal joints respectively).

❑ 4. It is worth noting that the location of the muscle bellies of the Tom, Dick and Harry muscles in the posterior leg is, from medial to lateral, Dick, Tom and Harry (i.e., flexor digitorum longus, tibialis posterior and flexor hallucis longus).

❑ 5. The flexor digitorum longus is one of only a few muscles in the body that has a tendon that makes an abrupt turn of 90° or more. (Other muscles that do this are the obturator internus, fibularis longus, tibialis posterior, flexor hallucis longus, tensor palati and the superior oblique.)

❑ 6. The distal tendons of the flexor digitorum longus reach their attachment site on the distal phalanges in an unusual manner. The tendons of the flexor digitorum brevis lie superficial to the tendons of the flexor digitorum longus. The tendons of the flexor digitorum brevis split, and the tendons of the flexor digitorum longus then pass through this split to continue on to the distal phalanges. (This is essentially identical to the arrangement of the flexor digitorum superficialis and flexor digitorum profundus of the upper extremity.)

❑ 7. The flexor digitorum longus helps to support the arch (medial longitudinal arch) of the foot.

❑ FLEXOR HALLUCIS LONGUS

("HARRY" OF THE "TOM, DICK AND HARRY" MUSCLES AND IN THE DEEP POSTERIOR COMPARTMENT)

❑ **The name, flexor hallucis longus, tells us that this muscle flexes the big toe and is long (longer than the flexor hallucis brevis).**

DERIVATION ❑ flexor: L. *a muscle that flexes a body part.*
hallucis: L. *the big toe.*
longus: L. *long.*

PRONUNCIATION ❑ **fleks**-or hal-**oo**-sis **long**-us

ATTACHMENTS

❑ **Distal Posterior Fibula**

❑ the distal 2/3 of the posterior fibula
and the distal 2/3 of the interosseus membrane

to the

❑ **Plantar Surface of the Big Toe (Toe #1)**

❑ the distal phalanx

ACTIONS

❑ 1. **Flexion of the Big Toe (Toe #1)**

❑ 2. **Plantarflexion of the Foot**

❑ 3. **Inversion of the Foot**

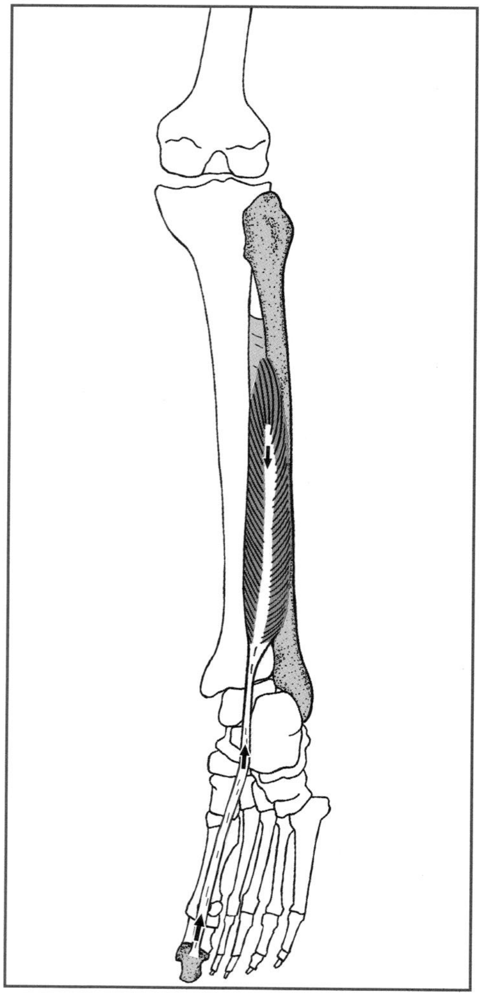

Posterior View of the Right Flexor Hallucis Longus
(with the foot plantarflexed)

INNERVATION ❑ The Tibial Nerve ❑ L5, **S1, 2**

ARTERIAL SUPPLY ❑ The Posterior Tibial Artery (A Terminal Branch of the Popliteal Artery)

PALPATION AND SUPPLEMENTARY TEXT

PALPATION

The distal tendon of the flexor hallucis longus is one of three tendons that are palpable posterior to the medial malleolus. The majority of the muscle belly of the flexor hallucis longus is very deep in the posterior leg and is difficult to palpate. However, a small part of it is superficial and easily palpable in the distal medial leg, between the fibula and the soleus (see illustration on page 415).

❑ **To palpate the distal tendon:**

- Have the client seated or supine.
- Place palpating hand approximately 1/2 to 1 inch (2 cm) posterior to the medial malleolus.
- Have the client actively flex the big toe and feel for the tensing of the distal tendon of the flexor hallucis longus.

  (Note: The tendons of the tibialis posterior and the flexor digitorum longus might also be palpable. The tendon of the flexor hallucis longus will be the farthest of the three from the medial malleolus, just anterior to the calcaneal tendon.)

❑ **To palpate the belly in the posterior leg:**

- Locate the soleus (see the palpation section for this muscle on page 438) and palpate between the soleus and the shaft of the fibula in the lateral leg.
- To further bring out the flexor hallucis longus, resistance may be added.

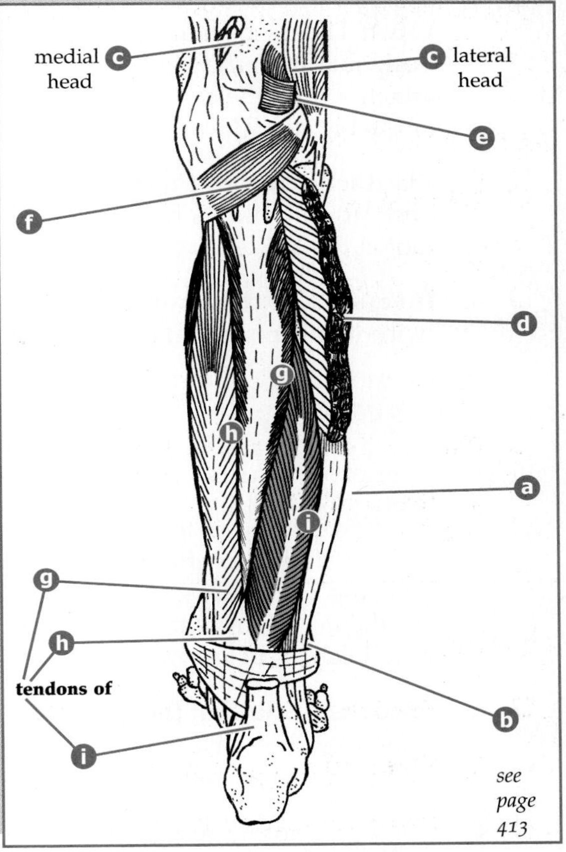

see page 413

Posterior View of the Right Leg (Deep)

a. Fibularis Longus
b. Fibularis Brevis
c. Gastrocnemius (cut)
d. Soleus (cut and reflected)
e. Plantaris (cut and reflected)
f. Popliteus
g. Tibialis Posterior
h. Flexor Digitorum Longus
i. **Flexor Hallucis Longus**

RELATIONSHIP TO OTHER MUSCULOSKELETAL STRUCTURES

❑ 1. The flexor hallucis longus, flexor digitorum longus and the tibialis posterior are the deepest muscles in the posterior leg. Where these muscles overlap, the tibialis posterior is the deepest of the three.

❑ 2. The flexor hallucis longus is deep to the soleus.

❑ 3. Deep to the flexor hallucis longus are the fibula and the interosseus membrane.

❑ 4. The flexor hallucis longus is lateral to the tibialis posterior and the flexor digitorum longus.

FLEXOR HALLUCIS LONGUS – continued

- ❑ 5. Lateral to the flexor hallucis longus is the fibularis longus.
- ❑ 6. The distal tendon of the flexor hallucis longus crosses posterior to the medial malleolus along with the distal tendons of the tibialis posterior and the flexor digitorum longus.

METHODOLOGY FOR LEARNING MUSCLE ACTIONS

- ❑ 1. **Flexion of the Big Toe (Toe #1) at the Metatarsophalangeal Joint and the Interphalangeal Joint:** The flexor hallucis longus crosses the big toe on the plantar side (with its fibers running horizontally in the sagittal plane); therefore, it flexes the big toe. Given that the flexor hallucis longus attaches onto the distal phalanx, it crosses both the metatarsophalangeal joint and interphalangeal joint of the big toe. Therefore, the flexor hallucis longus flexes the big toe at both of these joints.
- ❑ 2. **Plantarflexion of the Foot at the Ankle Joint:** The flexor hallucis longus crosses the ankle joint posteriorly (with its fibers running vertically in the sagittal plane); therefore, it plantarflexes the foot at the ankle joint.
- ❑ 3. **Inversion of the Foot at the Tarsal Joints:** The flexor hallucis longus crosses the foot medially (with its fibers running vertically in the frontal plane); therefore, it inverts the foot at the tarsal joints.

MISCELLANEOUS

- ❑ 1. The flexor hallucis longus is located in the deep posterior compartment of the leg.
- ❑ 2. The flexor **H**allucis longus is "**H**arry" of the "Tom, Dick and **H**arry" muscles. The Tom, Dick and Harry muscles are the tibialis posterior, flexor digitorum longus and flexor hallucis longus. Tom, Dick and Harry are grouped together because they are all deep in the posterior leg and all of their distal <u>tendons</u> cross posterior to the medial malleolus of the tibia (in order from anterior to posterior, Tom, Dick and Harry).
- ❑ 3. Since the tendons of the Tom, Dick and Harry group cross into the foot posterior to the medial malleolus, their line of pull is posteromedial. Therefore, all three Tom, Dick and Harry muscles plantarflex and invert the foot (at the ankle and tarsal joints respectively).
- ❑ 4. It is worth noting that the location of the muscle <u>bellies</u> of the Tom, Dick and Harry muscles in the posterior leg is, from medial to lateral, Dick, Tom and Harry (i.e., flexor digitorum longus, tibialis posterior and flexor hallucis longus).
- ❑ 5. The flexor hallucis longus is one of only a few muscles in the body that has a tendon that makes an abrupt turn of 90° or more. (Other muscles that do this are the obturator internus, fibularis longus, tibialis posterior, flexor digitorum longus, tensor palati and the superior oblique.)
- ❑ 6. The flexor hallucis longus is actually quite large and powerful; it is larger and stronger than the flexor digitorum longus. The reason for the size and strength of this muscle is to increase our propulsive force when we push off ("toe-off") the ground by flexing the big toe when walking and running.

INTRINSIC MUSCLES OF THE FOOT

OVERVIEW OF THE INTRINSIC MUSCLES OF THE FOOT

Intrinsic muscles of the foot are muscles that are confined to the foot, which means they originate and insert in the foot.

ANATOMICALLY, THE INTRINSIC MUSCLES OF THE FOOT CAN BE DIVIDED INTO TWO GROUPS: DORSAL AND PLANTAR. THE PLANTAR GROUP IS USUALLY FURTHER DIVIDED INTO FOUR LAYERS FROM SUPERFICIAL TO DEEP, RESPECTIVELY.

The Dorsal Side:

- Extensor Digitorum Brevis
- Extensor Hallucis Brevis

The Plantar Side:

Layer I:

- Abductor Hallucis
- Abductor Digiti Minimi Pedis
- Flexor Digitorum Brevis

Layer II:

- Quadratus Plantae
- Lumbricals Pedis

Layer III:

- Flexor Hallucis Brevis
- Flexor Digiti Minimi Pedis
- Adductor Hallucis

Layer IV:

- Plantar Interossei
- Dorsal Interossei Pedis

THE FOLLOWING MUSCLES ARE COVERED IN OTHER CHAPTERS OF THIS BOOK, BUT ARE ALSO PRESENT IN THE FOOT:

- Tibialis Anterior
- Extensor Digitorum Longus
- Extensor Hallucis Longus
- Fibularis Tertius
- Fibularis Longus
- Fibularis Brevis
- Gastrocnemius
- Soleus
- Plantaris
- Tibialis Posterior
- Flexor Digitorum Longus
- Flexor Hallucis Longus

The above classification is consistently used. However, like any classification, it can be overly simplistic. Please note the following:

- Some sources include the extensor hallucis brevis muscle as a part of the extensor digitorum brevis since they are one muscle at their proximal attachment. However, it is more consistent with naming to separate the portion of this muscle that goes to the big toe as a separate muscle, the extensor hallucis brevis. (This situation is similar to the extensor digitorum longus and the fibularis tertius.)
- Each plantar layer of muscles does not entirely cover the plantar surface of the foot. Therefore, some muscles of deeper layers may be partially superficial.
- In Layer I, the plantar fascia can also be found. (The plantar fascia is a layer of fascia that overlies the plantar surface of the foot. The thickened part of the plantar fascia near the midline of the foot is called the *plantar aponeurosis.*)
- In Layer II, the distal tendons of the flexor digitorum longus and the flexor hallucis longus are also found.
- In Layer IV, the distal tendons of the fibularis longus and the tibialis posterior are also found.

Functionally, the intrinsic muscles of the foot cross the toe joints. Therefore, intrinsic muscles of the foot move the toes. The following general rule regarding actions can be stated for the intrinsic muscles of the foot:

- If a muscle crosses the toe joint(s) on the plantar side, it can flex the toe at the toe joint(s).
- If a muscle crosses the toe joint(s) on the dorsal side, it can extend the toe at the toe joint(s).
- If a muscle crosses the toe joint(s) laterally, it can move the toe laterally. (This will be termed abduction or adduction, depending on the toe.)
- If a muscle crosses the toe joint(s) medially, it can move the toe medially. (This will be termed abduction or adduction, depending on the toe.)
- Functionally, all the intrinsic muscles of the foot on the plantar side, in addition to their specific actions, tend to contract as a group to stabilize the structure of the foot (maintain the arches), especially during propulsion.

Dorsal Digital Expansion

There is a dorsal digital expansion of the foot which is similar to the dorsal digital expansion of the hand (see Dorsal Digital Expansion of the Right Hand on page 636). The dorsal digital expansion of the foot is formed by the extensor digitorum longus and ultimately attaches onto the middle and distal phalanges of toes #2-5. The dorsal digital expansion of the foot serves as an attachment site for the lumbricals pedis, extensor digitorum brevis, dorsal interossei pedis and plantar interossei muscles. Note: Unlike the thumb, which has a dorsal digital expansion, the big toe has no dorsal digital expansion.

INNERVATION

- The intrinsic muscles of the foot on the dorsal side are innervated by the deep fibular nerve.
- The intrinsic muscles of the foot on the plantar side are innervated by the medial and/or lateral plantar nerves.

ARTERIAL SUPPLY

- The intrinsic muscles of the foot on the dorsal side receive their arterial supply from the dorsalis pedis artery.
- The intrinsic muscles of the foot on the plantar side receive their arterial supply from either branches of the medial and/or lateral plantar arteries or from branches of the anastamosis between the medial and lateral plantar arteries (the plantar arch).

A NOTE REGARDING REVERSE ACTIONS

As a rule, this book does not employ the terms "origin" and "insertion." However, it is useful to utilize these terms to describe the concept of "reverse actions." The action section of this book describes the action of a muscle by stating the movement of a body part that is created by a muscle's contraction. The body part that usually moves when a muscle contracts is called the insertion. The methodology section further states at which joint the movement of the insertion occurs. However, the other body part that the muscle attaches to, the origin, can also move at that joint. *This movement can be called the reverse action of the muscle.* Keep in mind that the reverse action of a muscle is always possible. The likelihood that a reverse action will occur is based upon the ability of the insertion to be fixed so that the origin moves (instead of the insertion moving) when the muscle contracts. For more information and examples of reverse actions, see page 702.

❑ DORSAL VIEW OF THE BONES AND BONY LANDMARKS OF THE RIGHT FOOT

Note: Usually, only muscular attachments and landmarks of this chapter are labeled. However, all tarsal bones have been labeled, even if they are not listed individually in this chapter.

First level attachments are indicated in **bold** print.

Second level attachments are indicated in non-bold print.

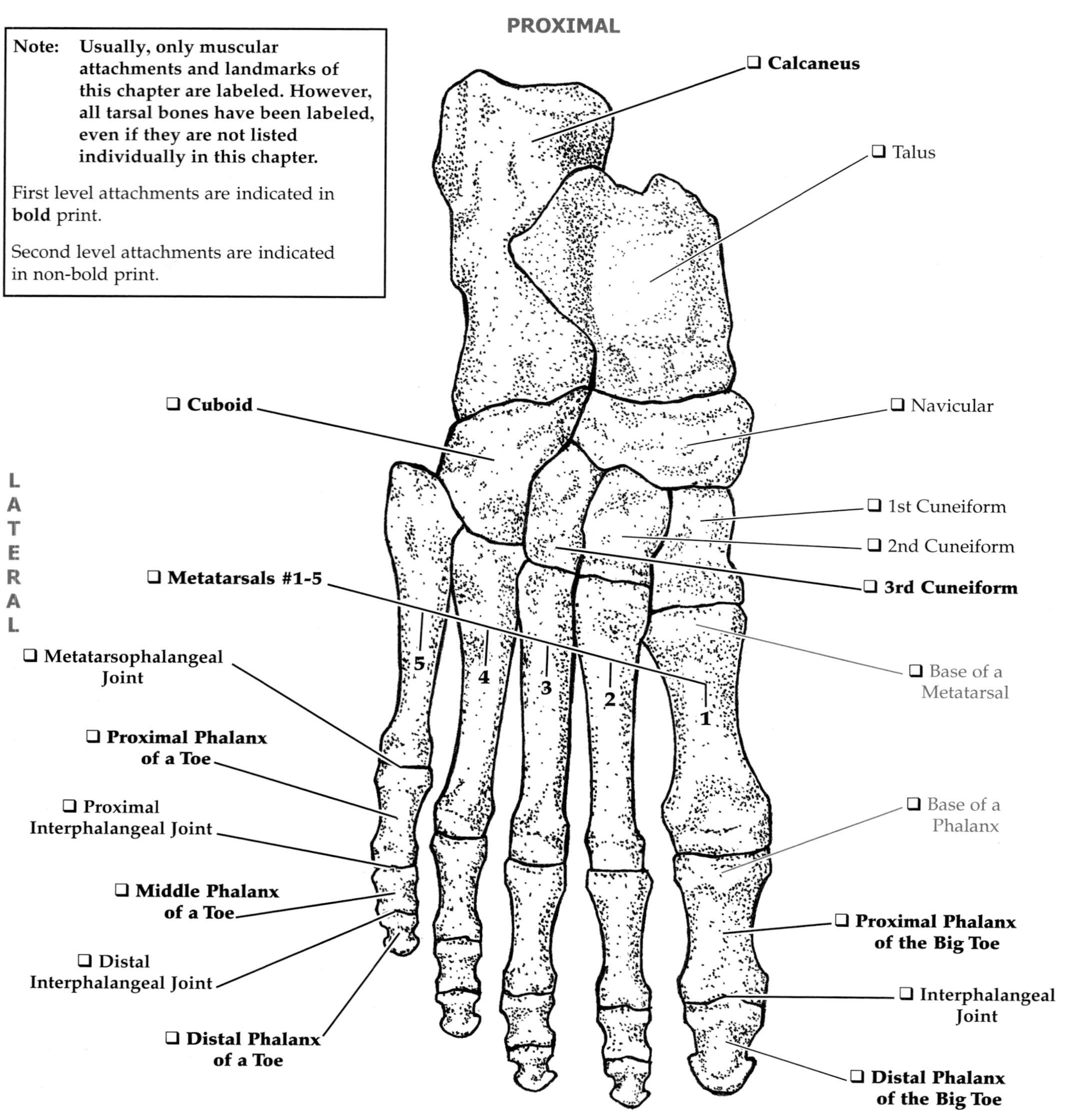

DORSAL VIEW OF THE BONY ATTACHMENTS OF THE RIGHT FOOT

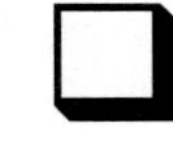

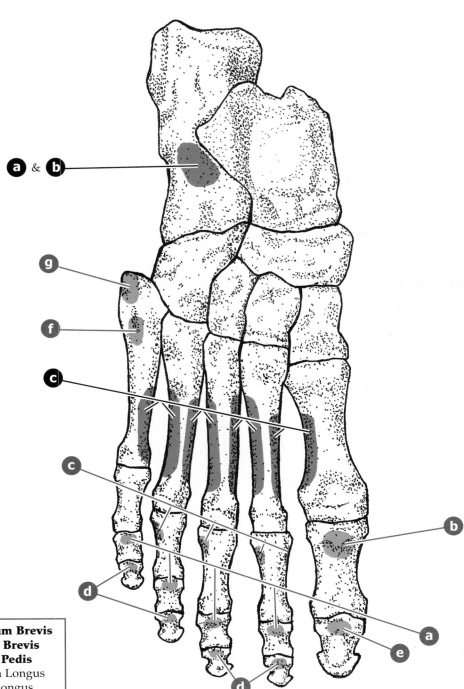

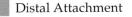

PROXIMAL

LATERAL

MEDIAL

a & b

g

f

c

c

b

d

a

e

d

DISTAL

a. **Extensor Digitorum Brevis**
b. **Extensor Hallucis Brevis**
c. **Dorsal Interossei Pedis**
d. Extensor Digitorum Longus
e. Extensor Hallucis Longus
f. Fibularis Tertius
g. Fibularis Brevis

Proximal Attachment

Distal Attachment

❑ PLANTAR VIEW OF THE BONES AND BONY LANDMARKS OF THE RIGHT FOOT

Note: Usually, only muscular attachments and landmarks of this chapter are labeled. However, all tarsal bones have been labeled, even if they are not listed individually in this chapter.

First level attachments are indicated in **bold** print.

Second level attachments are indicated in non-bold print.

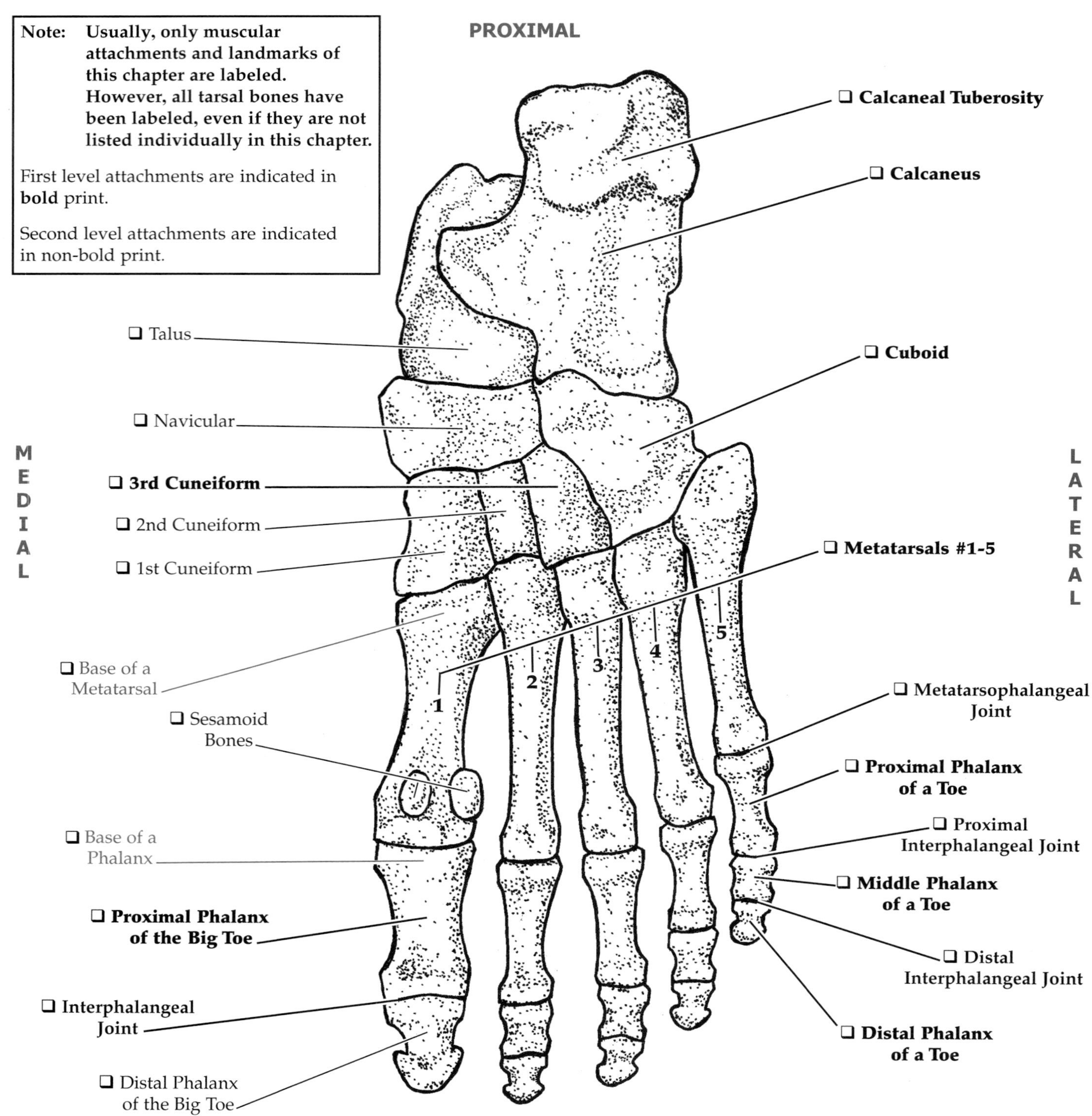

PLANTAR VIEW OF THE BONY ATTACHMENTS OF THE RIGHT FOOT

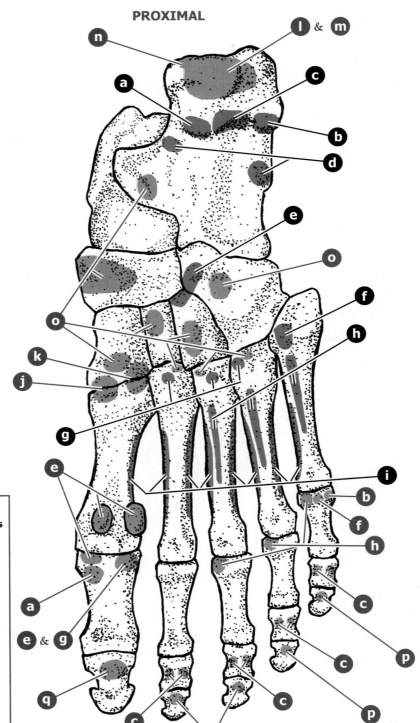

PROXIMAL

MEDIAL

LATERAL

a. **Abductor Hallucis**
b. **Abductor Digiti Minimi Pedis**
c. **Flexor Digitorum Brevis**
d **Quadratus Plantae**
e. **Flexor Hallucis Brevis**
f. **Flexor Digiti Minimi Pedis**
g. **Adductor Hallucis**
h. **Plantar Interossei**
i. **Dorsal Interossei Pedis**
j. Tibialis Anterior
k. Fibularis Longus
l Gastrocnemius
m. Soleus
n. Plantaris
o. Tibialis Posterior
p. Flexor Digitorum Longus
q. Flexor Hallucis Longus

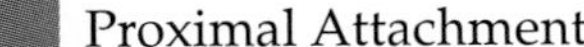

Proximal Attachment

Distal Attachment

DISTAL

DORSAL VIEW OF THE RIGHT FOOT

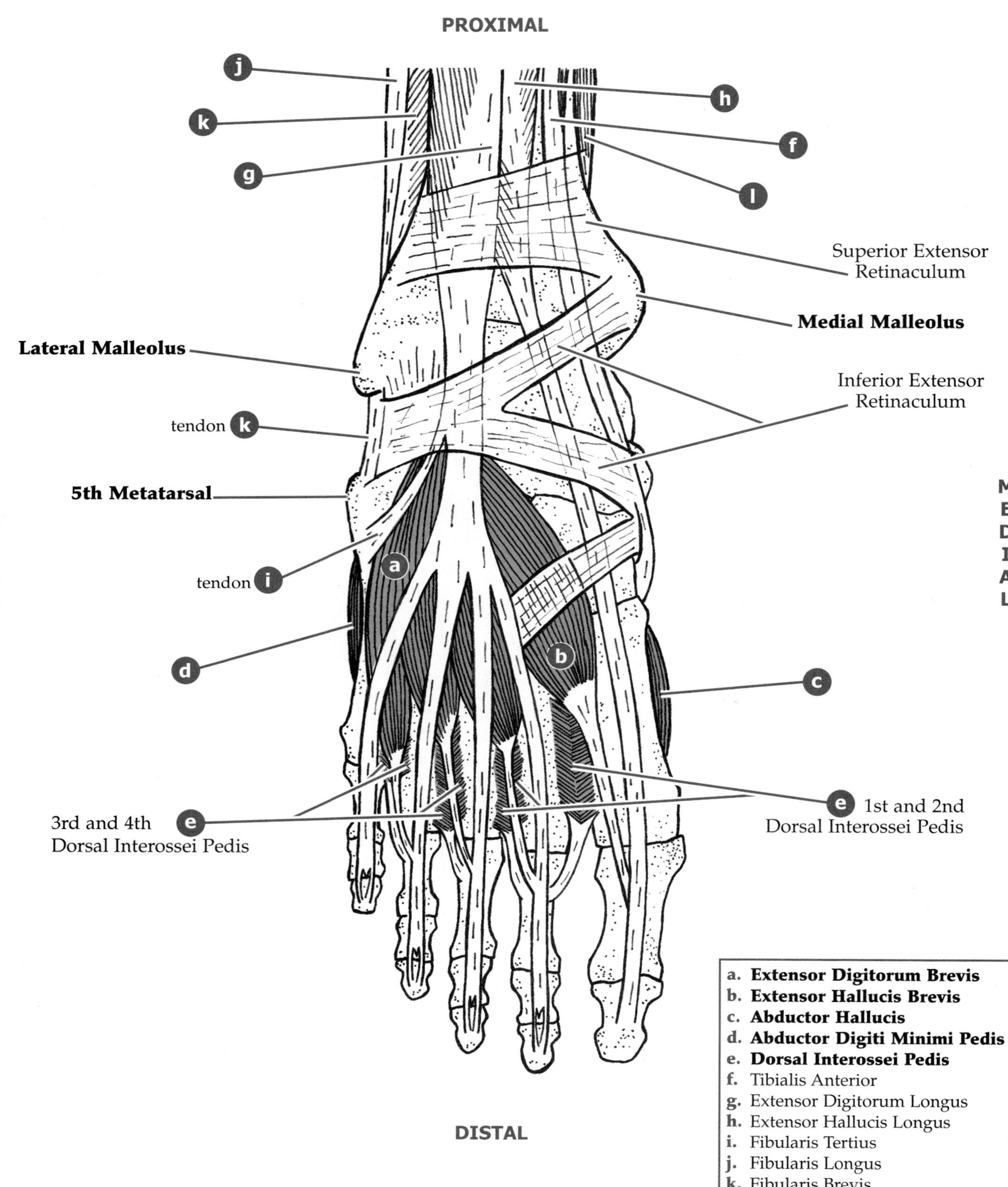

a. **Extensor Digitorum Brevis**
b. **Extensor Hallucis Brevis**
c. **Abductor Hallucis**
d. **Abductor Digiti Minimi Pedis**
e. **Dorsal Interossei Pedis**
f. Tibialis Anterior
g. Extensor Digitorum Longus
h. Extensor Hallucis Longus
i. Fibularis Tertius
j. Fibularis Longus
k. Fibularis Brevis
l. Soleus

PLANTAR VIEW OF THE RIGHT FOOT (SUPERFICIAL)

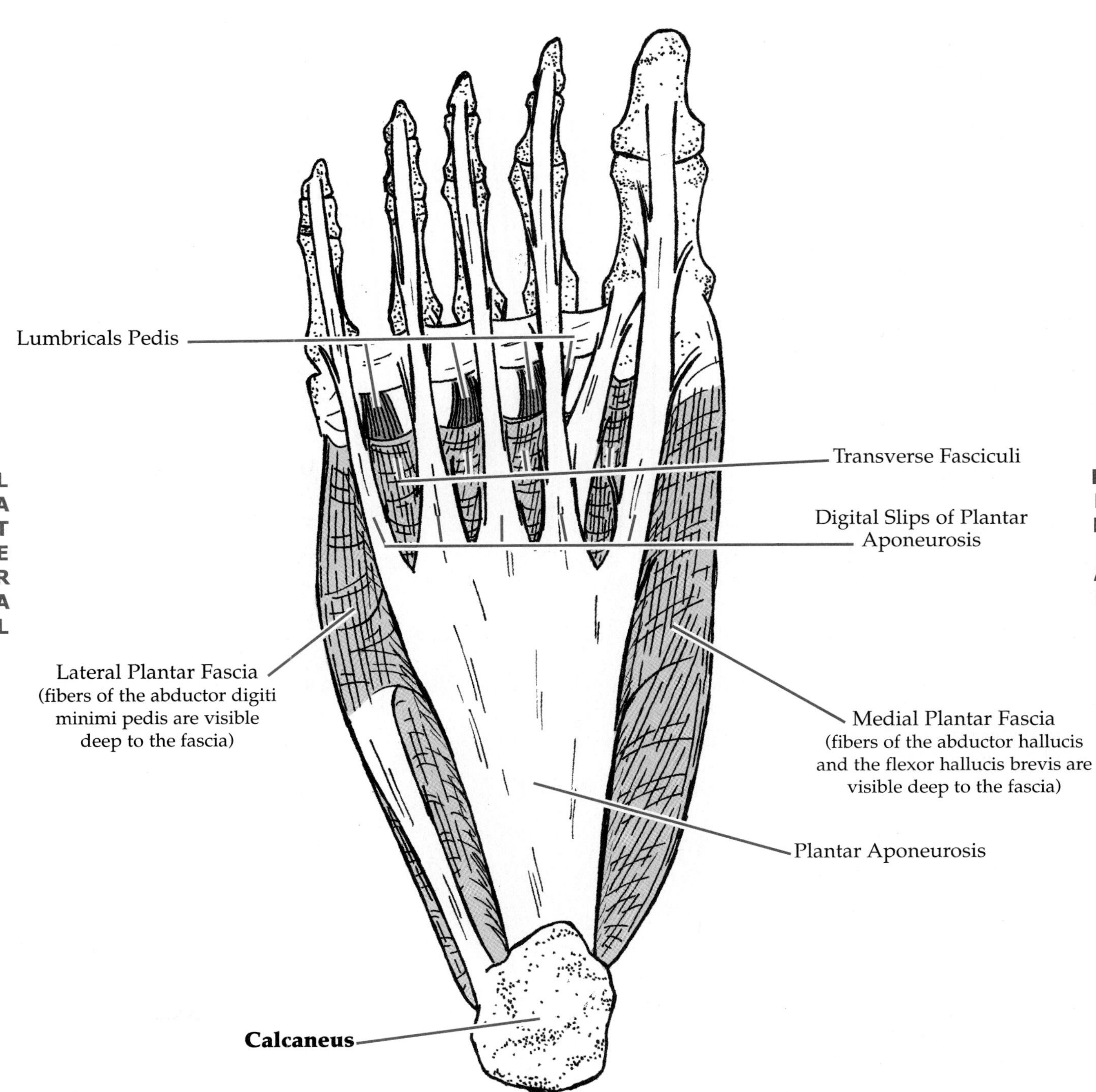

PLANTAR VIEW OF THE RIGHT FOOT (SUPERFICIAL MUSCULAR LAYER)

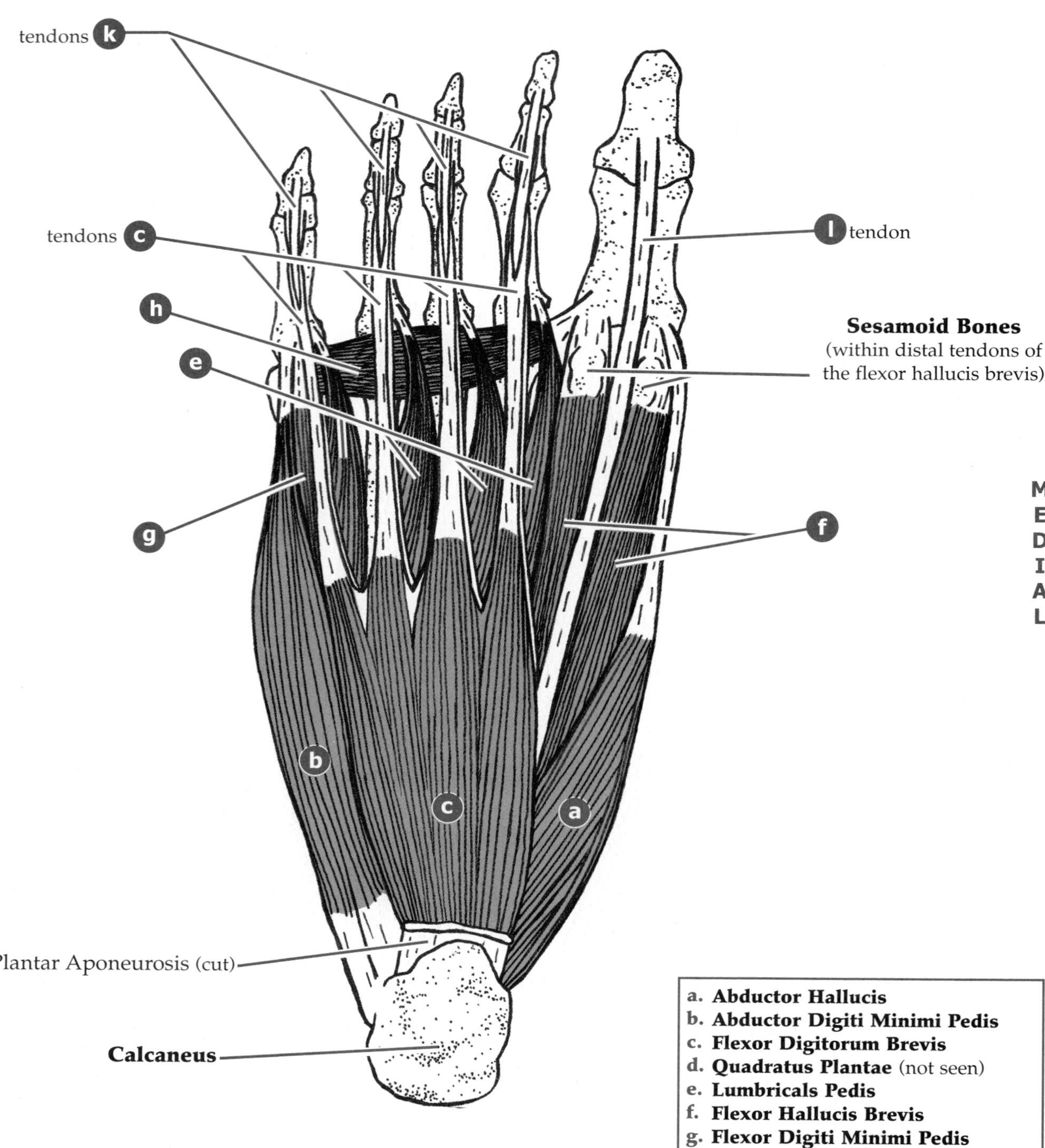

- a. **Abductor Hallucis**
- b. **Abductor Digiti Minimi Pedis**
- c. **Flexor Digitorum Brevis**
- d. **Quadratus Plantae** (not seen)
- e. **Lumbricals Pedis**
- f. **Flexor Hallucis Brevis**
- g. **Flexor Digiti Minimi Pedis**
- h. **Adductor Hallucis**
- i. **Plantar Interossei** (not seen)
- j. **Dorsal Interossei Pedis** (not seen)
- k. Flexor Digitorum Longus
- l. Flexor Hallucis Longus

PLANTAR VIEW OF THE RIGHT FOOT (INTERMEDIATE MUSCULAR LAYER)

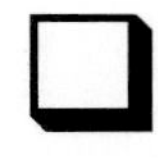

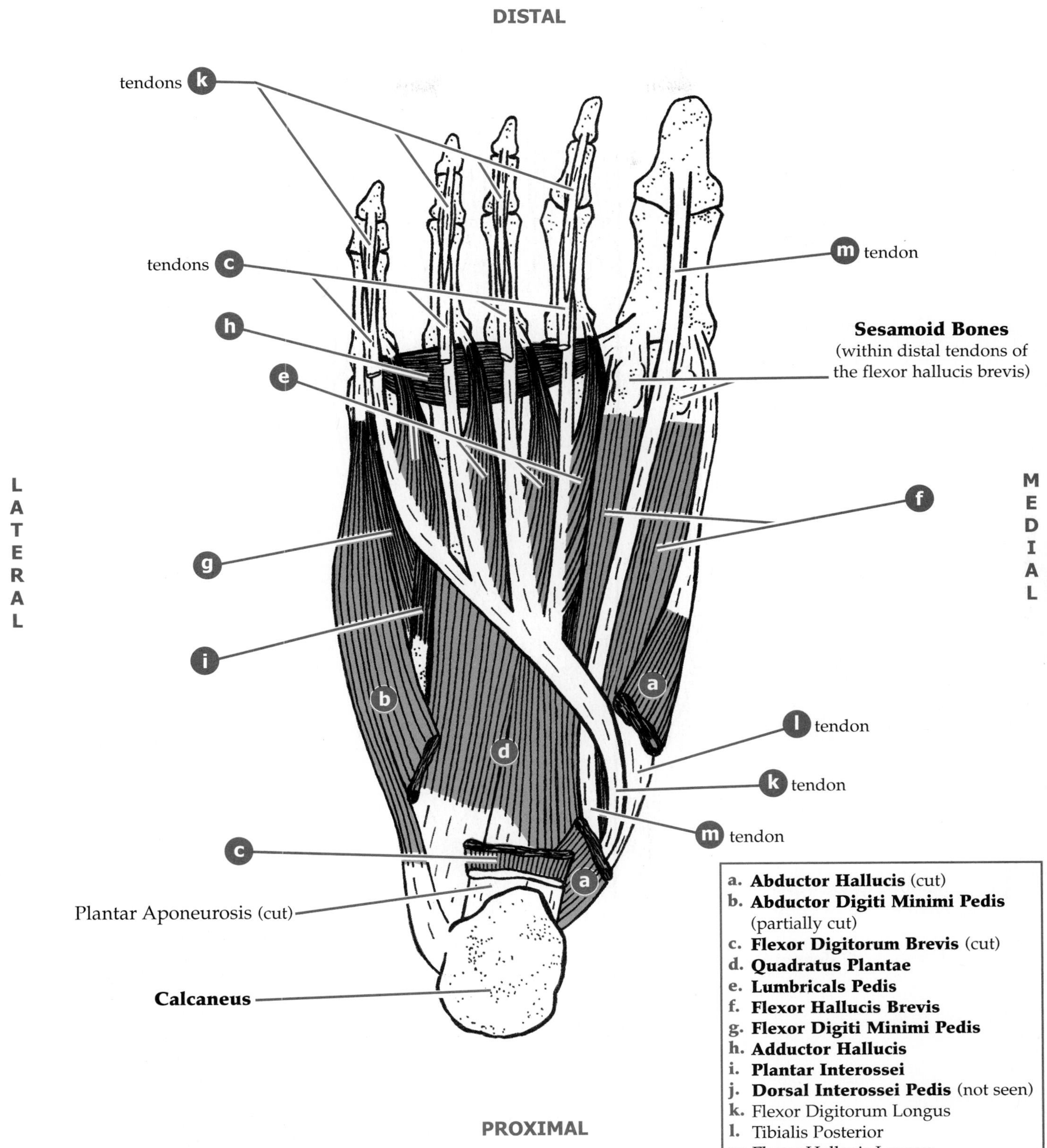

DISTAL

tendons k

tendons c

h

e

m tendon

Sesamoid Bones
(within distal tendons of the flexor hallucis brevis)

LATERAL

MEDIAL

f

g

i

a

b

d

l tendon

k tendon

m tendon

c

a

Plantar Aponeurosis (cut)

Calcaneus

PROXIMAL

a. **Abductor Hallucis** (cut)
b. **Abductor Digiti Minimi Pedis** (partially cut)
c. **Flexor Digitorum Brevis** (cut)
d. **Quadratus Plantae**
e. **Lumbricals Pedis**
f. **Flexor Hallucis Brevis**
g. **Flexor Digiti Minimi Pedis**
h. **Adductor Hallucis**
i. **Plantar Interossei**
j. **Dorsal Interossei Pedis** (not seen)
k. Flexor Digitorum Longus
l. Tibialis Posterior
m. Flexor Hallucis Longus

❑ PLANTAR VIEW OF THE RIGHT FOOT (DEEP MUSCULAR LAYER)

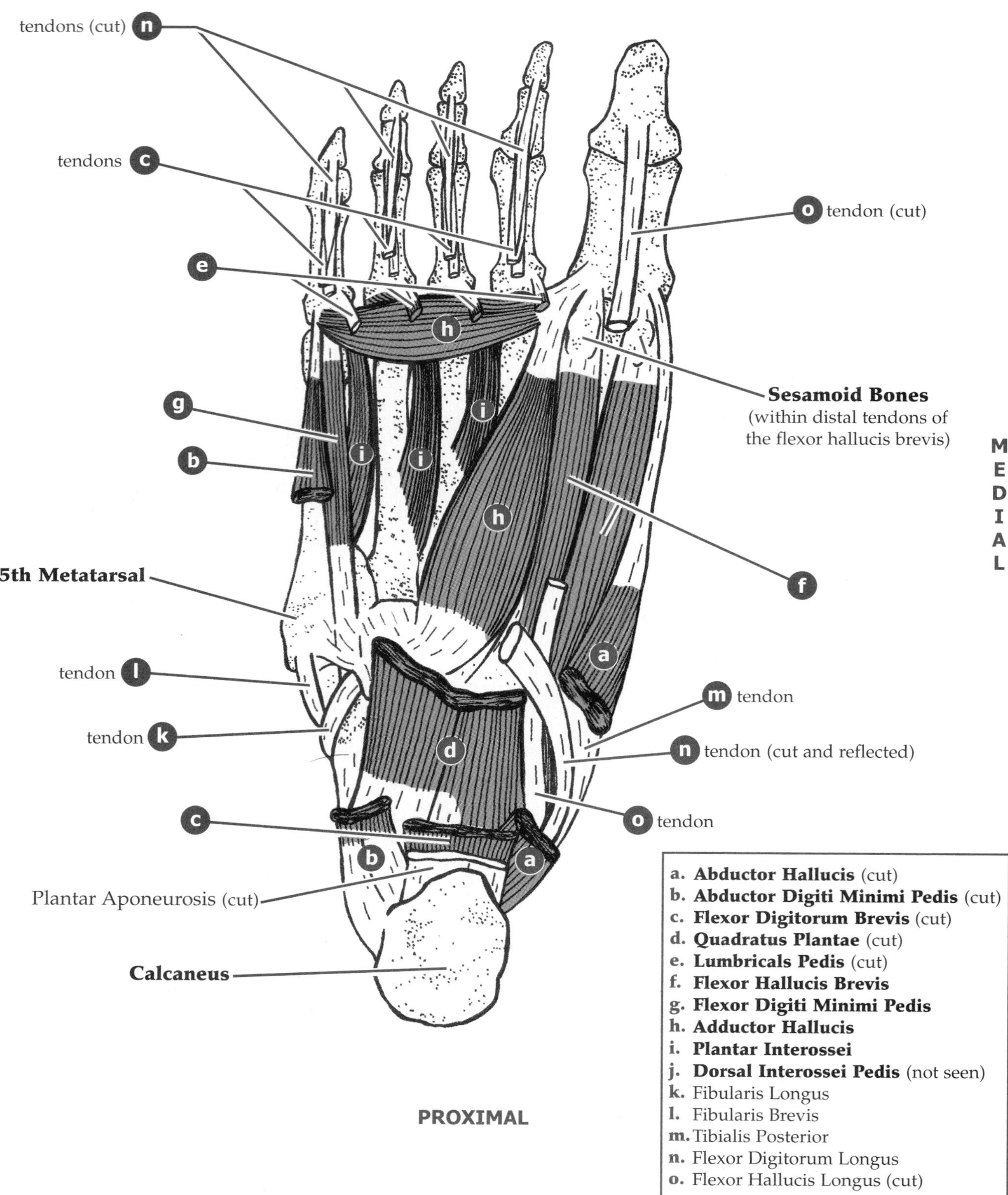

a. **Abductor Hallucis** (cut)
b. **Abductor Digiti Minimi Pedis** (cut)
c. **Flexor Digitorum Brevis** (cut)
d. **Quadratus Plantae** (cut)
e. **Lumbricals Pedis** (cut)
f. **Flexor Hallucis Brevis**
g. **Flexor Digiti Minimi Pedis**
h. **Adductor Hallucis**
i. **Plantar Interossei**
j. **Dorsal Interossei Pedis** (not seen)
k. Fibularis Longus
l. Fibularis Brevis
m. Tibialis Posterior
n. Flexor Digitorum Longus
o. Flexor Hallucis Longus (cut)

CROSS SECTION VIEW OF THE RIGHT FOOT THROUGH THE METATARSAL BONES

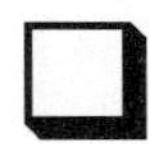

DORSAL

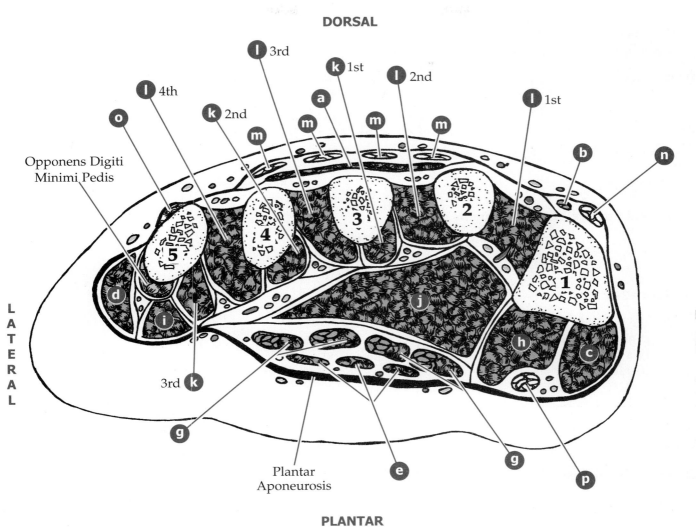

l 3rd
k 1st
l 2nd
l 4th
a
l 1st
k 2nd
o
m
m
m
m
b
n
Opponens Digiti Minimi Pedis
5
4
3
2
1
d
j
i
h
c
LATERAL
MEDIAL
3rd k
g
Plantar Aponeurosis
e
g
p

PLANTAR

Note: This is a Proximal View (looking from distal to proximal).

- a. **Extensor Digitorum Brevis**
- b. **Extensor Hallucis Brevis** (tendon)
- c. **Abductor Hallucis**
- d. **Abductor Digiti Minimi Pedis**
- e. **Flexor Digitorum Brevis** (tendons)
- f. **Quadratus Plantae** (not seen)
- g. **Lumbricals Pedis** (attached to tendons of flexor digitorum longus)
- h. **Flexor Hallucis Brevis**
- i. **Flexor Digiti Minimi Pedis**
- j. **Adductor Hallucis** (oblique head)
- k. **Plantar Interossei**
- l. **Dorsal Interossei Pedis**
- m. Extensor Digitorum Longus
- n. Extensor Hallucis Longus
- o. Fibularis Tertius
- p. Flexor Hallucis Longus

❑

EXTENSOR DIGITORUM BREVIS

(DORSAL SURFACE)

❑ **The name, extensor digitorum brevis, tells us that this muscle extends the digits, i.e., toes, and is short (shorter than the extensor digitorum longus).**

DERIVATION ❑ extensor: L. *a muscle that extends a body part.*
digitorum: L. *refers to a digit* (toe).
brevis: L. *short.*

PRONUNCIATION ❑ eks-**ten**-sor dij-i-**toe**-rum **bre**-vis

ATTACHMENTS

❑ **Dorsal Surface of the Calcaneus**

to the

❑ **Toes #2-4**

- ❑ the lateral side of the distal tendons of the extensor digitorum longus muscle of toes #2-4
(via the dorsal digital expansion into the middle and distal phalanges)

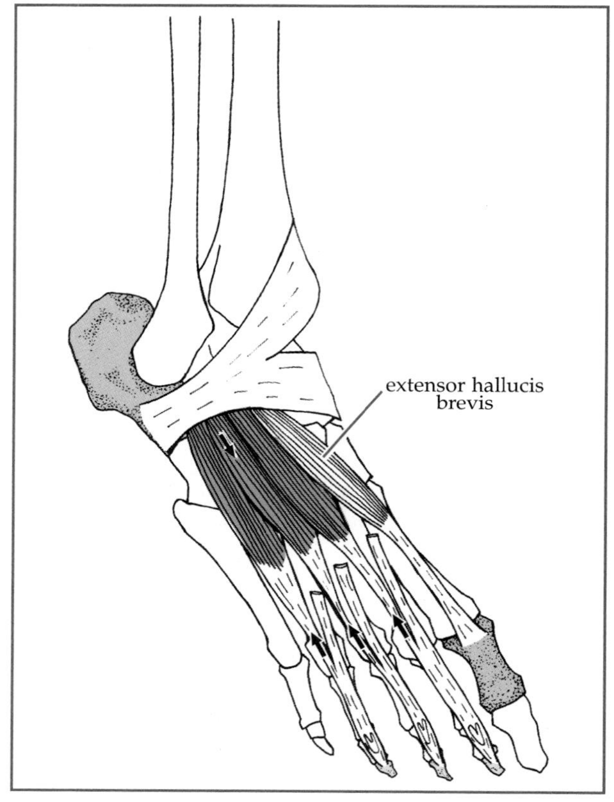

Dorsolateral View of the Right Extensor Digitorum Brevis

ACTION

❑ **Extension of Toes #2-4**

INNERVATION ❑ The Deep Fibular Nerve ❑ L5, S1

ARTERIAL SUPPLY ❑ The Dorsalis Pedis Artery (The Continuation of the Anterior Tibial Artery)

PALPATION AND SUPPLEMENTARY TEXT

PALPATION

- ❑ The extensor digitorum brevis is visible and palpable on the dorsum of the foot.
  - Have the client seated or supine.
  - Place palpating hand approximately one inch (2-3 cm) distal to the lateral malleolus on the dorsum of the foot.
  - Ask the client to actively extend the toes (#2-4) and feel for the contraction of the extensor digitorum brevis.

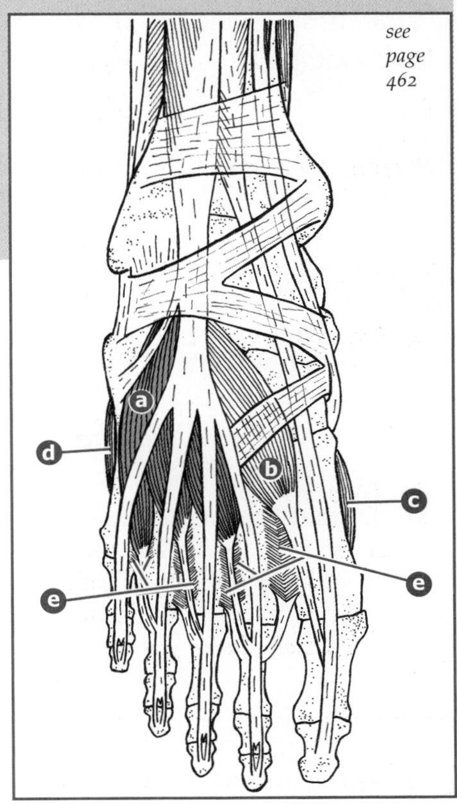

see page 462

Dorsal View of the Right Foot

a. Extensor Digitorum Brevis
b. Extensor Hallucis Brevis
c. Abductor Hallucis
d. Abductor Digiti Minimi Pedis
e. Dorsal Interossei Pedis

RELATIONSHIP TO OTHER MUSCULOSKELETAL STRUCTURES

❑ 1. The extensor digitorum brevis is superficial except where the distal tendons of the extensor digitorum longus and the fibularis tertius cross superficially to it.

❑ 2. Deep to the extensor digitorum brevis are the tarsal and metatarsal bones.

❑ 3. The extensor digitorum brevis is lateral to the extensor hallucis brevis.

METHODOLOGY FOR LEARNING MUSCLE ACTIONS

❑ **Extension of Toes #2-4 at the Metatarsophalangeal and Proximal and Distal Interphalangeal Joints:** The extensor digitorum brevis crosses toe joints #2-4 dorsally (with its fibers running horizontally in the sagittal plane); therefore, it extends toes #2-4. By attaching onto the distal tendon of the extensor digitorum longus of toes #2-4 (which attaches onto the distal phalanges of toes #2-4), the extensor digitorum brevis pulls these tendons as if the belly of the extensor digitorum longus muscle itself had contracted. Therefore, the extensor digitorum brevis has the same actions at toes #2-4 in the foot as the extensor digitorum longus muscle has, namely, extension of toes #2-4 at the metatarsophalangeal joint and the proximal and distal interphalangeal joints of toes #2-4.

MISCELLANEOUS

❑ 1. The extensor digitorum brevis and the extensor hallucis brevis are the only intrinsic foot muscles located on the dorsal side.

❑ 2. The most medial part of extensor digitorum brevis does not attach onto a "digit." Therefore, it is given a separate name, the extensor hallucis brevis (see pages 470-1). The term "digit" in the name of a muscle is usually reserved for toes #2-5, not toe #1, the big toe.

❑ EXTENSOR HALLUCIS BREVIS

(DORSAL SURFACE)

❑ **The name, extensor hallucis brevis, tells us that this muscle extends the big toe and is short (shorter than the extensor hallucis longus).**

DERIVATION ❑ extensor: L. *a muscle that extends a body part.*
hallucis: L. *refers to the big toe.*
brevis: L. *short.*

PRONUNCIATION ❑ eks-**ten**-sor hal-**oo**-sis **bre**-vis

ATTACHMENTS

❑ **Dorsal Surface of the Calcaneus**

to the

❑ **Dorsal Surface of the Big Toe (Toe #1)**

- ❑ the base of the proximal phalanx of the big toe

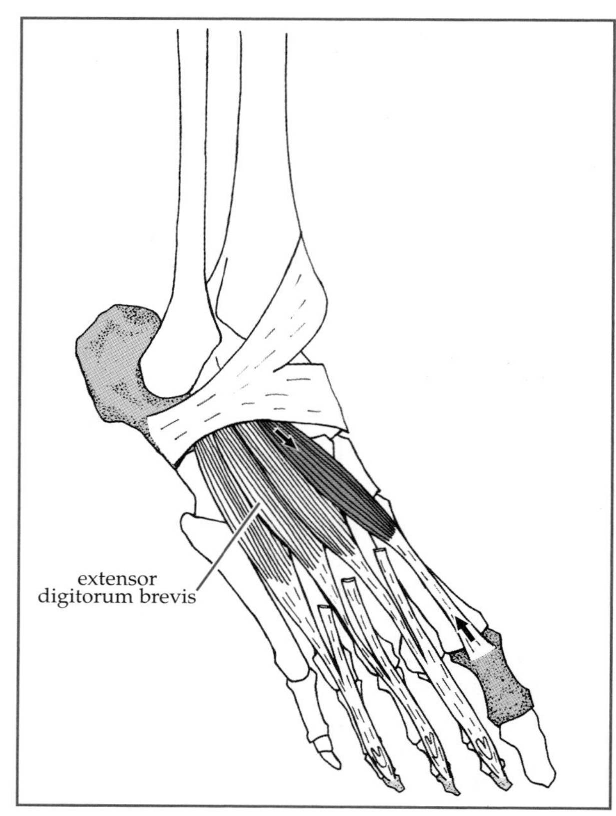

Dorsolateral View of the Right Extensor Hallucis Brevis

ACTION

❑ **Extension of the Big Toe (Toe #1)**

INNERVATION ❑ The Deep Fibular Nerve ❑ L5, S1

ARTERIAL SUPPLY ❑ The Dorsalis Pedis Artery (The Continuation of the Anterior Tibial Artery)

PALPATION AND SUPPLEMENTARY TEXT

PALPATION

- ❑ The extensor hallucis brevis is visible and palpable on the dorsum of the foot.
  - Have the client seated or supine.
  - Place palpating hand approximately one inch (2-3 cm) distal to the lateral malleolus on the dorsum of the foot.
  - Ask the client to actively extend the big toe and feel for the contraction of the extensor hallucis brevis. It will be medial to the extensor digitorum brevis.

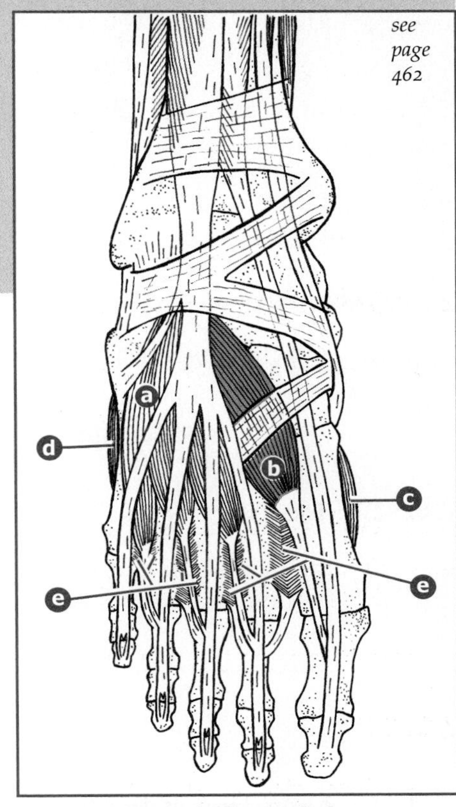

Dorsal View of the Right Foot

a. Extensor Digitorum Brevis
b. Extensor Hallucis Brevis
c. Abductor Hallucis
d. Abductor Digiti Minimi Pedis
e. Dorsal Interossei Pedis

RELATIONSHIP TO OTHER MUSCULOSKELETAL STRUCTURES

❑ 1. The extensor hallucis brevis is superficial except where the distal tendons of the extensor digitorum longus and the fibularis tertius cross superficially to it.

❑ 2. Deep to the extensor hallucis brevis are the tarsal and metatarsal bones.

❑ 3. The extensor hallucis brevis is medial to the extensor digitorum brevis.

METHODOLOGY FOR LEARNING MUSCLE ACTIONS

❑ **Extension of the Big Toe (Toe #1) at the Metatarsophalangeal Joint:** The extensor hallucis brevis crosses the metatarsophalangeal joint of the big toe dorsally (with its fibers running horizontally in the sagittal plane) to attach onto the proximal phalanx of the big toe. Therefore, it extends the big toe at the metatarsophalangeal joint.

MISCELLANEOUS

❑ 1. The extensor hallucis brevis and the extensor digitorum brevis are the only intrinsic foot muscles located on the dorsal side.

❑ 2. The extensor hallucis brevis is actually the most medial part of the extensor digitorum brevis (see pages 468-9). The extensor hallucis brevis is differentiated from the rest of the extensor digitorum brevis and given a separate name because this part of the muscle does not attach onto a "digit." Instead, the most medial part of the extensor digitorum brevis attaches onto the big toe (the hallux). Therefore, this portion of the extensor digitorum brevis is called the extensor hallucis brevis. The term "digit" in the name of a muscle is usually reserved for toes #2-5, not toe #1, the big toe.

❑ 3. Given that the extensor hallucis brevis crosses the metatarsophalangeal joint of the big toe from lateral on the foot to medial on the big toe, this muscle should have the ability to adduct the big toe at the metatarsophalangeal joint.

❑ ABDUCTOR HALLUCIS

(PLANTAR SURFACE – LAYER I)

❑ **The name, abductor hallucis, tells us that this muscle abducts the big toe.**

DERIVATION ❑ abductor: L. *a muscle that abducts a body part.*
hallucis: L. *refers to the big toe.*

PRONUNCIATION ❑ ab-**duk**-tor hal-**oo**-sis

ATTACHMENTS

❑ **Tuberosity of the Calcaneus**

- ❑ and the flexor retinaculum and plantar fascia

to the

❑ **Big Toe (Toe #1)**

- ❑ the medial plantar side of the base of the proximal phalanx

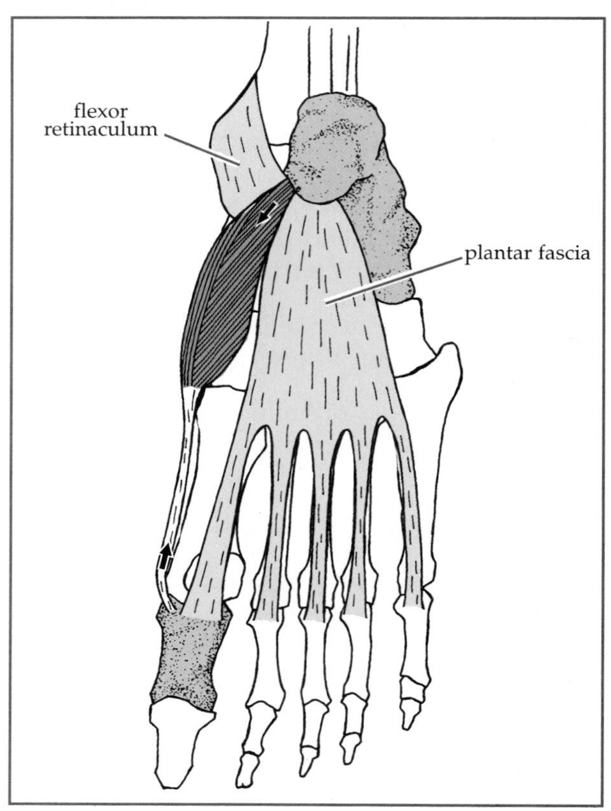

Plantar View of the Right Abductor Hallucis

ACTIONS

❑ **1. Abduction of the Big Toe (Toe #1)**

❑ **2.** Flexion of the Big Toe (Toe #1)

INNERVATION ❑ The Medial Plantar Nerve ❑ S1, 2

ARTERIAL SUPPLY ❑ The Medial Plantar Artery (A Branch of the Posterior Tibial Artery)

PALPATION AND SUPPLEMENTARY TEXT

PALPATION

- ❑ The abductor hallucis is superficial and palpable on the medial side of the plantar surface of the foot.
  - The client can be in any position.
  - Place palpating hand along the proximal half of the plantar foot on the medial side.
  - Ask the client to actively abduct the big toe at the metatarsophalangeal joint and feel for the contraction of the abductor hallucis.

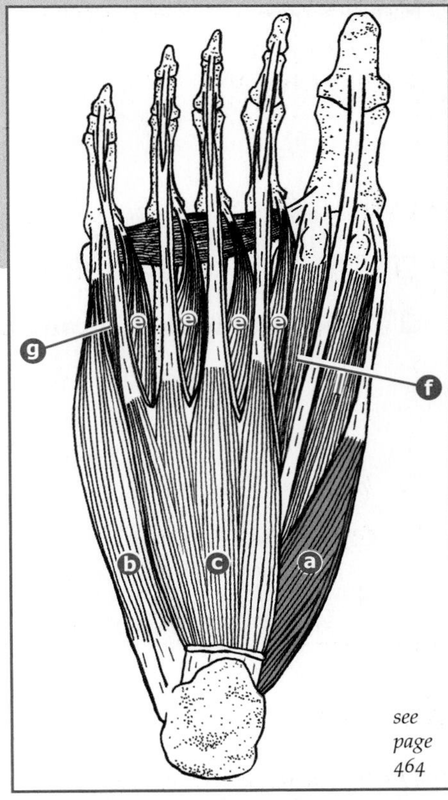

see page 464

Plantar View of the Right Foot (Superficial Muscular Layer)

a. **Abductor Hallucis**
b. Abductor Digiti Minimi Pedis
c. Flexor Digitorum Brevis
d. Quadratus Plantae (not seen)
e. Lumbricals Pedis
f. Flexor Hallucis Brevis
g. Flexor Digiti Minimi Pedis
h. Adductor Hallucis (not seen)
i. Plantar Interossei (not seen)
j. Dorsal Interossei Pedis (not seen)

RELATIONSHIP TO OTHER MUSCULOSKELETAL STRUCTURES

❑ 1. The abductor hallucis is located in the 1st layer of intrinsic muscles of the foot along with the abductor digiti minimi pedis and the flexor digitorum brevis (and the plantar fascia).

❑ 2. The abductor hallucis is medial to the plantar fascia and the flexor digitorum brevis (which is deep to the plantar fascia).

METHODOLOGY FOR LEARNING MUSCLE ACTIONS

❑ 1. **Abduction of the Big Toe (Toe #1) at the Metatarsophalangeal Joint:** The abductor hallucis crosses the metatarsophalangeal joint to attach onto the proximal phalanx of the big toe on the medial side (with its fibers running horizontally). Therefore, when the abductor hallucis contracts, it pulls the big toe medially away from the 2nd toe (which is the axis of abduction/adduction of the foot). Therefore, the abductor hallucis abducts the big toe at the metatarsophalangeal joint.

❑ 2. **Flexion of the Big Toe (Toe #1) at the Metatarsophalangeal Joint:** The abductor hallucis crosses the metatarsophalangeal joint to attach onto the proximal phalanx of the big toe on the plantar side (with its fibers running horizontally in the sagittal plane). Therefore, when the abductor hallucis pulls on the big toe, it flexes the big toe at the metatarsophalangeal joint.

MISCELLANEOUS

❑ All three muscles in the 1st layer of intrinsic muscles of the foot attach proximally onto the tuberosity of the calcaneus and the plantar fascia, and then attach distally onto the toes.

❑ ABDUCTOR DIGITI MINIMI PEDIS

(PLANTAR SURFACE – LAYER I)

❑ **The name, abductor digiti minimi pedis, tells us that this muscle abducts the little toe.**

DERIVATION ❑ abductor: L. *a muscle that abducts a body part.*
digiti: L. *refers to a digit* (toe).
minimi: L. *least.*
pedis: L. *refers to the foot.*

PRONUNCIATION ❑ ab-**duk**-tor **dij**-i-tee **min**-i-mee **peed**-us

ATTACHMENTS

❑ **Tuberosity of the Calcaneus**

❑ and the plantar fascia

to the

❑ **Little Toe (Toe #5)**

❑ the lateral plantar side of the base of the proximal phalanx

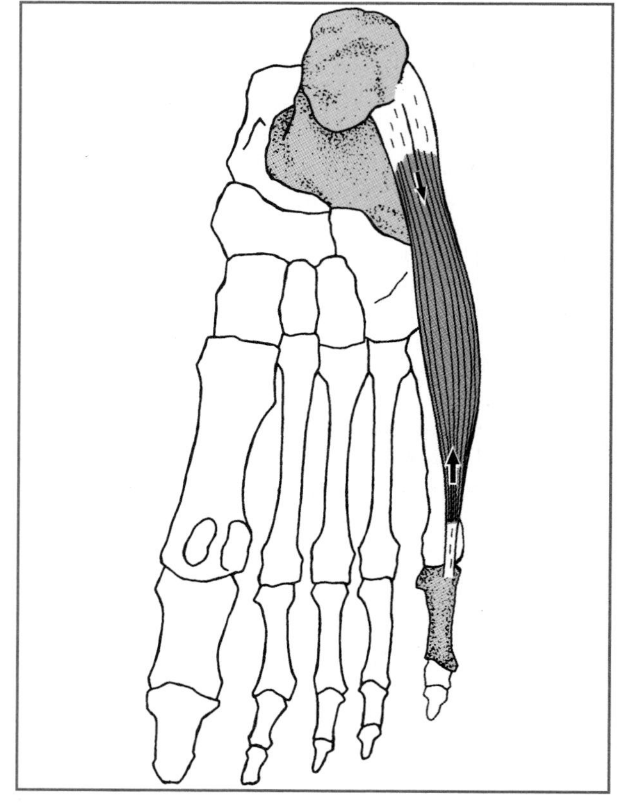

Plantar View of the Right Abductor Digiti Minimi Pedis

ACTIONS

❑ **1. Abduction of the Little Toe (Toe #5)**

❑ **2.** Flexion of the Little Toe (Toe #5)

INNERVATION ❑ The Lateral Plantar Nerve ❑ S2, 3

ARTERIAL SUPPLY ❑ The Lateral Plantar Artery (A Branch of the Posterior Tibial Artery)

PALPATION AND SUPPLEMENTARY TEXT

PALPATION

- ❑ The abductor digiti minimi pedis is superficial and palpable on the lateral side of the plantar surface of the foot.
  - The client can be in any position.
  - Place palpating hand on the lateral side of the plantar surface of the foot.
  - Ask the client to actively abduct the little toe and feel for the contraction of the abductor digiti minimi pedis.

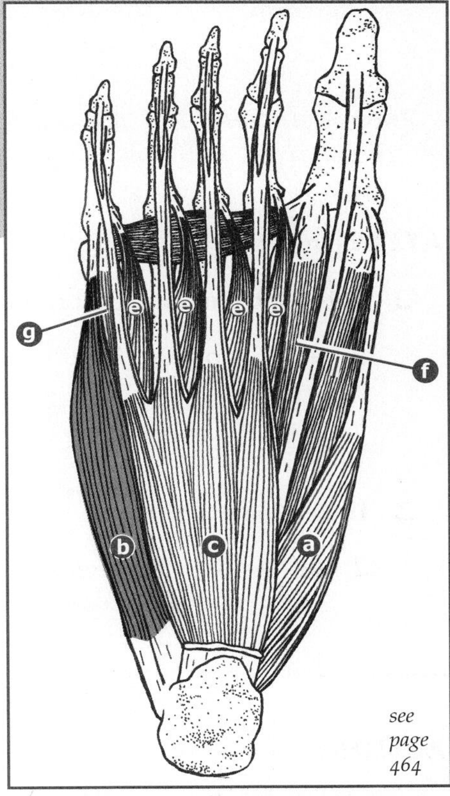

Plantar View of the Right Foot (Superficial Muscular Layer)

a. Abductor Hallucis
b. Abductor Digiti Minimi Pedis
c. Flexor Digitorum Brevis
d. Quadratus Plantae (not seen)
e. Lumbricals Pedis
f. Flexor Hallucis Brevis
g. Flexor Digiti Minimi Pedis
h. Adductor Hallucis (not seen)
i. Plantar Interossei (not seen)
j. Dorsal Interossei Pedis (not seen)

RELATIONSHIP TO OTHER MUSCULOSKELETAL STRUCTURES

❑ 1. The abductor digiti minimi pedis is located in the 1st layer of intrinsic muscles of the foot along with the abductor hallucis and the flexor digitorum brevis (and the plantar fascia).

❑ 2. The abductor digiti minimi pedis is lateral to the plantar fascia and the flexor digitorum brevis (which is deep to the plantar fascia).

METHODOLOGY FOR LEARNING MUSCLE ACTIONS

❑ **1. Abduction of the Little Toe (Toe #5) at the Metatarsophalangeal Joint:** The abductor digiti minimi pedis crosses the metatarsophalangeal joint to attach onto the proximal phalanx of the little toe on the lateral side (with its fibers running horizontally). When the abductor digiti minimi pedis contracts, it pulls the little toe laterally away from the 2nd toe (which is the axis of abduction/adduction of the foot); therefore, the abductor digiti minimi pedis abducts the little toe at the metatarsophalangeal joint.

❑ **2. Flexion of the Little Toe (Toe #5) at the Metatarsophalangeal Joint:** The abductor digiti minimi pedis crosses the metatarsophalangeal joint to attach onto the proximal phalanx of the little toe on the plantar side (with its fibers running horizontally in the sagittal plane); therefore, when it pulls on the little toe, the abductor digiti minimi pedis flexes the little toe at the metatarsophalangeal joint.

MISCELLANEOUS

❑ 1. The abductor digiti minimi pedis is also known as the *abductor digiti minimi*. However, this allows for confusion with the abductor digiti minimi manus of the hand, which abducts the little finger of the hand.

❑ 2. All three muscles in the 1st layer of intrinsic muscles of the foot attach proximally onto the tuberosity of the calcaneus and the plantar fascia, and then attach distally onto the toes.

❑

FLEXOR DIGITORUM BREVIS
(PLANTAR SURFACE – LAYER I)

❑ **The name, flexor digitorum brevis, tells us that this muscle flexes the digits, i.e., toes, and is short (shorter than the flexor digitorum longus).**

DERIVATION ❑ flexor: L. *a muscle that flexes a body part.*
digitorum: L. *refers to a digit* (toe).
brevis: L. *short.*

PRONUNCIATION ❑ **fleks**-or dij-i-**toe**-rum **bre**-vis

ATTACHMENTS

❑ **Tuberosity of the Calcaneus**

❑ and the plantar fascia

to the

❑ **Toes #2-5**

❑ the medial and lateral sides of the middle phalanges

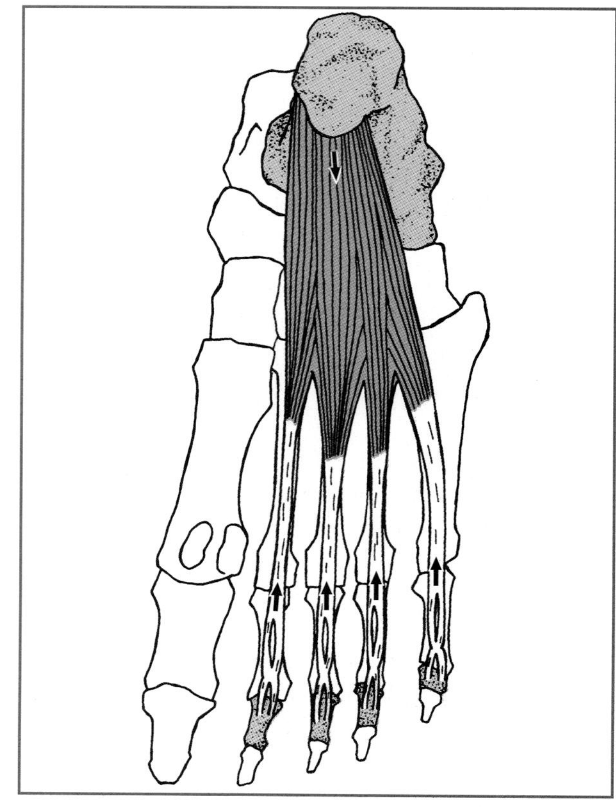

Plantar View of the Right Flexor Digitorum Brevis

ACTION

❑ **Flexion of Toes #2-5**

INNERVATION ❑ The Medial Plantar Nerve ❑ S1, 2

ARTERIAL SUPPLY ❑ The Medial and Lateral Plantar Arteries (Terminal Branches of the Posterior Tibial Artery)

PALPATION AND SUPPLEMENTARY TEXT

PALPATION

- ❑ The flexor digitorum brevis is directly deep to the center of the plantar fascia. Given the thickness of the plantar fascia, it can be difficult to distinguish the musculature that is deep to it.
  - Have the client prone or supine.
  - Place palpating hand on the midline of the plantar side of the foot.
  - Ask the client to actively flex toes #2-5 and feel for the contraction of the flexor digitorum brevis deep to the plantar fascia.

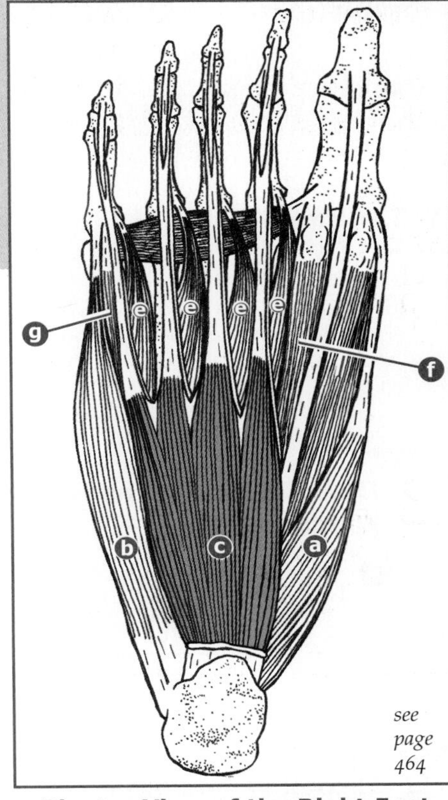

see page 464

Plantar View of the Right Foot (Superficial Muscular Layer)

a. Abductor Hallucis
b. Abductor Digiti Minimi Pedis
c. **Flexor Digitorum Brevis**
d. Quadratus Plantae (not seen)
e. Lumbricals Pedis
f. Flexor Hallucis Brevis
g. Flexor Digiti Minimi Pedis
h. Adductor Hallucis (not seen)
i. Plantar Interossei (not seen)
j. Dorsal Interossei Pedis (not seen)

RELATIONSHIP TO OTHER MUSCULOSKELETAL STRUCTURES

❑ 1. The flexor digitorum brevis is located in the 1st layer of intrinsic muscles of the foot along with the abductor hallucis and the abductor digiti minimi pedis (and the plantar fascia).

❑ 2. The flexor digitorum brevis is lateral to the abductor hallucis, medial to the abductor digiti minimi pedis and deep to the plantar fascia.

❑ 3. Deep to the belly of the flexor digitorum brevis is the quadratus plantae.

❑ 4. The tendons of the flexor digitorum brevis are superficial to the tendons of the flexor digitorum longus.

METHODOLOGY FOR LEARNING MUSCLE ACTIONS

❑ **Flexion of Toes #2-5 at the Metatarsophalangeal and the Proximal Interphalangeal Joints:** The flexor digitorum brevis crosses both the metatarsophalangeal joint and the proximal interphalangeal joint of toes #2-5 on the plantar side (with its fibers running horizontally in the sagittal plane) to then attach onto the medial and lateral sides of the middle phalanx of toes #2-5. Since the flexor digitorum brevis crosses these joints on the plantar side, it flexes the metatarsophalangeal and the proximal interphalangeal joints of toes #2-5.

MISCELLANEOUS

❑ 1. All three muscles in the 1st layer of intrinsic muscles of the foot attach proximally onto the tuberosity of the calcaneus and the plantar fascia, and then attach distally onto the toes.

❑ 2. Every distal tendon of the flexor digitorum brevis splits to allow passage for the flexor digitorum longus' distal tendon to attach onto the distal phalanx of toes #2-5. (This arrangement is essentially identical to that of the splitting of every distal tendon of the flexor digitorum superficialis to allow passage for the flexor digitorum profundus' distal tendon onto the distal phalanx of fingers #2-5 in the upper extremity.)

QUADRATUS PLANTAE
(PLANTAR SURFACE – LAYER II)

❑ **The name, quadratus plantae, tells us that this muscle has a square shape and is located on the plantar side of the foot.**

DERIVATION ❑ quadratus: L. *squared.*
plantae: L. *refers to the plantar surface of the foot.*

PRONUNCIATION ❑ kwod-**ray**-tus **plan**-tee

ATTACHMENTS

❑ **The Calcaneus**

❑ the medial and lateral sides

to the

❑ **Distal Tendon of the Flexor Digitorum Longus Muscle**

❑ the lateral margin

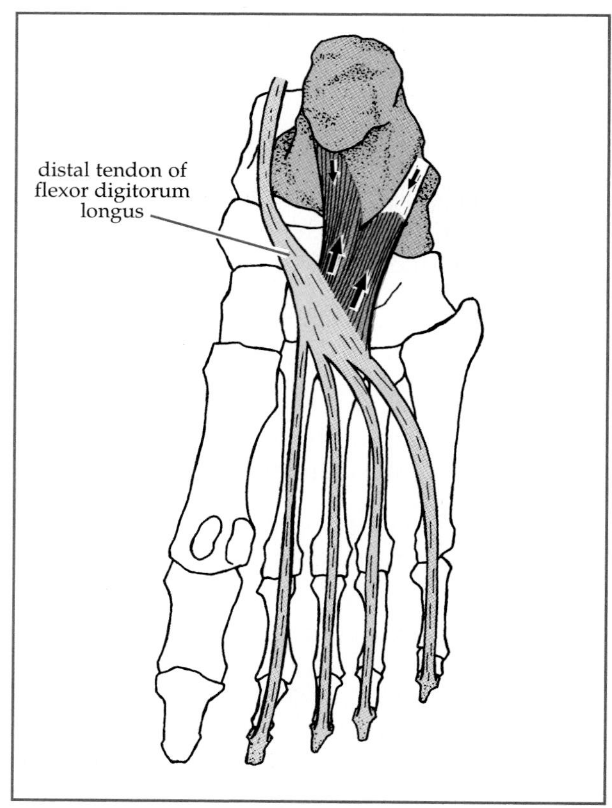

Plantar View of the Right Quadratus Plantae

ACTION

❑ **Flexion of Toes #2-5**

INNERVATION ❑ The Lateral Plantar Nerve ❑ S2, 3

ARTERIAL SUPPLY ❑ The Medial and Lateral Plantar Arteries (Terminal Branches of the Posterior Tibial Artery)

PALPATION AND SUPPLEMENTARY TEXT

PALPATION

- ❑ The quadratus plantae is directly deep to the center of the plantar fascia in the proximal foot. Given the thickness of the plantar fascia, it can be difficult to distinguish the musculature that is deep to it.
  - Have the client prone or supine.
  - Place palpating hand on the midline of the proximal half of the plantar side of the foot and feel for the quadratus plantae deep to the plantar fascia and flexor digitorum brevis.
  - To further bring out the quadratus plantae, resist the client from actively flexing toes #2-5. Keep in mind that this will cause the more superficial flexor digitorum brevis to contract as well.

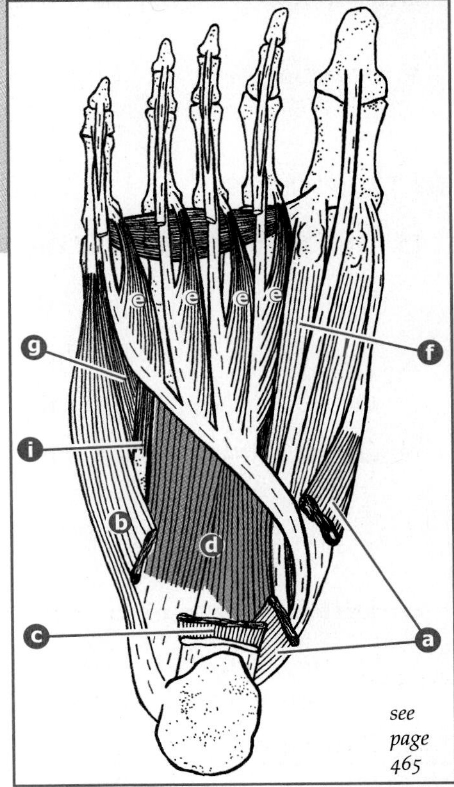

see page 465

Plantar View of the Right Foot (Intermediate Muscular Layer)

a. Abductor Hallucis (cut)
b. Abductor Digiti Minimi Pedis (partially cut)
c. Flexor Digitorum Brevis (cut)
d. Quadratus Plantae
e. Lumbricals Pedis
f. Flexor Hallucis Brevis
g. Flexor Digiti Minimi Pedis
h. Adductor Hallucis (not seen)
i. Plantar Interossei
j. Dorsal Interossei Pedis (not seen)

RELATIONSHIP TO OTHER MUSCULOSKELETAL STRUCTURES

❑ 1. The quadratus plantae is in the 2nd layer of intrinsic muscles of the foot along with the lumbricals pedis.

❑ 2. The quadratus plantae is deep to the flexor digitorum brevis.

❑ 3. Deep to the quadratus plantae are the tarsal bones.

METHODOLOGY FOR LEARNING MUSCLE ACTIONS

❑ **Flexion of Toes #2-5 at the Metatarsophalangeal and the Proximal and Distal Interphalangeal Joints:** The quadratus plantae (with its fibers running horizontally in the sagittal plane) attaches into the distal tendon of the flexor digitorum longus muscle. When the quadratus plantae contracts, it pulls on that tendon in the same way as if the belly of the flexor digitorum longus muscle itself had contracted. Therefore, the quadratus plantae muscle has the same actions as the flexor digitorum longus muscle (in the foot), namely, flexion of toes #2-5. Given that the attachments are onto the distal phalanx of these toes, the metatarsophalangeal joint and the proximal and distal interphalangeal joints are all crossed and, therefore, are all flexed.

MISCELLANEOUS

❑ 1. Proximally, the quadratus plantae has two heads. The medial head attaches onto the medial side of the calcaneus and the lateral head attaches onto the lateral side of the calcaneus.

❑ 2. The quadratus plantae, given its assistance to the flexor digitorum longus, is also known as the *flexor accessorius* or the *flexor digitorum accessorius*. The quadratus plantae not only assists by adding further strength, but also assists by affecting (straightening out) the line of pull of the flexor digitorum longus muscle. If not for the quadratus plantae's assistance, the contraction of the flexor digitorum longus would pull the toes medially as it flexed them.

LUMBRICALS PEDIS

(PLANTAR SURFACE – LAYER II)

(There are four lumbrical pedis muscles, named #1, #2, #3 and #4.)

- ❑ **The name, lumbricals pedis, tells us that these muscles are shaped like earthworms and located in the foot.**

DERIVATION ❑ lumbricals: L. *earthworms.*
pedis: L. *refers to the foot.*

PRONUNCIATION ❑ **lum**-bri-kuls **peed**-us

ATTACHMENTS

- ❑ **The Distal Tendons of the Flexor Digitorum Longus**
  - ❑ **#1**: medial border of the tendon to toe #2
  - ❑ **#2**: adjacent sides of the tendons to toes #2 and #3
  - ❑ **#3**: adjacent sides of the tendons to toes #3 and #4
  - ❑ **#4**: adjacent sides of the tendons to toes #4 and #5

to the

- ❑ **Distal Tendons of the Extensor Digitorum Longus**
  - ❑ the medial side of the tendons merging into the dorsal digital expansion

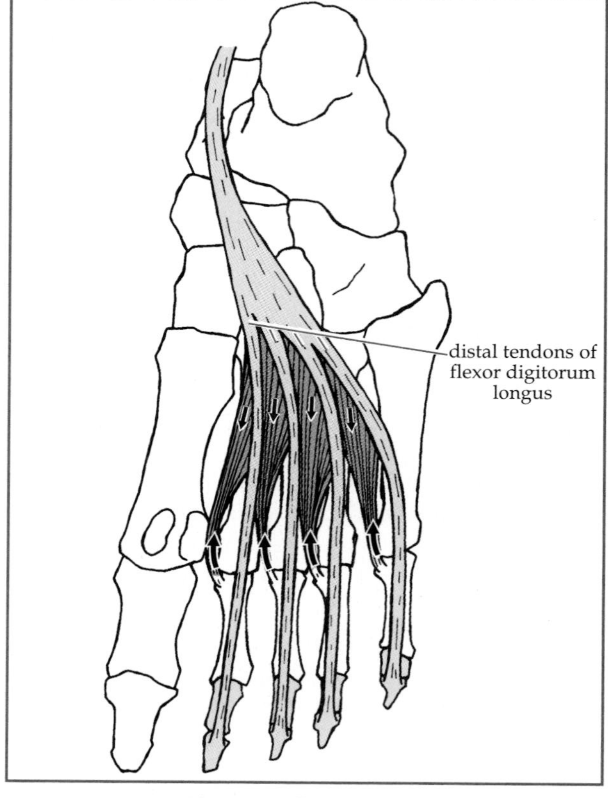

Plantar View of the Right Lumbricals Pedis

ACTIONS

- ❑ 1. **Extension of Toes #2-5 at the Interphalangeal Joints**
- ❑ 2. **Flexion of Toes #2-5 at the Metatarsophalangeal Joint**

INNERVATION ❑ The Medial and Lateral Plantar Nerves
- ❑ S1, 2, 3
- ❑ medial plantar nerve to lumbrical pedis #1
- ❑ lateral plantar nerve to lumbricals pedis #2-4

ARTERIAL SUPPLY ❑ The Medial and Lateral Plantar Arteries (Terminal Branches of the Posterior Tibial Artery)
- ❑ branches of the plantar arch (an anastomosis between the lateral plantar artery and the dorsalis pedis artery)

PALPATION AND SUPPLEMENTARY TEXT

PALPATION

- ❑ The lumbricals pedis are directly deep to the plantar fascia in the distal foot. Given the thickness of the plantar fascia, it can be difficult to distinguish the musculature that is deep to it.
  - Have the client prone or supine.
  - Place palpating hand distally on the plantar surface of the foot and feel for the lumbricals pedis between the metatarsal bones.
  - To further bring out the lumbricals pedis, resist the client from actively flexing the metatarsophalangeal joint (with the interphalangeal joints extended) of toes #2-5.

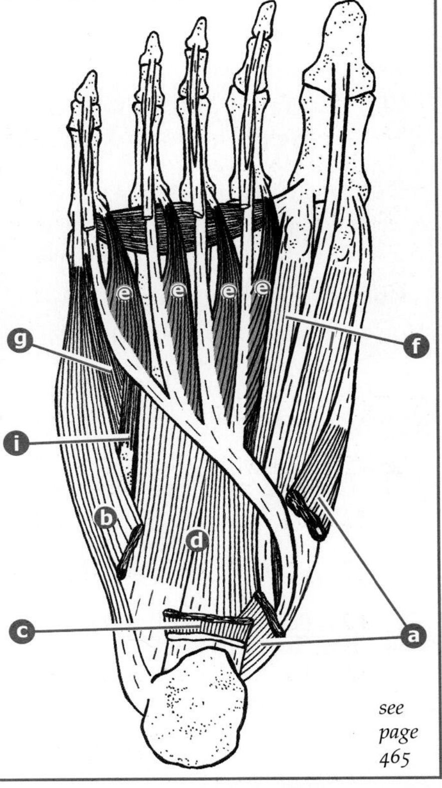

see page 465

Plantar View of the Right Foot (Intermediate Muscular Layer)

a. Abductor Hallucis (cut)
b. Abductor Digiti Minimi Pedis (partially cut)
c. Flexor Digitorum Brevis (cut)
d. Quadratus Plantae
e. **Lumbricals Pedis**
f. Flexor Hallucis Brevis
g. Flexor Digiti Minimi Pedis
h. Adductor Hallucis (not seen)
i. Plantar Interossei
j. Dorsal Interossei Pedis (not seen)

RELATIONSHIP TO OTHER MUSCULOSKELETAL STRUCTURES

❑ 1. The lumbricals pedis are in the 2nd layer of the intrinsic muscles of the foot along with the quadratus plantae.

❑ 2. The lumbricals pedis are located between the distal tendons of the flexor digitorum longus in the distal foot.

❑ 3. The lumbricals pedis are deep to the plantar aponeurosis. No muscles are superficial to the lumbricals pedis except, perhaps, a small part of the flexor digitorum brevis.

❑ 4. Deep to the lumbricals pedis are the metatarsals and the plantar interossei and dorsal interossei pedis muscles.

METHODOLOGY FOR LEARNING MUSCLE ACTIONS

❑ 1. **Extension of Toes #2-5 at the Proximal and Distal Interphalangeal Joints:** The lumbricals pedis, by attaching into the tendons of the extensor digitorum longus (after the metatarsophalangeal joint but before the interphalangeal joints of the toes), in effect exert their pull at the attachments of the extensor digitorum longus, which are the middle and distal phalanges of toes #2-5. The lumbricals pedis, in effect, cross the proximal and distal interphalangeal joints on the dorsal side (with their pull being exerted horizontally in the sagittal plane); therefore, they extend both the proximal and distal interphalangeal joints of toes #2-5.

❑ 2. **Flexion of Toes #2-5 at the Metatarsophalangeal Joint:** The lumbricals pedis cross the metatarsophalangeal joint of toes #2-5 on the plantar side (with their fibers running horizontally in the sagittal plane); therefore, they flex toes #2-5 at the metatarsophalangeal joint.

MISCELLANEOUS

❑ 1. The lumbricals pedis are actually four small separate muscles named from the medial side: #1, #2, #3, and #4.

❑ 2. The lumbricals pedis are usually known as the *lumbricals.* However, this allows for confusion with the lumbricals manus of the hand.

❑ 3. The lumbricals manus of the hand have similar actions in that they flex the fingers at the metacarpophalangeal joints and extend the fingers at the proximal and distal interphalangeal joints.

❑

FLEXOR HALLUCIS BREVIS
(PLANTAR SURFACE – LAYER III)

❑ **The name, flexor hallucis brevis, tells us that this muscle flexes the big toe and is short (shorter than the flexor hallucis longus).**

DERIVATION ❑ flexor: L. *a muscle that flexes a body part.*
hallucis: L. *refers to the big toe.*
brevis: L. *short.*

PRONUNCIATION ❑ **fleks**-or hal-**oo**-sis **bre**-vis

ATTACHMENTS

❑ **Cuboid and the 3rd Cuneiform**

to the

❑ **Big Toe (Toe #1)**

- ❑ the medial and lateral sides of the plantar surface of the base of the proximal phalanx

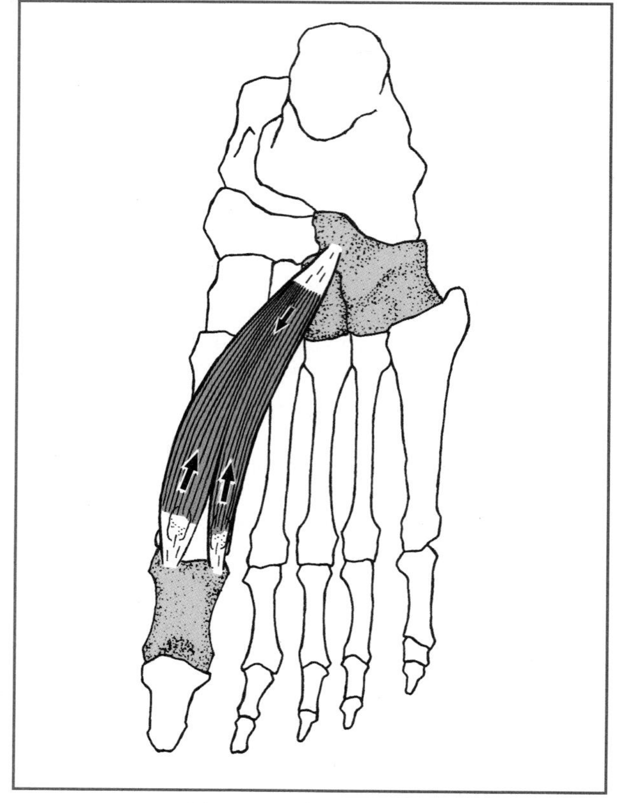

Plantar View of the Right Flexor Hallucis Brevis

ACTION

❑ **Flexion of the Big Toe (Toe #1)**

INNERVATION ❑ The Medial Plantar Nerve ❑ S1, 2

ARTERIAL SUPPLY ❑ The Medial Plantar Artery (A Branch of the Posterior Tibial Artery)

PALPATION AND SUPPLEMENTARY TEXT

PALPATION

- ❑ The flexor hallucis brevis is directly deep to the plantar fascia in the medial distal foot. Given the thickness of the plantar fascia, it can be difficult to distinguish the musculature that is deep to it.
  - Have the client prone or supine.
  - Place palpating hand distally on the medial side of the plantar surface of the foot and feel for the flexor hallucis brevis.
  - To further bring out the flexor hallucis brevis, resist the client from actively flexing the big toe.

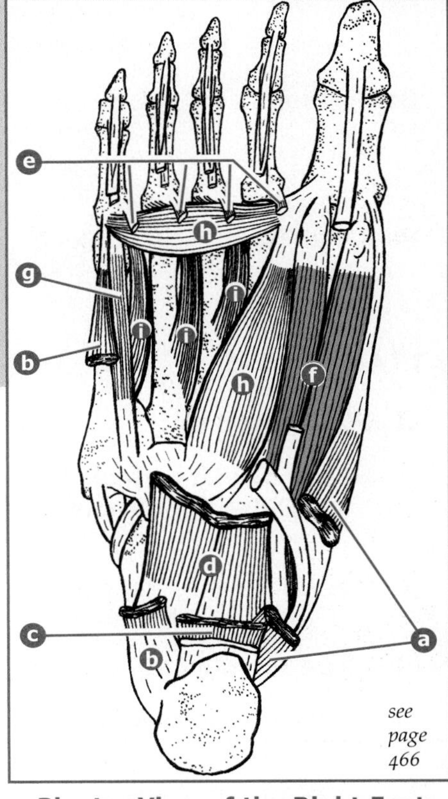

Plantar View of the Right Foot (Deep Muscular Layer)

a. Abductor Hallucis (cut)
b. Abductor Digiti Minimi Pedis (cut)
c. Flexor Digitorum Brevis (cut)
d. Quadratus Plantae (cut)
e. Lumbricals Pedis(cut)
f. **Flexor Hallucis Brevis**
g. Flexor Digiti Minimi Pedis
h. Adductor Hallucis
i. Plantar Interossei
j. Dorsal Interossei Pedis (not seen)

RELATIONSHIP TO OTHER MUSCULOSKELETAL STRUCTURES

- ❑ 1. The flexor hallucis brevis is located in the 3rd layer of intrinsic muscles of the foot along with the flexor digiti minimi pedis and the adductor hallucis.
- ❑ 2. The flexor hallucis brevis is medial to the oblique head of the adductor hallucis and lateral to the abductor hallucis.
- ❑ 3. Even though the flexor hallucis brevis is in the 3rd layer, it is relatively superficial, as there is no belly of any other muscle directly superficial to it. Only the tendon of the flexor hallucis longus is superficial to it, as well as the plantar fascia.
- ❑ 4. Deep to the flexor hallucis brevis is the 1st metatarsal and the 1st dorsal interosseus pedis muscle.

METHODOLOGY FOR LEARNING MUSCLE ACTIONS

- ❑ **Flexion of the Big Toe (Toe #1) at the Metatarsophalangeal Joint:** The flexor hallucis brevis crosses the metatarsophalangeal joint of the big toe on the plantar side (with its fibers running horizontally in the sagittal plane) to attach onto the proximal phalanx of the big toe. Therefore, the flexor hallucis brevis flexes the big toe at the metatarsophalangeal joint.

MISCELLANEOUS

- ❑ 1. The flexor hallucis brevis splits distally to attach onto the medial and lateral sides of the proximal phalanx of the big toe. The medial head of the flexor hallucis brevis crosses the metatarsophalangeal joint medially to attach onto the proximal phalanx of the big toe, so it can pull the big toe medially away from the 2nd toe (abduction). The lateral head of the flexor hallucis brevis crosses the metatarsophalangeal joint laterally to attach onto the proximal phalanx of the big toe, so it can pull the big toe laterally toward the 2nd toe (adduction). Since the 2nd toe is the axis for abduction/adduction of the foot, the flexor hallucis brevis can both abduct and adduct the big toe at the metatarsophalangeal joint.
- ❑ 2. Distally, there is a sesamoid bone in the medial and lateral tendons of the flexor hallucis brevis.

❑

FLEXOR DIGITI MINIMI PEDIS

(PLANTAR SURFACE – LAYER III)

❑ **The name, flexor digiti minimi pedis, tells us that this muscle flexes the little toe.**

DERIVATION ❑ flexor: L. *a muscle that flexes a body part.*
digiti: L. *refers to a digit* (toe).
minimi: L. *least.*
pedis: L. *refers to the foot.*

PRONUNCIATION ❑ **fleks**-or **dij**-i-tee **min**-i-mee **peed**-us

ATTACHMENTS

❑ **5th Metatarsal**

❑ the plantar surface of the base of the 5th metatarsal and the distal tendon of the fibularis longus

to the

❑ **Little Toe (Toe #5)**

❑ the plantar surface of the proximal phalanx

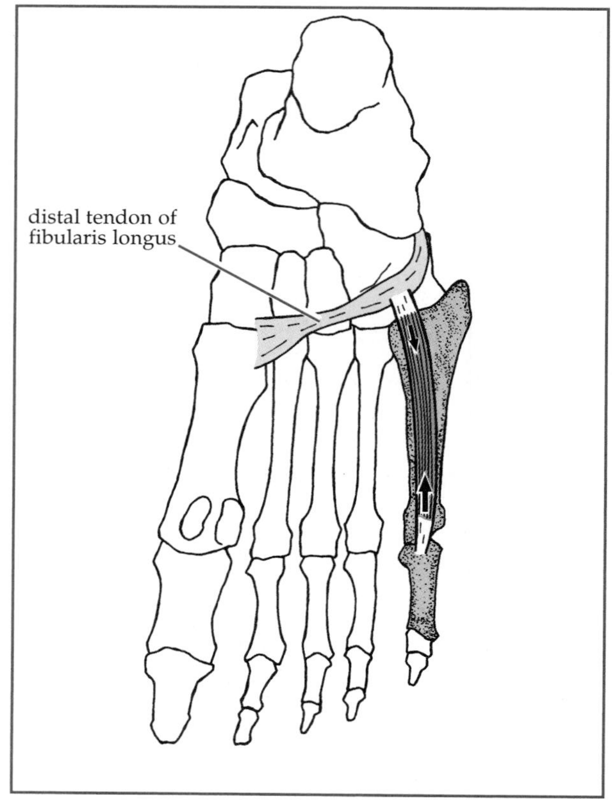

Plantar View of the Right Flexor Digiti Minimi Pedis

ACTION

❑ **Flexion of the Little Toe (Toe #5)**

INNERVATION ❑ The Lateral Plantar Nerve ❑ S2, 3

ARTERIAL SUPPLY ❑ The Lateral Plantar Artery (A Branch of the Posterior Tibial Artery)

PALPATION AND SUPPLEMENTARY TEXT

PALPATION

- ❑ The flexor digiti minimi pedis is directly deep to the plantar fascia in the lateral distal foot. Given the thickness of the plantar fascia, it can be difficult to distinguish the musculature that is deep to it.
  - Have the client prone or supine.
  - Place palpating hand distally on the lateral side of the plantar surface of the foot (just medial to the abductor digiti minimi pedis, see the palpation section for this muscle on page 475) and feel for the flexor digiti minimi.
  - To further bring out the flexor digiti minimi, resist the client from actively flexing the little toe at the metatarsophalangeal joint.

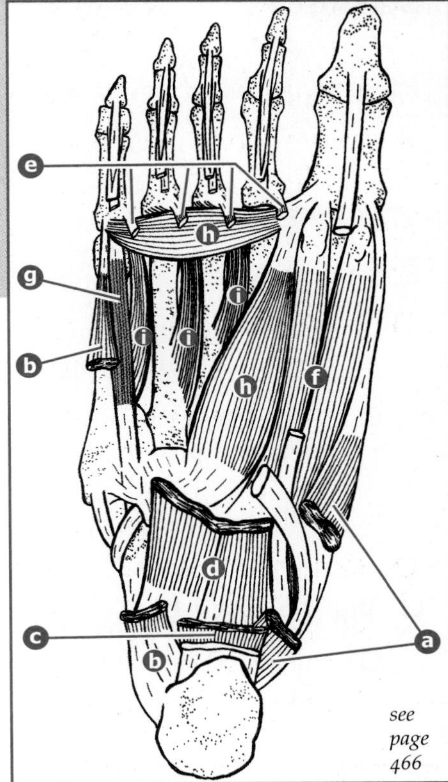

Plantar View of the Right Foot (Deep Muscular Layer)

a. Abductor Hallucis (cut)
b. Abductor Digiti Minimi Pedis (cut)
c. Flexor Digitorum Brevis (cut)
d. Quadratus Plantae (cut)
e. Lumbricals Pedis (cut)
f. Flexor Hallucis Brevis
g. Flexor Digiti Minimi Pedis
h. Adductor Hallucis
i. Plantar Interossei
j. Dorsal Interossei Pedis (not seen)

RELATIONSHIP TO OTHER MUSCULOSKELETAL STRUCTURES

❑ 1. The flexor digiti minimi pedis is in the 3rd layer of intrinsic muscles of the foot along with the flexor hallucis brevis and the adductor hallucis.

❑ 2. The flexor digiti minimi pedis lies directly medial to the abductor digiti minimi and lateral to the 4th lumbrical pedis muscle.

❑ 3. Even though the flexor digiti minimi pedis is in the 3rd layer, it is relatively superficial, as there is no belly of any other muscle directly superficial to it. It is deep only to the plantar fascia.

❑ 4. Deep to the flexor digiti minimi pedis is the 5th metatarsal (and a small portion of the 3rd plantar interosseus and the 4th dorsal interosseus pedis).

METHODOLOGY FOR LEARNING MUSCLE ACTIONS

❑ **Flexion of the Little Toe (Toe #5) at the Metatarsophalangeal Joint:** The flexor digiti minimi pedis crosses the metatarsophalangeal joint of the little toe (toe #5) on the plantar side (with its fibers running horizontally in the sagittal plane) to attach onto the proximal phalanx of the little toe. Therefore, the flexor digiti minimi pedis flexes the little toe at the metatarsophalangeal joint.

MISCELLANEOUS

❑ 1. The flexor digiti minimi pedis is also known as the *flexor digiti minimi*. However, this allows for confusion with the flexor digiti minimi manus of the hand, which flexes the little finger.

❑ 2. The flexor digiti minimi pedis is also known as the *flexor digiti minimi brevis*, although the addition of the word "brevis" at the end does not make sense in this case. Usually, the word brevis at the end of a muscle's name is added to distinguish the muscle from a longer muscle that does the same action. In this case, there is no flexor digiti minimi longus.

❑ 3. The flexor digiti minimi pedis occasionally has attachments that range from the tarsals proximally, onto the 5th metatarsal distally. When this occurs, this muscle has the ability to oppose the little toe toward the other toes; therefore, it is named the *opponens digiti minimi pedis* (see illustration on page 467.) This muscle is commonly found in apes whose feet are more "handy" than ours. ☺

ADDUCTOR HALLUCIS
(PLANTAR SURFACE – LAYER III)

❑ **The name, adductor hallucis, tells us that this muscle adducts the big toe.**

DERIVATION ❑ adductor: L. *a muscle that adducts a body part.*
hallucis: L. *refers to the big toe.*

PRONUNCIATION ❑ ad-**duk**-tor hal-**oo**-sis

ATTACHMENTS

❑ **Metatarsals**

- ❑ OBLIQUE HEAD: from the base of metatarsals #2-4 and the distal tendon of the fibularis longus .
- ❑ TRANSVERSE HEAD: arises from the plantar metatarsophalangeal ligaments #3, 4, and 5

to the

❑ **Big Toe (Toe #1)**

- ❑ the lateral side of the base of the proximal phalanx

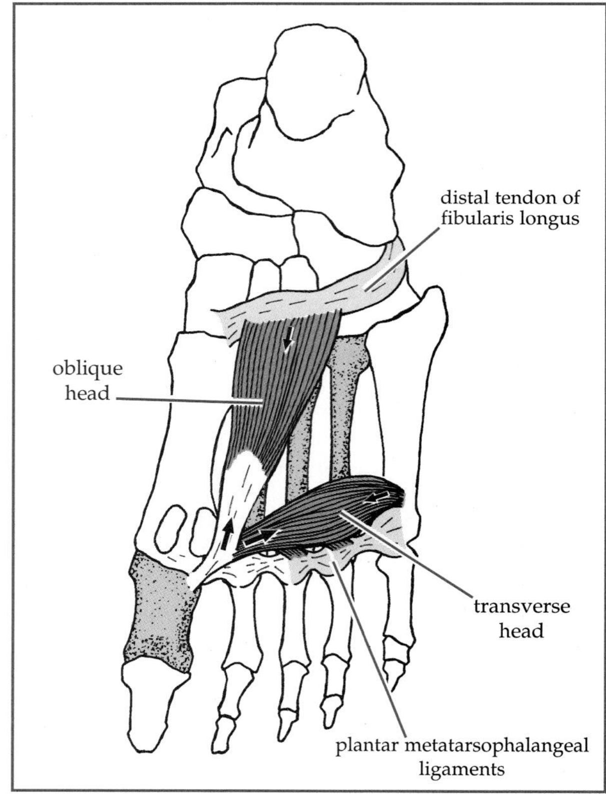

Plantar View of the Right Adductor Hallucis

ACTIONS

❑ 1. **Adduction of the Big Toe (Toe #1)**

❑ 2. Flexion of the Big Toe (Toe #1)

INNERVATION ❑ The Lateral Plantar Nerve ❑ S2, 3

ARTERIAL SUPPLY ❑ Branches of the Plantar Arch (An Anastomosis between the Lateral Plantar Artery and the Dorsalis Pedis Artery)

PALPATION AND SUPPLEMENTARY TEXT

PALPATION

❑ The adductor hallucis is located on the plantar surface of the foot, overlying the 2nd, 3rd and 4th metatarsals. Given the thickness of the plantar fascia, and the depth of the adductor hallucis, it is extremely difficult to palpate.

- Have the client prone or supine.
- Place palpating hand on the plantar surface of the foot over the 2nd, 3rd and 4th metatarsals.
- Ask the client to actively adduct the big toe and feel for the contraction of the adductor hallucis.

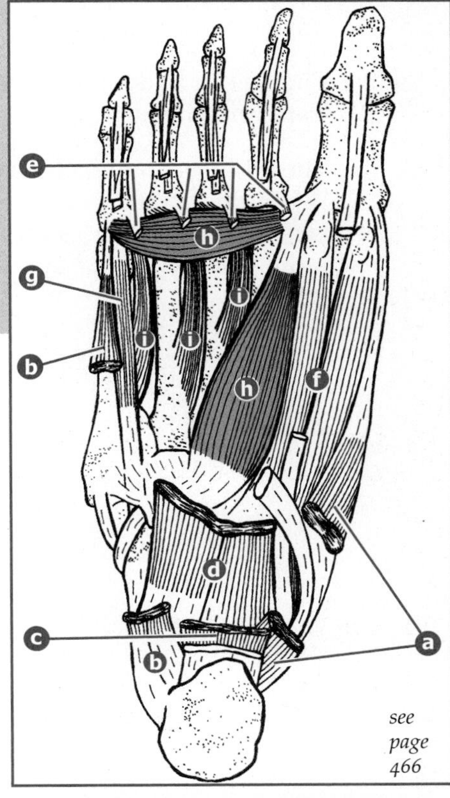

see page 466

Plantar View of the Right Foot (Deep Muscular Layer)

a. Abductor Hallucis (cut)
b. Abductor Digiti Minimi Pedis (cut)
c. Flexor Digitorum Brevis (cut)
d. Quadratus Plantae (cut)
e. Lumbricals Pedis (cut)
f. Flexor Hallucis Brevis
g. Flexor Digiti Minimi Pedis
h. Adductor Hallucis
i. Plantar Interossei
j. Dorsal Interossei Pedis (not seen)

RELATIONSHIP TO OTHER MUSCULOSKELETAL STRUCTURES

❑ 1. The adductor hallucis is located in the 3rd layer of intrinsic muscles of the foot along with the flexor hallucis brevis and the flexor digiti minimi pedis.

❑ 2. The oblique head of the adductor hallucis is directly lateral to the flexor hallucis brevis.

❑ 3. The oblique head of the adductor hallucis is deep to the lumbricals pedis and the quadratus plantae.

❑ 4. The transverse head of the adductor hallucis is deep to the flexor digitorum longus and brevis tendons.

❑ 5. Deep to the adductor hallucis are the interossei muscles and the metatarsals.

METHODOLOGY FOR LEARNING MUSCLE ACTIONS

❑ **1. Adduction of the Big Toe (Toe #1) at the Metatarsophalangeal Joint:** The adductor hallucis crosses the metatarsophalangeal joint of the big toe on the lateral side (with its fibers running horizontally) to attach onto the proximal phalanx of the big toe. When the adductor hallucis contracts, it pulls the big toe laterally toward the 2nd toe (which is the axis for abduction/adduction of the foot). Therefore, the adductor hallucis adducts the big toe at the metatarsophalangeal joint.

❑ **2. Flexion of the Big Toe (Toe #1) at the Metatarsophalangeal Joint:** The adductor hallucis crosses the metatarsophalangeal joint of the big toe on the plantar side (with its fibers running horizontally in the sagittal plane) to attach to the proximal phalanx of the big toe. Therefore, the adductor hallucis flexes the big toe at the metatarsophalangeal joint.

ADDUCTOR HALLUCIS – continued

MISCELLANEOUS

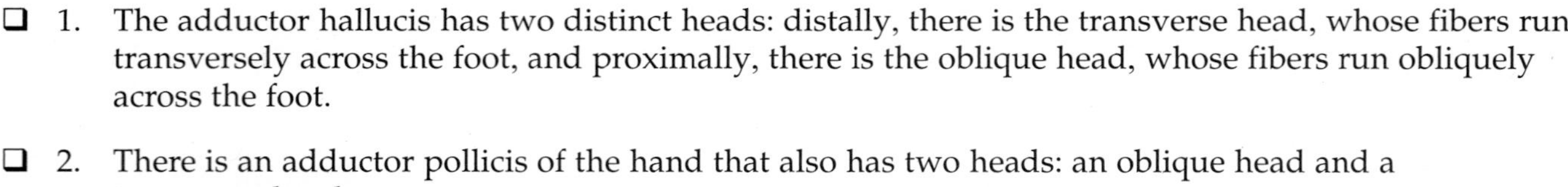

- ❑ 1. The adductor hallucis has two distinct heads: distally, there is the transverse head, whose fibers run transversely across the foot, and proximally, there is the oblique head, whose fibers run obliquely across the foot.
- ❑ 2. There is an adductor pollicis of the hand that also has two heads: an oblique head and a transverse head.
- ❑ 3. The adductor hallucis occasionally has attachments that attach distally onto the 1st metatarsal. When this occurs, this muscle has the ability to oppose the big toe toward the other toes, and is named the *opponens hallucis* of the foot. (This arrangement is common in apes, whose feet are more "handy" than ours. ☺)
- ❑ 4. The oblique head of the adductor hallucis often blends with the flexor hallucis brevis.

PLANTAR INTEROSSEI

(PLANTAR SURFACE – LAYER IV)

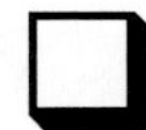

(There are three plantar interossei, named #1, #2 and #3.)

❑ **The name, plantar interossei, tells us that these muscles are located between bones (metatarsals) on the plantar side.**

DERIVATION ❑ plantar: L. *refers to the plantar side of the foot.*
interossei: L. *between bones.*

PRONUNCIATION ❑ **plan**-tar in-ter-**oss**-ee-eye

ATTACHMENTS

❑ **Metatarsals**

❑ the medial side ("2nd Toe Side") of metatarsals #3-5:

❑ **#1**: attaches onto metatarsal #3

❑ **#2**: attaches onto metatarsal #4

❑ **#3**: attaches onto metatarsal #5

to the

❑ **Sides of the Phalanges and the Distal Tendons of the Extensor Digitorum Longus**

❑ the base of the proximal phalanges (on the "2nd Toe Side") and the dorsal digital expansion:

❑ **#1**: attaches to toe #3

❑ **#2**: attaches to toe #4

❑ **#3**: attaches to toe #5

Plantar View of the Right Plantar Interossei

ACTIONS

❑ 1. **Adduction of Toes #3-5**

❑ 2. **Flexion of Toes #3-5 at the Metatarsophalangeal Joint**

❑ 3. **Extension of Toes #3-5 at the Interphalangeal Joints**

INNERVATION ❑ The Lateral Plantar Nerve ❑ S2, 3

ARTERIAL SUPPLY ❑ Branches of the Plantar Arch
(An Anastomosis between the Lateral Plantar Artery and the Dorsalis Pedis Artery)

PLANTAR INTEROSSEI – PALPATION AND SUPPLEMENTARY TEXT

PALPATION

- ❑ Given the thickness of the plantar fascia and the depth of the plantar interossei, it is difficult to distinguish them from other deep muscles of the foot on the plantar side.

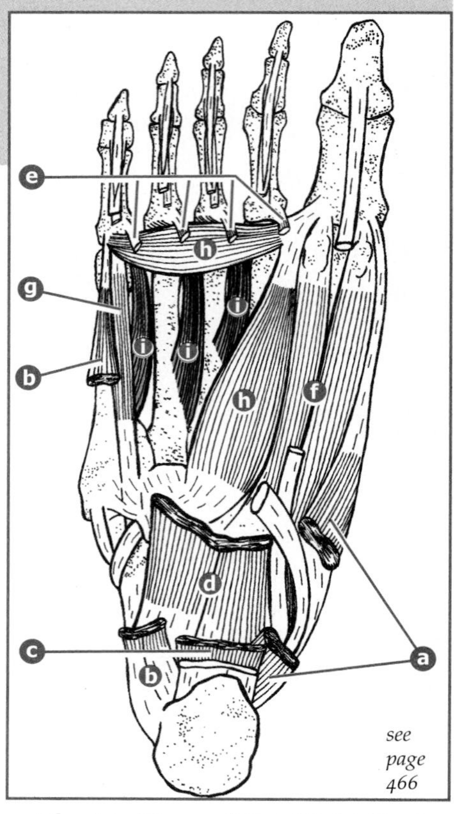

Plantar View of the Right Foot (Deep Muscular Layer)

a. Abductor Hallucis (cut)
b. Abductor Digiti Minimi Pedis (cut)
c. Flexor Digitorum Brevis (cut)
d. Quadratus Plantae (cut)
e. Lumbricals Pedis (cut)
f. Flexor Hallucis Brevis
g. Flexor Digiti Minimi Pedis
h. Adductor Hallucis
i. **Plantar Interossei**
j. Dorsal Interossei Pedis (not seen)

RELATIONSHIP TO OTHER MUSCULOSKELETAL STRUCTURES

❑ 1. The plantar interossei are in the 4th layer of intrinsic muscles of the foot along with the dorsal interossei pedis (and the distal tendons of the fibularis longus and tibialis posterior).

❑ 2. From the plantar perspective, the plantar interossei are deep to the lumbricals pedis.

❑ 3. From the plantar perspective, the plantar interossei are somewhat superficial (partially overlap) the metatarsals and the dorsal interossei pedis.

METHODOLOGY FOR LEARNING MUSCLE ACTIONS

❑ 1. **Adduction of Toes #3-5 at the Metatarsophalangeal Joint:** The plantar interossei cross the metatarsophalangeal joint of toes #3-5 medially (with their fibers running horizontally) and pull toes #3-5 medially toward the 2nd toe (which is the axis for abduction/adduction of the foot). Therefore, the plantar interossei adduct toes #3-5 at the metatarsophalangeal joint.

❑ 2. **Flexion of Toes #3-5 at the Metatarsophalangeal Joint:** The plantar interossei cross the metatarsophalangeal joint of toes #3-5 on the plantar side (with their fibers running horizontally in the sagittal plane); therefore, they flex toes #3-5 at the metatarsophalangeal joint.

❑ 3. **Extension of Toes #3-5 at the Proximal and Distal Interphalangeal Joints:** The plantar interossei, by attaching into the tendon of the extensor digitorum longus muscle (after the metatarsophalangeal joint, but before the interphalangeal joints of the toes), exert their pull at the attachments of the extensor digitorum longus, the distal phalanx of toes #3-5. The plantar interossei, in effect, cross the proximal and distal interphalangeal joints on the dorsal side (with their fibers running horizontally in the sagittal plane); therefore, the plantar interossei extend both the proximal and distal interphalangeal joints of toes #3-5.

MISCELLANEOUS

❑ 1. There are three separate plantar interossei. They are named from the medial side: #1, #2 and #3.

PLANTAR INTEROSSEI – continued

- ☐ 2. The 1st plantar interosseus attaches to the 3rd digit of the foot and moves the 3rd toe. Similarly, the 2nd plantar interosseus attaches onto and moves the 4th toe, and the 3rd plantar interosseus attaches onto and moves the 5th toe.
- ☐ 3 The plantar interossei have the same actions as the lumbricals pedis of the foot (flexion of the metatarsophalangeal joint and extension of the proximal and distal interphalangeal joints) as well as adduction of toes #3-5 at the metatarsophalangeal joint.
- ☐ 4. There are also palmar interossei of the hand that have essentially identical actions (adduction of the fingers at the metacarpophalangeal joint, flexion of the fingers at the metacarpophalangeal joint and extension of the fingers at the proximal and distal interphalangeal joints) to the plantar interossei of the foot.
- ☐ 5. A mnemonic for remembering the actions of the plantar interossei and dorsal interossei pedis muscles is **"DAB"** and **"PAD."** The **D**orsals **AB**duct, and the **P**lantars **AD**duct.

❑ DORSAL INTEROSSEI PEDIS

(PLANTAR SURFACE – LAYER IV)

(There are four dorsal interossei pedis muscles, named #1, #2, #3 and #4.)

❑ **The name, dorsal interossei pedis, tells us that these muscles are located between bones (metatarsals) on the dorsal side and located in the foot.**

DERIVATION ❑ dorsal: L. *refers to the dorsal side.*
interossei: L. *between bones.*
pedis: L. *refers to the foot.*

PRONUNCIATION ❑ **plan**-tar in-ter-**oss**-ee-eye **peed**-us

ATTACHMENTS

❑ **Metatarsals**

- ❑ each one arises from the adjacent sides of two metatarsals:
  - ❑ **#1**: attaches onto metatarsals #1 and #2
  - ❑ **#2**: attaches onto metatarsals #2 and #3
  - ❑ **#3**: attaches onto metatarsals #3 and #4
  - ❑ **#4**: attaches onto metatarsals #4 and #5

to the

❑ **Sides of the Phalanges and the Distal Tendons of the Extensor Digitorum Longus**

- ❑ the bases of the proximal phalanges (on the sides away from the center of the 2nd toe) and the dorsal digital expansion:
  - ❑ **#1**: attaches to the medial side of toe #2
  - ❑ **#2**: attaches to the lateral side of toe #2
  - ❑ **#3**: attaches to the lateral side of toe #3
  - ❑ **#4**: attaches to the lateral side of toe #4

Dorsolateral View of the Right Dorsal Interossei Pedis

ACTIONS

❑ 1. **Abduction of Toes #2-4**

❑ 2. **Flexion of Toes #2-4 at the Metatarsophalangeal Joint**

❑ 3. **Extension of Toes #2-4 at the Interphalangeal Joints**

INNERVATION ❑ The Lateral Plantar Nerve ❑ S2, 3

ARTERIAL SUPPLY ❑ Branches of the Plantar Arch (An Anastomosis between the Lateral Plantar Artery and the Dorsalis Pedis Artery)

DORSAL INTEROSSEI PEDIS – PALPATION AND SUPPLEMENTARY TEXT

PALPATION

❑ The dorsal interossei pedis may be palpated between the metatarsals on the dorsal side of the foot.

- Have the client supine.
- Place palpating fingers on the dorsal side of the foot between the 1st and 2nd metatarsal bones.
- Ask the client to actively abduct the 2nd toe toward the big toe (tibial abduction) and feel for the contraction of the 1st dorsal interosseus pedis.
- Repeat between the 2nd and 3rd metatarsal bones with fibular abduction of the 2nd toe and feel for the contraction of the 2nd dorsal interosseus pedis.
- Repeat between metatarsals #3-4 and #4-5 with abduction of the 3rd and 4th toes and feel for the contraction of the 3rd and 4th dorsal interossei pedis respectively.

RELATIONSHIP TO OTHER MUSCULOSKELETAL STRUCTURES

❑ 1. The dorsal interossei pedis are in the 4th layer of intrinsic muscles of the foot along with the plantar interossei (and the distal tendons of the fibularis longus and tibialis posterior).

❑ 2. The dorsal interossei pedis are located between the metatarsals; hence, they are bordered on either side by the metatarsal bones.

❑ 3. From the dorsal perspective, the dorsal interossei pedis are deep to the tendons of the extensor digitorum longus and extensor digitorum brevis.

❑ 4. From the plantar perspective, the dorsal interossei pedis are adjacent, and deep to (partially overlapped by), the plantar interossei.

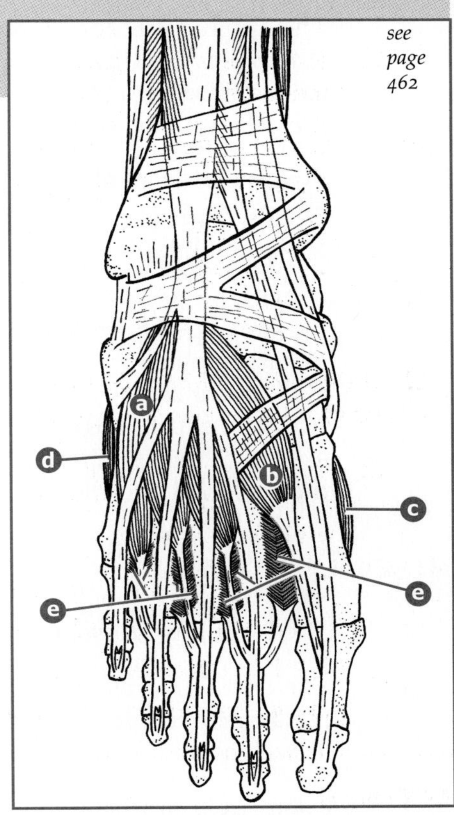

see page 462

Dorsal View of the Right Foot

a. Extensor Digitorum Brevis
b. Extensor Hallucis Brevis
c. Abductor Hallucis
d. Abductor Digiti Minimi Pedis
e. **Dorsal Interossei Pedis**

DORSAL INTEROSSEI PEDIS – continued

METHODOLOGY FOR LEARNING MUSCLE ACTIONS

❑ **1. Abduction of Toes #2-4 at the Metatarsophalangeal Joint:** All the dorsal interossei pedis cross the metatarsophalangeal joint to attach onto the proximal phalanx of toes #2-4 (with their fibers running horizontally).

The 1st dorsal interosseus pedis attaches onto the medial side of the 2nd toe. When the 1st dorsal interosseus pedis contracts, it pulls the 2nd toe medially away from the axis of abduction/adduction of the foot (which is an imaginary line drawn through the 2nd toe). Therefore, the 1st dorsal interosseus pedis performs "tibial abduction" of the 2nd toe at the metatarsophalangeal joint.

The 2nd dorsal interosseus pedis attaches onto the lateral side of the 2nd toe. When the 2nd dorsal interosseus pedis contracts, it pulls the 2nd toe laterally away from the axis of abduction/adduction of the foot (which is an imaginary line drawn through the 2nd toe). Therefore, the 2nd dorsal interosseus pedis performs "fibular abduction" of the 2nd toe at the metatarsophalangeal joint.

The 3rd and 4th dorsal interossei pedis attach onto the lateral side of the 3rd and 4th toes respectively. When they contract, they pull the 3rd and 4th toes laterally away from the 2nd toe (which is the axis for abduction/adduction of the foot). Therefore, the 3rd and 4th dorsal interossei pedis abduct the 3rd and 4th toes at the metatarsophalangeal joint.

❑ **2. Flexion of Toes #2-4 at the Metatarsophalangeal Joint:** The dorsal interossei pedis cross the metatarsophalangeal joint of toes #2-4 on the plantar side (with their fibers running horizontally in the sagittal plane); therefore, they flex toes #2-4 at the metatarsophalangeal joint.

❑ **3. Extension of Toes #2-4 at the Proximal and Distal Interphalangeal Joints:** The dorsal interossei pedis, by attaching into the tendons of the extensor digitorum longus muscle (after the metatarsophalangeal joint but before the interphalangeal joints of the toes), exert their pull at the attachment of the extensor digitorum longus (at the distal phalanx of toes #2-4). The dorsal interossei pedis, in effect, cross the proximal and distal interphalangeal joints on the dorsal side (essentially exerting their pull horizontally in the sagittal plane); therefore, the dorsal interossei pedis extend both the proximal and the distal interphalangeal joints of toes #2-4.

MISCELLANEOUS

❑ 1. There are four dorsal interossei pedis muscles named from the medial side: #1, #2, #3 and #4.

❑ 2. The dorsal interossei pedis have the same actions as the lumbricals pedis (flexion of the metatarsophalangeal joint and extension of the proximal and distal interphalangeal joints) as well as abduction of toes #2-4 at the metatarsophalangeal joint.

❑ 3. There are four dorsal interossei manus of the hand, which have essentially identical actions (abduction of the fingers at the metacarpophalangeal joint, flexion of the fingers at the metacarpophalangeal joint and extension of the fingers at the proximal and distal interphalangeal joints) to the dorsal interossei pedis of the foot.

❑ 4. A mnemonic for remembering the actions of the dorsal interossei pedis and plantar interossei muscles is **"DAB"** and **"PAD."** The **D**orsals **AB**duct and the **P**lantars **AD**duct.

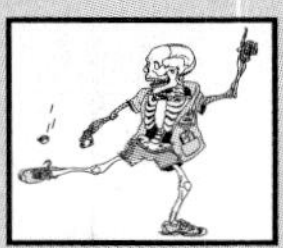

PART THREE – MUSCLES OF THE UPPER EXTREMITY

MUSCLES OF THE SCAPULA/ARM

MUSCLES OF THE FOREARM

INTRINSIC MUSCLES OF THE HAND

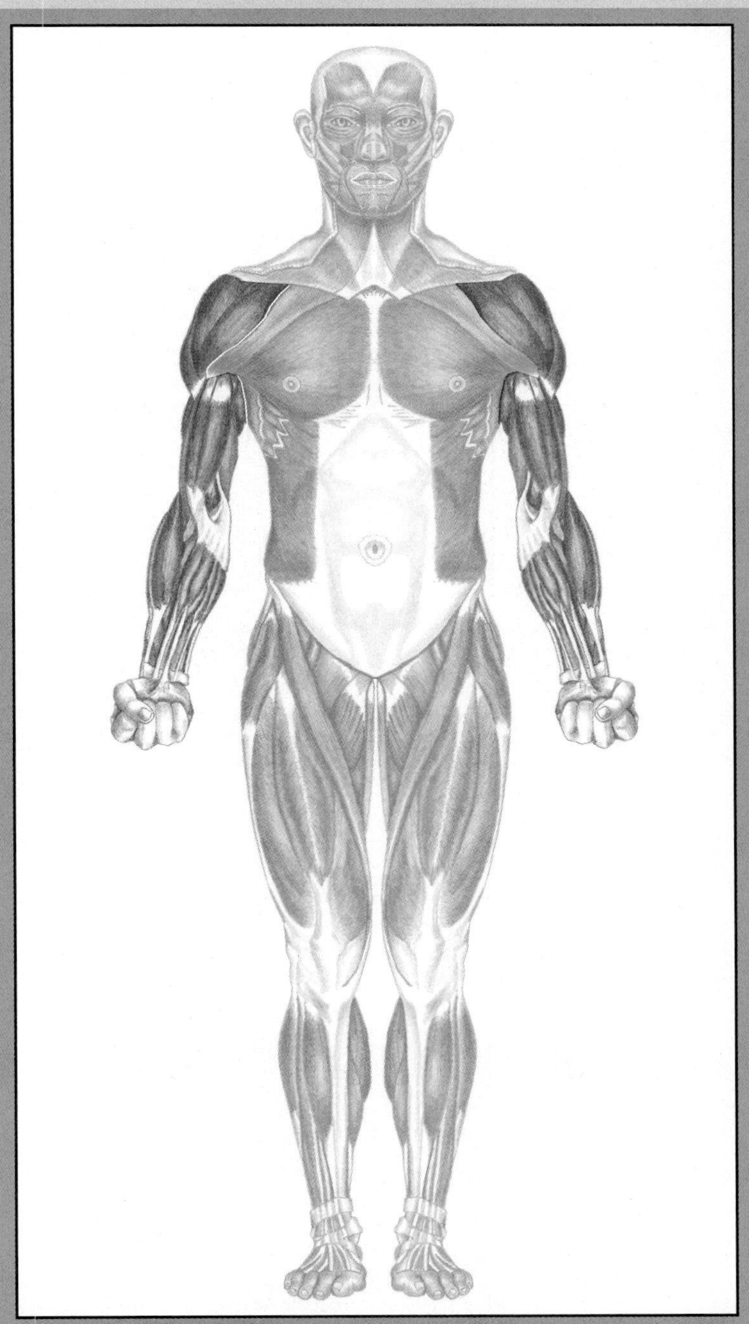

UPPER EXTREMITY

MUSCLES OF THE SCAPULA/ARM

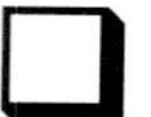

OVERVIEW OF THE MUSCLES OF THE SCAPULA/ARM

ANATOMICALLY, THE MUSCLES OF THE SCAPULA/ARM CAN BE DIVIDED INTO TWO GROUPS:

Muscles of the Scapula:

Rotator Cuff Muscles

- Supraspinatus
- Infraspinatus
- Teres Minor
- Subscapularis

- Teres Major

Muscles of the Arm:

- Deltoid
- Coracobrachialis
- Biceps Brachii
- Brachialis
- Triceps Brachii

THE FOLLOWING MUSCLES ARE COVERED IN OTHER CHAPTERS OF THIS BOOK, BUT ARE ALSO PRESENT IN THE SCAPULA/ARM:

Scapula

- Trapezius
- Levator Scapulae
- Omohyoid
- Latissimus Dorsi
- Rhomboids Major and Minor
- Serratus Anterior
- Pectoralis Minor

Arm

- Pectoralis Major
- Latissimus Dorsi
- Pronator Teres
- Flexor Carpi Radialis
- Palmaris Longus
- Flexor Carpi Ulnaris
- Flexor Digitorum Superficialis
- Brachioradialis
- Flexor Pollicis Longus
- Anconeus
- Extensor Carpi Radialis Longus
- Extensor Carpi Radialis Brevis
- Extensor Digitorum
- Extensor Digiti Minimi
- Extensor Carpi Ulnaris
- Supinator

This classification of the muscles of the scapula/arm is based primarily upon the location of the bellies of these muscles. However, other classifications are often used. Based upon certain actions or attachment sites, some of these muscles could be organized and grouped into other categories:

- As movers of the arm, the rotator cuff muscles are primarily important as rotators (as their name implies) of the arm at the shoulder joint.
- In addition to their role as movers, the rotator cuff muscles are also important as fixators (stabilizers) of the arm at the shoulder joint.
- Of the muscles in the arm, the deltoid and the coracobrachialis primarily move the arm at the shoulder joint.
- Of the muscles in the arm, the biceps brachii, brachialis and the triceps brachii primarily move the forearm at the elbow joint.

Functionally, the muscles of the scapula/arm cross either the shoulder joint and/or the elbow joint and/or the scapulocostal joint. Therefore, the muscles of the scapula/arm have their actions at these joints. The following general rules regarding actions can be stated for muscles of the scapula/arm:

- If a muscle crosses the shoulder joint anteriorly, it can flex the arm at the shoulder joint.
- If a muscle crosses the shoulder joint posteriorly, it can extend the arm at the shoulder joint.
- If a muscle crosses the shoulder joint laterally (superiorly, over the top of the joint), it can abduct the arm at the shoulder joint.
- If a muscle crosses the shoulder joint medially (inferiorly, below the center of the joint), it can adduct the arm at the shoulder joint.
- Medial rotators of the arm wrap around the humerus from medial to lateral, anterior to the shoulder joint.
- Lateral rotators of the arm wrap around the humerus from medial to lateral, posterior to the shoulder joint.
- If a muscle crosses the elbow joint anteriorly, it can flex the forearm at the elbow joint.
- If a muscle crosses the elbow joint posteriorly, it can extend the forearm at the elbow joint.

INNERVATION

- The three muscles of the anterior arm (coracobrachialis, biceps brachii and the brachialis) are innervated by the musculocutaneous nerve.
- The triceps brachii in the posterior arm is innervated by the radial nerve.

ARTERIAL SUPPLY

- The rotator cuff muscles receive their arterial supply almost entirely from the suprascapular artery and the circumflex scapular artery.
- The three muscles of the anterior arm (coracobrachialis, biceps brachii and the brachialis) receive their arterial supply primarily from the brachial artery.
- The triceps brachii in the posterior arm receives its arterial supply primarily from the deep brachial artery.

A NOTE REGARDING REVERSE ACTIONS

As a rule, this book does not employ the terms "origin" and "insertion." However, it is useful to utilize these terms to describe the concept of "reverse actions." The action section of this book describes the action of a muscle by stating the movement of a body part that is created by a muscle's contraction. The body part that usually moves when a muscle contracts is called the insertion. The methodology section further states at which joint the movement of the insertion occurs. However, the other body part that the muscle attaches to, the origin, can also move at that joint. *This movement can be called the reverse action of the muscle.* Keep in mind that the reverse action of a muscle is always possible. The likelihood that a reverse action will occur is based upon the ability of the insertion to be fixed so that the origin moves (instead of the insertion moving) when the muscle contracts. For more information and examples of reverse actions, see page 702.

❑ ANTERIOR VIEW OF THE BONES AND BONY LANDMARKS OF THE RIGHT SCAPULA/ARM

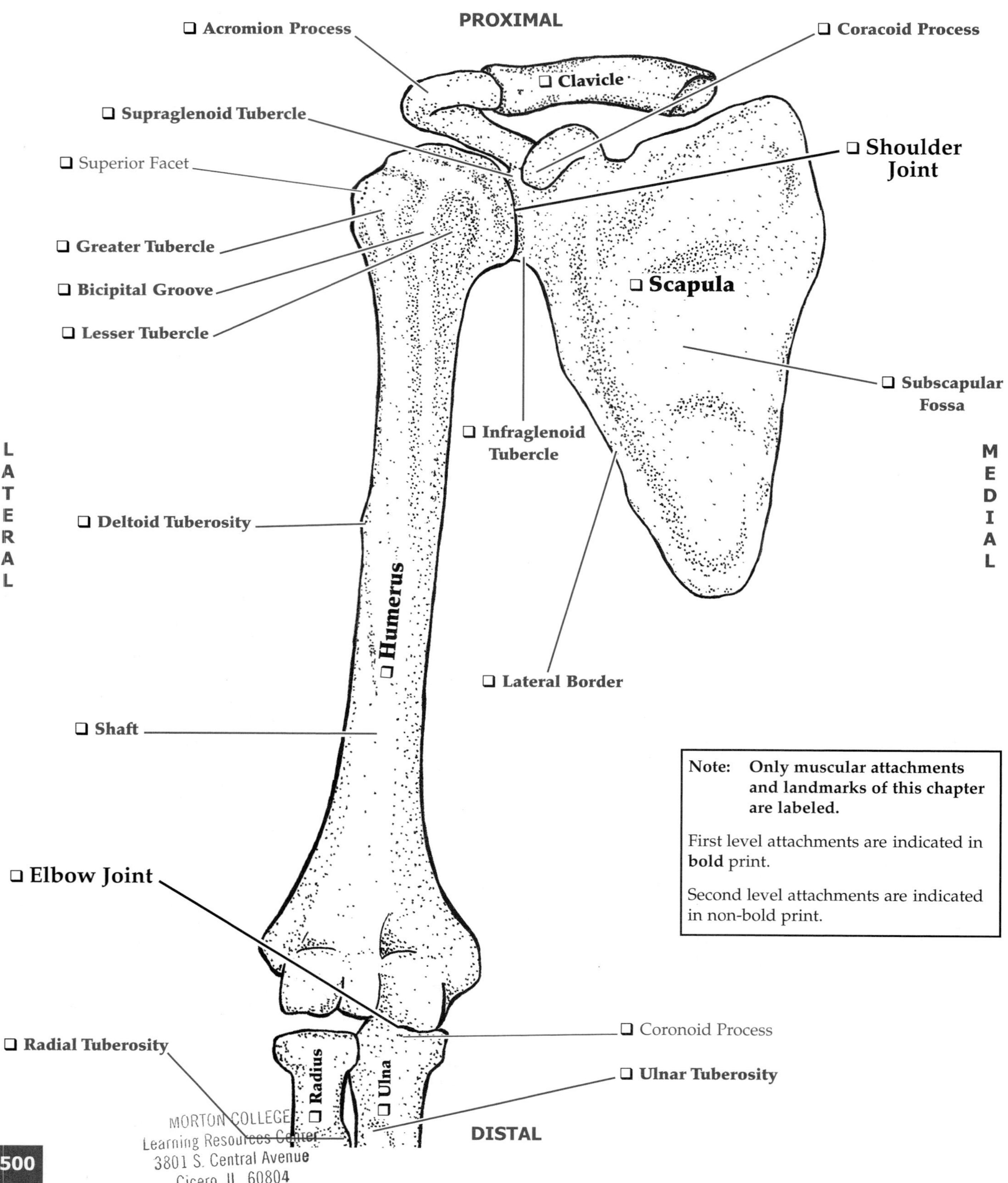

Note: **Only muscular attachments and landmarks of this chapter are labeled.**

First level attachments are indicated in **bold** print.

Second level attachments are indicated in non-bold print.

ANTERIOR VIEW OF THE BONY ATTACHMENTS OF THE RIGHT SCAPULA/ARM

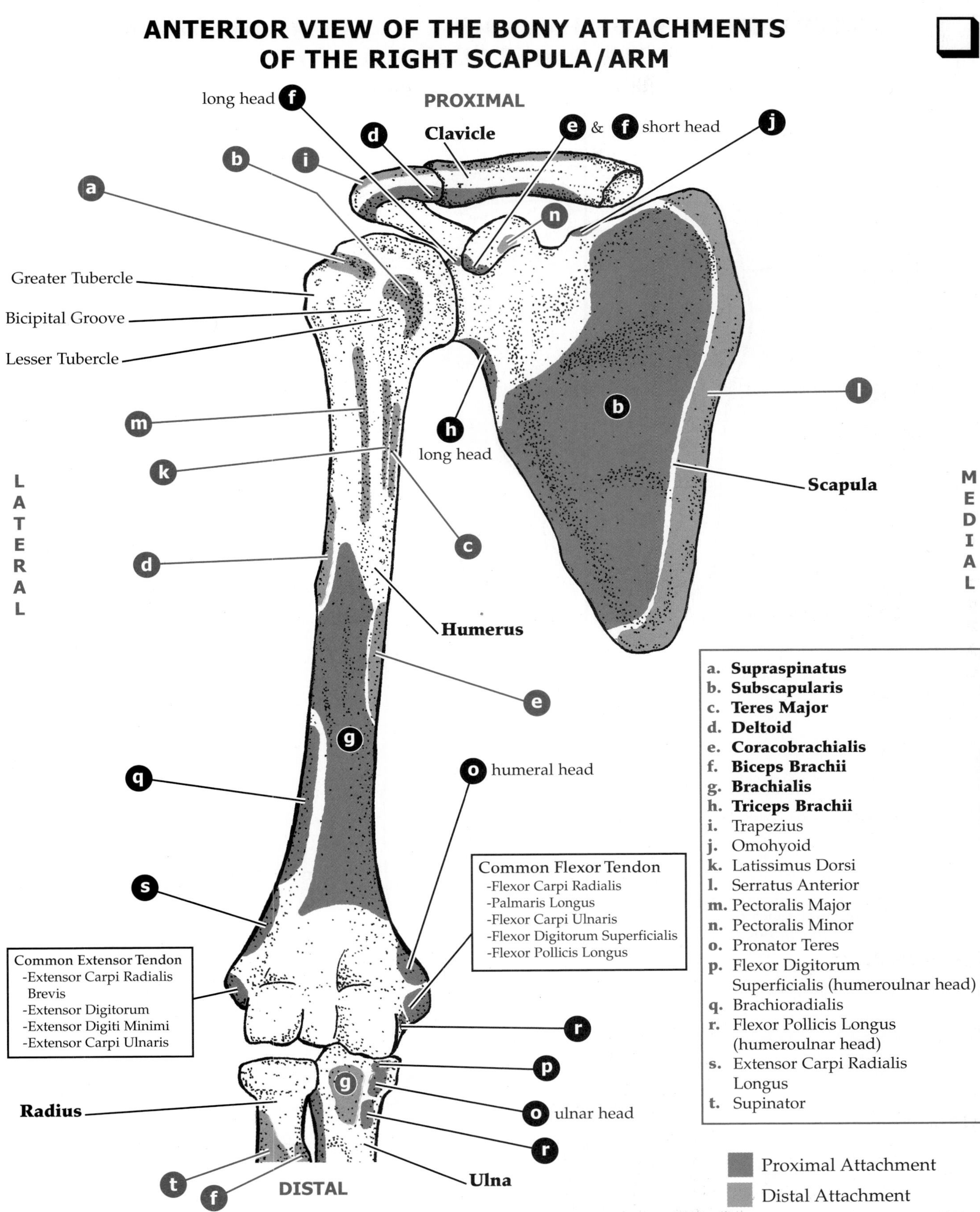

a. **Supraspinatus**
b. **Subscapularis**
c. **Teres Major**
d. **Deltoid**
e. **Coracobrachialis**
f. **Biceps Brachii**
g. **Brachialis**
h. **Triceps Brachii**
i. Trapezius
j. Omohyoid
k. Latissimus Dorsi
l. Serratus Anterior
m. Pectoralis Major
n. Pectoralis Minor
o. Pronator Teres
p. Flexor Digitorum Superficialis (humeroulnar head)
q. Brachioradialis
r. Flexor Pollicis Longus (humeroulnar head)
s. Extensor Carpi Radialis Longus
t. Supinator

Proximal Attachment
Distal Attachment

POSTERIOR VIEW OF THE BONES AND BONY LANDMARKS OF THE RIGHT SCAPULA/ARM

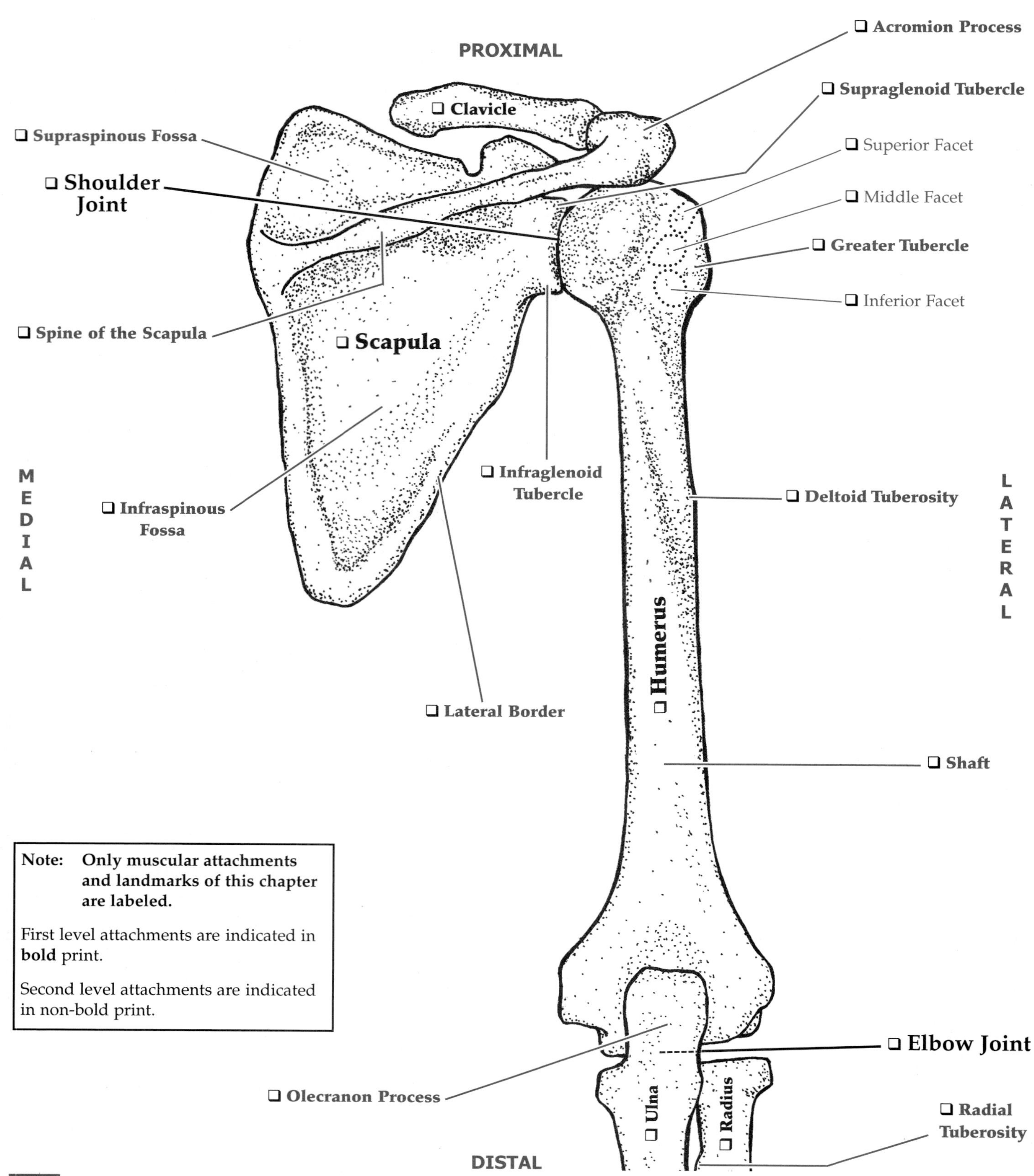

Note: **Only muscular attachments and landmarks of this chapter are labeled.**

First level attachments are indicated in **bold** print.

Second level attachments are indicated in non-bold print.

POSTERIOR VIEW OF THE BONY ATTACHMENTS OF THE RIGHT SCAPULA/ARM

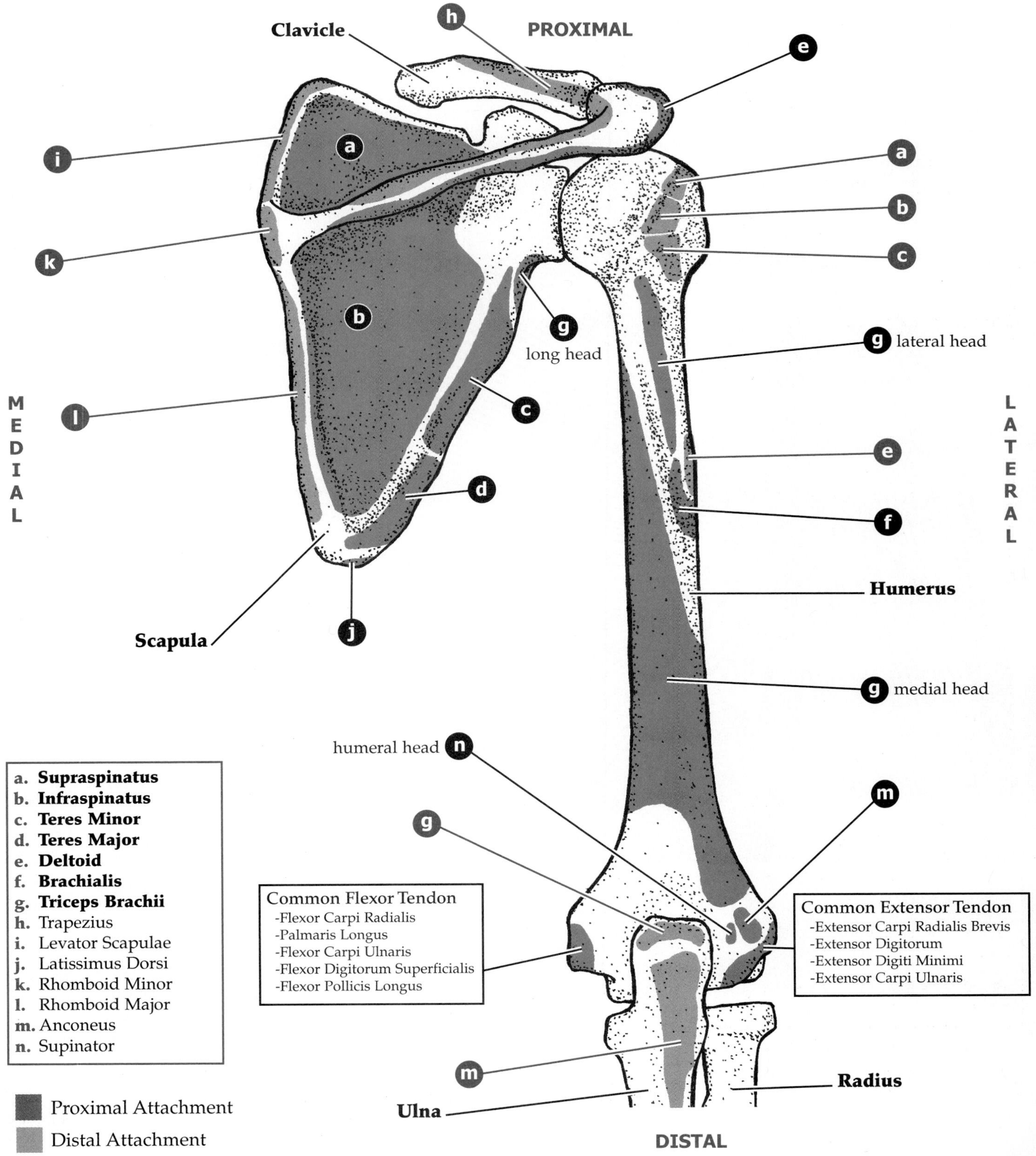

a. **Supraspinatus**
b. **Infraspinatus**
c. **Teres Minor**
d. **Teres Major**
e. **Deltoid**
f. **Brachialis**
g. **Triceps Brachii**
h. Trapezius
i. Levator Scapulae
j. Latissimus Dorsi
k. Rhomboid Minor
l. Rhomboid Major
m. Anconeus
n. Supinator

Proximal Attachment

Distal Attachment

ANTERIOR VIEW OF THE RIGHT SHOULDER

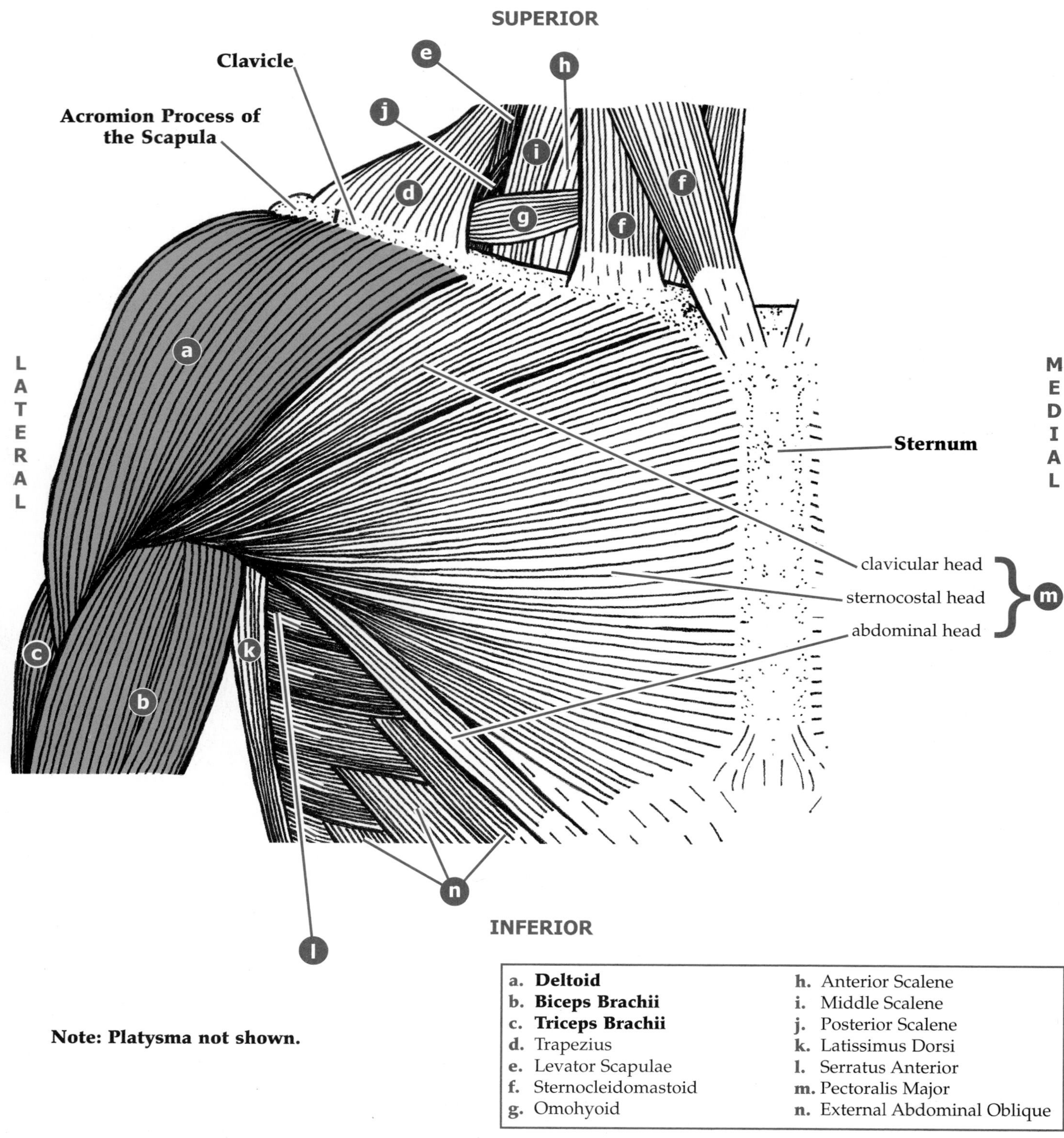

Note: Platysma not shown.

- **a. Deltoid**
- **b. Biceps Brachii**
- **c. Triceps Brachii**
- d. Trapezius
- e. Levator Scapulae
- f. Sternocleidomastoid
- g. Omohyoid
- h. Anterior Scalene
- i. Middle Scalene
- j. Posterior Scalene
- k. Latissimus Dorsi
- l. Serratus Anterior
- m. Pectoralis Major
- n. External Abdominal Oblique

POSTERIOR VIEW OF THE SHOULDERS (SUPERFICIAL AND INTERMEDIATE)

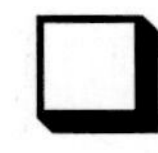

SUPERIOR

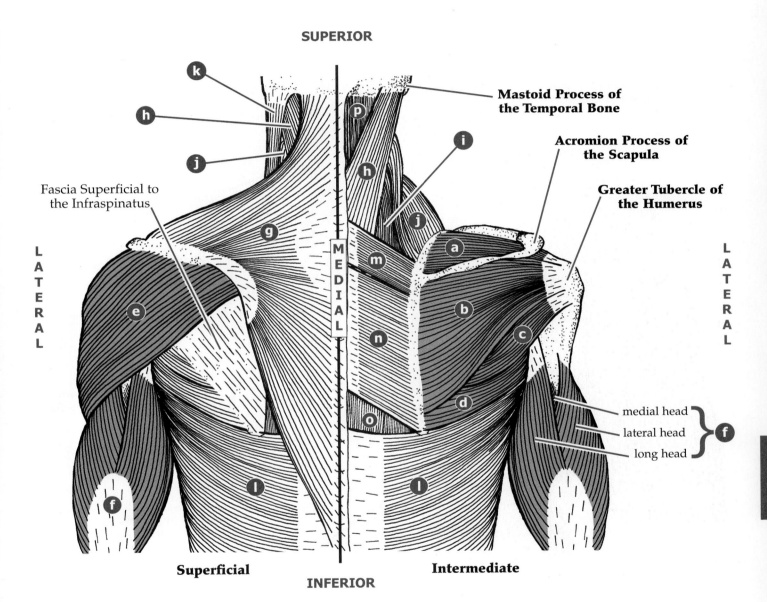

k
h
j
Fascia Superficial to the Infraspinatus
g
e
f
l
p
h
i
j
m
n
o
a
b
c
d
l
Mastoid Process of the Temporal Bone
Acromion Process of the Scapula
Greater Tubercle of the Humerus
LATERAL
MEDIAL
LATERAL
medial head
lateral head
long head
f

Superficial

INFERIOR

Intermediate

a. **Supraspinatus**
b. **Infraspinatus**
c. **Teres Minor**
d. **Teres Major**
e. **Deltoid**
f. **Triceps Brachii**
g. Trapezius
h. Splenius Capitis
i. Splenius Cervicis
j. Levator Scapulae
k. Sternocleidomastoid
l. Latissimus Dorsi
m. Rhomboid Minor
n. Rhomboid Major
o. Erector Spinae
p. Semispinalis Capitis (of Transversospinalis)

☐ ANTERIOR VIEWS OF THE RIGHT GLENOHUMERAL JOINT

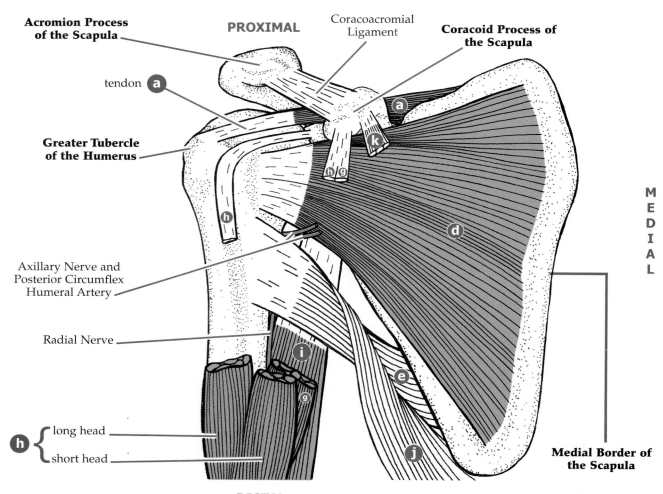

Acromion Process of the Scapula

PROXIMAL

Coracoacromial Ligament

Coracoid Process of the Scapula

tendon a

Greater Tubercle of the Humerus

LATERAL

MEDIAL

Axillary Nerve and Posterior Circumflex Humeral Artery

Radial Nerve

h { long head / short head

Medial Border of the Scapula

DISTAL

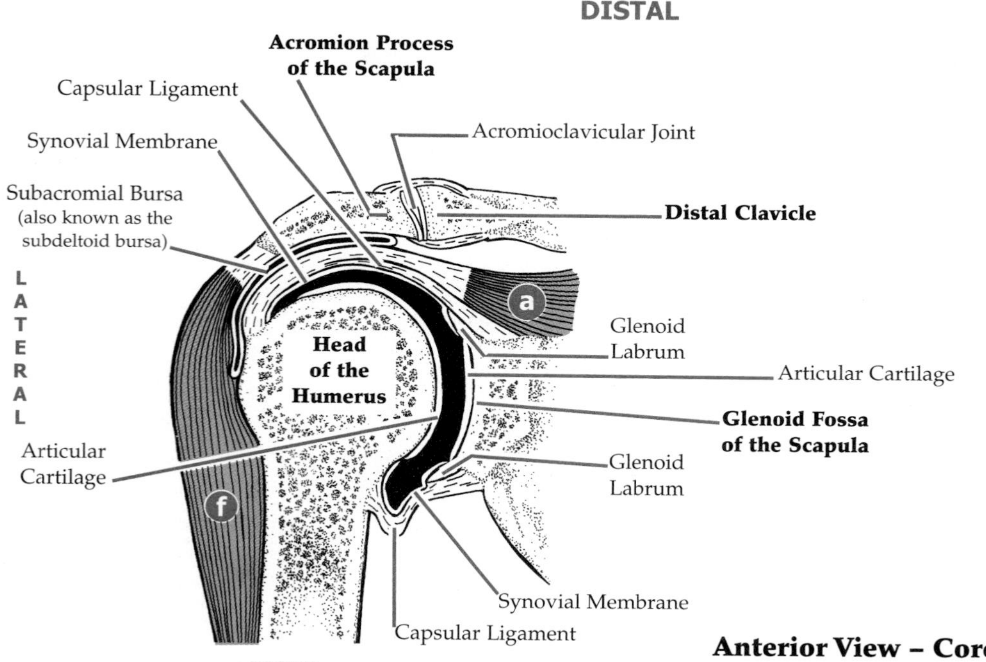

a. **Supraspinatus**
b. **Infraspinatus** (not seen)
c. **Teres Minor** (not seen)
d. **Subscapularis**
e. **Teres Major**
f. **Deltoid**
g. **Coracobrachialis** (cut)
h. **Biceps Brachii** (cut)
i. **Triceps Brachii**
j. Latissimus Dorsi
k. Pectoralis Minor (cut)

Anterior View – Coronal Section Through the Joint

POSTERIOR VIEW OF THE RIGHT GLENOHUMERAL JOINT

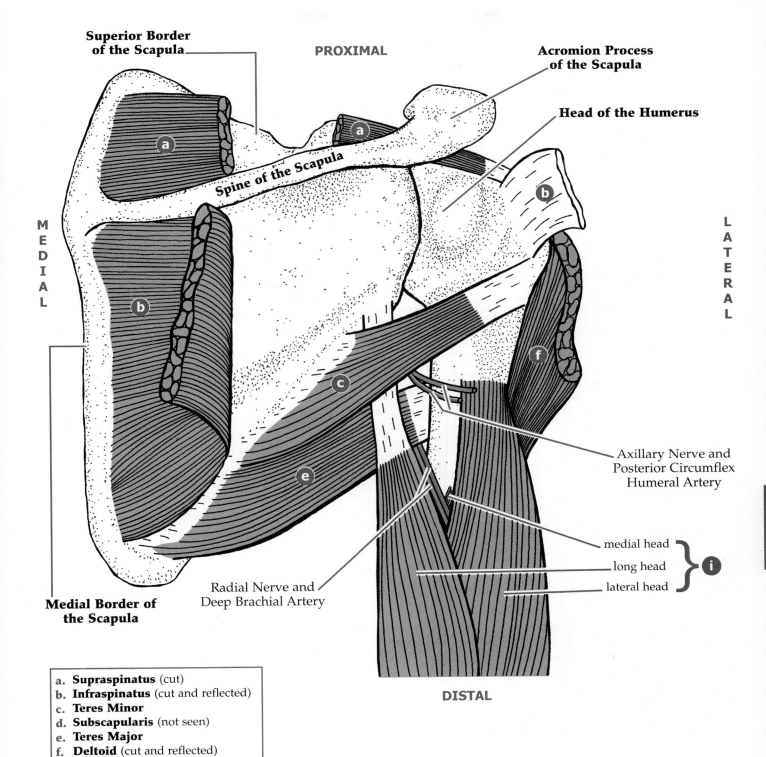

a. **Supraspinatus** (cut)
b. **Infraspinatus** (cut and reflected)
c. **Teres Minor**
d. **Subscapularis** (not seen)
e. **Teres Major**
f. **Deltoid** (cut and reflected)
g. **Coracobrachialis** (not seen)
h. **Biceps Brachii** (not seen)
i. **Triceps Brachii**
j. Latissimus Dorsi (not seen)
k. Pectoralis Minor (not seen)

☐ ANTERIOR VIEW OF THE RIGHT ARM (SUPERFICIAL)

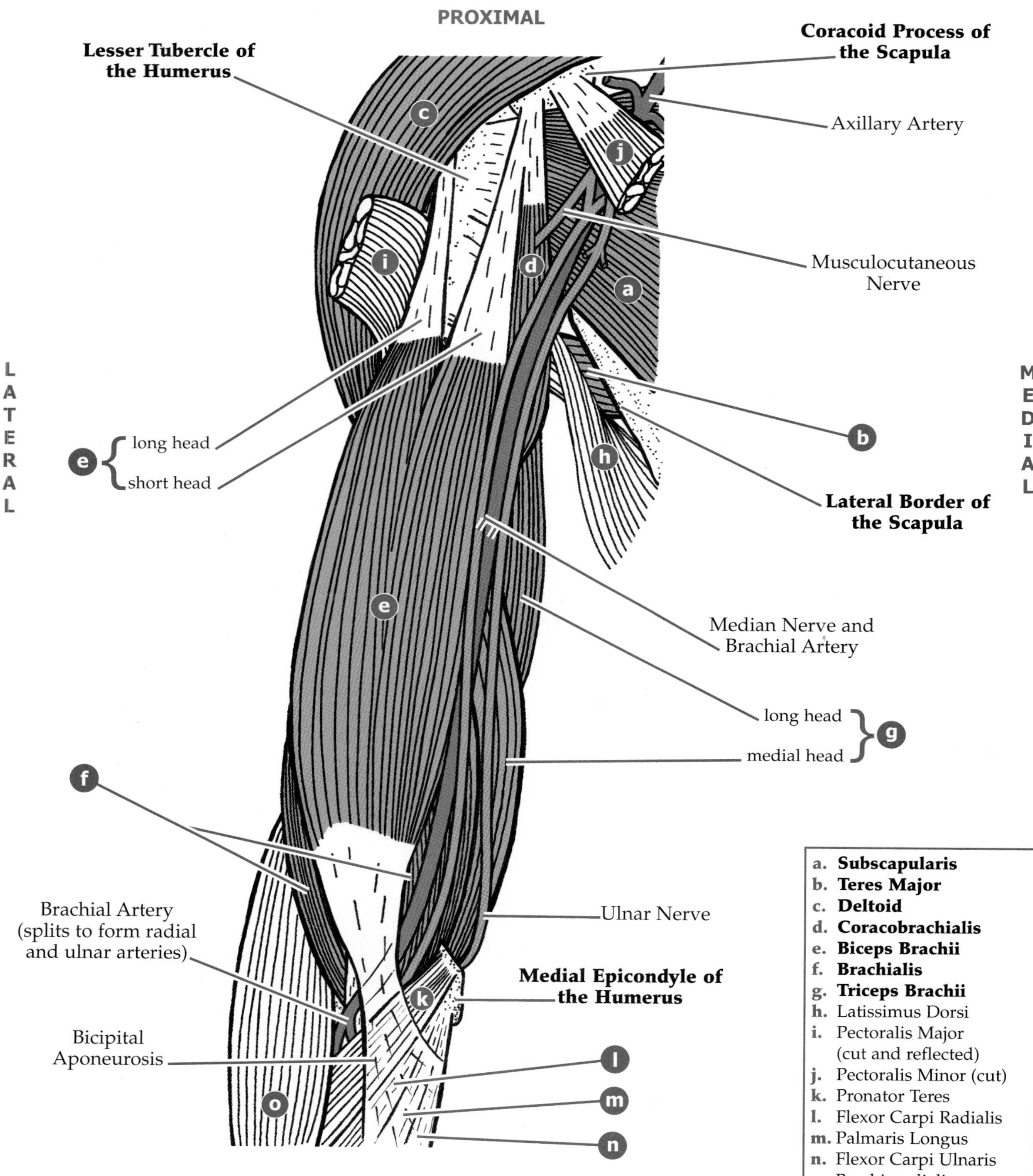

PROXIMAL
Lesser Tubercle of the Humerus
Coracoid Process of the Scapula
Axillary Artery
Musculocutaneous Nerve
LATERAL
MEDIAL
e long head
short head
b
Lateral Border of the Scapula
Median Nerve and Brachial Artery
long head
medial head
g
f
Brachial Artery (splits to form radial and ulnar arteries)
Ulnar Nerve
Medial Epicondyle of the Humerus
Bicipital Aponeurosis
l
m
n
DISTAL
a. Subscapularis
b. Teres Major
c. Deltoid
d. Coracobrachialis
e. Biceps Brachii
f. Brachialis
g. Triceps Brachii
h. Latissimus Dorsi
i. Pectoralis Major (cut and reflected)
j. Pectoralis Minor (cut)
k. Pronator Teres
l. Flexor Carpi Radialis
m. Palmaris Longus
n. Flexor Carpi Ulnaris
o. Brachioradialis

ANTERIOR VIEW OF THE RIGHT ARM (DEEP)

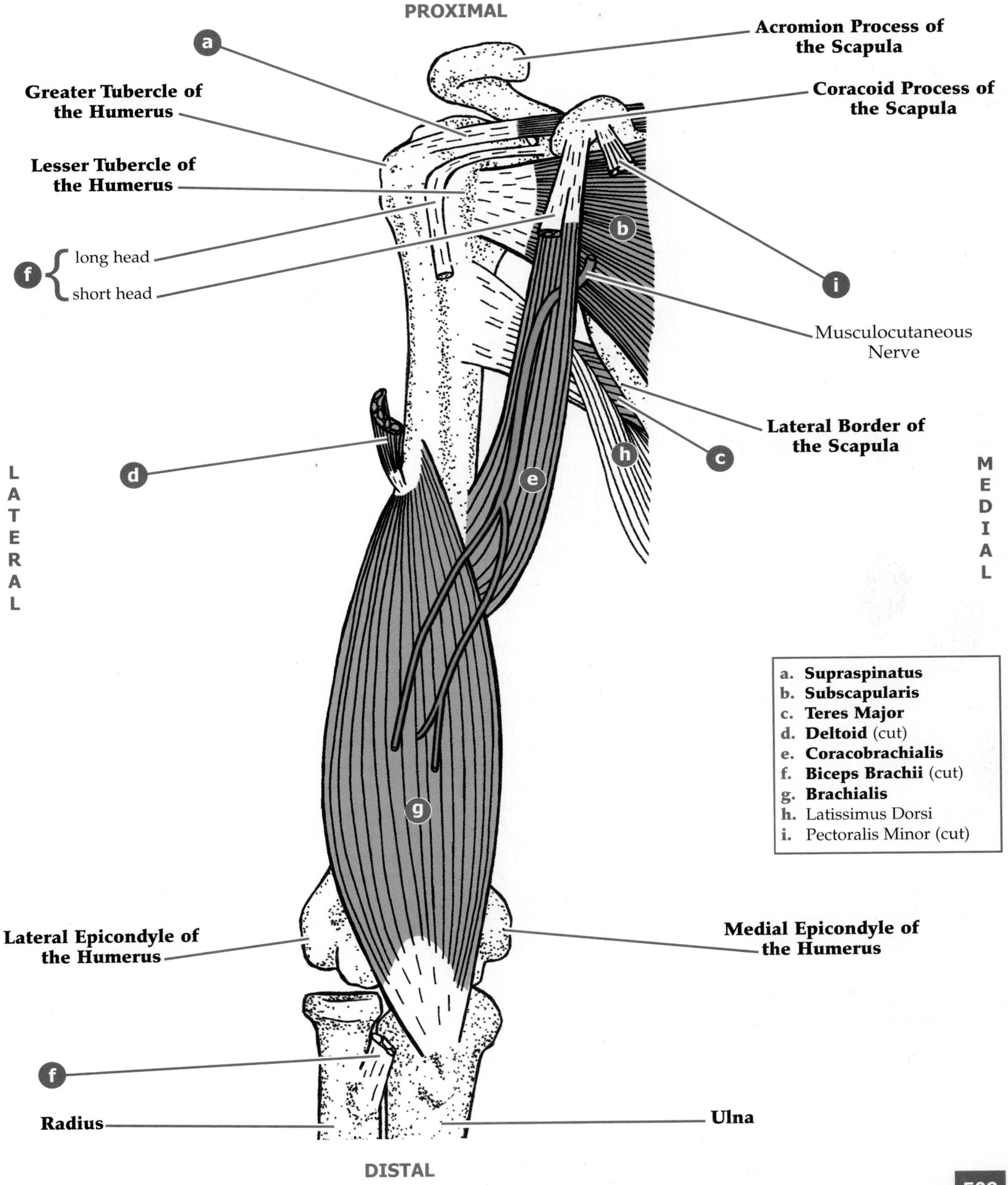

a. **Supraspinatus**
b. **Subscapularis**
c. **Teres Major**
d. **Deltoid** (cut)
e. **Coracobrachialis**
f. **Biceps Brachii** (cut)
g. **Brachialis**
h. Latissimus Dorsi
i. Pectoralis Minor (cut)

POSTERIOR VIEW OF THE RIGHT ARM

PROXIMAL

Acromion Process of the Scapula

Greater Tubercle of the Humerus

Axillary Nerve and Posterior Circumflex Humeral Artery

f lateral head

MEDIAL

LATERAL

Radial Nerve and Deep Brachial Artery

f { medial head
long head
medial head

Medial Epicondyle of the Humerus

Ulnar Nerve

Olecranon Process of the Ulna

Lateral Epicondyle of the Humerus

a. **Supraspinatus**
b. **Infraspinatus**
c. **Teres Minor**
d. **Teres Major**
e. **Deltoid** (cut and reflected)
f. **Triceps Brachii**
g. Brachioradialis
h. Extensor Carpi Radialis Longus
i. Extensor Carpi Radialis Brevis
j. Extensor Digitorum
k. Extensor Digiti Minimi
l. Extensor Carpi Ulnaris
m. Anconeus
n. Flexor Carpi Ulnaris

DISTAL

MEDIAL VIEW OF THE RIGHT ARM

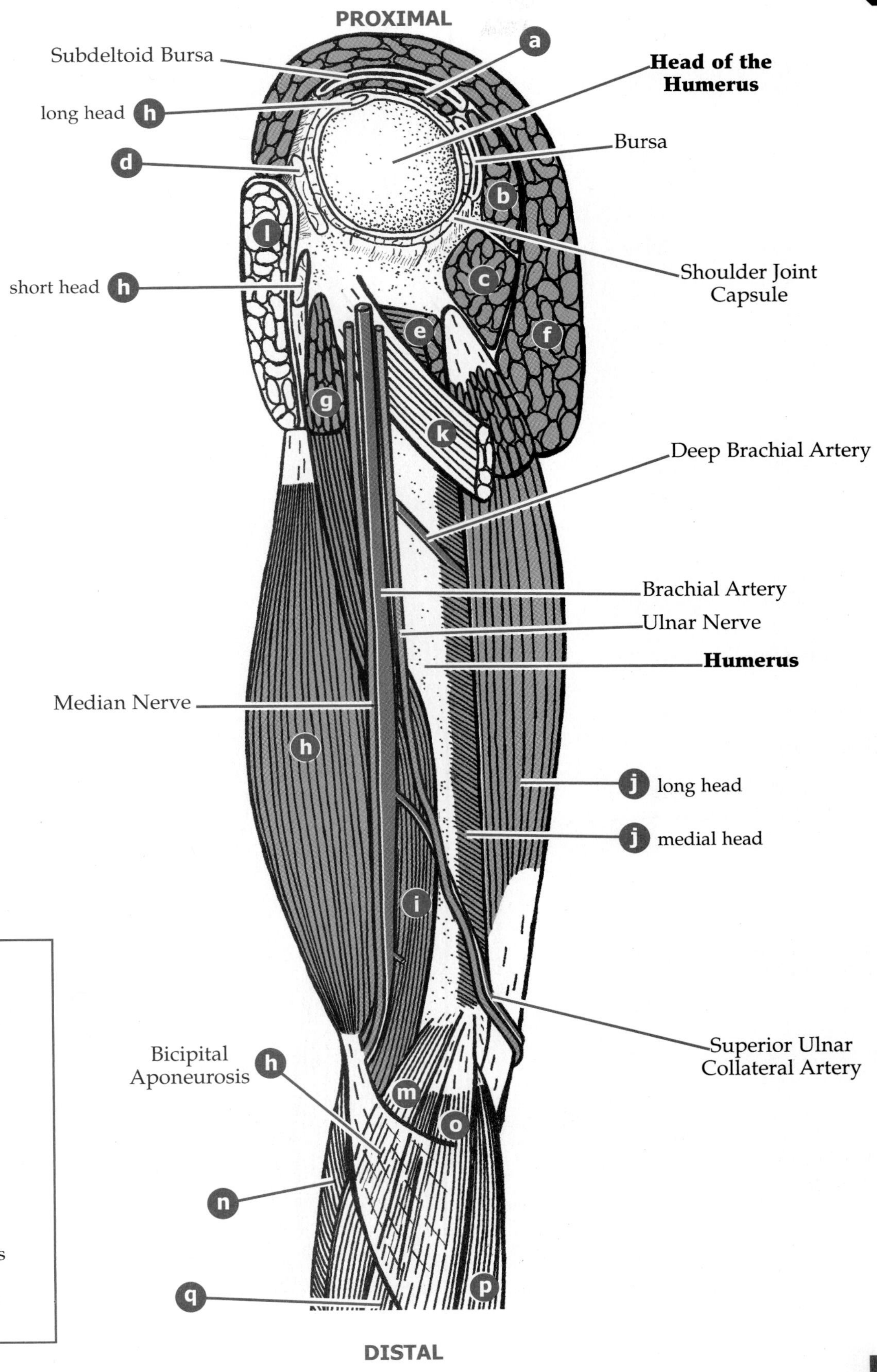

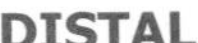

a. **Supraspinatus**
b. **Infraspinatus**
c. **Teres Minor**
d. **Subscapularis**
e. **Teres Major**
f. **Deltoid**
g. **Coracobrachialis**
h. **Biceps Brachii**
i. **Brachialis**
j. **Triceps Brachii**
k. Latissimus Dorsi
l. Pectoralis Major
m. Pronator Teres
n. Flexor Carpi Radialis
o. Palmaris Longus
p. Flexor Carpi Ulnaris
q. Brachioradialis

LATERAL VIEW OF THE RIGHT ARM

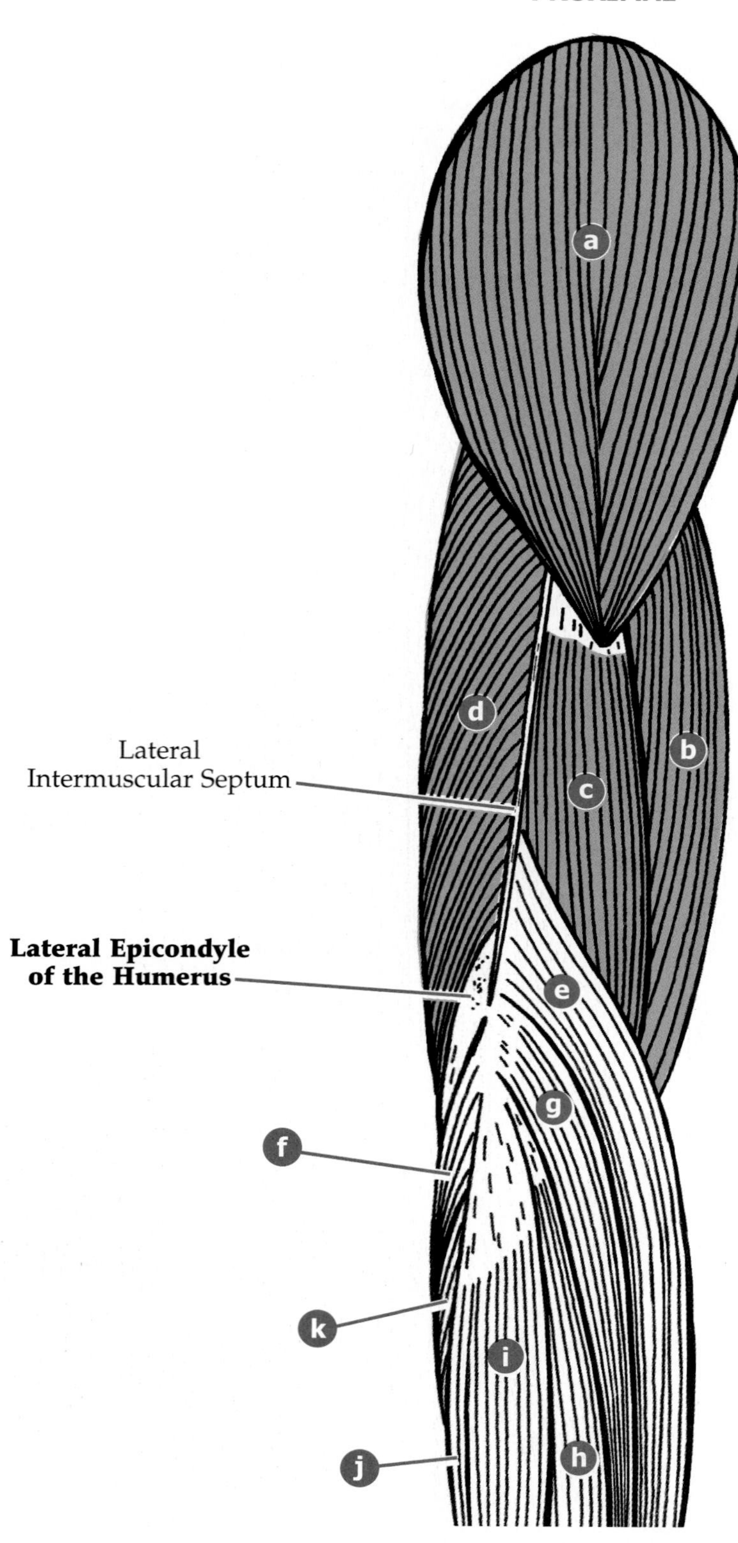

a. **Deltoid**
b. **Biceps Brachii**
c. **Brachialis**
d. **Triceps Brachii**
e. Brachioradialis
f. Anconeus
g. Extensor Carpi Radialis Longus
h. Extensor Carpi Radialis Brevis
i. Extensor Digitorum
j. Extensor Digiti Minimi
k. Extensor Carpi Ulnaris

CROSS SECTION VIEWS OF THE RIGHT ARM

Muscles
- a. **Teres Major**
- b. **Deltoid**
- c. **Coracobrachialis**
- d. **Biceps Brachii**
- e. **Brachialis**
- f. **Triceps Brachii**
- g. Pectoralis Major
- h. Latissimus Dorsi
- i. Brachioradialis
- j. Extensor Carpi Radialis Longus

Nerves
- N1. **Median**
- N2. **Musculocutaneous**
- N3. **Ulnar**
- N4. **Radial**
- N5. **Medial Brachial Cutaneous**
- N6. **Medial Antebrachial Cutaneous**
- N7. **Lateral Antebrachial Cutaneous**
- N8. **Posterior Antebrachial Cutaneous**

Arteries
- A1. **Brachial**
- A2. **Deep Brachial**
- A3. **Radial Collateral**
- A4. **Middle Collateral**
- A5. **Superior Ulnar Collateral**

Veins
- V1. **Cephalic**
- V2. **Basilic**
- V3. **Brachial**

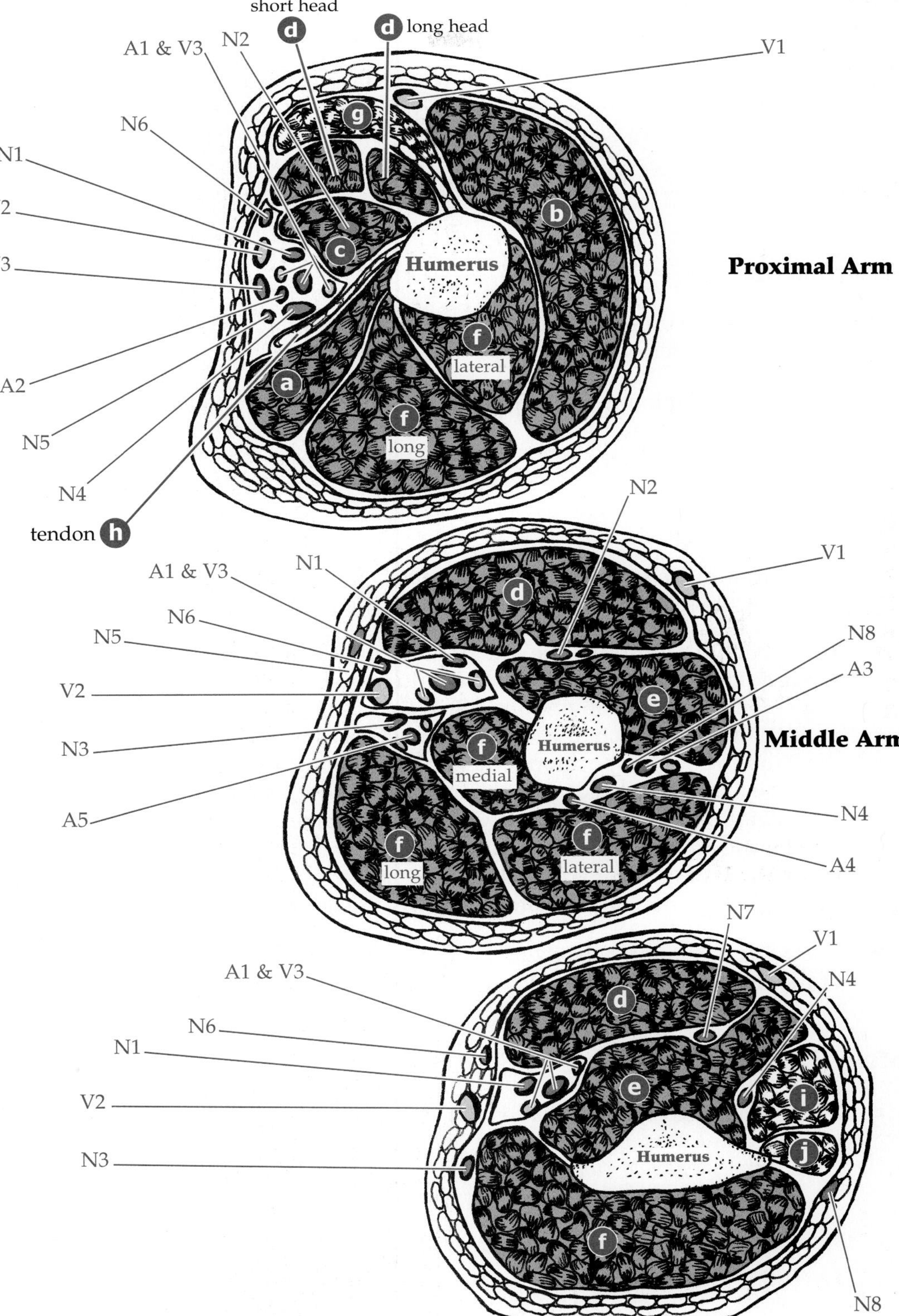

Perspective:
Right is lateral and left is medial.
Top is anterior and bottom is posterior.

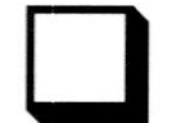

THE ROTATOR CUFF MUSCLES

The rotator cuff is a group of four muscles that attach from the scapula to the humerus.

THERE ARE FOUR ROTATOR CUFF MUSCLES:	
Supraspinatus Infraspinatus	Teres Minor Subscapularis

Attachments:

- These four muscles are grouped together as the rotator "cuff" group because their distal tendons all conjoin to form a cuff across the tubercles of the humerus.
  - The supraspinatus, infraspinatus and the teres minor all attach to the greater tubercle of the humerus.
  - The subscapularis attaches to the lesser tubercle of the humerus.

Actions:

- These four muscles are designated as the "rotator" cuff group because when they act as movers of the humerus, three of the four muscles rotate the humerus.
- Functionally, as a group, the rotator cuff muscles are extremely important because they act to fix (stabilize) the head of the humerus into the glenoid fossa of the scapula whenever the distal humerus is elevated from anatomical position. When the distal humerus is elevated (which can occur with flexion, extension, abduction and adduction of the arm), it is desirable to elevate only the distal end of the humerus to bring the hand to a higher position. When this occurs, the proximal end of the humerus (the head of the humerus) must be fixed (stabilized) down into the glenoid fossa of the scapula. This is accomplished principally by the rotator cuff group. Given that flexion, extension, abduction and adduction of the humerus may all involve elevation of the distal humerus, the rotator cuff muscles are actually more active as fixators (stabilizers) of the humerus than as movers. Of the four rotator cuff muscles, the two most active in this regard are the infraspinatus and the subscapularis.
- Their role as fixators (stabilizers) is especially important and necessary because the ligamentous structure of the shoulder joint is very lax and more stability must be provided by the muscles of the shoulder.

Miscellaneous:

- There is a bursa located between the supraspinatus portion of the rotator cuff tendon and the acromion process of the scapula and deltoid muscle superior to it. This bursa is known as the *subacromial bursa* and/or the *subdeltoid bursa*.

INNERVATION The rotator cuff muscles are innervated by the suprascapular, axillary and upper and lower subscapular nerves.

♥ **ARTERIAL SUPPLY** The rotator cuff muscles receive their arterial supply almost entirely from the suprascapular and circumflex scapular arteries.

VIEWS OF THE ROTATOR CUFF MUSCLES

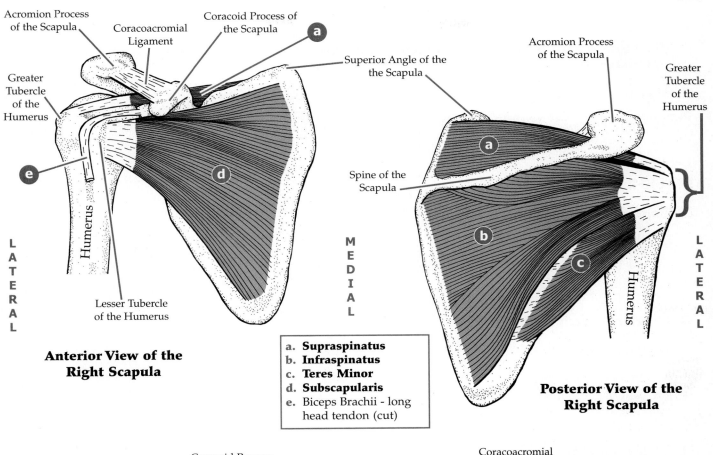

Acromion Process of the Scapula
Coracoacromial Ligament
Coracoid Process of the Scapula
a
Superior Angle of the the Scapula
Greater Tubercle of the Humerus
e
d
Humerus
LATERAL
Lesser Tubercle of the Humerus
MEDIAL

Anterior View of the Right Scapula

Acromion Process of the Scapula
Greater Tubercle of the Humerus
a
Spine of the Scapula
b
c
Humerus
LATERAL

Posterior View of the Right Scapula

a. **Supraspinatus**
b. **Infraspinatus**
c. **Teres Minor**
d. **Subscapularis**
e. Biceps Brachii - long head tendon (cut)

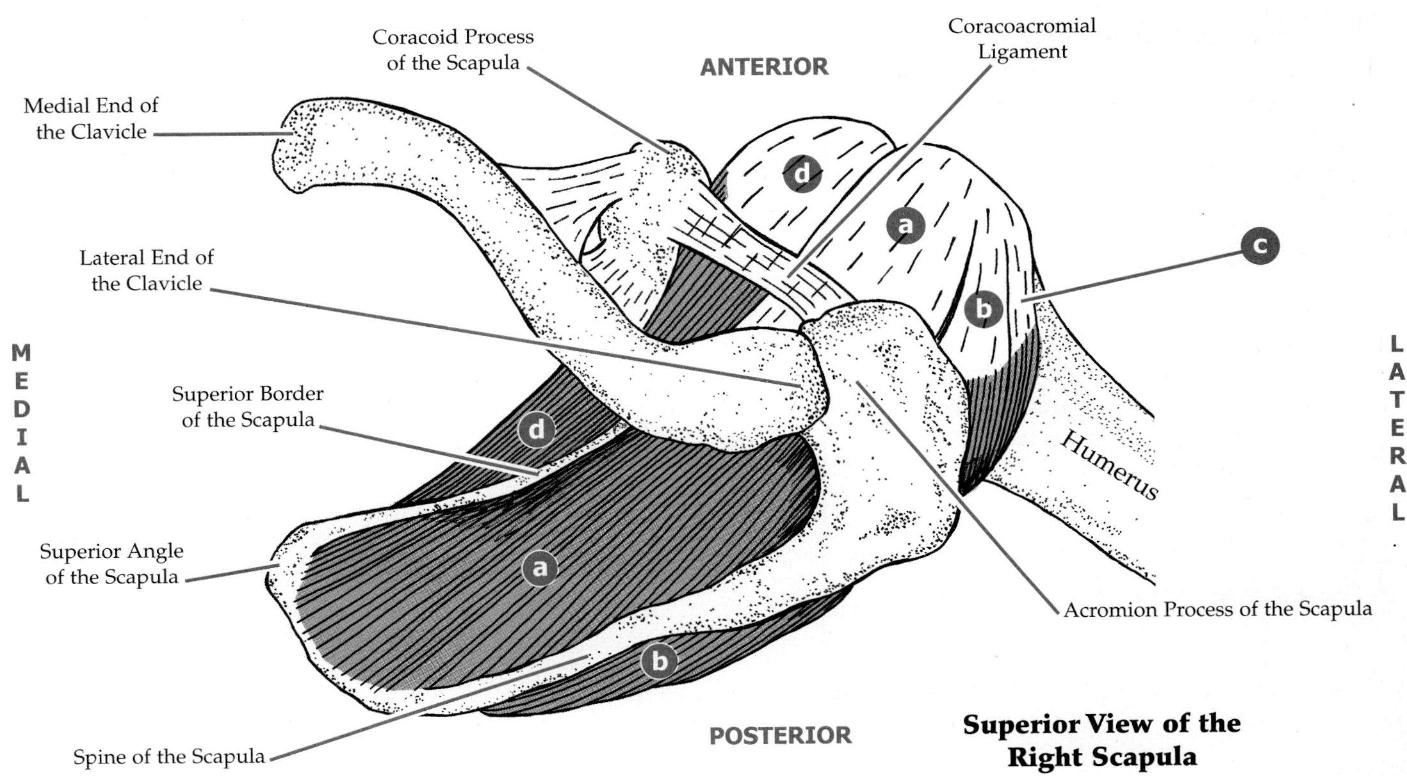

Superior View of the Right Scapula

❑

SUPRASPINATUS
(OF THE ROTATOR CUFF GROUP)

❑ **The name, supraspinatus, tells us that one of this muscle's attachments is the supraspinous fossa of the scapula.**

DERIVATION ❑ supraspinatus: L. *above the spine* (of the scapula).

PRONUNCIATION ❑ **soo**-pra-spy-**nay**-tus

ATTACHMENTS

❑ **Supraspinous Fossa of the Scapula**

- ❑ the medial 2/3

to the

❑ **Greater Tubercle of the Humerus**

- ❑ the superior facet

ACTION

❑ **Abduction of the Arm**

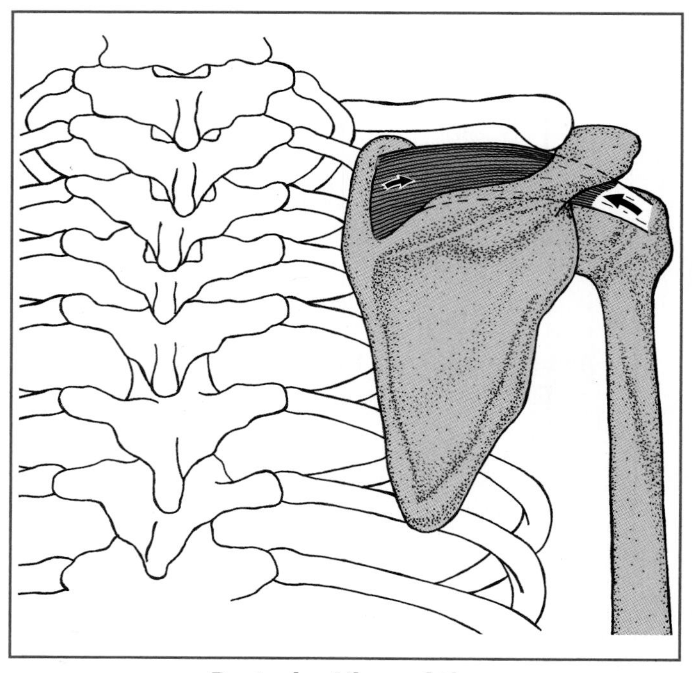

Posterior View of the Right Supraspinatus

INNERVATION ❑ The Suprascapular Nerve ❑ **C5**, 6

ARTERIAL SUPPLY ❑ The Suprascapular Artery (A Branch of the Thyrocervical Artery)

PALPATION AND SUPPLEMENTARY TEXT

PALPATION

The supraspinatus is deep to the trapezius and may be palpable superior to the spine of the scapula if the trapezius is relaxed.

❑ **Seated:**

- Have the client seated with the arm medially rotated at the shoulder joint and hanging at the side.
- Place palpating hand just superior to the spine of the scapula.
- Ask the client to perform a short, quick range of motion of active abduction of the arm at the shoulder joint and feel for the contraction of the supraspinatus. (The contraction is done in this manner to prevent the upper trapezius from contracting to perform upward rotation of the scapula, a coupled action of humeral abduction, which will block palpation of the underlying supraspinatus.)

❑ **To palpate the distal attachment of the supraspinatus, which is deep to the deltoid:**

- Have the client seated with the arm medially rotated at the shoulder joint and hanging at the side.
- Place palpating finger off the acromion process onto the greater tubercle of the humerus and feel for the tendon of the supraspinatus. (It can be difficult to distinguish the distal tendon of the supraspinatus from the more superficial deltoid.)
- To further bring out the tendon of the supraspinatus, have the client abduct the arm.

❑ **Prone:**

- Have the client prone with the arm hanging off the table. (This will put the scapula into a position of partial upward rotation so that abduction of the humerus will not require the trapezius to contract as much.)
- Place palpating hand just superior to the spine of the scapula.
- Ask the client to perform a short, quick range of motion of active abduction of the arm at the shoulder joint and feel for the contraction of the supraspinatus. (Note: Abduction of the arm in this position will involve moving the hand parallel to the table up toward the head.)

Note: During the above palpations, it may be desirable to have the client actively move the arm halfway between abduction and flexion at the shoulder joint (instead of pure abduction) because the recruitment of the trapezius will be less during flexion efforts and there will still be plenty of supraspinatus contraction to palpate. Further, adding in medial rotation of the arm at the shoulder joint will cause scapular protraction (at the scapulocostal joint), which will further decrease the recruitment of the trapezius.

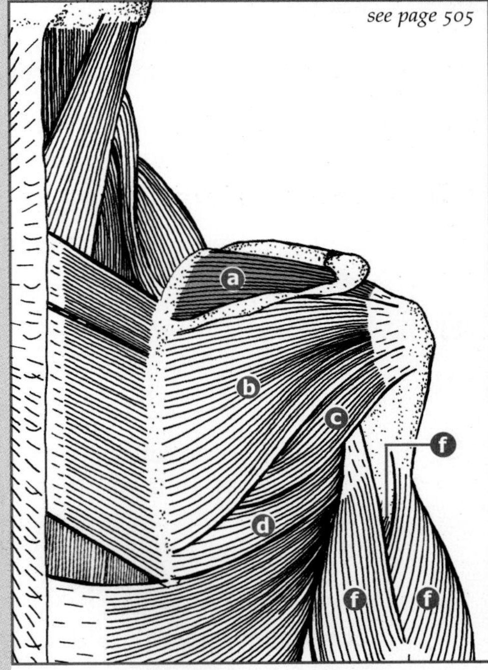

see page 505

Posterior View of the Right Shoulder (Intermediate)

a. Supraspinatus
b. Infraspinatus
c. Teres Minor
d. Teres Major
e. Deltoid (not seen)
f. Triceps Brachii

SUPRASPINATUS – continued

RELATIONSHIP TO OTHER MUSCULOSKELETAL STRUCTURES

- ❑ 1. The supraspinatus is superior to the spine of the scapula.
- ❑ 2. The proximal attachment of the supraspinatus is deep to the trapezius.
- ❑ 3. The distal tendon of the supraspinatus courses deep to the acromion process of the scapula to then attach distally onto the greater tubercle of the humerus.
- ❑ 4. The distal attachment of the supraspinatus is deep to the deltoid.

METHODOLOGY FOR LEARNING MUSCLE ACTIONS

- ❑ **Abduction of the Arm at the Shoulder Joint:** The supraspinatus crosses the shoulder joint over the top of the joint (with its fibers running first horizontally and then vertically in the frontal plane); therefore, it abducts the arm at the shoulder joint. (Note the similarity of the direction of fibers of the supraspinatus to the direction of fibers of the middle deltoid.)

MISCELLANEOUS

- ❑ 1. The supraspinatus is one of the four rotator cuff muscles. The rotator cuff muscles are the supraspinatus, infraspinatus, teres minor and the subscapularis. Sometimes the rotator cuff muscles are called the "SITS" muscles; each of the four letters stands for the first letter of the four rotator cuff muscles. **S**upraspinatus is the first "**S**" of "**S**ITS."
- ❑ 2. The supraspinatus is one of three muscles that attach onto the greater tubercle of the humerus. The two other muscles that attach here are the infraspinatus and the teres minor.
- ❑ 3. The distal tendon of the supraspinatus adheres to the capsule of the shoulder joint (glenohumeral joint), which is deep to the supraspinatus (see coronal section of the glenohumeral joint illustration on page 506).
- ❑ 4. The acromion process and the deltoid are superior to the supraspinatus. There is a bursa called the *subacromial* and/or *subdeltoid bursa* that is located between the supraspinatus and these two other structures.
- ❑ 5. For quite some time, it was believed that the supraspinatus could only initiate abduction of the arm at the shoulder joint and that the deltoid would have to complete this motion. However, recent research has shown that the supraspinatus is capable of moving the arm through the entire range of motion of abduction at the shoulder joint. Of course, the supraspinatus does not have the strength of the deltoid.
- ❑ 6. Some sources state that the supraspinatus can also contribute to both flexion and horizontal extension of the arm at the shoulder joint.
- ❑ 7. The supraspinatus is the only one of the four rotator cuff muscles that does not contribute to rotation of the arm at the shoulder joint.
- ❑ 8. A main function of the supraspinatus is to act as a fixator (stabilizer) of the shoulder joint.
- ❑ 9. The supraspinatus' distal tendon is the most commonly injured tendon of the rotator cuff musculature. In fact, the distal tendon of the supraspinatus is sometimes referred to as the "critical zone" of the rotator cuff tendon.

INFRASPINATUS
(OF THE ROTATOR CUFF GROUP)

❑ **The name, infraspinatus, tells us that one of this muscle's attachments is the infraspinous fossa of the scapula.**

DERIVATION ❑ infraspinatus: L. *below the spine* (of the scapula).

PRONUNCIATION ❑ **in**-fra-spy-**nay**-tus

ATTACHMENTS

❑ **Infraspinous Fossa of the Scapula**

❑ the medial 2/3

to the

❑ **Greater Tubercle of the Humerus**

❑ the middle facet

ACTION

❑ **Lateral Rotation of the Arm**

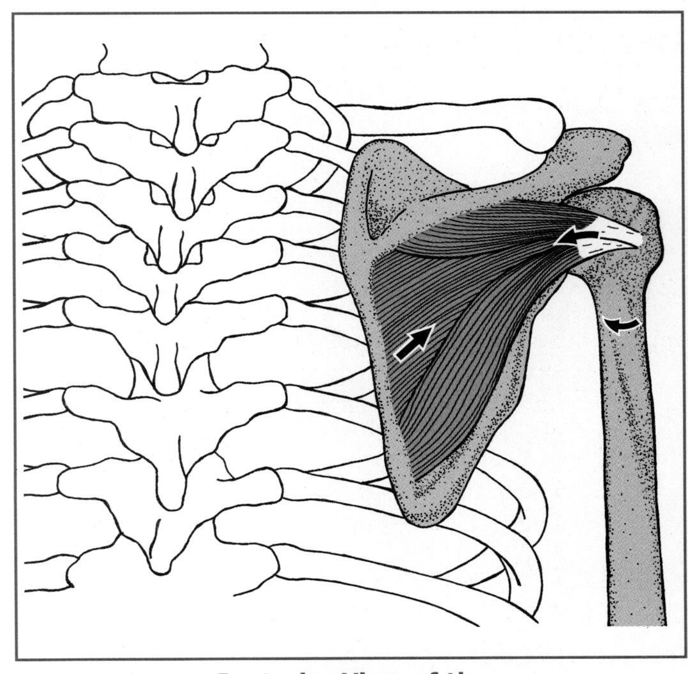

Posterior View of the Right Infraspinatus

INNERVATION ❑ The Suprascapular Nerve ❑ **C5**, 6

ARTERIAL SUPPLY ❑ The Suprascapular Artery (A Branch of the Thyrocervical Artery)
❑ and the circumflex scapular artery (a branch of the subscapular artery)

INFRASPINATUS – PALPATION AND SUPPLEMENTARY TEXT

PALPATION

Much of the muscle belly and distal tendon of the infraspinatus are superficial and palpable inferior to the posterior deltoid.

❑ **To palpate the muscle belly:**

- Have the client prone with the arm hanging off the table.
- Place palpating hand on the infraspinous fossa. (Make sure you are just inferior to the deltoid.)
- Ask the client to actively laterally rotate the arm at the shoulder joint through a small range of motion and feel for the contraction of the infraspinatus. (Given that the infraspinatus and teres minor have the same fiber direction and therefore the same actions, they will contract together. Differentiating them can be difficult; the teres minor will be more inferior and somewhat lateral.)

❑ **To palpate the distal tendon:**

- Have the client prone with the arm hanging off the table.
- Support the client's arm in passive flexion (to relax the deltoid).
- Place palpating finger on the greater tubercle of the humerus and proceed somewhat inferiorly along the posterior margin of the humerus.
- Ask the client to actively laterally rotate the arm at the shoulder joint and feel for the tensing of the tendon of the infraspinatus.

see page 505

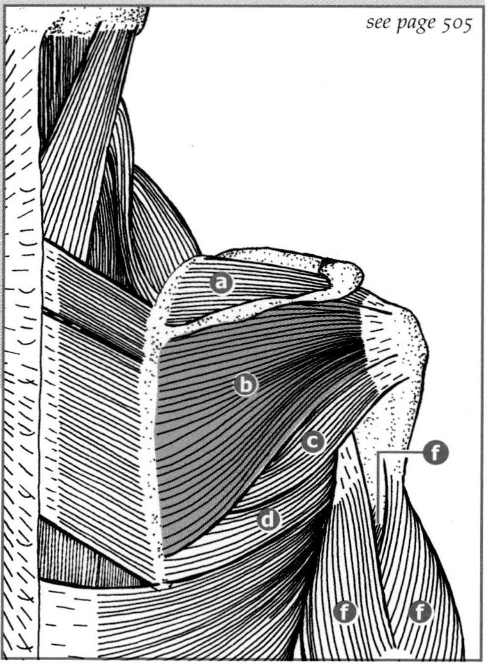

Posterior View of the Right Shoulder (Intermediate)

a. Supraspinatus
b. **Infraspinatus**
c. Teres Minor
d. Teres Major
e. Deltoid (not seen)
f. Triceps Brachii

RELATIONSHIP TO OTHER MUSCULOSKELETAL STRUCTURES

❑ 1. The infraspinatus is inferior to the spine of the scapula.

❑ 2. Inferior to the infraspinatus are the teres minor and teres major.

❑ 3. Most of the infraspinatus is superficial in the infraspinous fossa.

❑ 4. Medially, a small portion of the infraspinatus lies deep to the trapezius. Distally, the infraspinatus is deep to the deltoid.

METHODOLOGY FOR LEARNING MUSCLE ACTIONS

❑ **Lateral Rotation of the Arm at the Shoulder Joint:** The infraspinatus crosses the shoulder joint posteriorly from medial to lateral (with its fibers running horizontally in the transverse plane). However, it does not attach onto the first aspect of the humerus that it reaches, but rather wraps around the humerus to attach onto the greater tubercle. Therefore, when the infraspinatus contracts and the humeral attachment is pulled toward the scapular attachment, the posterior side of the humerus moves medially. This movement is called lateral rotation of the arm at the shoulder joint because the anterior side of the humerus rotates laterally. (Note the similarity of the direction of fibers of the infraspinatus to the direction of fibers of the teres minor.)

INFRASPINATUS – continued

MISCELLANEOUS

- ❑ 1. The infraspinatus is one of the four rotator cuff muscles. The rotator cuff muscles are the supraspinatus, infraspinatus, teres minor and the subscapularis. Sometimes the rotator cuff muscles are called the "SITS" muscles; each of the four letters stands for the first letter of the four rotator cuff muscles. **I**nfraspinatus is the "**I**" of "S**I**TS."
- ❑ 2. The infraspinatus is one of three muscles that attach onto the greater tubercle of the humerus. The two other muscles that attach here are the supraspinatus and the teres minor.
- ❑ 3. The distal tendon of the infraspinatus adheres to the capsule of the shoulder joint (glenohumeral joint), which is deep to the infraspinatus.
- ❑ 4. Sometimes there is a bursa located between the infraspinatus and the glenohumeral joint capsule.
- ❑ 5. There is usually a thick layer of fascia overlying the infraspinatus muscle (see the posterior view of the shoulder illustration on page 505).
- ❑ 6. Sometimes the infraspinatus blends with the teres minor.
- ❑ 7. The infraspinatus can also horizontally extend the arm at the shoulder joint.
- ❑ 8. There is controversy regarding whether the infraspinatus can abduct or adduct the arm at the shoulder joint. Some sources state that the upper fibers can abduct the arm and the lower fibers can adduct the arm. Other sources state that whether one or the other occurs is due to the position of the glenohumeral joint at the time. In either case, due to the poor lever arm, the infraspinatus has little strength as an abductor or adductor of the arm at the shoulder joint.
- ❑ 9. The infraspinatus is a very active muscle because so many arm movements also involve lateral rotation of the arm at the shoulder joint.
- ❑ 10. A main function of the infraspinatus is to act as a fixator (stabilizer) of the shoulder joint.

TERES MINOR
(OF THE ROTATOR CUFF GROUP)

❑ **The name, teres minor, tells us that this muscle is round and small (smaller than the teres major).**

DERIVATION ❑ teres: L. *round.*
minor: L. *small.*

PRONUNCIATION ❑ **te**-reez **my**-nor

ATTACHMENTS

❑ **Superior Lateral Border of the Scapula**

- ❑ the superior 2/3 of the dorsal surface

to the

❑ **Greater Tubercle of the Humerus**

- ❑ the inferior facet

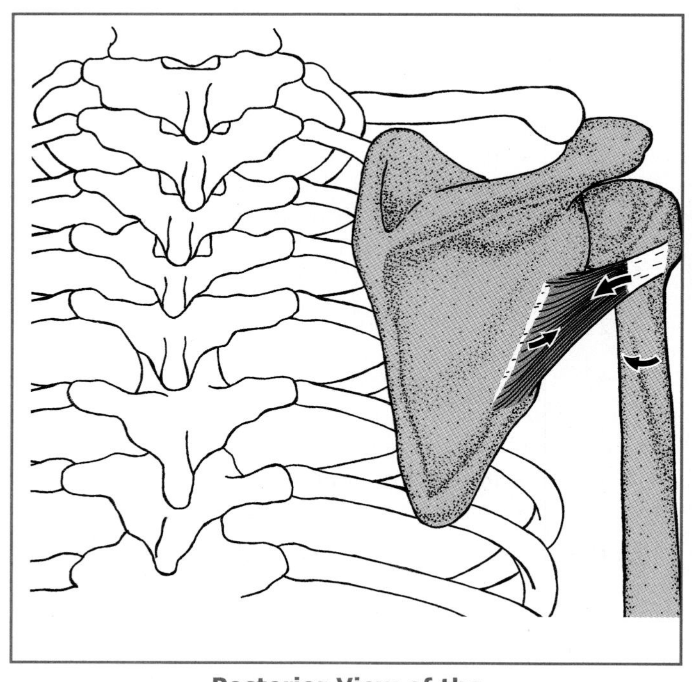

Posterior View of the Right Teres Minor

ACTION

❑ **1. Lateral Rotation of the Arm**

❑ **2.** Adduction of the Arm

INNERVATION ❑ The Axillary Nerve ❑ **C5**, 6

ARTERIAL SUPPLY ❑ The Circumflex Scapular Artery (A Branch of the Subscapular Artery)
❑ and the posterior circumflex humeral artery (a branch of the axillary artery)

PALPATION AND SUPPLEMENTARY TEXT

PALPATION

The teres minor is a small muscle that is largely superficial and located between the infraspinatus and teres major.

❑ **To palpate the muscle belly:**

- Have the client prone with the arm hanging off the table.
- Place palpating hand just lateral to the lateral border of the scapula and feel for the round belly of the teres minor.
- To bring out the teres minor, ask the client to actively laterally rotate the arm at the shoulder joint. (Given that the infraspinatus and teres minor have the same fiber direction and therefore the same actions, they will contract together. Differentiating them can be difficult; the teres minor will be more inferior and somewhat lateral.)
- To differentiate the teres minor from the teres major, which is inferior to it, place palpating hand on the lateral border of the scapula. Have the client alternately perform lateral and then medial rotation of the arm at the shoulder joint. The teres minor will be felt to contract with lateral rotation of the arm; the teres major will be felt to contract with medial rotation of the arm.

❑ **To palpate the distal attachment:**

- Have the client prone with the arm hanging off the table.
- Support the client's arm in passive flexion (to relax the deltoid).
- Place palpating finger on the greater tubercle of the humerus and proceed to the most posterior and inferior aspect of the greater tubercle.
- Ask the client to actively laterally rotate the arm at the shoulder joint and feel for the tensing of the tendon of the teres minor.

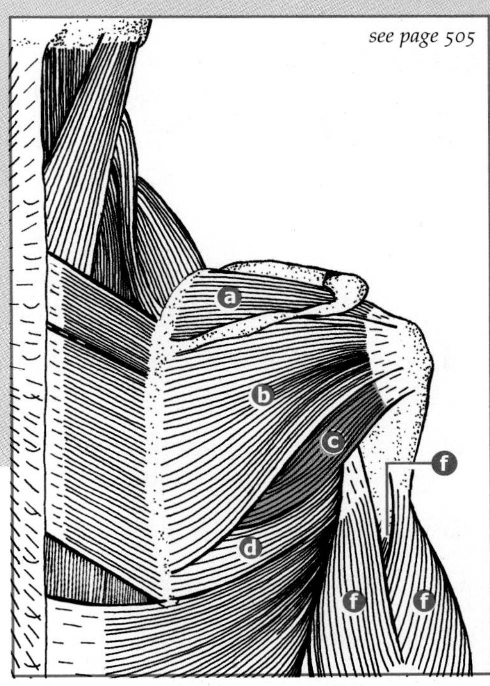

see page 505

Posterior View of the Right Shoulder (Intermediate)

a. Supraspinatus
b. Infraspinatus
c. **Teres Minor**
d. Teres Major
e. Deltoid (not seen)
f. Triceps Brachii

RELATIONSHIP TO OTHER MUSCULOSKELETAL STRUCTURES

❑ 1. The medial portion of the teres minor is superficial and is located at the lateral border of the scapula. The lateral portion of the teres minor is deep to the deltoid.

❑ 2. On the scapula, the teres minor attaches just superior to the attachment of the teres major.

❑ 3. The teres minor lies between the infraspinatus (which is superior to it) and the teres major (which is inferior to it).

TERES MINOR – CONTINUED

METHODOLOGY FOR LEARNING MUSCLE ACTIONS

- ❑ **1. Lateral Rotation of the Arm at the Shoulder Joint:** The teres minor crosses the shoulder joint posteriorly from medial to lateral (with its fibers running horizontally in the transverse plane). However, it does not attach onto the first aspect of the humerus that it reaches, but rather wraps around the humerus to attach onto the greater tubercle. Therefore, when the teres minor contracts and the humeral attachment is pulled toward the scapular attachment, the posterior side of the humerus moves medially. This movement is called lateral rotation of the arm at the shoulder joint because the anterior side of the humerus rotates laterally. (Note the similarity of the direction of fibers of the teres minor to the direction of fibers of the infraspinatus.)
- ❑ **2. Adduction of the Arm at the Shoulder Joint:** The teres minor crosses the shoulder joint posteriorly, from medial on the scapula to lateral on the humerus (with fibers running horizontally in the frontal plane). Therefore, when the lateral attachment, the humerus, is pulled toward the medial attachment, the scapula, the humerus is pulled toward the midline. Therefore, the teres minor adducts the arm at the shoulder joint.

MISCELLANEOUS

- ❑ 1. The teres minor is one of the four rotator cuff muscles. The rotator cuff muscles are the supraspinatus, infraspinatus, teres minor and the subscapularis. Sometimes the rotator cuff muscles are called the "SITS" muscles; each of the four letters stands for the first letter of the four rotator cuff muscles. **T**eres minor is the "**T**" of "SI**T**S."
- ❑ 2. The teres minor is one of three muscles that attach onto the greater tubercle of the humerus. The other two muscles that attach here are the supraspinatus and the infraspinatus.
- ❑ 3 Although the teres minor and the teres major share the word "teres" in their name (because they are both round in shape) and sit next to each other, they wrap around the humerus in opposite directions and therefore, have opposite rotary actions. The teres minor wraps around to the posterior side of the shoulder joint to attach onto the humerus and therefore laterally rotates the arm at the shoulder joint; the teres major wraps around to the anterior side of the shoulder joint to attach onto the humerus and therefore medially rotates the arm at the shoulder joint.
- ❑ 4. The teres major and the teres minor, due to their different rotary actions of the arm, are in different functional groups. These two muscles are also innervated by different nerves.
- ❑ 5. The distal tendon of the teres minor adheres to the capsule of the shoulder joint (glenohumeral joint), which is deep to the teres minor.
- ❑ 6. Sometimes the teres minor blends with the infraspinatus.
- ❑ 7. The teres minor can also horizontally extend the arm at the shoulder joint.
- ❑ 8. The teres minor is a very active muscle because so many arm movements also involve lateral rotation of the arm at the shoulder joint.
- ❑ 9. There is some controversy regarding whether or not the teres minor can adduct the arm at the shoulder joint. However, the humeral attachment seems clearly distal enough in order for it to perform adduction.
- ❑ 10. As part of the rotator cuff group, the teres minor has classically been considered to have an important role as a fixator (stabilizer) of the shoulder joint during most motions. However, recent evidence seems to indicate that this is not true. Most likely this is because the teres minor has an adduction action which would oppose any abduction movement, and its posterior location would oppose flexion movements as well.

SUBSCAPULARIS

(OF THE ROTATOR CUFF GROUP)

❑ **The name, subscapularis, tells us that one of this muscle's attachments is the subscapular fossa of the scapula.**

DERIVATION ❑ subscapularis: L. *refers to the subscapular fossa.*

PRONUNCIATION ❑ sub-skap-u-**la**-ris

ATTACHMENTS

❑ **Subscapular Fossa of the Scapula**

to the

❑ **Lesser Tubercle of the Humerus**

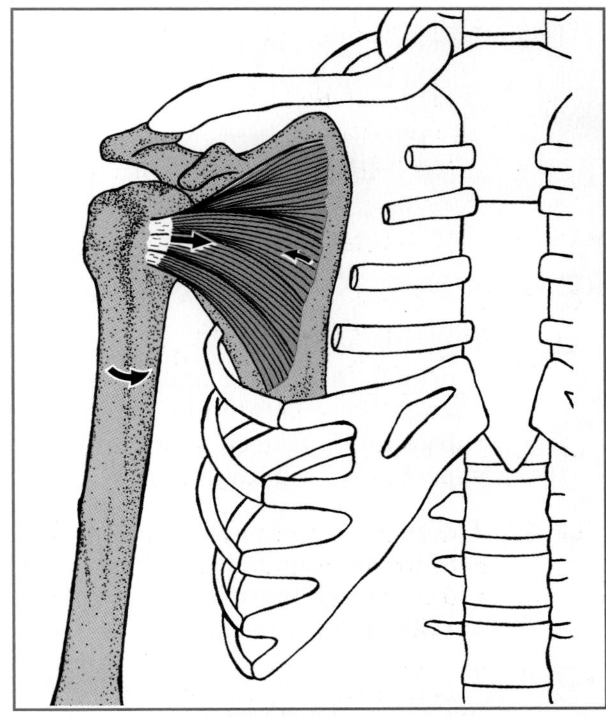

Anterior View of the Right Subscapularis (superior ribs cut and removed)

ACTION

❑ **Medial Rotation of the Arm**

INNERVATION ❑ The Upper and Lower Subscapular Nerves ❑ C5, **6**

ARTERIAL SUPPLY ❑ The Circumflex Scapular Artery (A Branch of the Subscapular Artery) and the Dorsal Scapular and Suprascapular Arteries (Both Either Direct or Indirect Branches of the Subclavian Artery)
❑ and the lateral thoracic artery (a branch of the axillary artery)

SUBSCAPULARIS – PALPATION AND SUPPLEMENTARY TEXT

PALPATION

Given its location, the subscapularis is difficult to palpate. There are two methods (standing or sidelying) in which to attempt to palpate this muscle.

- ❑ **Standing:** Have the client standing with the trunk flexed (and/or with the pelvis anteriorly tilted at the hip joints to incline the trunk forward). This causes the scapula to be passively protracted due to the weight of the arm.
- ❑ **Sidelying:** Have the client sidelying with the client's arm supported in a position of flexion. This will cause the scapula to protract and allow for better access to the subscapularis.
  - From either position, place palpating fingers anterior to the latissimus dorsi (the posterior axillary fold of tissue) toward the anterior surface of the scapula.
  - Ask the client to actively medially rotate the arm at the shoulder joint and feel for the contraction of the belly of the subscapularis.

RELATIONSHIP TO OTHER MUSCULOSKELETAL STRUCTURES

❑ 1. From the posterior perspective, the subscapularis is deep to the scapula and superficial to the ribcage. From the anterior perspective, the subscapularis is deep to the entire ribcage and superficial to the scapula.

❑ 2. The anterior wall of the subscapularis faces the serratus anterior. Both the subscapularis and the serratus anterior are located between the scapula and the ribcage.

❑ 3. The distal tendon of the subscapularis is deep to the proximal tendons of the short head of the biceps brachii and the coracobrachialis.

❑ 4. The distal tendon of the subscapularis attaches onto the lesser tubercle of the humerus. Therefore, it lies between the humeral attachments of the supraspinatus and the latissimus dorsi.

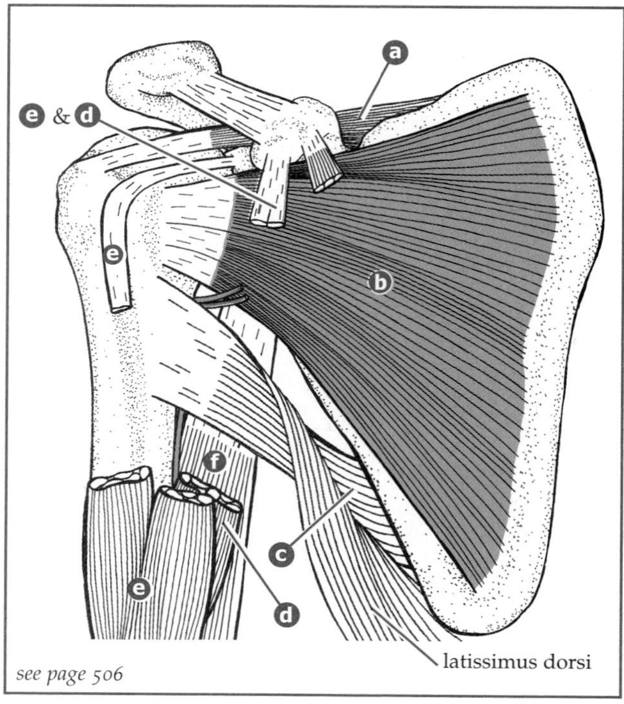

see page 506

Anterior View of the Right Glenohumeral Joint

a. Supraspinatus
b. **Subscapularis**
c. Teres Major
d. Coracobrachialis (cut)
e. Biceps Brachii (cut)
f. Triceps Brachii

SUBSCAPULARIS – CONTINUED

METHODOLOGY FOR LEARNING MUSCLE ACTIONS

- ❑ **Medial Rotation of the Arm at the Shoulder Joint:** The subscapularis crosses the shoulder joint anteriorly from medial to lateral (with its fibers running horizontally in the transverse plane). However, it does not attach onto the first aspect of the humerus that it reaches, but rather wraps around the humerus to attach onto the lesser tubercle. Therefore, when the subscapularis contracts and the humeral attachment is pulled toward the scapular attachment, the anterior side of the humerus moves medially. This movement is called medial rotation of the arm at the shoulder joint because the anterior side of the humerus rotates medially. (Note the similarity of the direction of fibers of the subscapularis to the direction of fibers of the latissimus dorsi and teres major.)

MISCELLANEOUS

❑ 1. The subscapularis is one of the four rotator cuff muscles. The rotator cuff muscles are the supraspinatus, infraspinatus, teres minor and the subscapularis. Sometimes the rotator cuff muscles are called the "SITS" muscles; each of the four letters stands for the first letter of the four rotator cuff muscles. **S**ubscapularis is the last "**S**" of "SIT**S**."

❑ 2. The subscapularis (along with the latissimus dorsi and teres major) is located in the "posterior axillary fold" of tissue, which borders the axilla (armpit) posteriorly.

❑ 3. The distal tendon of the subscapularis adheres to the capsule of the shoulder joint (glenohumeral joint), which is deep to the subscapularis.

❑ 4. There is controversy regarding whether or not the subscapularis can perform other actions of the arm at the shoulder joint. Some sources state that depending upon the position of the arm, the subscapularis adducts, abducts, flexes or extends the arm. However, given that its attachment site is so far proximal on the humerus, its lever arm would be very poor. If these actions did occur, they would be very weak.

❑ 5. There is a bursa located between the subscapularis muscle and the scapula called the *subscapular bursa*.

❑ 6. A main function of the subscapularis is to act as a fixator (stabilizer) of the shoulder joint.

TERES MAJOR

❑ **The name, teres major, tells us that this muscle is round and large (larger than the teres minor).**

DERIVATION ❑ teres: L. *round.*
major: L. *large.*

PRONUNCIATION ❑ **te**-reez **may**-jor

ATTACHMENTS

❑ **Inferior Lateral Border of the Scapula**

- ❑ the inferior 1/3 of the dorsal surface

to the

❑ **Medial Lip of the Bicipital Groove of the Humerus**

ACTIONS

❑ 1. **Medial Rotation of the Arm**

❑ 2. **Adduction of the Arm**

❑ 3. **Extension of the Arm**

❑ 4. Upward Rotation of the Scapula

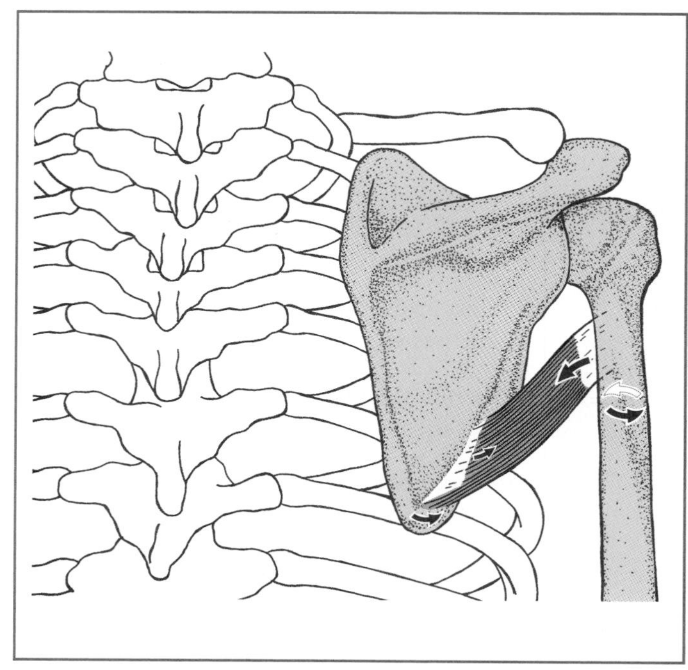

Posterior View of the Right Teres Major

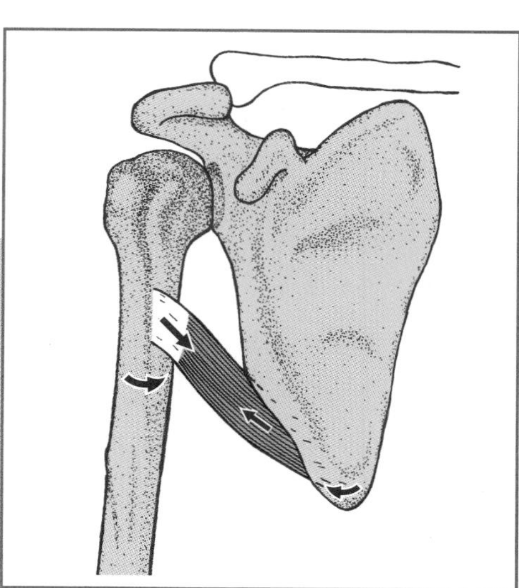

Anterior View of the Right Teres Major

INNERVATION ❑ The Lower Subscapular Nerve
- ❑ C5, **6**, 7

ARTERIAL SUPPLY ❑ The Circumflex Scapular Artery (A Branch of the Subscapular Artery)
- ❑ and the thoracodorsal artery (a continuation of the subscapular artery)

PALPATION AND SUPPLEMENTARY TEXT

PALPATION

Palpating the belly of the teres major is fairly easy, but it can be difficult to distinguish the distal tendon of the teres major from the distal tendon of the latissimus dorsi.

❑ **Prone:**

- Have the client prone with the arm hanging off the table.
- Place palpating hand on the lower 1/2 of the lateral border of the scapula.
- Ask the client to actively medially rotate the arm at the shoulder joint and feel for the contraction of the teres major.
- To distinguish the teres major from the teres minor (just superior to it), have the client alternately medially and laterally rotate the arm at the shoulder joint. The teres major will be felt to contract during medial rotation of the arm; the teres minor will be felt to contract during lateral rotation of the arm.

❑ **Standing:**

- Have the client standing with the trunk flexed (and/or with the pelvis anteriorly tilted at the hip joints to incline the trunk forward). This causes the scapula to be passively protracted due to the weight of the arm. Follow the above steps to palpate the teres major with the client standing.

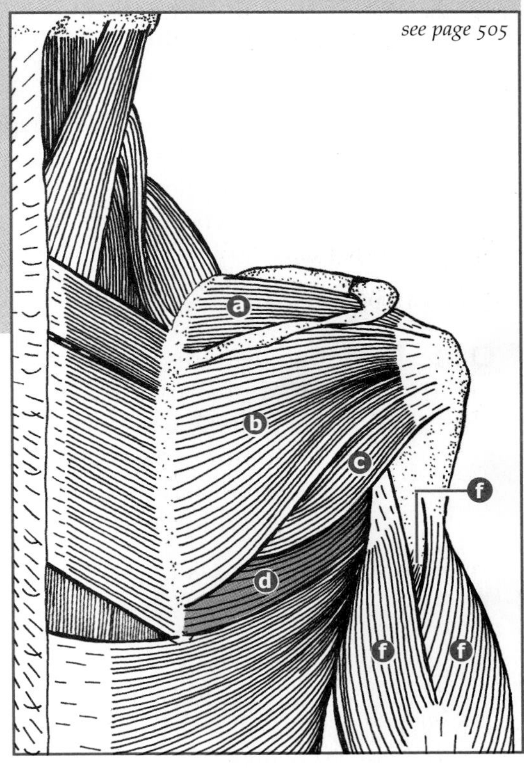

see page 505

Posterior View of the Right Shoulder (Intermediate)

a. Supraspinatus
b. Infraspinatus
c. Teres Minor
d. **Teres Major**
e. Deltoid (not seen)
f. Triceps Brachii

RELATIONSHIP TO OTHER MUSCULOSKELETAL STRUCTURES

❑ 1. The teres major lies inferior to the infraspinatus and the teres minor.

❑ 2. The long head of the triceps brachii runs between the teres minor and the teres major.

❑ 3. The distal tendon of the teres major runs parallel to the distal tendon of the latissimus dorsi.

❑ 4. The teres major and the latissimus dorsi both attach onto the medial lip of the bicipital groove of the humerus. On the medial lip, the teres major attaches posterior to the latissimus dorsi.

❑ 5. Deep to the teres major is the scapula.

TERES MAJOR – CONTINUED

METHODOLOGY FOR LEARNING MUSCLE ACTIONS

- ❑ **1. Medial Rotation of the Arm at the Shoulder Joint:** The teres major crosses the shoulder joint from medial on the scapula to lateral on the humerus (with its fibers oriented somewhat horizontally in the transverse plane). However, it does not attach onto the first aspect on the humerus that it reaches, but rather wraps around to the anterior side of the humerus to attach onto the medial lip of the bicipital groove of the humerus. Therefore, when the teres major contracts and the humeral attachment is pulled toward the scapular attachment, the anterior side of the humerus moves medially. This movement is called medial rotation of the arm at the shoulder joint because the anterior side of the humerus rotates medially. (Note the similarity of the direction of fibers of the teres major to the direction of fibers of the latissimus dorsi.)
- ❑ **2. Adduction of the Arm at the Shoulder Joint:** The teres major crosses the shoulder joint posteriorly, from medial on the scapula to lateral on the humerus (with fibers running horizontally in the frontal plane). Therefore, when the lateral attachment, the humerus, is pulled toward the medial attachment, the scapula, the humerus is pulled toward the midline. Therefore, the teres major adducts the arm at the shoulder joint.
- ❑ **3. Extension of the Arm at the Shoulder Joint:** The teres major crosses the shoulder joint posteriorly (with the fibers running somewhat vertically in the sagittal plane); therefore, it extends the arm at the shoulder joint.
- ❑ **4. Upward Rotation of the Scapula at the Scapulocostal Joint:** When the teres major pulls on the scapula, it pulls the scapula in such a way that the inferior angle swings up toward the arm anteriorly. This causes the glenoid fossa to orient upward; therefore, the teres major upwardly rotates the scapula at the scapulocostal joint.

MISCELLANEOUS

- ❑ 1. Although the teres major and the teres minor share the word "teres" in their name (because they are both round in shape) and sit next to each other, they wrap around the humerus in opposite directions and therefore have opposite rotary actions. The teres major wraps around to the anterior side of the shoulder joint to attach onto the humerus and therefore medially rotates the arm at the shoulder joint; the teres minor wraps around to the posterior side of the shoulder joint to attach onto the humerus and therefore laterally rotates the arm at the shoulder joint.
- ❑ 2. The teres major and the teres minor, due to their different rotary actions of the arm, are in different functional groups. These two muscles are also innervated by different nerves.
- ❑ 3. The latissimus dorsi and the teres major make up the majority of the "posterior axillary fold" of tissue which borders the axilla (armpit) posteriorly.
- ❑ 4. The belly and/or distal tendon of the teres major sometimes blend with the latissimus dorsi.
- ❑ 5. The teres major is sometimes called the "little brother" or the "little helper" of the latissimus dorsi because they run together between the scapula and the humerus, they attach together onto the medial lip of the bicipital groove of the humerus and they have the same direction of muscle fibers and therefore, the same actions of the arm at the shoulder joint (medial rotation, adduction and extension). Perhaps a better name for the teres major would be the "fat little brother" or "fat little helper" because this muscle is extremely thick, hence the name teres "major." ☺

DELTOID

❑ The name, deltoid, tells us that this muscle has a triangular shape like the Greek letter delta (Δ).

DERIVATION ❑ delta: Gr. *the letter delta* (Δ).
oid: Gr. *resemblance.*

PRONUNCIATION ❑ **del**-toid

ATTACHMENTS

❑ **Lateral Clavicle, Acromion Process and the Spine of the Scapula**

❑ the lateral 1/3 of the clavicle

to the

❑ **Deltoid Tuberosity of the Humerus**

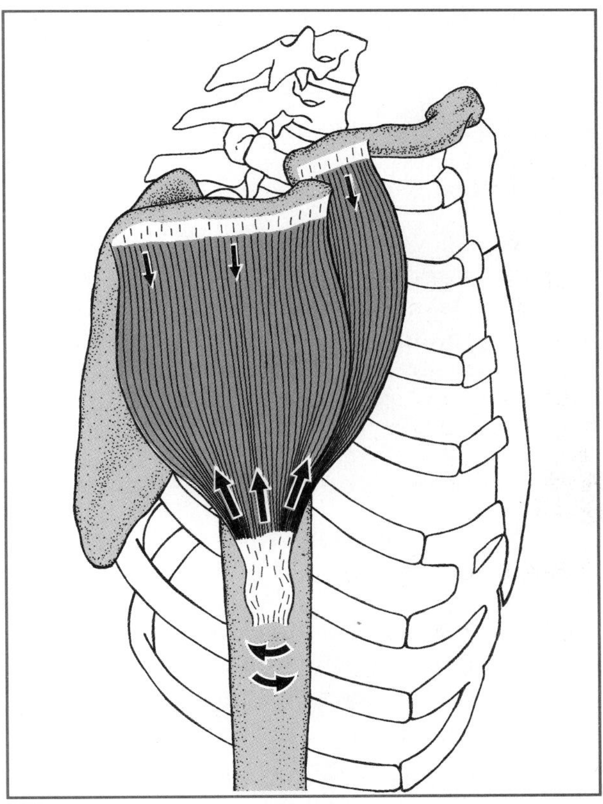

Lateral View of the Right Deltoid

ACTIONS

❑ **1. Abduction of the Arm (entire muscle)**

❑ **2. Flexion of the Arm (anterior deltoid)**

❑ **3. Extension of the Arm (posterior deltoid)**

❑ **4. Medial Rotation of the Arm (anterior deltoid)**

❑ **5. Lateral Rotation of the Arm (posterior deltoid)**

❑ **6.** Downward Rotation of the Scapula (entire muscle)

❑ **7.** Ipsilateral Rotation of the Trunk (anterior deltoid)

❑ **8.** Contralateral Rotation of the Trunk (posterior deltoid)

INNERVATION ❑ The Axillary Nerve ❑ **C5**, 6

ARTERIAL SUPPLY ❑ The Anterior and Posterior Circumflex Humeral Arteries (Branches of the Axillary Artery)

❑ and the pectoral and deltoid branches of the thoracoacromial trunk (a branch of the axillary artery)

DELTOID – PALPATION AND SUPPLEMENTARY TEXT

PALPATION

The deltoid is superficial and easy to palpate from attachment to attachment.

- Have the client seated or standing.

❑ **Middle deltoid:**

- Place palpating hand just proximal to the deltoid tuberosity.
- Ask the client to actively abduct the arm and feel for the contraction of the middle deltoid.
- Continue palpating the middle deltoid toward the acromion process.

❑ **Anterior deltoid:**

- Place palpating hand on the anterior shoulder.
- Ask the client to actively horizontally flex the arm at the shoulder joint and feel for the contraction of the anterior deltoid.

❑ **Posterior deltoid:**

- Place palpating hand just inferior to the spine of the scapula.
- Ask the client to actively horizontally extend the arm at the shoulder joint and feel for the contraction of the posterior deltoid.

In all cases, resistance may be added.

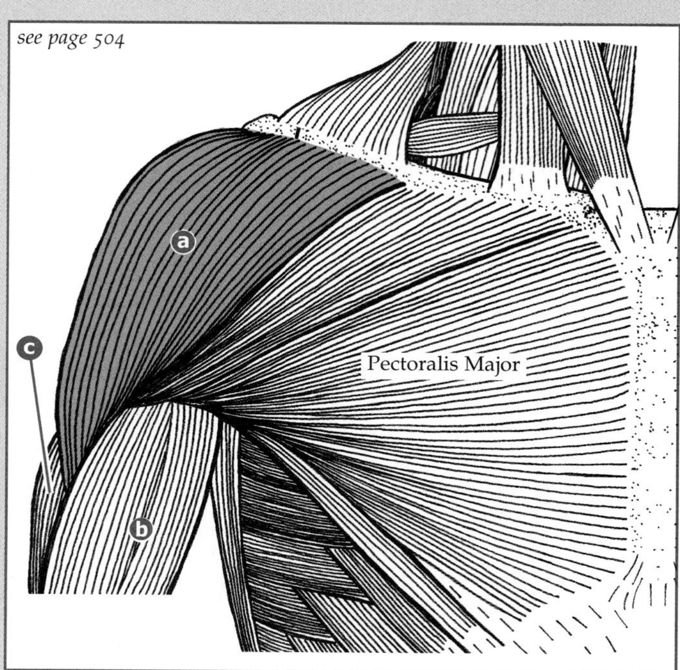

Anterior View of the Right Shoulder

a. **Deltoid**
b. Biceps Brachii
c. Triceps Brachii

RELATIONSHIP TO OTHER MUSCULOSKELETAL STRUCTURES

❑ 1. The deltoid is superficial and found at the anterior, lateral and posterior shoulder. It gives the shoulder its characteristic shape.

❑ 2. The anterior deltoid lies next to the clavicular head of the pectoralis major.

❑ 3. Posterior to the deltoid are the infraspinatus, teres minor, teres major and the triceps brachii.

❑ 4. The following muscles all have tendons that are deep to the deltoid: pectoralis minor, coracobrachialis and the short head of the biceps brachii (all attaching to the coracoid process of the scapula); the supraspinatus, infraspinatus, teres minor and the subscapularis (rotator cuff muscles attaching to the greater and lesser tubercles of the humerus); and the pectoralis major, long head of the biceps brachii and the long and lateral heads of the triceps brachii.

DELTOID – CONTINUED

METHODOLOGY FOR LEARNING MUSCLE ACTIONS

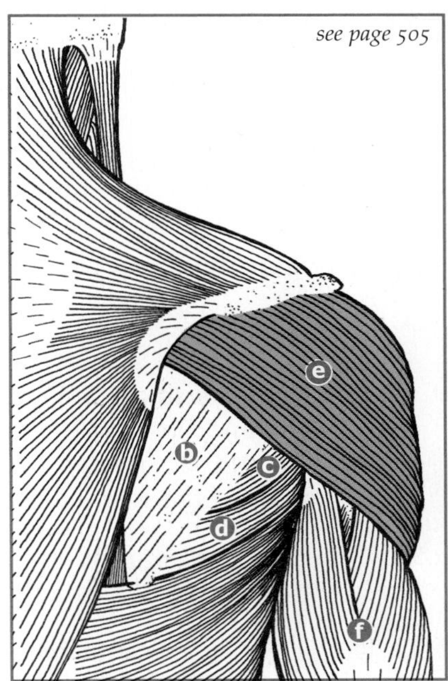

Posterior View of the Right Shoulder (Superficial)

a. Supraspinatus (not seen)
b. Infraspinatus (deep to fascia)
c. Teres Minor
d. Teres Major
e. **Deltoid**
f. Triceps Brachii

❑ 1. **Abduction of the Arm at the Shoulder Joint (entire muscle):** The deltoid crosses over the top of the shoulder joint on the lateral side (with its fibers running vertically in the frontal plane); therefore, it abducts the arm at the shoulder joint. (Note: The anterior and posterior parts of the deltoid can abduct the arm at the shoulder joint, but the fibers of the middle deltoid have the best line of pull for this action.)

❑ 2. **Flexion of the Arm at the Shoulder Joint (anterior deltoid):** The anterior deltoid crosses the shoulder joint anteriorly (with its fibers running vertically in the sagittal plane); therefore, it flexes the arm at the shoulder joint.

❑ 3. **Extension of the Arm at the Shoulder Joint (posterior deltoid):** The posterior deltoid crosses the shoulder joint posteriorly (with its fibers running vertically in the sagittal plane); therefore, it extends the arm at the shoulder joint.

❑ 4. **Medial Rotation of the Arm at the Shoulder Joint (anterior deltoid):** The anterior deltoid crosses the shoulder joint anteriorly from medial on the clavicle, to more lateral on the humerus (with its fibers running somewhat horizontally in the transverse plane). However, it does not attach onto the first aspect of the humerus that it reaches, but rather wraps around the humerus to attach onto the deltoid tuberosity. Therefore, when the anterior deltoid contracts and the humeral attachment is pulled toward the clavicular attachment, the humerus moves anteromedially. This movement is called medial rotation of the arm at the shoulder joint because the anterior side of the humerus rotates medially.

❑ 5. **Lateral Rotation of the Arm at the Shoulder Joint (posterior deltoid):** The posterior deltoid crosses the shoulder joint posteriorly from medial on the scapula, to more lateral on the humerus (with its fibers running somewhat horizontally in the transverse plane). However, it does not attach onto the first aspect of the humerus that it reaches, but rather wraps around the humerus to attach onto the deltoid tuberosity. Therefore, when the posterior deltoid contracts and the humeral attachment is pulled toward the scapular attachment, the humerus moves posteromedially. This movement is called lateral rotation of the arm at the shoulder joint because the anterior side of the humerus rotates laterally.

❑ 6. **Downward Rotation of the Scapula at the Scapulocostal Joint (entire muscle):** When the arm is fixed and the deltoid contracts, the deltoid pulls directly on the scapula (and indirectly on the scapula by pulling on the lateral clavicle), pulling the acromion process inferiorly toward the humerus. This causes the inferior angle to swing up toward the vertebral column and causes the glenoid fossa to orient downward. Therefore, the deltoid downwardly rotates the scapula.

❑ 7. **Ipsilateral Rotation of the Trunk at the Shoulder Joint (anterior deltoid):** When the humeral attachment of the deltoid is fixed and the trunk moves, the anterior deltoid pulls the trunk toward the humerus (anteriorly). This causes the anterior trunk to rotate toward the same side of the body that the deltoid is attached (since the fibers are running somewhat horizontally in the transverse plane). Therefore, the anterior deltoid ipsilaterally rotates the trunk at the shoulder joint.

DELTOID – CONTINUED

- ❑ 8. **Contralateral Rotation of the Trunk at the Shoulder Joint (posterior deltoid):** When the humeral attachment of the deltoid is fixed and the trunk moves, the posterior deltoid pulls the trunk toward the humerus (posteriorly). This causes the anterior trunk to rotate toward the opposite side of the body from the side of the body that the deltoid is attached (since the fibers are running somewhat horizontally in the transverse plane). Therefore, the posterior deltoid contralaterally rotates the trunk at the shoulder joint.

MISCELLANEOUS

- ❑ 1. The deltoid is considered to have three parts: anterior, middle and posterior.
- ❑ 2. The anterior deltoid crosses the shoulder joint anteriorly and attaches to the lateral clavicle proximally. The middle deltoid crosses the shoulder joint laterally and attaches to the acromion process of the scapula proximally. The posterior deltoid crosses the shoulder joint posteriorly and attaches to the spine of the scapula proximally.
- ❑ 3. The most anterior and posterior fibers of the deltoid (crossing below the center of the shoulder joint) are capable of adducting the arm at the shoulder joint.
- ❑ 4. The proximal attachments of the deltoid are the same as the lateral attachments of the trapezius, namely, the lateral clavicle, acromion process and the spine of the scapula.
- ❑ 5. The anterior deltoid is a strong horizontal flexor and the posterior deltoid is a strong horizontal extensor of the arm at the shoulder joint.
- ❑ 6. Although the deltoid can abduct the arm at the shoulder joint throughout its entire range of motion, the deltoid's activity is strongest between 90° and 120°.
- ❑ 7. The anterior deltoid is considered to be the prime mover of flexion of the arm at the shoulder joint.
- ❑ 8. Please note how the deltoid fans around the shoulder joint. It crosses the shoulder joint anteriorly, laterally and posteriorly. This orientation is similar to the orientation of the gluteus medius to the hip joint. Therefore, both of these muscles can do the same actions at their respective joints. The deltoid abducts, flexes, extends, medially rotates and laterally rotates the arm at the shoulder joint. The gluteus medius abducts, flexes, extends, medially rotates and laterally rotates the thigh at the hip joint.
- ❑ 9. **Clavicular Actions:** Although the clavicle often moves passively by accompanying scapular movement, the clavicle can be directly acted upon by musculature and therefore actively moved. The anterior deltoid attaches from the lateral clavicle to the humerus. When the humeral attachment is fixed, the anterior deltoid can depress, downwardly rotate and/or protract the clavicle (at the sternocostal joint) toward the humerus.

CORACOBRACHIALIS ❑

❑ **The name, coracobrachialis, tells us that this muscle is related to the coracoid process and the brachium (the arm), hence its attachments onto the coracoid process of the scapula and the humerus.**

DERIVATION ❑ coraco: Gr. *refers to the coracoid process of the scapula.*
brachialis: L. *refers to the arm.*

PRONUNCIATION ❑ **kor**-a-ko-**bra**-key-**al**-is

ATTACHMENTS

❑ **Coracoid Process of the Scapula**

- ❑ the apex

to the

❑ **Medial Shaft of the Humerus**

- ❑ the middle 1/3

ACTIONS

❑ **1. Flexion of the Arm**

❑ **2. Adduction of the Arm**

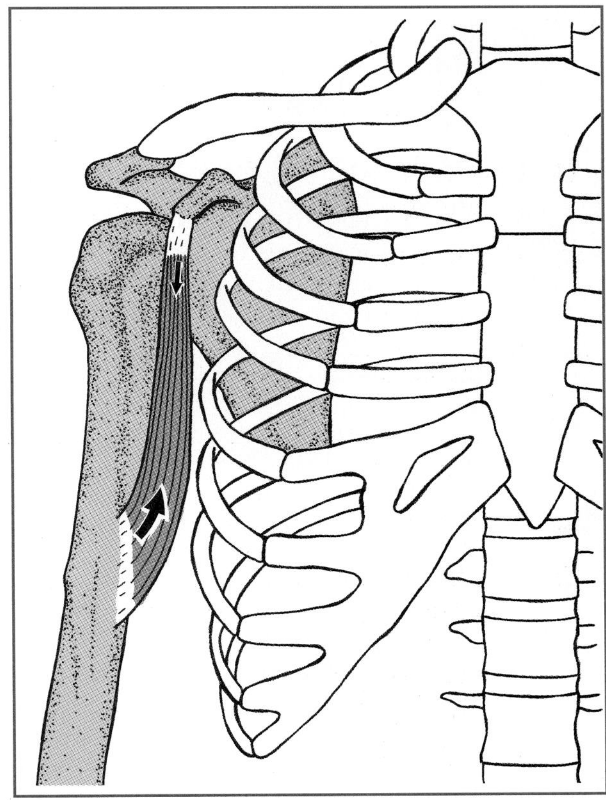

Anterior View of the Right Coracobrachialis

INNERVATION ❑ The Musculocutaneous Nerve ❑ C5, 6, 7

ARTERIAL SUPPLY ❑ The Muscular Branches of the Brachial Artery (The Continuation of the Axillary Artery)
❑ and the anterior circumflex humeral artery (a branch of the axillary artery)

CORACOBRACHIALIS – PALPATION AND SUPPLEMENTARY TEXT

PALPATION

- ❑ The coracobrachialis is palpable just posterior to the pectoralis major, but it can be difficult to distinguish from the biceps brachii.
  - Have the client seated with the arm partially abducted and laterally rotated at the shoulder joint.
  - Locate the pectoralis major (see page 260), which forms the anterior wall of the axilla.
  - Place palpating hand just posterior to the pectoralis major and feel for the coracobrachialis and short head of the biceps brachii. The coracobrachialis will feel like a slender, rounded muscle.
  - To further bring out the coracobrachialis, as well as the biceps brachii, resist the client from adducting the arm. (Since these muscles are located directly next to each other and both adduct the arm, distinguishing between the two can be difficult.)
  - Palpate more posteriorly for the coracobrachialis.
  - Another way to distinguish the biceps brachii from the coracobrachialis is to ask the client to actively flex the forearm at the elbow joint against resistance. This will cause the biceps brachii to contract, but not the coracobrachialis.

(Note: Be careful with palpation in the medial arm because the median nerve and brachial artery are superficial here.)

RELATIONSHIP TO OTHER MUSCULOSKELETAL STRUCTURES

❑ 1. From an anterior perspective, the coracobrachialis lies deep to the deltoid and the pectoralis major.

❑ 2. Proximally, the coracobrachialis lies medial to the short head of the biceps brachii. More distally, the coracobrachialis is deep to the short head of the biceps brachii.

❑ 3. The coracobrachialis attaches onto the shaft of the humerus on the medial side between the attachments of the brachialis and the triceps brachii (medial head).

❑ 4. The proximal attachment of the coracobrachialis is the coracoid process of the scapula. The short head of the biceps brachii and the pectoralis minor also attach to the coracoid process.

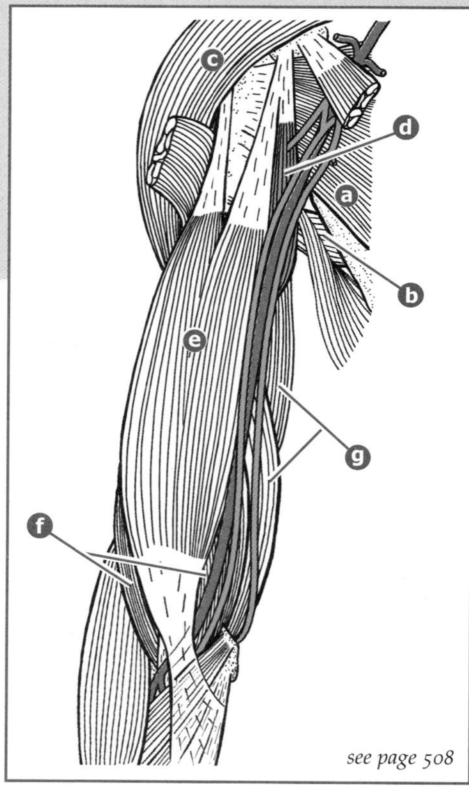

see page 508

Anterior View of the Right Arm (Superficial)

a. Subscapularis
b. Teres Major
c. Deltoid
d. **Coracobrachialis**
e. Biceps Brachii
f. Brachialis
g. Triceps Brachii

CORACOBRACHIALIS – CONTINUED

METHODOLOGY FOR LEARNING MUSCLE ACTIONS

❑ **1. Flexion of the Arm at the Shoulder Joint:** The coracobrachialis crosses the shoulder joint anteriorly (with its fibers running vertically in the sagittal plane); therefore, it flexes the arm at the shoulder joint.

❑ **2. Adduction of the Arm at the Shoulder Joint:** The coracobrachialis crosses the shoulder joint medially below the center of the joint (with the fibers running somewhat horizontally in the frontal plane); therefore, it adducts the arm at the shoulder joint.

MISCELLANEOUS

❑ 1. The proximal attachment of the coracobrachialis blends with the proximal attachment of the short head of the biceps brachii.

❑ 2. Scapular Tilt Actions: In addition to its other actions, the scapula can also tilt.

When the coracobrachialis pulls on the coracoid process, it pulls the scapula in such a manner that the lateral border of the scapula is pulled in toward the lateral body wall and the medial border of the scapula moves away from the posterior body wall. The medial border of the scapula coming away from the body wall is called lateral tilt. Therefore, the coracobrachialis laterally tilts the scapula (at the scapulocostal joint).

When the coracobrachialis pulls on the coracoid process, it pulls the scapula in such a manner that the scapula is pulled inferiorly and toward the anterior body wall, and the inferior angle of the scapula moves superiorly and away from the posterior body wall. The inferior angle of the scapula coming away from the body wall is called upward tilt. Therefore, the coracobrachialis upwardly tilts the scapula (at the scapulocostal joint).

❑ 3. The coracobrachialis is also a strong horizontal flexor of the arm at the shoulder joint.

❑ 4. The musculocutaneous nerve pierces through the coracobrachialis.

❑ BICEPS BRACHII

❑ **The name, biceps brachii, tells us that this muscle has two heads and lies over the brachium (the arm).**

DERIVATION ❑ biceps: L. *two heads.*
brachii: L. *refers to the arm.*

PRONUNCIATION ❑ **by**-seps **bray**-key-eye

ATTACHMENTS

❑ **LONG HEAD: Supraglenoid Tubercle of the Scapula**

❑ **SHORT HEAD: Coracoid Process of the Scapula**

- ❑ the apex

to the

❑ **Radial Tuberosity**

- ❑ and the bicipital aponeurosis into deep fascia overlying the common flexor tendon

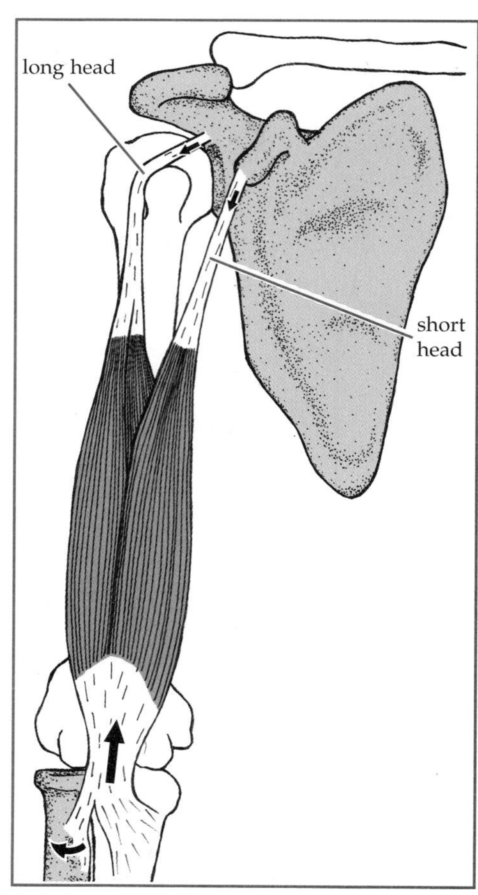

Anterior View of the Right Biceps Brachii

ACTIONS

❑ **1. Flexion of the Forearm (entire muscle)**

❑ **2. Supination of the Forearm (entire muscle)**

❑ **3. Flexion of the Arm (entire muscle)**

❑ 4. Abduction of the Arm (long head)

❑ 5. Adduction of the Arm (short head)

INNERVATION ❑ The Musculocutaneous Nerve ❑ C5, 6

ARTERIAL SUPPLY ❑ The Muscular Branches of the Brachial Artery (The Continuation of the Axillary Artery)

- ❑ and the anterior circumflex humeral artery (a branch of the axillary artery)

PALPATION AND SUPPLEMENTARY TEXT

PALPATION

- ❑ The biceps brachii is superficial, visible and easy to palpate. The muscle belly can be palpated while relaxed or contracted. (To palpate the proximal portion of the short head of the biceps brachii, follow the palpation guidelines for the coracobrachialis on page 536).
  - Have the client seated or supine with the forearm supinated.
  - Place palpating hand on the anterior arm and feel for the biceps brachii.
  - Continue palpating the biceps brachii proximally and distally toward its attachments.
  - To palpate the biceps brachii while contracted, ask the client to actively flex the forearm at the elbow joint (with the forearm fully supinated) against resistance.

(Note: Be careful with palpation in the medial arm because the median nerve and brachial artery are superficial here.)

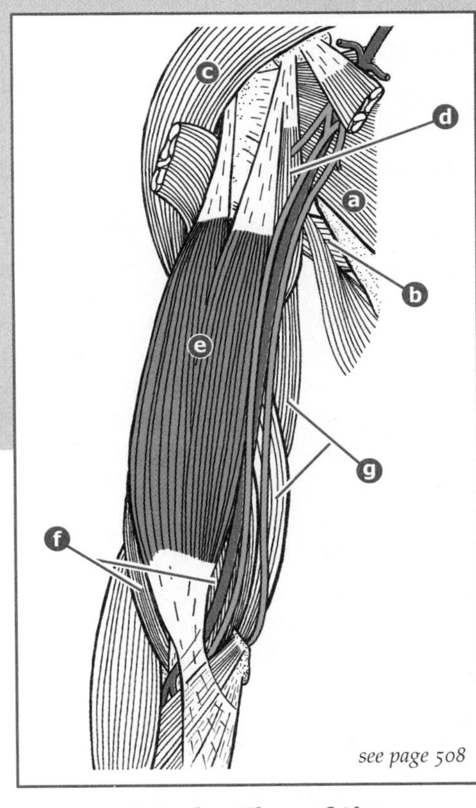

see page 508

Anterior View of the Right Arm (Superficial)

a. Subscapularis
b. Teres Major
c. Deltoid
d. Coracobrachialis
e. **Biceps Brachii**
f. Brachialis
g. Triceps Brachii

RELATIONSHIP TO OTHER MUSCULOSKELETAL STRUCTURES

❑ 1. Proximally, the biceps brachii is deep to the deltoid and deep to the distal tendon of the pectoralis major. The remainder of the biceps brachii is superficial.

❑ 2. The brachialis lies deep to the biceps brachii.

❑ 3. The short head of the biceps brachii lies lateral to the coracobrachialis.

❑ 4. The proximal attachment of the short head of the biceps brachii is the coracoid process of the scapula. The coracobrachialis and the pectoralis minor also attach to the coracoid process.

❑ 5. The long head of the biceps brachii courses through the bicipital groove of the humerus. The long head of the biceps brachii then courses through the joint cavity of the shoulder joint (glenohumeral joint); therefore, it is intra-articular.

❑ 6. Directly medial to the belly and distal tendon of the biceps brachii are the brachial artery and the median nerve.

❑ 7. The bicipital aponeurosis is superficial to the common flexor tendon.

METHODOLOGY FOR LEARNING MUSCLE ACTIONS

❑ **1. Flexion of the Forearm at the Elbow Joint (entire muscle):** The biceps brachii crosses the elbow joint anteriorly (with its fibers running vertically in the sagittal plane); therefore, it flexes the forearm at the elbow joint.

BICEPS BRACHII – continued

- ❑ **2. Supination of the Forearm at the Radioulnar Joints (entire muscle):** When the forearm is pronated, the biceps brachii attachment onto the radial tuberosity is deep between the radius and the ulna. Thus, the fibers wrap around the medial side of the proximal radius. When the biceps brachii pulls at the radial tuberosity, the head of the radius will laterally rotate and the distal radius will move around the distal ulna. This movement of the radius is called supination. Therefore, the biceps brachii supinates the forearm at the radioulnar joints.
- ❑ **3. Flexion of the Arm at the Shoulder Joint (entire muscle):** The biceps brachii crosses the shoulder joint anteriorly (with its fibers running vertically in the sagittal plane); therefore, it flexes the arm at the shoulder joint.
- ❑ **4. Abduction of the Arm at the Shoulder Joint (long head):** The long head of the biceps brachii crosses over the top of the shoulder joint (with its fibers running somewhat vertically in the frontal plane); therefore, it abducts the arm at the shoulder joint. (Note the similarity of the direction of fibers of the biceps brachii to the direction of fibers of the middle deltoid.)
- ❑ **5. Adduction of the Arm at the Shoulder Joint (short head):** The short head of the biceps brachii crosses the shoulder joint below the center of the joint, from medial on the trunk, to lateral on the upper extremity (with its fibers running somewhat horizontally in the frontal plane). Therefore, when the upper extremity is pulled toward the trunk, the arm is adducted at the shoulder joint. (Note the similarity of the direction of fibers of the short head of the biceps brachii to the direction of fibers of the coracobrachialis.)

MISCELLANEOUS

- ❑ 1. The bicipital groove of the humerus is named the "bicipital" groove because the long head of the biceps brachii courses through it. (The bicipital groove of the humerus is also known as the *intertubercular groove* because it is located between the two tubercles of the humerus.)
- ❑ 2. The proximal attachment of the short head of the biceps brachii blends with the proximal attachment of the coracobrachialis at the coracoid process of the scapula.
- ❑ 3. The bicipital aponeurosis is also known as the *lacertus fibrosis*.
- ❑ 4. Scapular Tilt Actions: In addition to its other actions, the scapula can also tilt.

  When the biceps brachii pulls on the coracoid process, it pulls the scapula in such a manner that the lateral border of the scapula is pulled in toward the lateral body wall and the medial border of the scapula moves away from the posterior body wall. The medial border of the scapula coming away from the body wall is called lateral tilt. Therefore, the biceps brachii laterally tilts the scapula (at the scapulocostal joint).

  When the biceps brachii pulls on the coracoid process, it pulls the scapula in such a manner that the scapula is pulled inferiorly and toward the anterior body wall and the inferior angle of the scapula moves superiorly and away from the posterior body wall. The inferior angle of the scapula coming away from the body wall is called upward tilt. Therefore, the biceps brachii upwardly tilts the scapula (at the scapulocostal joint).
- ❑ 5. The biceps brachii also contributes to horizontal flexion of the arm at the shoulder joint.
- ❑ 6. The biceps brachii can flex the forearm at the elbow joint regardless of the position of pronation/supination of the radioulnar joints. However, the biceps brachii is strongest with regard to flexion of the forearm when the forearm is fully supinated.
- ❑ 7. The biceps brachii can supinate the forearm at the radioulnar joints regardless of the position of flexion/extension of the elbow joint. However, the biceps brachii is strongest with regard to supination of the forearm when the forearm is partially flexed.

BRACHIALIS

❑ **The name, brachialis, tells us that this muscle attaches to the brachium (the arm).**

DERIVATION ❑ brachialis: L. *refers to the arm.* **PRONUNCIATION** ❑ **bray**-key-**al**-is

ATTACHMENTS

❑ **Distal 1/2 of the Anterior Shaft of the Humerus**

to the

❑ **Ulnar Tuberosity**

- ❑ and the coronoid process of the ulna

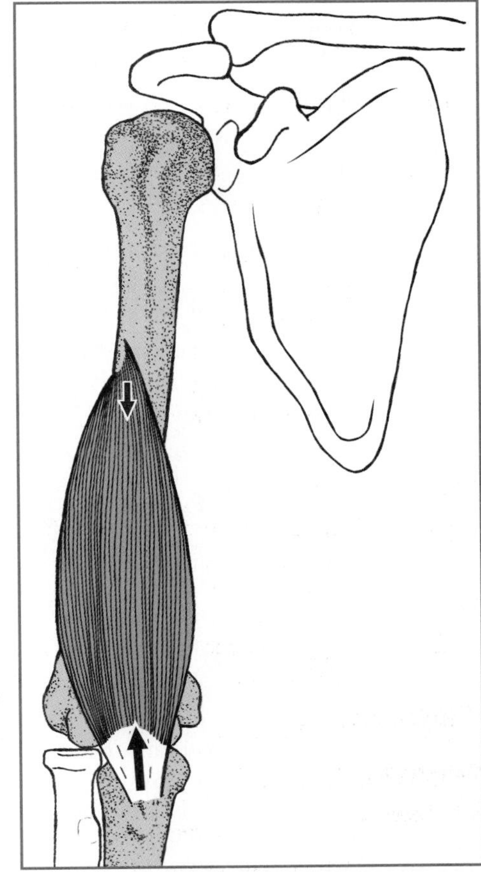

Anterior View of the Right Brachialis

ACTION

❑ **Flexion of the Forearm**

INNERVATION ❑ The Musculocutaneous Nerve ❑ C5, **6**, 7

ARTERIAL SUPPLY ❑ Muscular Branches of the Brachial Artery (The Continuation of the Axillary Artery)

BRACHIALIS – PALPATION AND SUPPLEMENTARY TEXT

PALPATION

Much of the brachialis is deep to the biceps brachii and not easily palpable. However, two areas of the brachialis are superficial and palpable: the distal end, on either side of the distal tendon of the biceps brachii, and the lateral margin, posterior to the lateral margin of the biceps brachii.

❑ **To palpate the distal end:**

- With the client seated or supine, locate the distal tendon of the biceps brachii by having the client actively flex the forearm at the elbow joint with the forearm fully supinated (see the palpation section for the biceps brachii on page 539).
- Now have the client partially passively flex and pronate the forearm. (The position of pronation will lessen the contraction of the biceps brachii.)
- Place palpating fingers on either side of the distal tendon of the biceps brachii.
- Ask the client to flex the forearm further with a short, quick range of motion and feel for the contraction of the brachialis.
  (Note: Be careful with palpation in the distal medial arm because the median nerve and brachial artery are superficial here.)

❑ **To palpate the lateral margin:**

- Have the client seated or supine.
- Locate the posterolateral margin of the biceps brachii by having the client flex the forearm while fully supinated (see the palpation section for the biceps brachii on page 539).
- Now locate the anterolateral margin of the triceps brachii on the lateral arm by having the client extend the arm (see the palpation section for the triceps brachii on page 545).
- Palpate between these two areas.
- Once you have located the lateral margin of the brachialis, its contraction may be felt by having the client actively flex the forearm with the forearm pronated.

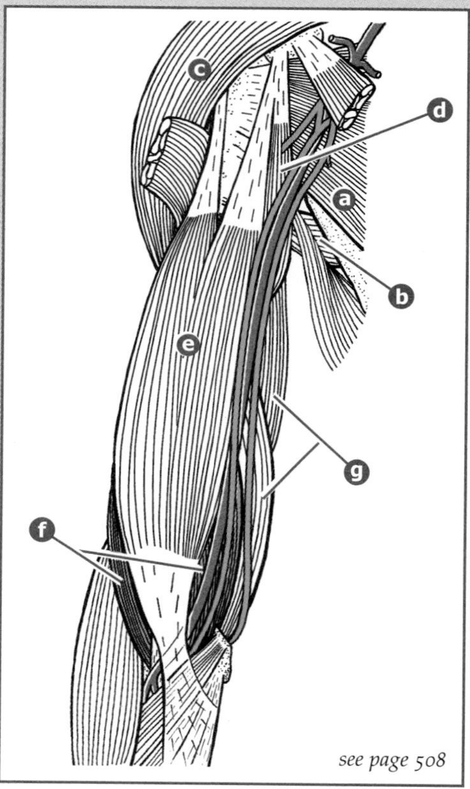

see page 508

Anterior View of the Right Arm (Superficial)

a. Subscapularis
b. Teres Major
c. Deltoid
d. Coracobrachialis
e. Biceps Brachii
f. **Brachialis**
g. Triceps Brachii

RELATIONSHIP TO OTHER MUSCULOSKELETAL STRUCTURES

❑ 1. Although most of the brachialis is deep to the biceps brachii, the lateral margin of the brachialis is superficial between the biceps brachii and the triceps brachii. More distally, the brachialis is superficial on both sides of the biceps brachii's distal tendon.

❑ 2. Deep to the brachialis is the shaft of the humerus.

BRACHIALIS – continued

- ❑ 3. The proximal attachment of the brachialis forms a "V" shape and surrounds the distal attachment of the deltoid.
- ❑ 4. On the medial side, the triceps brachii is posterior to the brachialis.
- ❑ 5. On the lateral side, the triceps brachii is posterior to the brachialis proximally; the brachioradialis is posterior to the brachialis distally.

METHODOLOGY FOR LEARNING MUSCLE ACTIONS

- ❑ **Flexion of the Forearm at the Elbow Joint:** The brachialis crosses the elbow joint anteriorly (with its fibers running vertically in the sagittal plane); therefore, it flexes the forearm at the elbow joint.

MISCELLANEOUS

- ❑ 1. The brachialis is a strong and fairly large muscle, which accounts for much of the contour of the biceps brachii being so visible. ("Behind every great biceps brachii is a great brachialis."☺)
- ❑ 2. The brachialis is the prime mover of flexion of the forearm at the elbow joint.

TRICEPS BRACHII

❑ **The name, triceps brachii, tells us that this muscle has three heads and lies over the brachium (the arm).**

DERIVATION ❑ triceps: L. *three heads.*
brachii: L. *refers to the arm.*

PRONUNCIATION ❑ **try**-seps **bray**-key-eye

ATTACHMENTS

❑ **LONG HEAD: Infraglenoid Tubercle of the Scapula**

❑ **LATERAL HEAD: Posterior Shaft of the Humerus**

- ❑ the proximal 1/2

❑ **MEDIAL HEAD: Posterior Shaft of the Humerus**

- ❑ the distal 1/2

to the

❑ **Olecranon Process of the Ulna**

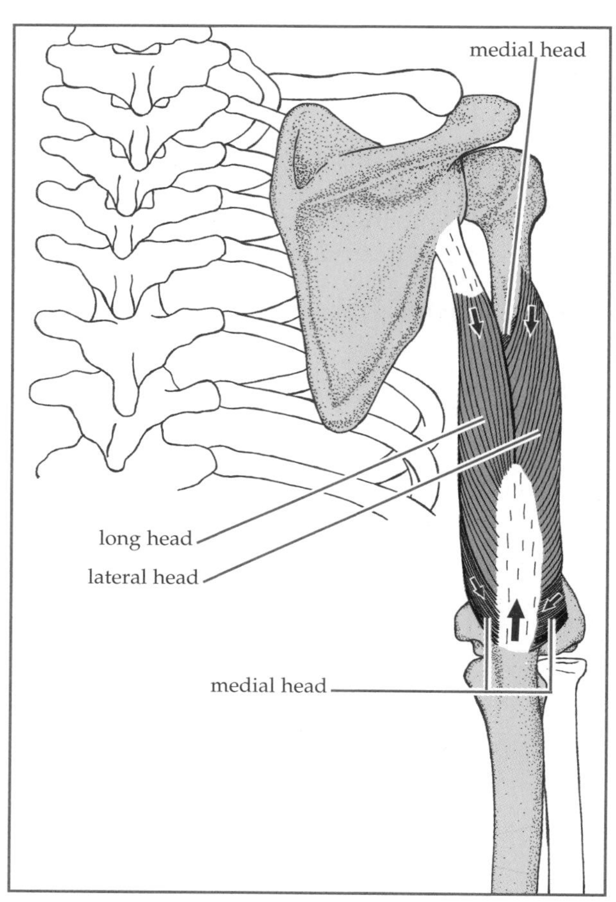

Posterior View of the Right Triceps Brachii

ACTIONS

❑ **1. Extension of the Forearm (entire muscle)**

❑ **2.** Adduction of the Arm (long head)

❑ **3.** Extension of the Arm (long head)

INNERVATION ❑ The Radial Nerve ❑ C6, **7**, 8

ARTERIAL SUPPLY ❑ The Deep Brachial Artery (A Branch of the Brachial Artery)
❑ and the circumflex scapular artery (a branch of the subscapular artery)

PALPATION AND SUPPLEMENTARY TEXT

PALPATION

The triceps brachii is mostly superficial and easily palpable.

❑ **To palpate the muscle belly:**

- Have the client seated with the arm partially flexed at the shoulder joint and the forearm partially flexed at the elbow joint.
- Place palpating hand just proximal to the olecranon process and resist the client from extending the forearm.
- Continue palpating the triceps brachii proximally toward the posterior deltoid.

❑ **To palpate the long head:**

- Except for the portion that is deep to the posterior deltoid, the long head of the triceps brachii is superficial and easily palpable in the proximal medial 2/3 of the arm.

❑ **To palpate the medial head:**

- Most of the medial head of the triceps brachii is deep to the other two heads. The best location to palpate the medial head is distally on the medial side just proximal to the medial epicondyle of the humerus. The medial head is also palpable on the lateral side, just proximal to the lateral epicondyle of the humerus.

❑ **To palpate the lateral head:**

- Except for the portion that is deep to the posterior deltoid, the lateral head of the triceps brachii is superficial and easily palpable in the proximal lateral 2/3 of the arm.

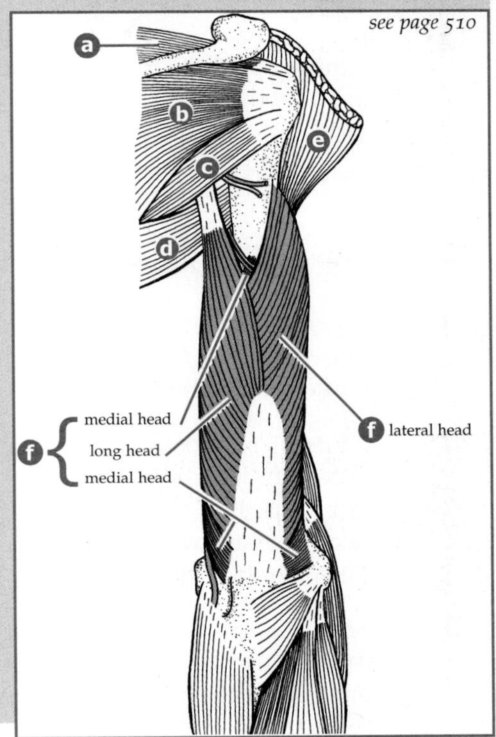

Posterior View of the Right Arm

a. Supraspinatus
b. Infraspinatus
c. Teres Minor
d. Teres Major
e. Deltoid (cut and reflected)
f. **Triceps Brachii**

RELATIONSHIP TO OTHER MUSCULOSKELETAL STRUCTURES

❑ 1. The triceps brachii is superficial in the posterior arm except for the proximal attachments of the long head and the lateral head, which are deep to the deltoid.

❑ 2. On the lateral side, the triceps brachii borders the brachialis proximally and the brachioradialis and the extensor carpi radialis longus distally.

❑ 3. On the medial side, the triceps brachii borders the coracobrachialis and the brachialis.

❑ 4. The long head of the triceps brachii runs between the teres minor and the teres major.

TRICEPS BRACHII – continued

METHODOLOGY FOR LEARNING MUSCLE ACTIONS

- ❑ **1. Extension of the Forearm at the Elbow Joint (entire muscle):** The triceps brachii crosses the elbow joint posteriorly (with its fibers running vertically in the sagittal plane); therefore, it extends the forearm at the elbow joint.
- ❑ **2. Adduction of the Arm at the Shoulder Joint (long head):** The long head of the triceps brachii crosses the shoulder joint posteriorly on the medial side below the center of the joint (with its fibers running somewhat horizontally in the frontal plane); therefore, it adducts the arm at the shoulder joint.
- ❑ **3. Extension of the Arm at the Shoulder Joint (long head):** The long head of the triceps brachii crosses the shoulder joint posteriorly (with the fibers running vertically in the sagittal plane); therefore, it extends the arm at the shoulder joint.

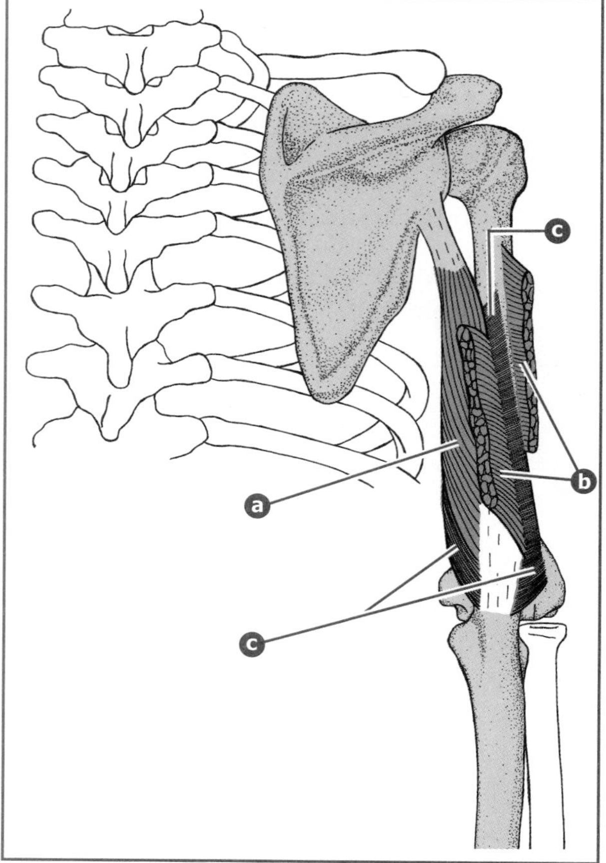

Posterior View of the Right Triceps Brachii (lateral head cut and reflected to better view the medial head)

a. Long Head
b. Lateral Head (cut and reflected)
c. Medial Head

MISCELLANEOUS

- ❑ 1. From the posterior perspective, the medial head of the triceps brachii lies deep to the other two heads.
- ❑ 2. The medial head of the triceps brachii is sometimes known as the *deep head* (which probably is a better name for this head of the triceps brachii).
- ❑ 3. At its proximal end, the medial head of the triceps brachii attaches to the medial proximal humerus. However, more distally, the medial head crosses over to also attach to the lateral distal shaft of the humerus.
- ❑ 4. **Scapular Tilt Actions:** In addition to its other actions, the scapula can also tilt. When the long head of the triceps brachii pulls on the infraglenoid tubercle of the scapula, it pulls the scapula in such a manner that the lateral border of the scapula is pulled in toward the lateral body wall and the medial border of the scapula moves away from the posterior body wall. The medial border of the scapula coming away from the body wall is called lateral tilt. Therefore, the triceps brachii laterally tilts the scapula (at the scapulocostal joint).
- ❑ 5. The triceps brachii long head can also horizontally extend the arm at the shoulder joint.
- ❑ 6. The triceps brachii is the prime mover of extension of the forearm at the elbow joint.
- ❑ 7. The medial head of the triceps brachii is the most active of the three heads but the lateral head is the strongest.
- ❑ 8. The radial nerve runs between the medial and lateral heads of the triceps brachii. Due to its location here, the radial nerve is often injured.

MUSCLES OF THE FOREARM

OVERVIEW OF THE MUSCLES OF THE FOREARM

ANATOMICALLY, THE MUSCLES OF THE FOREARM CAN BE DIVIDED INTO TWO GROUPS:	
The Anterior Group:	**The Posterior Group:**
Superficial ▪ Pronator Teres ▪ Flexor Carpi Radialis ▪ Palmaris Longus ▪ Flexor Carpi Ulnaris ▪ Brachioradialis *Intermediate* ▪ Flexor Digitorum Superficialis *Deep* ▪ Flexor Digitorum Profundus ▪ Flexor Pollicis Longus ▪ Pronator Quadratus	*Superficial* ▪ Anconeus ▪ Extensor Carpi Radialis Longus ▪ Extensor Carpi Radialis Brevis ▪ Extensor Digitorum ▪ Extensor Digiti Minimi ▪ Extensor Carpi Ulnaris *Deep* ▪ Supinator ▪ Abductor Pollicis Longus ▪ Extensor Pollicis Brevis ▪ Extensor Pollicis Longus ▪ Extensor Indicis

THE FOLLOWING MUSCLES ARE COVERED IN OTHER CHAPTERS OF THIS BOOK, BUT ARE ALSO PRESENT IN THE FOREARM:	
▪ Coracobrachialis	▪ Brachialis
▪ Biceps Brachii	▪ Triceps Brachii

The above classification, like any classification, may be overly simplistic. Please note the following:

- The brachioradialis, extensor carpi radialis longus and the extensor carpi radialis brevis are often grouped together as the *radial group* because they constitute a distinct group of muscles located at the radial side of the forearm.
- Six muscles of the posterior forearm attach onto the lateral epicondyle of the humerus: the extensor carpi radialis brevis, extensor digitorum, extensor digiti minimi, the extensor carpi ulnaris (all via the common extensor tendon) and the anconeus and the supinator. (The brachioradialis and the extensor carpi radialis longus both attach onto the lateral supracondylar ridge of the humerus.)
- Six muscles of the anterior forearm attach onto the medial epicondyle of the humerus: the pronator teres, flexor carpi radialis, palmaris longus, flexor carpi ulnaris, flexor digitorum superficialis (all via the common flexor tendon) and the flexor pollicis longus. (The pronator teres also attaches onto the medial supracondylar ridge of the humerus.)
- The flexor carpi radialis, palmaris longus and the flexor carpi ulnaris are often grouped together as the *wrist flexors*.
- The extensor carpi radialis longus, extensor carpi radialis brevis and the extensor carpi ulnaris are often grouped together as the *wrist extensors*.

Functionally, the muscles of the forearm cross either the wrist joint and/or the elbow joint and/or the radioulnar joints. Therefore, the muscles of the forearm have their actions at these joints. The following general rules regarding actions can be stated for muscles of the forearm:

- If a muscle crosses the elbow joint anteriorly, it can flex the forearm at the elbow joint.
- If a muscle crosses the elbow joint posteriorly, it can extend the forearm at the elbow joint.
- If a muscle crosses the wrist joint anteriorly, it can flex the hand at the wrist joint.
- If a muscle crosses the wrist joint posteriorly, it can extend the hand at the wrist joint.
- If a muscle crosses the wrist joint radially (laterally), it can radially deviate (abduct) the hand at the wrist joint.
- If a muscle crosses the wrist joint on the ulnar side (medially), it can ulnar deviate (adduct) the hand at the wrist joint.
- If a muscle crosses the radioulnar joints anteriorly with a horizontal orientation to its fibers, it will pronate the forearm at the radioulnar joints; if it crosses the radioulnar joints posteriorly with a horizontal direction to its fibers, it will supinate the forearm at the radioulnar joints.
- Some muscles of the forearm also cross joints in the hand and can move the fingers (at the carpometacarpal and/or metacarpophalangeal and interphalangeal joints.)

INNERVATION

- The muscles of the posterior forearm and the brachioradialis are innervated by the radial nerve.
- The muscles of the anterior forearm are innervated by the median nerve (except the flexor carpi ulnaris and part of the flexor digitorum profundus, which are innervated by the ulnar nerve).

ARTERIAL SUPPLY

- The superficial and intermediate muscles of the anterior forearm (except the brachioradialis) receive their arterial supply from the ulnar and radial arteries.
- The deep muscles of the anterior forearm receive their arterial supply from the ulnar, radial and anterior interosseus arteries.
- The lateral group (radial group) of forearm muscles (brachioradialis, extensor carpi radialis longus and extensor carpi radialis brevis) receive their arterial supply from the brachial and radial arteries.
- The extensor digitorum, extensor digiti minimi and the extensor carpi ulnaris receive their arterial supply from the posterior interosseus artery.
- The majority of the arterial supply to the muscles of the deep posterior forearm is supplied by the posterior interosseus artery.

A NOTE REGARDING REVERSE ACTIONS

As a rule, this book does not employ the terms "origin" and "insertion." However, it is useful to utilize these terms to describe the concept of "reverse actions." The action section of this book describes the action of a muscle by stating the movement of a body part that is created by a muscle's contraction. The body part that usually moves when a muscle contracts is called the insertion. The methodology section further states at which joint the movement of the insertion occurs. However, the other body part that the muscle attaches to, the origin, can also move at that joint. *This movement can be called the reverse action of the muscle.* Keep in mind that the reverse action of a muscle is always possible. The likelihood that a reverse action will occur is based upon the ability of the insertion to be fixed so that the origin moves (instead of the insertion moving) when the muscle contracts. For more information and examples of reverse actions, see page 702.

❑ ANTERIOR VIEW OF THE BONES AND BONY LANDMARKS OF THE RIGHT FOREARM

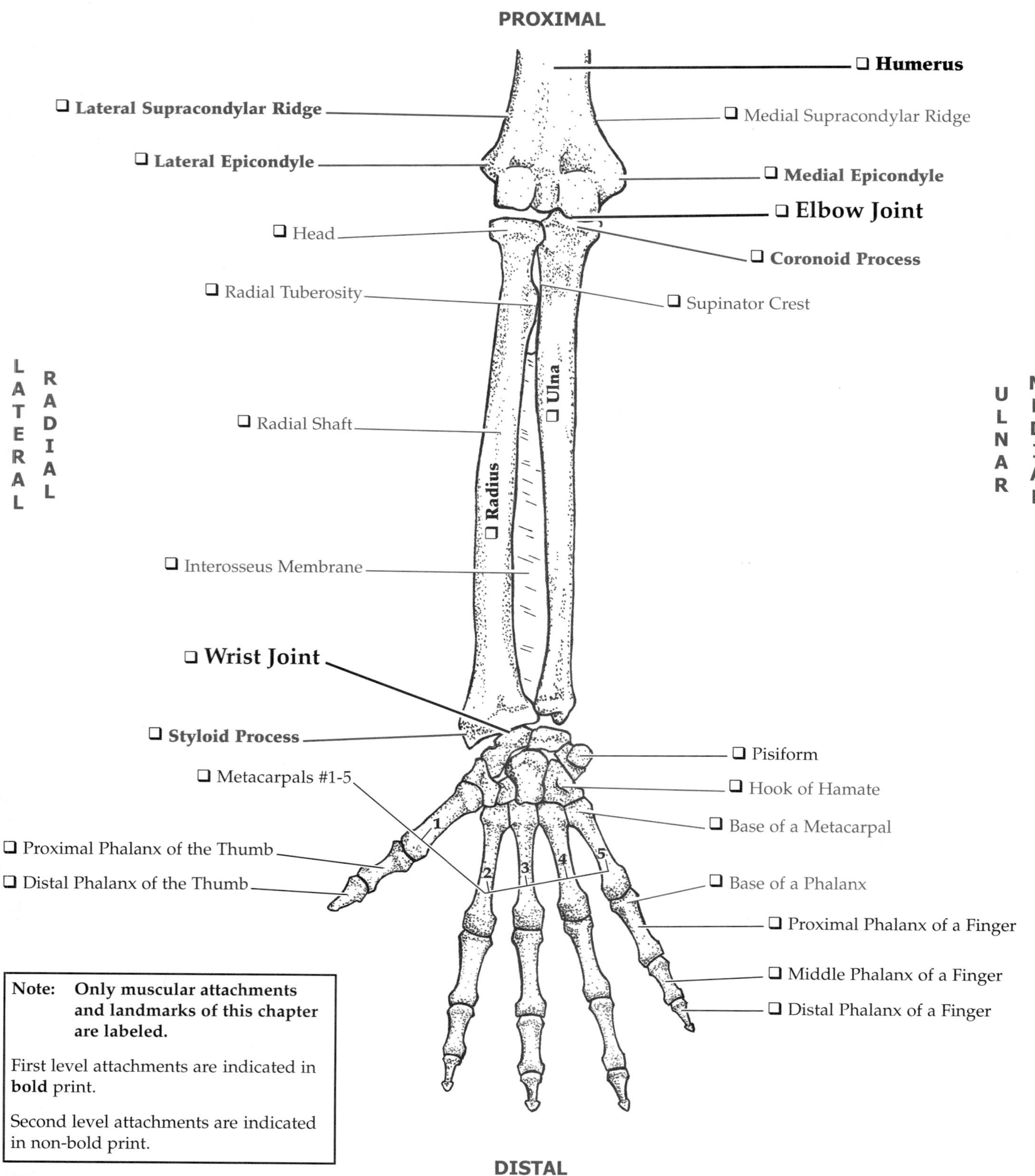

Note: **Only muscular attachments and landmarks of this chapter are labeled.**

First level attachments are indicated in **bold** print.

Second level attachments are indicated in non-bold print.

ANTERIOR VIEW OF THE BONY ATTACHMENTS OF THE RIGHT FOREARM

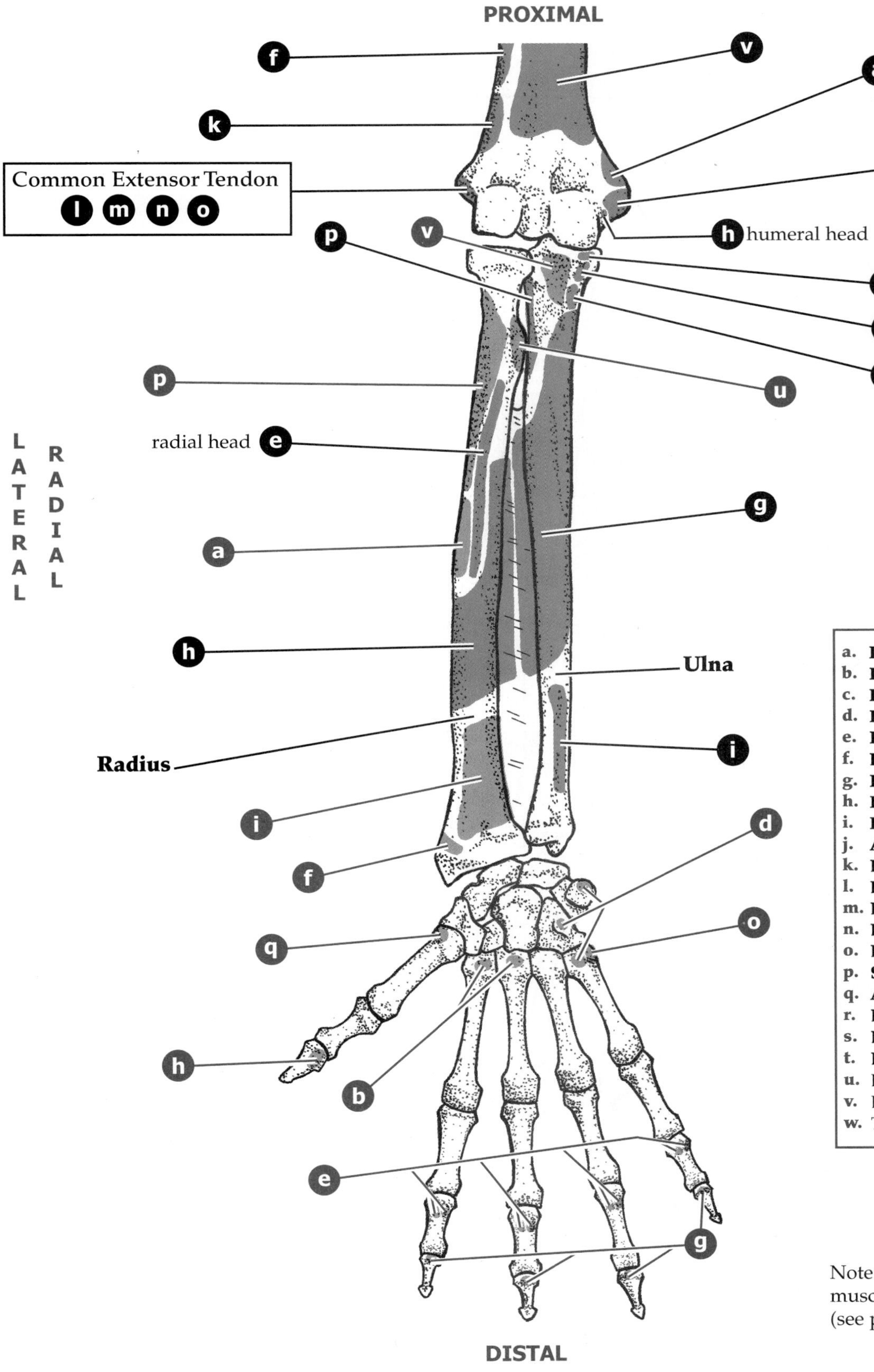

a. **Pronator Teres**
b. **Flexor Carpi Radialis**
c. **Palmaris Longus**
d. **Flexor Carpi Ulnaris**
e. **Flexor Digitorum Superficialis**
f. **Brachioradialis**
g. **Flexor Digitorum Profundus**
h. **Flexor Pollicis Longus**
i. **Pronator Quadratus**
j. **Anconeus** (not seen)
k. **Extensor Carpi Radialis Longus**
l. **Extensor Carpi Radialis Brevis**
m. **Extensor Digitorum**
n. **Extensor Digiti Minimi**
o. **Extensor Carpi Ulnaris**
p. **Supinator**
q. **Abductor Pollicis Longus**
r. **Extensor Pollicis Brevis** (not seen)
s. **Extensor Pollicis Longus** (not seen)
t. **Extensor Indicis** (not seen)
u. Biceps Brachii
v. Brachialis
w. Triceps Brachii (not seen)

Proximal Attachment
Distal Attachment

Note: The attachments of the intrinsic muscles of the hand are not shown (see page 629).

POSTERIOR VIEW OF THE BONES AND BONY LANDMARKS OF THE RIGHT FOREARM

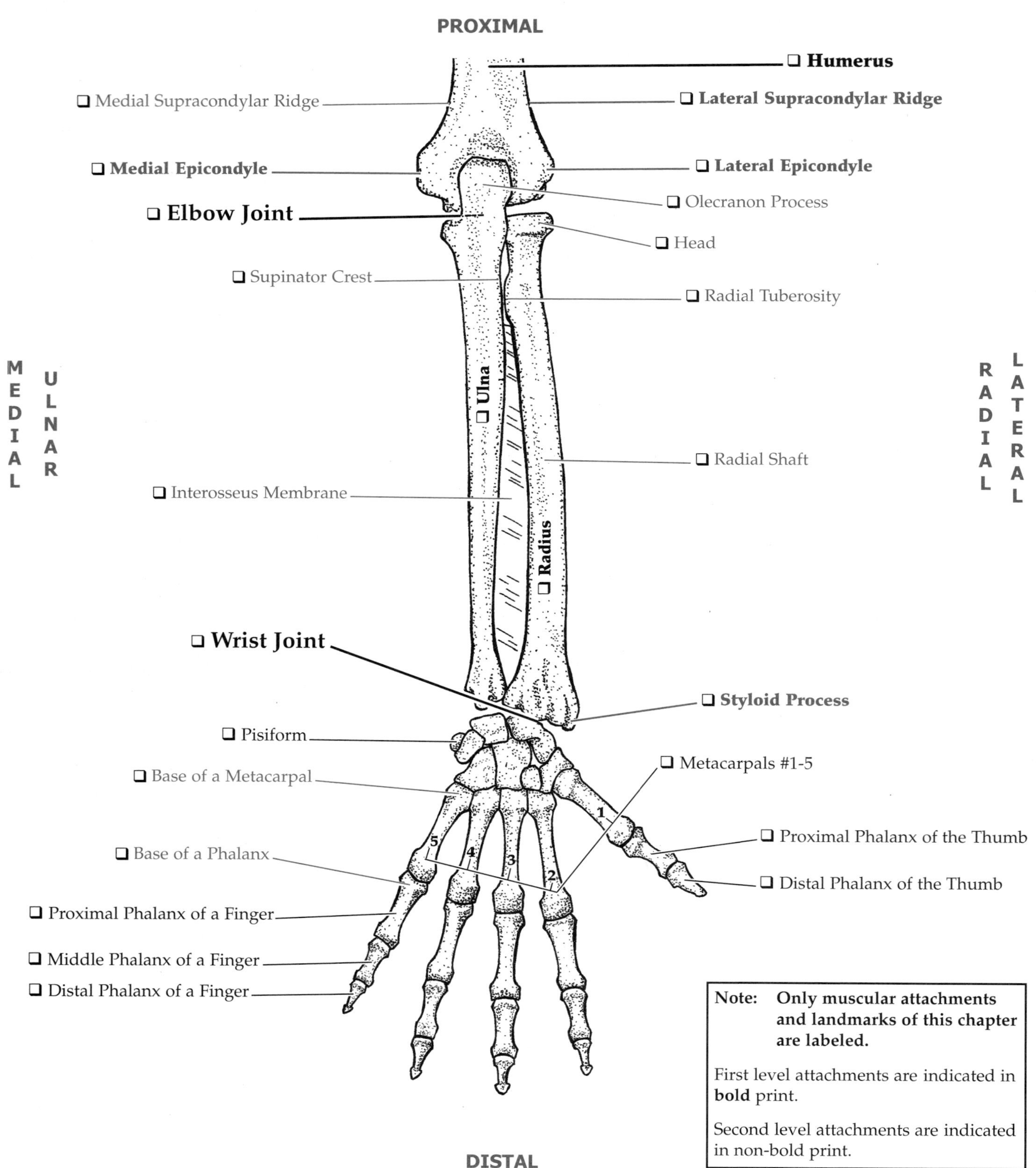

Note: Only muscular attachments and landmarks of this chapter are labeled.

First level attachments are indicated in **bold** print.

Second level attachments are indicated in non-bold print.

POSTERIOR VIEW OF THE BONY ATTACHMENTS OF THE RIGHT FOREARM

a. **Pronator Teres**
b. **Flexor Carpi Radialis** (not seen)
c. **Palmaris Longus** (not seen)
d. **Flexor Carpi Ulnaris**
e. **Flexor Digitorum Superficialis** (not seen)
f. **Brachioradialis**
g. **Flexor Digitorum Profundus**
h. **Flexor Pollicis Longus** (not seen)
i. **Pronator Quadratus** (not seen)
j. **Anconeus**
k. **Extensor Carpi Radialis Longus**
l. **Extensor Carpi Radialis Brevis**
m. **Extensor Digitorum**
n. **Extensor Digiti Minimi**
o. **Extensor Carpi Ulnaris**
p. **Supinator**
q. **Abductor Pollicis Longus**
r. **Extensor Pollicis Brevis**
s. **Extensor Pollicis Longus**
t. **Extensor Indicis**
u. Biceps Brachii
v. Brachialis (not seen)
w. Triceps Brachii

Proximal Attachment
Distal Attachment

Note: The attachments of the intrinsic muscles of the hand are not shown (see page 631).

ANTERIOR VIEW OF THE RIGHT FOREARM (SUPERFICIAL)

PROXIMAL

p

o (deep to median nerve and brachial artery from this view)

Median Nerve and Brachial Artery

Radial Artery

Medial Epicondyle of the Humerus

n Bicipital Aponeurosis

j

LATERAL RADIAL

ULNAR MEDIAL

c

k

e

h

i

m

g

Ulnar Nerve and Artery

Radial Artery

Median Nerve

Transverse Fibers of Palmar Aponeurosis

Thenar Musculature

Hypothenar Musculature

DISTAL

Palmar Aponeurosis

a. **Pronator Teres**
b. **Flexor Carpi Radialis**
c. **Palmaris Longus**
d. **Flexor Carpi Ulnaris**
e. **Flexor Digitorum Superficialis**
f. **Brachioradialis**
g. **Flexor Digitorum Profundus**
h. **Flexor Pollicis Longus**
i. **Pronator Quadratus**
j. **Extensor Carpi Radialis Longus**
k. **Extensor Carpi Radialis Brevis**
l. **Supinator** (not seen)
m. **Abductor Pollicis Longus**
n. Biceps Brachii
o. Brachialis
p. Triceps Brachii (medial head)

ANTERIOR VIEW OF THE RIGHT FOREARM (INTERMEDIATE)

a. **Pronator Teres** (cut)
b. **Flexor Carpi Radialis** (cut)
c. **Palmaris Longus** (cut)
d. **Flexor Carpi Ulnaris**
e. **Flexor Digitorum Superficialis**
f. **Brachioradialis**
g. **Flexor Digitorum Profundus**
h. **Flexor Pollicis Longus**
i. **Pronator Quadratus**
j. **Extensor Carpi Radialis Longus** (not seen)
k. **Extensor Carpi Radialis Brevis** (not seen)
l. **Supinator**
m. **Abductor Pollicis Longus**
n. Biceps Brachii
o. Brachialis
p. Triceps Brachii (medial head)

ANTERIOR VIEW OF THE RIGHT FOREARM (DEEP)

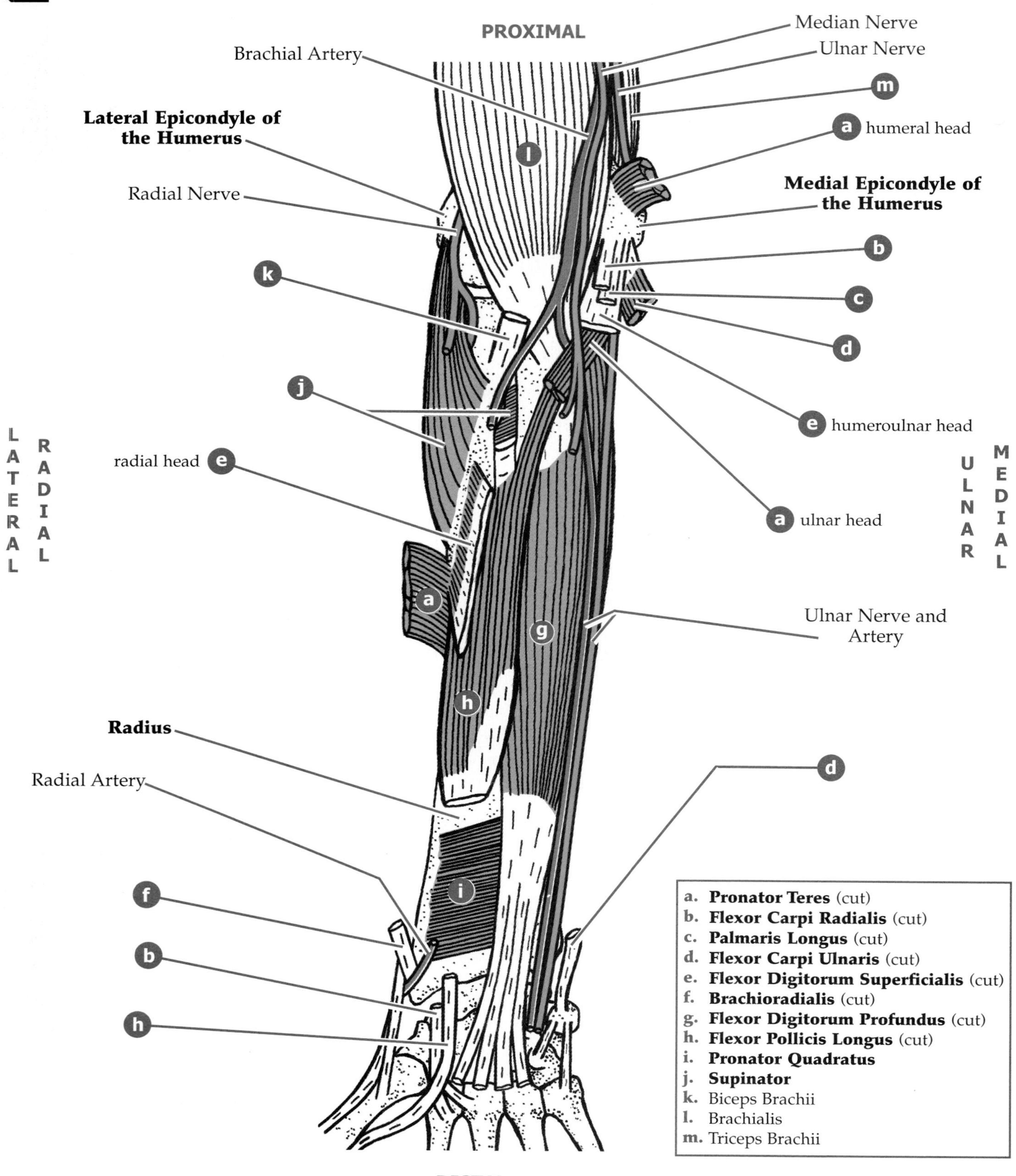
PROXIMAL
Brachial Artery
Median Nerve
Ulnar Nerve
m
a humeral head
Lateral Epicondyle of the Humerus
Medial Epicondyle of the Humerus
Radial Nerve
l
b
k
c
d
j
e humeroulnar head
LATERAL
RADIAL
radial head e
ULNAR
MEDIAL
a ulnar head
a
g
Ulnar Nerve and Artery
h
Radius
d
Radial Artery
i
f
b
h
DISTAL
a. Pronator Teres (cut)
b. Flexor Carpi Radialis (cut)
c. Palmaris Longus (cut)
d. Flexor Carpi Ulnaris (cut)
e. Flexor Digitorum Superficialis (cut)
f. Brachioradialis (cut)
g. Flexor Digitorum Profundus (cut)
h. Flexor Pollicis Longus (cut)
i. Pronator Quadratus
j. Supinator
k. Biceps Brachii
l. Brachialis
m. Triceps Brachii

ANTERIOR VIEWS OF THE PRONATORS AND SUPINATOR OF THE RIGHT RADIUS

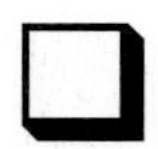

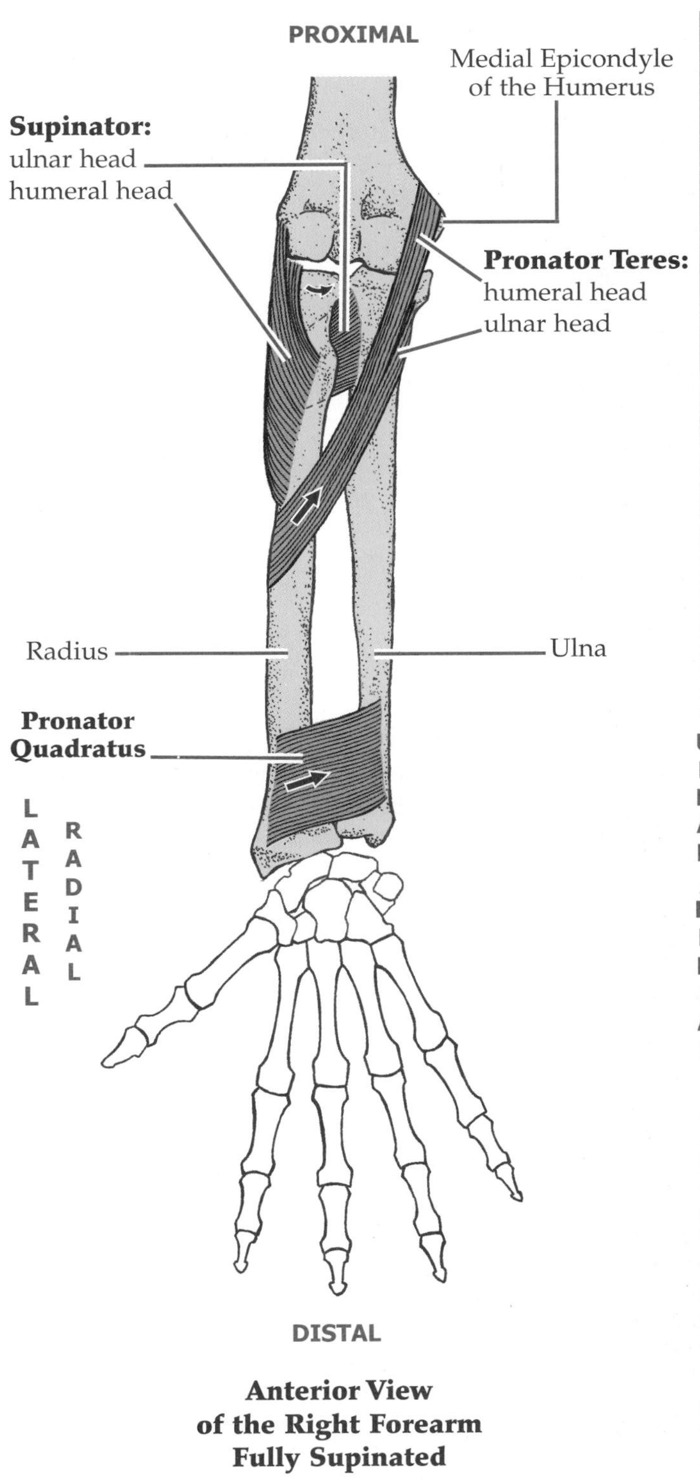

Anterior View of the Right Forearm Fully Supinated

ULNAR/MEDIAL

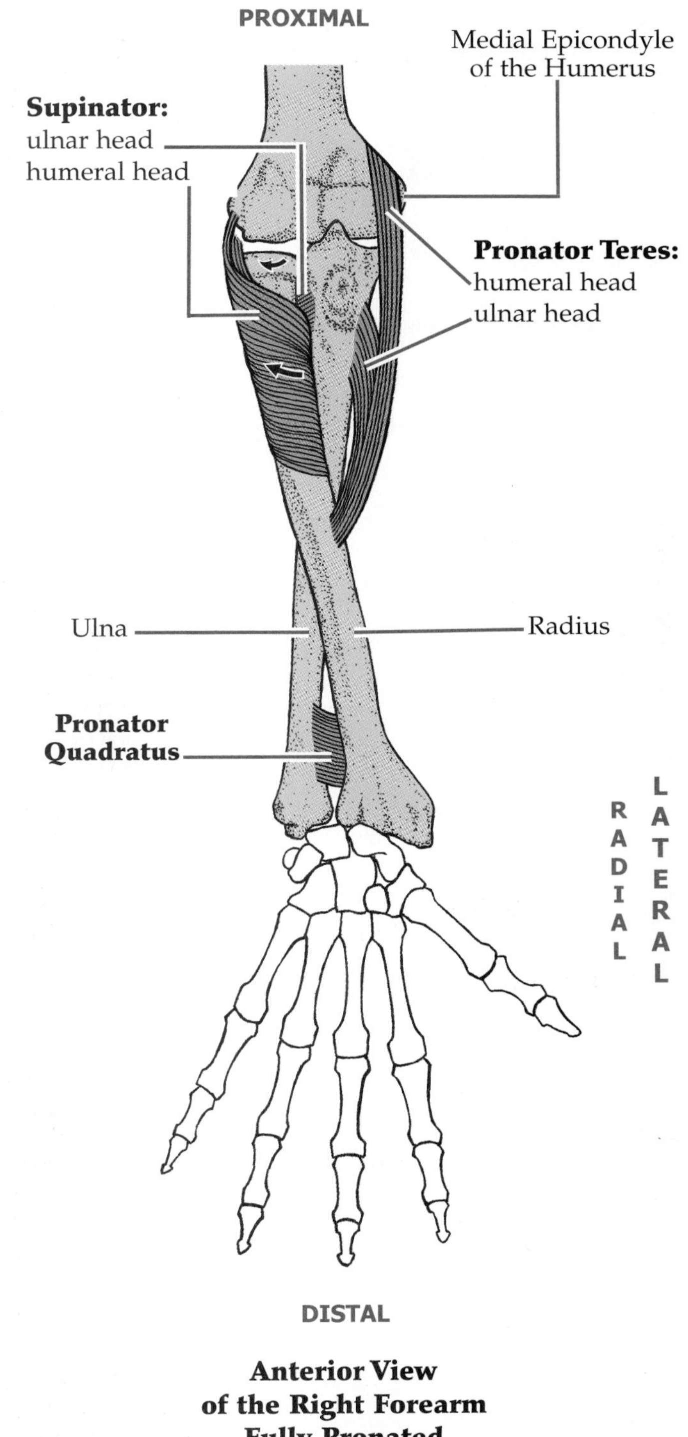

Anterior View of the Right Forearm Fully Pronated

❑ POSTERIOR VIEW OF THE RIGHT FOREARM (SUPERFICIAL)

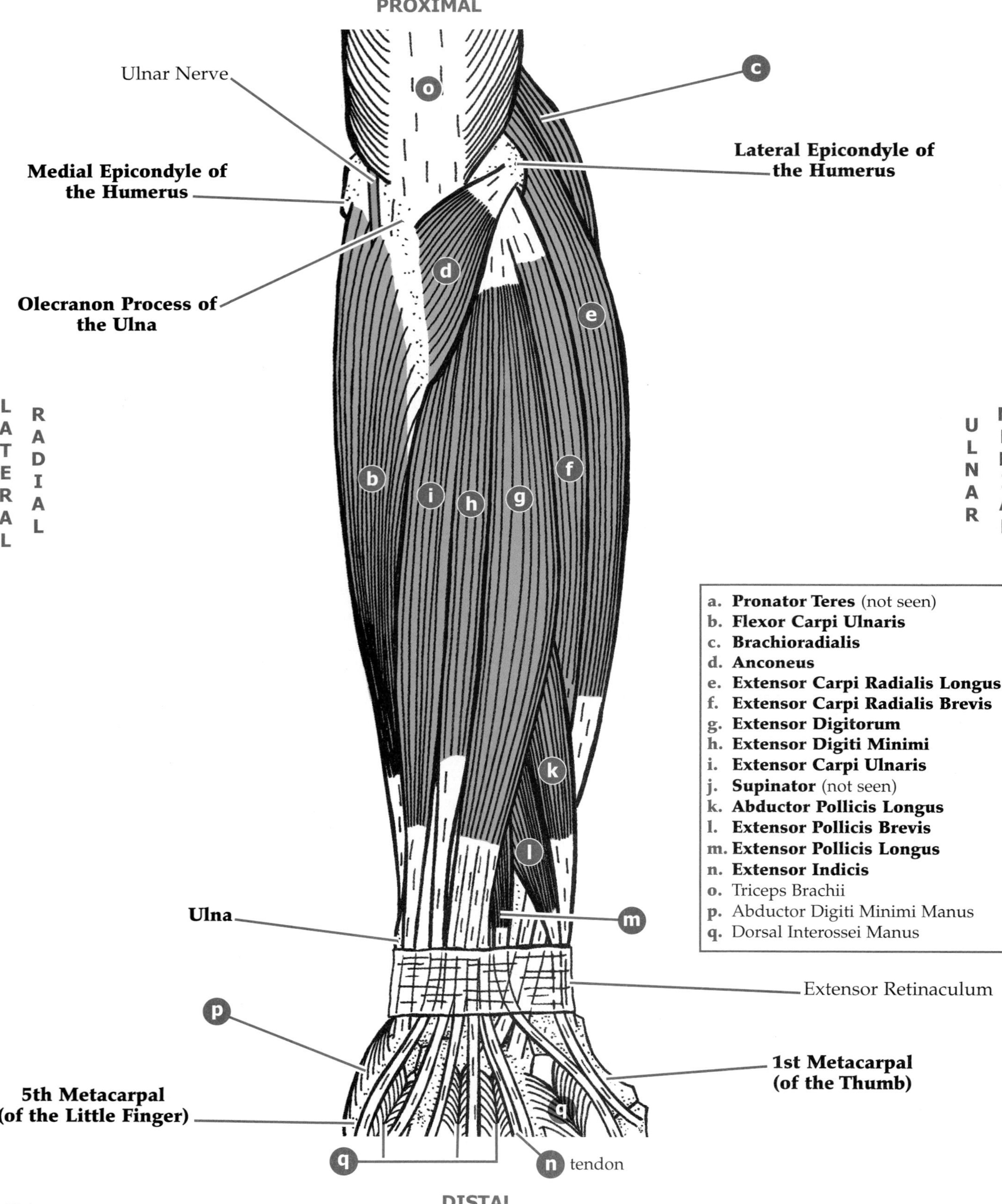
PROXIMAL
Ulnar Nerve
Medial Epicondyle of the Humerus
Olecranon Process of the Ulna
Lateral Epicondyle of the Humerus
LATERAL
RADIAL
ULNAR
MEDIAL
o
c
d
e
b
i
h
g
f
k
l
m
Ulna
Extensor Retinaculum
p
1st Metacarpal (of the Thumb)
5th Metacarpal (of the Little Finger)
q
n tendon
DISTAL
a. Pronator Teres (not seen)
b. Flexor Carpi Ulnaris
c. Brachioradialis
d. Anconeus
e. Extensor Carpi Radialis Longus
f. Extensor Carpi Radialis Brevis
g. Extensor Digitorum
h. Extensor Digiti Minimi
i. Extensor Carpi Ulnaris
j. Supinator (not seen)
k. Abductor Pollicis Longus
l. Extensor Pollicis Brevis
m. Extensor Pollicis Longus
n. Extensor Indicis
o. Triceps Brachii
p. Abductor Digiti Minimi Manus
q. Dorsal Interossei Manus

POSTERIOR VIEW OF THE RIGHT FOREARM (DEEP)

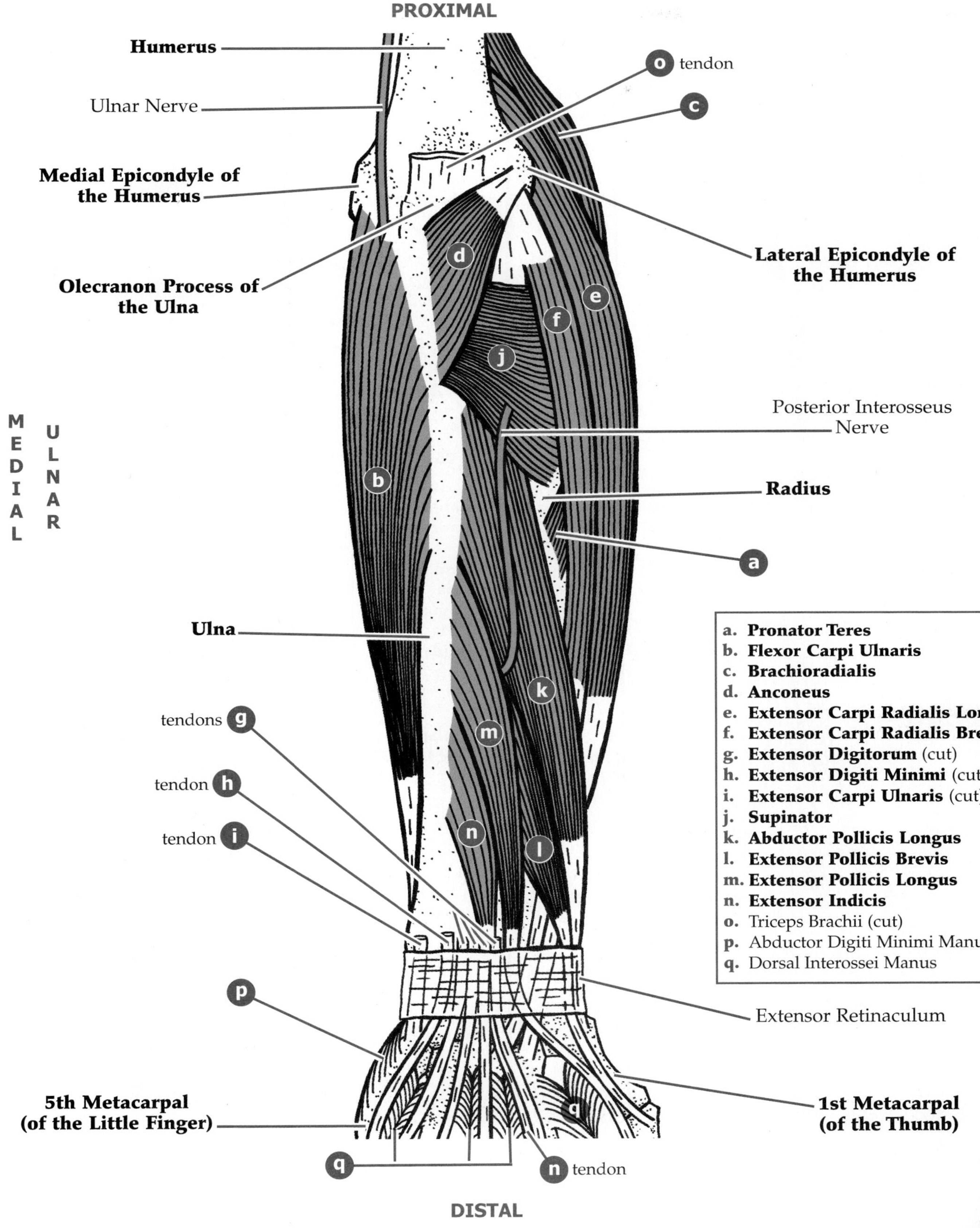

PROXIMAL

Humerus

Ulnar Nerve

Medial Epicondyle of the Humerus

Olecranon Process of the Ulna

o tendon

c

Lateral Epicondyle of the Humerus

d e f j b

MEDIAL ULNAR

Posterior Interosseus Nerve

Radius

a

RADIAL LATERAL

Ulna

tendons g

tendon h

tendon i

k m n l

- a. **Pronator Teres**
- b. **Flexor Carpi Ulnaris**
- c. **Brachioradialis**
- d. **Anconeus**
- e. **Extensor Carpi Radialis Longus**
- f. **Extensor Carpi Radialis Brevis**
- g. **Extensor Digitorum** (cut)
- h. **Extensor Digiti Minimi** (cut)
- i. **Extensor Carpi Ulnaris** (cut)
- j. **Supinator**
- k. **Abductor Pollicis Longus**
- l. **Extensor Pollicis Brevis**
- m. **Extensor Pollicis Longus**
- n. **Extensor Indicis**
- o. Triceps Brachii (cut)
- p. Abductor Digiti Minimi Manus
- q. Dorsal Interossei Manus

p

Extensor Retinaculum

5th Metacarpal (of the Little Finger)

1st Metacarpal (of the Thumb)

q

q

n tendon

DISTAL

❑ POSTERIOR VIEWS OF THE RIGHT FOREARM AND HAND

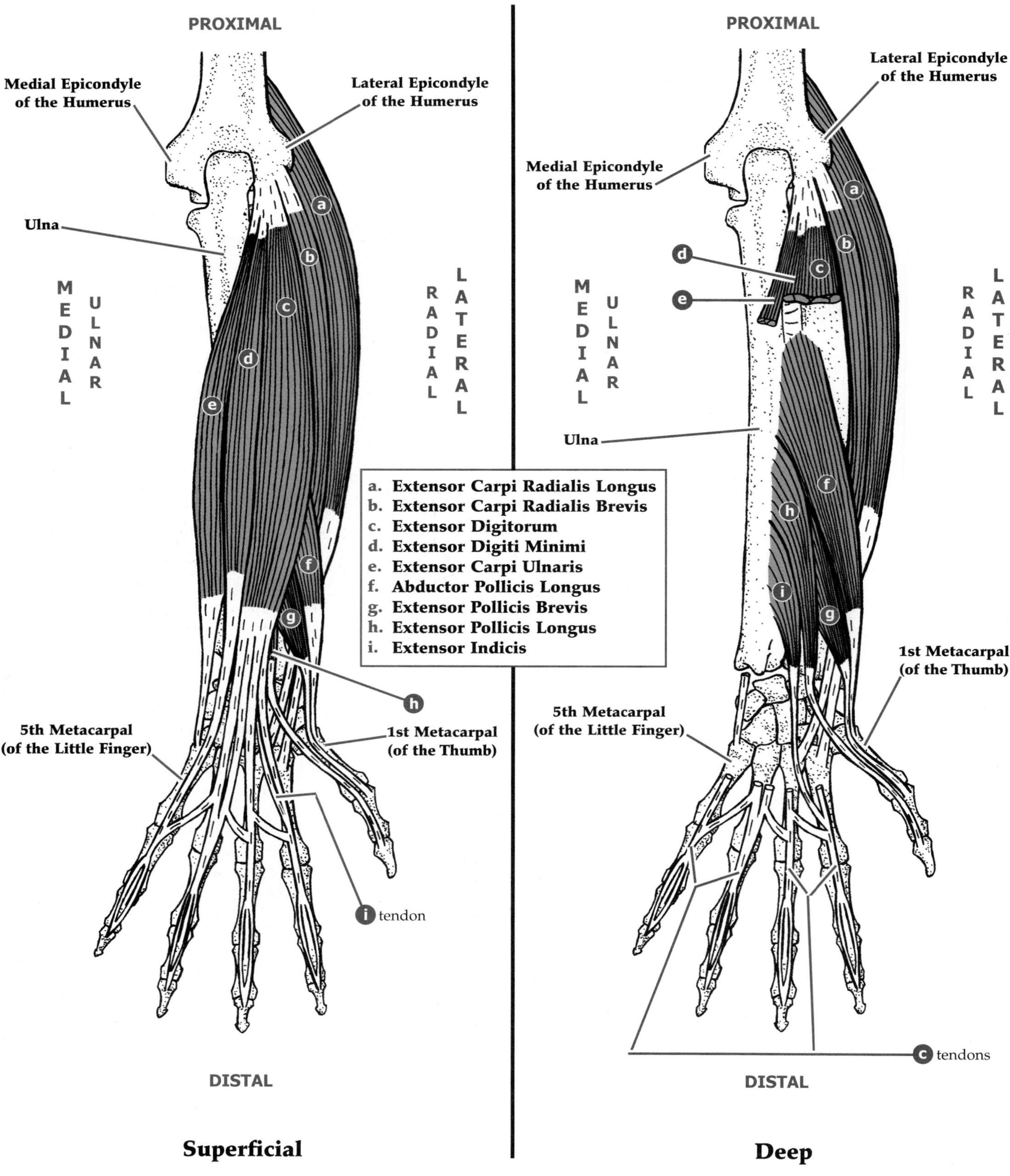

a. Extensor Carpi Radialis Longus
b. Extensor Carpi Radialis Brevis
c. Extensor Digitorum
d. Extensor Digiti Minimi
e. Extensor Carpi Ulnaris
f. Abductor Pollicis Longus
g. Extensor Pollicis Brevis
h. Extensor Pollicis Longus
i. Extensor Indicis

Superficial **Deep**

CROSS SECTION VIEWS OF THE RIGHT FOREARM

Muscles
- a. **Pronator Teres**
- b. **Flexor Carpi Radialis**
- c. **Palmaris Longus**
- d. **Flexor Carpi Ulnaris**
- e. **Flexor Digitorum Superficialis**
- f. **Brachioradialis**
- g. **Flexor Digitorum Profundus**
- h. **Flexor Pollicis Longus**
- i. **Pronator Quadratus**
- j. **Anconeus**
- k. **Extensor Carpi Radialis Longus**
- l. **Extensor Carpi Radialis Brevis**
- m. **Extensor Digitorum**
- n. **Extensor Digiti Minimi**
- o. **Extensor Carpi Ulnaris**
- p. **Supinator**
- q. **Abductor Pollicis Longus**
- r. **Extensor Pollicis Brevis**
- s. **Extensor Pollicis Longus**
- t. **Extensor Indicis**

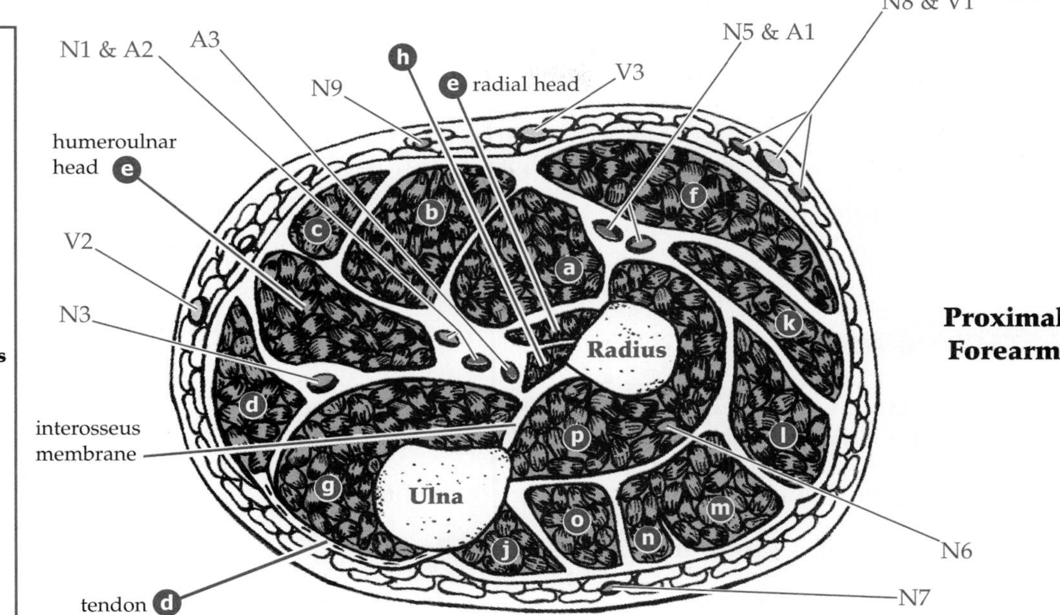

Nerves
- N1. **Median**
- N2. **Anterior Interosseus**
- N3. **Ulnar**
- N4. **Dorsal Branch of Ulnar**
- N5. **Superficial Branch of Radial**
- N6. **Posterior Interosseus**
- N7. **Posterior Antebrachial Cutaneous**
- N8. **Lateral Antebrachial Cutaneous**
- N9. **Anterior Branch of Medial Antebrachial Cutaneous**

Arteries
- A1. **Radial**
- A2. **Ulnar**
- A3. **Common Interosseus**
- A4. **Anterior Interosseus**
- A5. **Posterior Interosseus**

Veins
- V1. **Cephalic**
- V2. **Basilic**
- V3. **Median Antebrachial**

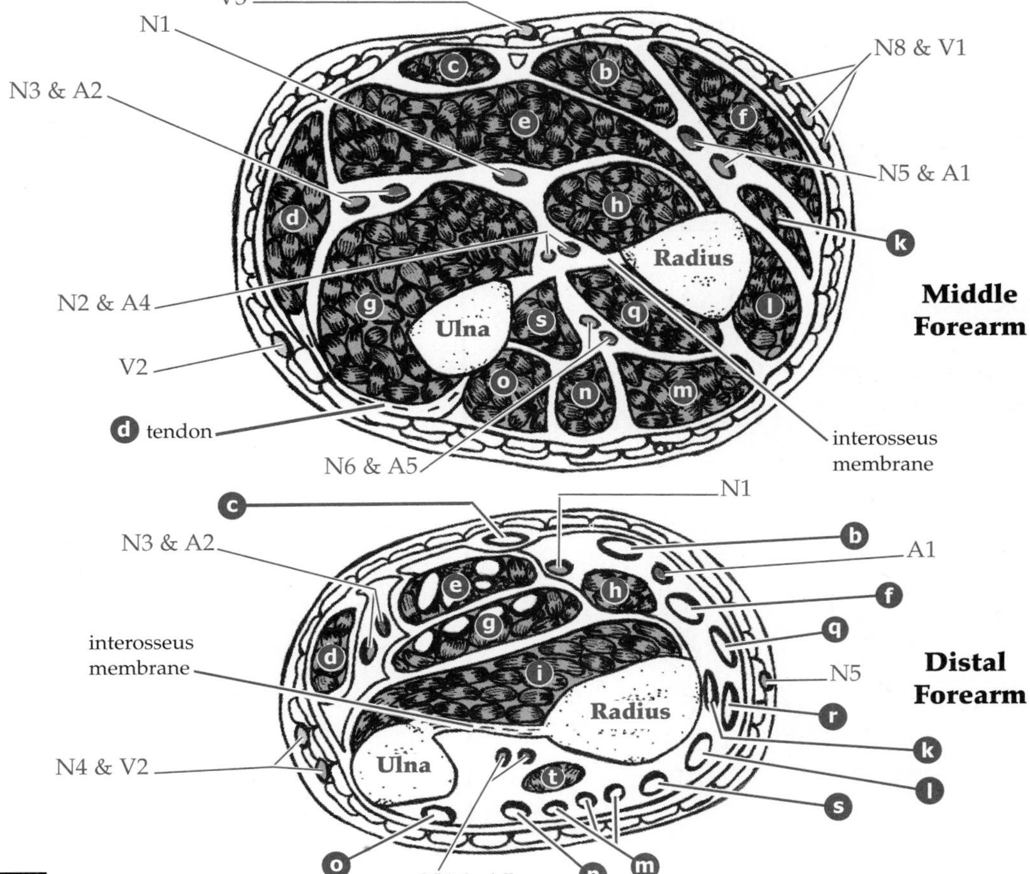

Perspective:
Left is medial and right is lateral.
Top is anterior and bottom is posterior.

PRONATOR TERES

❑ **The name, pronator teres, tells us that this muscle pronates the forearm and is round in shape.**

DERIVATION ❑ pronator: L. *a muscle that pronates a body part.*
teres: L. *round.*

PRONUNCIATION ❑ pro-**nay**-tor **te**-reez

ATTACHMENTS

❑ **HUMERAL HEAD: Medial Epicondyle of the Humerus (via the Common Flexor Tendon)**

❑ and the medial supracondylar ridge of the humerus

❑ **ULNAR HEAD: Coronoid Process of the Ulna**

❑ the medial surface

to the

❑ **Lateral Radius**

❑ the middle 1/3

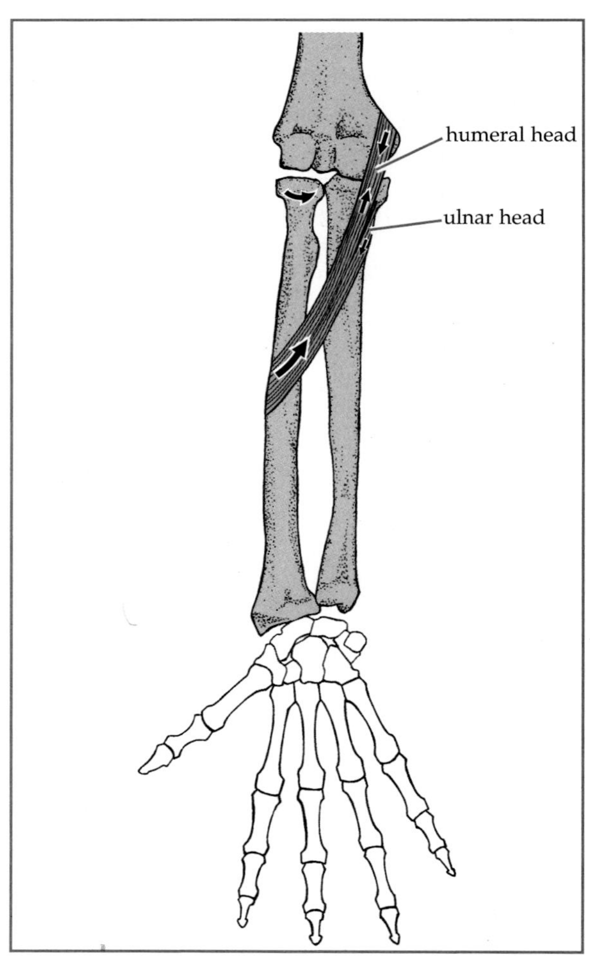

Anterior View of the Right Pronator Teres

ACTIONS

❑ 1. **Pronation of the Forearm**

❑ 2. **Flexion of the Forearm**

INNERVATION ❑ The Median Nerve ❑ C6, **7**

ARTERIAL SUPPLY ❑ The Ulnar Artery (A Terminal Branch of the Brachial Artery)
❑ and the radial artery (a terminal branch of the brachial artery)

PALPATION AND SUPPLEMENTARY TEXT

PALPATION

- ❑ The proximal attachment and the muscle belly of the pronator teres are superficial and easy to palpate, but the distal attachment is deep to the brachioradialis.
  - Have the client seated with the forearm partially flexed at the elbow joint and pronated at the radioulnar joints to a midpoint between full pronation and full supination.
  - Place palpating hand on the lateral forearm.
  - Ask the client to further flex or pronate the forearm and feel for the contraction of the pronator teres. The entire humeral head will be palpable.
  - Continue palpating the pronator teres proximally toward the medial epicondyle of the humerus and distally toward the lateral radius.
  - To further bring out the pronator teres, resistance may be added.

see page 554

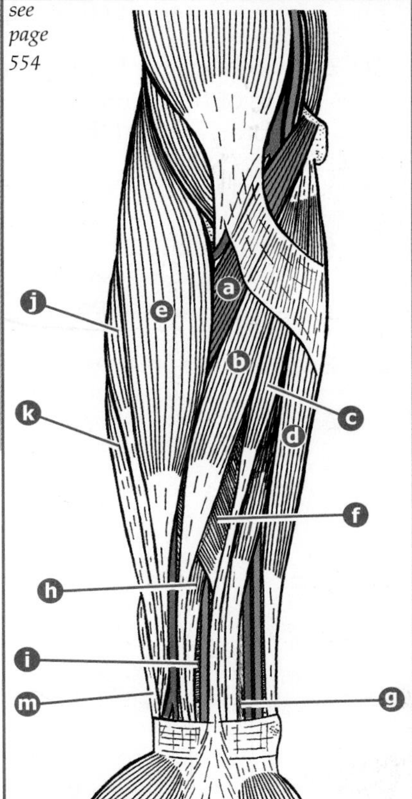

Anterior View of the Right Forearm (Superficial)

a. Pronator Teres
b. Flexor Carpi Radialis
c. Palmaris Longus
d. Flexor Carpi Ulnaris
e. Brachioradialis
f. Flexor Digitorum Superficialis
g. Flexor Digitorum Profundus
h. Flexor Pollicis Longus
i. Pronator Quadratus
j. Extensor Carpi Radialis Longus
k. Extensor Carpi Radialis Brevis
l. Supinator (not seen)
m. Abductor Pollicis Longus

RELATIONSHIP TO OTHER MUSCULOSKELETAL STRUCTURES

❑ 1. The proximal part of the pronator teres is superficial in the proximal anterior forearm, but the distal attachment is deep to the brachioradialis.

❑ 2. The ulnar head of the pronator teres is entirely deep or nearly entirely deep to the humeral head of the pronator teres.

❑ 3. The pronator teres is lateral to the flexor carpi radialis.

❑ 4. The pronator teres is largely superficial to the flexor digitorum superficialis.

METHODOLOGY FOR LEARNING MUSCLE ACTIONS

❑ **1. Pronation of the Forearm at the Radioulnar Joints:** The pronator teres crosses from the medial elbow region to the lateral (radial) side of the forearm onto the radius (with its fibers running somewhat horizontally in the transverse plane), crossing the radioulnar joints anteriorly. When it contracts, it pulls the lateral attachment (the radius) anteromedially. This causes the head of the radius to medially rotate and the distal radius to cross in front of the ulna. This movement of the radius is called pronation. Therefore, the pronator teres pronates the forearm at the radioulnar joints.

❑ **2. Flexion of the Forearm at the Elbow Joint:** The pronator teres crosses the elbow joint anteriorly (with its fibers running running vertically in the sagittal plane); therefore, it flexes the forearm at the elbow joint.

PRONATOR TERES – continued

MISCELLANEOUS

- ❑ 1. The humeral head of the pronator teres arises proximally from the medial epicondyle of the humerus by the *common flexor tendon.* The common flexor tendon is the common proximal attachment of five muscles: the pronator teres, flexor carpi radialis, palmaris longus, flexor carpi ulnaris and the flexor digitorum superficialis.
- ❑ 2. Although the humeral head of the pronator teres is part of the common flexor tendon, the actual attachment site of the humeral head of the pronator teres onto the medial epicondyle of the humerus is slightly more proximal than the attachment of the other four muscles of the common flexor tendon.
- ❑ 3. The humeral head of the pronator teres is by far the larger of the two heads.
- ❑ 4. The median nerve courses between the humeral head and the ulnar head of the pronator teres, making it a possible entrapment site of the median nerve. When the median nerve is entrapped there, it is termed *pronator teres syndrome* (and may mimic symptoms of *carpal tunnel syndrome*).
- ❑ 5. Irritation and inflammation of the medial epicondyle and/or the common flexor tendon is known as *medial epicondylitis* and is usually called *golfer's elbow* (and occasionally called *tennis elbow).*

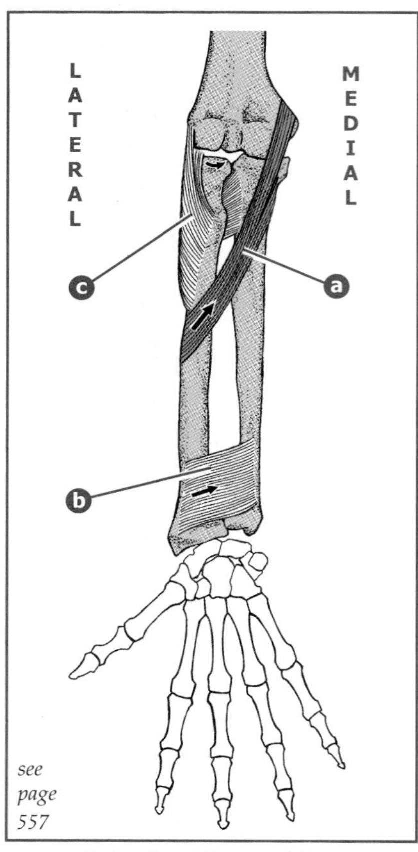

see page 557

Anterior View of the Right Forearm Fully Supinated

a. **Pronator Teres**
b. Pronator Quadratus
c. Supinator

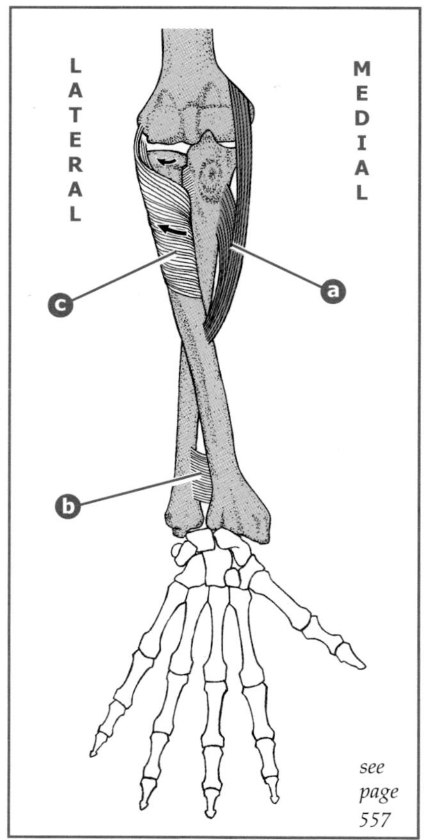

see page 557

Anterior View of the Right Forearm Fully Pronated

a. **Pronator Teres**
b. Pronator Quadratus
c. Supinator

FLEXOR CARPI RADIALIS
(OF THE WRIST FLEXOR GROUP)

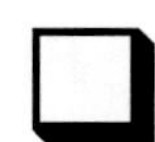

❑ **The name, flexor carpi radialis, tells us two of its actions: "flexor" tells us that this muscle performs flexion and "radialis" tells us that this muscle performs radial deviation (abduction). Both of these actions occur at the wrist; "carpi" means wrist.**

DERIVATION ❑ flexor: L. *a muscle that flexes a body part.*
carpi: L. *wrist.*
radialis: L. *refers to the radial side* (of the forearm).

PRONUNCIATION ❑ **fleks**-or **kar**-pie **ray**-dee-**a**-lis

ATTACHMENTS

❑ **Medial Epicondyle of the Humerus (via the Common Flexor Tendon)**

to the

❑ **Radial Hand on the Anterior Side**

- ❑ the anterior side of the bases of the 2nd and 3rd metacarpals

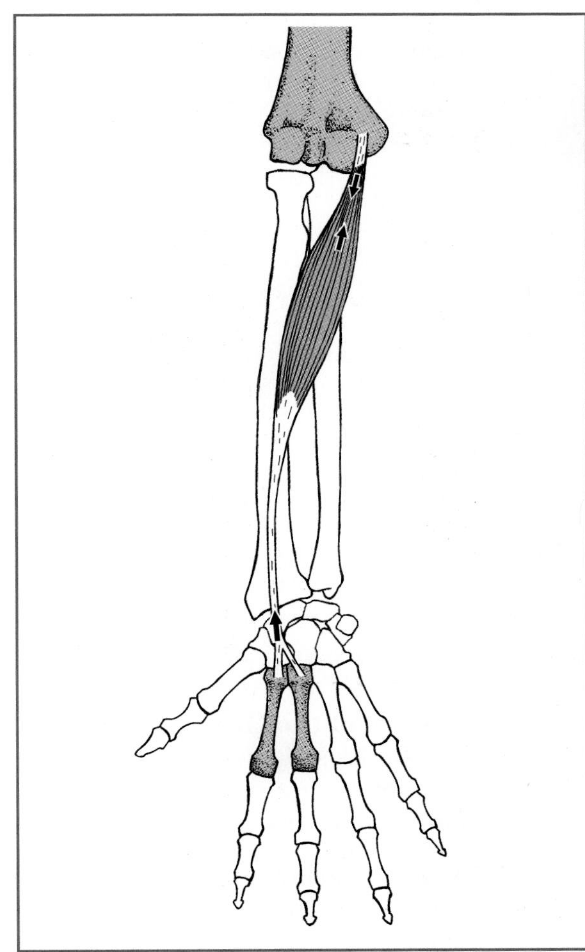

Anterior View of the Right Flexor Carpi Radialis

ACTIONS

❑ **1. Flexion of the Hand**

❑ **2. Radial Deviation (Abduction) of the Hand**

❑ **3.** Flexion of the Forearm

❑ **4.** Pronation of the Forearm

INNERVATION ❑ The Median Nerve ❑ C6, 7

ARTERIAL SUPPLY ❑ The Ulnar and Radial Arteries (Terminal Branches of the Brachial Artery)

FLEXOR CARPI RADIALIS – PALPATION AND SUPPLEMENTARY TEXT

PALPATION

❑ The distal tendon of the flexor carpi radialis is easy to palpate in the distal forearm and wrist. However, the distal attachment at the 2nd and 3rd metacarpals is extremely difficult to palpate because it runs deep to the oblique head of the adductor pollicis.

- Have the client seated or supine.
- Place palpating hand across the anterior wrist.
- Ask the client to actively flex and radially deviate (abduct) the hand at the wrist joint and feel for the distal tendon of the flexor carpi radialis on the radial (lateral) side (lateral to the distal tendon of the palmaris longus, see the palpation section for this muscle on page 569).
- Continue palpating the flexor carpi radialis proximally toward the medial epicondyle of the humerus.
- To further bring out the flexor carpi radialis, resistance may be added.

see page 554

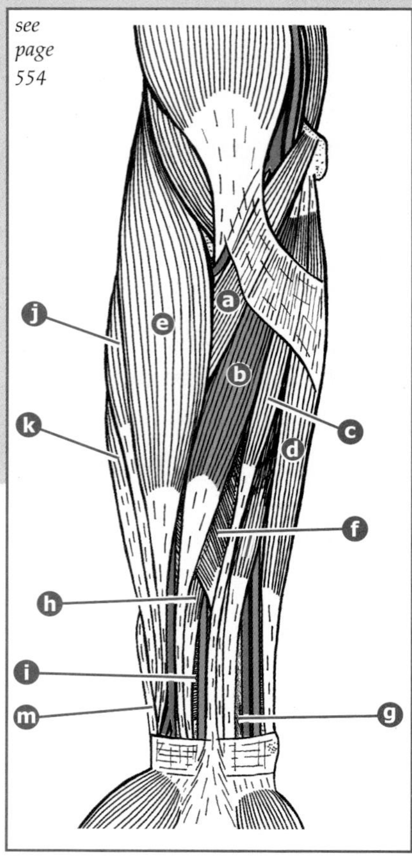

Anterior View of the Right Forearm (Superficial)

a. Pronator Teres
b. **Flexor Carpi Radialis**
c. Palmaris Longus
d. Flexor Carpi Ulnaris
e. Brachioradialis
f. Flexor Digitorum Superficialis
g. Flexor Digitorum Profundus
h. Flexor Pollicis Longus
i. Pronator Quadratus
j. Extensor Carpi Radialis Longus
k. Extensor Carpi Radialis Brevis
l. Supinator (not seen)
m. Abductor Pollicis Longus

RELATIONSHIP TO OTHER MUSCULOSKELETAL STRUCTURES

❑ 1. The flexor carpi radialis is superficial in the anterior forearm.

❑ 2. Proximally, the flexor carpi radialis is medial to the pronator teres. More distally, the flexor carpi radialis is medial to the brachioradialis.

❑ 3. The flexor carpi radialis is lateral to the palmaris longus.

❑ 4. The flexor carpi radialis is superficial to the flexor digitorum superficialis.

METHODOLOGY FOR LEARNING MUSCLE ACTIONS

❑ 1. **Flexion of the Hand at the Wrist Joint:** The flexor carpi radialis crosses the wrist on the anterior side (with its fibers running vertically in the sagittal plane); therefore, it flexes the hand at the wrist joint.

❑ 2. **Radial Deviation (Abduction) of the Hand at the Wrist Joint:** The flexor carpi radialis crosses the wrist on the radial (lateral) side to attach onto the hand (with its fibers running vertically in the frontal plane); therefore, it radially deviates (abducts) the hand at the wrist joint.

❑ 3. **Flexion of the Forearm at the Elbow Joint:** The flexor carpi radialis crosses the elbow joint anteriorly (with its fibers running vertically in the sagittal plane); therefore, it flexes the forearm at the elbow joint.

FLEXOR CARPI RADIALIS – continued

- ❑ **4. Pronation of the Forearm at the Radioulnar Joints:** The flexor carpi radialis crosses from the medial elbow region to the lateral (radial) side of the hand (with its fibers running somewhat horizontally in the transverse plane). It crosses the radioulnar joints anteriorly in such a way that when it pulls at the lateral hand attachment, it pulls the radial side of the hand anteromedially, thereby pulling the distal radius around the distal ulna (and causing the head of the radius to medially rotate). Therefore, the flexor carpi radialis pronates the forearm at the radioulnar joints.

MISCELLANEOUS

- ❑ 1. The flexor carpi radialis arises proximally from the medial epicondyle of the humerus by the *common flexor tendon*. The common flexor tendon is the common proximal attachment of five muscles: the pronator teres, flexor carpi radialis, palmaris longus, flexor carpi ulnaris and the flexor digitorum superficialis.
- ❑ 2. All three muscles of the wrist flexor group (flexor carpi radialis, palmaris longus and flexor carpi ulnaris) can also flex the forearm at the elbow joint since they cross the elbow joint anteriorly.
- ❑ 3. All three muscles of the wrist flexor group (flexor carpi radialis, palmaris longus and flexor carpi ulnaris) as well as the muscles of the wrist extensor group (extensor carpi radialis longus, extensor carpi radialis brevis and extensor carpi ulnaris) can flex the forearm at the elbow joint except the extensor carpi ulnaris, which extends the forearm at the elbow joint.
- ❑ 4. Irritation and inflammation of the medial epicondyle and/or the common flexor tendon is known as *medial epicondylitis* and is usually called *golfer's elbow* (and occasionally called *tennis elbow).*

PALMARIS LONGUS
(OF THE WRIST FLEXOR GROUP)

❑ **The name, palmaris longus, tells us that this muscle attaches into the palm of the hand and is long (longer than the palmaris brevis).**

DERIVATION ❑ palmaris: L. *refers to the palm.* longus: L. *long.*

PRONUNCIATION ❑ pall-**ma**-ris **long**-us

ATTACHMENTS

❑ **Medial Epicondyle of the Humerus (via the Common Flexor Tendon)**

to the

❑ **Palm of the Hand**

- ❑ the palmar aponeurosis and the flexor retinaculum

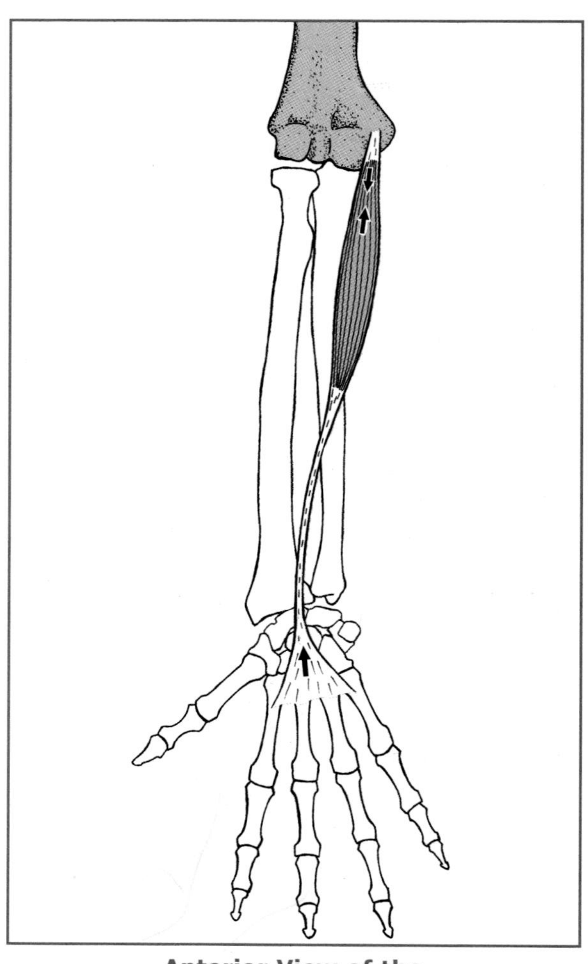

Anterior View of the Right Palmaris Longus

ACTIONS

❑ **1. Flexion of the Hand**

❑ **2.** Flexion of the Forearm

❑ **3.** Pronation of the Forearm

❑ **4.** Wrinkles the Skin of the Palm

INNERVATION ❑ The Median Nerve ❑ C7, 8

ARTERIAL SUPPLY ❑ The Ulnar Artery (A Terminal Branch of the Brachial Artery)

PALPATION AND SUPPLEMENTARY TEXT

PALPATION

- ❑ The palmaris longus is superficial and easy to palpate.
  - Have the client seated or supine.
  - Place palpating hand on the anterior wrist.
  - Ask the client to strongly flex the hand at the wrist joint with the fingers fully extended and feel for the distal tendon of the palmaris longus in the center of the anterior wrist. (Having the fingers extended will cause the flexor digitorum superficialis to relax.)
  - Continue palpating the palmaris longus distally into the palmar fascia and proximally toward the medial epicondyle of the humerus.
  - To further bring out the palmaris longus, resistance may be added.

see page 554

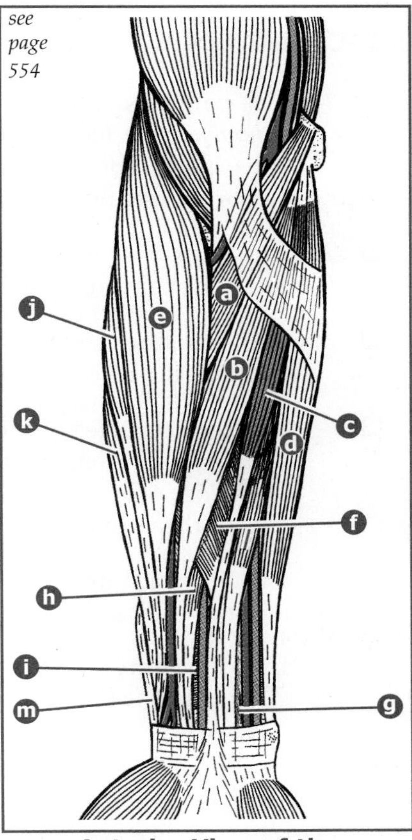

Anterior View of the Right Forearm (Superficial)

a. Pronator Teres
b. Flexor Carpi Radialis
c. **Palmaris Longus**
d. Flexor Carpi Ulnaris
e. Brachioradialis
f. Flexor Digitorum Superficialis
g. Flexor Digitorum Profundus
h. Flexor Pollicis Longus
i. Pronator Quadratus
j. Extensor Carpi Radialis Longus
k. Extensor Carpi Radialis Brevis
l. Supinator (not seen)
m. Abductor Pollicis Longus

RELATIONSHIP TO OTHER MUSCULOSKELETAL STRUCTURES

❑ 1. The palmaris longus is superficial in the anteromedial forearm.

❑ 2. The palmaris longus is medial to the flexor carpi radialis.

❑ 3. Proximally, the palmaris longus is lateral to the flexor carpi ulnaris. More distally, the palmaris longus is lateral to the flexor digitorum superficialis.

METHODOLOGY FOR LEARNING MUSCLE ACTIONS

❑ **1. Flexion of the Hand at the Wrist Joint:** The palmaris longus crosses the wrist on the anterior side (with its fibers running vertically in the sagittal plane); therefore, it flexes the hand at the wrist joint.

❑ **2. Flexion of the Forearm at the Elbow Joint:** The palmaris longus crosses the elbow joint anteriorly (with its fibers running vertically in the sagittal plane); therefore, it flexes the forearm at the elbow joint.

❑ **3. Pronation of the Forearm at the Radioulnar Joints:** The palmaris longus crosses from the medial elbow region to attach more laterally into the palm of the hand. It crosses the radioulnar joints anteriorly in such a way that when it pulls at the more lateral hand attachment, it pulls the radial side of the hand anteromedially, thereby pulling the distal radius around the distal ulna (and causing the head of the radius to medially rotate). Therefore, the palmaris longus pronates the forearm at the radioulnar joints.

❑ **4. Wrinkles the Skin of the Palm:** The palmaris longus attaches distally into the palmar aponeurosis of the hand. When the palmaris longus pulls on the palmar aponeurosis, it causes the skin of the hand to wrinkle. Wrinkling of the skin of the hand helps to create a slightly stronger grip on an object that is being held.

PALMARIS LONGUS – continued

MISCELLANEOUS

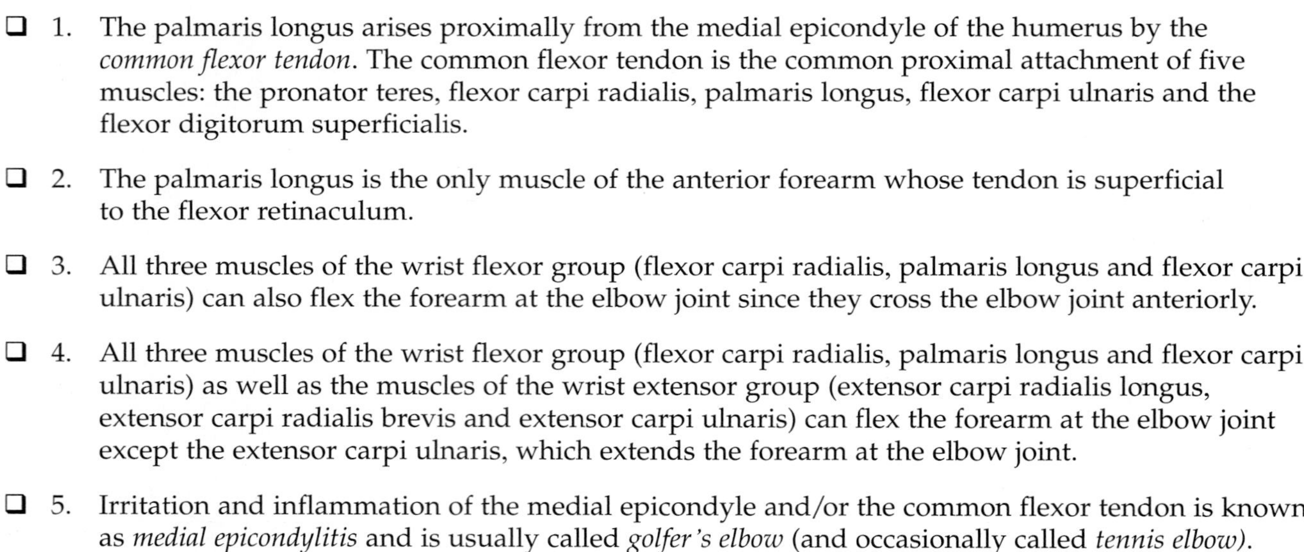

- ❑ 1. The palmaris longus arises proximally from the medial epicondyle of the humerus by the *common flexor tendon*. The common flexor tendon is the common proximal attachment of five muscles: the pronator teres, flexor carpi radialis, palmaris longus, flexor carpi ulnaris and the flexor digitorum superficialis.
- ❑ 2. The palmaris longus is the only muscle of the anterior forearm whose tendon is superficial to the flexor retinaculum.
- ❑ 3. All three muscles of the wrist flexor group (flexor carpi radialis, palmaris longus and flexor carpi ulnaris) can also flex the forearm at the elbow joint since they cross the elbow joint anteriorly.
- ❑ 4. All three muscles of the wrist flexor group (flexor carpi radialis, palmaris longus and flexor carpi ulnaris) as well as the muscles of the wrist extensor group (extensor carpi radialis longus, extensor carpi radialis brevis and extensor carpi ulnaris) can flex the forearm at the elbow joint except the extensor carpi ulnaris, which extends the forearm at the elbow joint.
- ❑ 5. Irritation and inflammation of the medial epicondyle and/or the common flexor tendon is known as *medial epicondylitis* and is usually called *golfer's elbow* (and occasionally called *tennis elbow)*.
- ❑ 6. In many individuals, the palmaris longus is bilaterally absent and sometimes unilaterally absent.

FLEXOR CARPI ULNARIS

(OF THE WRIST FLEXOR GROUP)

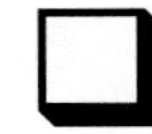

❑ **The name, flexor carpi ulnaris, tells us two of its actions: "flexor" tells us that this muscle performs flexion and "ulnaris" tells us that this muscle performs ulnar deviation (adduction). Both of these actions occur at the wrist; "carpi" means wrist.**

DERIVATION ❑ flexor: L. *a muscle that flexes a body part.*
carpi: L. *wrist.*
ulnaris: L. *refers to the ulnar side* (of the forearm).

PRONUNCIATION ❑ **fleks**-or **kar**-pie ul-**na**-ris

ATTACHMENTS

❑ **HUMERAL HEAD: Medial Epicondyle of the Humerus (via the Common Flexor Tendon) and the Ulna**

- ❑ the medial margin of the olecranon and the posterior proximal 2/3 of the ulna

to the

❑ **Ulnar Hand on the Anterior Side**

- ❑ the pisiform, the hook of the hamate and the base of the 5th metacarpal

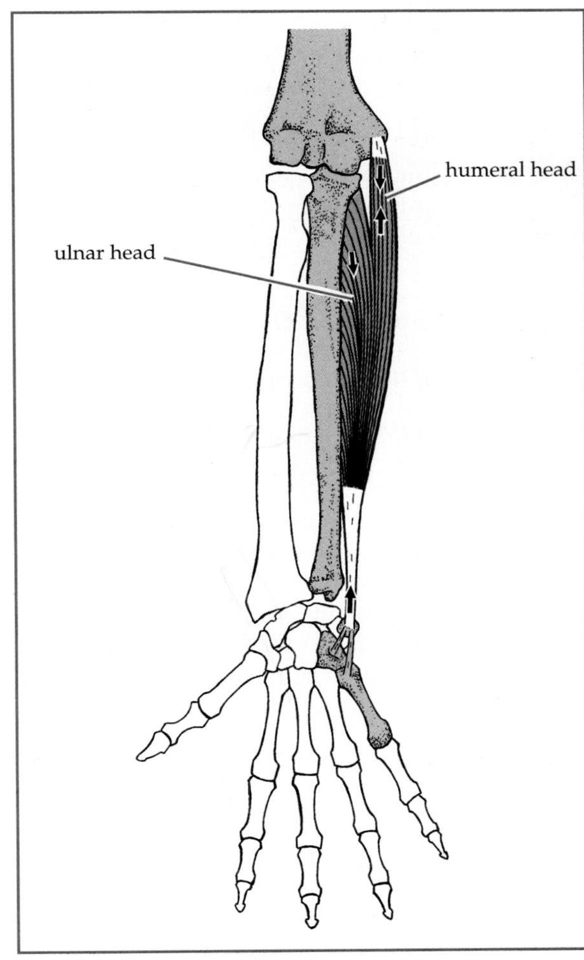

Anterior View of the Right Flexor Carpi Ulnaris

ACTIONS

❑ 1. **Flexion of the Hand**

❑ 2. **Ulnar Deviation (Adduction) of the Hand**

❑ 3. Flexion of the Forearm

INNERVATION ❑ The Ulnar Nerve ❑ **C7**, 8

ARTERIAL SUPPLY ❑ The Ulnar Artery (A Terminal Branch of the Brachial Artery)

FLEXOR CARPI ULNARIS – PALPATION AND SUPPLEMENTARY TEXT

PALPATION

- ❑ The flexor carpi ulnaris is superficial and easy to palpate on the ulnar (medial) side of the anterior wrist, but it is not as visible as the flexor carpi radialis and the palmaris longus.

  - Have the client seated or supine.
  - Place palpating hand across the anterior wrist.
  - Ask the client to actively flex and ulnar deviate (adduct) the hand at the wrist joint and feel for the distal tendon of the flexor carpi ulnaris on the ulnar (medial) side of the anterior wrist. (Make sure that the client keeps the fingers extended to lessen the contraction of the flexor digitorum superficialis.)
  - Continue palpating the flexor carpi ulnaris distally toward the pisiform and proximally toward the medial epicondyle of the humerus and to the posterior ulna.
  - To further bring out the flexor carpi ulnaris, resistance may be added.

see page 554

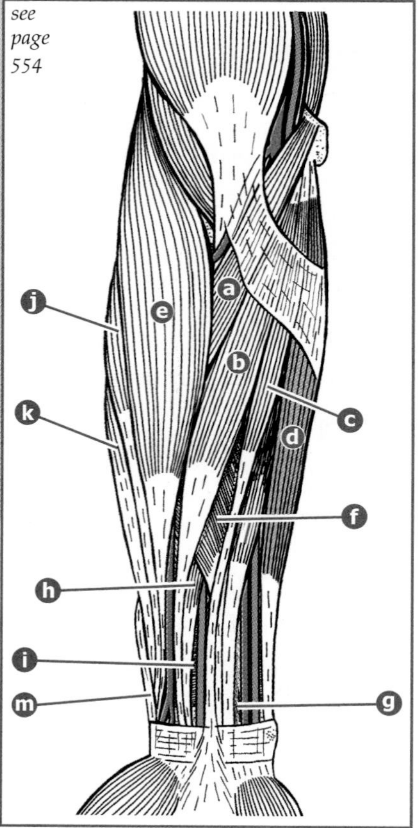

Anterior View of the Right Forearm (Superficial)

a. Pronator Teres
b. Flexor Carpi Radialis
c. Palmaris Longus
d. Flexor Carpi Ulnaris
e. Brachioradialis
f. Flexor Digitorum Superficialis
g. Flexor Digitorum Profundus
h. Flexor Pollicis Longus
i. Pronator Quadratus
j. Extensor Carpi Radialis Longus
k. Extensor Carpi Radialis Brevis
l. Supinator (not seen)
m. Abductor Pollicis Longus

RELATIONSHIP TO OTHER MUSCULOSKELETAL STRUCTURES

❑ 1. The flexor carpi ulnaris is superficial in the medial forearm.

❑ 2. The flexor carpi ulnaris is anterior to the extensor carpi ulnaris.

❑ 3. Proximally, the flexor carpi ulnaris is medial to the palmaris longus. More distally, the flexor carpi ulnaris is medial to the flexor digitorum superficialis.

❑ 4. From the medial perspective, the flexor carpi ulnaris is superficial to the flexor digitorum superficialis and the flexor digitorum profundus.

METHODOLOGY FOR LEARNING MUSCLE ACTIONS

❑ **1. Flexion of the Hand at the Wrist Joint:** The flexor carpi ulnaris crosses the wrist on the anterior side (with its fibers running vertically in the sagittal plane); therefore, it flexes the hand at the wrist joint.

❑ **2. Ulnar Deviation (Adduction) of the Hand at the Wrist Joint:** The flexor carpi ulnaris crosses the wrist on the ulnar (medial) side to attach onto the hand (with its fibers running vertically in the frontal plane); therefore, it ulnar deviates (adducts) the hand at the wrist joint.

❑ **3. Flexion of the Forearm at the Elbow Joint:** The flexor carpi ulnaris crosses the elbow joint anteriorly (with its fibers running vertically in the sagittal plane); therefore, it flexes the forearm at the elbow joint.

FLEXOR CARPI ULNARIS – continued

MISCELLANEOUS

- ☐ 1. The flexor carpi ulnaris arises proximally from the medial epicondyle of the humerus by the *common flexor tendon*. The common flexor tendon is the common proximal attachment of five muscles: the pronator teres, flexor carpi radialis, palmaris longus, flexor carpi ulnaris and the flexor digitorum superficialis.
- ☐ 2. The flexor carpi ulnaris has two heads: a humeral head and an ulnar head.
- ☐ 3. The ulnar head attachment of the flexor carpi ulnaris blends with the ulnar attachments of the extensor carpi ulnaris and the flexor digitorum profundus.
- ☐ 4. Some sources describe the distal tendon of the flexor carpi ulnaris ending at the pisiform, with the pull of its contraction passing onto the hamate and the 5th metacarpal via the pisohamate and pisometacarpal ligaments.
- ☐ 5. All three muscles of the wrist flexor group (flexor carpi radialis, palmaris longus and flexor carpi ulnaris) can also flex the forearm at the elbow joint since they cross the elbow joint anteriorly.
- ☐ 6. All three muscles of the wrist flexor group (flexor carpi radialis, palmaris longus and flexor carpi ulnaris) as well as the muscles of the wrist extensor group (extensor carpi radialis longus, extensor carpi radialis brevis and extensor carpi ulnaris) can flex the forearm at the elbow joint except the extensor carpi ulnaris, which extends the forearm at the elbow joint.
- ☐ 7. The ulnar nerve passes between the two heads of the flexor carpi ulnaris.
- ☐ 8. The flexor carpi ulnaris is the only muscle of the anterior forearm that is innervated by the ulnar nerve instead of the median nerve. (The flexor digitorum profundus is innervated by both the median and ulnar nerves.)
- ☐ 9. Irritation and inflammation of the medial epicondyle and/or the common flexor tendon is known as *medial epicondylitis* and is usually called *golfer's elbow* (and occasionally called *tennis elbow)*.

❑

BRACHIORADIALIS

(OF THE RADIAL GROUP)

❑ **The name, brachioradialis, tells us that this muscle attaches onto the brachium (the arm) and the radius.**

DERIVATION ❑ brachio: L. *refers to the arm.*
radialis: L. *radius.*

PRONUNCIATION ❑ **bray**-key-o-**ray**-dee-**al**-is

ATTACHMENTS

❑ **Lateral Supracondylar Ridge of the Humerus**

- ❑ the proximal 2/3

to the

❑ **Styloid Process of the Radius**

- ❑ the lateral side

ACTIONS

❑ **1. Flexion of the Forearm**

❑ **2.** Supination of the Forearm

❑ **3.** Pronation of the Forearm

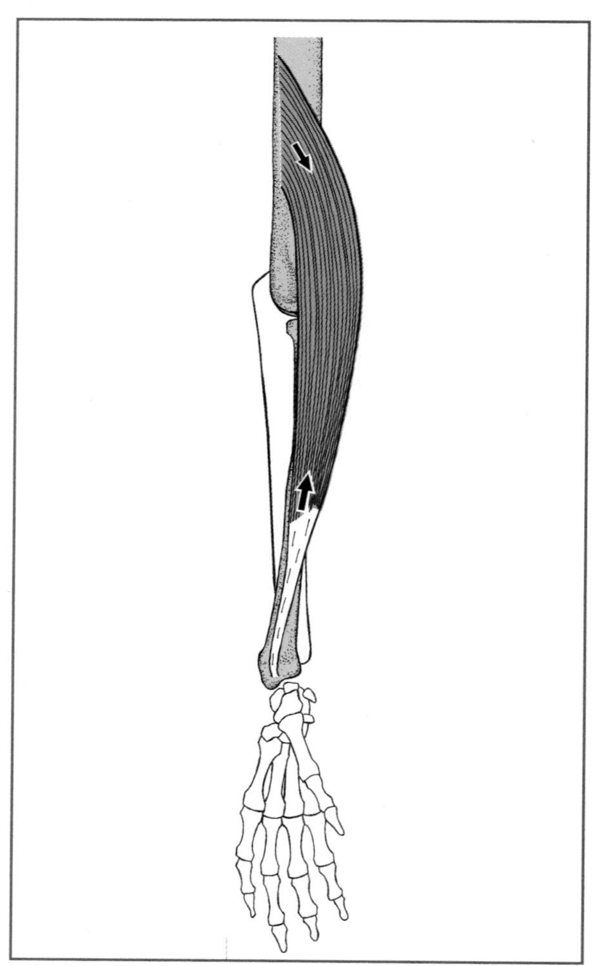

Lateral View of the Right Brachioradialis

INNERVATION ❑ The Radial Nerve ❑ C5, **6**

ARTERIAL SUPPLY ❑ Branches of the Brachial Artery (The Continuation of the Axillary Artery) and the Radial Artery (A Terminal Branch of the Brachial Artery)

PALPATION AND SUPPLEMENTARY TEXT

PALPATION

- ❑ The brachioradialis is superficial, visible and easy to palpate (except at its distal tendon, where it is deep to the abductor pollicis longus and the extensor pollicis brevis).
  - Have the client seated or supine with the forearm flexed at the elbow joint to 90° and in a position halfway between full pronation and full supination.
  - Place palpating hand on the lateral forearm.
  - Resist the client from further flexing the forearm and feel for the contraction of the brachioradialis.
  - Continue palpating the brachioradialis proximally toward the lateral supracondylar ridge of the humerus and distally toward the styloid process of the radius.

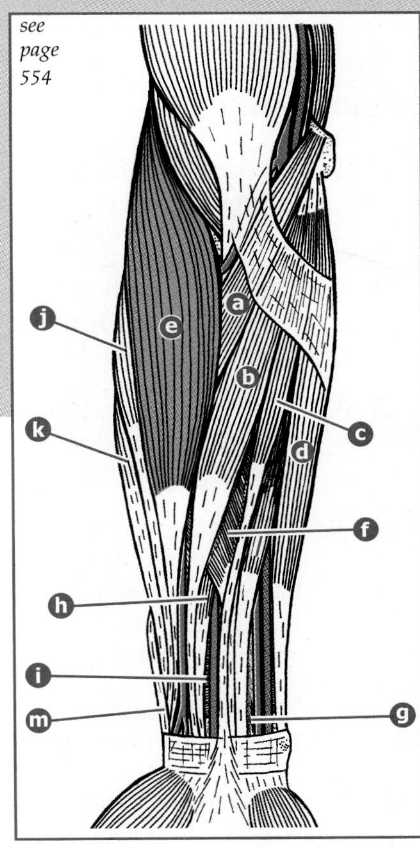

Anterior View of the Right Forearm (Superficial)

a. Pronator Teres
b. Flexor Carpi Radialis
c. Palmaris Longus
d. Flexor Carpi Ulnaris
e. **Brachioradialis**
f. Flexor Digitorum Superficialis
g. Flexor Digitorum Profundus
h. Flexor Pollicis Longus
i. Pronator Quadratus
j. Extensor Carpi Radialis Longus
k. Extensor Carpi Radialis Brevis
l. Supinator (not seen)
m. Abductor Pollicis Longus

RELATIONSHIP TO OTHER MUSCULOSKELETAL STRUCTURES

❑ 1. The brachioradialis is superficial in the lateral forearm, except at its distal end, where the abductor pollicis longus and the extensor pollicis brevis cross over it superficially.

❑ 2. The proximal tendon of the brachioradialis is found between the brachialis and the lateral head of the triceps brachii.

❑ 3. The belly of the brachioradialis is directly anterior to the extensor carpi radialis longus.

METHODOLOGY FOR LEARNING MUSCLE ACTIONS

❑ **1. Flexion of the Forearm at the Elbow Joint:**
The brachioradialis crosses the elbow joint anteriorly (with its fibers running vertically in the sagittal plane); therefore, it flexes the forearm at the elbow joint.

❑ **2. Supination of the Forearm at the Radioulnar Joints:**
When the brachioradialis shortens, it attempts to bring its two attachments toward each other. If the forearm is fully pronated, the brachioradialis will supinate the pronated forearm (at the radioulnar joints) until a position halfway between full pronation and full supination of the forearm is attained. That position will have the two attachments of the brachioradialis, the styloid process of the radius and the lateral supracondylar ridge of the humerus, as close to each other as possible.

BRACHIORADIALIS – continued

❑ **3. Pronation of the Forearm at the Radioulnar Joints:** When the brachioradialis shortens, it attempts to bring its two attachments toward each other. If the forearm is fully supinated, the brachioradialis will pronate the supinated forearm (at the radioulnar joints) until a position halfway between full pronation and full supination of the forearm is attained. That position will have the two attachments of the brachioradialis, the styloid process of the radius and the lateral supracondylar ridge of the humerus, as close to each other as possible.

MISCELLANEOUS

❑ 1. The brachioradialis, the extensor carpi radialis longus and the extensor carpi radialis brevis are often grouped together as the *radial group* of forearm muscles. (They are also sometimes known as the *wad of three.)*

❑ 2. The brachioradialis is sometimes nicknamed the *hitchhiker muscle* for the characteristic action of flexing the forearm in a position halfway between full pronation and full supination (with the thumb up) when hitchhiking. (Keep in mind that the brachioradialis has no action upon the thumb itself.)

❑ 3. The brachioradialis can only supinate the forearm to a position that is halfway between full pronation and full supination, and can only pronate the forearm to a position that is halfway between full pronation and full supination as explained in the methodology section.

❑ 4. The brachioradialis is an excellent example of a muscle in the human body that has one line of pull, but can have two opposite actions at the same joint (pronation and supination at the radioulnar joints) based upon the position that the joint is in when the muscle contracts. Although the brachioradialis may be the best known example of this concept, it is by no means the only muscle that can change its action at a joint when the position of the joint changes. ☺

❑ 5. The brachioradialis is most effective as a forearm flexor when the forearm is in a position that is halfway between full pronation and full supination.

❑ 6. The brachioradialis is a flexor of the forearm at the elbow joint, but it is innervated by the radial nerve, which innervates all the forearm extensors.

FLEXOR DIGITORUM SUPERFICIALIS

❑ **The name, flexor digitorum superficialis, tells us that this muscle flexes the digits, i.e., fingers, and is superficial (superficial to the flexor digitorum profundus).**

DERIVATION ❑ flexor: L. *a muscle that flexes a body part.*
digitorum: L. *refers to a digit* (finger).
superficialis: L. *superficial* (near the surface).

PRONUNCIATION ❑ **fleks**-or dij-i-**toe**-rum **soo**-per-fish-ee-**a**-lis

ATTACHMENTS

❑ **Medial Epicondyle of the Humerus (via the Common Flexor Tendon) and the Anterior Ulna, and the Radius**

- ❑ HUMEROULNAR HEAD: medial epicondyle of the humerus (via the common flexor tendon) and the coronoid process of the ulna
- ❑ RADIAL HEAD: proximal 1/2 of the anterior shaft of the radius (starting just distal to the radial tuberosity)

to the

❑ **Anterior Surfaces of Fingers #2-5**

- ❑ the four tendons each divide into two slips that attach onto the sides of the anterior surfaces of the middle phalanges

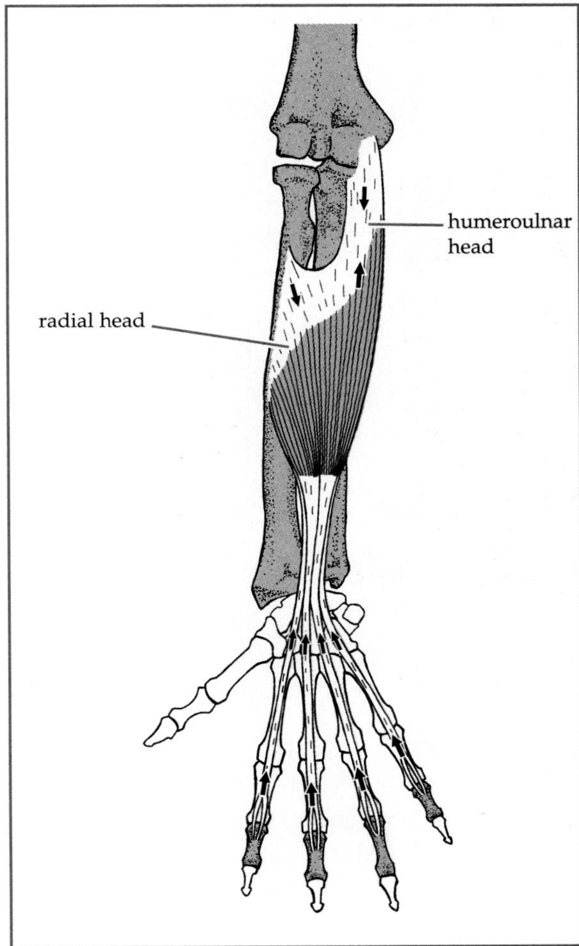

Anterior View of the Right Flexor Digitorum Superficialis

ACTIONS

❑ 1. **Flexion of Fingers #2-5**

❑ 2. **Flexion of the Hand**

❑ 3. Flexion of the Forearm

INNERVATION ❑ The Median Nerve ❑ C7, **8**, T1

ARTERIAL SUPPLY ❑ The Ulnar and Radial Arteries (Terminal Branches of the Brachial Artery)

FLEXOR DIGITORUM SUPERFICIALIS PALPATION AND SUPPLEMENTARY TEXT

PALPATION

The belly of the flexor digitorum superficialis is found medially in the proximal anterior forearm; it is deep to the wrist flexor group (flexor carpi radialis, palmaris longus and flexor carpi ulnaris) and superficial to the flexor digitorum profundus. The distal tendons of the flexor digitorum superficialis are found between the distal tendons of the palmaris longus and flexor carpi ulnaris.

❑ **To palpate the distal tendons:**

- Have the client seated or supine.
- Place palpating hand on the distal anterior forearm.
- Ask the client to make a tight fist (flex the fingers) and then resist the client from flexing the hand at the wrist joint.
- Palpate the distal tendons of the flexor digitorum superficialis between the tendons of palmaris longus and flexor carpi ulnaris (see the palpation sections for these muscles on pages 569 and 572). The ring and the middle fingers' tendons are the most easily palpable.
- Continue palpating the flexor digitorum superficialis proximally as far as possible.

❑ **To palpate the muscle belly:**

- Have the client seated or supine.
- Place palpating hand on the medial side of the proximal anterior forearm approximately 1/2 inch (1 cm) anterior to the shaft of the ulna.
- Ask the client to actively flex the fingers (make a fist) and feel for the contraction of the flexor digitorum superficialis.

  (Note: Flexing the fingers will also cause the flexor digitorum profundus to contract. Two methods that can be used to relax the flexor digitorum profundus so that the flexor digitorum superficialis will be more easily palpable and distinguished from the flexor digitorum profundus are listed below.)

  1. When flexion of the fingers is performed, make sure that the distal interphalangeal joint is extended.
  2. If a fist is made by flexing the fingers, make sure that the wrist joint is partially flexed or in a neutral position.

see page 555

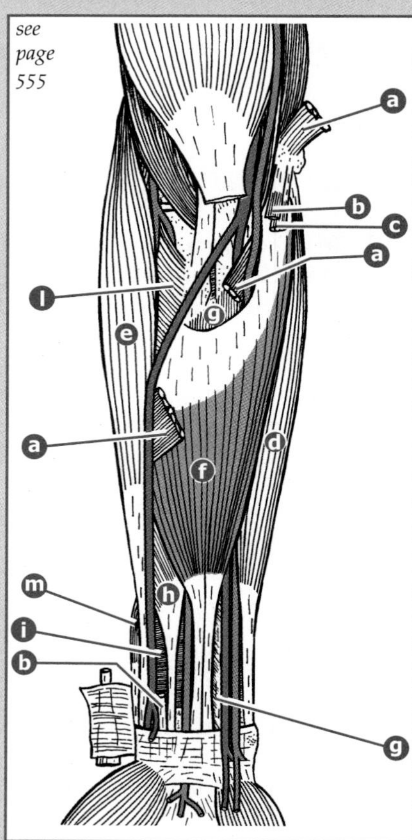

Anterior View of the Right Forearm (Intermediate)

- **a.** Pronator Teres (cut)
- **b.** Flexor Carpi Radialis (cut)
- **c.** Palmaris Longus (cut)
- **d.** Flexor Carpi Ulnaris
- **e.** Brachioradialis
- **f.** **Flexor Digitorum Superficialis**
- **g.** Flexor Digitorum Profundus
- **h.** Flexor Pollicis Longus
- **i.** Pronator Quadratus
- **j.** Extensor Carpi Radialis Longus (not seen)
- **k.** Extensor Carpi Radialis Brevis (not seen)
- **l.** Supinator
- **m.** Abductor Pollicis Longus

FLEXOR DIGITORUM SUPERFICIALIS – continued

RELATIONSHIP TO OTHER MUSCULOSKELETAL STRUCTURES

❑ 1. The flexor digitorum superficialis is located in the anterior forearm, directly deep to the flexor carpi radialis, palmaris longus and the flexor carpi ulnaris.

❑ 2. Deep to the flexor digitorum superficialis are the flexor digitorum profundus and flexor pollicis longus.

❑ 3. The four tendons of the flexor digitorum superficialis travel through the carpal tunnel medial to the median nerve and superficial to the four tendons of the flexor digitorum profundus.

METHODOLOGY FOR LEARNING MUSCLE ACTIONS

❑ **1. Flexion of Fingers #2-5 at the Metacarpophalangeal and Proximal Interphalangeal Joints:** The flexor digitorum superficialis crosses the metacarpophalangeal joint and the proximal interphalangeal joint of fingers #2-5 on the anterior side (with its fibers running vertically in the sagittal plane). Therefore, the flexor digitorum superficialis flexes fingers #2-5 at the metacarpophalangeal and the proximal interphalangeal joints. (Note: This muscle cannot flex the distal interphalangeal joint of the fingers.)

❑ **2. Flexion of the Hand at the Wrist Joint:** The flexor digitorum superficialis crosses the wrist joint anteriorly (with its fibers running vertically in the sagittal plane); therefore, it flexes the hand at the wrist joint.

❑ **3. Flexion of the Forearm at the Elbow Joint**: The humeroulnar head of the flexor digitorum superficialis crosses the elbow joint anteriorly (with its fibers running vertically in the sagittal plane); therefore, it flexes the forearm at the elbow joint.

MISCELLANEOUS

❑ 1. The flexor digitorum superficialis is also known as the *flexor digitorum sublimis.*

❑ 2. The four distal tendons of the flexor digitorum superficialis are arranged in two layers, with the tendons going to the middle and ring fingers superficially and the tendons going to the little finger and index finger deeply. (If you take your own little finger and index finger and you make them touch behind the middle and ring fingers, you will have the arrangement that these tendons are in when they travel through the carpal tunnel.)

❑ 3. The distal tendons of the flexor digitorum superficialis attach onto the middle phalanges in an unusual manner. Since the distal tendons of the flexor digitorum profundus are deeper and yet they must ultimately attach further distally onto the distal phalanges, the tendons of the flexor digitorum superficialis must split to allow passage for the tendons of the flexor digitorum profundus through to the distal phalanges. Each one of the split distal tendons of the flexor digitorum superficialis then attaches onto both sides of the anterior surface of the middle phalanx. (This arrangement is essentially identical to that of the splitting of each of the distal tendons of the flexor digitorum brevis' distal tendon to allow passage of the flexor digitorum longus' distal tendon onto the distal phalanx of toes #2-5 in the lower extremity.)

❑ 4. The major action of the flexor digitorum superficialis is flexion of the middle phalanx of fingers #2-5 at the proximal interphalangeal joint.

❑ 5. The median nerve and ulnar artery travel between the two heads of the flexor digitorum superficialis.

❑ 6. Irritation of the synovial sheaths of the flexor digitorum superficialis and/or the flexor digitorum profundus in the carpal tunnel can press on the median nerve and cause *carpal tunnel syndrome.*

❑ 7. Irritation and inflammation of the medial epicondyle and/or the common flexor tendon is known as *medial epicondylitis* and is usually called *golfer's elbow* (and occasionally called *tennis elbow*).

❑ FLEXOR DIGITORUM PROFUNDUS

❑ **The name, flexor digitorum profundus, tells us that this muscle flexes the digits, i.e., fingers, and is deep (deep to the flexor digitorum superficialis).**

DERIVATION ❑ flexor: L. *a muscle that flexes a body part.*
digitorum: L. *refers to a digit* (finger).
profundus: L. *deep.*

PRONUNCIATION ❑ **fleks**-or dij-i-**toe**-rum pro-**fun**-dus

ATTACHMENTS

❑ **Medial and Anterior Ulna**

❑ the proximal 1/2 (starting distal to the coronoid process) and the interosseus membrane

to the

❑ **Anterior Surfaces of Fingers #2-5**

❑ the distal phalanges

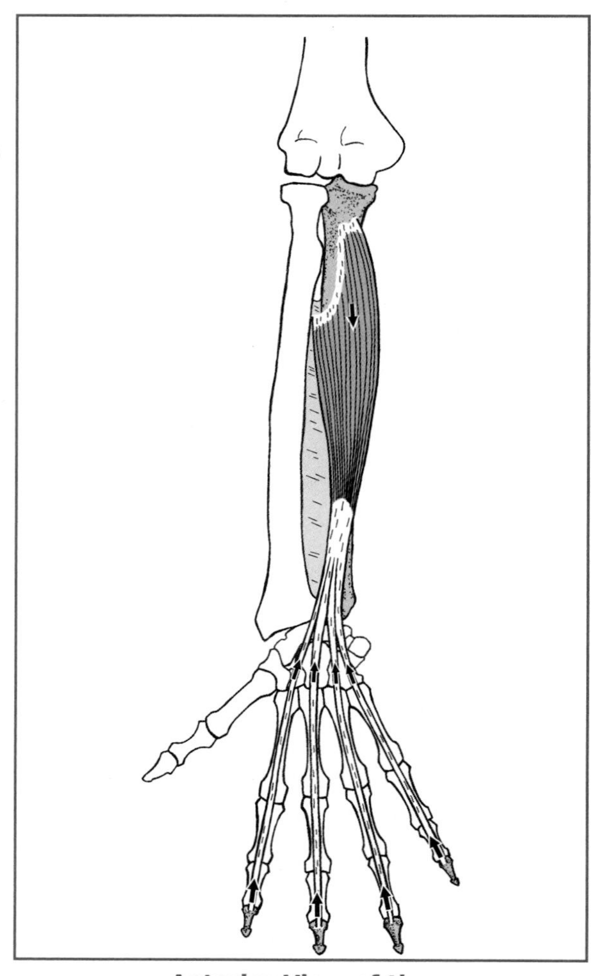

Anterior View of the Right Flexor Digitorum Profundus

ACTIONS

❑ 1. **Flexion of Fingers #2-5**

❑ 2. **Flexion of the Hand**

INNERVATION ❑ The Median and the Ulnar Nerves ❑ C8, T1
❑ the anterior interosseus branch of the median nerve

ARTERIAL SUPPLY ❑ The Ulnar and Radial Arteries (Terminal Branches of the Brachial Artery) and the Anterior Interosseus Artery (A Branch of the Ulnar Artery)

PALPATION AND SUPPLEMENTARY TEXT

PALPATION

❑ The flexor digitorum profundus is deep but palpable. However, it is difficult to distinguish it from the flexor digitorum superficialis.

- Have the client seated or supine.
- Place palpating hand on the medial side of the proximal forearm just anterior to the shaft of the ulna.
- Place your other hand across the anterior surface of the client's middle phalanges.
- Ask the client to flex the distal phalanges at the distal interphalangeal joint and feel for the contraction of the flexor digitorum profundus.
- Another method in which to palpate the flexor digitorum profundus is to ask the client to flex the fingers (make a fist) with the wrist joint in extension. Palpate as instructed above.

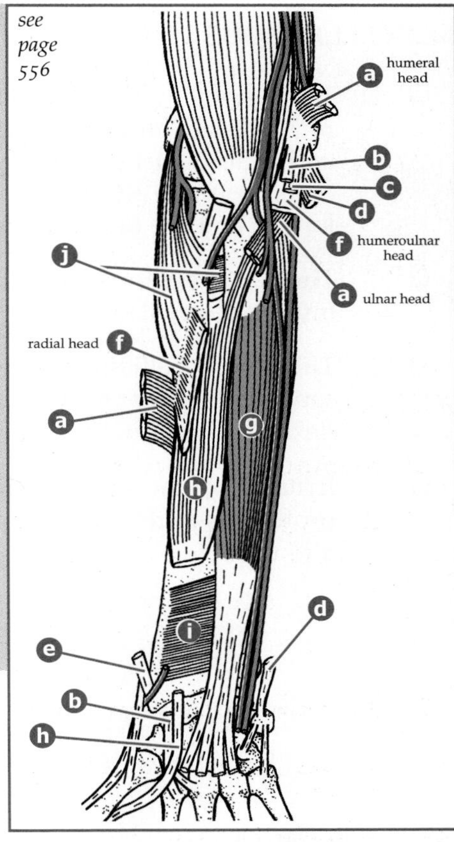

Anterior View of the Right Forearm (Deep)

a. Pronator Teres (cut)
b. Flexor Carpi Radialis (cut)
c. Palmaris Longus (cut)
d. Flexor Carpi Ulnaris (cut)
e. Brachioradialis (cut)
f. Flexor Digitorum Superficialis (cut)
g. **Flexor Digitorum Profundus** (cut)
h. Flexor Pollicis Longus (cut)
i. Pronator Quadratus
j. Supinator

RELATIONSHIP TO OTHER MUSCULOSKELETAL STRUCTURES

❑ 1. The flexor digitorum profundus is deep to the flexor digitorum superficialis.

❑ 2. The flexor digitorum profundus is medial to the flexor pollicis longus.

❑ 3. Deep to the flexor digitorum profundus are the ulna and the interosseus membrane.

METHODOLOGY FOR LEARNING MUSCLE ACTIONS

❑ **1. Flexion of Fingers #2-5 at the Metacarpophalangeal and Proximal and Distal Interphalangeal Joints:** The flexor digitorum profundus crosses the metacarpophalangeal and the proximal and distal interphalangeal joints of fingers #2-5 on the anterior side (with its fibers running vertically in the sagittal plane). Therefore, the flexor digitorum profundus flexes fingers #2-5 at the metacarpophalangeal and the proximal and distal interphalangeal joints.

❑ **2. Flexion of the Hand at the Wrist Joint:** The flexor digitorum profundus crosses the wrist joint anteriorly (with its fibers running vertically in the sagittal plane); therefore, it flexes the hand at the wrist joint.

FLEXOR DIGITORUM PROFUNDUS – continued

MISCELLANEOUS

- ❑ 1. The distal tendons of the flexor digitorum profundus reach their attachment site on the distal phalanges in an unusual manner. The tendons of the flexor digitorum superficialis are superficial and split; the tendons of the flexor digitorum profundus then pass through this split to continue onto the distal phalanges. (This is essentially identical to the arrangement of the flexor digitorum longus and the flexor digitorum brevis of the lower extremity.)
- ❑ 2. The flexor digitorum profundus is the only muscle that can flex the distal phalanges at the distal interphalangeal joints.
- ❑ 3. The muscle bellies for each individual finger of the flexor digitorum profundus are not well separated (except for the index finger). Therefore, it is difficult to isolate distal interphalangeal flexion of one finger.
- ❑ 4. Irritation of the synovial sheaths of the flexor digitorum superficialis and/or the flexor digitorum profundus in the carpal tunnel can press on the median nerve and cause *carpal tunnel syndrome.*

FLEXOR POLLICIS LONGUS

❑ **The name, flexor pollicis longus, tells us that this muscle flexes the thumb and is long (longer than the flexor pollicis brevis).**

DERIVATION ❑ flexor: L. *a muscle that flexes a body part.*
pollicis: L. *thumb.*
longus: L. *long.*

PRONUNCIATION ❑ **fleks**-or **pol**-i-sis **long**-us

ATTACHMENTS

❑ **Anterior Surface of the Radius**

❑ and the interosseus membrane, the medial epicondyle of the humerus and the coronoid process of the ulna

to the

❑ **Thumb**

❑ the anterior aspect of the base of the distal phalanx

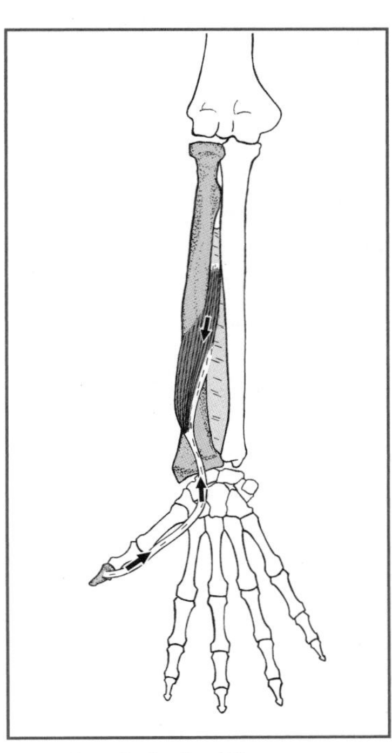

Anterior View: common variation - no humeroulnar head

Anterior View of the Right Flexor Pollicis Longus

ACTIONS

❑ 1. **Flexion of the Thumb**

❑ 2. **Flexion of the Hand**

❑ 3. Flexion of the Forearm

INNERVATION ❑ The Median Nerve
❑ the anterior interosseus branch of the median nerve; C7, **8**

ARTERIAL SUPPLY ❑ The Radial Artery (A Terminal Branch of the Brachial Artery) and the Anterior Interosseus Artery (A Branch of the Ulnar Artery)

FLEXOR POLLICIS LONGUS – PALPATION AND SUPPLEMENTARY TEXT

PALPATION

- ❑ The majority of the flexor pollicis longus is deep and not easily palpated. However, the distal belly and tendon can be palpated in the distal anterior forearm on the radial side between the tendons of the flexor carpi radialis and the brachioradialis.
  - Have the client seated or supine.
  - Locate the tendons of the flexor carpi radialis and the brachioradialis (see the palpation sections for these muscles on pages 566 and 575).
  - Ask the client to actively flex the distal phalanx of the thumb at the interphalangeal joint and palpate between the tendons of the flexor carpi radialis and the brachioradialis to locate the flexor pollicis longus.
  - Follow the flexor pollicis longus' muscle belly proximally until it can no longer be felt, deep to the brachioradialis and the flexor digitorum superficialis.

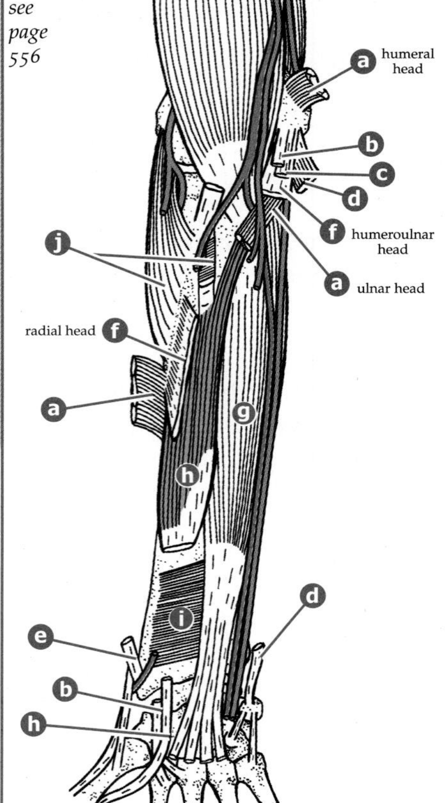

Anterior View of the Right Forearm (Deep)

a. Pronator Teres (cut)
b. Flexor Carpi Radialis (cut)
c. Palmaris Longus (cut)
d. Flexor Carpi Ulnaris (cut)
e. Brachioradialis (cut)
f. Flexor Digitorum Superficialis (cut)
g. Flexor Digitorum Profundus (cut)
h. **Flexor Pollicis Longus** (cut)
i. Pronator Quadratus
j. Supinator

RELATIONSHIP TO OTHER MUSCULOSKELETAL STRUCTURES

❑ 1. The flexor pollicis longus is a deep muscle of the anterior forearm. The majority of it is directly deep to the flexor digitorum superficialis. However, a small part of the flexor pollicis longus is superficial in the distal forearm on the medial side (and to a lesser extent, the lateral side) of the distal tendon of the flexor carpi radialis.

❑ 2. The flexor pollicis longus is found lateral to the flexor digitorum profundus.

❑ 3. Deep to the flexor pollicis longus are the radius and the interosseus membrane.

METHODOLOGY FOR LEARNING MUSCLE ACTIONS

❑ 1. **Flexion of the Thumb at the Carpometacarpal, Metacarpophalangeal and the Interphalangeal Joints:** The flexor pollicis longus crosses the carpometacarpal joint of the thumb medially (on the ulnar side) to attach onto the distal phalanx of the thumb (with its fibers running vertically in the frontal plane). When the flexor pollicis longus contracts, it pulls the thumb medially (in an ulnar direction) within the plane of the palm of the hand (frontal plane) toward the index finger. This action is called flexion of the thumb. Therefore, the flexor pollicis longus flexes the thumb by flexing the metacarpal of the thumb at the 1st carpometacarpal joint. The flexor pollicis longus also crosses the metacarpophalangeal and the interphalangeal joints of the thumb medially (on the ulnar side) to attach onto the distal phalanx of the thumb. Therefore, the flexor pollicis longus also flexes the proximal and distal phalanges of the thumb at these joints as well. (Note: Due to the rotational development of the thumb embryologically, the named actions of flexion and extension of the thumb occur within the frontal plane. For more details, see the Muscular System Manual, Volume I.)

FLEXOR POLLICIS LONGUS – continued

- ❑ 2. **Flexion of the Hand at the Wrist Joint:** The flexor pollicis longus crosses the wrist joint anteriorly (with its fibers running vertically in the sagittal plane); therefore, it flexes the hand at the wrist joint.
- ❑ 3. **Flexion of the Forearm at the Elbow Joint:** If the flexor pollicis longus attaches onto the medial epicondyle of the humerus (this attachment is variable and often absent), then it would cross the elbow joint anteriorly (with its fibers running vertically in the sagittal plane). Therefore, the flexor pollicis longus would flex the forearm at the elbow joint.

MISCELLANEOUS

- ❑ 1. The distal tendon of the flexor pollicis longus travels through the carpal tunnel lateral to the median nerve.
- ❑ 2. The humeroulnar head of the flexor pollicis longus is very small. Therefore, it does not contribute much strength toward the joint actions of this muscle.
- ❑ 3. The proximal attachments of the flexor pollicis longus are variable. The medial epicondylar attachment is often missing. Sometimes the coronoid process attachment is on the medial side of the coronoid process, sometimes it is on the lateral side and other times it is missing altogether.
- ❑ 4. The flexor pollicis longus is the only muscle that can flex the distal phalanx of the thumb at the interphalangeal joint.

❑ PRONATOR QUADRATUS

❑ **The name, pronator quadratus, tells us that this muscle pronates the forearm and has a square shape.**

DERIVATION ❑ pronator: L. *a muscle that pronates a body part.*
quadratus: L. *squared.*

PRONUNCIATION ❑ pro-**nay**-tor kwod-**ray**-tus

ATTACHMENTS

❑ **Anterior Distal Ulna**

- ❑ the distal 1/4

to the

❑ **Anterior Distal Radius**

- ❑ the distal 1/4

ACTION

❑ **Pronation of the Forearm**

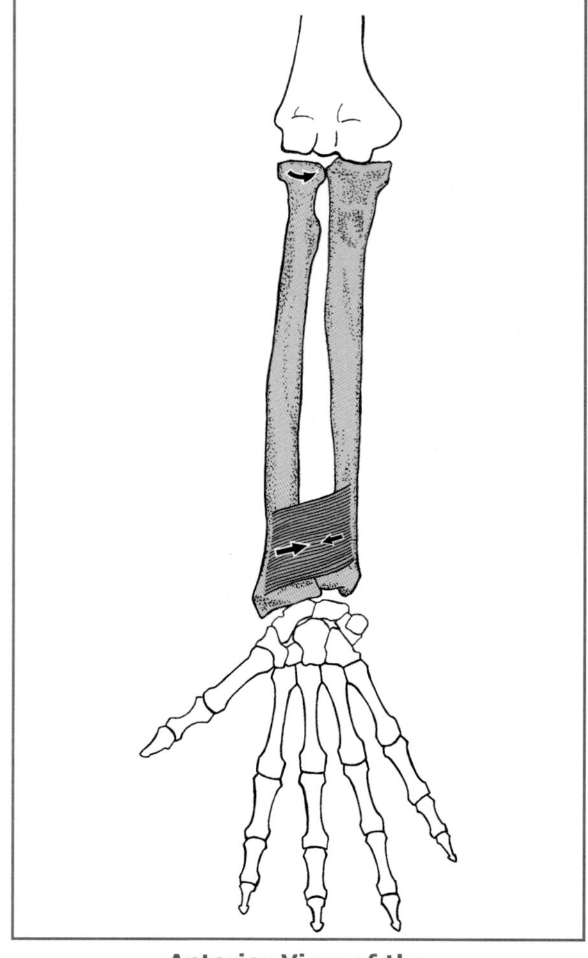

Anterior View of the Right Pronator Quadratus

INNERVATION ❑ The Median Nerve ❑ anterior interosseus nerve, C7, **8**

ARTERIAL SUPPLY ❑ The Anterior Interosseus Artery (A Branch of the Ulnar Artery)

PALPATION AND SUPPLEMENTARY TEXT

PALPATION

- ❑ The pronator quadratus is very deep and difficult to palpate. The only part that is superficial is a small part far distal in the anterior forearm on the lateral (radial) side between the flexor carpi radialis and the brachioradialis, and distal to the belly of the flexor pollicis longus. However, the radial artery is located here and care must be taken to not palpate directly over it with too much pressure.
  - Have the client seated or supine.
  - Place palpating hand distally on the lateral anterior forearm.
  - Find the radial pulse to locate the radial artery and then palpate on either side of it to locate the pronator quadratus.
  - Resist the client from actively pronating the forearm at the radioulnar joints and feel for the contraction of the pronator quadratus.

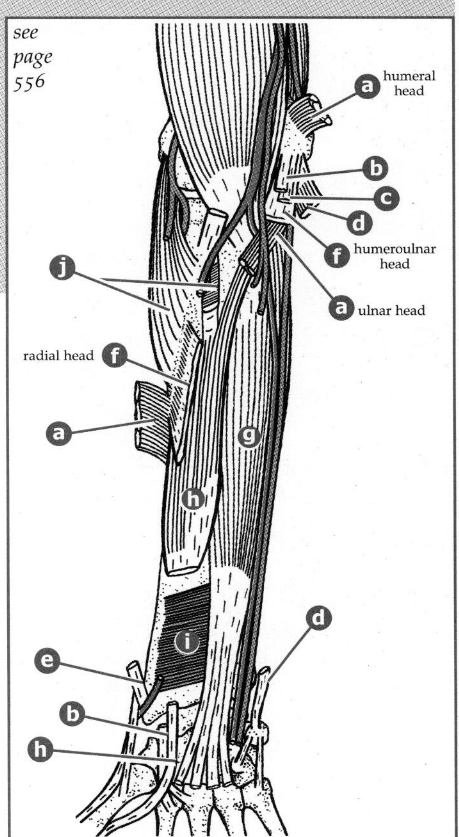

Anterior View of the Right Forearm (Deep)

- **a.** Pronator Teres (cut)
- **b.** Flexor Carpi Radialis (cut)
- **c.** Palmaris Longus (cut)
- **d.** Flexor Carpi Ulnaris (cut)
- **e.** Brachioradialis (cut)
- **f.** Flexor Digitorum Superficialis (cut)
- **g.** Flexor Digitorum Profundus (cut)
- **h.** Flexor Pollicis Longus (cut)
- **i.** **Pronator Quadratus**
- **j.** Supinator

RELATIONSHIP TO OTHER MUSCULOSKELETAL STRUCTURES

- ❑ 1. The pronator quadratus is the deepest muscle in the anterior forearm.
- ❑ 2. Every structure that crosses the wrist on the anterior side is superficial to the pronator quadratus.
- ❑ 3. Deep to the pronator quadratus are the radius, ulna and the interosseus membrane.

METHODOLOGY FOR LEARNING MUSCLE ACTIONS

- ❑ **Pronation of the Forearm at the Radioulnar Joints:** The pronator quadratus crosses the distal anterior forearm from the ulna to the radius (with its fibers running horizontally in the transverse plane). When the pronator quadratus contracts, it pulls the distal radius anteromedially. This causes the distal radius to cross in front of the distal ulna (and the head of the radius to medially rotate). This movement of the radius is called pronation. Therefore, the pronator quadratus pronates the forearm at the radioulnar joints.

MISCELLANEOUS

- ❑ According to most sources, the pronator quadratus is the prime mover of forearm pronation at the radioulnar joints even though the pronator teres is much larger and bulkier. This is due to the pronator quadratus' excellent leverage at the distal radius.

PRONATOR QUADRATUS – continued

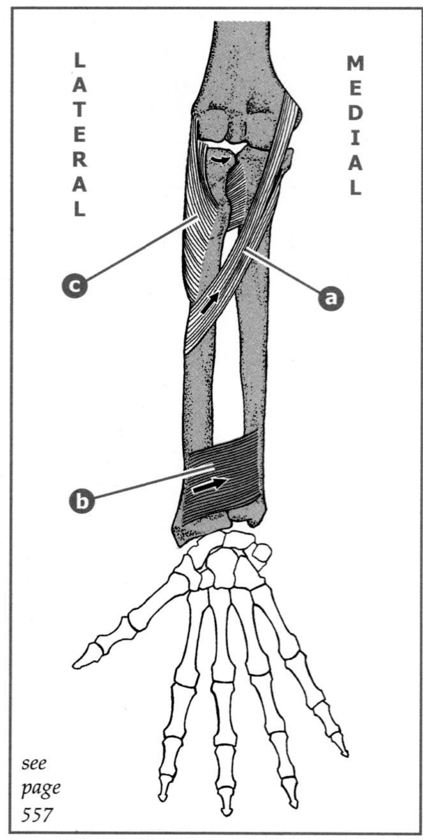

see page 557

Anterior View of the Right Forearm Fully Supinated

a. Pronator Teres
b. Pronator Quadratus
c. Supinator

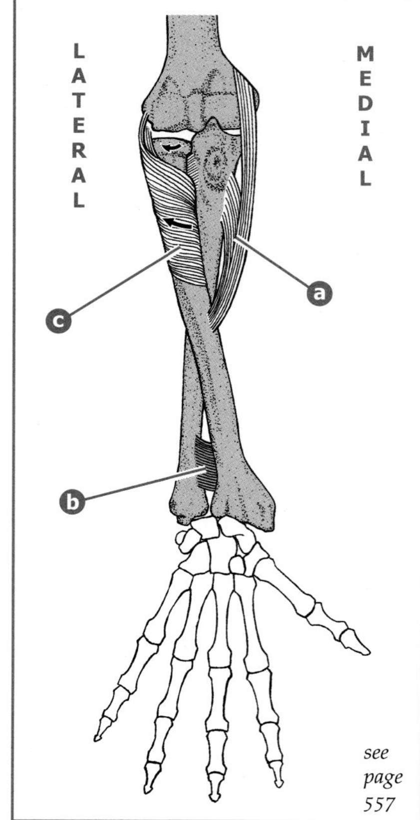

see page 557

Anterior View of the Right Forearm Fully Pronated

a. Pronator Teres
b. Pronator Quadratus
c. Supinator

ANCONEUS

❑ **The name, anconeus, tells us that this muscle is involved with the elbow.**

DERIVATION ❑ anconeus: Gr. *elbow.*

PRONUNCIATION ❑ an-**ko**-nee-us

ATTACHMENTS

❑ **Lateral Epicondyle of the Humerus**

to the

❑ **Posterior Ulna**

- ❑ the lateral side of the olecranon process of the ulna and the proximal 1/4 of the posterior ulna

ACTION

❑ **Extension of the Forearm**

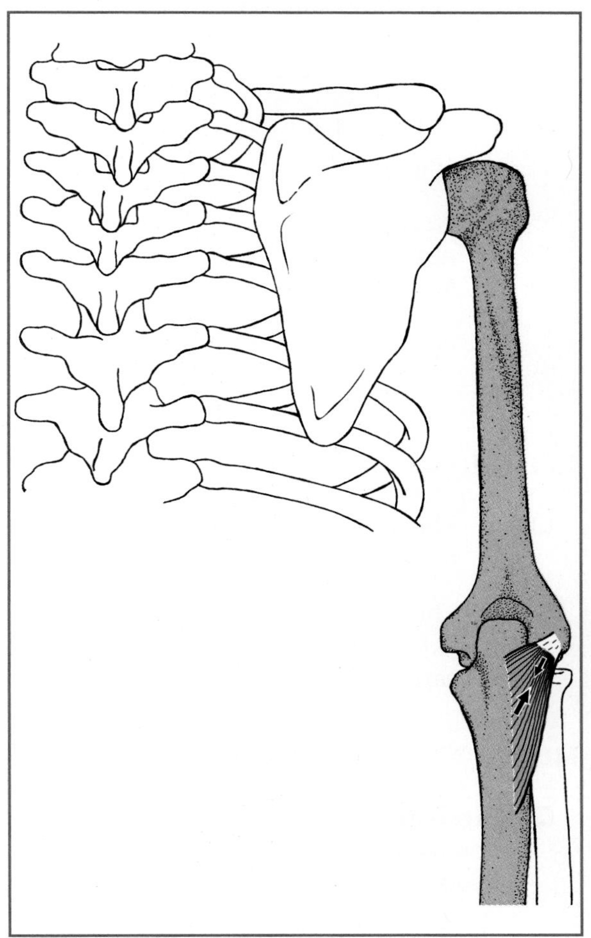

Posterior View of the Right Anconeus

INNERVATION ❑ The Radial Nerve ❑ C6, 7, 8

ARTERIAL SUPPLY ❑ The Deep Brachial Artery (A Branch of the Brachial Artery)

ANCONEUS – PALPATION AND SUPPLEMENTARY TEXT

PALPATION

- The anconeus is superficial and easy to palpate.
  - Have the client seated.
  - To locate the anconeus, place one finger on the olecranon process of the ulna and another finger on the lateral epicondyle of the humerus. Now place your palpating finger halfway between the first two fingers and move approximately 1/2 inch (1 cm) distal.
  - Ask the client to actively extend the forearm at the elbow joint against resistance and feel for the contraction of the anconeus.
  - Be careful to distinguish the anconeus from the extensor carpi ulnaris, which lies very close to the anconeus and can assist with forearm extension. To eliminate the extensor carpi ulnaris from contracting, have the client flex and/or radially deviate (abduct) the hand at the wrist joint.

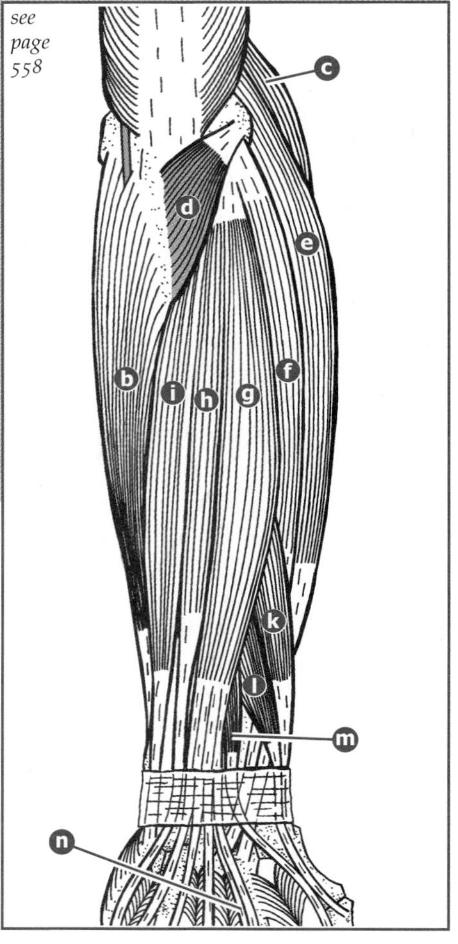

Posterior View of the Right Forearm (Superficial)

a. Pronator Teres (not seen)
b. Flexor Carpi Ulnaris
c. Brachioradialis
d. Anconeus
e. Extensor Carpi Radialis Longus
f. Extensor Carpi Radialis Brevis
g. Extensor Digitorum
h. Extensor Digiti Minimi
i. Extensor Carpi Ulnaris
j. Supinator (not seen)
k. Abductor Pollicis Longus
l. Extensor Pollicis Brevis
m. Extensor Pollicis Longus
n. Extensor Indicis

RELATIONSHIP TO OTHER MUSCULOSKELETAL STRUCTURES

1. The anconeus is superficial and located in the proximal posterior forearm on the lateral side.
2. The anconeus is proximal to the extensor carpi radialis brevis, extensor digitorum, extensor digiti minimi and the extensor carpi ulnaris.

METHODOLOGY FOR LEARNING MUSCLE ACTIONS

- **Extension of the Forearm at the Elbow Joint:** The anconeus crosses the elbow joint posteriorly (with its fibers running vertically in the sagittal plane); therefore, it extends the forearm at the elbow joint.

MISCELLANEOUS

1. Besides the anconeus, the supinator attaches proximally to the lateral epicondyle of the humerus. Also arising from the lateral epicondyle are four other muscles that share the common extensor tendon attachment onto the lateral epicondyle of the humerus (the extensor carpi radialis brevis, extensor digitorum, extensor digiti minimi and the extensor carpi ulnaris).
2. The anconeus often blends with the triceps brachii.
3. Irritation and inflammation of the lateral epicondyle and/or the common extensor tendon is known as *lateral epicondylitis* or *tennis elbow.*

EXTENSOR CARPI RADIALIS LONGUS

(OF THE WRIST EXTENSOR GROUP – AND – THE RADIAL GROUP)

❑ **The name, extensor carpi radialis longus, tells us two of its actions: "extensor" tells us that this muscle performs extension and "radialis" tells us that this muscle performs radial deviation (abduction). Both of these actions occur at the wrist; "carpi" means wrist. "Longus" tells us that this muscle is long (longer than the extensor carpi radialis brevis).**

DERIVATION ❑ extensor: L. *a muscle that extends a body part.*
carpi: L. *wrist.*
radialis: L. *refers to the radial side* (of the forearm).
longus: L. *long.*

PRONUNCIATION ❑ eks-**ten**-sor **kar**-pie ray-dee-**a**-lis **long**-us

ATTACHMENTS

❑ **Lateral Supracondylar Ridge of the Humerus**

- ❑ the distal 1/3

to the

❑ **Radial Hand on the Posterior Side**

- ❑ the posterior side of the base of the 2nd metacarpal

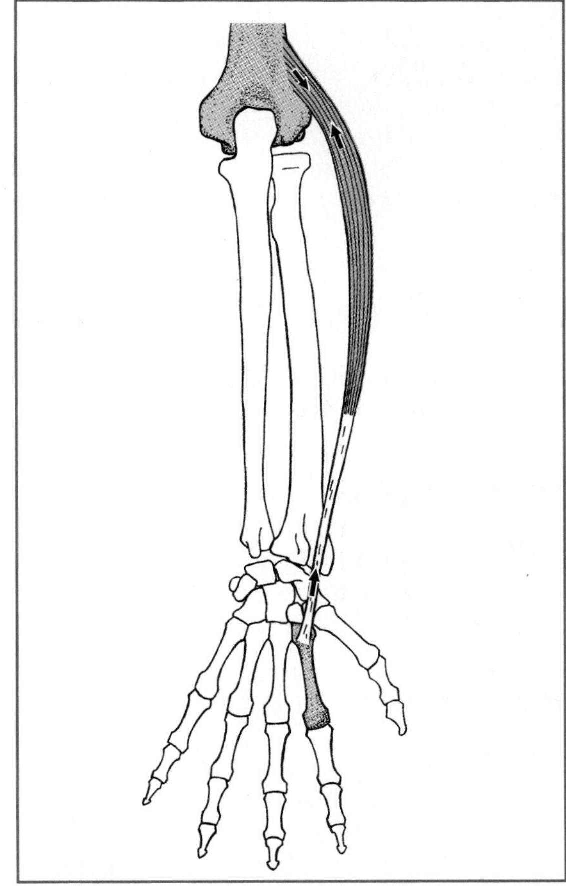

Posterior View of the Right Extensor Carpi Radialis Longus

ACTIONS

❑ **1. Extension of the Hand**

❑ **2. Radial Deviation (Abduction) of the Hand**

❑ **3.** Flexion of the Forearm

❑ **4.** Pronation of the Forearm

INNERVATION ❑ The Radial Nerve ❑ C5, **6**

ARTERIAL SUPPLY ❑ Branches of the Brachial Artery (The Continuation of the Axillary Artery) and the Radial Artery (A Terminal Branch of the Brachial Artery)

EXTENSOR CARPI RADIALIS LONGUS PALPATION AND SUPPLEMENTARY TEXT

PALPATION

- ❑ The belly of the extensor carpi radialis longus is superficial and located between the brachioradialis and the extensor carpi radialis brevis. The distal tendon is visible and palpable at the posterior wrist when the client makes a fist (flexes the fingers) with the wrist in neutral position.

  - Have the client seated or supine.
  - Place palpating hand posterior to the brachioradialis (see the palpation section for this muscle on page 575).
  - Ask the client to make a fist with the hand extended at the wrist joint and feel for the contraction of the belly of the extensor carpi radialis longus.
  - Continue palpating the extensor carpi radialis longus distally all the way to the 2nd metacarpal and proximally toward the lateral supracondylar ridge. Its distal tendon of the extensor carpi radialis longus is visible and palpable on the radial (lateral) side of the posterior wrist (especially if the wrist is in neutral position).

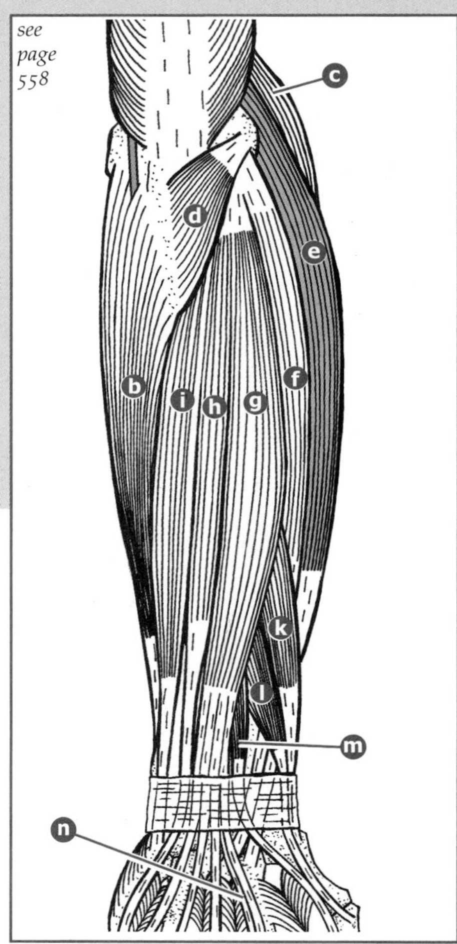

Posterior View of the Right Forearm (Superficial)

a. Pronator Teres (not seen)
b. Flexor Carpi Ulnaris
c. Brachioradialis
d. Anconeus
e. **Extensor Carpi Radialis Longus**
f. Extensor Carpi Radialis Brevis
g. Extensor Digitorum
h. Extensor Digiti Minimi
i. Extensor Carpi Ulnaris
j. Supinator (not seen)
k. Abductor Pollicis Longus
l. Extensor Pollicis Brevis
m. Extensor Pollicis Longus
n. Extensor Indicis

RELATIONSHIP TO OTHER MUSCULOSKELETAL STRUCTURES

❑ 1. The extensor carpi radialis longus lies directly posterior to the brachioradialis and directly anterior to the extensor carpi radialis brevis.

❑ 2. The extensor carpi radialis longus is superficial except for a small part that is deep to the brachioradialis proximally, and a portion of its distal tendon, which is deep to the abductor pollicis longus, extensor pollicis brevis and the extensor pollicis longus.

METHODOLOGY FOR LEARNING MUSCLE ACTIONS

❑ 1. **Extension of the Hand at the Wrist Joint:** The extensor carpi radialis longus crosses the wrist joint posteriorly (with its fibers running vertically in the sagittal plane); therefore, it extends the hand at the wrist joint.

❑ 2. **Radial Deviation (Abduction) of the Hand at the Wrist Joint:** The extensor carpi radialis longus crosses the wrist joint on the radial (lateral) side to attach onto the hand (with its fibers running vertically in the frontal plane). Therefore, the extensor carpi radialis longus radially deviates (abducts) the hand at the wrist joint.

EXTENSOR CARPI RADIALIS LONGUS – continued

- ❑ 3. **Flexion of the Forearm at the Elbow Joint:** The extensor carpi radialis longus crosses the elbow joint anteriorly (with its fibers running vertically in the sagittal plane); therefore, it flexes the forearm at the elbow joint.
- ❑ 4. **Pronation of the Forearm at the Radioulnar Joints:** When the extensor carpi radialis longus shortens, it attempts to bring its two attachments toward each other. If the forearm is fully supinated, the extensor carpi radialis longus will pronate the supinated forearm (at the radioulnar joints) until a position halfway between full pronation and full supination of the forearm is attained. That position will have the two attachments of the extensor carpi radialis longus, the 2nd metacarpal and the lateral supracondylar ridge of the humerus, as close to each other as possible. (Note the similarity of the direction of fibers of the extensor carpi radialis longus to the direction of fibers of the brachioradialis.)

MISCELLANEOUS

- ❑ 1. The extensor carpi radialis longus, extensor carpi radialis brevis and the extensor carpi ulnaris are often grouped together as the *wrist extensor group* of the forearm.
- ❑ 2. All three muscles of the wrist flexor group (flexor carpi radialis, palmaris longus and flexor carpi ulnaris) as well as the muscles of the wrist extensor group (extensor carpi radialis longus, extensor carpi radialis brevis and extensor carpi ulnaris) can flex the forearm at the elbow joint except the extensor carpi ulnaris, which extends the forearm at the elbow joint.
- ❑ 3. The extensor carpi radialis longus, extensor carpi radialis brevis and the brachioradialis are often grouped together as the *radial group* of forearm muscles. (They are also sometimes known as the *wad of three.)*
- ❑ 4. Making a strong grip (i.e., flexing the fingers) requires the wrist extensor muscles to contract as fixators (stabilizers) of the wrist to prevent wrist flexion that the flexor digitorum superficialis and flexor digitorum profundus would produce if they were unopposed. Make a fist while palpating the common extensor tendon region near the lateral epicondyle of the humerus and the contraction of the wrist extensors can be felt.

❑ EXTENSOR CARPI RADIALIS BREVIS

(OF THE WRIST EXTENSOR GROUP – AND – THE RADIAL GROUP)

❑ **The name, extensor carpi radialis brevis, tells us two of its actions: "extensor" tells us that this muscle performs extension and "radialis" tells us that this muscle performs radial deviation (abduction). Both of these actions occur at the wrist; "carpi" means wrist. "Brevis" tells us that this muscle is short (shorter than the extensor carpi radialis longus).**

DERIVATION ❑ extensor: L. *a muscle that extends a body part.*
carpi: L. *wrist.*
radialis: L. *refers to the radial side* (of the forearm).
brevis: L. *short.*

PRONUNCIATION ❑ eks-**ten**-sor **kar**-pie **ray**-dee-**a**-lis **bre**-vis

ATTACHMENTS

❑ **Lateral Epicondyle of the Humerus (via the Common Extensor Tendon)**

to the

❑ **Radial Hand on the Posterior Side**

- ❑ the posterior side of the base of the 3rd metacarpal

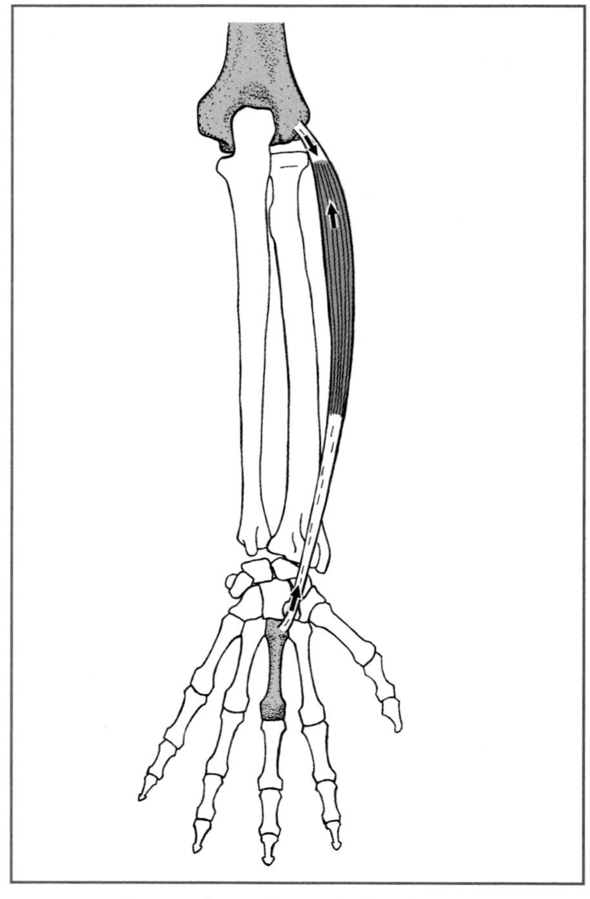

Posterior View of the Right Extensor Carpi Radialis Brevis

ACTIONS

❑ 1. **Extension of the Hand**

❑ 2. **Radial Deviation (Abduction) of the Hand**

❑ 3. Flexion of the Forearm

INNERVATION ❑ The Radial Nerve ❑ posterior interosseus nerve, **C7**, 8

ARTERIAL SUPPLY ❑ Branches of the Brachial Artery (The Continuation of the Axillary Artery) and the Radial Artery (A Terminal Branch of the Brachial Artery)

PALPATION AND SUPPLEMENTARY TEXT

PALPATION

The extensor carpi radialis brevis is the most posterior of the three muscles of the radial group of the forearm. The distal tendon can be difficult to palpate and distinguish from the extensor carpi radialis longus.

❑ **To palpate the belly:**

- Have the client seated or supine.
- Pinch the radial group of the forearm muscles (brachioradialis, extensor carpi radialis longus and extensor carpi radialis brevis) with your thumb on one side and your fingers on the other side and pull it slightly away from the forearm. The fingers on the posterior aspect of the radial group are on the extensor carpi radialis brevis.
- Ask the client to actively extend and/or radially deviate the hand at the wrist joint and feel for the contraction of the extensor carpi radialis brevis.

  (Note: These actions will also bring out the extensor carpi radialis longus.)

❑ **To palpate the distal tendon:** The distal tendon of the extensor carpi radialis brevis can sometimes be felt slightly medial to the distal tendon of the extensor carpi radialis longus (see the palpation section for this muscle on page 592). To palpate the distal tendon of the extensor carpi radialis brevis, locate the distal tendon of the extensor carpi radialis longus and palpate just medial to it.

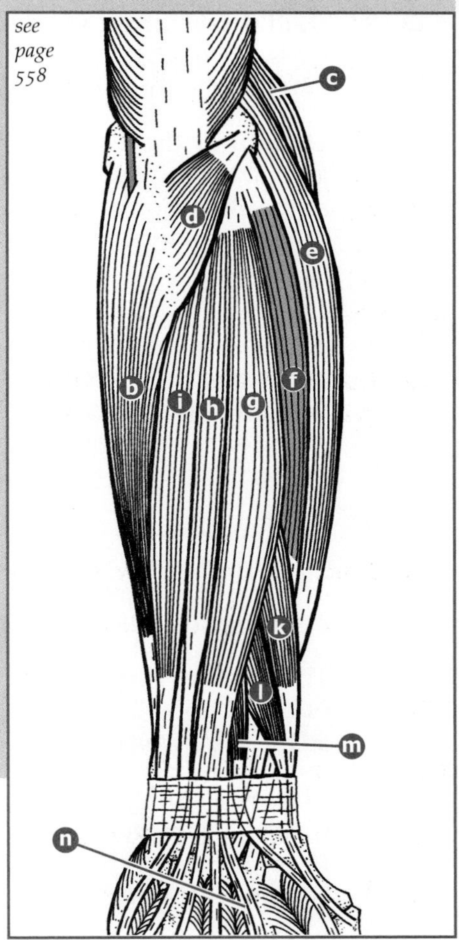

Posterior View of the Right Forearm (Superficial)

a. Pronator Teres (not seen)
b. Flexor Carpi Ulnaris
c. Brachioradialis
d. Anconeus
e. Extensor Carpi Radialis Longus
f. Extensor Carpi Radialis Brevis
g. Extensor Digitorum
h. Extensor Digiti Minimi
i. Extensor Carpi Ulnaris
j. Supinator (not seen)
k. Abductor Pollicis Longus
l. Extensor Pollicis Brevis
m. Extensor Pollicis Longus
n. Extensor Indicis

RELATIONSHIP TO OTHER MUSCULOSKELETAL STRUCTURES

❑ 1. The extensor carpi radialis brevis is superficial except for a small part that is deep to the brachioradialis and the extensor carpi radialis longus proximally, and a portion of its distal tendon, which is deep to the abductor pollicis longus, extensor pollicis brevis and the extensor pollicis longus. The actual distal attachment onto the 3rd metacarpal is deep to the distal tendon of the extensor indicis.

❑ 2. The extensor carpi radialis brevis lies directly posterior to the extensor carpi radialis longus.

❑ 3. The extensor carpi radialis brevis lies directly anterior to the extensor digitorum.

EXTENSOR CARPI RADIALIS BREVIS – continued

METHODOLOGY FOR LEARNING MUSCLE ACTIONS

- ❑ **1. Extension of the Hand at the Wrist Joint:** The extensor carpi radialis brevis crosses the wrist joint posteriorly (with its fibers running vertically in the sagittal plane); therefore, it extends the hand at the wrist joint.
- ❑ **2. Radial Deviation (Abduction) of the Hand at the Wrist Joint:** The extensor carpi radialis brevis crosses the wrist joint on the radial (lateral) side to attach onto the hand (with its fibers running vertically in the frontal plane); therefore it radially deviates (abducts) the hand at the wrist joint.
- ❑ **3. Flexion of the Forearm at the Elbow Joint:** The extensor carpi radialis brevis crosses the elbow joint anteriorly (with its fibers running vertically in the sagittal plane); therefore it flexes the forearm at the elbow joint.

MISCELLANEOUS

- ❑ 1. The extensor carpi radialis brevis arises proximally from the lateral epicondyle of the humerus by the *common extensor tendon*. The common extensor tendon is the common proximal attachment of four muscles: the extensor carpi radialis brevis, extensor digitorum, extensor digiti minimi and the extensor carpi ulnaris. The anconeus and the supinator also arise from the lateral epicondyle of the humerus (but not from the common extensor tendon).
- ❑ 2. All three muscles of the wrist flexor group (flexor carpi radialis, palmaris longus and flexor carpi ulnaris) as well as the muscles of the wrist extensor group (extensor carpi radialis longus, extensor carpi radialis brevis and extensor carpi ulnaris) can flex the forearm at the elbow joint except the extensor carpi ulnaris, which extends the forearm at the elbow joint.
- ❑ 3. The extensor carpi radialis brevis, the extensor carpi radialis longus and the brachioradialis are often grouped together as the *radial group* of forearm muscles. (They are also sometimes known as the *wad of three.)*
- ❑ 4. Making a strong grip (i.e., flexing the fingers) requires the wrist extensor muscles to contract as fixators (stabilizers) of the wrist to prevent wrist flexion that the flexor digitorum superficialis and flexor digitorum profundus would produce if they were unopposed. Make a fist while palpating the common extensor tendon region near the lateral epicondyle of the humerus and the contraction of the wrist extensors can be felt.
- ❑ 5. Irritation and inflammation of the lateral epicondyle and/or the common extensor tendon is known as *lateral epicondylitis* or *tennis elbow.*

EXTENSOR DIGITORUM ❑

❑ **The name, extensor digitorum, tells us that this muscle extends the digits, i.e., fingers.**

DERIVATION ❑ extensor: L. *a muscle that extends a body part.*
digitorum: L. *refers to a digit* (finger).

PRONUNCIATION ❑ eks-**ten**-sor dij-i-**toe**-rum

ATTACHMENTS

❑ **Lateral Epicondyle of the Humerus (via the Common Extensor Tendon)**

to the

❑ **Phalanges of Fingers #2-5**

- ❑ via its dorsal digital expansion onto the posterior surface of the middle and distal phalanges

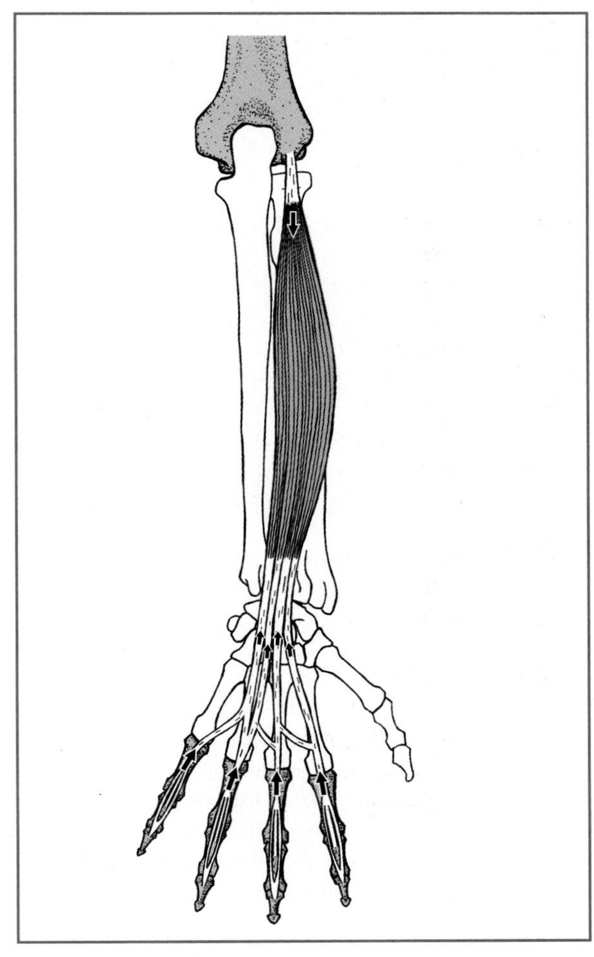

Posterior View of the Right Extensor Digitorum

ACTIONS

❑ 1. **Extension of Fingers #2-5**

❑ 2. **Extension of the Hand**

❑ 3. Medial Rotation of the Little Finger (Finger #5)

❑ 4. Extension of the Forearm

INNERVATION ❑ The Radial Nerve ❑ posterior interosseus nerve, C7, 8

ARTERIAL SUPPLY ❑ The Posterior Interosseus Artery (A Branch of the Ulnar Artery)

EXTENSOR DIGITORUM – PALPATION AND SUPPLEMENTARY TEXT

PALPATION

- ❑ The belly of the extensor digitorum is superficial and located in the posterior forearm. The distal tendons are superficial, visible and palpable in the distal posterior forearm and posterior hand.
  - Have the client seated or supine.
  - Place palpating hand between the extensor carpi radialis muscles and the extensor carpi ulnaris (and the extensor digiti minimi) to locate the extensor digitorum. (See the palpation sections for these muscles on pages 592, 595, 604 and 601.)
  - Ask the client to actively extend fingers #2-5 (at the metacarpophalangeal and interphalangeal joints) and feel for the contraction of the extensor digitorum.
  - To further bring out the extensor digitorum, resistance may be added.

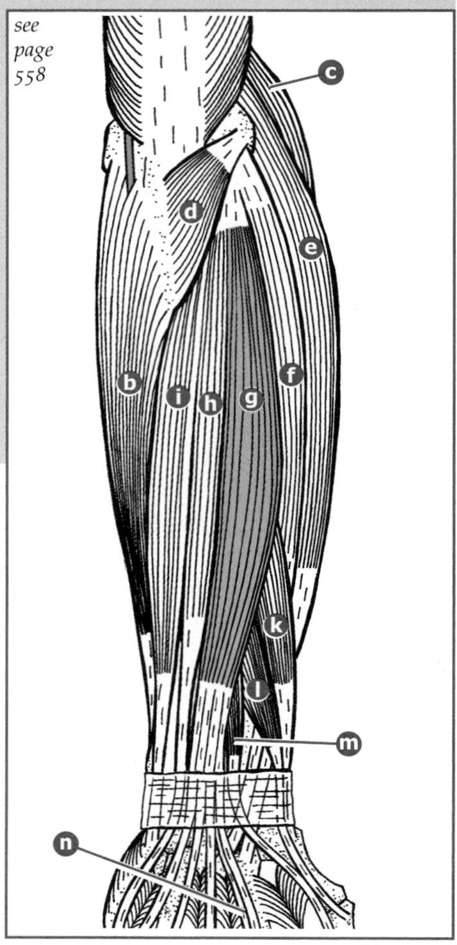

Posterior View of the Right Forearm (Superficial)

a. Pronator Teres (not seen)
b. Flexor Carpi Ulnaris
c. Brachioradialis
d. Anconeus
e. Extensor Carpi Radialis Longus
f. Extensor Carpi Radialis Brevis
g. **Extensor Digitorum**
h. Extensor Digiti Minimi
i. Extensor Carpi Ulnaris
j. Supinator (not seen)
k. Abductor Pollicis Longus
l. Extensor Pollicis Brevis
m. Extensor Pollicis Longus
n. Extensor Indicis

RELATIONSHIP TO OTHER MUSCULOSKELETAL STRUCTURES

❑ 1. The extensor digitorum is located medial to the extensor carpi radialis brevis and extensor carpi radialis longus and lateral to the extensor digiti minimi and the extensor carpi ulnaris.

❑ 2. The extensor digitorum is superficial. Deep to the extensor digitorum is the deeper layer of posterior forearm muscles, which includes the supinator, abductor pollicis longus, extensor pollicis brevis, extensor pollicis longus and the extensor indicis.

METHODOLOGY FOR LEARNING MUSCLE ACTIONS

❑ 1. **Extension of Fingers #2-5 at the Metacarpophalangeal and Proximal and Distal Interphalangeal Joints:** The extensor digitorum crosses the metacarpophalangeal joint and the interphalangeal joints posteriorly to finally attach onto the distal phalanges of fingers #2-5, i.e., the index, middle, ring and little fingers (with its fibers running vertically in the sagittal plane). Therefore, the extensor digitorum extends fingers #2-5 at the metacarpophalangeal and the proximal and distal interphalangeal joints.

❑ 2. **Extension of the Hand at the Wrist Joint:** The extensor digitorum crosses the wrist joint posteriorly (with its fibers running vertically in the sagittal plane); therefore, it extends the hand at the wrist joint.

EXTENSOR DIGITORUM – continued

- ❑ **3. Medial Rotation of the Little Finger (Finger #5) at the Carpometacarpal Joint:** The tendon of the extensor digitorum that goes to the little finger crosses the 5th carpometacarpal joint posteriorly from lateral on the lateral epicondyle to attach more medially onto the phalanges of the little finger (with its fibers running slightly horizontally in the transverse plane). When the extensor digitorum contracts, it pulls the posterior side of the little finger laterally. This is medial rotation of the little finger because the anterior side of the little finger rotates medially. Therefore, the extensor digitorum medially rotates the metacarpal of the little finger at the 5th carpometacarpal joint.
- ❑ **4. Extension of the Forearm at the Elbow Joint:** The extensor digitorum crosses the elbow joint posteriorly (with its fibers running vertically in the sagittal plane); therefore, it extends the forearm at the elbow joint.

MISCELLANEOUS

- ❑ 1. The extensor digitorum is sometimes called the *extensor digitorum communis.*
- ❑ 2. The extensor digitorum arises proximally from the lateral epicondyle of the humerus by the *common extensor tendon.* The common extensor tendon is the common proximal attachment of four muscles: the extensor carpi radialis brevis, extensor digitorum, extensor digiti minimi and the extensor carpi ulnaris. The anconeus and the supinator also arise from the lateral epicondyle of the humerus (but not from the common extensor tendon).
- ❑ 3. Distally, the tendons of the extensor digitorum are somewhat tied together by intertendinous connections. These interconnections make independent movement of an individual finger more difficult.
- ❑ 4. The distal attachment of the extensor digitorum spreads out to become a fibrous aponeurotic expansion that covers the posterior, medial and lateral sides of the proximal phalanx. It then continues distally to attach onto the posterior sides of the middle and distal phalanges. This structure is called the *dorsal digital expansion* (see pages 636-7).
- ❑ 5. The dorsal digital expansion is also known as the *extensor expansion* and/or the *dorsal hood.*
- ❑ 6. The dorsal digital expansion is sometimes called the dorsal hood because one of its purposes is to serve as a movable hood of tissue when the fingers flex and extend.
- ❑ 7. The dorsal digital expansion also serves as an attachment site for the lumbricals manus, palmar interossei, dorsal interossei manus and the abductor digiti minimi manus muscles. Given that the dorsal digital expansion crosses the proximal and distal interphalangeal joints posteriorly, these muscles can extend the middle and distal phalanges at these joints.
- ❑ 8. Irritation and inflammation of the lateral epicondyle and/or the common extensor tendon is known as *lateral epicondylitis* or *tennis elbow.*

❑ EXTENSOR DIGITI MINIMI

❑ **The name, extensor digiti minimi, tells us that this muscle extends the little finger.**

DERIVATION ❑ extensor: L. *a muscle that extends a body part.*
digiti: L. *refers to a digit* (finger).
minimi: L. *least.*

PRONUNCIATION ❑ eks-**ten**-sor **dij**-i-tee **min**-i-mee

ATTACHMENTS

❑ **Lateral Epicondyle of the Humerus (via the Common Extensor Tendon)**

to the

❑ **Phalanx of the Little Finger (Finger #5)**

- ❑ attaches into the ulnar side of the tendon of the extensor digitorum muscle (to attach onto the posterior surface of the middle and distal phalanges of the little finger via the dorsal digital expansion)

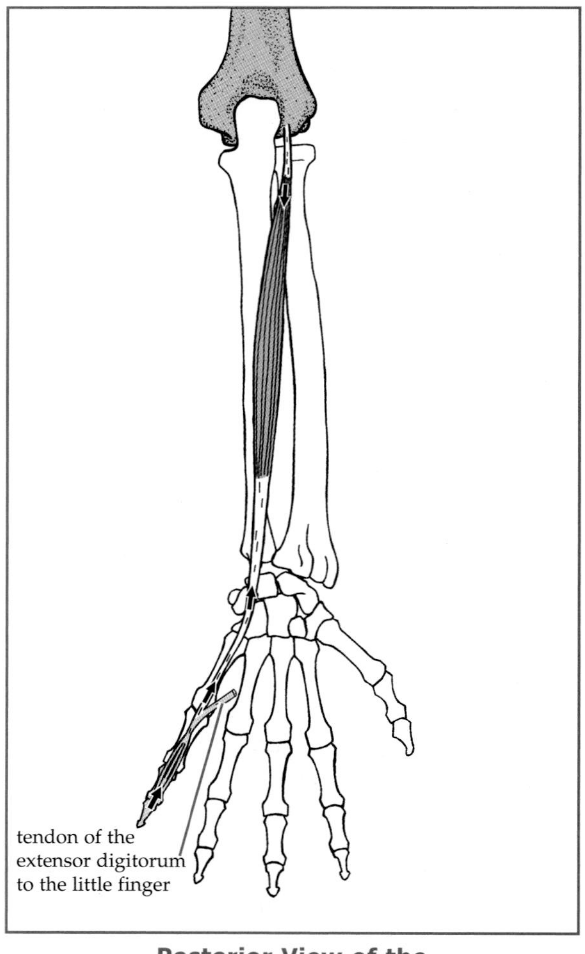

Posterior View of the Right Extensor Digiti Minimi

ACTIONS

❑ 1. **Extension of the Little Finger (Finger #5)**

❑ 2. **Extension of the Hand**

❑ 3. Medial Rotation of the Little Finger (Finger #5)

❑ 4. Extension of the Forearm

INNERVATION ❑ The Radial Nerve ❑ posterior interosseus nerve, **C7**, 8

ARTERIAL SUPPLY ❑ The Posterior Interosseus Artery (A Branch of the Ulnar Artery)

PALPATION AND SUPPLEMENTARY TEXT

PALPATION

- ❑ It is difficult to distinguish the extensor digiti minimi from the medial fibers of the extensor digitorum.
  - Have the client seated or supine.
  - Place palpating hand just lateral to the extensor carpi ulnaris (see the palpation section for this muscle on page 604) to locate the extensor digiti minimi.
  - Ask the client to actively extend the little finger at the 5th metacarpophalangeal and interphalangeal joints and feel for the contraction of the extensor digiti minimi.
  - To further bring out the extensor digiti minimi, resistance may be added.

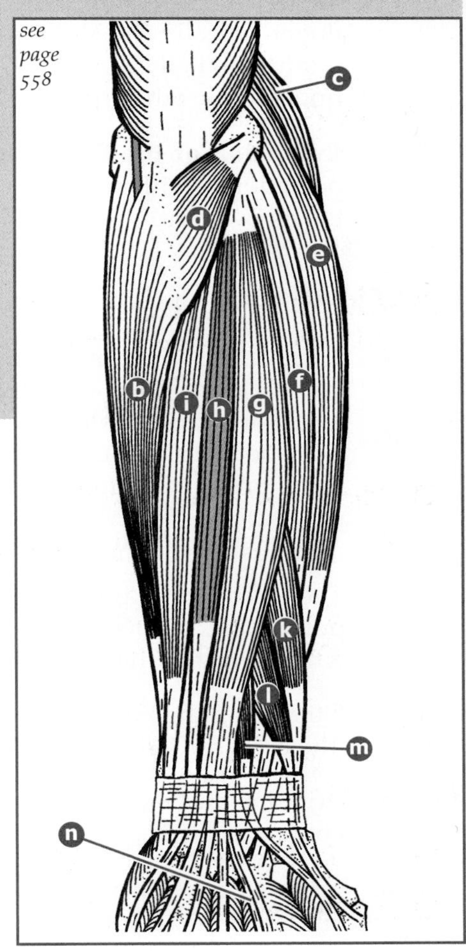

Posterior View of the Right Forearm (Superficial)

- **a.** Pronator Teres (not seen)
- **b.** Flexor Carpi Ulnaris
- **c.** Brachioradialis
- **d.** Anconeus
- **e.** Extensor Carpi Radialis Longus
- **f.** Extensor Carpi Radialis Brevis
- **g.** Extensor Digitorum
- **h.** **Extensor Digiti Minimi**
- **i.** Extensor Carpi Ulnaris
- **j.** Supinator (not seen)
- **k.** Abductor Pollicis Longus
- **l.** Extensor Pollicis Brevis
- **m.** Extensor Pollicis Longus
- **n.** Extensor Indicis

RELATIONSHIP TO OTHER MUSCULOSKELETAL STRUCTURES

❑ 1. The extensor digiti minimi is superficial and located between the extensor digitorum (which is lateral to it) and the extensor carpi ulnaris (which is medial to it).

❑ 2. The extensor digiti minimi is superficial to the deeper layer of posterior forearm muscles, which includes the supinator, abductor pollicis longus, extensor pollicis brevis, extensor pollicis longus and the extensor indicis.

METHODOLOGY FOR LEARNING MUSCLE ACTIONS

❑ 1. **Extension of the Little Finger (Finger #5) at the Metacarpophalangeal and Proximal and Distal Interphalangeal Joints:** The extensor digiti minimi crosses the 5th metacarpophalangeal joint (of the little finger) before it attaches into the distal tendon of the extensor digitorum muscle of the little finger. Since the extensor digiti minimi crosses this joint posteriorly (with its fibers running vertically in the sagittal plane), it extends the little finger at the 5th metacarpophalangeal joint. Furthermore, by attaching into the distal tendon of the extensor digitorum, the extensor digiti minimi pulls on that tendon in the same manner as if the belly of the extensor digitorum muscle itself had contracted. Therefore, the extensor digiti minimi has the same actions at the little finger as the extensor digitorum muscle, namely, extension of the middle and distal phalanges of the little finger at the proximal and distal interphalangeal joints.

❑ 2. **Extension of the Hand at the Wrist Joint:** The extensor digiti minimi crosses the wrist joint posteriorly (with its fibers running vertically in the sagittal plane); therefore, it extends the hand at the wrist joint.

EXTENSOR DIGITI MINIMI – continued

- ❑ **3. Medial Rotation of the Little Finger (Finger #5) at the Carpometacarpal Joint:** The extensor digiti minimi crosses the 5th carpometacarpal joint posteriorly from lateral on the lateral epicondyle to attach more medially onto the little finger (with its fibers running slightly horizontally in the transverse plane). When the extensor digiti minimi contracts, it pulls the posterior side of the little finger laterally. This is medial rotation of the little finger because the anterior side of the little finger rotates medially. Therefore, the extensor digiti minimi medially rotates the metacarpal of the little finger at the 5th carpometacarpal joint.
- ❑ **4. Extension of the Forearm at the Elbow Joint:** The extensor digiti minimi crosses the elbow joint posteriorly (with its fibers running vertically in the sagittal plane); therefore, it extends the forearm at the elbow joint.

MISCELLANEOUS

- ❑ 1. The extensor digiti minimi arises proximally from the lateral epicondyle of the humerus by the *common extensor tendon*. The common extensor tendon is the common proximal attachment of four muscles: the extensor carpi radialis brevis, extensor digitorum, extensor digiti minimi and the extensor carpi ulnaris. The anconeus and the supinator also arise from the lateral epicondyle of the humerus (but not from the common extensor tendon).
- ❑ 2. The extensor digiti minimi sometimes blends with the extensor digitorum.
- ❑ 3. The extensor digiti minimi, by attaching into the distal tendon of the extensor digitorum, exerts a pull upon the dorsal digital expansion of the little finger. (This is similar to the extensor indicis, which attaches into the distal tendon of the extensor digitorum of the index finger.)
- ❑ 4. Other than the little finger and the thumb, only the index finger has a second extensor muscle (the extensor indicis).
- ❑ 5. Irritation and inflammation of the lateral epicondyle and/or the common extensor tendon is known as *lateral epicondylitis* or *tennis elbow*.
- ❑ 6. The extensor indicis of the index finger also attaches into the ulnar side of the tendon of the extensor digitorum (that goes to the index finger).

EXTENSOR CARPI ULNARIS
(OF THE WRIST EXTENSOR GROUP)

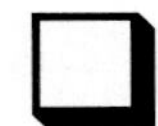

❑ **The name, extensor carpi ulnaris, tells us two of its actions: "extensor" tells us that this muscle performs extension and "ulnaris" tells us that this muscle performs ulnar deviation (adduction). Both of these actions occur at the wrist; "carpi" means wrist.**

DERIVATION ❑ extensor: L. *a muscle that extends a body part.*
carpi: L. *wrist.*
ulnaris: L. *refers to the ulnar side* (of the forearm).

PRONUNCIATION ❑ eks-**ten**-sor **kar**-pie ul-**na**-ris

ATTACHMENTS

❑ **Lateral Epicondyle of the Humerus (via the Common Extensor Tendon) and the Ulna**

❑ the posterior middle 1/3 of the ulna

to the

❑ **Ulnar Hand on the Posterior Side**

❑ the posterior side of the base of the 5th metacarpal

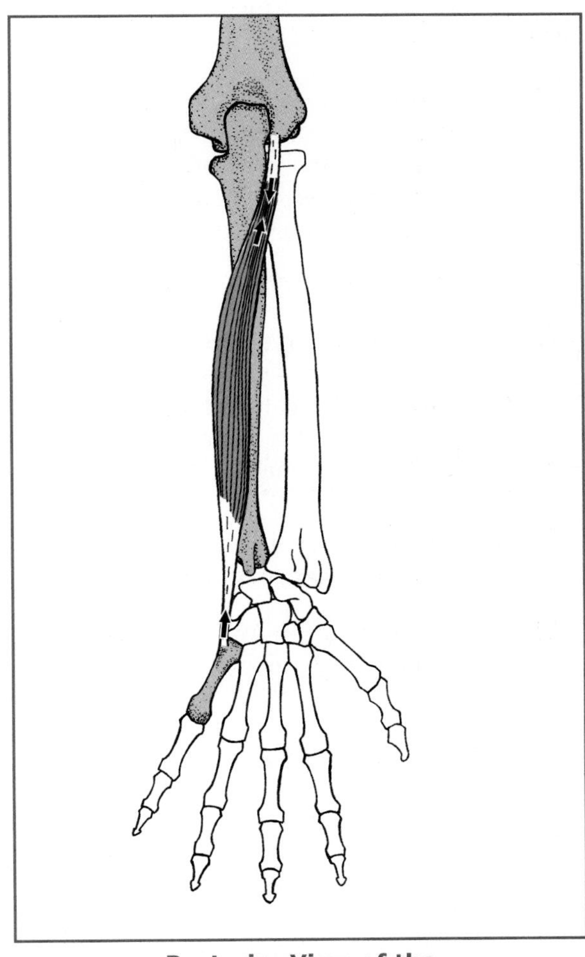

Posterior View of the Right Extensor Carpi Ulnaris

ACTIONS

❑ 1. **Extension of the Hand**

❑ 2. **Ulnar Deviation (Adduction) of the Hand**

❑ 3. Extension of the Forearm

INNERVATION ❑ The Radial Nerve ❑ posterior interosseus nerve, **C7**, 8

ARTERIAL SUPPLY ❑ The Posterior Interosseus Artery (A Branch of the Ulnar Artery)

EXTENSOR CARPI ULNARIS – PALPATION AND SUPPLEMENTARY TEXT

PALPATION

- ❑ The belly of the extensor carpi ulnaris is located directly posterior to the shaft of the ulna. The distal tendon is easily palpable where it crosses the wrist just lateral to the styloid process of the ulna.
  - Have the client seated or supine.
  - Place palpating hand directly posterior to the shaft of the ulna and feel for the belly of the extensor carpi ulnaris.
  - Continue palpating the extensor carpi ulnaris proximally toward the lateral epicondyle of the humerus and distally toward the 5th metacarpal.

    (Note: The distal tendon is easily palpable just lateral to the styloid process of the ulna.)
  - To further bring out the extensor carpi ulnaris, ask the client to actively extend and ulnar deviate (adduct) the hand at the wrist joint (with the fingers gently flexed to relax the extensor digitorum).

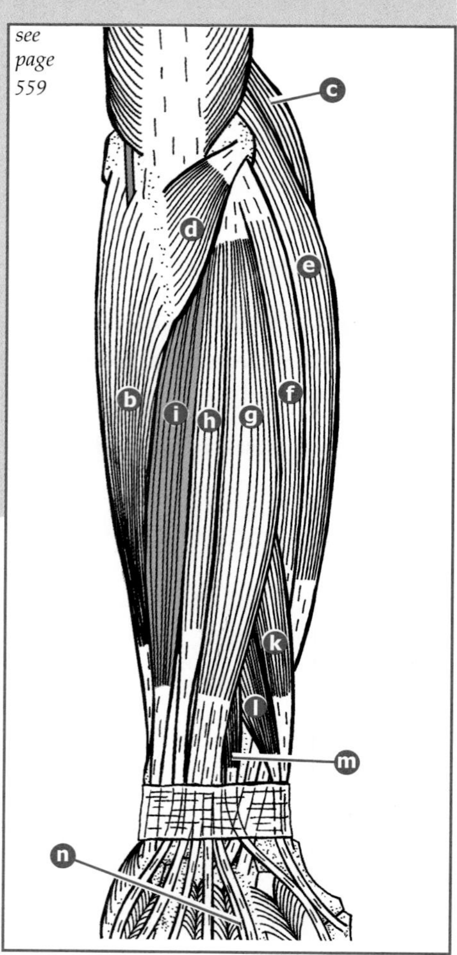

Posterior View of the Right Forearm (Superficial)

- **a.** Pronator Teres (not seen)
- **b.** Flexor Carpi Ulnaris
- **c.** Brachioradialis
- **d.** Anconeus
- **e.** Extensor Carpi Radialis Longus
- **f.** Extensor Carpi Radialis Brevis
- **g.** Extensor Digitorum
- **h.** Extensor Digiti Minimi
- **i.** **Extensor Carpi Ulnaris**
- **j.** Supinator (not seen)
- **k.** Abductor Pollicis Longus
- **l.** Extensor Pollicis Brevis
- **m.** Extensor Pollicis Longus
- **n.** Extensor Indicis

RELATIONSHIP TO OTHER MUSCULOSKELETAL STRUCTURES

- ❑ 1. The extensor carpi ulnaris is superficial in the posterior forearm and is medial to the extensor digiti minimi and lateral to the flexor carpi ulnaris.
- ❑ 2. The anconeus is proximal to the extensor carpi ulnaris.
- ❑ 3. The extensor carpi ulnaris is superficial to the shaft of the ulna and the deeper layer of posterior forearm muscles, which includes the supinator, abductor pollicis longus, extensor pollicis brevis, extensor pollicis longus and the extensor indicis.

METHODOLOGY FOR LEARNING MUSCLE ACTIONS

- ❑ **1. Extension of the Hand at the Wrist Joint:** The extensor carpi ulnaris crosses the wrist joint posteriorly (with its fibers running vertically in the sagittal plane); therefore, it extends the hand at the wrist joint.
- ❑ **2. Ulnar Deviation (Adduction) of the Hand at the Wrist Joint:** The extensor carpi ulnaris crosses the wrist joint on the ulnar (medial) side to attach onto the hand (with its fibers running vertically in the frontal plane); therefore, it ulnar deviates (adducts) the hand at the wrist joint.
- ❑ **3. Extension of the Forearm at the Elbow Joint:** The extensor carpi ulnaris crosses the elbow joint posteriorly (with its fibers running vertically in the sagittal plane); therefore, it extends the forearm at the elbow joint.

EXTENSOR CARPI ULNARIS – continued

MISCELLANEOUS

- ❑ 1. The extensor carpi ulnaris arises proximally from the lateral epicondyle of the humerus by the *common extensor tendon.* The common extensor tendon is the common proximal attachment of four muscles: the extensor carpi radialis brevis, extensor digitorum, extensor digiti minimi and the extensor carpi ulnaris. The anconeus and the supinator also arise from the lateral epicondyle of the humerus (but not from the common extensor tendon).
- ❑ 2. The extensor carpi ulnaris has two heads: a humeral head and an ulnar head.
- ❑ 3. The attachment of the extensor carpi ulnaris onto the ulna blends with the ulnar attachment of the flexor carpi ulnaris and the flexor digitorum profundus.
- ❑ 4. All three muscles of the wrist flexor group (flexor carpi radialis, palmaris longus and flexor carpi ulnaris) as well as the muscles of the wrist extensor group (extensor carpi radialis longus, extensor carpi radialis brevis and extensor carpi ulnaris) can flex the forearm at the elbow joint except the extensor carpi ulnaris, which extends the forearm at the elbow joint.
- ❑ 5. Making a strong grip (i.e., flexing the fingers) requires the wrist extensor muscles to contract as fixators (stabilizers) of the wrist to prevent wrist flexion that the flexor digitorum superficialis and flexor digitorum profundus would produce if they were unopposed. Make a fist while palpating the common extensor tendon region near the lateral epicondyle of the humerus and the contraction of the wrist extensors can be felt.
- ❑ 6. Irritation and inflammation of the lateral epicondyle and/or the common extensor tendon is known as *lateral epicondylitis* or *tennis elbow.*

❑ SUPINATOR

❑ **The name, supinator, tells us that this muscle supinates the forearm.**

DERIVATION ❑ supinator: L. *a muscle that supinates a body part.*

PRONUNCIATION ❑ **sue**-pin-**a**-tor

ATTACHMENTS

❑ **Lateral Epicondyle of the Humerus and the Proximal Ulna**

❑ the supinator crest of the ulna

to the

❑ **Proximal Radius**

❑ the proximal 1/3 of the posterior, lateral and anterior sides

ACTION

❑ **Supination of the Forearm**

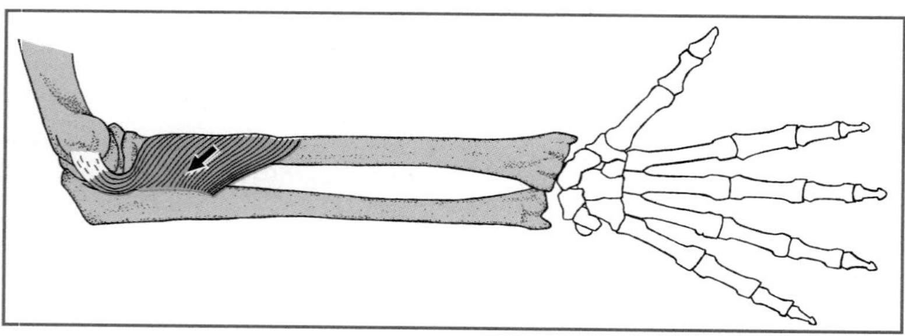

Lateral View of the Right Supinator
(with the forearm halfway between full pronation and full supination)

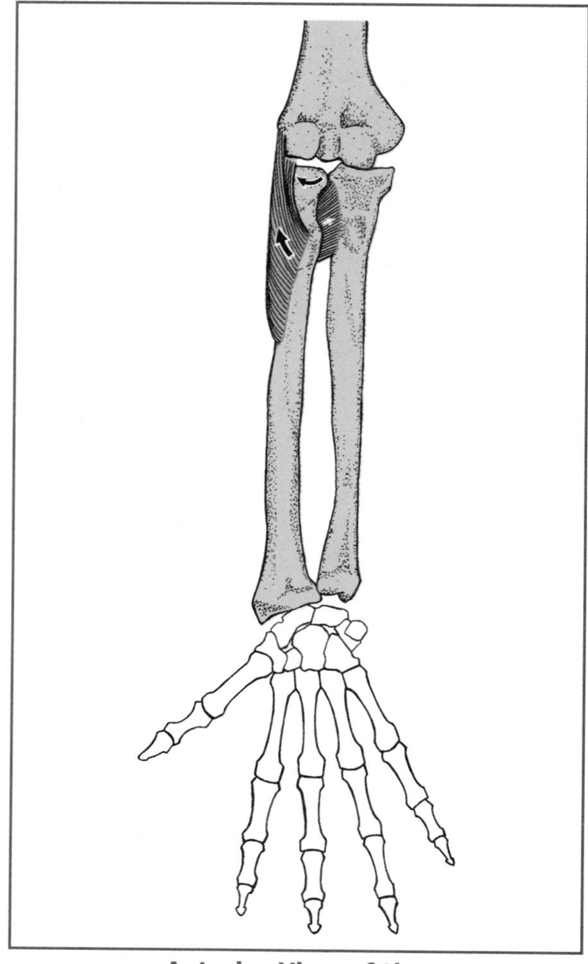

Anterior View of the Right Supinator

INNERVATION ❑ The Radial Nerve ❑ **C6**, 7

ARTERIAL SUPPLY ❑ Branches of the Radial Artery (A Terminal Branch of the Brachial Artery) and the Interosseus Recurrent and Posterior Interosseus Arteries (Branches of the Ulnar Artery)

PALPATION AND SUPPLEMENTARY TEXT

PALPATION

- ❑ The supinator is deep but not too difficult to palpate.
  - Have the client seated with the forearm passively flexed, pronated and resting comfortably on the lap.
  - Pinch the radial group of the forearm muscles (brachioradialis, extensor carpi radialis longus and extensor carpi radialis brevis) with your thumb on one side and your fingers on the other side.
  - Palpate deeper against the radius between the radial group of the forearm and the extensor digitorum to locate the radial attachment of the supinator.
  - Ask the client to slowly supinate the forearm at the radioulnar joints and feel for the contraction of the supinator.

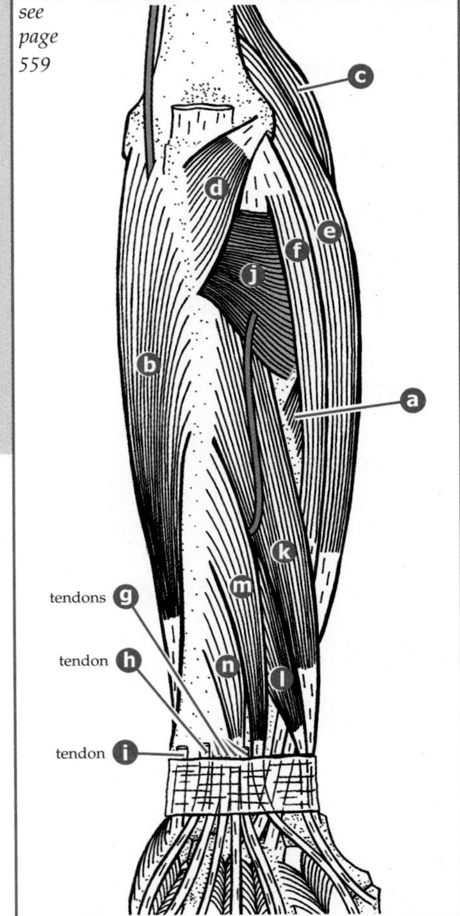

Posterior View of the Right Forearm (Deep)

a. Pronator Teres
b. Flexor Carpi Ulnaris
c. Brachioradialis
d. Anconeus
e. Extensor Carpi Radialis Longus
f. Extensor Carpi Radialis Brevis
g. Extensor Digitorum
h. Extensor Digiti Minimi
i. Extensor Carpi Ulnaris
j. Supinator
k. Abductor Pollicis Longus
l. Extensor Pollicis Brevis
m. Extensor Pollicis Longus
n. Extensor Indicis

RELATIONSHIP TO OTHER MUSCULOSKELETAL STRUCTURES

❑ 1. The supinator is a deep muscle in the proximal posterior forearm. The supinator lies deep to the anconeus, extensor digitorum, extensor digiti minimi, extensor carpi radialis brevis, extensor carpi radialis longus and the brachioradialis.

❑ 2. The distal tendon of the supinator attaches onto the radius next to the distal attachment of the pronator teres.

METHODOLOGY FOR LEARNING MUSCLE ACTIONS

❑ **Supination of the Forearm at the Radioulnar Joints:**
The supinator crosses from the proximal posterior ulna to the proximal posterolateral radius; thus, it wraps around the posterior forearm. When the supinator pulls the radius toward the ulna on the posterior side, it causes the head of the radius to laterally rotate and the distal radius to move posterolaterally around the distal ulna. This movement of the radius is called supination. Therefore, the supinator supinates the forearm at the radioulnar joints.

MISCELLANEOUS

❑ 1. Besides the supinator, the anconeus attaches proximally to the lateral epicondyle of the humerus. Also arising from the lateral epicondyle are four other muscles that share the common extensor tendon attachment onto the lateral epicondyle of the humerus (the extensor carpi radialis brevis, extensor digitorum, extensor digiti minimi and the extensor carpi ulnaris).

❑ 2. Proximally, the supinator muscle has two layers: a superficial layer and a deep layer.

SUPINATOR – continued

- ❑ 3. The posterior interosseus nerve, a deep branch of the radial nerve, runs between the two layers of the supinator and may be entrapped there. (Most sources state that the posterior interosseus nerve can also be called the *deep branch of the radial nerve*. However, other sources state that the posterior interosseus nerve is the continuation of the deep branch of the radial nerve after it has emerged from the supinator muscle.)
- ❑ 4. The supinator has some fibers that cross the elbow joint (running vertically in the sagittal plane). Given that these fibers cross slightly anterior to the center of the joint, the supinator should have a weak ability to flex the forearm at the elbow joint.
- ❑ 5. The supinator crest is located deep between the two bones of the forearm on the lateral side of the ulna.
- ❑ 6. Irritation and inflammation of the lateral epicondyle and/or the common extensor tendon is known as *lateral epicondylitis* or *tennis elbow*.

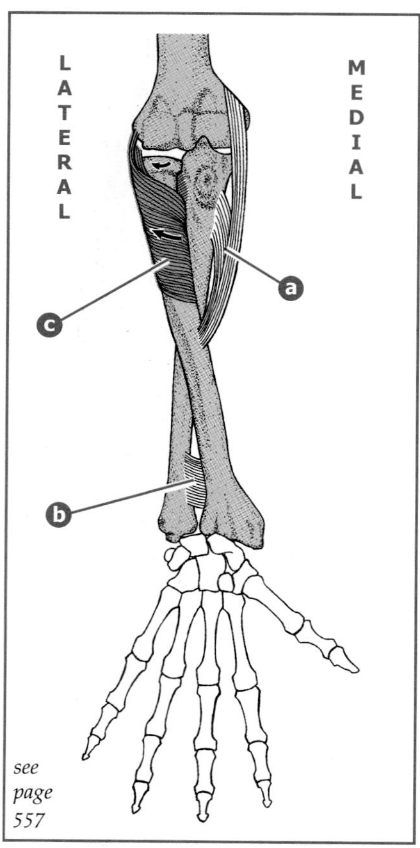

see page 557

Anterior View of the Right Forearm Fully Pronated

a. Pronator Teres
b. Pronator Quadratus
c. **Supinator**

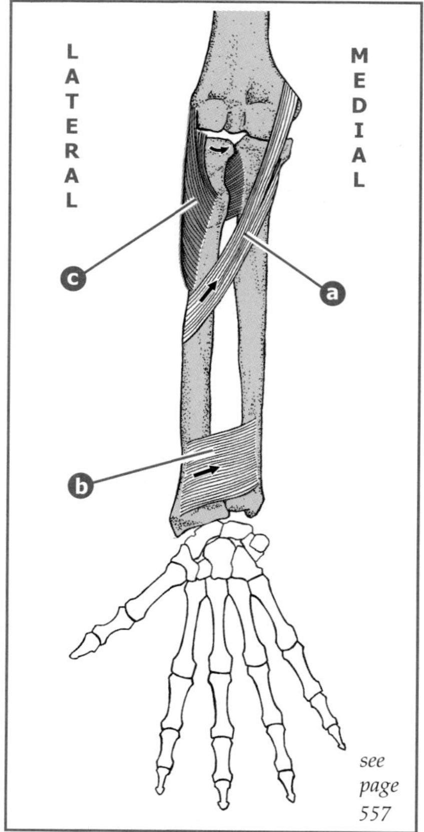

see page 557

Anterior View of the Right Forearm Fully Supinated

a. Pronator Teres
b. Pronator Quadratus
c. **Supinator**

ABDUCTOR POLLICIS LONGUS

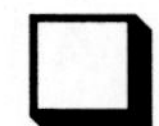

❑ **The name, abductor pollicis longus, tells us that this muscle abducts the thumb and is long (longer than the abductor pollicis brevis).**

DERIVATION ❑ abductor: L. *a muscle that abducts a body part.*
pollicis: L. *thumb.*
longus: L. *long.*

PRONUNCIATION ❑ ab-**duk**-tor **pol**-i-sis **long**-us

ATTACHMENTS

❑ **Posterior Radius and Ulna**

- ❑ approximately the middle 1/3 of the radius, ulna and interosseus membrane

to the

❑ **Thumb**

- ❑ the lateral side of the base of the 1st metacarpal

ACTIONS

❑ **1. Abduction of the Thumb**

❑ 2. Extension of the Thumb

❑ 3. Lateral Rotation of the Thumb

❑ 4. Radial Deviation (Abduction) of the Hand

❑ 5. Flexion of the Hand

❑ 6. Supination of the Forearm

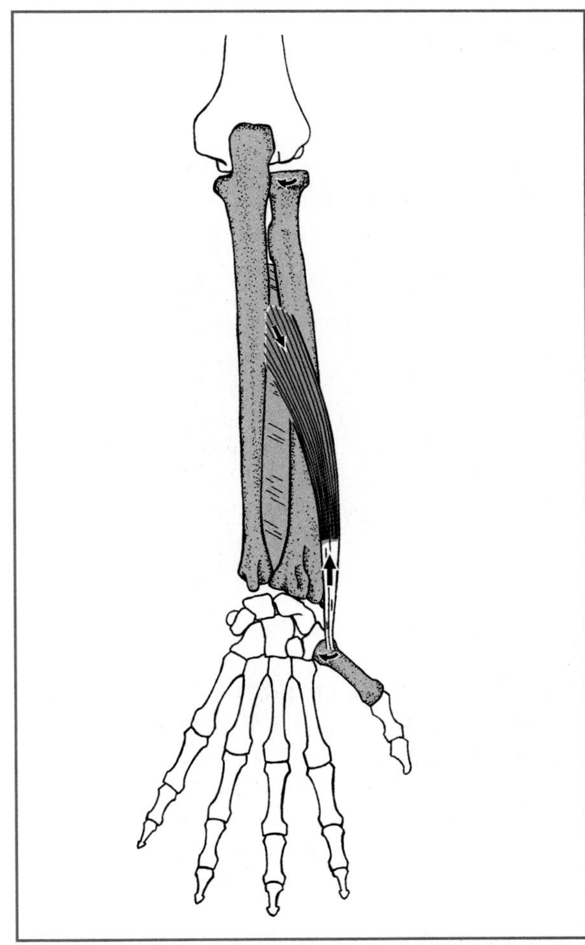

Posterior View of the Right Abductor Pollicis Longus

INNERVATION ❑ The Radial Nerve ❑ posterior interosseus nerve, **C7**, 8

ARTERIAL SUPPLY ❑ The Posterior Interosseus Artery (A Branch of the Ulnar Artery)
❑ and the perforating branches of the anterior interosseus artery (a branch of the ulnar artery)

ABDUCTOR POLLICIS LONGUS – PALPATION AND SUPPLEMENTARY TEXT

PALPATION

- ❑ The distal bellies and tendons of the abductor pollicis longus and extensor pollicis brevis are visible as an oblique elevation in the distal posterolateral forearm and border the anatomical snuffbox on the radial (lateral) side.
  - Have the client seated with the forearm in a position halfway between pronation and supination.
  - Place palpating hand on the lateral wrist.
  - Ask the client to actively abduct and extend the thumb at the 1st carpometacarpal joint and feel for the distal tendons of the abductor pollicis longus and extensor pollicis brevis. They will both become clearly visible bordering the anatomical snuffbox on the radial (lateral) side.
  - Continue palpating the abductor pollicis longus and extensor pollicis brevis proximally until the muscles dive deep to the extensor digitorum and are no longer palpable.
  - Continue palpating the abductor pollicis longus tendon distally until it attaches into the 1st metacarpal.
  - It may be necessary to gently place a fingernail between the tendons of the abductor pollicis longus and extensor pollicis brevis to clearly see that there are in fact two tendons very close together and parallel to each other. The abductor pollicis longus is the more anterolateral one of the two.

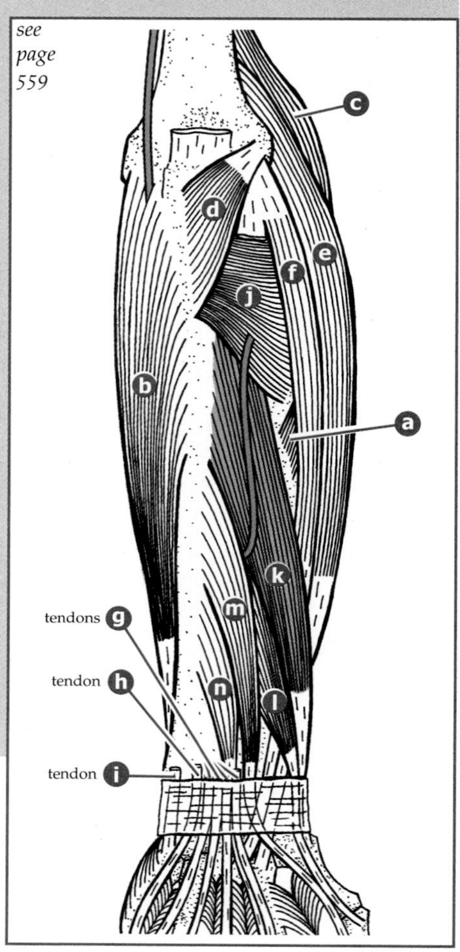

Posterior View of the Right Forearm (Deep)

a. Pronator Teres
b. Flexor Carpi Ulnaris
c. Brachioradialis
d. Anconeus
e. Extensor Carpi Radialis Longus
f. Extensor Carpi Radialis Brevis
g. Extensor Digitorum
h. Extensor Digiti Minimi
i. Extensor Carpi Ulnaris
j. Supinator
k. Abductor Pollicis Longus
l. Extensor Pollicis Brevis
m. Extensor Pollicis Longus
n. Extensor Indicis

RELATIONSHIP TO OTHER MUSCULOSKELETAL STRUCTURES

❑ 1. The abductor pollicis longus is one of four deep muscles found in the distal posterior forearm (the abductor pollicis longus, extensor pollicis brevis, extensor pollicis longus and the extensor indicis). Most of the belly of the abductor pollicis longus is deep to the extensor digitorum, the extensor digiti minimi and the extensor carpi ulnaris.

❑ 2. The abductor pollicis longus is directly lateral to the extensor pollicis longus and the extensor pollicis brevis.

❑ 3. The distal belly and tendon of the abductor pollicis longus become superficial (along with the extensor pollicis brevis) in the distal posterolateral forearm and lie superficial to the radial group of muscles (the brachioradialis, extensor carpi radialis longus and the extensor carpi radialis brevis).

ABDUCTOR POLLICIS LONGUS – continued

METHODOLOGY FOR LEARNING MUSCLE ACTIONS

- ❑ 1. **Abduction of the Thumb at the Carpometacarpal Joint:** The abductor pollicis longus crosses the 1st carpometacarpal joint anteriorly to attach onto the 1st metacarpal of the thumb (with its fibers running vertically in the sagittal plane). When the abductor pollicis longus contracts, it pulls the metacarpal of the thumb anteriorly (in the sagittal plane, in a direction that is perpendicular to and away from the plane of the palm of the hand). This action is called abduction of the thumb. Therefore, the abductor pollicis longus abducts the thumb by abducting the metacarpal of the thumb at the 1st carpometacarpal joint. (Note: Due to the rotational development of the thumb embryologically, the named actions of abduction and adduction of the thumb occur within the sagittal plane. For more details, see the Muscular System Manual, Volume I.)

- ❑ 2. **Extension of the Thumb at the Carpometacarpal Joint:** The abductor pollicis longus crosses the 1st carpometacarpal joint laterally (radially) to attach onto the 1st metacarpal of the thumb (with its fibers running vertically in the frontal plane). When the abductor pollicis longus contracts, it pulls the metacarpal of the thumb laterally (i.e., radially, in the frontal plane, within the plane of the palm of the hand away from the index finger). This action is called extension of the thumb. Therefore, the abductor pollicis longus extends the thumb by extending the metacarpal of the thumb at the 1st carpometacarpal joint. (Note: Due to the rotational development of the thumb embryologically, the named actions of flexion and extension of the thumb occur within the frontal plane. For more details, see the Muscular System Manual, Volume I.)

- ❑ 3. **Lateral Rotation of the Thumb at the Carpometacarpal Joint:** The abductor pollicis longus crosses the 1st carpometacarpal joint posteriorly from medial in the forearm to attach more laterally onto the thumb (with its fibers running slightly horizontally in the transverse plane). When the abductor pollicis longus contracts, it pulls the thumb posterolaterally. This is lateral rotation of the thumb because the anterior side of the thumb rotates laterally. Therefore, the abductor pollicis longus laterally rotates the thumb at the 1st carpometacarpal joint.

- ❑ 4. **Radial Deviation (Abduction) of the Hand at the Wrist Joint:** The abductor pollicis longus crosses the wrist on the radial (lateral) side (with it fibers running vertically in the frontal plane); therefore, it radially deviates (abducts) the hand at the wrist joint.

- ❑ 5. **Flexion of the Hand at the Wrist Joint:** The abductor pollicis longus crosses the wrist slightly anteriorly (with its fibers running vertically in the sagittal plane); therefore, it flexes the hand at the wrist joint.

- ❑ 6. **Supination of the Forearm at the Radioulnar Joints:** The abductor pollicis longus crosses the ulna and radius in the posterior forearm with an ulnar to radial orientation to its fibers (hence its fibers are running somewhat horizontally in the transverse plane). When the thumb and the hand are fixed to the forearm, and the abductor pollicis longus pulls at its distal attachment, the distal forearm moves. If the forearm is in a position of pronation, then the abductor pollicis longus' line of pull causes the distal radius to be pulled in a posterolateral direction around the distal ulna (and the head of the radius to laterally rotate). This movement of the radius is called supination. Therefore, the abductor pollicis longus supinates the forearm at the radioulnar joints.

ABDUCTOR POLLICIS LONGUS – continued

MISCELLANEOUS

- ❑ 1. The distal tendon of the abductor pollicis longus, along with the distal tendon of the extensor pollicis brevis, make up the lateral border of the *anatomical snuffbox*. These two tendons are very close together and can be difficult to distinguish from each other. The abductor pollicis longus will be the more anterolateral one of the two. (Note: The medial border of the anatomical snuffbox is made up of the extensor pollicis longus.)
- ❑ 2. The distal tendon of the abductor pollicis longus often splits to also attach onto the trapezium.
- ❑ 3. The abductor pollicis longus and the extensor pollicis brevis share a common synovial sheath. With excessive movements of the thumb, the friction between the tendons of the abductor pollicis longus and/or the extensor pollicis brevis and the styloid process of the radius can cause a tenosynovitis (inflammation of the synovial sheath). This condition is known as *de Quervain's Disease.*
- ❑ 4. All four deep distal muscles of the posterior forearm (abductor pollicis longus, extensor pollicis brevis, extensor pollicis longus and extensor indicis) can do supination of the forearm at the radioulnar joints.

EXTENSOR POLLICIS BREVIS

❑ **The name, extensor pollicis brevis, tells us that this muscle extends the thumb and is short (shorter than the extensor pollicis longus).**

DERIVATION ❑ extensor: L. *a muscle that extends a body part.*
pollicis: L. *thumb.*
brevis: L. *short.*

PRONUNCIATION ❑ eks-**ten**-sor **pol**-i-sis **bre**-vis

ATTACHMENTS

❑ **Posterior Radius**

- ❑ the distal 1/3 and the adjacent interosseus membrane

to the

❑ **Thumb**

- ❑ the posterolateral base of the proximal phalanx

ACTIONS

❑ 1. **Extension of the Thumb**

❑ 2. Abduction of the Thumb

❑ 3. Lateral Rotation of the Thumb

❑ 4. Radial Deviation (Abduction) of the Hand

❑ 5. Supination of the Forearm

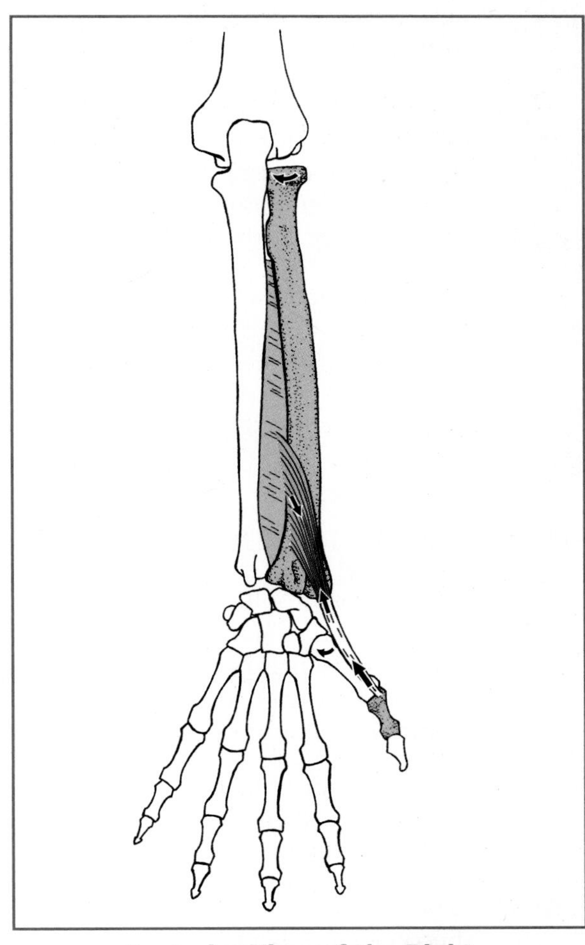

Posterior View of the Right Extensor Pollicis Brevis

INNERVATION ❑ The Radial Nerve ❑ the posterior interosseus nerve, **C7**, 8

ARTERIAL SUPPLY ❑ The Posterior Interosseus Artery (A Branch of the Ulnar Artery)
❑ and the perforating branches of the anterior interosseus artery (a branch of the ulnar artery)

EXTENSOR POLLICIS BREVIS – PALPATION AND SUPPLEMENTARY TEXT

PALPATION

- [ ] The distal bellies and tendons of the extensor pollicis brevis and abductor pollicis longus are visible as an oblique elevation in the distal posterolateral forearm and border the anatomical snuffbox on the radial (lateral) side.

  - Have the client seated with the forearm in a position halfway between pronation and supination.
  - Place palpating hand on the lateral wrist.
  - Ask the client to actively abduct and extend the thumb at the 1st carpometacarpal joint and feel for the distal tendons of the extensor pollicis brevis and abductor pollicis longus. They will both become clearly visible bordering the anatomical snuffbox on the radial (lateral) side.
  - Continue palpating the extensor pollicis brevis and abductor pollicis longus proximally until the muscles dive deep to the extensor digitorum and are no longer palpable.
  - It may be necessary to gently place a fingernail between the tendons of the extensor pollicis brevis and abductor pollicis longus to clearly see that there are in fact two tendons very close together and parallel to each other. The extensor pollicis brevis is the more posteromedial one of the two.

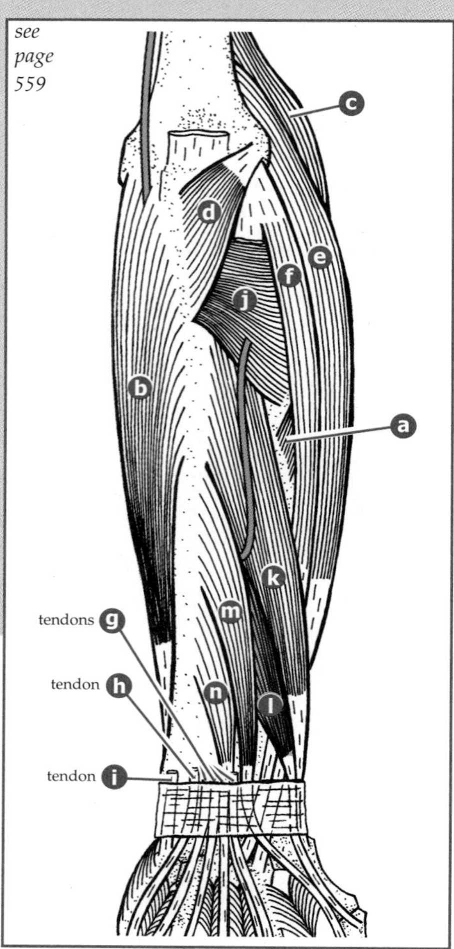

Posterior View of the Right Forearm (Deep)

a. Pronator Teres
b. Flexor Carpi Ulnaris
c. Brachioradialis
d. Anconeus
e. Extensor Carpi Radialis Longus
f. Extensor Carpi Radialis Brevis
g. Extensor Digitorum
h. Extensor Digiti Minimi
i. Extensor Carpi Ulnaris
j. Supinator
k. Abductor Pollicis Longus
l. **Extensor Pollicis Brevis**
m. Extensor Pollicis Longus
n. Extensor Indicis

RELATIONSHIP TO OTHER MUSCULOSKELETAL STRUCTURES

- [ ] 1. The extensor pollicis brevis is one of four deep muscles found in the distal posterior forearm (the abductor pollicis longus, extensor pollicis brevis, extensor pollicis longus and the extensor indicis). Most of the belly of the extensor pollicis brevis is deep to the extensor digitorum.
- [ ] 2. The extensor pollicis brevis lies directly medial to the abductor pollicis longus and directly lateral to the extensor pollicis longus.
- [ ] 3. The distal belly and tendon of the extensor pollicis brevis become superficial (along with the abductor pollicis longus) in the distal posterolateral forearm and lie superficial to the radial group of muscles (the brachioradialis, extensors carpi radialis longus and brevis).
- [ ] 4. The tendon of the extensor pollicis brevis turns around a bony fulcrum called the *dorsal tubercle* of the radius (also known as *Lister's tubercle*) that alters its line of pull.

EXTENSOR POLLICIS BREVIS – continued

METHODOLOGY FOR LEARNING MUSCLE ACTIONS

- ❑ 1. **Extension of the Thumb at the Carpometacarpal and Metacarpophalangeal Joints:** The extensor pollicis brevis crosses the 1st carpometacarpal joint of the thumb laterally (radially) to attach onto the proximal phalanx of the thumb (with its fibers running vertically in the frontal plane). When the extensor pollicis brevis contracts, it pulls the proximal phalanx of the thumb laterally (radially) within the plane of the hand (frontal plane), away from the index finger. This action is called extension of the thumb. Therefore, the extensor pollicis brevis extends the thumb by extending the metacarpal of the thumb at the 1st carpometacarpal joint. Additionally, the extensor pollicis brevis also crosses the 1st metacarpophalangeal joint of the thumb laterally (radially). Therefore, it extends the proximal phalanx of the thumb at this joint as well. (Note: Due to the rotational development of the thumb embryologically, the named actions of flexion and extension of the thumb occur within the frontal plane. For more details, see the **Muscular System Manual, Volume I.**)

- ❑ 2. **Abduction of the Thumb at the Carpometacarpal Joint:** The extensor pollicis brevis crosses the 1st carpometacarpal joint of the thumb anteriorly to attach onto the proximal phalanx of the thumb (with its fibers running vertically in the sagittal plane). When the extensor pollicis brevis contracts, it pulls the proximal phalanx of the thumb in a direction that is perpendicular to and away from the plane of the palm of the hand (sagittal plane). This action is called abduction of the thumb. Therefore, the extensor pollicis brevis abducts the thumb by abducting the metacarpal of the thumb at the 1st carpometacarpal joint. The extensor pollicis brevis also crosses the 1st metacarpophalangeal joint of the thumb anteriorly; however, this joint does not allow abduction. (Note: Due to the rotational development of the thumb embryologically, the named actions of abduction and adduction of the thumb occur within the sagittal plane. For more details, see the **Muscular System Manual, Volume I.**)

- ❑ 3. **Lateral Rotation of the Thumb at the Carpometacarpal Joint:** The extensor pollicis brevis crosses the 1st carpometacarpal joint posteriorly from medial in the forearm to attach more laterally onto the thumb (with its fibers running slightly horizontally in the transverse plane). When the extensor pollicis brevis contracts, it pulls the thumb posterolaterally. This is lateral rotation of the thumb because the anterior side of the thumb rotates laterally. Therefore, the extensor pollicis brevis laterally rotates the thumb at the 1st carpometacarpal joint.

- ❑ 4. **Radial Deviation (Abduction) of the Hand at the Wrist Joint:** The extensor pollicis brevis crosses the wrist on the radial (lateral) side (with it fibers running vertically in the frontal plane); therefore, it radially deviates (abducts) the hand at the wrist joint.

- ❑ 5. **Supination of the Forearm at the Radioulnar Joints:** The extensor pollicis brevis crosses the ulna and radius in the posterior forearm with an ulnar to radial orientation to its fibers (hence its fibers are running somewhat horizontally in the transverse plane). When the thumb and the hand are fixed to the forearm, and the extensor pollicis brevis pulls at its distal attachment, the distal forearm moves. If the forearm is in a position of pronation, then the extensor pollicis brevis' line of pull causes the distal radius to be pulled in a posterolateral direction around the distal ulna (and the head of the radius to laterally rotate). This movement of the radius is called supination. Therefore, the extensor pollicis brevis can supinate the forearm at the radioulnar joints.

EXTENSOR POLLICIS BREVIS – continued

MISCELLANEOUS

- ❑ 1. The distal tendon of the extensor pollicis brevis, along with the distal tendon of the abductor pollicis longus, make up the lateral border of the *anatomical snuffbox.* These two tendons are very close together and can be difficult to distinguish from each other. The extensor pollicis brevis will be the more posteromedial one of the two. (Note: The medial border of the anatomical snuffbox is made up of the extensor pollicis longus.)
- ❑ 2. The extensor pollicis brevis and the abductor pollicis longus share a common synovial sheath. With excessive movements of the thumb, the friction between the tendons of the extensor pollicis brevis and/or the abductor pollicis longus and the styloid process of the radius can cause a tenosynovitis (inflammation of the synovial sheath). This condition is known as *de Quervain's Disease.*
- ❑ 3. All four deep distal muscles of the posterior forearm (abductor pollicis longus, extensor pollicis brevis, extensor pollicis longus and extensor indicis) can do supination of the forearm at the radioulnar joints.

EXTENSOR POLLICIS LONGUS

❑ **The name, extensor pollicis longus, tells us that this muscle extends the thumb and is long (longer than the extensor pollicis brevis).**

DERIVATION ❑ extensor: L. *a muscle that extends a body part.*
pollicis: L. *thumb.*
longus: L. *long.*

PRONUNCIATION ❑ eks-**ten**-sor **pol**-i-sis **long**-us

ATTACHMENTS

❑ **Posterior Ulna**

- ❑ the middle 1/3 and the interosseus membrane

to the

❑ **Thumb**

- ❑ via its dorsal digital expansion onto the posterior surface of the distal phalanx of the thumb

ACTIONS

❑ **1. Extension of the Thumb**

❑ **2.** Lateral Rotation of the Thumb

❑ **3.** Extension of the Hand

❑ **4.** Radial Deviation (Abduction) of the Hand

❑ **5.** Supination of the Forearm

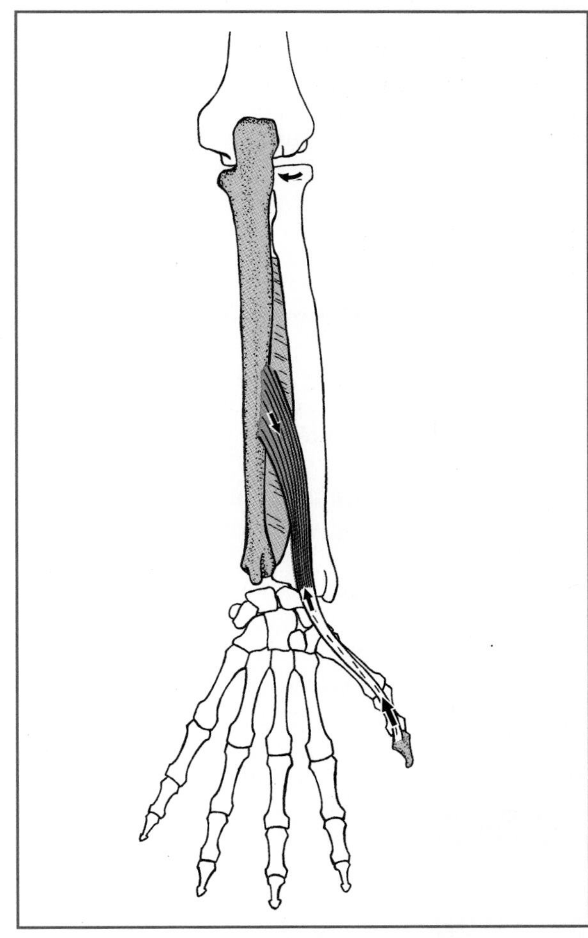

Posterior View of the Right Extensor Pollicis Longus

INNERVATION ❑ The Radial Nerve ❑ posterior interosseus nerve, **C7**, 8

ARTERIAL SUPPLY ❑ The Posterior Interosseus Artery (A Branch of the Ulnar Artery)
❑ and the perforating branches of the anterior interosseus artery (a branch of the ulnar artery)

EXTENSOR POLLICIS LONGUS – PALPATION AND SUPPLEMENTARY TEXT

PALPATION

The distal tendon of the extensor pollicis longus is visible and easy to palpate. It borders the anatomical snuffbox on the ulnar (medial) side. The belly of the extensor pollicis longus is deep to the extensor digitorum, but it can be palpated if the extensor digitorum is relaxed.

❑ **To palpate the distal tendon:**

- Have the client seated with the forearm in a position halfway between pronation and supination.
- Place palpating hand on the lateral wrist.
- Ask the client to actively abduct and extend the thumb at the 1st carpometacarpal joint, the 1st metacarpophalangeal joint and the 1st interphalangeal joint and feel for tensing of the distal tendon of the extensor pollicis longus. It will be clearly visible bordering the anatomical snuffbox on the ulnar (medial) side.

❑ **To palpate the muscle belly:**

- Have the client seated with the forearm resting across the lap in a position of pronation with the fingers passively flexed (which relaxes the extensor digitorum).
- Place palpating hand on the middle 1/3 of the posterior forearm between the radius and the ulna.
- Ask the client to alternately contract and relax the extensor pollicis longus (by extending and abducting the thumb and then relaxing) and feel for the contraction of the extensor pollicis longus. (Be careful that you are not too medial and over the extensor pollicis brevis and/or the abductor pollicis longus.)
- Continue palpating extensor pollicis longus toward its proximal attachment on the radial (lateral) surface of the ulna.

see page 559

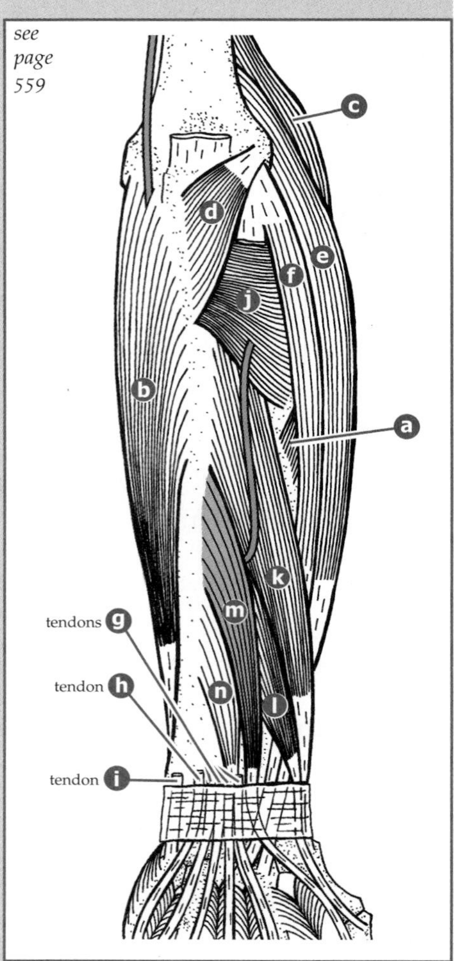

Posterior View of the Right Forearm (Deep)

a. Pronator Teres
b. Flexor Carpi Ulnaris
c. Brachioradialis
d. Anconeus
e. Extensor Carpi Radialis Longus
f. Extensor Carpi Radialis Brevis
g. Extensor Digitorum
h. Extensor Digiti Minimi
i. Extensor Carpi Ulnaris
j. Supinator
k. Abductor Pollicis Longus
l. Extensor Pollicis Brevis
m. Extensor Pollicis Longus
n. Extensor Indicis

RELATIONSHIP TO OTHER MUSCULOSKELETAL STRUCTURES

❑ 1. The extensor pollicis longus is one of four deep muscles found in the distal posterior forearm (the abductor pollicis longus, extensor pollicis brevis, extensor pollicis longus and the extensor indicis). Most of the belly of the extensor pollicis longus is deep to the extensor digitorum, extensor digiti minimi and the extensor carpi ulnaris.

EXTENSOR POLLICIS LONGUS – continued

- ❑ 2. The extensor pollicis longus' proximal attachment onto the posterior ulna is located between the abductor pollicis longus and the extensor indicis, it is distal to the abductor pollicis longus and proximal to the extensor indicis.
- ❑ 3. The extensor pollicis longus is superficial to the proximal attachment of the extensor pollicis brevis.
- ❑ 4. The bellies of the abductor pollicis longus and the extensor pollicis brevis lie just lateral to the belly of the extensor pollicis longus.
- ❑ 5. The distal belly and tendon of the extensor pollicis longus become superficial in the posterior wrist. It is superficial to the extensor carpi radialis longus and the extensor carpi radialis brevis.

METHODOLOGY FOR LEARNING MUSCLE ACTIONS

- ❑ **1. Extension of the Thumb at the Carpometacarpal, Metacarpophalangeal and the Interphalangeal Joints:** The extensor pollicis longus crosses the 1st carpometacarpal joint of the thumb laterally (radially) to attach onto the distal phalanx of the thumb (with its fibers running vertically in the frontal plane). When the extensor pollicis longus contracts, it pulls the distal phalanx of the thumb laterally (radially) within the plane of the palm of the hand (frontal plane), away from the index finger. This action is called extension of the thumb. Therefore, the extensor pollicis longus extends the thumb by extending the metacarpal of the thumb at the 1st carpometacarpal joint. Additionally, the extensor pollicis longus also crosses the 1st metacarpophalangeal and the 1st interphalangeal joints of the thumb laterally (radially). Therefore, it also extends the phalanges of the thumb at these joints as well. (Note: Due to the rotational development of the thumb embryologically, the named actions of flexion and extension of the thumb occur within the frontal plane. For more details, see the **Muscular System Manual, Volume I.**)
- ❑ **2. Lateral Rotation of the Thumb at the Carpometacarpal Joint:** The extensor pollicis longus crosses the 1st carpometacarpal joint posteriorly from medial in the forearm to attach more laterally onto the thumb (with its fibers running slightly horizontally in the transverse plane). When the extensor pollicis longus contracts, it pulls the thumb posterolaterally. This is lateral rotation of the thumb because the anterior side of the thumb rotates laterally. Therefore, the extensor pollicis longus laterally rotates the thumb at the 1st carpometacarpal joint.
- ❑ **3. Extension of the Hand at the Wrist Joint:** The extensor pollicis longus crosses the wrist posteriorly (with its fibers running vertically in the sagittal plane); therefore, it extends the hand at the wrist joint.
- ❑ **4. Radial Deviation (Abduction) of the Hand at the Wrist Joint:** The extensor pollicis longus crosses the wrist on the radial (lateral) side (with it fibers running vertically in the frontal plane); therefore, it radially deviates (abducts) the hand at the wrist joint.
- ❑ **5. Supination of the Forearm at the Radioulnar Joints:** The extensor pollicis longus crosses the ulna and radius in the posterior forearm with an ulnar to radial orientation to its fibers (hence its fibers are running somewhat horizontally in the transverse plane). When the thumb and the hand are fixed to the forearm, and the extensor pollicis longus pulls at its distal attachment, the distal forearm moves. If the forearm is in a position of pronation, then the extensor pollicis longus' line of pull causes the distal radius to be pulled in a posterolateral direction around the distal ulna (and the head of the radius to laterally rotate). This movement of the radius is called supination. Therefore, the extensor pollicis longus supinates the forearm at the radioulnar joints.

EXTENSOR POLLICIS LONGUS – continued

MISCELLANEOUS

- ❑ 1. The distal tendon of the extensor pollicis longus makes up the medial border of the *anatomical snuffbox.* (Note: The lateral border is made up of the abductor pollicis longus and the extensor pollicis brevis.)
- ❑ 2. If the thumb begins in an extended position, then the line of pull of the extensor pollicis longus relative to the carpometacarpal joint of the thumb is such that it can adduct the thumb.
- ❑ 3. The distal attachment of the extensor pollicis longus spreads out to become a fibrous aponeurotic expansion that covers the posterior, medial and lateral sides of the proximal phalanx of the thumb. It then continues distally to attach onto the posterior side of the distal phalanx. This structure is called the *dorsal digital expansion.*
- ❑ 4. The dorsal digital expansion is also known as the *extensor expansion* and/or the *dorsal hood.*
- ❑ 5. One purpose of the dorsal digital expansion is to serve as a movable hood of tissue when the fingers flex and extend (hence its other name, the dorsal hood).
- ❑ 6. The dorsal digital expansion of the thumb also serves as an attachment site for the abductor pollicis longus and adductor pollicis (and the palmar interosseus muscle of the thumb, if present). Given that the dorsal digital expansion of the thumb crosses the interphalangeal joint posteriorly, these muscles can all extend the distal phalanx at this joint.
- ❑ 7. All four deep distal muscles of the posterior forearm (abductor pollicis longus, extensor pollicis brevis, extensor pollicis longus and extensor indicis) can do supination of the forearm at the radioulnar joints.

EXTENSOR INDICIS

❑ **The name, extensor indicis, tells us that this muscle extends the index finger.**

DERIVATION ❑ extensor: L. *a muscle that extends a body part.*
indicis: L. *index finger* (finger #2).

PRONUNCIATION ❑ eks-**ten**-sor **in**-di-sis

ATTACHMENTS

❑ **Posterior Ulna**

- ❑ the distal 1/3 and the interosseus membrane

to the

❑ **Index Finger (Finger #2)**

- ❑ attaches into the ulnar side of the tendon of the extensor digitorum muscle (to attach onto the posterior surface of the middle and distal phalanges of the index finger via the dorsal digital expansion)

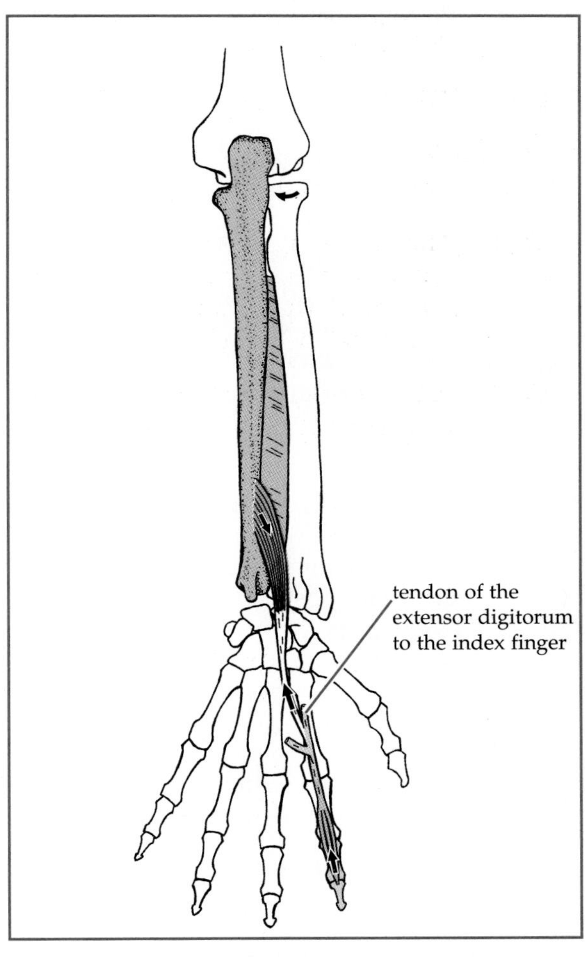

Posterior View of the Right Extensor Indicis

ACTIONS

❑ **1. Extension of the Index Finger (Finger #2)**

❑ **2. Extension of the Hand**

❑ 3. Adduction of the Index Finger (Finger #2)

❑ 4. Supination of the Forearm

INNERVATION ❑ The Radial Nerve ❑ posterior interosseus nerve, C7, 8

ARTERIAL SUPPLY ❑ The Posterior Interosseus Artery (A Branch of the Ulnar Artery)
❑ and the perforating branches of the anterior interosseus artery (a branch of the ulnar artery)

EXTENSOR INDICIS – PALPATION AND SUPPLEMENTARY TEXT

PALPATION

❑ The belly of the extensor indicis is deep to the bellies of the extensor digitorum and the extensor carpi ulnaris. Given that part of the extensor digitorum can also extend the index finger, it can be difficult to distinguish the extensor indicis from the extensor digitorum. However, the majority of the extensor indicis lies further medially on the ulna than the fibers of the extensor digitorum that extend the index finger.

- Have the client seated with the forearm fully pronated at the radioulnar joints.
- Place palpating hand on the distal 1/3 of the ulna on the posterior side.
- Ask the client to actively extend the index finger at the 2nd metacarpophalangeal and interphalangeal joints and feel for the contraction of the extensor indicis.
- Continue palpating the extensor indicis distally for the distal tendon of the extensor indicis. It may be difficult to distinguish the distal tendon of the extensor indicis from the distal tendon of the extensor digitorum that goes to the index finger. If the two can be felt, the extensor indicis will be the more medial one of the two.

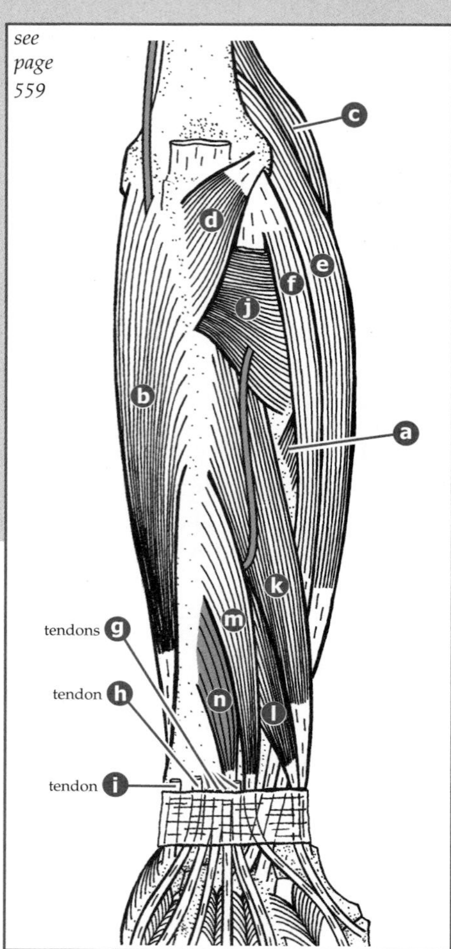

Posterior View of the Right Forearm (Deep)

a. Pronator Teres
b. Flexor Carpi Ulnaris
c. Brachioradialis
d. Anconeus
e. Extensor Carpi Radialis Longus
f. Extensor Carpi Radialis Brevis
g. Extensor Digitorum
h. Extensor Digiti Minimi
i. Extensor Carpi Ulnaris
j. Supinator
k. Abductor Pollicis Longus
l. Extensor Pollicis Brevis
m. Extensor Pollicis Longus
n. **Extensor Indicis**

RELATIONSHIP TO OTHER MUSCULOSKELETAL STRUCTURES

❑ 1. The extensor indicis is one of four deep muscles found in the distal posterior forearm (the abductor pollicis longus, extensor pollicis brevis, extensor pollicis longus and the extensor indicis). Most of the belly of the extensor indicis is deep to the extensor digitorum, the extensor digiti minimi and the extensor carpi ulnaris.

❑ 2. The extensor indicis attaches onto the posterior ulna just distal to the attachment of the extensor pollicis longus.

❑ 3. The belly of the extensor pollicis longus lies just lateral to the belly of the extensor indicis.

❑ 4. The distal tendon of the extensor indicis becomes superficial in the posterior hand and lies just medial (ulnar) to the tendon of the extensor digitorum that attaches onto the index finger.

EXTENSOR INDICIS – continued

METHODOLOGY FOR LEARNING MUSCLE ACTIONS

- ❑ 1. **Extension of the Index Finger (Finger #2) at the Metacarpophalangeal and Proximal and Distal Interphalangeal Joints:** The extensor indicis crosses the 2nd metacarpophalangeal joint (of the index finger) before it attaches into the distal tendon of the extensor digitorum muscle of the index finger. Since the extensor indicis crosses this joint posteriorly (with its fibers running vertically in the sagittal plane), it extends the index finger at the 2nd metacarpophalangeal joint. Further, by attaching into the distal tendon of the extensor digitorum, the extensor indicis pulls on that tendon the same as if the belly of the extensor digitorum muscle itself had contracted and pulled on its own tendon. Therefore, the extensor indicis has the same actions at the index finger as the extensor digitorum muscle has, namely, extension of the index finger at the proximal and distal interphalangeal joints.
- ❑ 2. **Extension of the Hand at the Wrist Joint:** The extensor indicis crosses the wrist posteriorly (with its fibers running vertically in the sagittal plane); therefore, it extends the hand at the wrist joint.
- ❑ 3. **Adduction of the Index Finger (Finger #2) at the Metacarpophalangeal Joint:** The extensor indicis attaches from the ulna to the index finger, crossing the 2nd metacarpophalangeal joint from medial to lateral (with its fibers running somewhat horizontally in the frontal plane). When the extensor indicis pulls on the index finger, it pulls the index finger medially toward the ulna, i.e., toward the middle finger. Therefore, the extensor indicis can adduct the index finger at the 2nd metacarpophalangeal joint.
- ❑ 4. **Supination of the Forearm at the Radioulnar Joints:** The extensor indicis crosses the ulna and radius in the posterior forearm with an ulnar to radial orientation to its fibers (hence its fibers are running somewhat horizontally in the transverse plane). When the index finger and the hand are fixed to the forearm, and the extensor indicis pulls at its distal attachment, the distal forearm moves. If the forearm is in a position of pronation, then the extensor indicis' line of pull causes the distal radius to be pulled in a posterolateral direction around the distal ulna (and the head of the radius to laterally rotate). This movement of the radius is called supination. Therefore, the extensor indicis supinates the forearm at the radioulnar joints.

MISCELLANEOUS

- ❑ 1. The extensor indicis, by attaching into the distal tendon of the extensor digitorum, exerts its pull upon the dorsal digital expansion of the index finger. (This is similar to the extensor digiti minimi, which attaches into the distal tendon of the extensor digitorum of the little finger.)
- ❑ 2. The extensor indicis is another extensor muscle (besides the extensor digitorum) of the index finger. This muscle helps us to point out things (or indicate, hence the name "indicis").
- ❑ 3. Other than the index finger and the thumb, only the little finger has a second extensor muscle (the extensor digiti minimi).
- ❑ 4. The extensor digiti minimi of the little finger also attaches into the ulnar (medial) side of the tendon of the extensor digitorum (that goes to the little finger).
- ❑ 5. All four deep distal muscles of the posterior forearm (abductor pollicis longus, extensor pollicis brevis, extensor pollicis longus and extensor indicis) can do supination of the forearm at the radioulnar joints.

INTRINSIC MUSCLES OF THE HAND

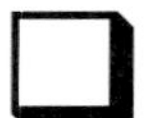

OVERVIEW OF THE INTRINSIC MUSCLES OF THE HAND

Intrinsic muscles of the hand are muscles that are confined to the hand, which means they originate and insert in the hand.

ANATOMICALLY, THE INTRINSIC MUSCLES OF THE HAND CAN BE DIVIDED INTO FOUR GROUPS:	
Superficial Fascial Muscle: ▪ Palmaris Brevis **Thenar Eminence** ▪ Abductor Pollicis Brevis ▪ Flexor Pollicis Brevis ▪ Opponens Pollicis	**Hypothenar Eminence** ▪ Abductor Digiti Minimi Manus ▪ Flexor Digiti Minimi Manus ▪ Opponens Digiti Minimi **Central Compartment:** ▪ Adductor Pollicis ▪ Lumbricals Manus ▪ Palmar Interossei ▪ Dorsal Interossei Manus

THE FOLLOWING MUSCLES ARE COVERED IN OTHER CHAPTERS OF THIS BOOK, BUT ARE ALSO PRESENT IN THE HAND:	
▪ Flexor Carpi Radialis ▪ Palmaris Longus ▪ Flexor Carpi Ulnaris ▪ Flexor Digitorum Superficialis ▪ Flexor Digitorum Profundus ▪ Flexor Pollicis Longus ▪ Extensor Carpi Radialis Longus ▪ Extensor Carpi Radialis Brevis	▪ Extensor Digitorum ▪ Extensor Digiti Minimi ▪ Extensor Carpi Ulnaris ▪ Abductor Pollicis Longus ▪ Extensor Pollicis Brevis ▪ Extensor Pollicis Longus ▪ Extensor Indicis

This is how the intrinsic muscles of the hand are usually classified. Please note the following:

- The palmaris brevis is superficial in the subcutaneous fascia over the hypothenar eminence.
- All three thenar muscles attach proximally onto the flexor retinaculum and the carpals. Distally, they attach onto the thumb.
- All three hypothenar muscles attach proximally onto the flexor retinaculum and/or the carpals. Distally, they attach onto the little finger (finger #5).
- The muscles of the central compartment generally constitute a deeper layer of musculature in the hand.

Functionally, the intrinsic muscles of the hand cross the finger joints. Therefore, intrinsic muscles of the hand move the fingers. The following general rules regarding actions can be stated for muscles of the hand:

- ► All three thenar muscles move the thumb.
- ► All three hypothenar muscles move the little finger.
- ► The adductor pollicis' major action is adduction of the thumb.

- The interossei are involved with adduction/abduction of the fingers at the metacarpophalangeal joint.
- The lumbricals manus and the interossei muscles flex the metacarpophalangeal joint and extend the interphalangeal joints of the fingers.

Miscellaneous:

- Dorsal Digital Expansion: There is a structure in the hand called the *dorsal digital expansion*. (For details, see pages 636-7.)
- There are analogous lumbrical and interossei muscles of the foot.

INNERVATION

- The three thenar muscles are innervated by the median nerve.
- The three hypothenar muscles are innervated by the ulnar nerve.
- The muscles of the central compartment of the hand are innervated by the ulnar nerve.

ARTERIAL SUPPLY

- The three thenar muscles receive their arterial supply from the radial artery.
- The three hypothenar muscles receive their arterial supply from the ulnar artery.
- The muscles of the central compartment of the hand receive their arterial supply from the radial and/or ulnar arteries.

A NOTE REGARDING THE PALMAR INTEROSSEUS MUSCLES

There is a great deal of confusion regarding the naming of the intrinsic hand muscles of the thumb. Some sources state that there are four palmar interossei muscles, one of which goes to the thumb; other sources state that there are only three palmar interossei muscles, none of which attach to the thumb. Some sources state that the flexor pollicis brevis has only one part to it; others state that it has superficial and deep heads. While all sources agree that the adductor pollicis has a transverse head and an oblique head, some state the deep head of the flexor pollicis brevis is actually part of the oblique head of the adductor pollicis and others state that the deep head of the flexor pollicis brevis is separate from the adductor pollicis. The reason for this confusion is due to the great deal of variation that occurs in this region. From one body to another, the anatomy of the musculature varies, leading to confusion as to how to name the structures that are present. This manual adheres to the following organization: there are three palmar interossei muscles, and the flexor pollicis brevis has two parts, a superficial head and a deep head. When another fasciculus (group of muscle fibers) is present in this region, it may be a true 4th palmar interosseus muscle (known as the *palmar interosseus of Henle*). It may also be another fasciculus of the deep head of the flexor pollicis brevis, or another fasciculus of the oblique head of the adductor pollicis.

A NOTE REGARDING REVERSE ACTIONS

As a rule, this book does not employ the terms "origin" and "insertion." However, it is useful to utilize these terms to describe the concept of "reverse actions." The action section of this book describes the action of a muscle by stating the movement of a body part that is created by a muscle's contraction. The body part that usually moves when a muscle contracts is called the insertion. The methodology section further states at which joint the movement of the insertion occurs. However, the other body part that the muscle attaches to, the origin, can also move at that joint. *This movement can be called the reverse action of the muscle.* Keep in mind that the reverse action of a muscle is always possible. The likelihood that a reverse action will occur is based upon the ability of the insertion to be fixed so that the origin moves (instead of the insertion moving) when the muscle contracts. For more information and examples of reverse actions, see page 702.

❑ PALMAR VIEW OF THE BONES AND BONY LANDMARKS OF THE RIGHT HAND

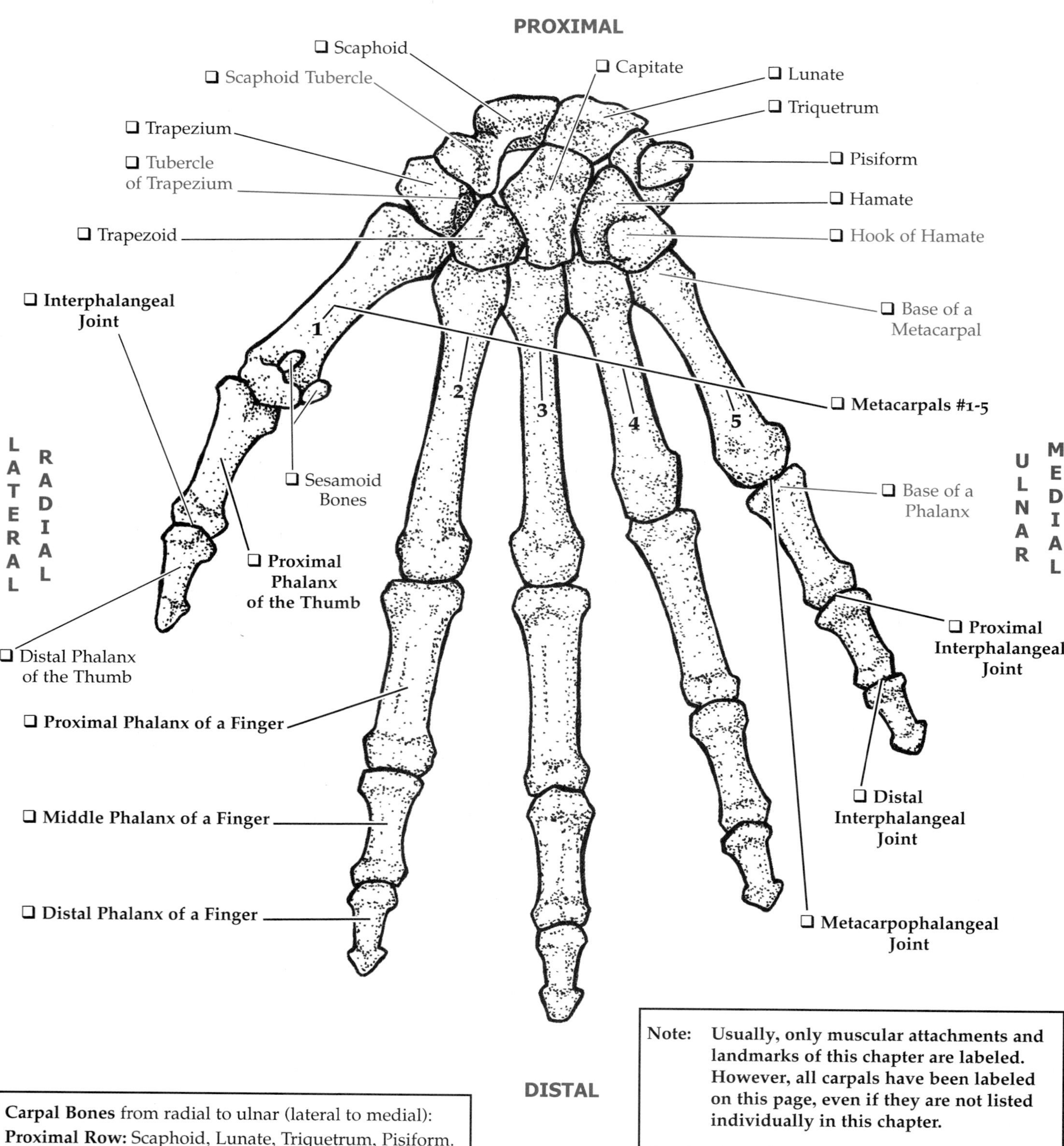

Carpal Bones from radial to ulnar (lateral to medial):
Proximal Row: Scaphoid, Lunate, Triquetrum, Pisiform.
Distal Row: Trapezium, Trapezoid, Capitate, Hamate.

Note: **Usually, only muscular attachments and landmarks of this chapter are labeled. However, all carpals have been labeled on this page, even if they are not listed individually in this chapter.**

First level attachments are indicated in **bold** print.

Second level attachments are indicated in non-bold print.

PALMAR VIEW OF THE BONY ATTACHMENTS OF THE RIGHT HAND

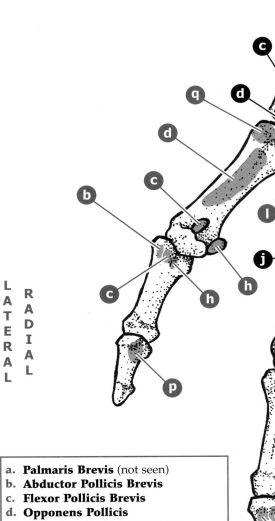

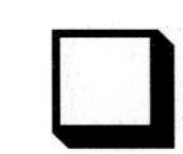

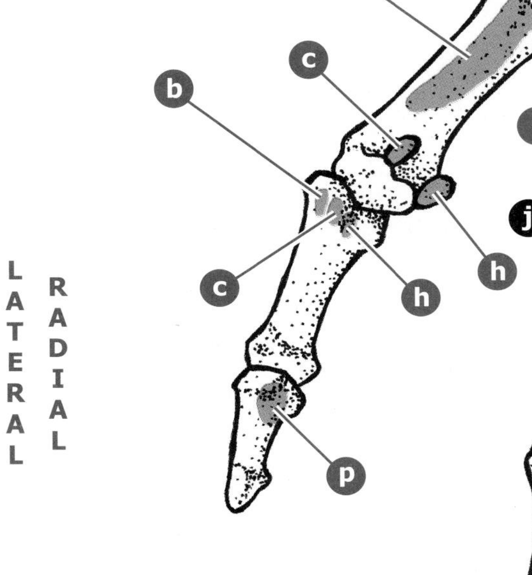

- a. **Palmaris Brevis** (not seen)
- b. **Abductor Pollicis Brevis**
- c. **Flexor Pollicis Brevis**
- d. **Opponens Pollicis**
- e. **Abductor Digiti Minimi Manus**
- f. **Flexor Digiti Minimi Manus**
- g. **Opponens Digiti Minimi**
- h. **Adductor Pollicis**
- i. **Lumbricals Manus** (not seen)
- j. **Palmar Interossei**
- k. **Dorsal Interossei Manus** (not seen)
- l. Flexor Carpi Radialis
- m. Flexor Carpi Ulnaris
- n. Flexor Digitorum Superficialis
- o. Flexor Digitorum Profundus
- p. Flexor Pollicis Longus
- q. Abductor Pollicis Longus

Proximal Attachment

Distal Attachment

❑ DORSAL VIEW OF THE BONES AND BONY LANDMARKS OF THE RIGHT HAND

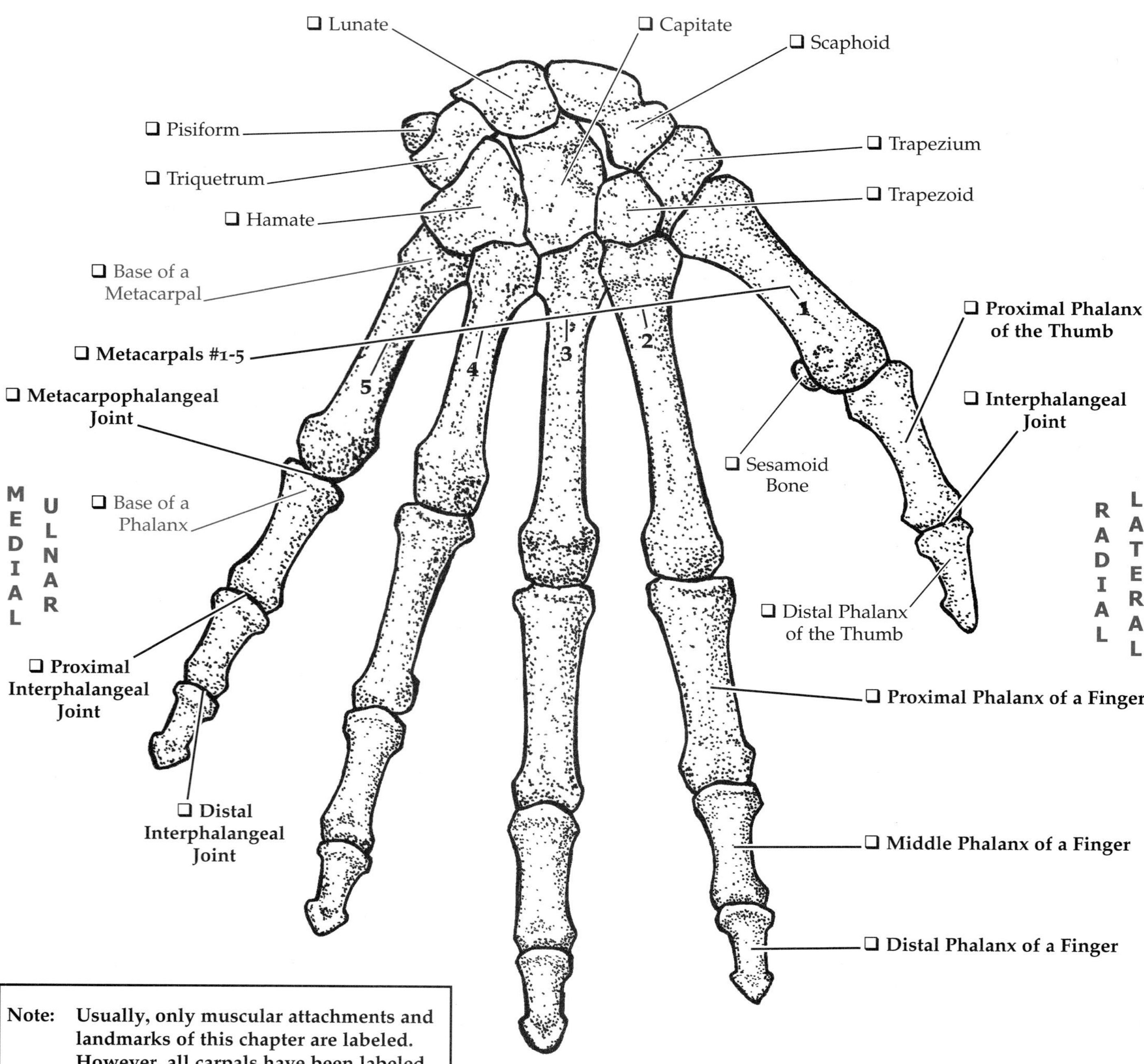

Note: Usually, only muscular attachments and landmarks of this chapter are labeled. However, all carpals have been labeled on this page, even if they are not listed individually in this chapter.

First level attachments are indicated in **bold** print.

Second level attachments are indicated in non-bold print.

Carpal Bones from radial to ulnar (lateral to medial):
Proximal Row: Scaphoid, Lunate, Triquetrum, Pisiform.
Distal Row: Trapezium, Trapezoid, Capitate, Hamate.

DORSAL VIEW OF THE BONY ATTACHMENTS OF THE RIGHT HAND

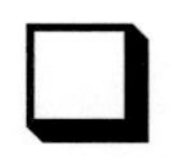

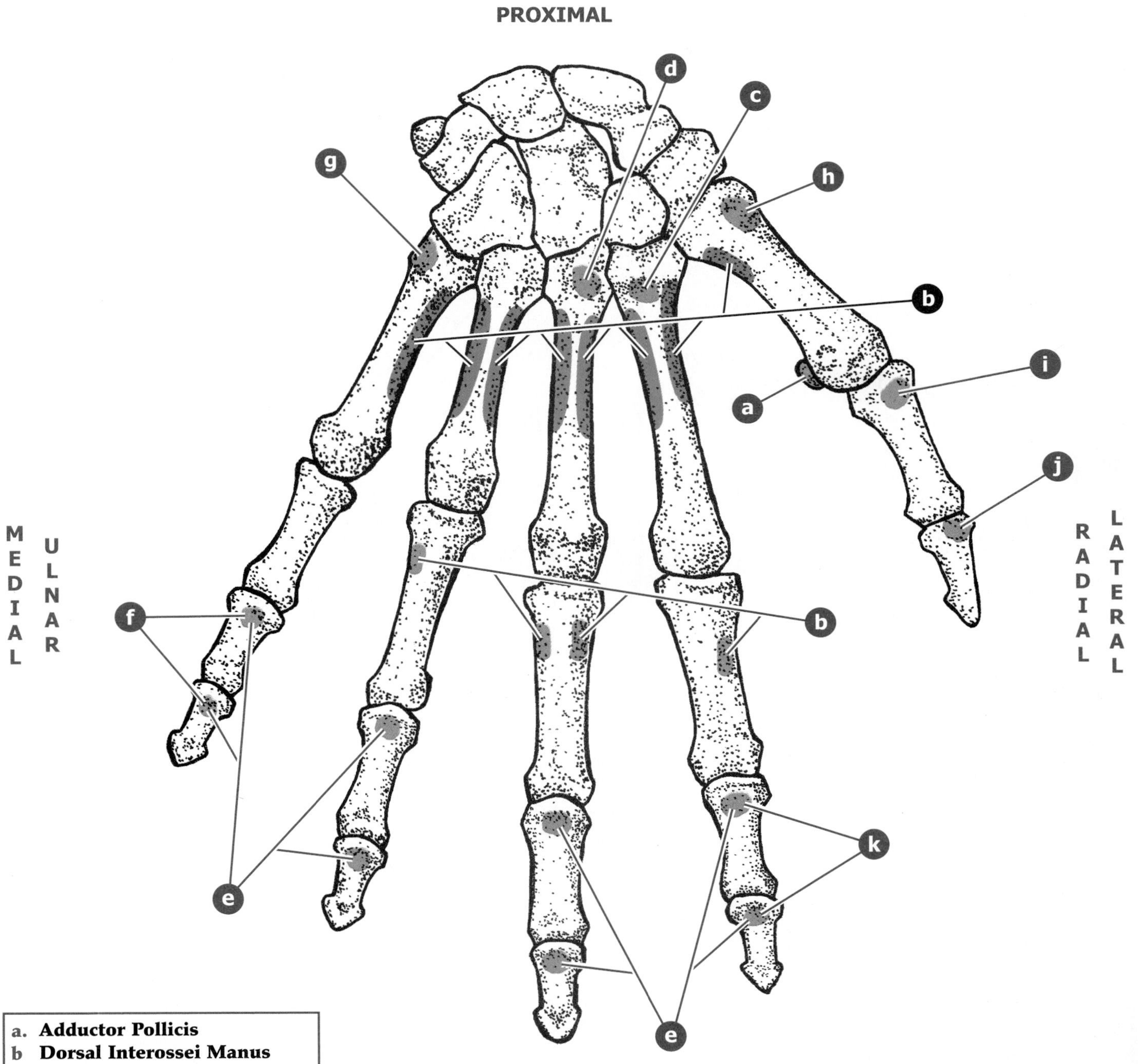

a. **Adductor Pollicis**
b **Dorsal Interossei Manus**
c. Extensor Carpi Radialis Longus
d Extensor Carpi Radialis Brevis
e. Extensor Digitorum
f. Extensor Digiti Minimi
g. Extensor Carpi Ulnaris
h. Abductor Pollicis Longus
i. Extensor Pollicis Brevis
j. Extensor Pollicis Longus
k. Extensor Indicis

Proximal Attachment
Distal Attachment

PALMAR VIEW OF THE RIGHT HAND (SUPERFICIAL)

tendon j

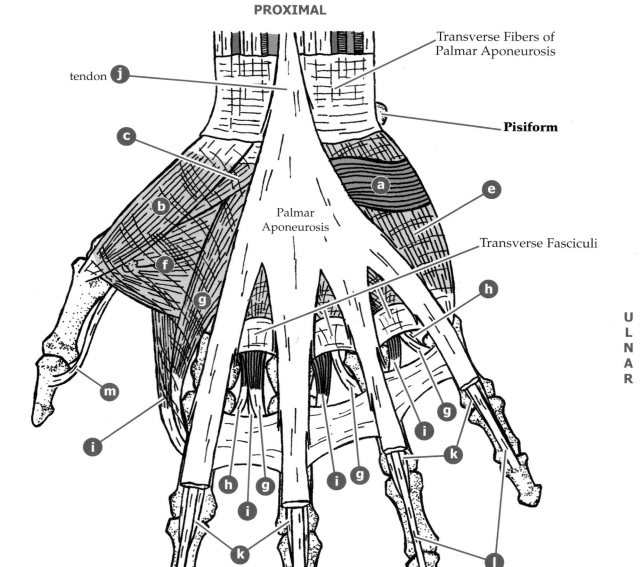

Transverse Fibers of Palmar Aponeurosis

Pisiform

Palmar Aponeurosis

Transverse Fasciculi

LATERAL RADIAL

ULNAR MEDIAL

DISTAL

a. **Palmaris Brevis**
b. **Abductor Pollicis Brevis** (deep to fascia)
c. **Flexor Pollicis Brevis** (deep to fascia)
d. **Opponens Pollicis** (not seen)
e. **Hypothenar Muscle Group** (deep to fascia)
f. **Adductor Pollicis** (deep to fascia)
g. **Lumbricals Manus** (partially deep to fascia)
h. **Palmar Interossei** (2nd not seen)
i. **Dorsal Interossei Manus**
j. Palmaris Longus
k. Flexor Digitorum Superficialis
l. Flexor Digitorum Profundus
m. Flexor Pollicis Longus

PALMAR VIEW OF THE RIGHT HAND (SUPERFICIAL MUSCULAR LAYER)

PROXIMAL

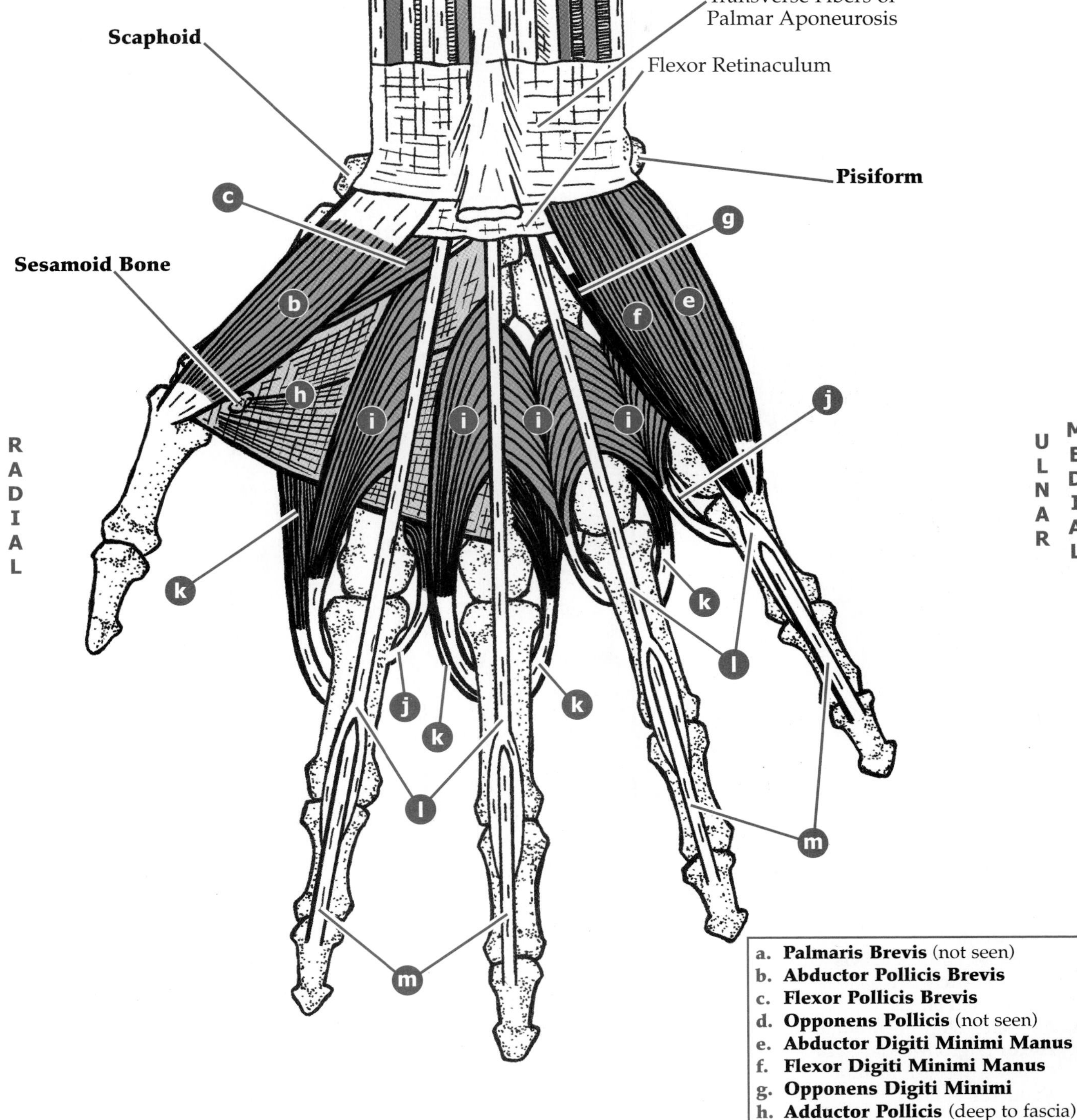

DISTAL

a. **Palmaris Brevis** (not seen)
b. **Abductor Pollicis Brevis**
c. **Flexor Pollicis Brevis**
d. **Opponens Pollicis** (not seen)
e. **Abductor Digiti Minimi Manus**
f. **Flexor Digiti Minimi Manus**
g. **Opponens Digiti Minimi**
h. **Adductor Pollicis** (deep to fascia)
i. **Lumbricals Manus**
j. **Palmar Interossei** (2nd not seen)
k. **Dorsal Interossei Manus**
l. Flexor Digitorum Superficialis
m. Flexor Digitorum Profundus

☐ PALMAR VIEW OF THE RIGHT HAND (DEEP MUSCULAR LAYER)

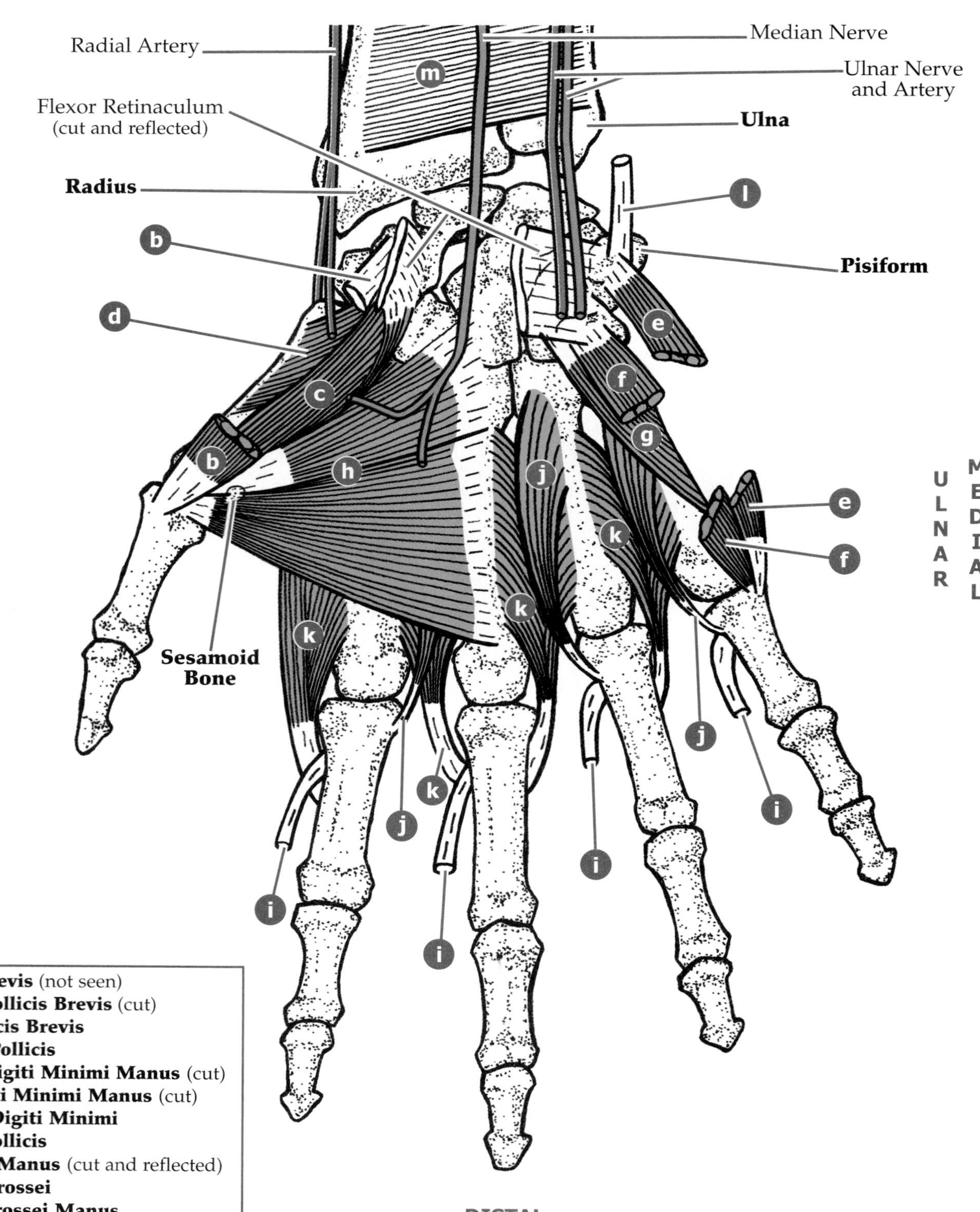

a. **Palmaris Brevis** (not seen)
b. **Abductor Pollicis Brevis** (cut)
c. **Flexor Pollicis Brevis**
d. **Opponens Pollicis**
e. **Abductor Digiti Minimi Manus** (cut)
f. **Flexor Digiti Minimi Manus** (cut)
g. **Opponens Digiti Minimi**
h. **Adductor Pollicis**
i. **Lumbricals Manus** (cut and reflected)
j. **Palmar Interossei**
k. **Dorsal Interossei Manus**
l. Flexor Carpi Ulnaris
m. Pronator Quadratus

DORSAL VIEW OF THE RIGHT HAND

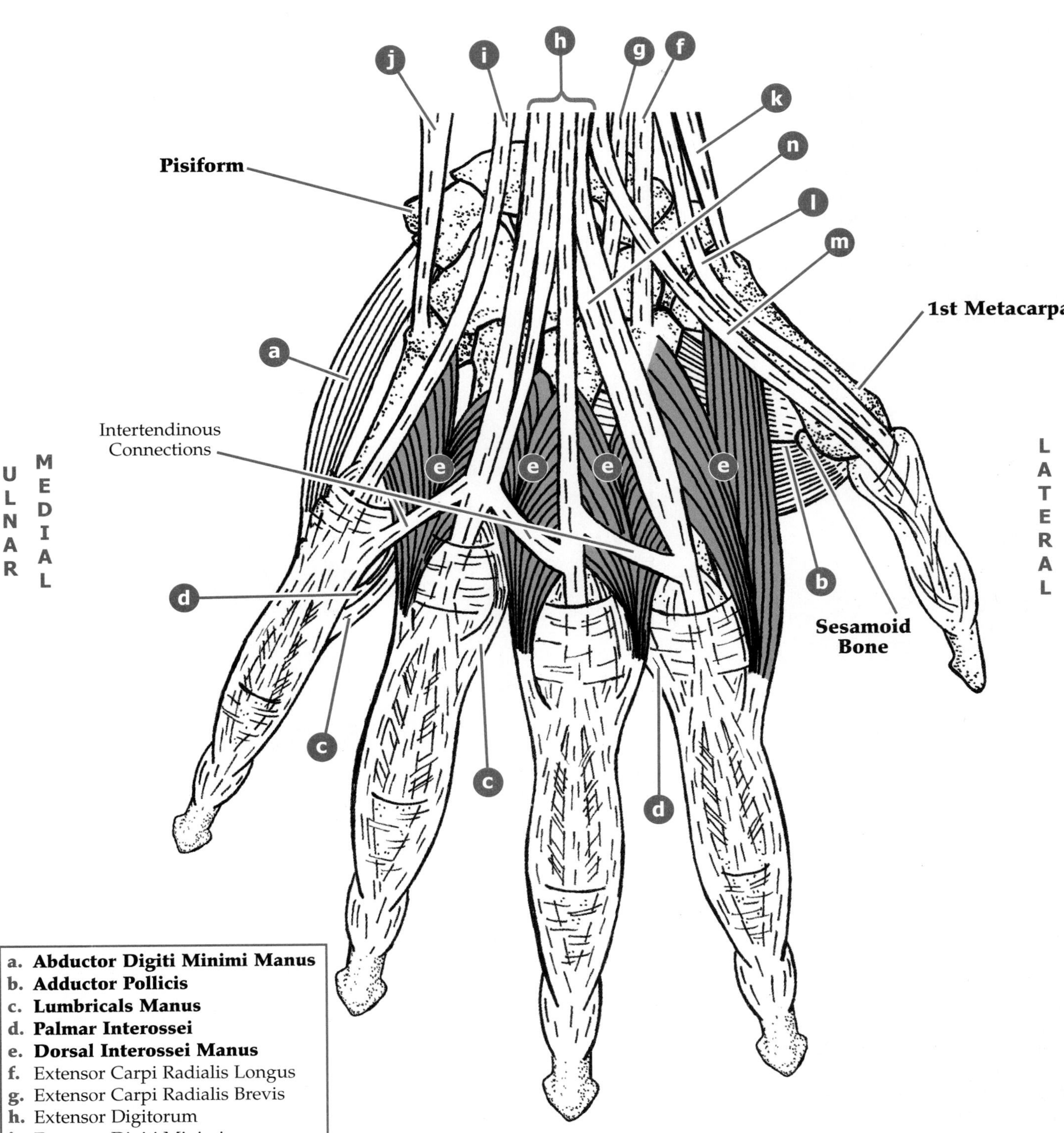

- **a. Abductor Digiti Minimi Manus**
- **b. Adductor Pollicis**
- **c. Lumbricals Manus**
- **d. Palmar Interossei**
- **e. Dorsal Interossei Manus**
- **f.** Extensor Carpi Radialis Longus
- **g.** Extensor Carpi Radialis Brevis
- **h.** Extensor Digitorum
- **i.** Extensor Digiti Minimi
- **j.** Extensor Carpi Ulnaris
- **k.** Abductor Pollicis Longus
- **l.** Extensor Pollicis Brevis
- **m.** Extensor Pollicis Longus
- **n.** Extensor Indicis

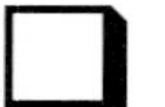

THE DORSAL DIGITAL EXPANSION OF THE RIGHT HAND

DORSAL DIGITAL EXPANSION

The dorsal digital expansion is an attachment site for the lumbricals manus, palmar interossei, dorsal interossei manus and the abductor digiti minimi manus muscles, which attach into it from the sides. The dorsal digital expansion is actually a fibrous aponeurotic expansion of the distal attachment of the extensor digitorum muscle on the fingers (index, middle, ring and little fingers) that serves as a movable hood of tissue when the fingers flex and extend. The dorsal digital expansion begins on the dorsal, lateral and medial sides of the proximal phalanx of each finger and then ultimately attaches onto the dorsal side of the middle and distal phalanges. Since the dorsal digital expansion eventually attaches onto the dorsal (posterior) side of the middle and distal phalanges, any muscle that attaches into the dorsal digital expansion will cause extension of these phalanges at the interphalangeal joints. There is also a dorsal digital expansion of the thumb formed by the distal tendon of the extensor pollicis longus. The dorsal digital expansion is also known as the *extensor expansion* and/or the *dorsal hood*. (Note: There is also a dorsal digital expansion in the foot, see page 457.)

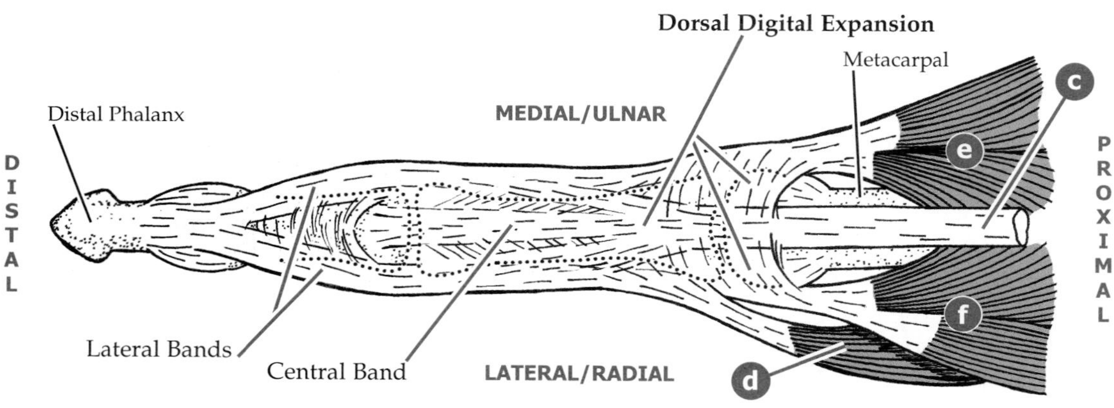

Dorsal View of the Right Index Finger in Full Extension

- **a.** Flexor Digitorum Superficialis (not seen)
- **b.** Flexor Digitorum Profundus (not seen)
- **c. Extensor Digitorum**
- **d. Lumbrical Manus**
- **e. Palmar Interosseus**
- **f. Dorsal Interosseus Manus**

VIEWS OF THE DORSAL DIGITAL EXPANSION OF THE RIGHT

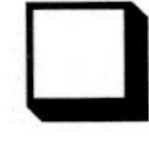

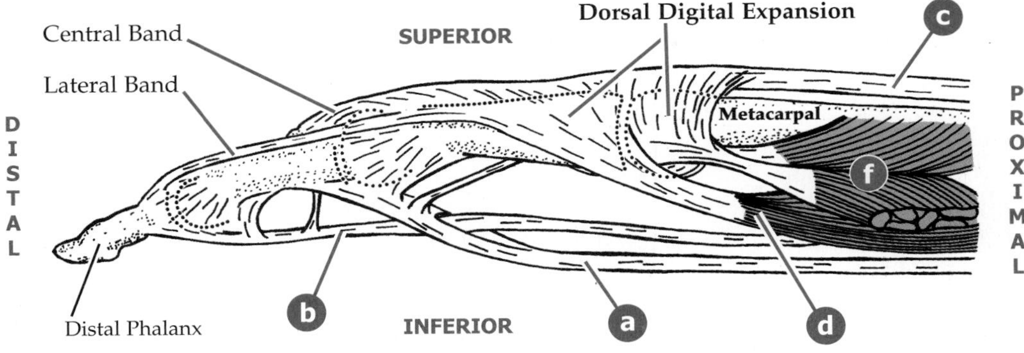

Lateral View of the Right Index Finger in Full Extension

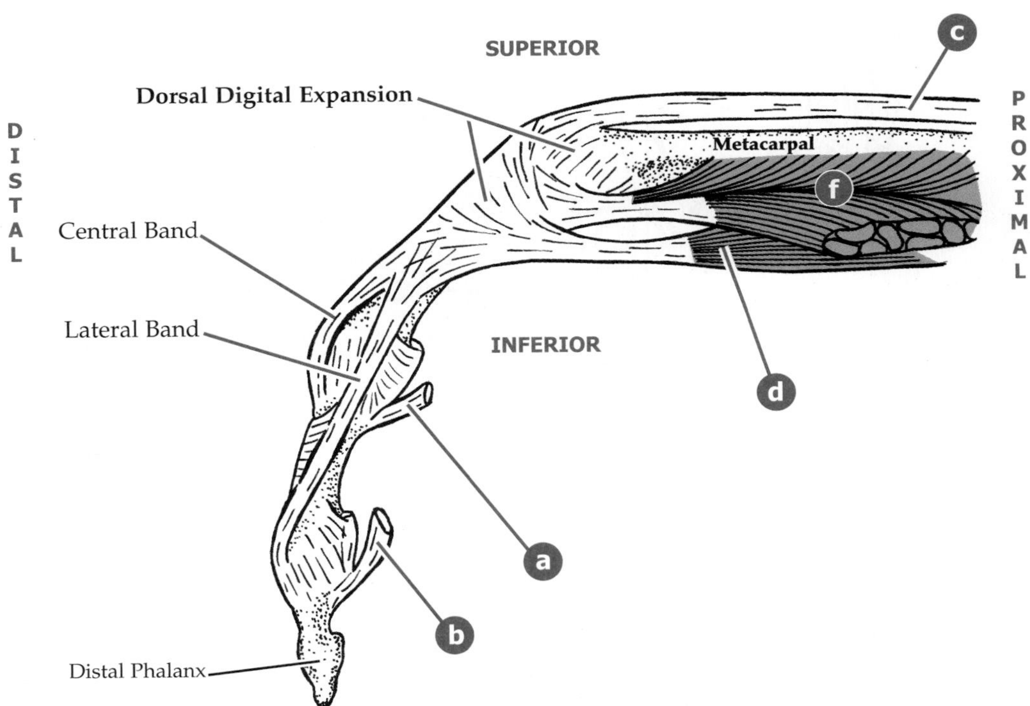

Lateral View of the Right Index Finger in Flexion

a. Flexor Digitorum Superficialis
b. Flexor Digitorum Profundus
c. **Extensor Digitorum**
d. **Lumbrical Manus**
e. **Palmar Interosseus** (not seen)
f. **Dorsal Interosseus Manus**

CROSS SECTION VIEW OF THE RIGHT WRIST

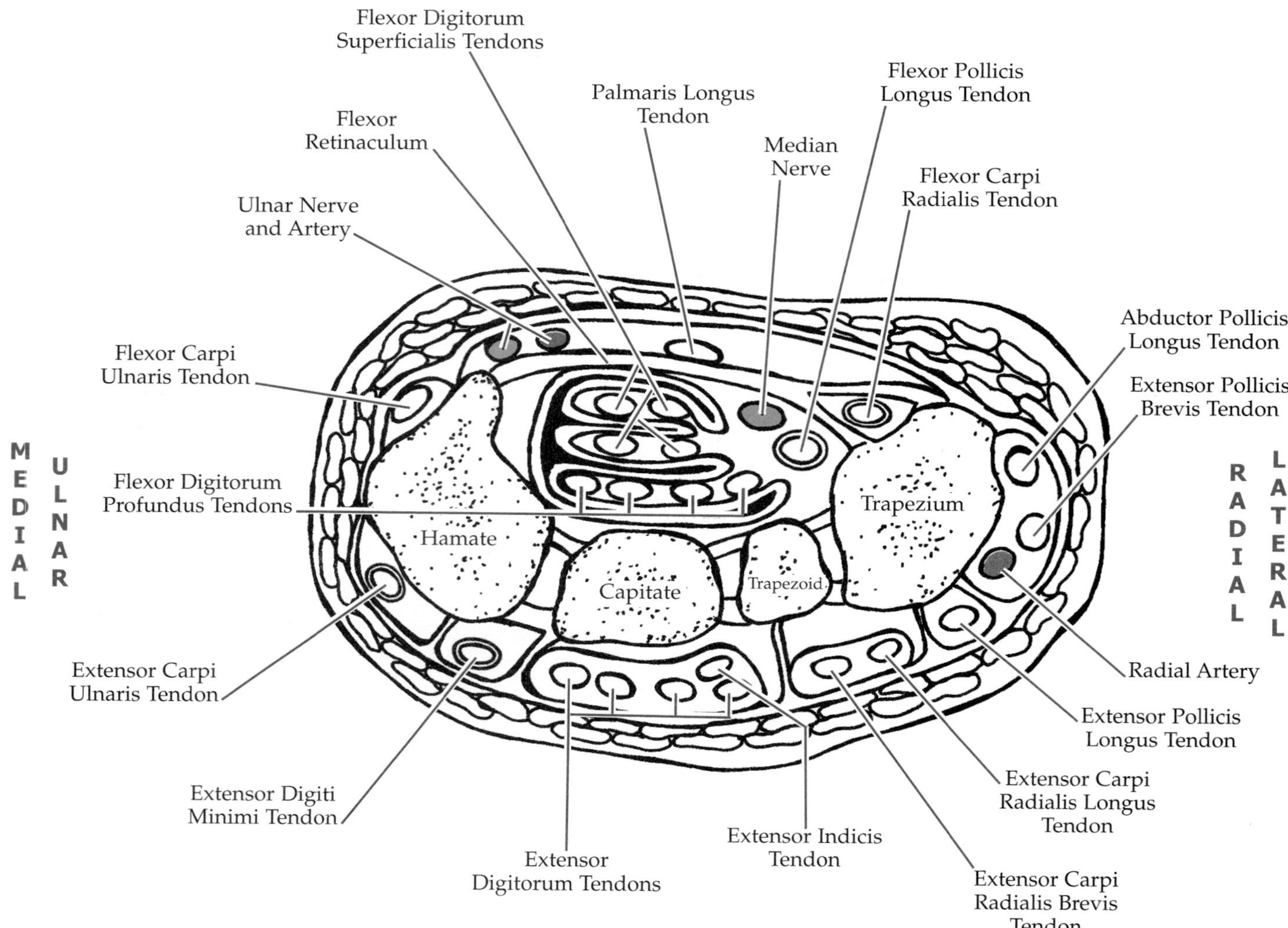

Note: **This is a Distal View (looking from proximal to distal).**

CROSS SECTION VIEW OF THE RIGHT HAND THROUGH THE METACARPAL BONES

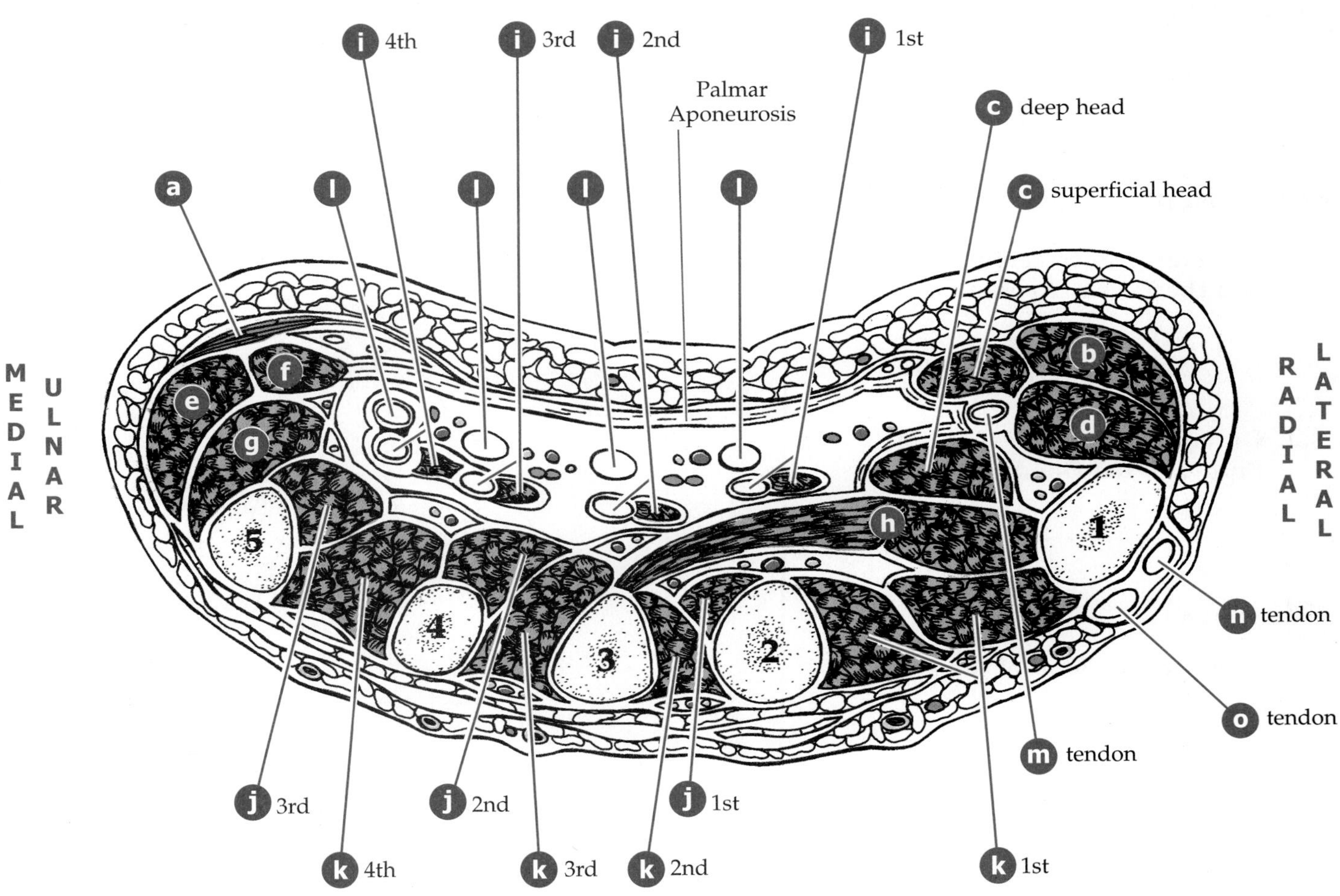

Note: This is a Distal View (looking from proximal to distal).

a. **Palmaris Brevis**	i. **Lumbricals Manus** (attached to flexor digitorum profundus tendons)
b. **Abductor Pollicis Brevis**	j. **Palmar Interossei**
c. **Flexor Pollicis Brevis**	k. **Dorsal Interossei Manus**
d. **Opponens Pollicis**	l. Flexor Digitorum Superficialis
e. **Abductor Digiti Minimi Manus**	m. Flexor Pollicis Longus
f. **Flexor Digiti Minimi Manus**	n. Extensor Pollicis Brevis
g. **Opponens Digiti Minimi**	
h. **Adductor Pollicis**	

PALMARIS BREVIS

❑ **The name, palmaris brevis, tells us that this muscle attaches into the palm of the hand and is short (shorter than the palmaris longus).**

DERIVATION ❑ palmaris: L. *refers to the palm.*
brevis: L. *short.*

PRONUNCIATION ❑ pall-**ma**-ris **bre**-vis

ATTACHMENTS

❑ **The Flexor Retinaculum and the Palmar Aponeurosis**

to the

❑ **Dermis of the Ulnar (Medial) Border of the Hand**

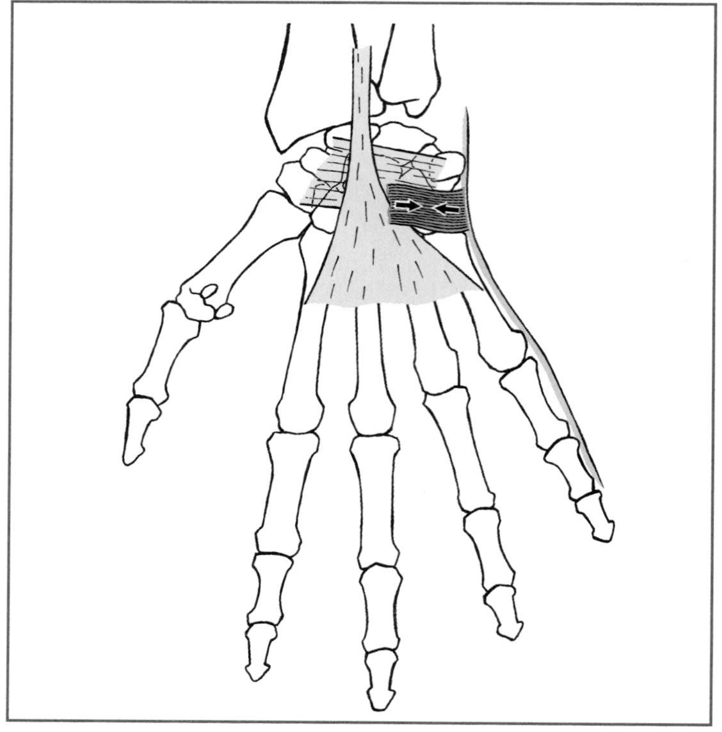

Anterior View of the Right Palmaris Brevis

ACTION

❑ **Wrinkles the Skin of the Palm**

INNERVATION ❑ The Ulnar Nerve ❑ C8, T1

ARTERIAL SUPPLY ❑ The Ulnar Artery (A Terminal Branch of the Brachial Artery) and the Superficial Palmar Branch of the Radial Artery

PALPATION AND SUPPLEMENTARY TEXT

PALPATION

- ❑ The palmaris brevis is located in the dermis proximally on the ulnar side of the palm, superficial to the hypothenar muscle group. However, it is too thin to palpate.

RELATIONSHIP TO OTHER MUSCULOSKELETAL STRUCTURES

- ❑ 1. The palmaris brevis is superficial in the medial (ulnar) side of the hand.
- ❑ 2. The hypothenar muscles are all deep to the palmaris brevis.

METHODOLOGY FOR LEARNING MUSCLE ACTIONS

- ❑ **Wrinkles the Skin of the Palm:** The palmaris brevis attaches from lateral to medial in the hand (with its fibers running horizontally). When the palmaris brevis contracts, it pulls its medial attachment, the dermis of the ulnar (medial) side of the hand, laterally toward the center of the palm of the hand; this causes the skin of the ulnar side of the hand to wrinkle. This wrinkling of the skin is thought to accentuate or increase the size of the hypothenar eminence. By so doing, it is believed to slightly contribute to the strength and security of the palmar grip.

MISCELLANEOUS

- ❑ 1. The palmaris brevis is a very thin, quadrilateral-shaped muscle.
- ❑ 2. The palmaris brevis overlies the hypothenar eminence. Like all the muscles of the hypothenar eminence, it is innervated by the ulnar nerve.

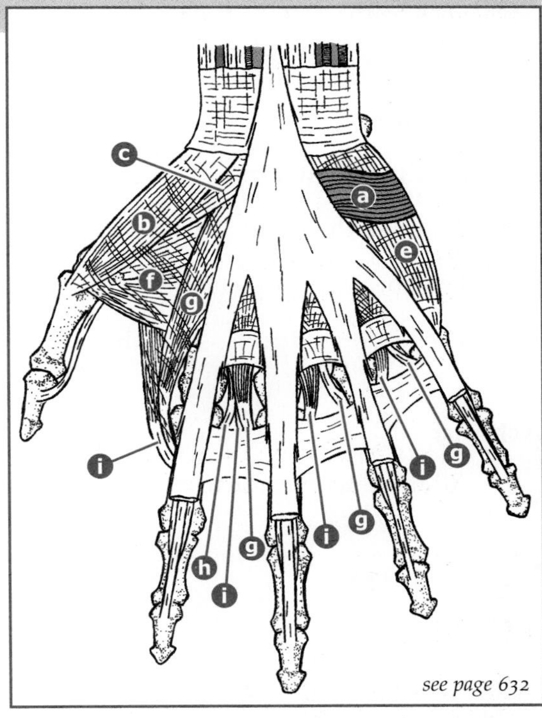

see page 632

Palmar View of the Right Hand (Superficial)

a. Palmaris Brevis
b. Abductor Pollicis Brevis (deep to fascia)
c. Flexor Pollicis Brevis (deep to fascia)
d. Opponens Pollicis (not seen)
e. Hypothenar Muscle Group (deep to fascia)
f. Adductor Pollicis (deep to fascia)
g. Lumbricals Manus (partially deep to fascia)
h. Palmar Interossei (2nd not seen)
i. Dorsal Interossei Manus

THE MUSCLES OF THE THENAR EMINENCE

The thenar eminence is an eminence of soft tissue located on the radial side of the palm of the hand.

THERE ARE THREE MUSCLES OF THE THENAR EMINENCE:		
Abductor Pollicis Brevis	Flexor Pollicis Brevis	Opponens Pollicis

Attachments:

- All three thenar muscles attach proximally onto the flexor retinaculum and carpal bones.
- All three thenar muscles attach distally onto the thumb.
- The abductor pollicis brevis and the flexor pollicis brevis attach onto the proximal phalanx of the thumb.
- The opponens pollicis attaches onto the 1st metacarpal (of the thumb).

Actions:

- All three thenar muscles move the thumb.

Miscellaneous:

- The layering of the thenar muscles is approximately as follows:
  - The abductor pollicis brevis is the most superficial of the three.
  - The flexor pollicis brevis is intermediate.
  - The opponens pollicis is the deepest of the three.
- There are three muscles located in the hypothenar eminence that are analogous to the thenar muscles. The three hypothenar muscles are the abductor digiti minimi manus, flexor digiti minimi manus and the opponens digiti minimi.

INNERVATION The three thenar muscles are innervated by the median nerve. (The ulnar nerve usually contributes to a small degree.)

ARTERIAL SUPPLY The three thenar muscles receive their arterial supply from the radial artery.

PALMAR VIEWS OF THE THENAR MUSCLES

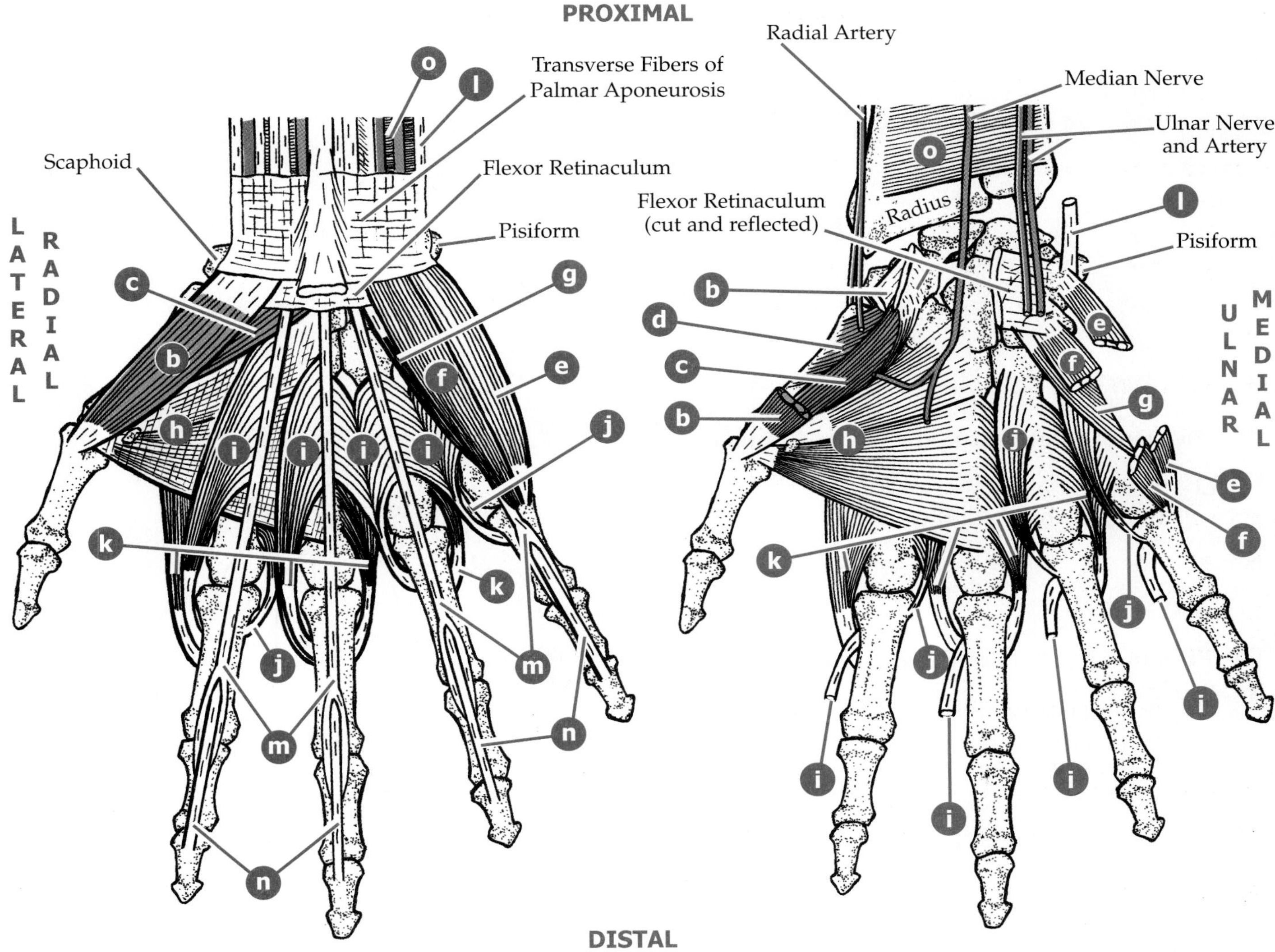

Palmar View of the Right Hand (Superficial Muscular Layer)

Palmar View of the Right Hand (Deep Muscular Layer)

- a. Palmaris Brevis (not seen)
- b. **Abductor Pollicis Brevis** (cut on our right)
- c. **Flexor Pollicis Brevis**
- d. **Opponens Pollicis** (not seen on our left)
- e. Abductor Digiti Minimi Manus (cut on our right)
- f. Flexor Digiti Minimi Manus (cut on our right)
- g. Opponens Digiti Minimi
- h. Adductor Pollicis (deep to fascia on our left)
- i. Lumbricals Manus (cut and reflected on our right)
- j. Palmar Interossei
- k. Dorsal Interossei Manus
- l. Flexor Carpi Ulnaris
- m. Flexor Digitorum Superficialis (not seen on our right)
- n. Flexor Digitorum Profundus (not seen on our right)
- o. Pronator Quadratus

❑ ABDUCTOR POLLICIS BREVIS

(OF THE THENAR EMINENCE)

❑ **The name, abductor pollicis brevis, tells us that this muscle abducts the thumb and is short (shorter than the abductor pollicis longus).**

DERIVATION ❑ abductor: L. *a muscle that abducts a body part.*
pollicis: L. *thumb.*
brevis: L. *short.*

PRONUNCIATION ❑ ab-**duk**-tor **pol**-i-sis **bre**-vis

ATTACHMENTS

❑ **The Flexor Retinaculum and the Carpals**

- ❑ the tubercle of the scaphoid and the tubercle of the trapezium

to the

❑ **Proximal Phalanx of the Thumb**

- ❑ the radial (lateral) side of the base of the proximal phalanx and the dorsal digital expansion

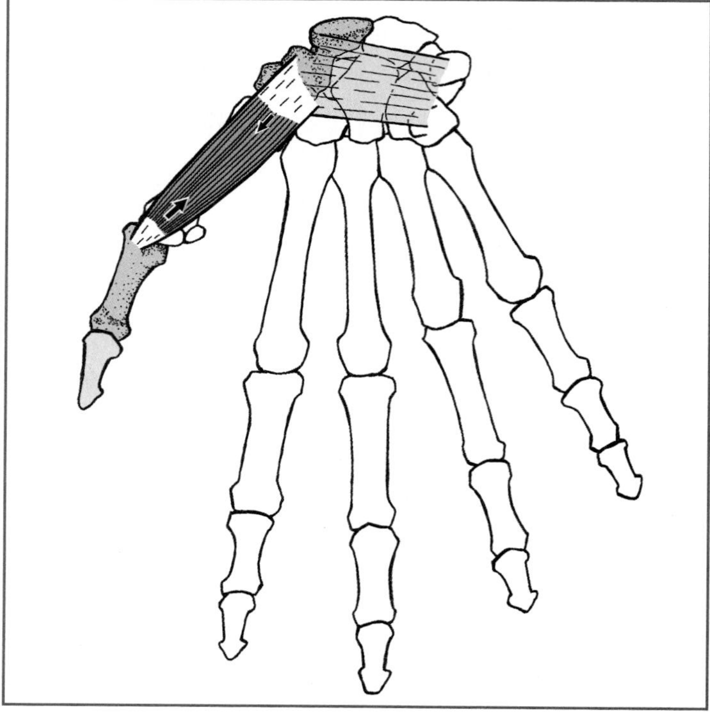

Anterior View of the Right Abductor Pollicis Brevis

ACTIONS

❑ **1. Abduction of the Thumb**

❑ **2.** Extension of the Thumb

❑ **3.** Flexion of the Thumb

INNERVATION ❑ The Median Nerve ❑ C8, **T1**

ARTERIAL SUPPLY ❑ Branches of the Radial Artery (A Terminal Branch of the Brachial Artery)

PALPATION AND SUPPLEMENTARY TEXT

PALPATION

- ❑ The belly of the abductor pollicis brevis is superficial and can be palpated in the lateral aspect of the thenar eminence.
    - Have the client seated or supine.
    - Place palpating fingers over the lateral aspect of the thenar eminence.
    - Ask the client to abduct the thumb at the 1st carpometacarpal joint against resistance and feel for the contraction of the abductor pollicis brevis. Distinguishing the ulnar (medial) border of the abductor pollicis brevis from the adjacent flexor pollicis brevis and the opponens pollicis can be difficult.

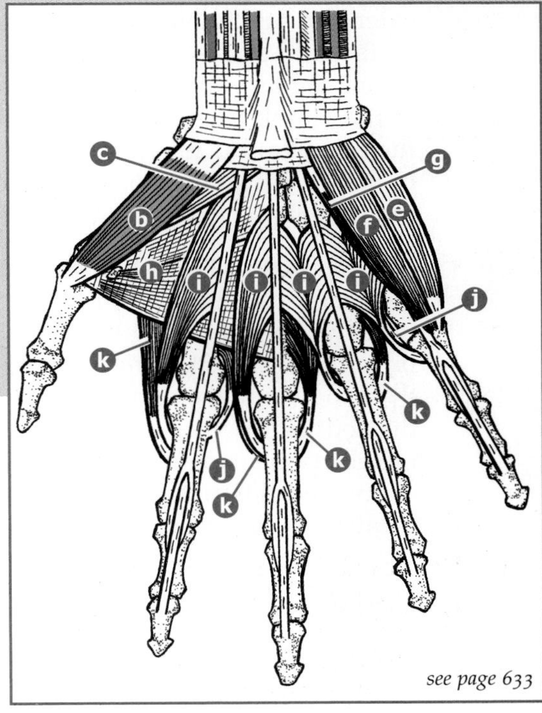

Palmar View of the Right Hand (Superficial Muscular Layer)

a. Palmaris Brevis (not seen)
b. **Abductor Pollicis Brevis**
c. Flexor Pollicis Brevis
d. Opponens Pollicis (not seen)
e. Abductor Digiti Minimi Manus
f. Flexor Digiti Minimi Manus
g. Opponens Digiti Minimi
h. Adductor Pollicis (deep to fascia)
i. Lumbricals Manus
j. Palmar Interossei (2nd not seen)
k. Dorsal Interossei Manus

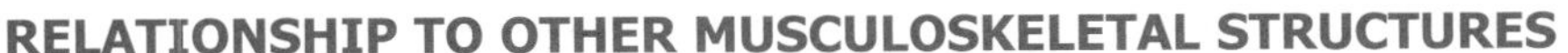

RELATIONSHIP TO OTHER MUSCULOSKELETAL STRUCTURES

❑ 1. The abductor pollicis brevis is superficial in the thenar eminence.

❑ 2. The abductor pollicis brevis is superficial and lateral to the flexor pollicis brevis. The lateral portion of the flexor pollicis brevis is covered by the abductor pollicis brevis. The abductor pollicis brevis is also superficial to the opponens pollicis.

METHODOLOGY FOR LEARNING MUSCLE ACTIONS

❑ 1. **Abduction of the Thumb at the Carpometacarpal Joint:** The abductor pollicis brevis crosses the 1st carpometacarpal joint of the thumb anteriorly to attach onto the proximal phalanx of the thumb (with its fibers running vertically in the sagittal plane). When the abductor pollicis brevis contracts, it pulls the metacarpal of the thumb in a direction that is perpendicular to and away from the plane of the palm of the hand (sagittal plane). This action is called abduction of the thumb. Therefore, the abductor pollicis brevis abducts the thumb by abducting the metacarpal of the thumb at the 1st carpometacarpal joint. Additionally, the abductor pollicis brevis also crosses the 1st metacarpophalangeal joint of the thumb, but this joint cannot abduct. (Note: Due to the rotational development of the thumb embryologically, the named actions of abduction and adduction of the thumb occur within the sagittal plane. For more details, see the Muscular System Manual, Volume I.)

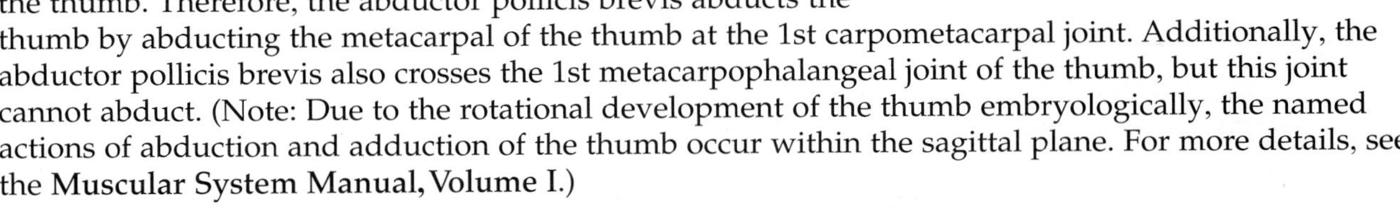

ABDUCTOR POLLICIS BREVIS – continued

- ❑ 2. **Extension of the Thumb at the Carpometacarpal and Interphalangeal Joints**: The abductor pollicis brevis crosses the 1st carpometacarpal joint laterally (radially) to attach onto the proximal phalanx of the thumb (with its fibers running vertically in the frontal plane). When the abductor pollicis brevis contracts, it pulls the metacarpal of the thumb in a lateral (radial) direction within the plane of the palm of the hand (frontal plane), away from the index finger. This action is called extension of the thumb. Therefore, the abductor pollicis brevis extends the thumb by extending the metacarpal of the thumb at the 1st carpometacarpal joint. Additionally, due to its attachment into the dorsal digital expansion of the thumb, the abductor pollicis brevis also crosses the interphalangeal joint of the thumb laterally (radially). Therefore, the abductor pollicis brevis extends the distal phalanx of the thumb at the interphalangeal joint of the thumb as well. (Note: Due to the rotational development of the thumb embryologically, the named actions of flexion and extension of the thumb occur within the frontal plane. For more details, see the Muscular System Manual, Volume I.)
- ❑ 3. **Flexion of the Thumb at the Metacarpophalangeal Joint**: The abductor pollicis brevis crosses the metacarpophalangeal joint of the thumb anteriorly to attach onto the proximal phalanx of the thumb (with its fibers running vertically in the frontal plane). When the abductor pollicis brevis contracts, it pulls the proximal phalanx of the thumb in a medial (ulnar) direction within the plane of the palm of the hand (frontal plane), toward the index finger. This action is called flexion of the thumb. Therefore, the abductor pollicis brevis flexes the thumb by flexing the proximal phalanx of the thumb at the metacarpophalangeal joint. (Note: Due to the rotational development of the thumb embryologically, the named actions of flexion and extension of the thumb occur within the frontal plane. For more details, see the Muscular System Manual, Volume I.)

MISCELLANEOUS

- ❑ 1. The three muscles of the thenar eminence are the abductor pollicis brevis, the flexor pollicis brevis and the opponens pollicis. (Note: There are three analogous hypothenar muscles. They are the abductor digiti minimi manus, the flexor digiti minimi manus and the opponens digiti minimi.)
- ❑ 2. All three thenar muscles attach onto and move the thumb. (Note: All three hypothenar muscles attach onto and move the little finger.)
- ❑ 3. Some sources state that the abductor pollicis brevis crosses the metacarpophalangeal joint of the thumb sufficiently anterior to flex the proximal phalanx of the thumb at this joint instead of extending it.

FLEXOR POLLICIS BREVIS
(OF THE THENAR EMINENCE)

❑ **The name, flexor pollicis brevis, tells us that this muscle flexes the thumb and is short (shorter than the flexor pollicis longus).**

DERIVATION ❑ flexor: L. *a muscle that flexes a body part.*
pollicis: L. *thumb.*
brevis: L. *short.*

PRONUNCIATION ❑ **fleks**-or **pol**-i-sis **bre**-vis

ATTACHMENTS

❑ **The Flexor Retinaculum and the Carpals**

- ❑ the trapezium

to the

❑ **Proximal Phalanx of the Thumb**

- ❑ the radial (lateral) side of the base of the proximal phalanx of the thumb

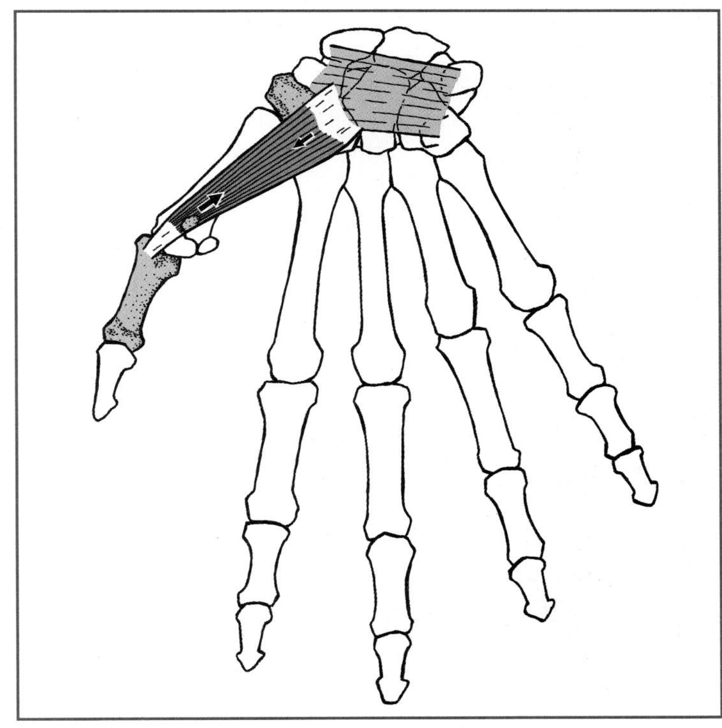

Anterior View of the Right Flexor Pollicis Brevis

ACTIONS

❑ 1. **Flexion of the Thumb**

❑ 2. Abduction of the Thumb

INNERVATION ❑ The Median and Ulnar Nerves
❑ C8, **T1**: (superficial head: the median nerve)
(deep head: the ulnar nerve)

ARTERIAL SUPPLY ❑ Branches of the Radial Artery (A Terminal Branch of the Brachial Artery)

FLEXOR POLLICIS BREVIS – PALPATION AND SUPPLEMENTARY TEXT

PALPATION

- ❑ The medial portion of the flexor pollicis brevis is superficial in the thenar eminence; the lateral portion of the flexor pollicis brevis is deep to the abductor pollicis brevis.
  - Have the client seated or supine.
  - Place palpating hand on the medial aspect of the thenar eminence.
  - Ask the client to flex the thumb at the 1st carpometacarpal joint and the 1st metacarpophalangeal joint against resistance and feel for the contraction of the medial portion of the flexor pollicis brevis.
  - Continue palpating the flexor pollicis brevis more laterally, deep to the abductor pollicis brevis. Distinguishing the lateral portion of the flexor pollicis brevis from the superficial abductor pollicis brevis can be difficult.

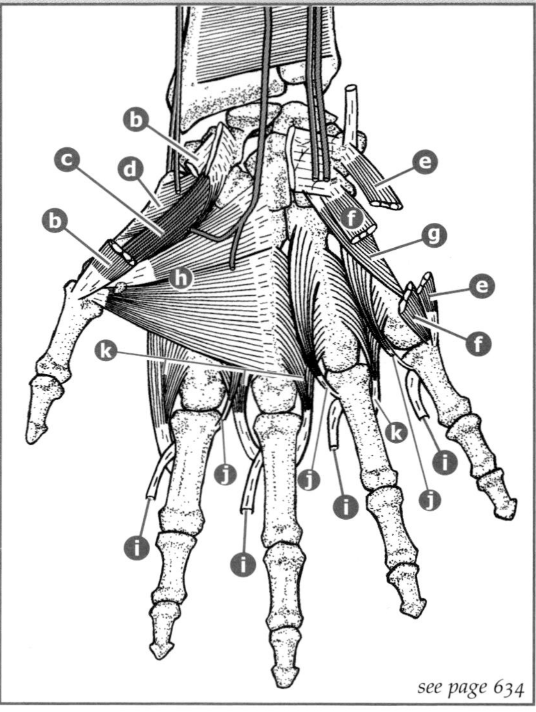

see page 634

Palmar View of the Right Hand (Deep Muscular Layer)

a. Palmaris Brevis (not seen)
b. Abductor Pollicis Brevis (cut)
c. **Flexor Pollicis Brevis**
d. Opponens Pollicis
e. Abductor Digiti Minimi Manus (cut)
f. Flexor Digiti Minimi Manus (cut)
g. Opponens Digiti Minimi
h. Adductor Pollicis
i. Lumbricals Manus (cut and reflected)
j. Palmar Interossei
k. Dorsal Interossei Manus

RELATIONSHIP TO OTHER MUSCULOSKELETAL STRUCTURES

❑ 1. The medial portion of the flexor pollicis brevis is superficial in the thenar eminence. The lateral portion of the flexor pollicis brevis is deep to the abductor pollicis brevis.

❑ 2. The superficial head of the flexor pollicis brevis is superficial to the medial portion of the opponens pollicis. The deep head of the flexor pollicis brevis is deep to the medial portion of the opponens pollicis. Hence, the medial portion of the opponens pollicis is sandwiched between the two heads of the flexor pollicis brevis.

❑ 3. The distal tendon of the flexor pollicis longus is sandwiched between the two heads of the flexor pollicis brevis.

METHODOLOGY FOR LEARNING MUSCLE ACTIONS

❑ **1. Flexion of the Thumb at the Carpometacarpal and the Metacarpophalangeal Joints:** The flexor pollicis brevis crosses the 1st carpometacarpal joint of the thumb medially (on the ulnar side) to attach onto the proximal phalanx of the thumb (with its fibers running vertically in the frontal plane). When the flexor pollicis brevis contracts, it pulls the metacarpal of the thumb in an medial (ulnar) direction within the plane of the palm of the hand (frontal plane), toward the index finger. This action is called flexion of the thumb. Therefore, the flexor pollicis brevis flexes the thumb by flexing the metacarpal of the thumb at the 1st carpometacarpal joint. Additionally, the flexor pollicis brevis also crosses the 1st metacarpophalangeal joint of the thumb medially (on the ulnar side). Therefore, the flexor pollicis brevis flexes the thumb by flexing the proximal phalanx of the thumb at the metacarpophalangeal joint as well. (Note: Due to the rotational development of the thumb embryologically, the named actions of flexion and extension of the thumb occur within the frontal plane. For more details, see the Muscular System Manual, Volume I.)

FLEXOR POLLICIS BREVIS – continued

- ❑ **2. Abduction of the Thumb at the Carpometacarpal Joint:** The flexor pollicis brevis crosses the 1st carpometacarpal joint of the thumb anteriorly to attach onto the proximal phalanx of the thumb (with its fibers running vertically in the sagittal plane). When the flexor pollicis brevis contracts, it pulls the metacarpal of the thumb in a direction that is perpendicular to and away from the plane of the palm of the hand (sagittal plane). This action is called abduction of the thumb. Therefore, the flexor pollicis brevis abducts the thumb by abducting the metacarpal of the thumb at the 1st carpometacarpal joint. Additionally, the flexor pollicis brevis also crosses the 1st metacarpophalangeal joint of the thumb, but this joint cannot abduct. (Note: Due to the rotational development of the thumb embryologically, the named actions of abduction and adduction of the thumb occur within the sagittal plane. For more details, see the Muscular System Manual, Volume I.)

MISCELLANEOUS

- ❑ 1. The three muscles of the thenar eminence are the abductor pollicis brevis, the flexor pollicis brevis and the opponens pollicis. (Note: There are three analogous hypothenar muscles. They are the abductor digiti minimi manus, the flexor digiti minimi manus and the opponens digiti minimi.)
- ❑ 2. All three thenar muscles attach onto and move the thumb. (Note: All three hypothenar muscles attach onto and move the little finger.)
- ❑ 3. Some sources state that the flexor pollicis brevis does not have a superficial and deep head, but rather has only one part to it.
- ❑ 4. What is called the deep head of the flexor pollicis brevis is considered by some sources to be part of the oblique head of the adductor pollicis, and by other sources to be a palmar interosseus muscle of the thumb (see note regarding the palmar interosseus muscles on page 627).
- ❑ 5. There is a sesamoid bone in the distal tendon of the flexor pollicis brevis. (Note: There is a second sesamoid bone of the thumb located in the distal tendon of the adductor pollicis.)

❑ OPPONENS POLLICIS
(OF THE THENAR EMINENCE)

❑ **The name, opponens pollicis, tells us that this muscle opposes the thumb.**

DERIVATION ❑ opponens: L. *opposing.*
pollicis: L. *thumb.*

PRONUNCIATION ❑ op-**po**-nens **pol**-i-sis

ATTACHMENTS

❑ **The Flexor Retinaculum and the Carpals**

- ❑ the tubercle of the trapezium

to the

❑ **1st Metacarpal (of the Thumb)**

- ❑ the anterior surface and lateral border

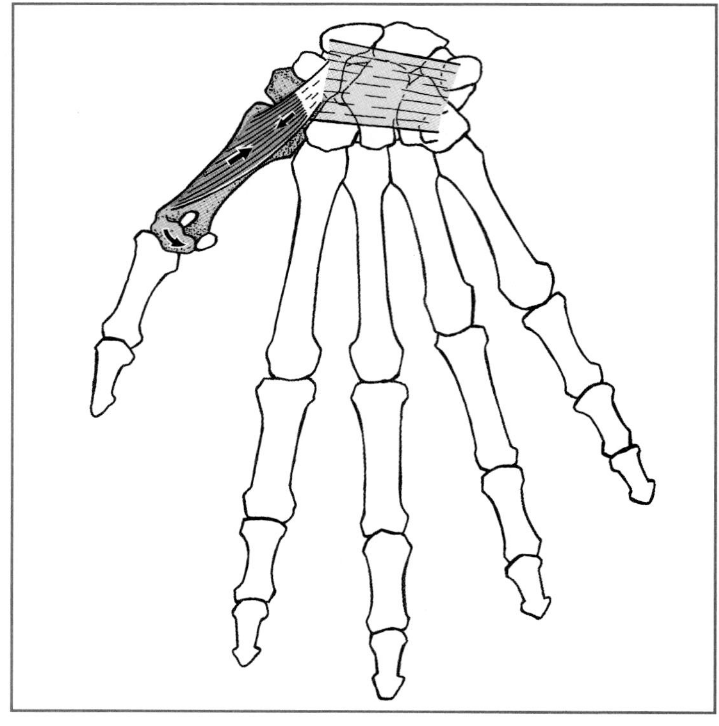

Anterior View of the
Right Opponens Pollicis

ACTIONS

❑ 1. **Opposition of the Thumb**

❑ 2. Flexion of the Thumb

❑ 3. Adduction of the Thumb

❑ 4. Medial Rotation of the Thumb

INNERVATION ❑ The Median and Ulnar Nerves ❑ C8, **T1**

ARTERIAL SUPPLY ❑ Branches of the Radial Artery (A Terminal Branch of the Brachial Artery)

PALPATION AND SUPPLEMENTARY TEXT

PALPATION

- ❑ The lateral portion of the opponens pollicis is palpable, deep to the abductor pollicis brevis. The medial portion is deep to the flexor pollicis brevis and difficult to palpate and distinguish from adjacent musculature.
  - Have the client seated or supine.
  - Place palpating fingers over the lateral portion of the thenar eminence.
  - Ask the client to flex the thumb at the 1st carpometacarpal joint against resistance and feel for the contraction of the lateral portion of the opponens pollicis. (Be sure that the client is not abducting the thumb at the same time or the abductor pollicis brevis will also contract and make palpation of the opponens pollicis impossible.)
  - Continue palpating the opponens pollicis more medially, deep to the flexor pollicis brevis. Distinguishing the opponens pollicis from the flexor pollicis brevis can be difficult. Since they both can flex the metacarpal of the thumb at the 1st carpometacarpal joint, the flexor pollicis brevis will contract whenever the opponens pollicis contracts.

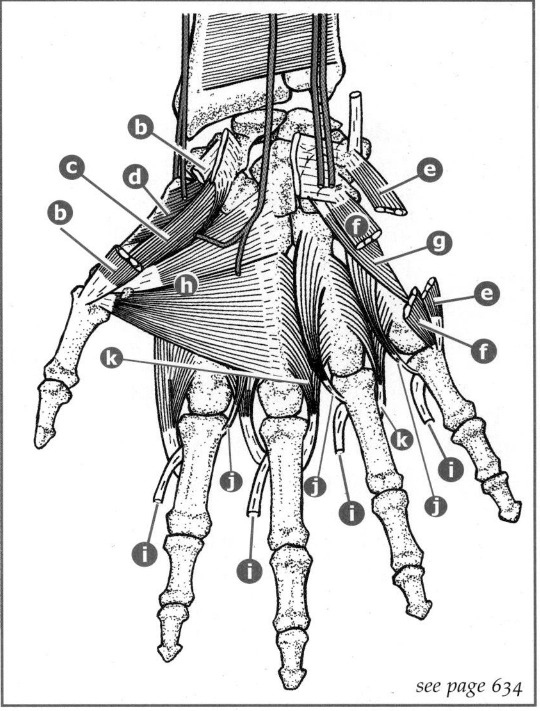

see page 634

Palmar View of the Right Hand (Deep Muscular Layer)

- **a.** Palmaris Brevis (not seen)
- **b.** Abductor Pollicis Brevis (cut)
- **c.** Flexor Pollicis Brevis
- **d.** **Opponens Pollicis**
- **e.** Abductor Digiti Minimi Manus (cut)
- **f.** Flexor Digiti Minimi Manus (cut)
- **g.** Opponens Digiti Minimi
- **h.** Adductor Pollicis
- **i.** Lumbricals Manus (cut and reflected)
- **j.** Palmar Interossei
- **k.** Dorsal Interossei Manus

RELATIONSHIP TO OTHER MUSCULOSKELETAL STRUCTURES

- ❑ 1. The opponens pollicis is the deepest of the three thenar muscles.
- ❑ 2. The opponens pollicis is deep to the abductor pollicis brevis and the flexor pollicis brevis.
- ❑ 3. Deep to the opponens pollicis is the distal attachment of the abductor pollicis longus.

METHODOLOGY FOR LEARNING MUSCLE ACTIONS

- ❑ 1. **Opposition of the Thumb at the Carpometacarpal Joint:** Opposition is not a specific action, but rather is the term given to a combination of actions that are required to bring the finger pad of the thumb against the finger pad of another finger. Due to its line of pull, the opponens pollicis is able to create all of these actions. (For more information, see miscellaneous #1 and methodologies #2-4.)

OPPONENS POLLICIS – continued

- ❑ 2. **Flexion of the Thumb at the Carpometacarpal Joint:** The opponens pollicis crosses the 1st carpometacarpal joint of the thumb medially (on the ulnar side) to attach onto the 1st metacarpal of the thumb (with its fibers running vertically in the frontal plane). When the opponens pollicis contracts, it pulls the metacarpal of the thumb in a medial (ulnar) direction within the plane of the palm of the hand (frontal plane), toward the index finger. This action is called flexion of the thumb. Therefore, the opponens pollicis flexes the thumb by flexing the metacarpal of the thumb at the 1st carpometacarpal joint. (Note: Due to the rotational development of the thumb embryologically, the named actions of flexion and extension of the thumb occur within the frontal plane. For more details, see the Muscular System Manual, Volume I.)

- ❑ 3. **Adduction of the Thumb at the Carpometacarpal Joint:** The opponens pollicis crosses the 1st carpometacarpal joint of the thumb posteriorly to attach more anteriorly onto the thumb (with its fibers running horizontally in the sagittal plane). When the thumb is first in a position of abduction, and the opponens pollicis contracts, it pulls the metacarpal of the thumb in a posterior direction, perpendicularly toward the plane of the palm. This action is called adduction of the thumb. Therefore, the adductor pollicis adducts the thumb by adducting the metacarpal of the thumb at the carpometacarpal joint. (Note: Due to the rotational development of the thumb embryologically, the named actions of flexion and extension of the thumb occur within the frontal plane. For more details, see the Muscular System Manual, Volume I.)

- ❑ 4. **Medial Rotation of the Thumb at the Carpometacarpal Joint:** The opponens pollicis crosses the 1st carpometacarpal joint on the anterior side from slightly medial on the flexor retinaculum to attach more laterally onto the 1st metacarpal of the thumb (with its fibers running somewhat horizontally in the transverse plane). When the opponens pollicis contracts, it rotates the 1st metacarpal anteromedially toward the little finger (finger #5) causing the anterior surface of the thumb to face somewhat medially. Therefore, the opponens pollicis medially rotates the thumb by medially rotating the metacarpal of the thumb at the carpometacarpal joint.

MISCELLANEOUS

- ❑ 1. Opposition is not a specific action, but rather is the term given to a combination of actions that are required to bring the finger pad of the thumb against the finger pad of another finger. Opposition of the thumb involves a combination of both flexion and adduction of the metacarpal of the thumb at the 1st carpometacarpal joint. (Depending upon which finger you are opposing the thumb to, the amount of flexion or adduction can vary. Relatively more flexion and less adduction are required to meet the little finger, and more adduction and less flexion are required to meet the index finger.) However, the additional movement that distinguishes and facilitates opposition is medial rotation of the metacarpal of the thumb at the 1st carpometacarpal joint. Flexion of the phalanges of the thumb at the metacarpophalangeal joint and/or the interphalangeal joint of the thumb may accompany opposition of the thumb.

- ❑ 2. The three muscles of the thenar eminence are the abductor pollicis brevis, the flexor pollicis brevis and the opponens pollicis. (Note: There are three analogous hypothenar muscles. They are the abductor digiti minimi manus, the flexor digiti minimi manus and the opponens digiti minimi.)

- ❑ 3. All three thenar muscles attach onto and move the thumb. (Note: All three hypothenar muscles attach onto and move the little finger.)

- ❑ 4. Both the opponens pollicis and the opponens digiti minimi attach onto their respective metacarpal bone (1st and 5th) and not onto the phalanges, as do all the other thenar and hypothenar muscles.

OPPONENS POLLICIS – continued

- ❑ 5. Some sources state that the opponens pollicis can also extend the thumb at the 1st metacarpophalangeal joint. If this were true, it would have to be the most lateral fibers that would create this action by pulling the thumb radially (laterally) away from the other fingers (in the plane of the palm of the hand). This action is called extension of the thumb at the 1st metacarpophalangeal joint.
- ❑ 6. There is some controversy regarding the ability of the opponens pollicis to abduct the thumb. Some sources state that the opponens pollicis can abduct the thumb at the 1st metacarpophalangeal joint instead of adduct it. This action would seem most likely if the thumb is already in a position of adduction.
- ❑ 7. The ulnar nerve component of the opponens pollicis is often absent.

THE MUSCLES OF THE HYPOTHENAR EMINENCE

The hypothenar eminence is an eminence of soft tissue located on the ulnar side of the palm of the hand.

THERE ARE THREE MUSCLES OF THE HYPOTHENAR EMINENCE:		
Abductor Digiti Minimi Manus	Flexor Digiti Minimi Manus	Opponens Digiti Minimi

Attachments:

- All three hypothenar muscles attach proximally onto the flexor retinaculum and/or the carpal bones.
- All three hypothenar muscles attach distally onto the little finger (finger #5).
- The abductor digiti minimi and flexor digiti minimi manus attach onto the proximal phalanx of the little finger.
- The opponens digiti minimi attaches onto the 5th metacarpal (of the little finger).

Actions:

- All three hypothenar muscles move the little finger.

Miscellaneous:

- The layering of the hypothenar muscles is approximately as follows:
  - The abductor digiti minimi manus is the most superficial of the three.
  - The flexor digiti minimi manus is intermediate.
  - The opponens digiti minimi is the deepest of the three.
- There are three muscles located in the thenar eminence that are analogous to the hypothenar muscles. The three thenar muscles are the abductor pollicis brevis, flexor pollicis brevis and the opponens pollicis.

INNERVATION The three hypothenar muscles are innervated by the ulnar nerve.

ARTERIAL SUPPLY The three hypothenar muscles receive their arterial supply from the ulnar artery.

VIEWS OF THE HYPOTHENAR MUSCLES

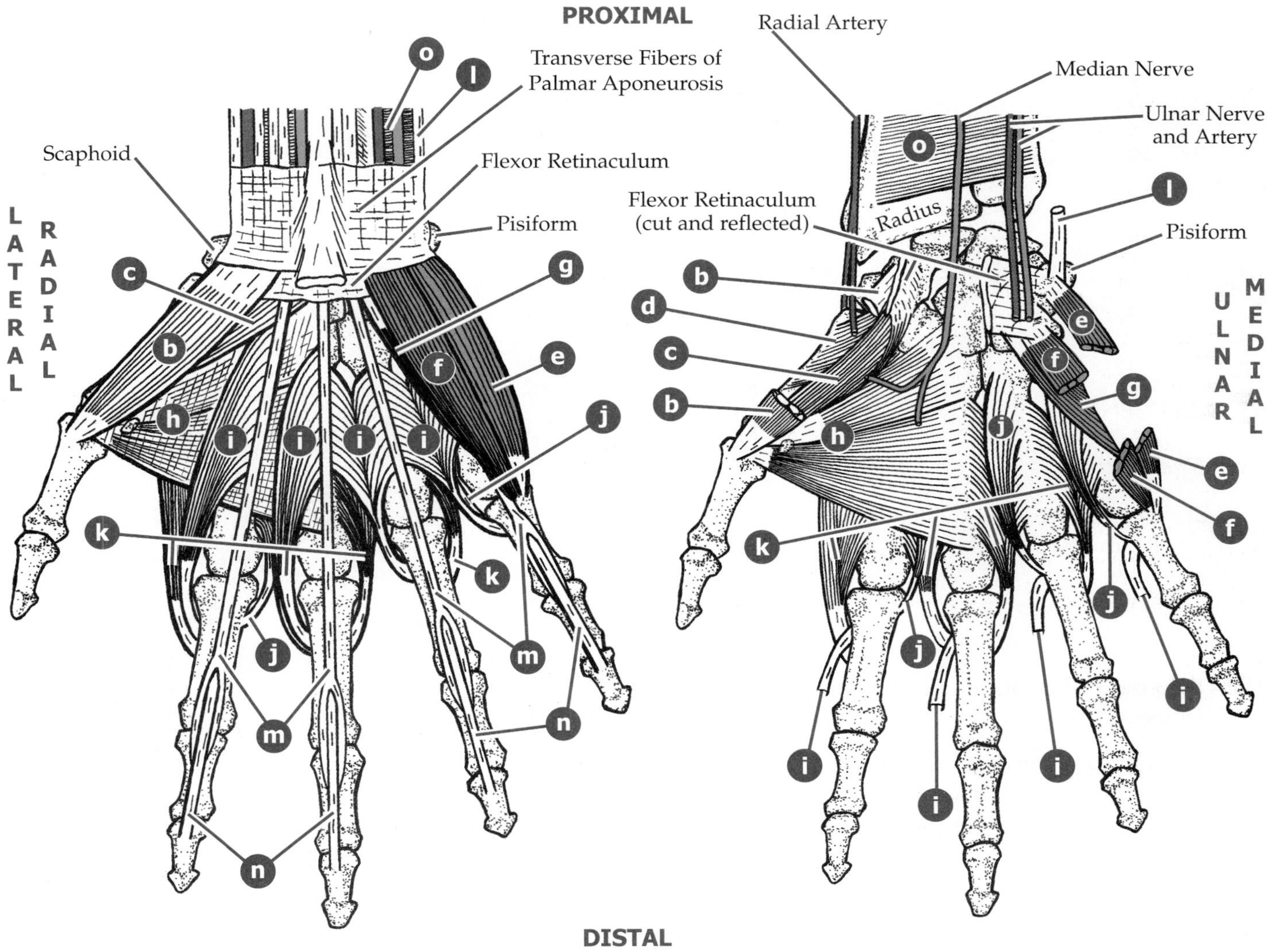

Palmar View of the Right Hand (Superficial Muscular Layer)

Palmar View of the Right Hand (Deep Muscular Layer)

a. Palmaris Brevis (not seen)
b. Abductor Pollicis Brevis (cut on our right)
c. Flexor Pollicis Brevis
d. Opponens Pollicis (not seen on our left)
e. **Abductor Digiti Minimi Manus** (cut on our right)
f. **Flexor Digiti Minimi Manus** (cut on our right)
g. **Opponens Digiti Minimi**
h. Adductor Pollicis (deep to fascia on our left)
i. Lumbricals Manus (cut and reflected on our right)
j. Palmar Interossei
k. Dorsal Interossei Manus
l. Flexor Carpi Ulnaris
m. Flexor Digitorum Superficialis (not seen on our right)
n. Flexor Digitorum Profundus (not seen on our right)
o. Pronator Quadratus

❑ ABDUCTOR DIGITI MINIMI MANUS

(OF THE HYPOTHENAR EMINENCE)

❑ **The name, abductor digiti minimi manus, tells us that this muscle abducts the little finger.**

DERIVATION ❑ abductor: L. *a muscle that abducts a body part.*
digiti: L. *refers to a digit* (finger).
minimi: L. *least.*
manus: L. *refers to the hand.*

PRONUNCIATION ❑ ab-**duk**-tor **dij**-i-tee **min**-i-mee **man**-us

ATTACHMENTS

❑ **The Carpals**

- ❑ the pisiform and the tendon of the flexor carpi ulnaris

to the

❑ **Proximal Phalanx of the Little Finger (Finger #5)**

- ❑ the ulnar (medial) side of the base of the proximal phalanx and the dorsal digital expansion

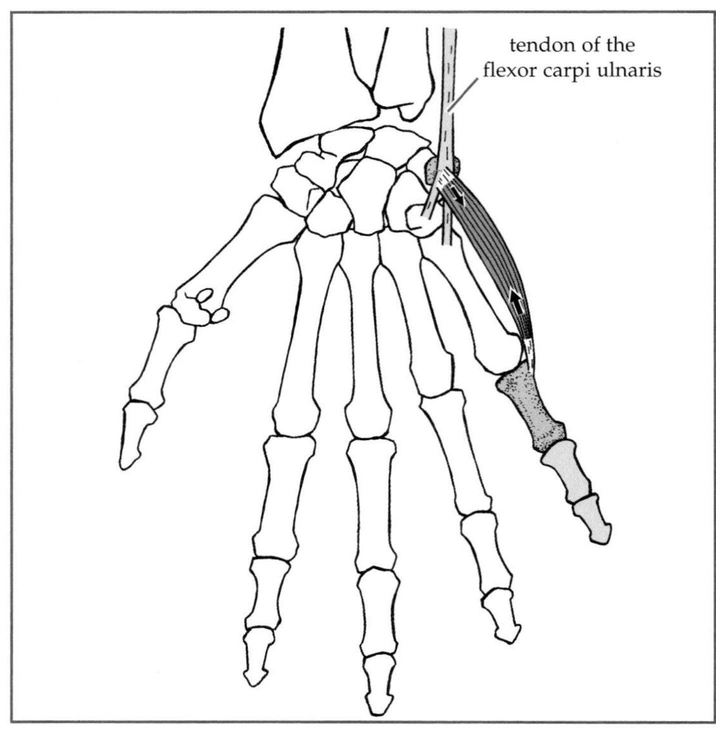

Anterior View of the Right Abductor Digiti Minimi Manus

ACTIONS

❑ 1. **Abduction of the Little Finger (Finger #5)**

❑ 2. Extension of the Little Finger (Finger #5)

INNERVATION ❑ The Ulnar Nerve ❑ C8, **T1**

ARTERIAL SUPPLY ❑ Branches of the Ulnar Artery (A Terminal Branch of the Brachial Artery)

PALPATION AND SUPPLEMENTARY TEXT

PALPATION

- ❑ The belly of the abductor digiti minimi manus is superficial and can be palpated in the medial aspect of the hypothenar eminence.
  - Have the client seated or supine.
  - Place palpating fingers on the medial aspect of the hypothenar eminence.
  - Ask the client to actively abduct the little finger at the 5th metacarpophalangeal joint and feel for the contraction of the belly of the abductor digiti minimi manus.
  - To further bring out the muscle belly, resistance may be added.

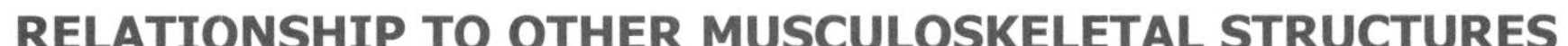

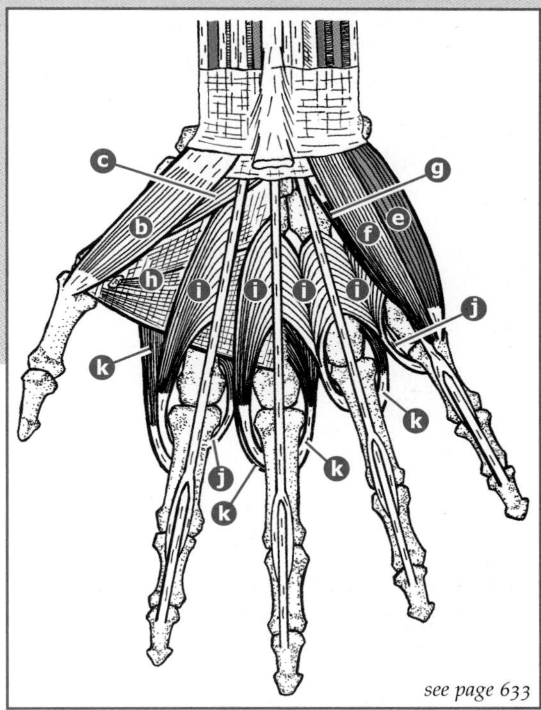

Palmar View of the Right Hand (Superficial Muscular Layer)

a. Palmaris Brevis (not seen)
b. Abductor Pollicis Brevis
c. Flexor Pollicis Brevis
d. Opponens Pollicis (not seen)
e. **Abductor Digiti Minimi Manus**
f. Flexor Digiti Minimi Manus
g. Opponens Digiti Minimi
h. Adductor Pollicis (deep to fascia)
i. Lumbricals Manus
j. Palmar Interossei (2nd not seen)
k. Dorsal Interossei Manus

RELATIONSHIP TO OTHER MUSCULOSKELETAL STRUCTURES

❑ 1. The abductor digiti minimi manus is superficial in the medial part of the hypothenar eminence.

❑ 2. The abductor digiti minimi manus is somewhat superficial to, and therefore somewhat overlies, the flexor digiti minimi manus.

METHODOLOGY FOR LEARNING MUSCLE ACTIONS

❑ **1. Abduction of the Little Finger (Finger #5) at the Metacarpophalangeal Joint:** The abductor digiti minimi manus crosses the 5th metacarpophalangeal joint of the little finger on the medial (ulnar) side to attach onto the little finger (with its fibers running vertically in the frontal plane). Therefore, the abductor digiti minimi manus pulls the proximal phalanx of the little finger medially (in an ulnar direction) away from the middle finger (finger #3) at the metacarpophalangeal joint, which is defined as abduction of the little finger. (Note: The abductor digiti minimi manus also crosses the carpometacarpal joint of the little finger laterally. However, this joint permits little or no movement in the frontal plane.)

❑ **2. Extension of the Little Finger (Finger #5) at the Proximal and Distal Interphalangeal Joints:** The abductor digiti minimi manus attaches into the dorsal digital expansion, which crosses the proximal and distal interphalangeal joints of the little finger on the posterior side (with the line of pull running vertically in the sagittal plane). Therefore, the abductor digiti minimi manus extends the middle and distal phalanges of the little finger at the proximal and distal interphalangeal joints of the little finger.

ABDUCTOR DIGITI MINIMI MANUS – continued

MISCELLANEOUS

- ❑ 1. The abductor digiti minimi manus is also known as the *abductor digiti minimi.* However, this allows for confusion with the abductor digiti minimi pedis of the foot, which abducts the little toe of the foot.
- ❑ 2. The three muscles of the hypothenar eminence are the abductor digiti minimi manus, the flexor digiti minimi manus and the opponens digiti minimi. (Note: There are three analogous thenar muscles. They are the abductor pollicis brevis, the flexor pollicis brevis and the opponens pollicis.)
- ❑ 3. All three hypothenar muscles attach onto and move the little finger. (Note: All three thenar muscles attach onto and move the thumb.)
- ❑ 4. The dorsal interossei manus muscles cross the metacarpophalangeal joint of the index, middle and ring fingers (fingers #2-4, respectively) on the side away from the middle finger; consequently, the dorsal interossei manus abduct the index, middle and ring fingers. The abductor digiti minimi manus also crosses the metacarpophalangeal joint of the little finger on the side away from the middle finger and abducts the little finger. Therefore, the abductor digiti minimi manus can be regarded as an analogous muscle to the dorsal interossei manus with respect to structure and function.

FLEXOR DIGITI MINIMI MANUS
(OF THE HYPOTHENAR EMINENCE)

❑ **The name, flexor digiti minimi manus, tells us that this muscle flexes the little finger.**

DERIVATION ❑ flexor: L. *a muscle that flexes a body part.*
digiti: L. *refers to a digit* (finger).
minimi: L. *least.*
manus: L. *refers to the hand.*

PRONUNCIATION ❑ **fleks**-or **dij**-i-tee **min**-i-mee **man**-us

ATTACHMENTS

❑ **The Flexor Retinaculum and the Carpals**

- ❑ the hook of the hamate

to the

❑ **Proximal Phalanx of the Little Finger (Finger #5)**

- ❑ the ulnar (medial) side of the base of the proximal phalanx

ACTION

❑ **Flexion of the Little Finger (Finger #5)**

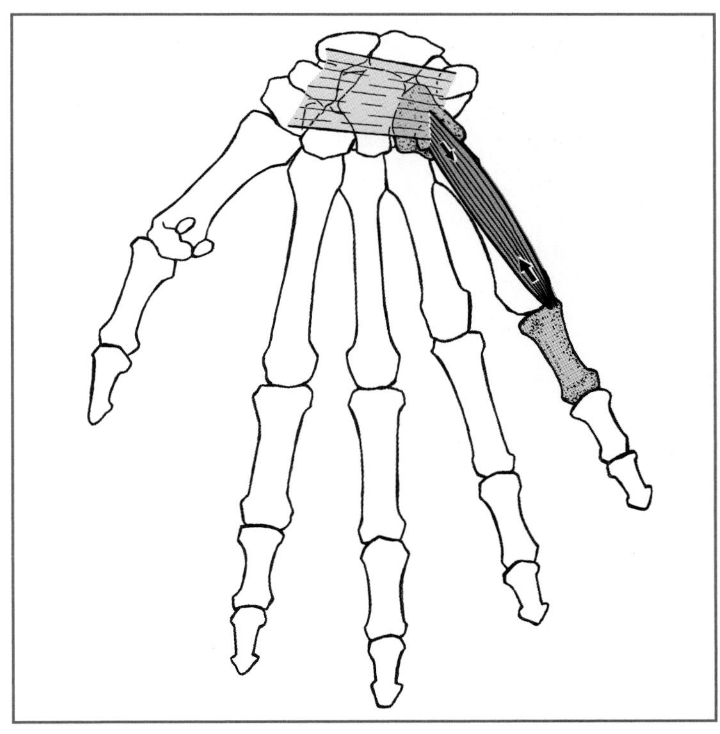

Anterior View of the Right Flexor Digiti Minimi Manus

INNERVATION ❑ The Ulnar Nerve ❑ C8, **T1**

ARTERIAL SUPPLY ❑ Branches of the Ulnar Artery (A Terminal Branch of the Brachial Artery)

FLEXOR DIGITI MINIMI MANUS PALPATION AND SUPPLEMENTARY TEXT

PALPATION

- ❑ The lateral portion of the flexor digiti minimi manus is superficial in the hypothenar eminence. The medial portion is deep to the abductor digiti minimi manus.
  - Have the client seated or supine.
  - Place palpating fingers in the middle of the hypothenar eminence.
  - Ask the client to actively flex the little finger at the 5th metacarpophalangeal joint and feel for the contraction of the lateral aspect of the belly of the flexor digit minimi.
  - A part of the medial portion of the flexor digiti minimi manus, deep to the abductor digiti minimi manus, can be palpated as you continue palpating medially as long as the abductor digiti minimi manus is relaxed. (Be sure that the client is not abducting the little finger at the same time or the abductor digiti minimi manus will also contract and make palpation of the flexor digiti minimi manus impossible.)
  - To further bring out the muscle belly, resistance may be added.

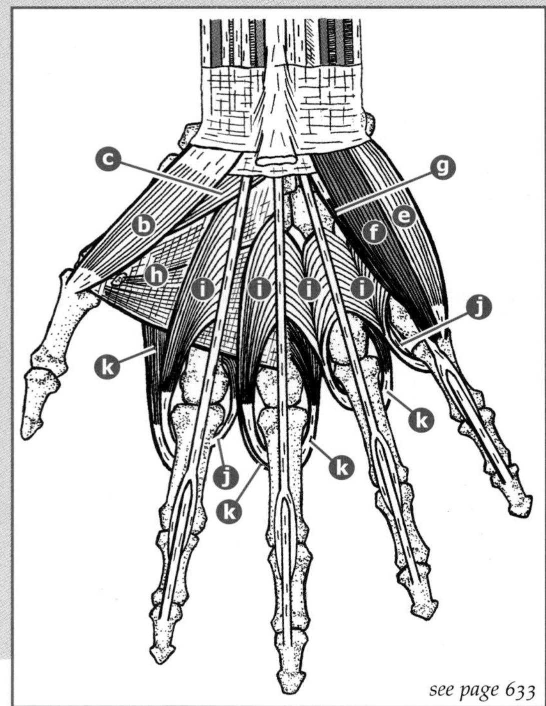

see page 633

Palmar View of the Right Hand (Superficial Muscular Layer)

a. Palmaris Brevis (not seen)
b. Abductor Pollicis Brevis
c. Flexor Pollicis Brevis
d. Opponens Pollicis (not seen)
e. Abductor Digiti Minimi Manus
f. Flexor Digiti Minimi Manus
g. Opponens Digiti Minimi
h. Adductor Pollicis (deep to fascia)
i. Lumbricals Manus
j. Palmar Interossei (2nd not seen)
k. Dorsal Interossei Manus

RELATIONSHIP TO OTHER MUSCULOSKELETAL STRUCTURES

- ❑ 1. The flexor digiti minimi manus lies in the hypothenar eminence, medial and partially deep to the abductor digiti minimi manus.
- ❑ 2. Partially deep to the flexor digiti minimi manus is the opponens digiti minimi.

METHODOLOGY FOR LEARNING MUSCLE ACTIONS

- ❑ **Flexion of the Little Finger (Finger #5) at the Metacarpophalangeal Joint:** The flexor digiti minimi manus crosses the 5th metacarpophalangeal joint of the little finger anteriorly (with its fibers running vertically in the sagittal plane); therefore, it flexes the proximal phalanx of the little finger at the metacarpophalangeal joint. (Note: The flexor digiti minimi manus also crosses the 5th carpometacarpal joint anteriorly; therefore, the flexor digiti minimi manus can also cause some flexion of the metacarpal of the little finger at the carpometacarpal joint. However, this motion is negligible because not much motion occurs at this joint.)

FLEXOR DIGITI MINIMI MANUS– continued

MISCELLANEOUS

- ☐ 1. The flexor digiti minimi manus is also known as the *flexor digiti minimi*. However, this allows for confusion with the flexor digiti minimi pedis of the foot, which flexes the little toe.
- ☐ 2. The flexor digiti minimi manus is also known as the *flexor digiti minimi brevis*. However, the addition of the word brevis at the end of the name is not necessary and does not make sense in this case. Usually, the word brevis at the end of a muscle's name is added to distinguish the muscle from a longer muscle that does the same action. In this case, there is no flexor digiti minimi longus.
- ☐ 3. The three muscles of the hypothenar eminence are the abductor digiti minimi manus, the flexor digiti minimi manus and the opponens digiti minimi. (Note: There are three analogous thenar muscles. They are the abductor pollicis brevis, the flexor pollicis brevis and the opponens pollicis.)
- ☐ 4. All three hypothenar muscles attach onto and move the little finger. (Note: All three thenar muscles attach onto and move the thumb.)
- ☐ 5. The flexor digiti minimi manus is the smallest of the three hypothenar muscles.
- ☐ 6. The flexor digiti minimi manus is often very small or entirely absent.

OPPONENS DIGITI MINIMI
(OF THE HYPOTHENAR EMINENCE)

❑ **The name, opponens digiti minimi, tells us that this muscle opposes the little finger.**

DERIVATION ❑ opponens: L. *opposing.*
digiti: L. *refers to a digit* (finger).
minimi: L. *least.*

PRONUNCIATION ❑ op-**po**-nens **dij**-i-tee **min**-i-mee

ATTACHMENTS

❑ **The Flexor Retinaculum and the Carpals**

- ❑ the hook of the hamate

to the

❑ **5th Metacarpal (of the Little Finger)**

- ❑ the anterior surface and the medial (ulnar) border of the 5th metacarpal

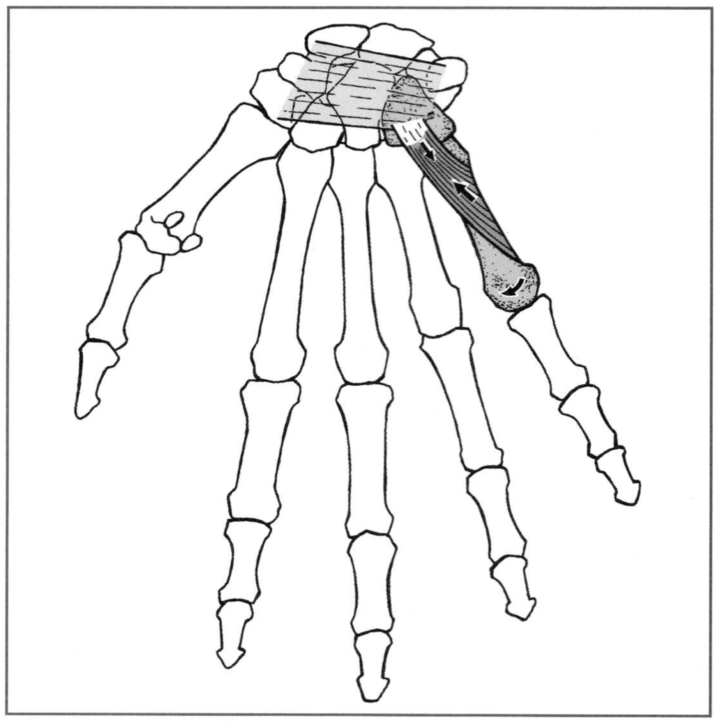

Anterior View of the Right Opponens Digiti Minimi

ACTIONS

❑ 1. **Opposition of the Little Finger (Finger #5)**

❑ 2. Flexion of the Little Finger (Finger #5)

❑ 3. Adduction of the Little Finger (Finger #5)

❑ 4. Lateral Rotation of the Little Finger (Finger #5)

INNERVATION ❑ The Ulnar Nerve ❑ C8, **T1**

ARTERIAL SUPPLY ❑ Branches of the Ulnar Artery (A Terminal Branch of the Brachial Artery)

PALPATION AND SUPPLEMENTARY TEXT

PALPATION

- ❑ The medial part of the opponens digiti minimi is deep to the abductor digiti minimi manus and flexor digiti minimi manus, but the lateral part is superficial and easy to palpate.
  - Have the client seated or supine.
  - Place palpating finger on the lateral aspect of the hypothenar eminence.
  - Ask the client to actively oppose the little finger at the 5th carpometacarpal joint (i.e., have the little finger meet the thumb) and feel for the contraction of the belly of the opponens digiti minimi.
  - Continue palpating the opponens digiti minimi medially and try to follow it deep to the flexor digiti minimi manus and the abductor digiti minimi manus.

    (Be sure to differentiate the contraction of the belly of the opponens digiti minimi from the contraction of the tendons of the flexors digitorum superficialis and profundus, which are just lateral to the opponens digiti minimi. The position of the tendons of the flexors digitorum superficialis and profundus can be determined by flexing the interphalangeal joints of the little finger without opposing the little finger to the thumb.)

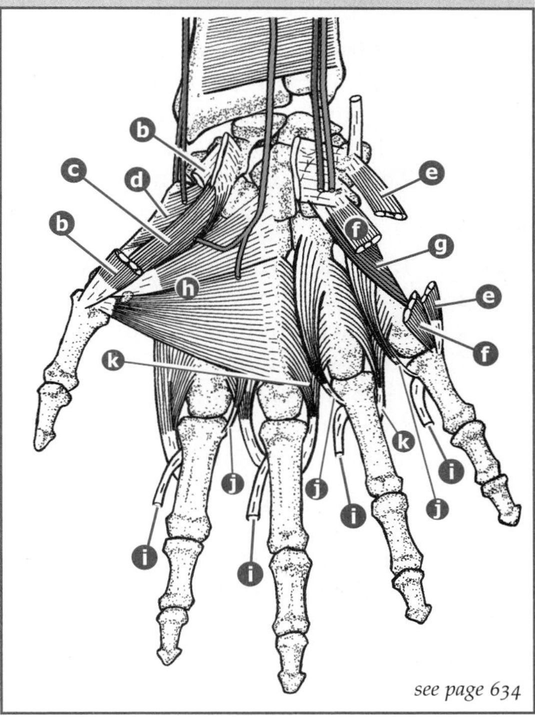

see page 634

Palmar View of the Right Hand (Deep Muscular Layer)

a. Palmaris Brevis (not seen)
b. Abductor Pollicis Brevis (cut)
c. Flexor Pollicis Brevis
d. Opponens Pollicis
e. Abductor Digiti Minimi Manus (cut)
f. Flexor Digiti Minimi Manus (cut)
g. **Opponens Digiti Minimi**
h. Adductor Pollicis
i. Lumbricals Manus (cut and reflected)
j. Palmar Interossei
k. Dorsal Interossei Manus

RELATIONSHIP TO OTHER MUSCULOSKELETAL STRUCTURES

❑ 1. The medial portion of the opponens digiti minimi is deep to the abductor digiti minimi manus and the flexor digiti minimi. A small part of the lateral portion of the opponens digiti minimi is superficial in the most lateral aspect of the hypothenar eminence.

❑ 2. The opponens digiti minimi is superficial to some of the more lateral tendons of the flexor digitorum superficialis and the flexor digitorum profundus.

METHODOLOGY FOR LEARNING MUSCLE ACTIONS

❑ 1. **Opposition of the Little Finger (Finger #5) at the Carpometacarpal Joint:** Opposition is not a specific action, but rather is the term given to a combination of actions that are required to bring the finger pad of the little finger against the finger pad of the thumb. Due to its line of pull, the opponens digiti minimi is able to create these actions. (For more information, see miscellaneous #1 and methodologies #2-3.)

OPPONENS DIGITI MINIMI – continued

- ❑ 2. **Flexion of the Little Finger (Finger #5) at the Carpometacarpal Joint:** The opponens digiti minimi crosses the 5th carpometacarpal joint anteriorly to attach onto the 5th metacarpal of the little finger (with its fibers running vertically in the sagittal plane). When the opponens digiti minimi contracts, it pulls the 5th metacarpal anteriorly into flexion. Therefore, the opponens digiti minimi flexes the little finger by flexing the metacarpal of the little finger at the carpometacarpal joint.

- ❑ 3. **Adduction of the Little Finger (Finger #5) at the Carpometacarpal Joint:** The opponens digiti minimi crosses the 5th carpometacarpal joint anteriorly from laterally at the wrist area to medially onto the 5th metacarpal of the little finger (with its fibers running slightly horizontally in the frontal plane). When the opponens digiti minimi contracts, it pulls the 5th metacarpal laterally into adduction. Therefore, the opponens digiti minimi adducts the little finger by adducting the metacarpal of the little finger at the carpometacarpal joint.

- ❑ 4. **Lateral Rotation of the Little Finger (Finger #5) at the Carpometacarpal Joint:** The opponens digiti minimi crosses the 5th carpometacarpal joint anteriorly from slightly more lateral on the flexor retinaculum to attach more medially onto the 5th metacarpal of the little finger (with its fibers running somewhat horizontally in the transverse plane). When the opponens digiti minimi contracts, it rotates the 5th metacarpal anterolaterally toward the thumb, causing the anterior surface of the little finger to face somewhat laterally. Therefore, the opponens digiti minimi laterally rotates the little finger by laterally rotating the metacarpal of the little finger at the carpometacarpal joint.

MISCELLANEOUS

- ❑ 1. Opposition of the little finger is not a specific action, but rather is the term given to a combination of actions that are required to bring the finger pad of the little finger against the finger pad of the thumb. Opposition of the little finger involves a combination of both flexion and adduction of the metacarpal of the little finger at the 5th carpometacarpal joint. However, the additional movement that distinguishes and facilitates opposition is lateral rotation of the metacarpal of the little finger at the 5th carpometacarpal joint. Flexion of the phalanges of the little finger at the metacarpophalangeal joint and/or the interphalangeal joints of the little finger as well as adduction of the proximal phalanx of the little finger at the metacarpophalangeal joint may accompany opposition of the little finger.

- ❑ 2. The three muscles of the hypothenar eminence are the abductor digiti minimi manus, the flexor digiti minimi manus and the opponens digiti minimi. (Note: There are three analogous thenar muscles. They are the abductor pollicis brevis, the flexor pollicis brevis and the opponens pollicis.)

- ❑ 3. All three hypothenar muscles attach onto and move the little finger. (Note: All three thenar muscles attach onto and move the thumb.)

- ❑ 4. Both the opponens digiti minimi and the opponens pollicis attach onto their respective metacarpal bone (5th and 1st) and not onto the phalanges, as do all the other thenar and hypothenar muscles.

- ❑ 5. The flexor digiti minimi manus, which overlies the opponens digiti minimi, is often very small or entirely absent. When this occurs, the opponens digiti minimi will have relatively more superficial exposure.

ADDUCTOR POLLICIS
(OF THE CENTRAL COMPARTMENT)

❑ **The name, adductor pollicis, tells us that this muscle adducts the thumb.**

DERIVATION ❑ adductor: L. *a muscle that adducts a body part.*
pollicis: L. *thumb.*

PRONUNCIATION ❑ ad-**duk**-tor **pol**-i-sis

ATTACHMENTS

❑ **3rd Metacarpal**

❑ OBLIQUE HEAD: the anterior bases of the 2nd and 3rd metacarpals and the capitate

❑ TRANSVERSE HEAD: the distal 2/3 of the anterior surface of the 3rd metacarpal

to the

❑ **Thumb**

❑ OBLIQUE HEAD: the medial side of the base of the proximal phalanx and the dorsal digital expansion

❑ TRANSVERSE HEAD: the medial side of the base of the proximal phalanx

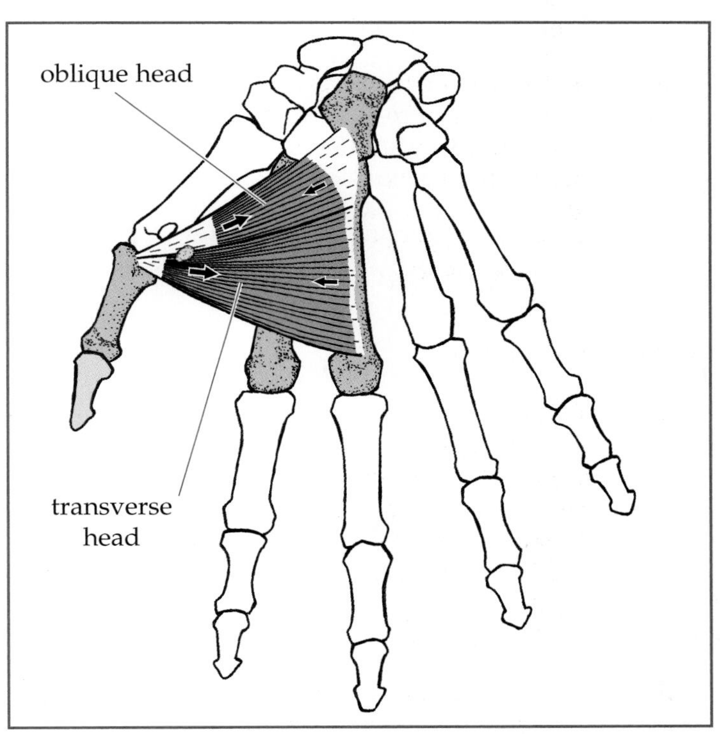

Anterior View of the Right Adductor Pollicis

ACTIONS

❑ 1. **Adduction of the Thumb**

❑ 2. Flexion of the Thumb

❑ 3. Extension of the Thumb

INNERVATION ❑ The Ulnar Nerve ❑ C8, T1

ARTERIAL SUPPLY ❑ Branches of the Radial Artery (A Terminal Branch of the Brachial Artery)

ADDUCTOR POLLICIS – PALPATION AND SUPPLEMENTARY TEXT

PALPATION

- ❑ Part of the adductor pollicis is superficial in the thumb web and easily palpable.
  - Have the client seated or supine.
  - Place palpating fingers in the middle of the thumb web of the hand. (Note: Be careful of your location because if you palpate too laterally toward the thumb, you will also be palpating the flexor pollicis brevis and the 1st dorsal interosseus manus muscles. If you palpate too medially toward the index finger, you will also be palpating the 1st lumbrical manus and the 1st dorsal interosseus manus muscles.)
  - Ask the client to actively adduct the thumb at the 1st carpometacarpal joint against resistance and feel for the contraction of the adductor pollicis.
  - Continue palpating the adductor pollicis as far lateral and medial as possible.

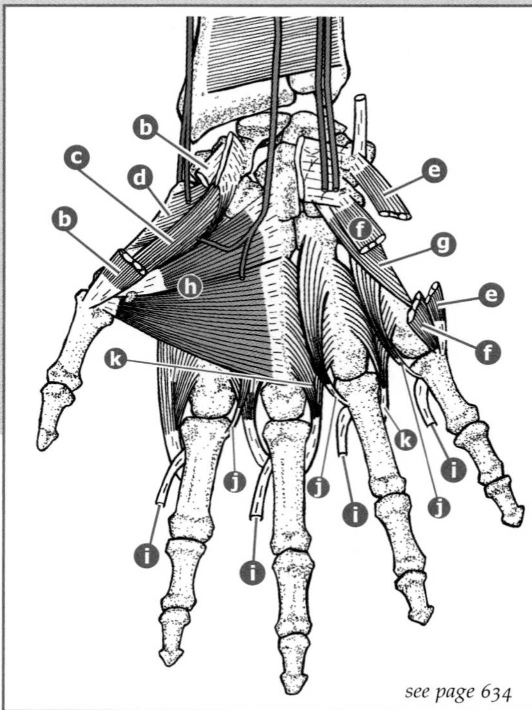

see page 634

Palmar View of the Right Hand (Deep Muscular Layer)

a. Palmaris Brevis (not seen)
b. Abductor Pollicis Brevis (cut)
c. Flexor Pollicis Brevis
d. Opponens Pollicis
e. Abductor Digiti Minimi Manus (cut)
f. Flexor Digiti Minimi Manus (cut)
g. Opponens Digiti Minimi
h. **Adductor Pollicis**
i. Lumbricals Manus (cut and reflected)
j. Palmar Interossei
k. Dorsal Interossei Manus

RELATIONSHIP TO OTHER MUSCULOSKELETAL STRUCTURES

❑ 1. Except for the part of the adductor pollicis that is superficial in the thumb web, the adductor pollicis is deeply situated in the hand. All the thenar muscles, the distal tendons of flexors digitorum superficialis and profundus (going to the 2nd and 3rd fingers), the distal tendon of the flexor pollicis longus and the 1st and 2nd lumbricals manus are superficial to the adductor pollicis.

❑ 2. Although somewhat deep to the thenar muscles, the adductor pollicis also lies medial to the flexor pollicis brevis and the opponens pollicis.

❑ 3. The distal attachment of the flexor carpi radialis and the shaft of the 2nd metacarpal bone are deep to the adductor pollicis.

❑ 4. From an anterior perspective, the 1st and 2nd dorsal interossei manus are also deep to the adductor pollicis.

METHODOLOGY FOR LEARNING MUSCLE ACTIONS

❑ **1. Adduction of the Thumb at the Carpometacarpal Joint:** The adductor pollicis crosses the 1st carpometacarpal joint of the thumb posteriorly by attaching from medially on the palm of the hand to laterally onto the thumb (with its fibers running horizontally in the sagittal plane). When the thumb is first in a position of abduction, and the adductor pollicis contracts, it pulls the thumb posteriorly, perpendicularly toward the plane of the palm. This action is called adduction of the thumb. Therefore, the adductor pollicis adducts the thumb by adducting the metacarpal of the thumb at the carpometacarpal joint. (Note: Due to the rotational development of the thumb embryologically, the named actions of abduction and adduction of the thumb occur within the sagittal plane. For more details, see the Muscular System Manual, Volume I.)

ADDUCTOR POLLICIS – continued

- ☐ 2. **Flexion of the Thumb at the Carpometacarpal and Metacarpophalangeal Joints:** The adductor pollicis crosses the 1st carpometacarpal joint of the thumb from medially on the hand to more laterally onto the 1st metacarpal of the thumb (with its fibers running horizontally in the frontal plane, especially the transverse head). When the adductor pollicis contracts, it pulls the thumb medially (in an ulnar direction) within the plane of the palm of the hand (frontal plane), toward its other attachment (the 3rd metacarpal). This action is called flexion of the thumb. Therefore, the adductor pollicis flexes the thumb by flexing the metacarpal of the thumb at the carpometacarpal joint. The adductor pollicis also crosses the 1st metacarpophalangeal joint of the thumb medially (with it fibers running somewhat vertically in the frontal plane, especially the oblique head). Therefore, the adductor pollicis flexes the thumb by flexing the proximal phalanx of the thumb at the 1st metacarpophalangeal joint. (Note: Due to the rotational development of the thumb embryologically, the named actions of flexion and extension of the thumb occur within the frontal plane. For more details, see the **Muscular System Manual, Volume I.**)

- ☐ 3. **Extension of the Thumb at the Interphalangeal Joint:** Due to its attachment into the dorsal digital expansion, which crosses the interphalangeal joint of the thumb on the lateral side (with its fibers running vertically in the frontal plane), the adductor pollicis can extend the thumb by extending the distal phalanx of the thumb at the interphalangeal joint. (Note: Due to the rotational development of the thumb embryologically, the named actions of flexion and extension of the thumb occur within the frontal plane. For more details, see the **Muscular System Manual, Volume I.**)

MISCELLANEOUS

- ☐ 1. The adductor pollicis has two heads: an *oblique head* and a *transverse head.* The oblique head runs more obliquely in the hand, i.e., its fiber direction is between vertical and horizontal in orientation. The transverse head runs transversely across the hand, i.e., its fiber direction is horizontal in orientation. (Note: The adductor hallucis of the foot also has two heads: an oblique head and a transverse head.)

- ☐ 2. There is a lot of variation and confusion regarding the region of the oblique head of the adductor pollicis. The oblique head often has a fasciculus (a group of muscle fibers) that joins with the flexor pollicis brevis and is called the *deep head* of the flexor pollicis brevis (see the note regarding the palmar interosseus muscles on page 627).

- ☐ 3. The oblique head of the adductor pollicis has a sesamoid bone located within it. (Note: There is a second sesamoid bone of the thumb located in the distal tendon of the flexor pollicis brevis.)

- ☐ 4. The majority of tissue of the thumb web of the hand is made up of the adductor pollicis and the 1st dorsal interosseus manus.

- ☐ 5. The attachment of the adductor pollicis into the dorsal digital expansion of the thumb is small and often absent. When it is absent, the adductor pollicis does not have the ability to extend the distal phalanx of the thumb at the interphalangeal joint of the thumb.

LUMBRICALS MANUS

(OF THE CENTRAL COMPARTMENT)

(There are four lumbrical manus muscles, named #1, #2, #3 and #4.)

❑ **The name, lumbricals manus, tells us that these muscles are shaped like earthworms and are located in the hand.**

DERIVATION ❑ lumbricals: L. *earthworms.*
manus: L. *refers to the hand.*

PRONUNCIATION ❑ **lum**-bri-kuls **man**-us

ATTACHMENTS

❑ **The Distal Tendons of the Flexor Digitorum Profundus**

- ❑ **#1**: the radial (lateral) side of the tendon of the index finger (finger #2)
- ❑ **#2**: the radial (lateral) side of the tendon of the middle finger (finger #3)
- ❑ **#3**: the ulnar (medial) side of the tendon of the middle finger (finger #3) and the radial (lateral) side of the tendon of the ring finger (finger #4)
- ❑ **#4**: the ulnar (medial) side of the tendon of the ring finger (finger #4) and the radial (lateral) side of the tendon of the little finger (finger #5)

to the

❑ **Distal Tendons of the Extensor Digitorum (the Dorsal Digital Expansion)**

- ❑ the radial (lateral) side of the tendons merging into the dorsal digital expansion
- ❑ **#1**: into the tendon of the index finger (finger #2)
- ❑ **#2**: into the tendon of the middle finger (finger #3)
- ❑ **#3**: into the tendon of the ring finger (finger #4)
- ❑ **#4**: into the tendon of the little finger (finger #5)

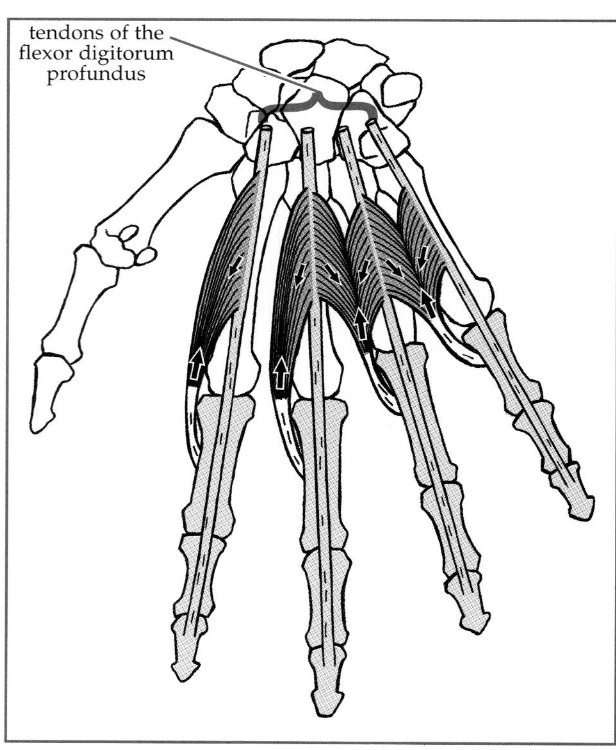

Anterior View of the Right Lumbricals Manus

ACTIONS

❑ 1. **Extension of Fingers #2-5 at the Interphalangeal Joints**

❑ 2. **Flexion of Fingers #2-5 at the Metacarpophalangeal Joint**

INNERVATION ❑ The Median and Ulnar Nerves
❑ C8, **T1** (1st and 2nd lumbricals manus: the median nerve)
(3rd and 4th lumbricals manus: the ulnar nerve)

ARTERIAL SUPPLY ❑ Branches of the Radial and Ulnar Arteries (Terminal Branches of the Brachial Artery)

PALPATION AND SUPPLEMENTARY TEXT

PALPATION

- ❑ The lumbricals manus are deep to the palmar fascia of the hand but palpable.
  - Have the client seated or supine.
  - Place palpating fingers on the lateral side of the metacarpal of the little finger.
  - Ask the client to actively flex the little finger at the 5th metacarpophalangeal joint with the interphalangeal joints fully extended and feel for the contraction of the 4th lumbrical manus.
  - To palpate the 1st, 2nd and 3rd lumbricals manus, follow the above procedure on the lateral sides of the index, middle and ring fingers respectively. It can be difficult to distinguish the border of a lumbrical manus from the flexor tendons of the flexors digitorum superficialis and profundus.

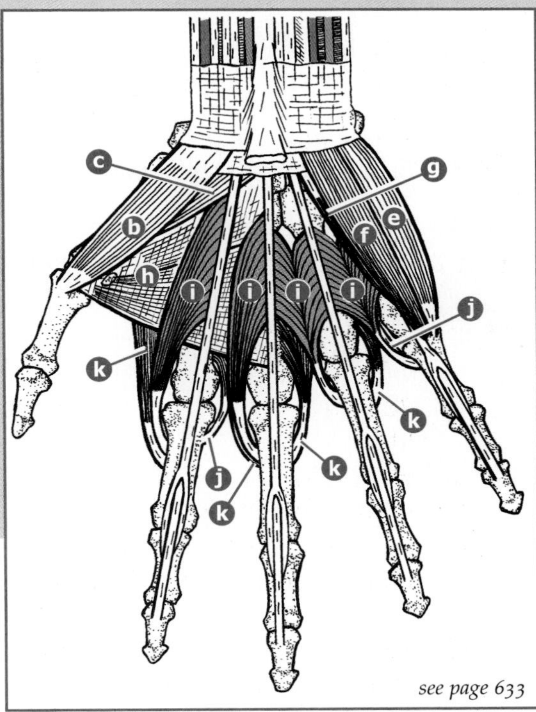

see page 633

Palmar View of the Right Hand (Superficial Muscular Layer)

a. Palmaris Brevis (not seen)
b. Abductor Pollicis Brevis
c. Flexor Pollicis Brevis
d. Opponens Pollicis (not seen)
e. Abductor Digiti Minimi Manus
f. Flexor Digiti Minimi Manus
g. Opponens Digiti Minimi
h. Adductor Pollicis (deep to fascia)
i. **Lumbricals Manus**
j. Palmar Interossei (2nd not seen)
k. Dorsal Interossei Manus

RELATIONSHIP TO OTHER MUSCULOSKELETAL STRUCTURES

❑ 1. The lumbricals manus are actually not that deep in the palm of the hand. In the palm, they are deep only to the palmar fascia. As the lumbricals manus approach the phalanges, they dive deeper (more posteriorly) to attach onto the tendons of the extensor digitorum, which is on the posterior side of the fingers.

❑ 2. The lumbricals manus are located between the distal tendons of the flexor digitorum profundus.

❑ 3. Directly deep to the 1st and 2nd lumbricals manus is the adductor pollicis. Directly deep to the 3rd and 4th lumbricals manus are the metacarpals and the palmar interossei.

METHODOLOGY FOR LEARNING MUSCLE ACTIONS

❑ **1. Extension of Fingers #2-5 at the Proximal and Distal Interphalangeal Joints:** The lumbricals manus, by attaching into the tendons of the extensor digitorum muscle (after the metacarpophalangeal joint but before the interphalangeal joints of the fingers), exert their pull on the distal attachments of the extensor digitorum, which are the distal phalanges of fingers #2-5. The lumbricals manus, in effect, cross the proximal and distal interphalangeal joints of fingers #2-5 posteriorly (with their pull exerted vertically in the sagittal plane) and, therefore, extend both the middle and distal phalanges at the proximal and distal interphalangeal joints of fingers #2-5.

❑ **2. Flexion of Fingers #2-5 at the Metacarpophalangeal Joint:** The lumbricals manus cross the metacarpophalangeal joint of fingers #2-5 anteriorly (with their fibers running vertically in the sagittal plane); therefore, they flex fingers #2-5 at the metacarpophalangeal joint.

LUMBRICALS MANUS – continued

MISCELLANEOUS

- ❑ 1. The lumbricals manus are actually four small separate muscles named from the lateral side: #1, #2, #3 and #4.
- ❑ 2. The lumbricals manus are usually known as the *lumbricals.* However, this allows for confusion with the lumbricals pedis of the foot.
- ❑ 3. The lumbricals pedis of the foot have similar actions in that they flex the toes at the metatarsophalangeal joints and extend the toes at the proximal and distal interphalangeal joints.
- ❑ 4. By flexing the metacarpophalangeal joint and simultaneously extending the proximal and distal interphalangeal joints, the lumbricals manus help to create a strong grip with the fingers opposed to the thumb.

PALMAR INTEROSSEI
(OF THE CENTRAL COMPARTMENT)

(There are three palmar interossei, named #1, #2 and #3.)

❑ **The name, palmar interossei, tells us that these muscles are located between bones (metacarpals) on the palmar (anterior) side.**

DERIVATION ❑ palmar: L. *refers to the palm.*
interossei: L. *between bones.*

PRONUNCIATION ❑ **pal**-mar **in**-ter-**oss**-ee-i

ATTACHMENTS

❑ **The Metacarpal of Fingers #2, #4 and #5**

- ❑ the anterior side and on the "middle finger side" of the metacarpals:
- ❑ **#1**: attaches to the metacarpal of the index finger (finger #2)
- ❑ **#2**: attaches to the metacarpal of the ring finger (finger #4)
- ❑ **#3**: attaches to the metacarpal of the little finger (finger #5)

to the

❑ **Proximal Phalanx of Fingers #2, #4 and #5 on the "Middle Finger Side"**

- ❑ the base of the proximal phalanx and the dorsal digital expansion:
- ❑ **#1**: attaches to the index finger (finger #2)
- ❑ **#2**: attaches to the ring finger (finger #4)
- ❑ **#3**: attaches to the little finger (finger #5)

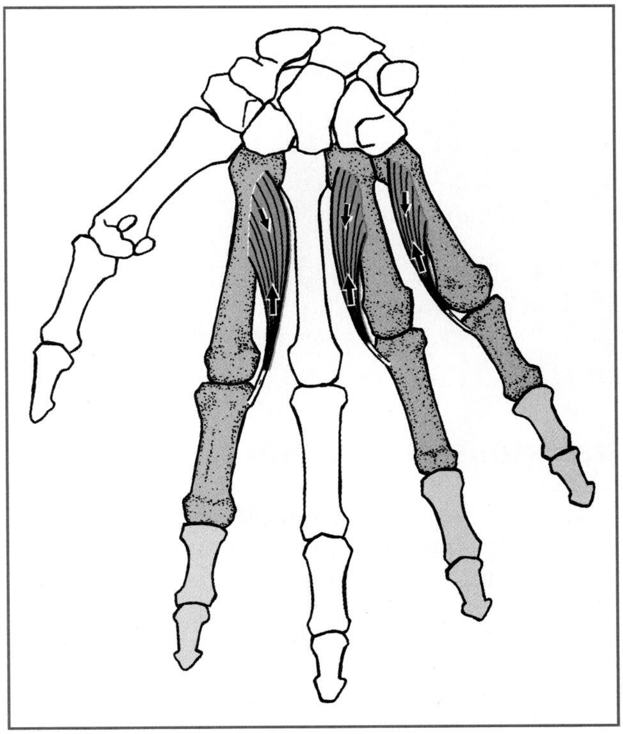

Anterior View of the Right Palmar Interossei

ACTIONS

❑ 1. **Adduction of Fingers #2, #4 and #5**

❑ 2. Flexion of Fingers #2, #4 and #5 at the Metacarpophalangeal Joint

❑ 3. Extension of Fingers #2, #4 and #5 at the Interphalangeal Joints

INNERVATION ❑ The Ulnar Nerve ❑ C8, **T1**; deep branch of the ulnar nerve

ARTERIAL SUPPLY ❑ Branches of the Radial and Ulnar Arteries (Terminal Branches of the Brachial Artery)

PALMAR INTEROSSEI – PALPATION AND SUPPLEMENTARY TEXT

PALPATION

❑ The palmar interossei are located deep within the palm but they are possible to palpate.

- Have the client seated or supine.
- To palpate the 1st palmar interosseus on the metacarpal of the index finger, have the client hold a pencil between the index and middle fingers. Holding the pencil in this position will require adduction of the index finger, causing the 1st palmar interosseus to contract.
- Place palpating fingers on the "middle finger side" (in this case, the medial side) of the 2nd metacarpal in the palm.
- Ask the client to forcefully adduct the index finger at the 2nd metacarpophalangeal joint toward the middle finger (against the pencil) and feel for the contraction of the 2nd palmar interosseus.
- To palpate the 2nd and 3rd palmar interossei, follow the above procedure on the middle finger side of the ring and little fingers, respectively.

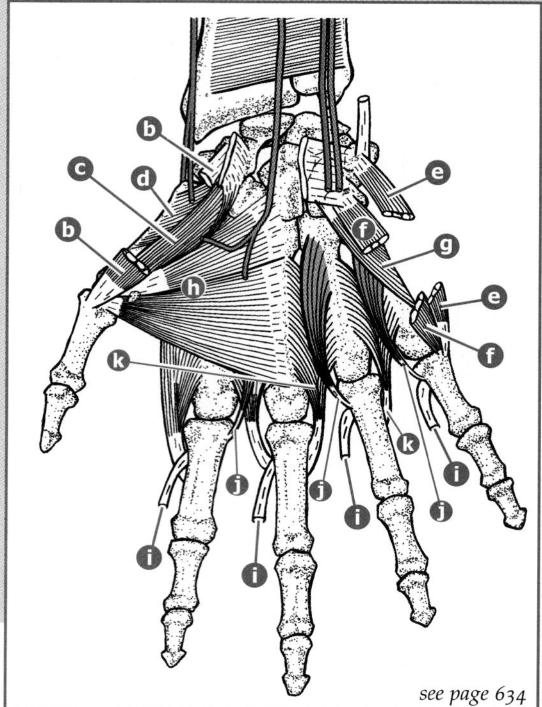

see page 634

Palmar View of the Right Hand (Deep Muscular Layer)

a. Palmaris Brevis (not seen)
b. Abductor Pollicis Brevis (cut)
c. Flexor Pollicis Brevis
d. Opponens Pollicis
e. Abductor Digiti Minimi Manus (cut)
f. Flexor Digiti Minimi Manus (cut)
g. Opponens Digiti Minimi
h. Adductor Pollicis
i. Lumbricals Manus (cut and reflected)
j. **Palmar Interossei**
k. Dorsal Interossei Manus

RELATIONSHIP TO OTHER MUSCULOSKELETAL STRUCTURES

❑ 1. The palmar interossei are located in a position that is palmar (anterior) on the metacarpals and slightly between the metacarpals.

❑ 2. Each palmar interosseus muscle is located on the side of the metacarpal that faces the middle finger. (The middle finger has no palmar interosseus muscle attached to it.)

❑ 3. From an anterior perspective, the palmar interossei are deep to all the other muscles of the anterior hand.

❑ 4. From the anterior perspective, the metacarpal bones and the dorsal interossei manus are deep to the palmar interossei.

METHODOLOGY FOR LEARNING MUSCLE ACTIONS

❑ **1. Adduction of Fingers #2, #4 and #5 at the Metacarpophalangeal Joint:** The 1st palmar interosseus muscle crosses the metacarpophalangeal joint of the index finger (fingers #2) on the medial side and therefore pulls the proximal phalanx of this finger medially, which is toward the middle finger (which is the axis for abduction/adduction in the hand). Therefore, the 1st palmar interosseus muscle adducts the index finger at the metacarpophalangeal joint.

PALMAR INTEROSSEI – continued

The 2nd and 3rd palmar interossei cross the metacarpophalangeal joint of the ring and little fingers (fingers #4 and 5) on the lateral side and therefore pull these fingers laterally, toward the middle finger (the axis for abduction/adduction in the hand). Therefore, the 2nd and 3rd palmar interossei adduct the ring finger and the little finger at the metacarpophalangeal joint.

Note: The palmar interossei are always on the "middle finger side" of the metacarpals and phalanges (with their fibers running vertically in the frontal plane); therefore, a palmar interosseus muscle always pulls the finger that it is attached to toward the middle finger. This action is defined as adduction of the finger.

❑ 2. **Flexion of Fingers #2, #4 and #5 at the Metacarpophalangeal Joint:** The palmar interossei cross the metacarpophalangeal joint on the palmar (anterior) side (with their fibers running vertically in the sagittal plane); therefore, they flex the proximal phalanx of fingers #2, 4 and 5 at the metacarpophalangeal joint.

❑ 3. **Extension of Fingers #2, #4 and #5 at the Proximal and Distal Interphalangeal Joints:** Due to their attachment into the dorsal digital expansion of the extensor digitorum, the palmar interossei exert their pull through the dorsal digital expansion, which crosses the proximal and distal interphalangeal joints of the fingers on the posterior side (with the line of pull running vertically in the sagittal plane). Therefore, the palmar interossei extend the middle and distal phalanges at the proximal and distal interphalangeal joints of fingers #2, 4 and 5.

MISCELLANEOUS

❑ 1. There are three palmar interossei muscles named from the lateral side: #1, #2 and #3.

❑ 2. There are three palmar interossei, one for each finger except the middle finger (and the thumb). It makes sense that the middle finger would not have a palmar interosseus muscle. The palmar interossei adduct the fingers, and the middle finger, by definition, cannot adduct because an imaginary line that runs through it is the axis for abduction/adduction of the fingers.

❑ 3. Many sources state that there is a 4th palmar interosseus muscle that attaches to the thumb. This would cause the naming of the palmar interossei muscles to change, since they are named from radial to ulnar (lateral to medial). Hence the palmar interosseus of the thumb would be #1, the 2nd palmar interosseus would attach to the index finger, the 3rd palmar interosseus would attach to the ring finger, and the 4th palmar interosseus would attach to the little finger. This palmar interosseus muscle that attaches to the thumb is also known as the *palmar interosseus of Henle.*

❑ 4. Whether or not a true 4th palmar interosseus muscle exists, even some of the time, is controversial. Some sources name this extra muscle, or bundle of muscle fibers, as part of the oblique head of the adductor pollicis, or as part of the deep head of the flexor pollicis brevis (see note regarding the palmar interosseus muscles on page 627).

❑ 5. A mnemonic for remembering the actions of the palmar interossei and the dorsal interossei manus muscles is **"DAB"** and **"PAD."** The **D**orsals **AB**duct and the **P**almars **AD**duct.

❑ 6. There are plantar interossei of the foot that have essentially identical actions (adduction of the toes at the metatarsophalangeal joint, flexion of the toes at the metatarsophalangeal joint and extension of the toes at the proximal and distal interphalangeal joints) to the palmar interossei of the hand.

DORSAL INTEROSSEI MANUS
(OF THE CENTRAL COMPARTMENT)

(There are four dorsal interossei manus muscles, named #1, #2, #3 and #4.)

❑ **The name, dorsal interossei manus, tells us that these muscles are located between bones (metacarpals) on the dorsal (posterior) side and located in the hand.**

DERIVATION ❑ dorsal: L. *back.*
interossei: L. *between bones.*
manus: L. *refers to the hand.*

PRONUNCIATION ❑ **dor**-sul **in**-ter-**oss**-ee-i **man**-us

ATTACHMENTS

❑ **The Metacarpal of Fingers #1-5**

- ❑ each one arises from the adjacent sides of two metacarpals:
- ❑ **#1**: attaches onto the metacarpal of the thumb and index finger (fingers #1 and #2)
- ❑ **#2**: attaches onto the metacarpal of the index and middle fingers (fingers #2 and #3)
- ❑ **#3**: attaches onto the metacarpal of the middle and ring fingers (fingers #3 and #4)
- ❑ **#4**: attaches onto the metacarpal of the ring and little fingers (fingers #4 and #5)

to the

❑ **Proximal Phalanx of Fingers #2, #3 and #4, on the Side Away From the Center of the Middle Finger**

- ❑ the base of the proximal phalanx and the dorsal digital expansion:
- ❑ **#1**: attaches to the lateral side of the index finger (finger #2)
- ❑ **#2**: attaches to the lateral side of the middle finger (finger #3)
- ❑ **#3**: attaches to the medial side of the middle finger (finger #3)
- ❑ **#4**: attaches to the medial side of the ring finger (finger #4)

Posterior View of the Right Dorsal Interossei Manus

ACTIONS

❑ 1. **Abduction of Fingers #2, #3 and #4**

❑ 2. Flexion of Fingers #2, #3 and #4 at the Metacarpophalangeal Joint

❑ 3. Extension of Fingers #2, #3 and #4 at the Interphalangeal Joints

INNERVATION ❑ The Ulnar Nerve ❑ C8, **T1**; deep branch of the ulnar nerve

ARTERIAL SUPPLY ❑ Branches of the Radial and Ulnar Arteries (Terminal Branches of the Brachial Artery)

PALPATION AND SUPPLEMENTARY TEXT

PALPATION

- ❑ The 1st dorsal interosseus manus muscle is easily palpated in the thumb web of the hand. Have the client seated or supine and resist the client from abducting the index finger and palpate in the thumb web, especially toward the metacarpal of the index finger. To palpate the other three dorsal interossei manus, palpate between the metacarpals from the dorsal side while resisting the client from abducting the finger to which the dorsal interosseus manus muscle is attached.

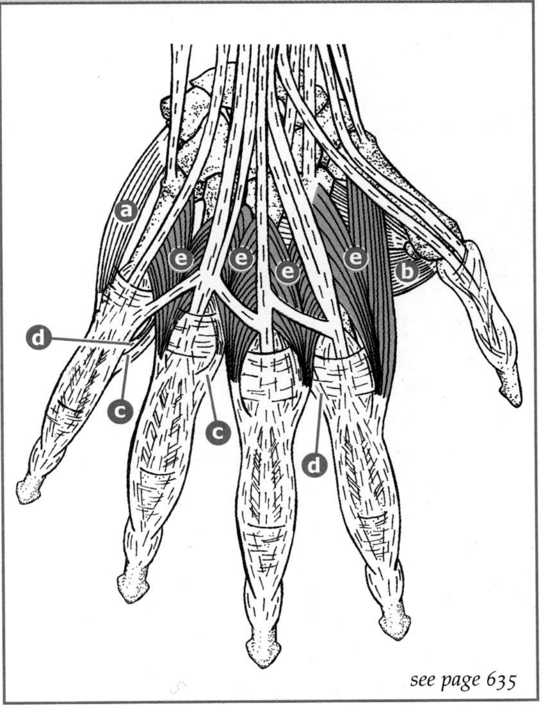

see page 635

Dorsal View of the Right Hand

a. Abductor Digiti Minimi Manus
b. Adductor Pollicis
c. Lumbricals Manus
d. Palmar Interossei
e. **Dorsal Interossei Manus**

RELATIONSHIP TO OTHER MUSCULOSKELETAL STRUCTURES

- ❑ 1. The dorsal interossei manus are located between the metacarpals toward the dorsal (posterior) side of the hand.
- ❑ 2. Each dorsal interosseus manus muscle is located on the side of the metacarpal that is away from the center of the middle finger. (The middle finger has two dorsal interossei manus muscles, one on each side.)
- ❑ 3. From the anterior perspective, the dorsal interossei manus are deep to the palmar interossei. The 1st dorsal interosseus manus muscle is mostly deep to the adductor pollicis.
- ❑ 4. From the posterior perspective, the dorsal interossei manus are superficial and located between the extensor digitorum tendons and between the metacarpal bones. The 1st dorsal interosseus manus muscle is superficial in the thumb web.

METHODOLOGY FOR LEARNING MUSCLE ACTIONS

- ❑ **1. Abduction of Fingers #2, #3 and #4 at the Metacarpophalangeal Joint:** The 1st and 2nd dorsal interossei manus cross the metacarpophalangeal joint of the index and middle fingers laterally. They pull the proximal phalanx of these fingers laterally, away from the axis of abduction/adduction, which is an imaginary line drawn through the middle of the middle finger. Therefore, the 1st dorsal interosseus manus muscle abducts the index finger and the 2nd dorsal interosseus manus muscle "radially abducts" the middle finger at the metacarpophalangeal joint.

  The 3rd and 4th dorsal interossei manus cross the metacarpophalangeal joint of the middle and ring fingers medially. They pull the proximal phalanx of these fingers medially, away from the axis of abduction/adduction, which is an imaginary line drawn through the middle of the middle finger. Therefore, the 3rd dorsal interosseus manus muscle "ulnar abducts" the middle finger and the 4th dorsal interosseus manus muscle abducts the ring finger at the metacarpophalangeal joint.

  Note: The dorsal interossei manus are always on the side of the metacarpals and phalanges (with their fibers running vertically in the frontal plane) away from the axis of abduction/adduction, which is an imaginary line drawn through the middle of the middle finger. Therefore, they always pull the fingers away from this axis, abducting the fingers.

DORSAL INTEROSSEI MANUS– continued

- ❑ 2. **Flexion of Fingers #2, #3 and #4 at the Metacarpophalangeal Joint:** The dorsal interossei manus cross the metacarpophalangeal joint anteriorly (with their fibers running vertically in the sagittal plane); therefore, they flex the proximal phalanx of the index, middle and ring fingers at the metacarpophalangeal joint.

- ❑ 3. **Extension of Fingers #2, #3 and #4 at the Proximal and Distal Interphalangeal Joints:** The dorsal interossei manus attach into the dorsal digital expansion, which crosses the proximal and distal interphalangeal joints of the fingers on the posterior side (with the line of pull running vertically in the sagittal plane). Therefore, the dorsal interossei manus extend the middle and distal phalanges at the proximal and distal interphalangeal joints of the index, middle and ring fingers.

MISCELLANEOUS

- ❑ 1. There are four dorsal interossei manus muscles named from the lateral side: #1, #2, #3 and #4.

- ❑ 2. There are four dorsal interossei manus muscles: one to abduct the index finger, one to abduct the ring finger and two to abduct the middle finger. The dorsal interossei manus muscle that attaches onto the radial side of the middle finger "radially abducts" the middle finger at the metacarpophalangeal joint; the dorsal interossei manus muscle that attaches onto the ulnar side of the middle finger "ulnar abducts" the middle finger at the metacarpophalangeal joint.

- ❑ 3. The 1st dorsal interosseus manus muscle (the largest) is sometimes known as the *abductor indicis*.

- ❑ 4. The dorsal interossei manus are bipenniform (fish-bone) in shape.

- ❑ 5. A mnemonic for remembering the actions of the dorsal interossei manus and the palmar interossei muscles is **"DAB"** and **"PAD**." The **D**orsals **AB**duct and the **P**almars **AD**duct.

- ❑ 6. Given that the abductor digiti minimi manus and the abductor pollicis brevis are intrinsic hand muscles that abduct the thumb and the little finger, they can be considered to be analogous to the dorsal interossei manus, which abduct the other three fingers (index, middle and ring fingers).

- ❑ 7. The majority of tissue of the thumb web of the hand is made up of the 1st dorsal interosseus manus muscle and the adductor pollicis.

- ❑ 8. There are four dorsal interossei pedis of the foot which have essentially identical actions (abduction of the toes at the metatarsophalangeal joint, flexion of the toes at the metatarsophalangeal joint and extension of the toes at the proximal and distal interphalangeal joints) to the dorsal interossei manus of the hand.

APPENDICES

APPENDIX A – ANATOMICAL POSITION AND PLANES OF THE BODY

ANATOMICAL POSITION

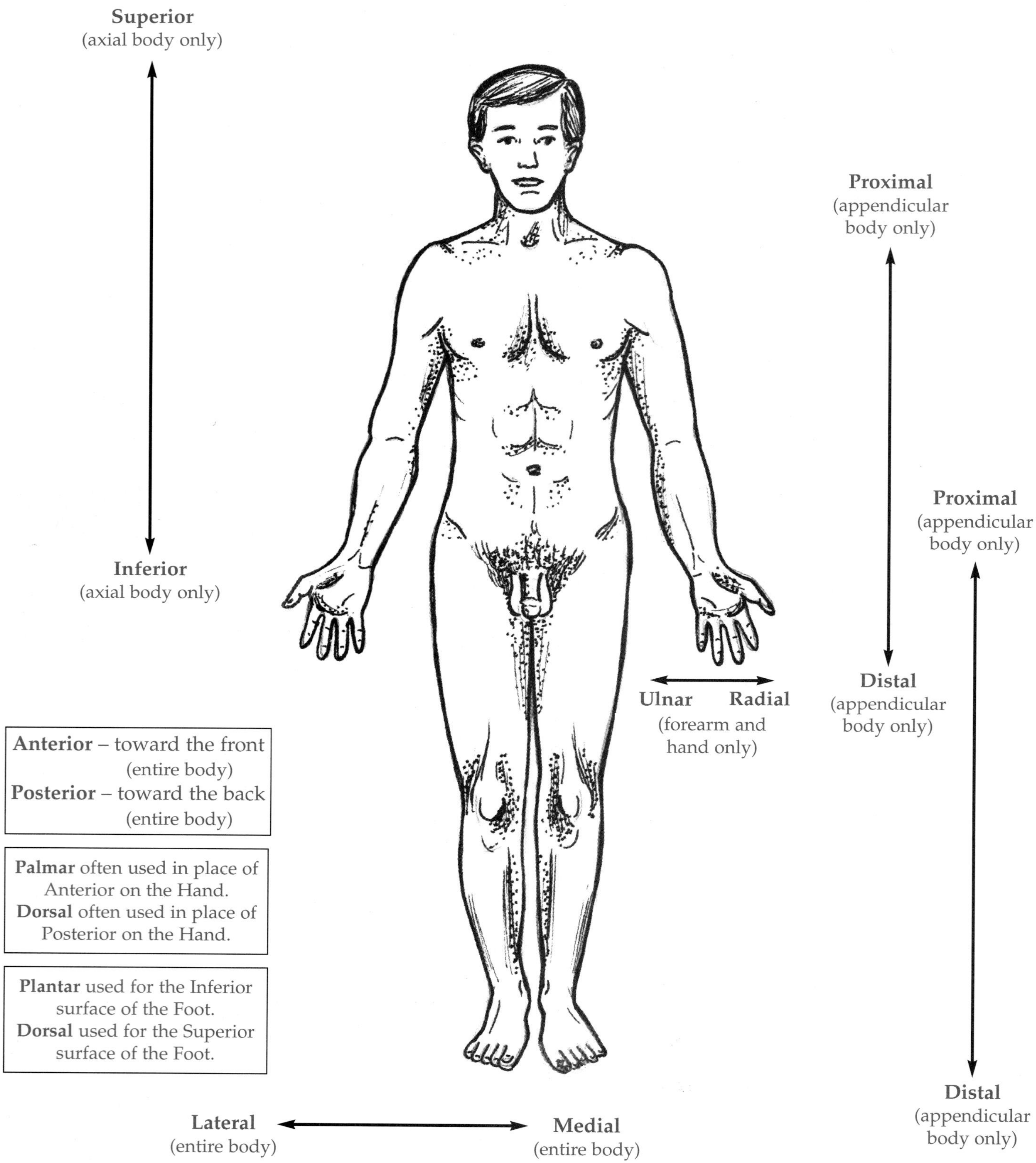

PLANES OF THE BODY

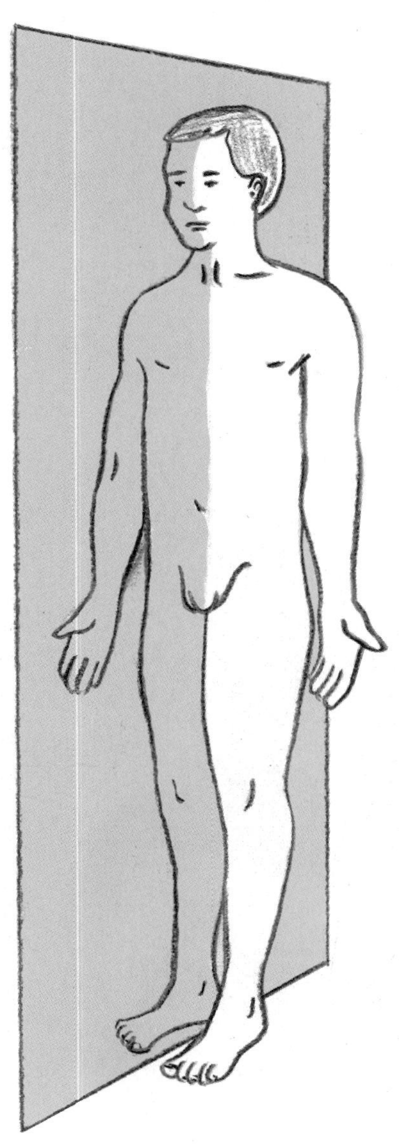

Sagittal Plane

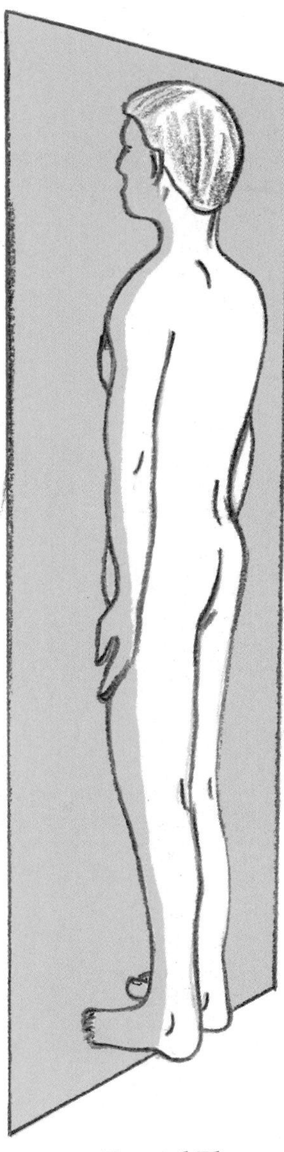

Frontal Plane
(Coronal Plane)

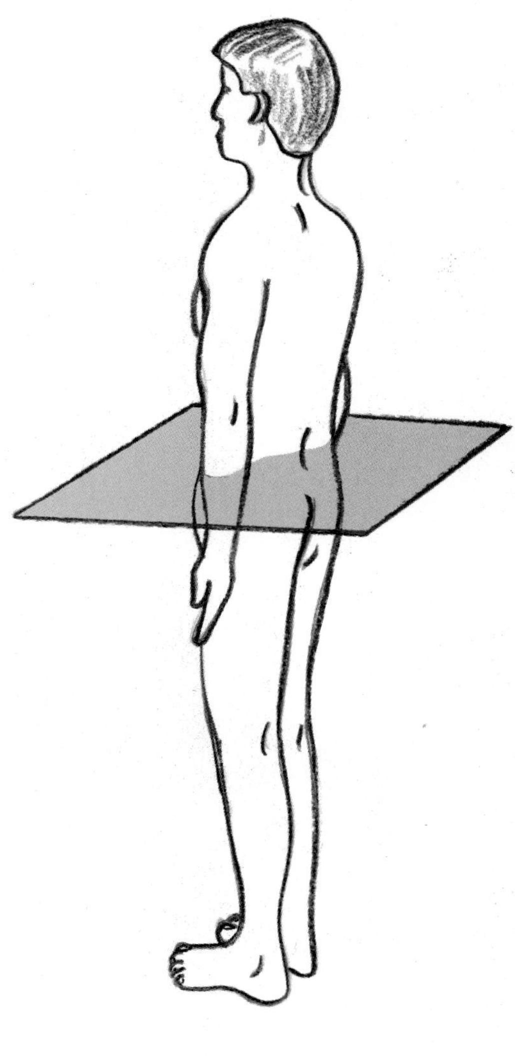

Transverse Plane

APPENDIX B – JOINT ACTIONS

PART ONE – JOINT ACTIONS OF THE AXIAL BODY

JOINT ACTIONS OF THE HEAD AT THE ATLANTO-OCCIPITAL JOINT

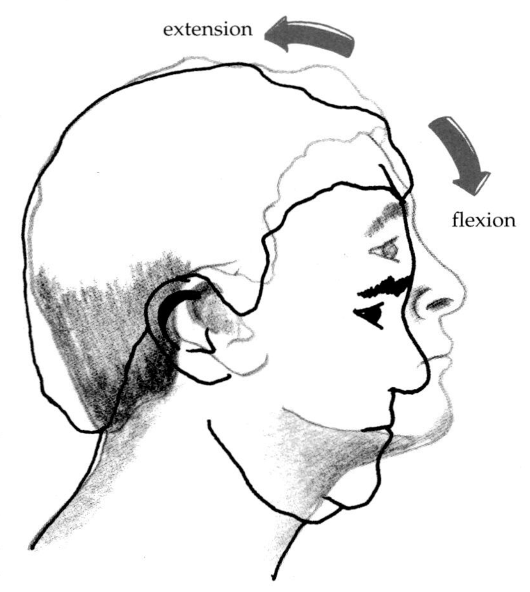

Extension and Flexion of the Head at the Atlanto-Occipital Joint

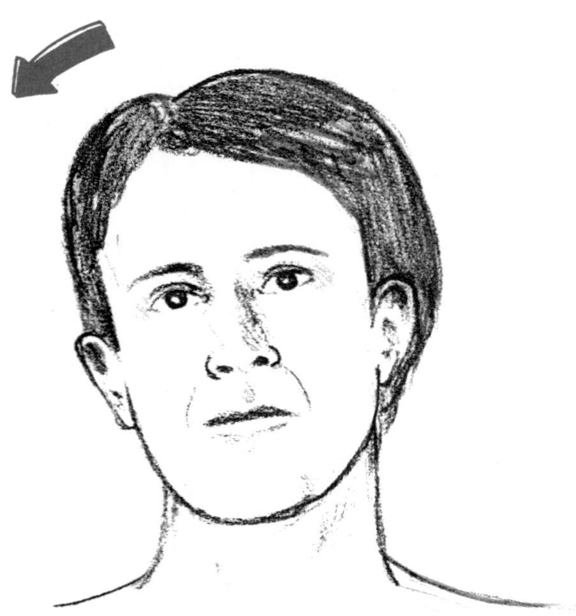

Right Lateral Flexion of the Head at the Atlanto-Occipital Joint

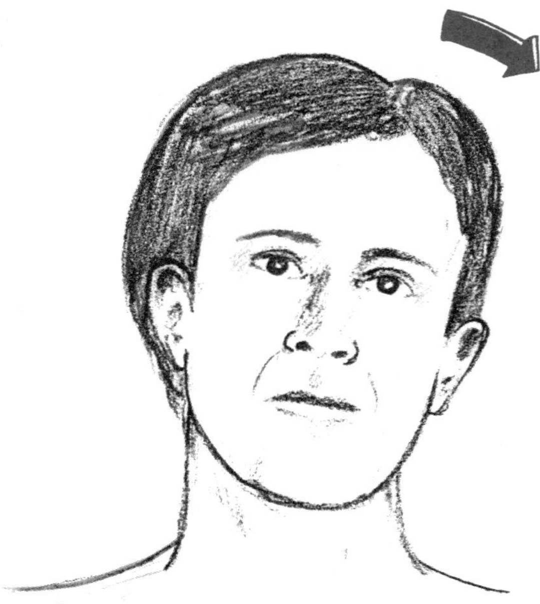

Left Lateral Flexion of the Head at the Atlanto-Occipital Joint

JOINT ACTIONS OF THE HEAD AT THE ATLANTO-OCCIPITAL JOINT

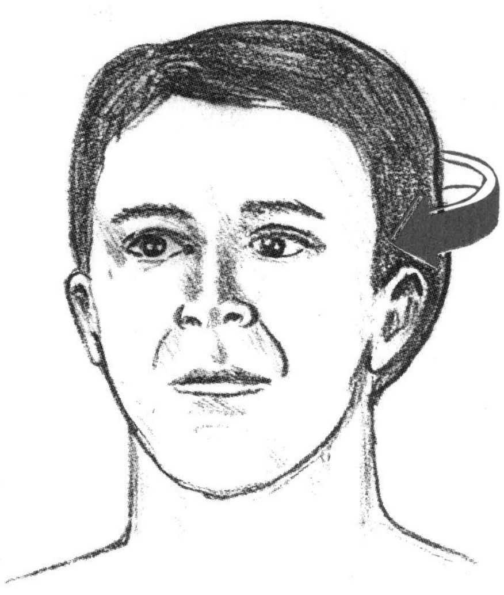

Right Rotation of the Head at the Atlanto-Occipital Joint

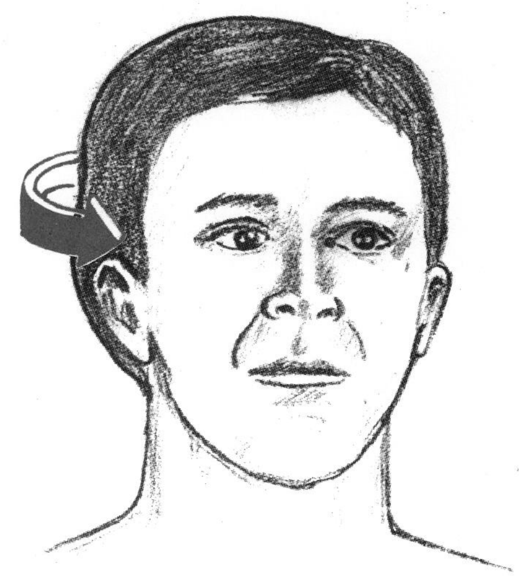

Left Rotation of the Head at the Atlanto-Occipital Joint

JOINT ACTIONS OF THE MANDIBLE AT THE TEMPOROMANDIBULAR JOINTS

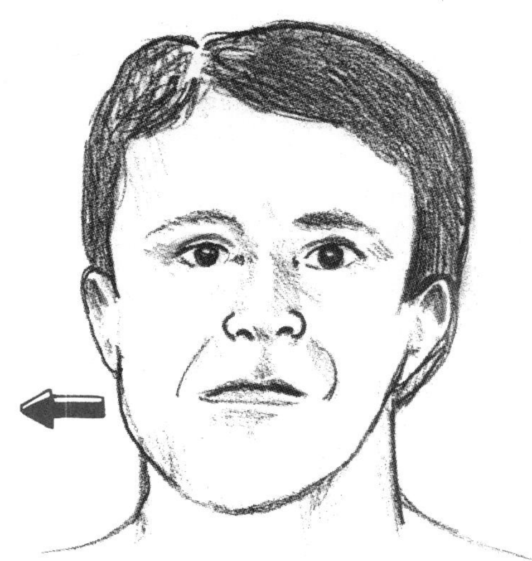

Right Lateral Deviation of the Mandible at the Temporomandibular Joint

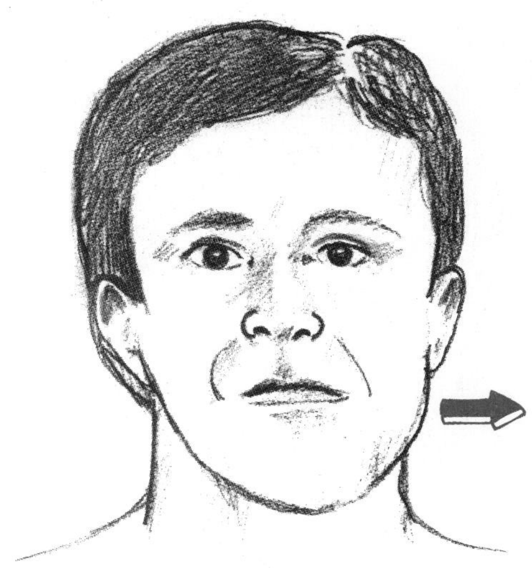

Left Lateral Deviation of the Mandible at the Temporomandibular Joint

JOINT ACTIONS OF THE MANDIBLE AT THE TEMPOROMANDIBULAR JOINTS

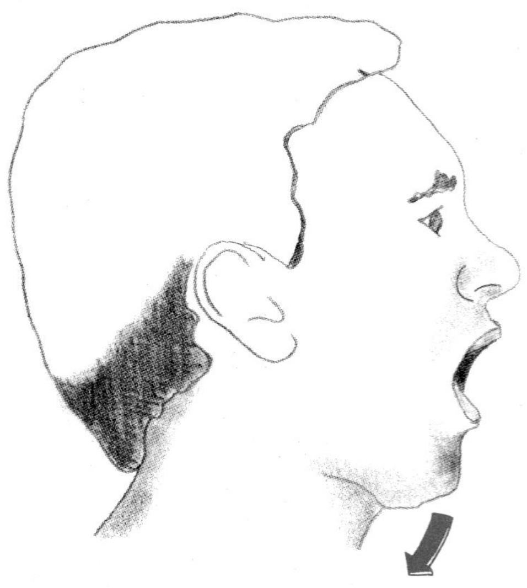

Depression of the Mandible at the Temporomandibular Joint

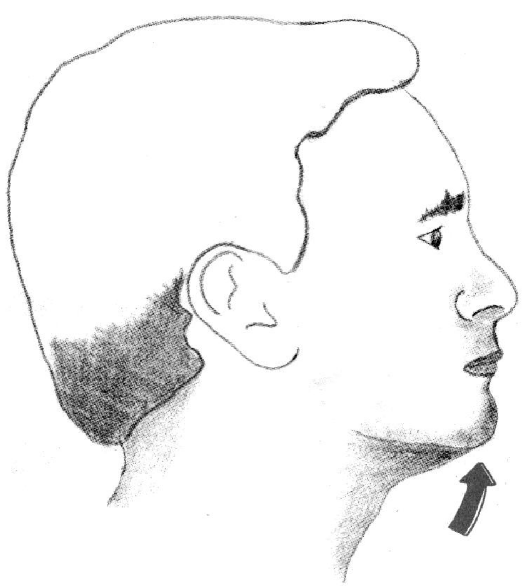

Elevation of the Mandible at the Temporomandibular Joint

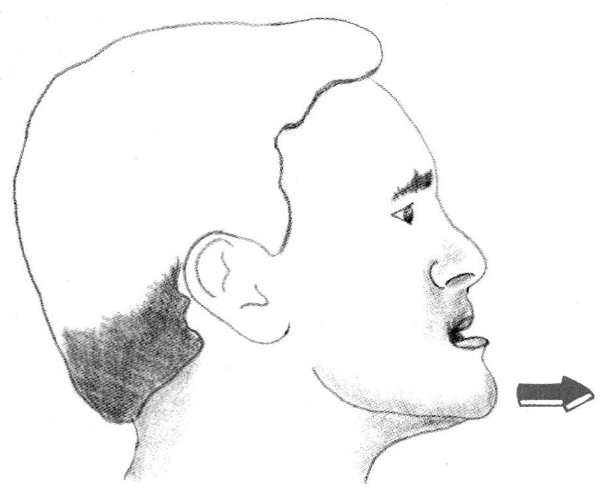

Protraction of the Mandible at the Temporomandibular Joint

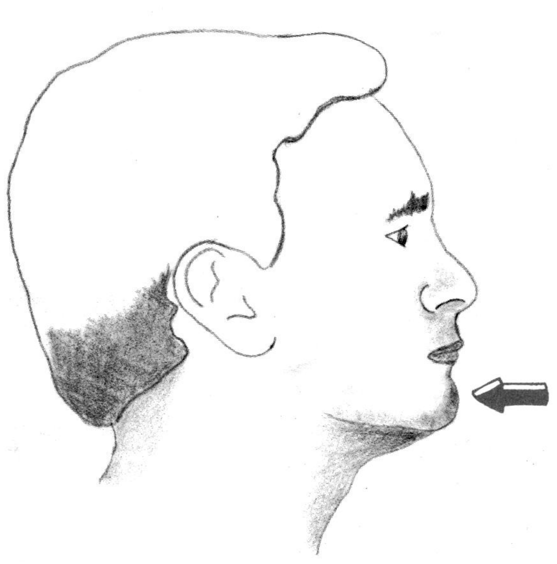

Retraction of the Mandible at the Temporomandibular Joint

JOINT ACTIONS OF THE NECK AT THE CERVICAL SPINAL JOINTS

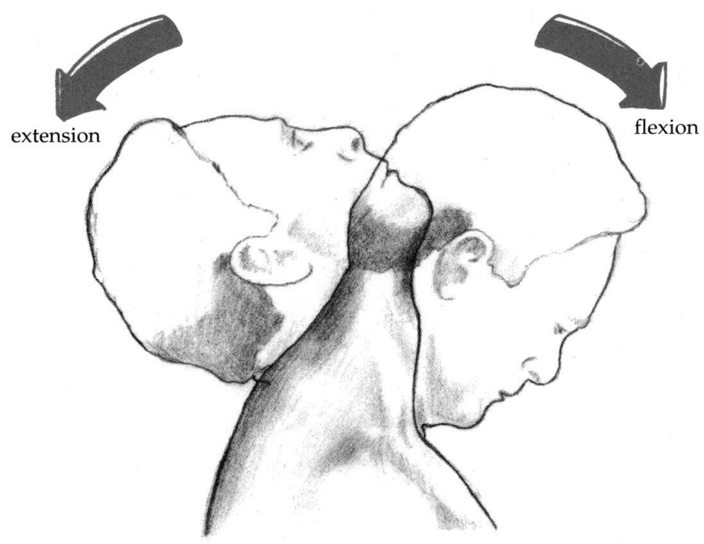

Extension and Flexion of the Neck at the Cervical Spinal Joints

---

JOINT ACTIONS OF THE NECK AT THE CERVICAL SPINAL JOINTS

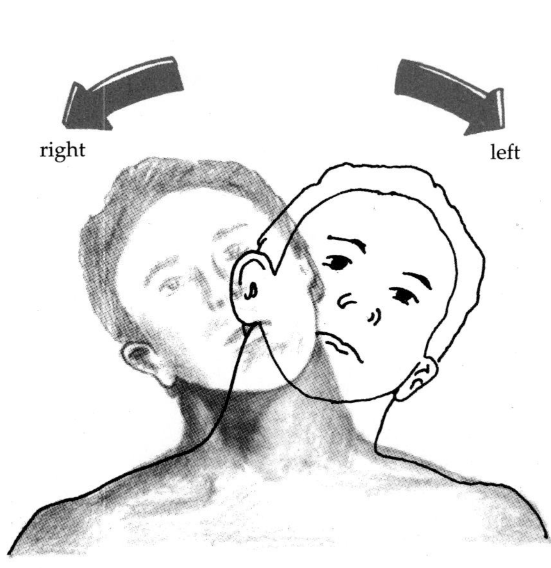

Right Lateral Flexion and Left Lateral Flexion of the Neck at the Cervical Spinal Joints

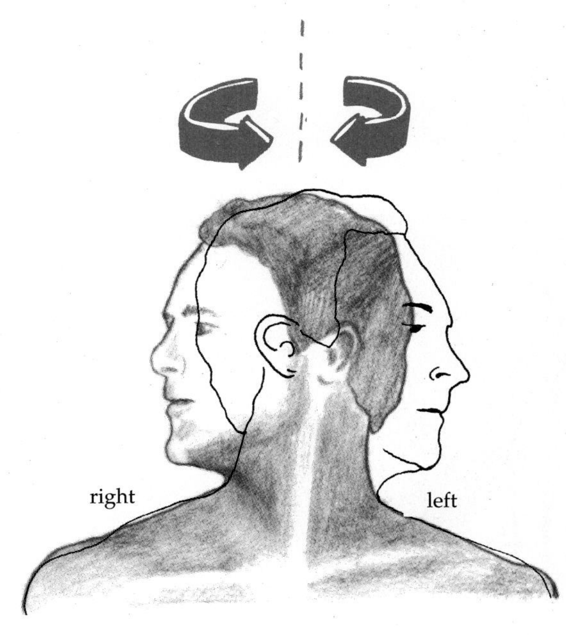

Right Rotation and Left Rotation of the Neck at the Cervical Spinal Joints

JOINT ACTIONS OF THE TRUNK AT THE SPINAL JOINTS

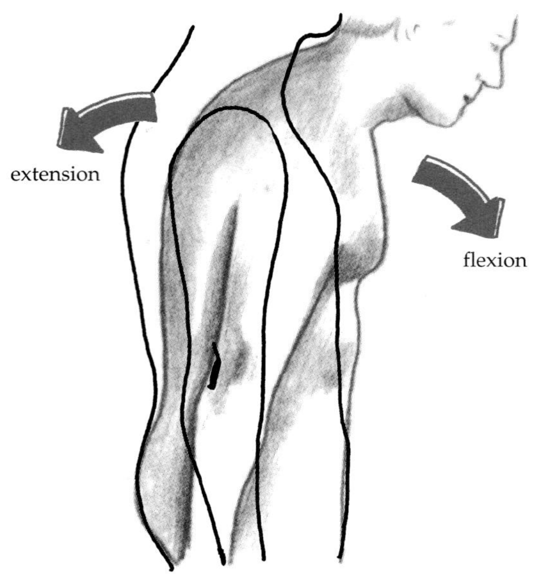

Extension and Flexion of the Trunk at the Spinal Joints

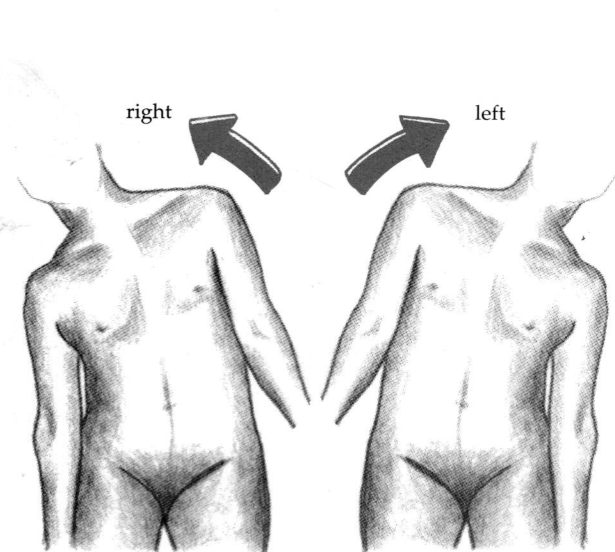

Right Lateral Flexion and Left Lateral Flexion of the Trunk at the Spinal Joints

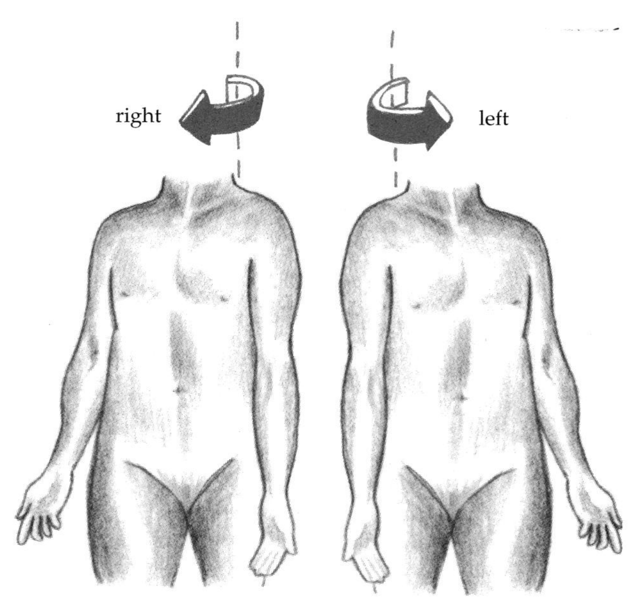

Right Rotation and Left Rotation of the Trunk at the Spinal Joints

JOINT ACTIONS OF THE TRUNK AT THE SHOULDER JOINT

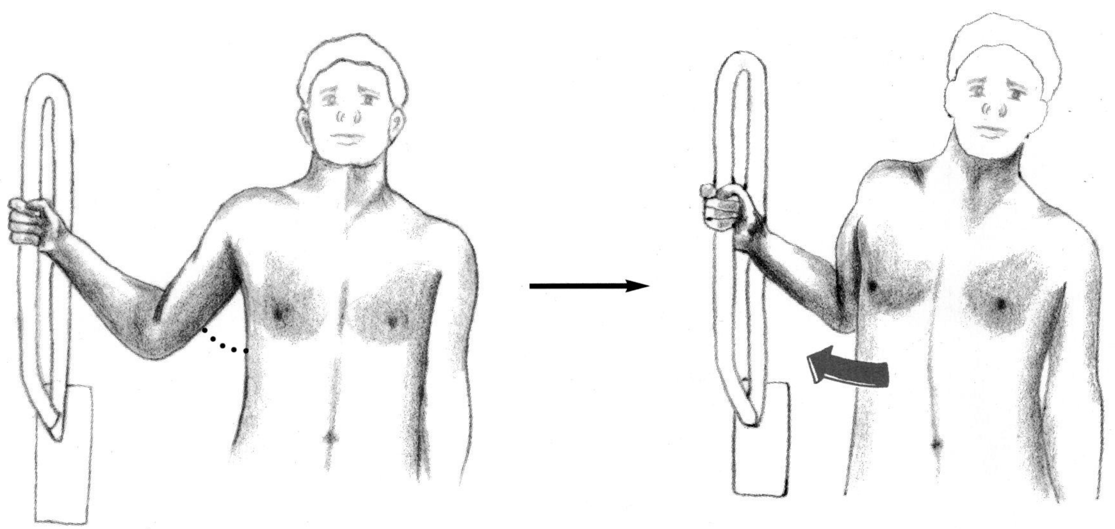

Neutral Position
(Angle between the arm and the trunk at the shoulder joint is indicated by the dotted line.)

Lateral Deviation of the Trunk at the Shoulder Joint
(Flexion of the arm at the elbow joint is also seen.)

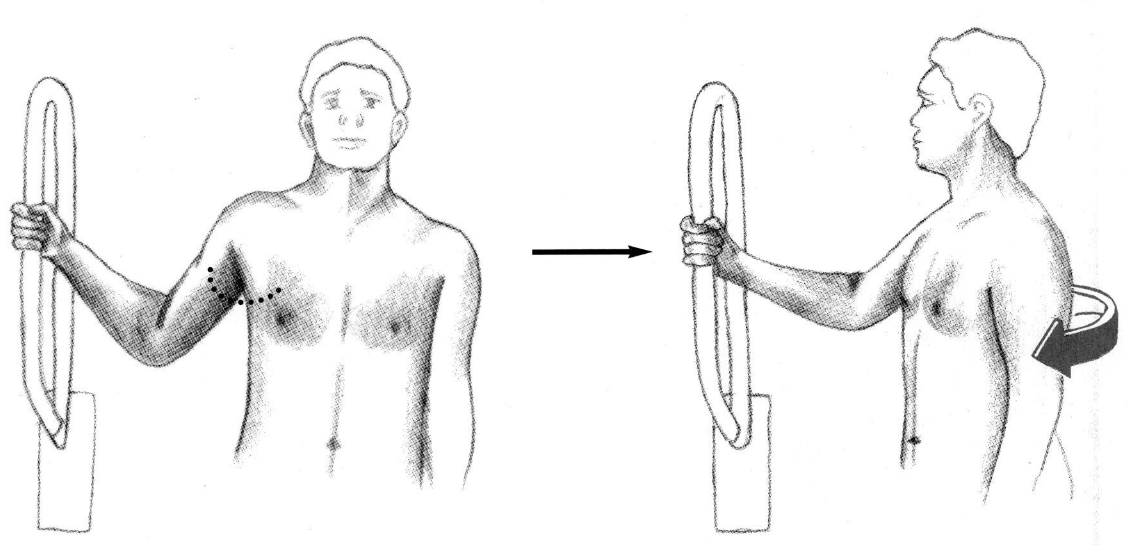

Neutral Position
(Angle between the arm and the trunk at the shoulder joint is indicated by the dotted line.)

Lateral (Right) Rotation of the Trunk at the Shoulder Joint

JOINT ACTIONS OF THE TRUNK AT THE SHOULDER JOINT

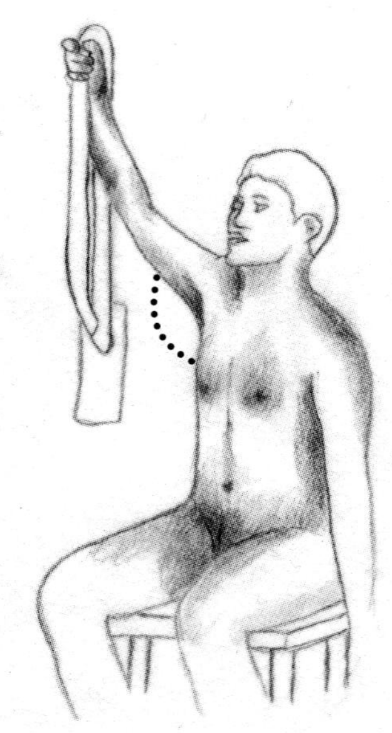

Neutral Position
(Angle between the arm and the trunk at the shoulder joint is indicated by the dotted line.)

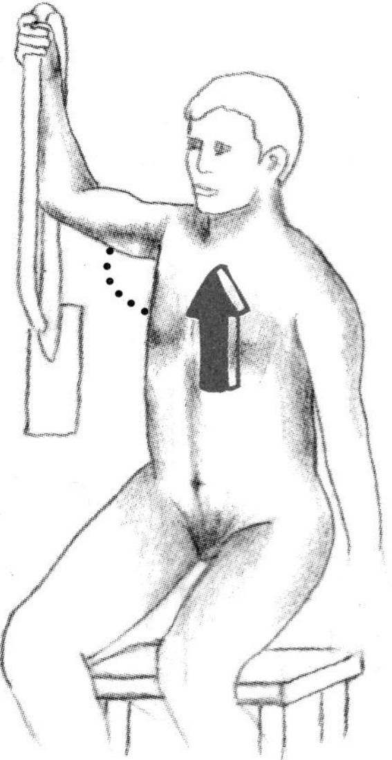

Elevation of the Trunk at the Shoulder Joint
(Angle between the arm and the trunk at the shoulder joint is indicated by the dotted line.)
(Flexion of the arm at the elbow joint is also seen.)

PART TWO – JOINT ACTIONS OF THE LOWER EXTREMITY

JOINT ACTIONS OF THE PELVIS AT THE LUMBOSACRAL AND HIP JOINTS

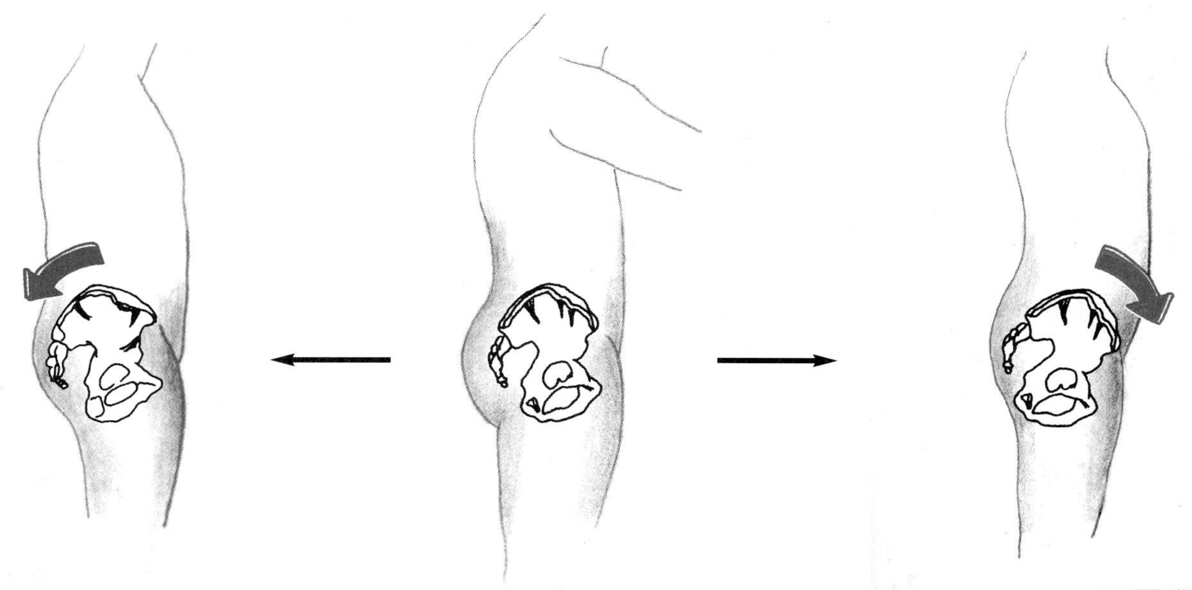

Posterior Tilt of the Pelvis at the Lumbosacral Joint and Hip Joints (with the person standing)

Neutral Position of the Pelvis at the Lumbosacral Joint and Hip Joints (with the person standing)

Anterior Tilt of the Pelvis at the Lumbosacral Joint and Hip Joints (with the person standing)

JOINT ACTIONS OF THE PELVIS AT THE LUMBOSACRAL JOINT

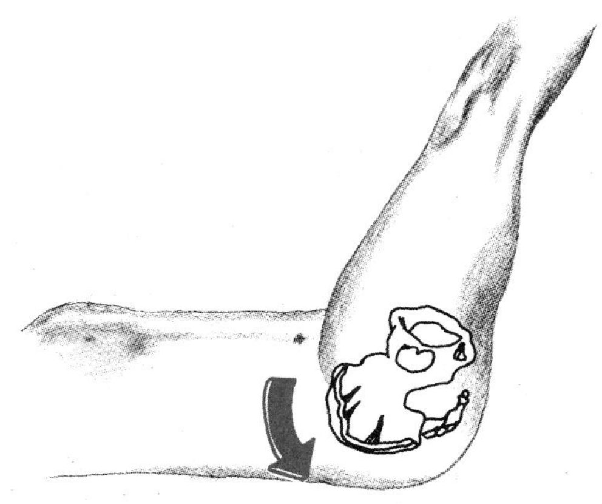

Posterior Tilt of the Pelvis at the Lumbosacral Joint (with the person supine)

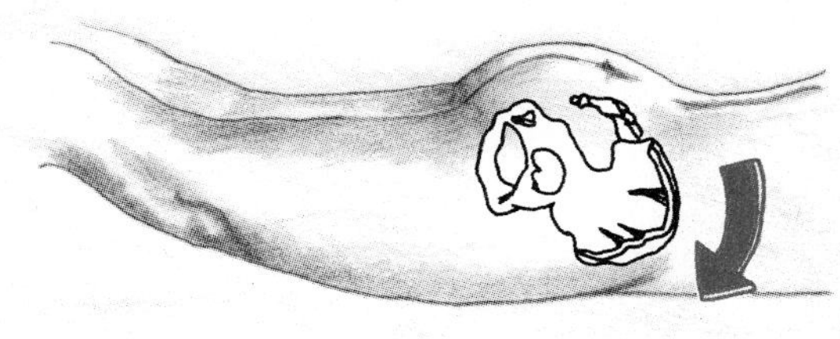

Anterior Tilt of the Pelvis at the Lumbosacral Joint (with the person prone)

JOINT ACTIONS OF THE PELVIS AT THE HIP JOINT

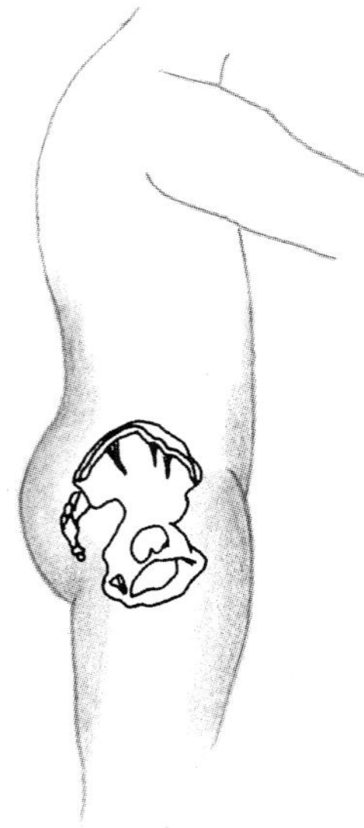

Neutral Position of the Pelvis at the Hip Joints

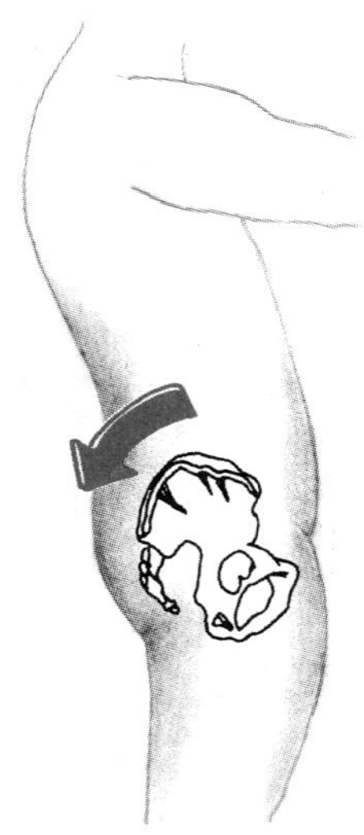

Posterior Tilt of the Pelvis at the Hip Joints Bilaterally (with the person standing)

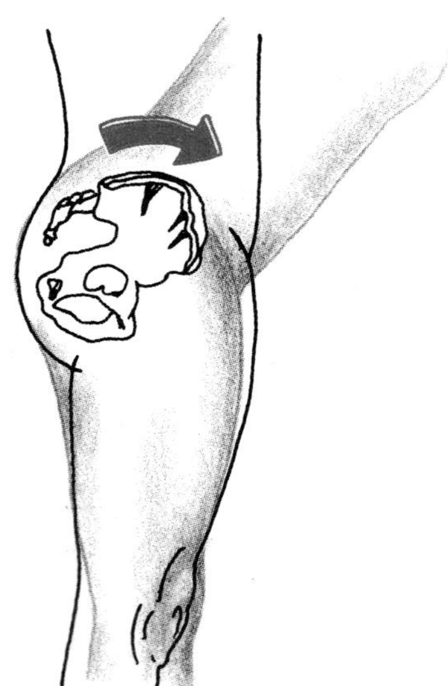

Anterior Tilt of the Pelvis at the Hip Joints Bilaterally (with the person standing)

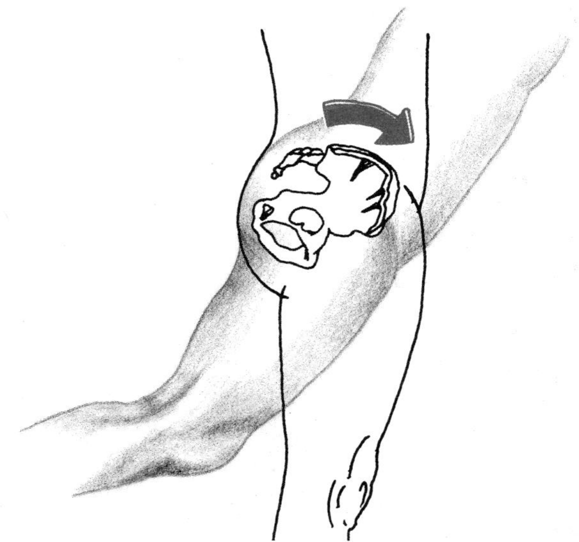

Anterior Tilt of the Pelvis at the Hip Joint Unilaterally (with the person standing)

JOINT ACTIONS OF THE PELVIS AT THE LUMBOSACRAL JOINT

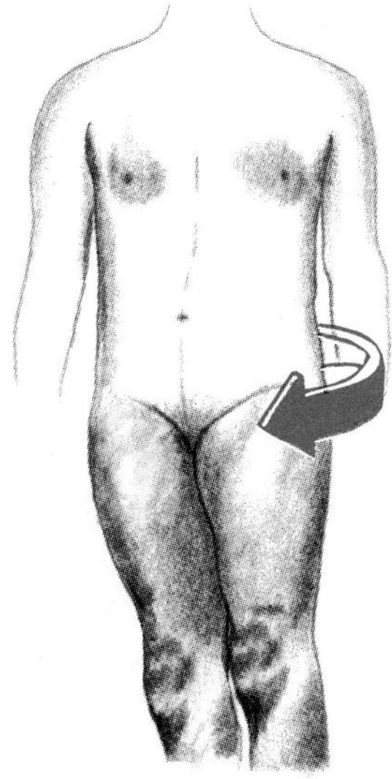

Right Rotation
of the Pelvis at the Lumbosacral Joint
(the thighs have stayed fixed to the pelvis)

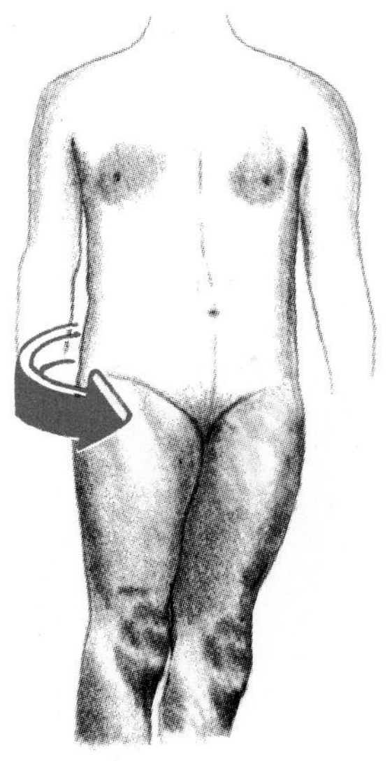

Left Rotation
of the Pelvis at the Lumbosacral Joint
(the thighs have stayed fixed to the pelvis)

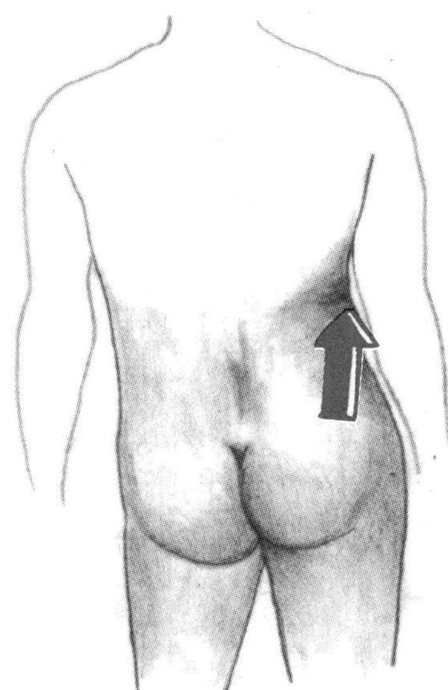

Elevation
of the Right Pelvis at the Lumbosacral Joint
(Relatively, the left pelvis is depressed, i.e., laterally tilted.)

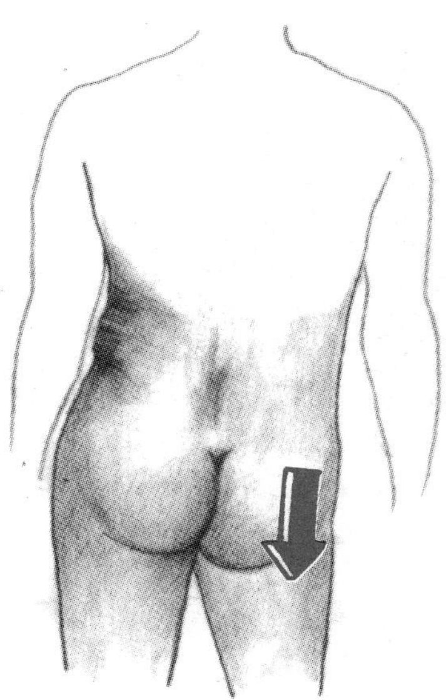

Depression (Lateral Tilt)
of the Right Pelvis at the Lumbosacral Joint
(Relatively, the left pelvis is elevated.)

JOINT ACTIONS OF THE PELVIS AT THE HIP JOINT

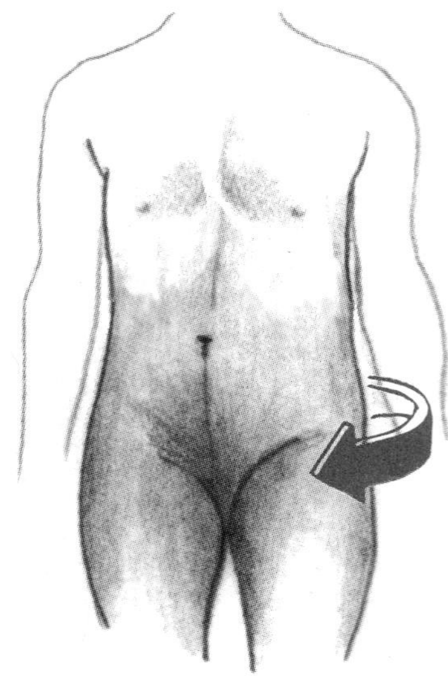

Right Rotation of the Pelvis at the Hip Joint
(the trunk has stayed fixed to the pelvis)

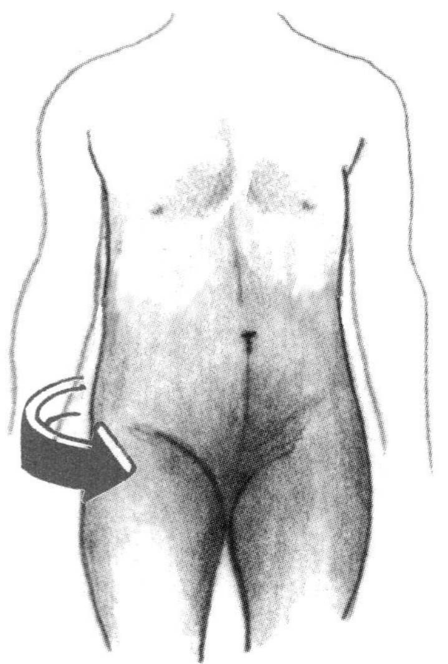

Left Rotation of the Pelvis at the Hip Joint
(the trunk has stayed fixed to the pelvis)

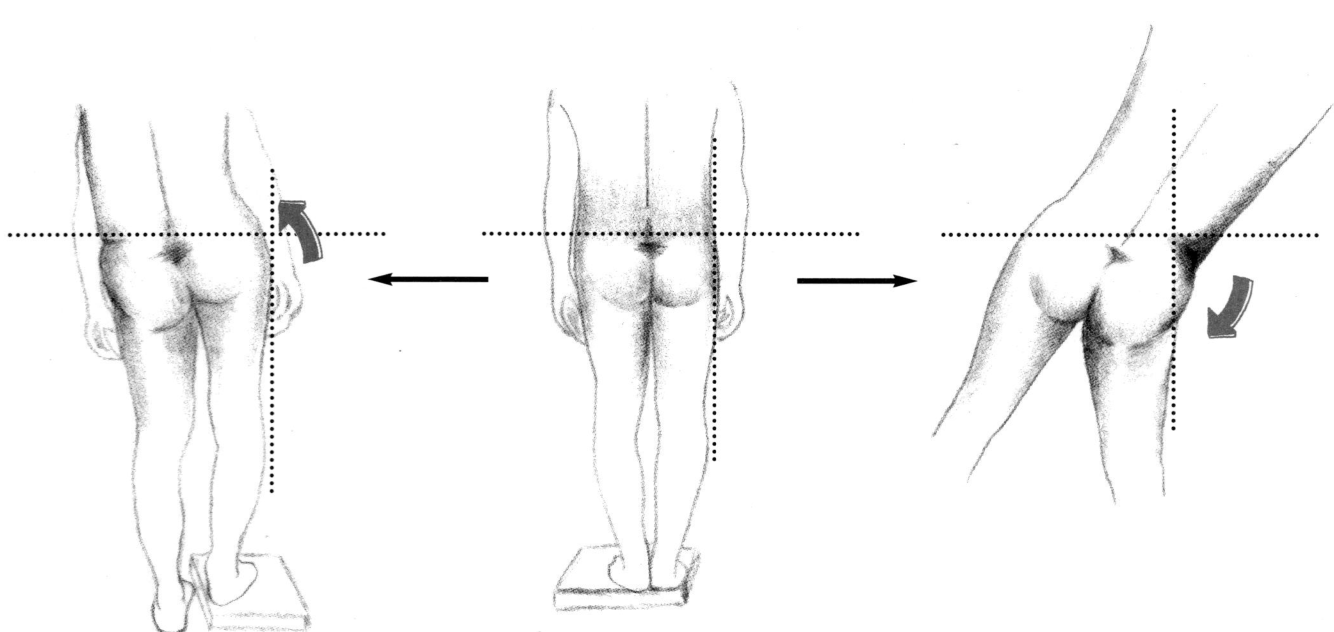

Elevation of the Right Pelvis at the Hip Joint
(Relatively, the left pelvis is depressed, i.e., laterally tilted.)

Neutral Position of the Pelvis at the Lumbosacral and Hip Joints

Depression (Lateral Tilt) of the Right Pelvis at the Hip Joint
(Relatively, the left pelvis is elevated.)

JOINT ACTIONS OF THE THIGH AT THE HIP JOINT

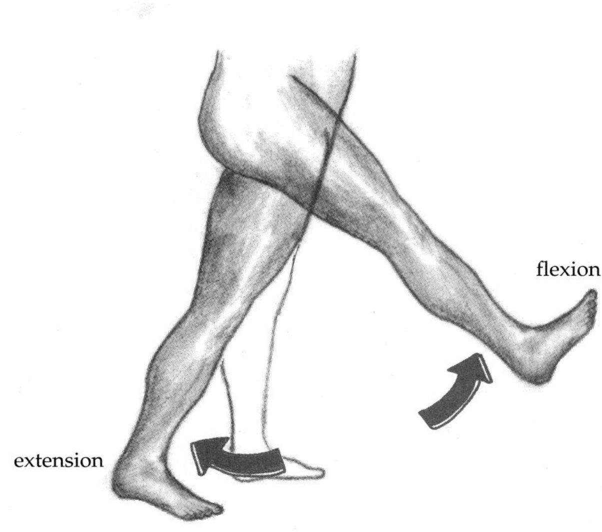

Extension and Flexion of the Thigh at the Hip Joint

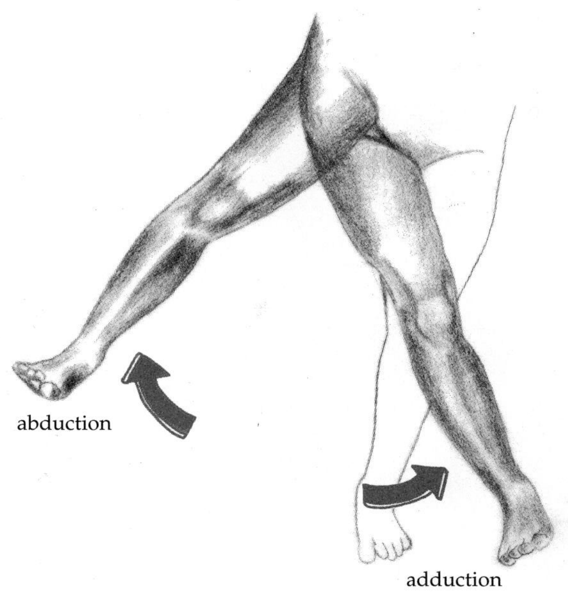

Abduction and Adduction of the Thigh at the Hip Joint

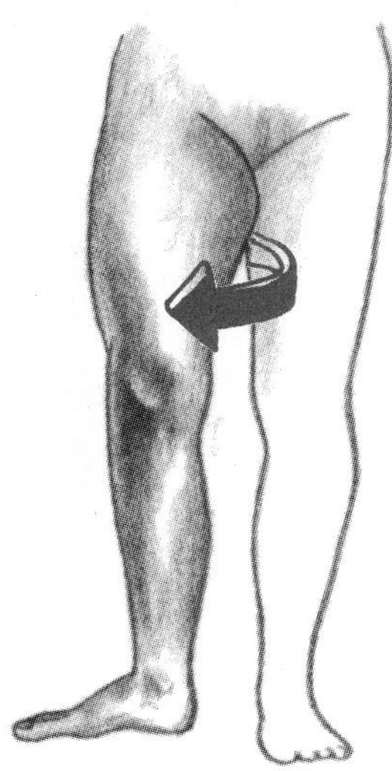

Lateral Rotation of the Thigh at the Hip Joint

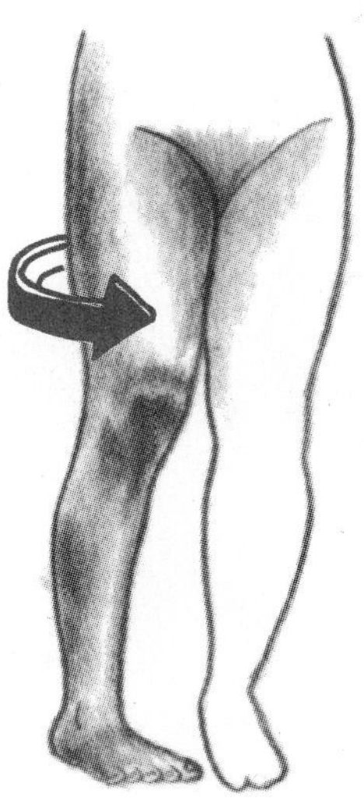

Medial Rotation of the Thigh at the Hip Joint

JOINT ACTIONS OF THE LEG AT THE KNEE JOINT

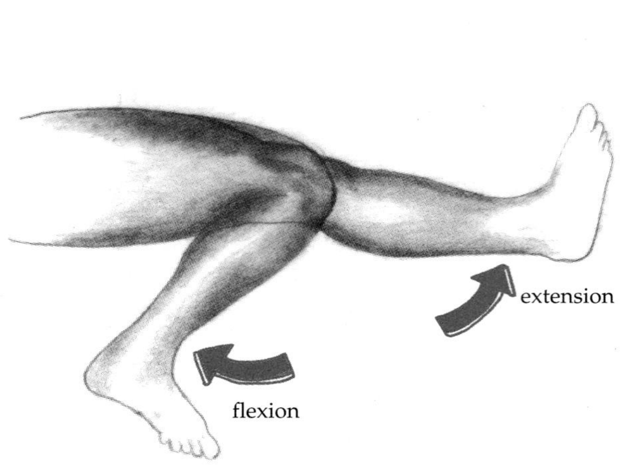

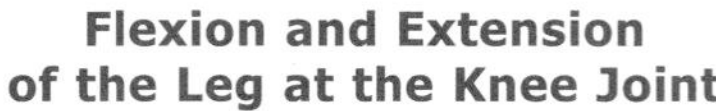
Flexion and Extension of the Leg at the Knee Joint

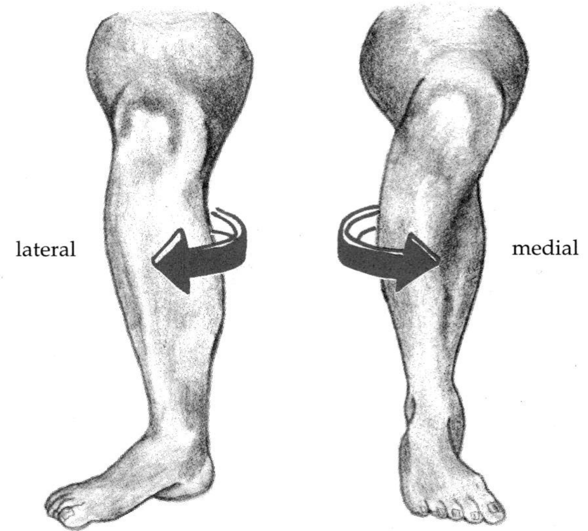

Lateral Rotation and Medial Rotation of the Leg at the Knee Joint
(note: the leg can only rotate at the knee joint if the knee joint is first flexed)

JOINT ACTIONS OF THE FOOT AT THE ANKLE AND TARSAL JOINTS

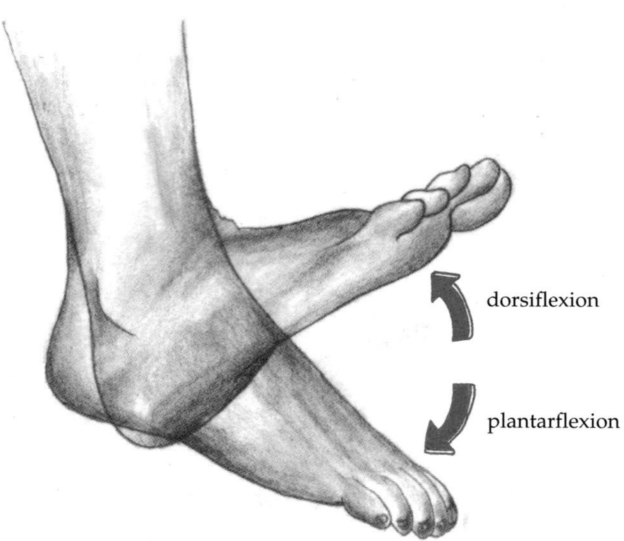

Dorsiflexion and Plantarflexion of the Foot at the Ankle Joint

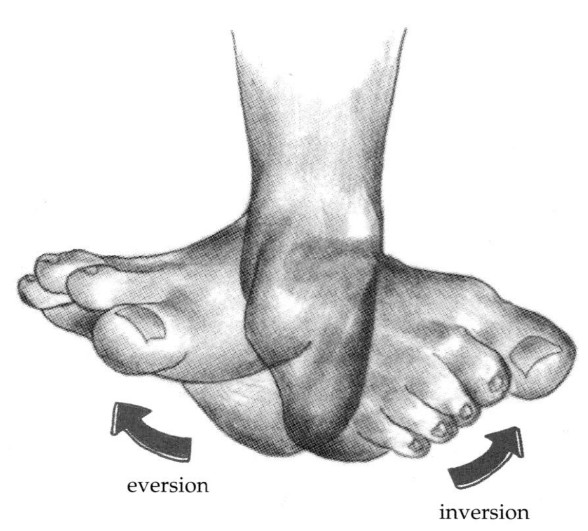

Eversion and Inversion of the Foot at the Tarsal Joints

JOINT ACTIONS OF THE TOES AT THE METATARSOPHALANGEAL JOINT (AND THE PROXIMAL AND DISTAL INTERPHALANGEAL JOINTS)

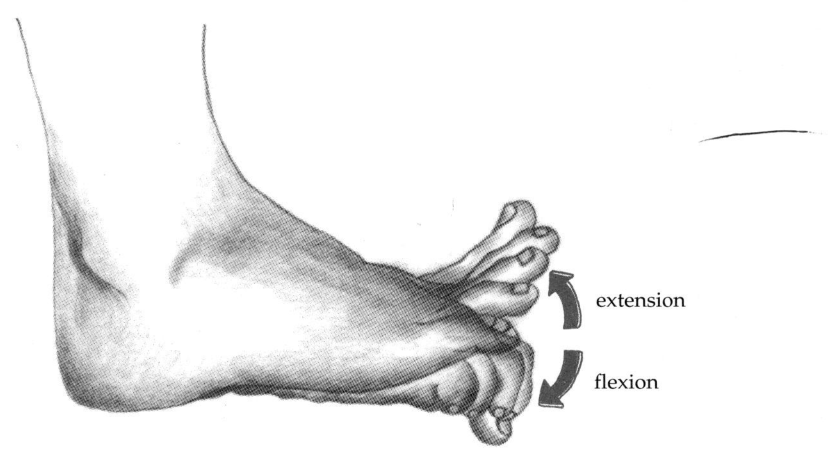

Flexion and Extension of the Toes at the Metatarsophalangeal Joint
(and the proximal and distal interphalangeal joints)

JOINT ACTIONS OF THE TOES AT THE METATARSOPHALANGEAL JOINT

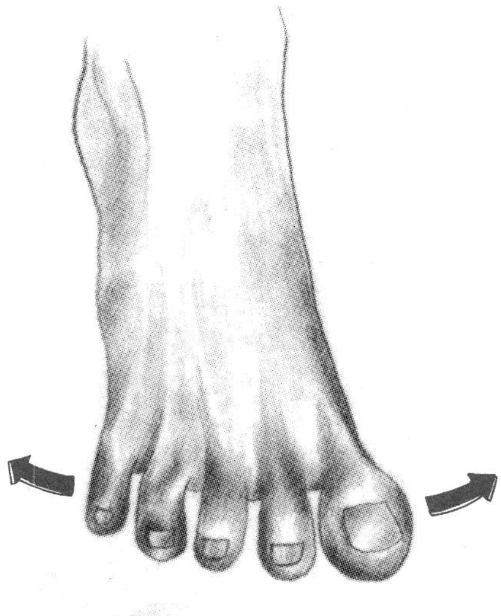

Abduction of the Toes at the Metatarsophalangeal Joint

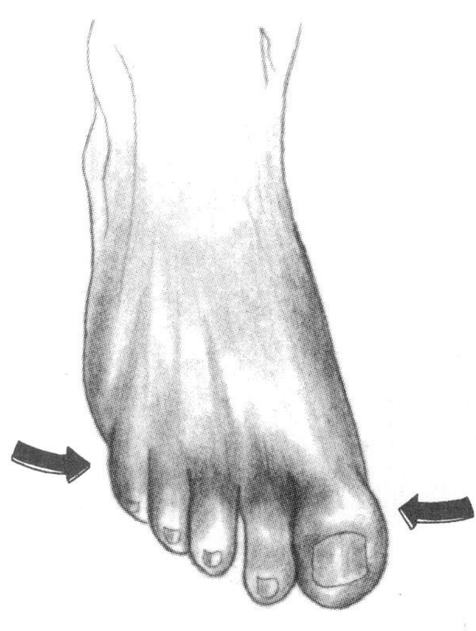

Adduction of the Toes at the Metatarsophalangeal Joint

JOINT ACTIONS OF THE SECOND TOE AT THE METATARSOPHALANGEAL JOINT

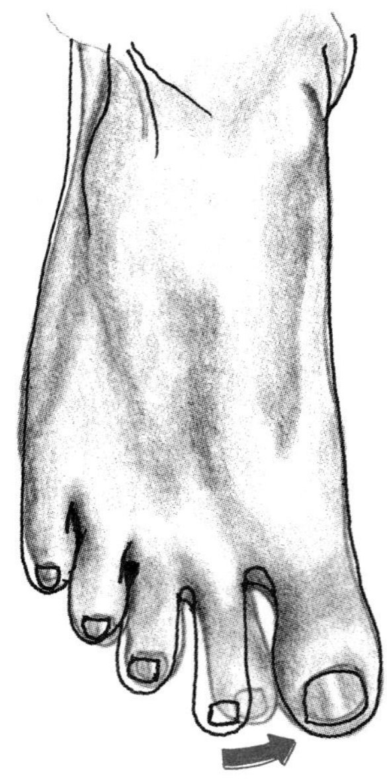

Tibial Abduction of the 2nd Toe at the Metatarsophalangeal Joint

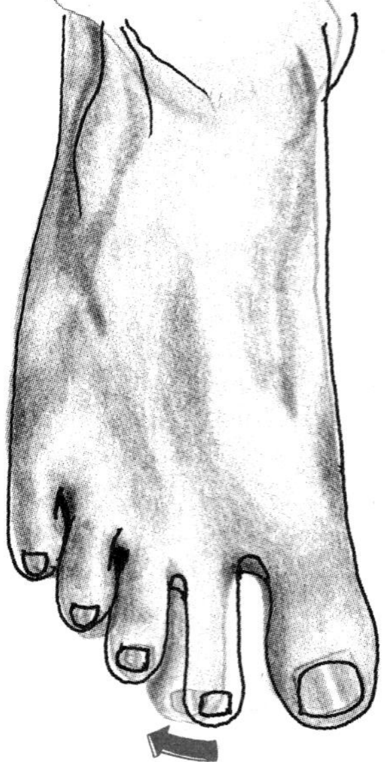

Fibular Abduction of the 2nd Toe at the Metatarsophalangeal Joint

PART THREE – JOINT ACTIONS OF THE UPPER EXTREMITY

JOINT ACTIONS OF THE SCAPULA AT THE SCAPULOCOSTAL JOINT

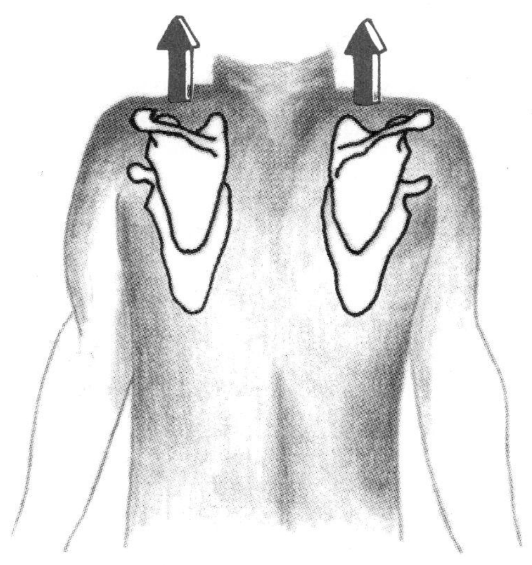

Elevation and Depression of the Scapula at the Scapulocostal Joint (Depression is a return to anatomical position.)

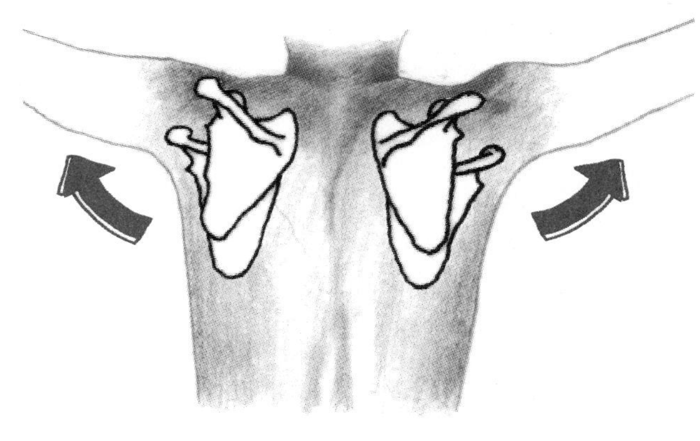

Upward Rotation and Downward Rotation of the Scapula at the Scapulocostal Joint (Downward rotation is a return to anatomical position.)

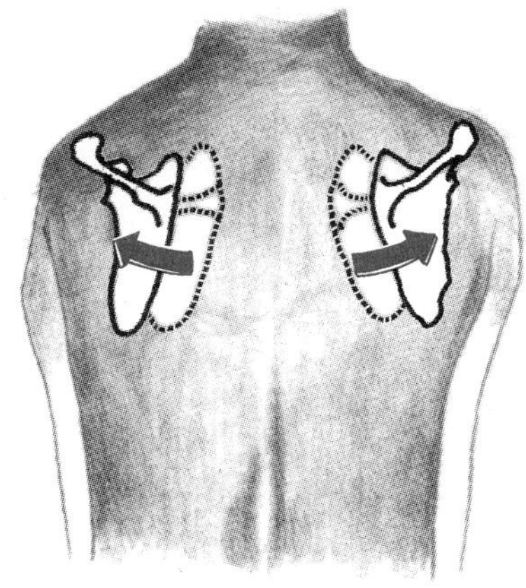

Protraction (Abduction) of the Scapula at the Scapulocostal Joint

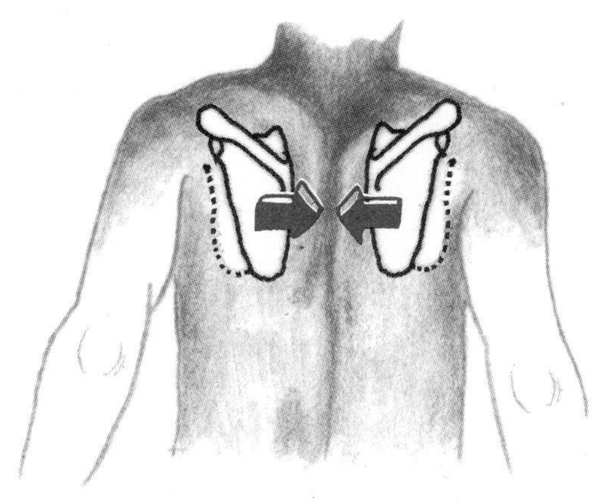

Retraction (Adduction) of the Scapula at the Scapulocostal Joint

JOINT ACTIONS OF THE SCAPULA AT THE SCAPULOCOSTAL JOINT

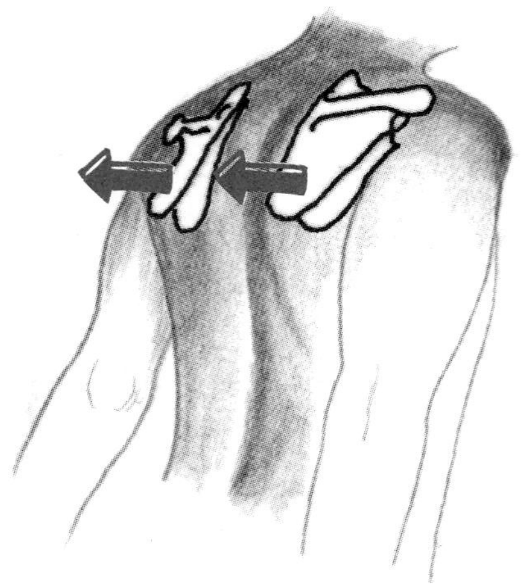

Upward Tilt and Downward Tilt of the Scapula at the Scapulocostal Joint
(Downward tilt is a return to anatomical position.)

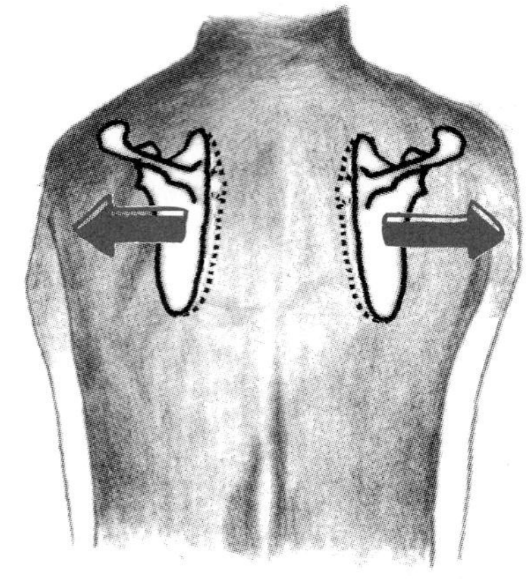

Lateral Tilt and Medial Tilt of the Scapula at the Scapulocostal Joint
(Medial tilt is a return to anatomical position.)

JOINT ACTIONS OF THE CLAVICLE AT THE STERNOCOSTAL JOINT

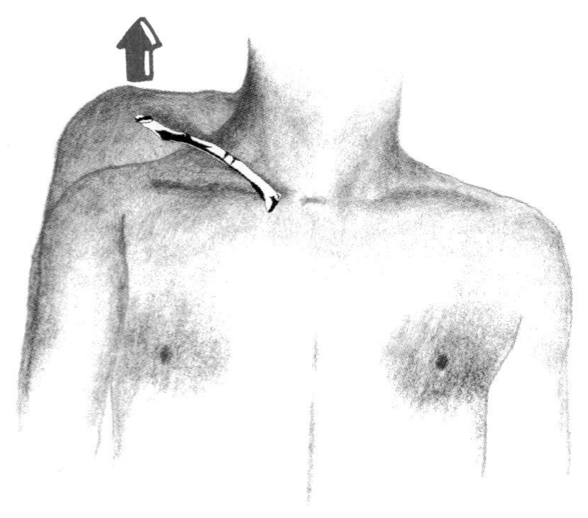

Elevation of the Clavicle at the Sternocostal Joint

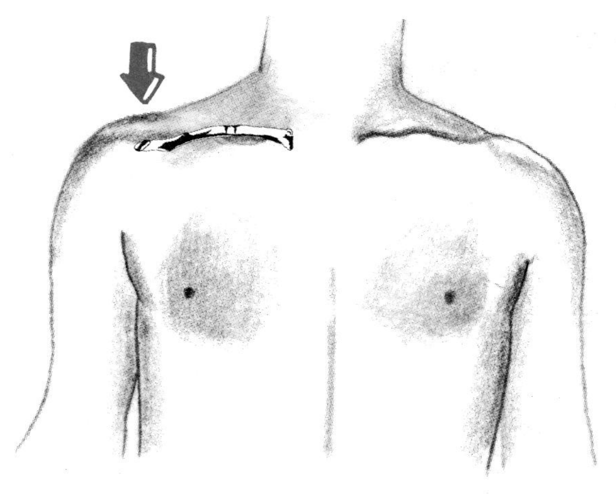

Depression of the Clavicle at the Sternocostal Joint

JOINT ACTIONS OF THE CLAVICLE AT THE STERNOCOSTAL JOINT

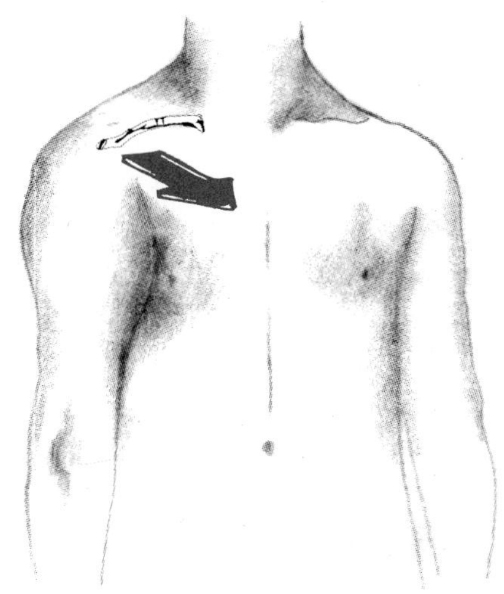

Protraction
of the Clavicle at the Sternocostal Joint

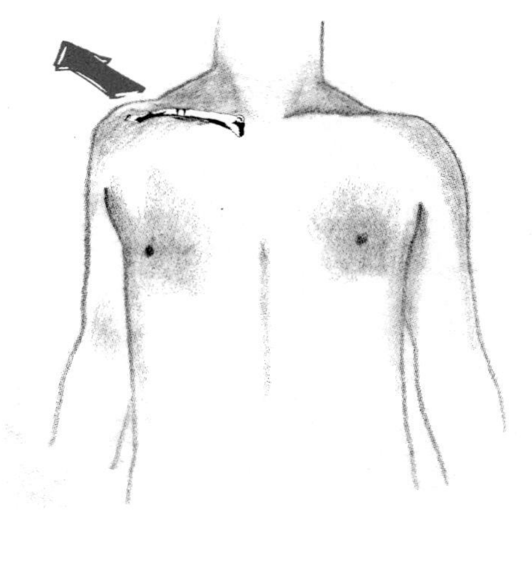

Retraction
of the Clavicle at the Sternocostal Joint

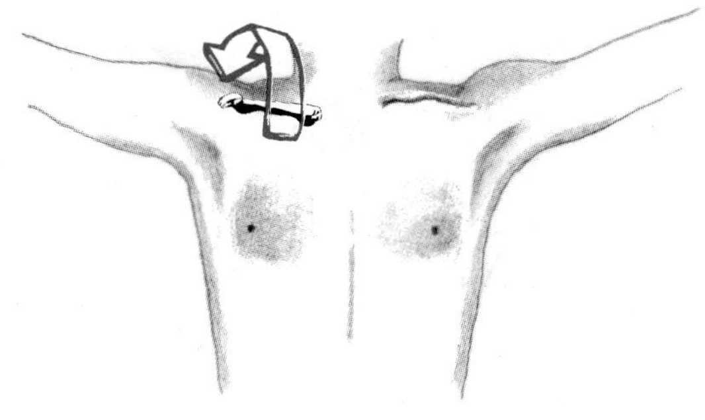

Upward Rotation
of the Clavicle at the Sternocostal Joint

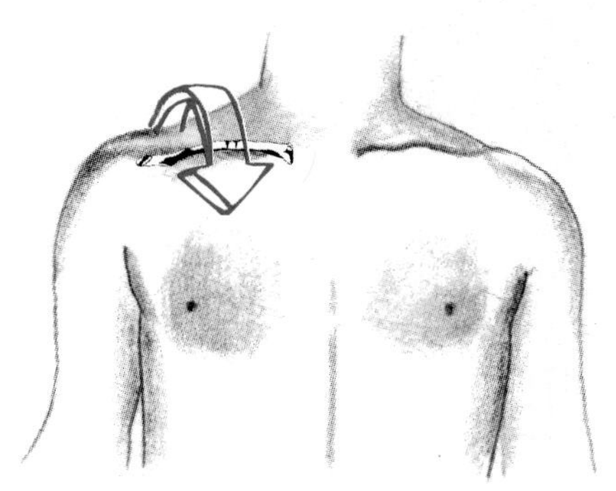

Downward Rotation
of the Clavicle at the Sternocostal Joint

JOINT ACTIONS OF THE ARM AT THE SHOULDER JOINT

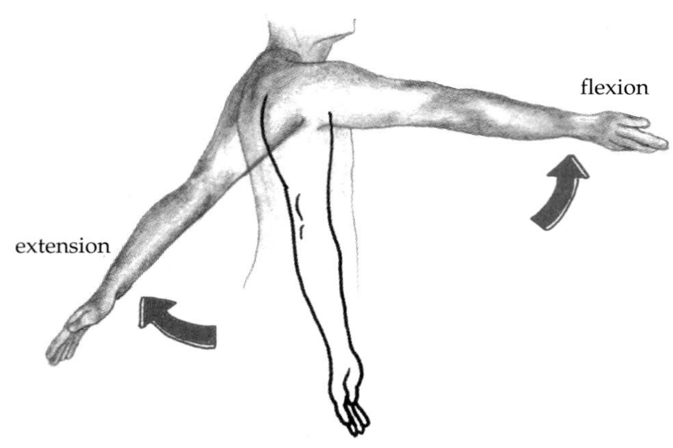

Extension and Flexion of the Arm at the Shoulder Joint

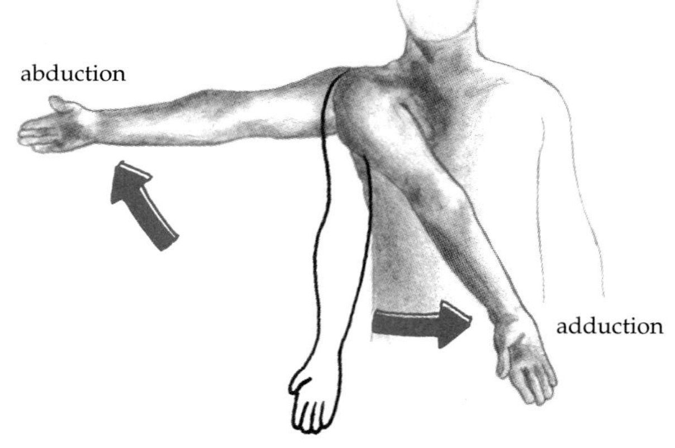

Abduction and Adduction of the Arm at the Shoulder Joint

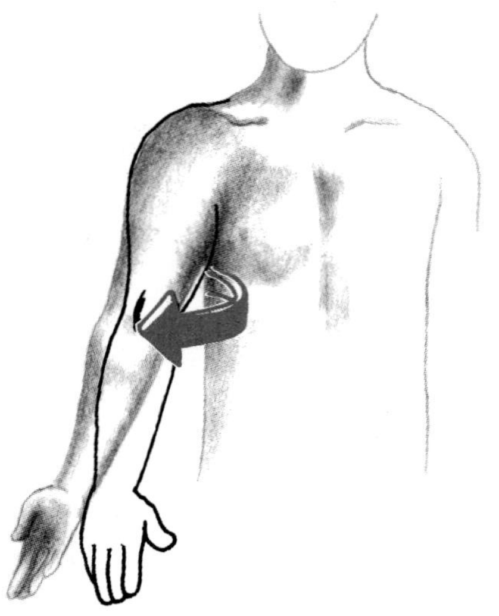

Lateral Rotation of the Arm at the Shoulder Joint

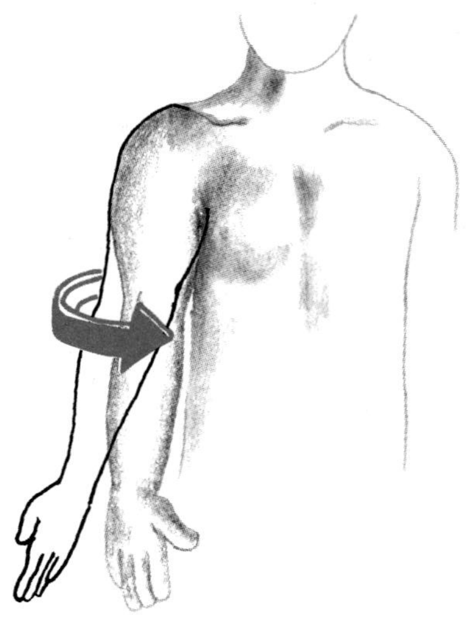

Medial Rotation of the Arm at the Shoulder Joint

JOINT ACTIONS OF THE FOREARM AT THE ELBOW AND RADIOULNAR JOINTS

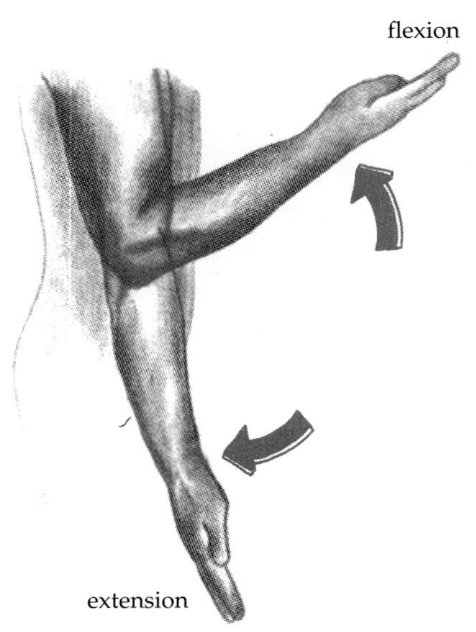

Extension and Flexion of the Forearm at the Elbow Joint

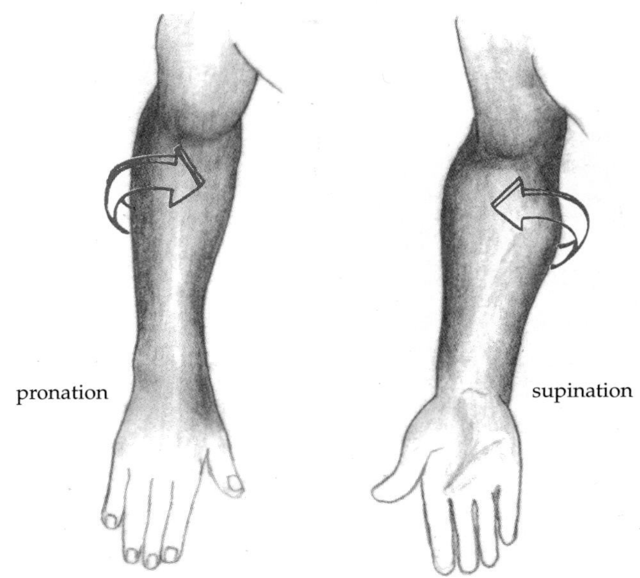

Pronation and Supination of the Forearm at the Radioulnar Joints

---

JOINT ACTIONS OF THE HAND AT THE WRIST JOINT

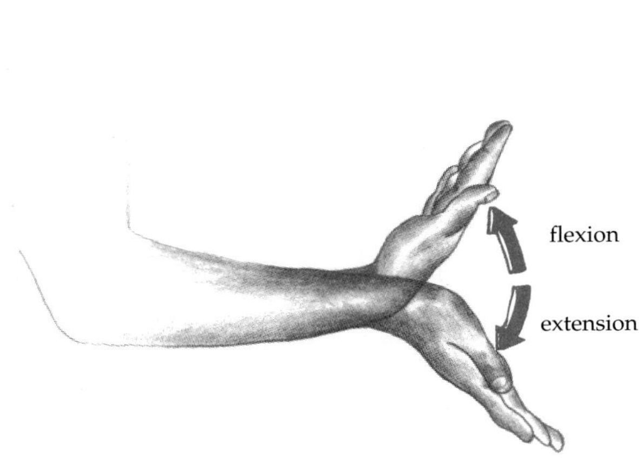

Flexion and Extension of the Hand at the Wrist Joint

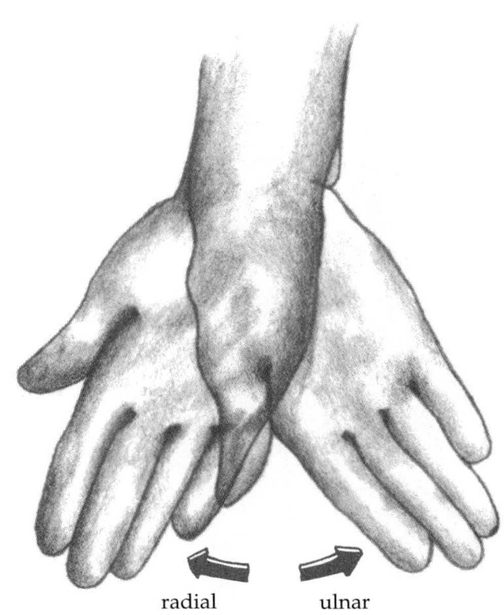

Radial Deviation (Abduction) and Ulnar Deviation (Adduction) of the Hand at the Wrist Joint

JOINT ACTIONS OF THE FINGERS AT THE METACARPOPHALANGEAL JOINT (AND THE PROXIMAL AND DISTAL INTERPHALANGEAL JOINTS)

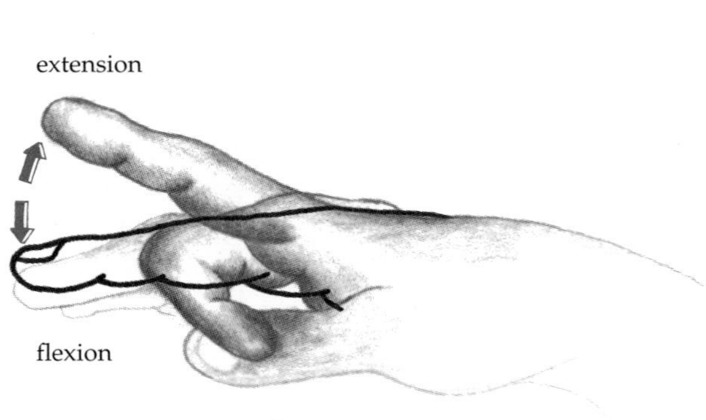

Extension and Flexion of a Finger at the Metacarpophalangeal Joint
(and the proximal and distal interphalangeal joints)

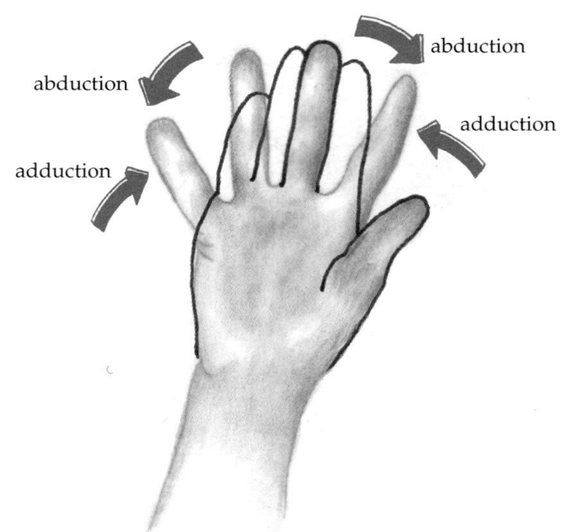

Abduction and Adduction of the Fingers at the Metacarpophalangeal Joint

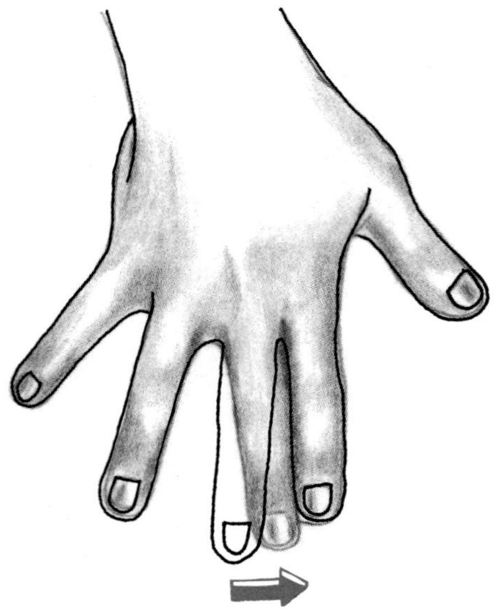

Radial Abduction of the Middle Finger at the Metacarpophalangeal Joint

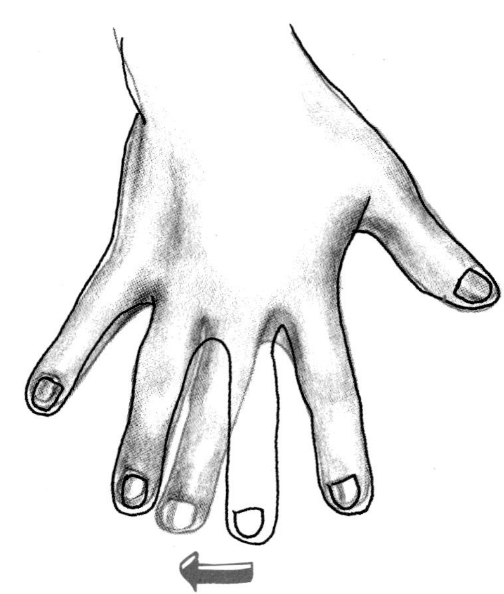

Ulnar Abduction of the Middle Finger at the Metacarpophalangeal Joint

JOINT ACTIONS OF THE THUMB AT THE 1ST CARPOMETACARPAL JOINT

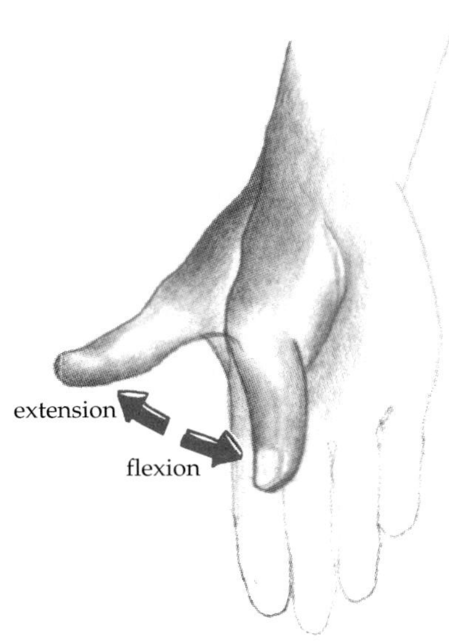

Extension and Flexion of the Thumb at the 1st Carpometacarpal Joint (flexion of the proximal phalanx at the metacarpophalangeal joint also visible)

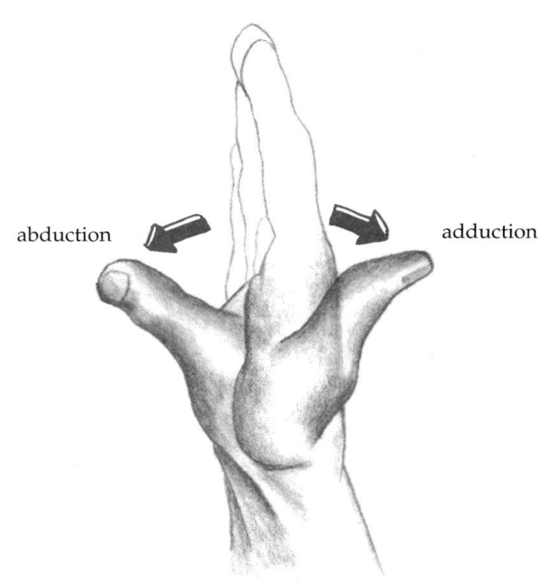

Abduction and Adduction of the Thumb at the 1st Carpometacarpal Joint

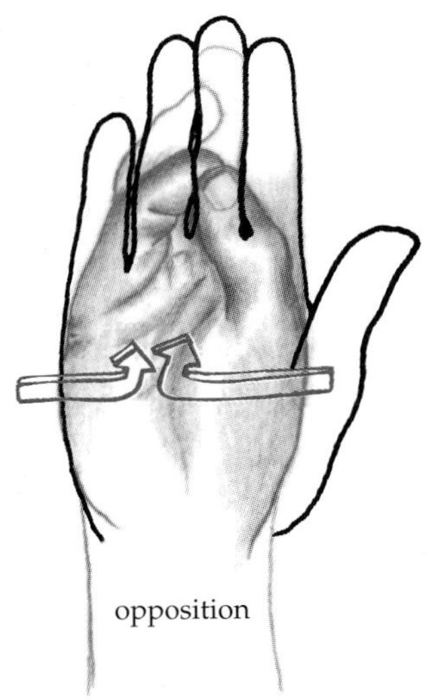

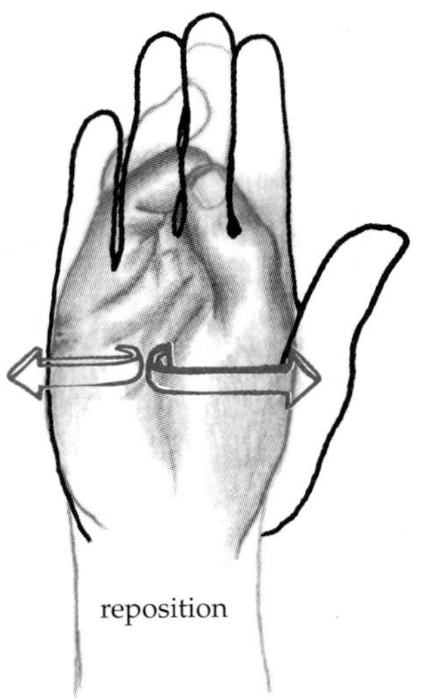

Opposition and Reposition of the Thumb at the 1st Carpometacarpal Joint and the Little Finger at the 5th Carpometacarpal Joint
(Flexion of the phalanges of the thumb at the metacarpophalangeal and interphalangeal joints and flexion of the phalanges of the little finger at the metacarpophalangeal and proximal and distal interphalangeal joints also visible.)

APPENDIX C – REVERSE ACTIONS

When a muscle concentrically contracts, either attachment will move toward the other. However, we often designate one attachment as the fixed "origin" and the other as the mobile "insertion." If we think of muscles this way, then we must keep in mind that the origin and insertion can switch; the attachment we designate as the insertion can stay fixed and the attachment we designate as the origin can move. When this type of action occurs, it is called a *reverse action*. Reverse actions occur quite often. Below are two examples of reverse actions.

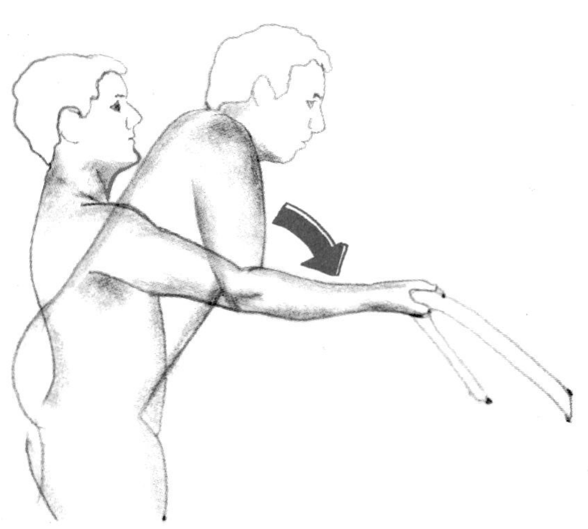

Flexion of the Arm at the Elbow Joint

In this example, muscles that cross the anterior elbow joint are contracting and creating flexion of the elbow joint. Typically, in this scenario, we would expect to see the arm (usually thought of as the origin) fixed and the forearm (usually thought of as the insertion) moving toward the arm. This action would be called "flexion of the forearm at the elbow joint." However, in this case, the forearm is fixed because the hand is holding onto a bar, so the arm moves instead. The elbow joint is still flexing, but since the arm is moving instead of the forearm, the action is termed "flexion of the arm at the elbow joint." This type of action is called a reverse action because the attachment that is usually thought of as the origin (the arm) moves and the attachment that is usually thought of as the insertion (the forearm) stays fixed. Doing a pull-up is another common example of a reverse action involving flexion of the elbow joint.

Reverse actions tend to happen less often than the typically thought of action. This is because the "origin" attachment is often the fixed attachment, as it is heavier and therefore less likely to move. In this case, not only is the arm heavier than the forearm, but for the arm to move, the trunk (along with the pelvis, head, neck and the upper extremity on the opposite side) must also move.

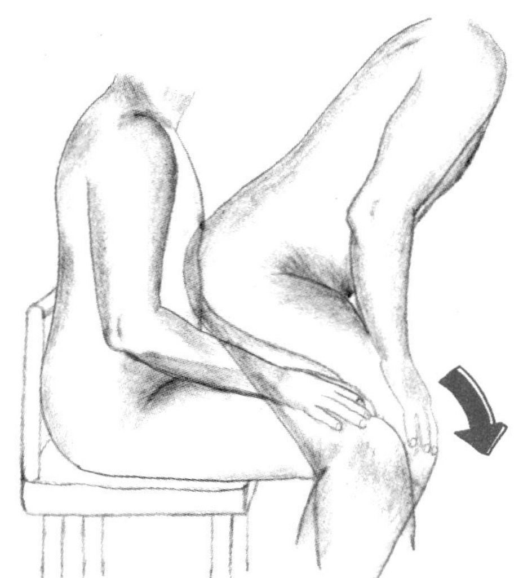

Extension of the Thigh at the Knee Joint

In this example, muscles that cross the anterior knee joint are contracting and creating extension of the knee joint. Typically, in this scenario, we would expect to see the thigh (usually thought of as the origin) fixed and the leg (usually thought of as the insertion) moving toward the thigh. This action would be called "extension of the leg at the knee joint." However, in this case, the leg is fixed because the feet are planted on the floor, so the thigh moves instead. The knee joint is still extending, but since the thigh is moving instead of the leg, the action is termed "extension of the thigh at the knee joint." This type of action is called a reverse action because the attachment that is usually thought of as the origin (the thigh) moves and the attachment that is usually thought of as the insertion (the leg) stays fixed.

Reverse actions tend to happen less often than the typically thought of action. This is because the "origin" attachment is often the fixed attachment, as it is heavier and therefore less likely to move. In this case, not only is the thigh heavier than the leg, but for the thigh to move, the trunk (along with the pelvis, head, neck and both upper extremities) must also move. This reverse action of the quadriceps is the main reason why the quadriceps group needs to be large and powerful.

APPENDIX D – MUSCLE ACTIONS BY GROUPS OF MOVERS

PART ONE – THE AXIAL BODY

HEAD

Scalp:

Drawn Anteriorly
Occipitofrontalis (frontalis)

Tightening the Scalp
Temporoparietalis
Auricularis muscles (anterior and superior)

Drawn Posteriorly
Occipitofrontalis (occipitalis)

Ear:

Drawn Anteriorly
Auricularis muscles (anterior)

Elevation (Drawn Superiorly)
Auricularis muscles (superior)
Temporoparietalis

Drawn Posteriorly
Auricularis muscles (posterior)

Eyebrow:

Elevation (Drawn Superiorly)
Occipitofrontalis (frontalis)
Procerus (medial eyebrow only)

Drawn Medially
Corrugator Supercilii

Depression (Drawn Inferiorly)
Corrugator Supercilii

Eye:

Closes and Squints the Eye
Orbicularis Oculi (orbital part)

Upper Eyelid

Elevation (Drawn Superiorly)
Levator Palpebrae Superioris

Lower Eyelid

Elevation (Drawn Superiorly)
Orbicularis Oculi (palpebral part)

Tear Transport and Drainage Assistance
Orbicularis Oculi (lacrimal part)

Depression (Drawn Inferiorly)
Orbicularis Oculi (palpebral part)

HEAD – continued

Nose:

Flares The Nostril
Nasalis
Levator Labii Superioris Alaeque Nasi

Wrinkles Skin
Procerus

Constriction of the Nostril
Depressor Septi Nasi

Upper Lip:

Elevation (Drawn Superiorly)
Levator Labii Superioris
Levator Labii Superioris Alaeque Nasi
Zygomaticus Minor

Eversion
Levator Labii Superioris
Levator Labii Superioris Alaeque Nasi
Zygomaticus Minor

Depression (Drawn Inferiorly)
Orbicularis Oris

Protraction (Protrusion)
Orbicularis Oris

Angle of the Mouth:

Elevation
Zygomaticus Major
Levator Anguli Oris

Drawn Laterally
Zygomaticus Major
Risorius
Depressor Anguli Oris

Depression
Depressor Anguli Oris

Lower Lip:

Depression (Drawn Inferiorly)
Depressor Labii Inferioris
Platysma

Drawn Laterally
Depressor Labii Inferioris
Platysma

Eversion
Depressor Labii Inferioris
Mentalis

Elevation (Drawn Superiorly)
Orbicularis Oris
Mentalis

Protraction (Protrusion)
Orbicularis Oris
Mentalis

Chin:

Wrinkles the Skin
Mentalis

HEAD – continued

Cheek:

Compression
Buccinator

Mandible at the Temporomandibular Joint:

Elevation
Temporalis
Masseter
Medial Pterygoid

Depression
Digastric
Mylohyoid
Geniohyoid
Platysma

Protraction
Medial Pterygoid
Lateral Pterygoid
Masseter

Retraction
Temporalis
Masseter
Digastric

Contralateral Deviation
Medial Pterygoid
Lateral Pterygoid

Head at the Atlanto-Occipital Joint:

Flexion
Longus Capitis
Rectus Capitis Anterior

Extension
Trapezius (upper)
Splenius Capitis
Erector Spinae Group
Spinalis
Longissimus
Transversospinalis Group
Semispinalis
Rectus Capitis Posterior Major
Rectus Capitis Posterior Minor
Obliquus Capitis Superior
Sternocleidomastoid

Lateral Flexion
Trapezius (upper)
Splenius Capitis
Sternocleidomastoid
Erector Spinae Group
Longissimus
Spinalis
Transversospinalis Group
Semispinalis
Rectus Capitis Posterior Major
Obliquus Capitis Superior
Longus Capitis
Rectus Capitis Lateralis

Ipsilateral Rotation
Splenius Capitis
Rectus Capitis Posterior Major
Erector Spinae Group
Longissimus
Spinalis

Contralateral Rotation
Trapezius (upper)
Sternocleidomastoid

NECK

Neck at the Spinal Joints:

Flexion
- Sternocleidomastoid
- Anterior Scalene
- Middle Scalene
- Longus Colli
- Longus Capitis

Extension
- Trapezius (upper)
- Splenius Capitis
- Splenius Cervicis
- Erector Spinae Group
  - Iliocostalis
  - Longissimus
  - Spinalis
- Transversospinalis Group
  - Semispinalis
  - Multifidus
  - Rotatores
- Levator Scapulae
- Rectus Capitis Posterior Major (C1 only)
- Interspinales

Lateral Flexion
- Trapezius (upper)
- Sternocleidomastoid
- Splenius Capitis
- Splenius Cervicis
- Scalene Group:
  - Anterior Scalene
  - Middle Scalene
  - Posterior Scalene
- Levator Scapulae
- Erector Spinae Group
  - Iliocostalis
  - Longissimus
  - Spinalis
- Transversospinalis Group
  - Semispinalis
  - Multifidus
- Longus Colli
- Longus Capitis
- Intertransversarii

Ipsilateral Rotation
- Splenius Capitis
- Splenius Cervicis
- Erector Spinae Group
  - Iliocostalis
  - Longissimus
  - Spinalis
- Obliquus Capitis Inferior (C1 only)
- Rectus Capitis Posterior Major (C1 only)
- Levator Scapulae

Contralateral Rotation
- Sternocleidomastoid
- Trapezius (upper)
- Transversospinalis Group
  - Semispinalis
  - Multifidus
  - Rotatores
- Anterior Scalene
- Longus Colli

Hyoid Bone:

Elevation
- Digastric
- Stylohyoid
- Mylohyoid
- Geniohyoid

Depression
- Sternohyoid
- Thyrohyoid
- Omohyoid

NECK – continued

Thyroid Cartilage:

Elevation
Thyrohyoid

Depression
Sternothyroid

Skin of the Neck:

Creates Ridges
Platysma

TRUNK

Trunk at the Spinal Joints:

Flexion
Rectus Abdominis
External Abdominal Oblique
Internal Abdominal Oblique
Psoas Major
Psoas Minor

Extension
Erector Spinae Group
- Iliocostalis
- Longissimus
- Spinalis

Transversospinalis Group
- Semispinalis
- Multifidus
- Rotatores

Quadratus Lumborum
Trapezius (middle and lower)
Interspinales
Levatores Costarum

Lateral Flexion
Erector Spinae Group
- Iliocostalis
- Longissimus
- Spinalis

Transversospinalis Group
- Semispinalis
- Multifidus

Psoas Major
Rectus Abdominis
External Abdominal Oblique
Internal Abdominal Oblique
Quadratus Lumborum
Intertransversarii
Levatores Costarum

Ipsilateral Rotation
Internal Abdominal Oblique
Erector Spinae Group
- Iliocostalis
- Longissimus
- Spinalis

Contralateral Rotation
External Abdominal Oblique
Transversospinalis Group
- Semispinalis
- Multifidus
- Rotatores

Psoas Major
Rhomboids Major and Minor

Levatores Costarum

TRUNK – continued

Trunk at the Shoulder Joint:

Lateral Deviation
Pectoralis Major
Latissimus Dorsi

Ipsilateral Rotation
Pectoralis Major
Deltoid (anterior deltoid)

Contralateral Rotation
Latissimus Dorsi
Deltoid (posterior deltoid)

Elevation
Pectoralis Major
Latissimus Dorsi

Ribs at the Costovertebral and Sternocostal Joints:

Elevation
External Intercostals (ribs #2-12 only)
Anterior Scalene (1st rib only)
Middle Scalene (1st rib only)
Posterior Scalene (2nd rib only)
Pectoralis Minor (ribs #3-5 only)
Serratus Posterior Superior (ribs #2-5 only)
Levatores Costarum
Subclavius (1st rib only)
Internal Intercostals (ribs #2-12 only)

Depression
Internal Intercostals (ribs #1-11 only)
Quadratus Lumborum (12th rib only)
Serratus Posterior Inferior (ribs #9-12)
Subcostales (ribs #8-10 only)
External Intercostals (ribs #1-11 only)
Transversus Thoracis (ribs #2-6 only)

Abdominal Contents:

Compression of
Rectus Abdominis
External Abdominal Oblique
Internal Abdominal Oblique
Transversus Abdominis

Other:

Draws up the Skin of the Superior Chest
Platysma

Increases the Volume of the Thoracic Cavity
Diaphragm

PART TWO – THE LOWER EXTREMITY

PELVIS

Pelvis at the Hip and/or Lumbosacral Joints:

Posterior Tilt
- Rectus Abdominis
- External Abdominal Oblique
- Internal Abdominal Oblique
- Biceps Femoris (long head)
- Semitendinosus
- Semimembranosus
- Gluteus Maximus
- Gluteus Medius (posterior fibers)
- Gluteus Minimus (posterior fibers)
- Adductor Magnus
- Psoas Minor

Anterior Tilt
- Erector Spinae Group
  - Iliocostalis
  - Longissimus
- Transversospinalis Group
  - Multifidus
- Quadratus Lumborum
- Latissimus Dorsi
- Psoas Major
- Iliacus
- Rectus Femoris
- Sartorius
- Tensor Fasciae Latae
- Gluteus Medius (anterior fibers)
- Gluteus Minimus (anterior fibers)
- Pectineus
- Adductor Longus
- Gracilis
- Adductor Brevis

Elevation
- Quadratus Lumborum
- Erector Spinae Group
  - Iliocostalis
  - Longissimus
- Transversospinalis Group
  - Multifidus
- Latissimus Dorsi

Depression (Lateral Tilt)
- Gluteus Medius (entire muscle)
- Gluteus Minimus (entire muscle)
- Tensor Fasciae Latae
- Sartorius

Ipsilateral Rotation
- External Abdominal Oblique
- Tensor Fasciae Latae
- Gluteus Medius (anterior fibers)
- Gluteus Minimus (anterior fibers)
- Transversospinalis Group
  - Multifidus

Contralateral Rotation
- Internal Abdominal Oblique
- Psoas Major
- Iliacus
- Sartorius
- Gluteus Maximus
- Gluteus Medius (posterior fibers)
- Gluteus Minimus (posterior fibers)
- Erector Spinae Group
  - Iliocostalis
  - Longissimus
- Piriformis
- Superior Gemellus
- Obturator Internus
- Inferior Gemellus
- Obturator Externus
- Quadratus Femoris

THIGH

Thigh at the Hip Joint:

Flexion
- Psoas Major
- Iliacus
- Sartorius
- Tensor Fasciae Latae
- Rectus Femoris
- Pectineus
- Adductor Longus
- Gracilis
- Adductor Brevis
- Gluteus Medius (anterior fibers)
- Gluteus Minimus (anterior fibers)

Extension
- Gluteus Maximus
- Hamstrings
  - Biceps Femoris (long head)
  - Semitendinosus
  - Semimembranosus
- Adductor Magnus
- Gluteus Medius (posterior fibers)
- Gluteus Minimus (posterior fibers)

Abduction
- Gluteus Medius (entire muscle)
- Gluteus Minimus (entire muscle)
- Tensor Fasciae Latae
- Sartorius
- Gluteus Maximus (upper 1/3)
- Piriformis
- Superior Gemellus
- Obturator Internus
- Inferior Gemellus

Adduction
- Pectineus
- Adductor Longus
- Gracilis
- Adductor Brevis
- Adductor Magnus
- Gluteus Maximus (lower 2/3)
- Biceps Femoris (long head)
- Quadratus Femoris

Lateral Rotation
- Gluteus Maximus
- Gluteus Medius (posterior fibers)
- Gluteus Minimus (posterior fibers)
- Piriformis
- Superior Gemellus
- Obturator Internus
- Inferior Gemellus
- Obturator Externus
- Quadratus Femoris
- Sartorius
- Psoas Major
- Iliacus
- Biceps Femoris (long head)
- Popliteus (at the knee joint)

Medial Rotation
- Gluteus Medius (anterior fibers)
- Gluteus Minimus (anterior fibers)
- Tensor Fasciae Latae
- Semitendinosus
- Semimembranosus
- Piriformis

LEG

Leg at the Knee Joint:

Flexion
- Hamstrings
  - Biceps Femoris
  - Semitendinosus
  - Semimembranosus
- Sartorius
- Gracilis
- Gastrocnemius
- Plantaris
- Popliteus

Extension
- Quadriceps Femoris
  - Vastus Lateralis
  - Vastus Medialis
  - Vastus Intermedius
  - Rectus Femoris
- Tensor Fasciae Latae
- Gluteus Maximus

LEG – continued

Leg at the Knee Joint continued:

Lateral Rotation
Biceps Femoris (entire muscle)
Semitendinosus
Popliteus
Sartorius
Gracilis

Medial Rotation
Semimembranosus

Tenses and Pulls the Knee Joint Capsule Proximally
Articularis Genus

FOOT

Foot at the Ankle Joint:

Plantarflexion (Flexion)
Gastrocnemius
Soleus
Fibularis Longus
Fibularis Brevis
Tibialis Posterior
Flexor Digitorum Longus
Flexor Hallucis Longus
Plantaris

Dorsiflexion (Extension)
Tibialis Anterior
Extensor Digitorum Longus
Extensor Hallucis Longus
Fibularis Tertius

Foot at the Tarsal Joints:

Inversion
Tibialis Posterior
Tibialis Anterior
Flexor Digitorum Longus
Flexor Hallucis Longus
Extensor Hallucis Longus
Gastrocnemius
Soleus

Eversion
Fibularis Longus
Fibularis Brevis
Fibularis Tertius
Extensor Digitorum Longus

Big Toe - Proximal Phalanx - at the Metatarsophalangeal Joint:

Flexion
Flexor Hallucis Longus
Flexor Hallucis Brevis
Abductor Hallucis
Adductor Hallucis

Extension
Extensor Hallucis Longus
Extensor Hallucis Brevis

Abduction
Abductor Hallucis

Adduction
Adductor Hallucis

Big Toe - Distal Phalanx - at the Interphalangeal Joint:

Flexion
Flexor Hallucis Longus

Extension
Extensor Hallucis Longus

FOOT – continued

Toes #2-5 - Proximal Phalanx - at the Metatarsophalangeal Joint:

Flexion
- Flexor Digitorum Longus
- Flexor Digitorum Brevis
- Flexor Digiti Minimi Pedis (5th toe only)
- Quadratus Plantae
- Abductor Digiti Minimi Pedis (5th toe only)
- Lumbricals Pedis
- Plantar Interossei (toes #3-5 only)
- Dorsal Interossei Pedis (toes #2-4 only)

Extension
- Extensor Digitorum Longus
- Extensor Digitorum Brevis (toes #2-4 only)

Abduction
- Dorsal Interossei Pedis (toes #2-4 only)
- Abductor Digiti Minimi Pedis (5th toe only)

Adduction
- Plantar Interossei (toes #3-5 only)

Toes #2-5 - Middle Phalanx - at the Proximal Interphalangeal Joint:

Flexion
- Flexor Digitorum Longus
- Flexor Digitorum Brevis
- Quadratus Plantae

Extension
- Extensor Digitorum Longus
- Extensor Digitorum Brevis (toes #2-4 only)
- Lumbricals Pedis
- Plantar Interossei (toes #3-5 only)
- Dorsal Interossei Pedis (toes #2-4 only)

Toes #2-5 -Distal Phalanx - at the Distal Interphalangeal Joint:

Flexion
- Flexor Digitorum Longus
- Quadratus Plantae

Extension
- Extensor Digitorum Longus
- Extensor Digitorum Brevis (toes #2-4 only)
- Lumbricals Pedis
- Plantar Interossei (toes #3-5 only)
- Dorsal Interossei Pedis (toes #2-4 only)

PART THREE – THE UPPER EXTREMITY

SCAPULA/ARM

Scapula at the Scapulocostal Joint:

Elevation
- Trapezius (upper)
- Levator Scapulae
- Rhomboids Major and Minor
- Serratus Anterior

Depression
- Trapezius (lower)
- Pectoralis Minor
- Latissimus Dorsi
- Pectoralis Major
- Serratus Anterior

Protraction (Abduction)
- Serratus Anterior
- Pectoralis Minor

Retraction (Adduction)
- Trapezius (entire muscle)
- Rhomboids Major and Minor
- Levator Scapulae

Upward Rotation
- Trapezius (upper and lower)
- Serratus Anterior
- Teres Major

Downward Rotation
- Rhomboids Major and Minor
- Pectoralis Minor
- Levator Scapulae
- Deltoid (entire muscle)

SCAPULA/ARM – continued

Scapula at the Scapulocostal Joint continued:

Upward Tilt
Pectoralis Minor
Levator Scapulae
Coracobrachialis
Biceps Brachii

Downward Tilt
Latissimus Dorsi
Serratus Anterior

Lateral Tilt
Pectoralis Minor
Coracobrachialis
Biceps Brachii
Triceps Brachii

Medial Tilt
Serratus Anterior
Rhomboids Major and Minor
Trapezius (middle and lower)
Latissimus Dorsi

Clavicle at the Sternoclavicular Joint:

Elevation
Sternocleidomastoid
Trapezius (upper)
Deltoid (anterior deltoid)

Depression
Subclavius
Pectoralis Major

Protraction
Subclavius
Pectoralis Major
Deltoid (anterior deltoid)

Retraction
Trapezius (upper)

Upward Rotation
Trapezius (upper)
Sternocleidomastoid
Deltoid (anterior deltoid)

Downward Rotation
Pectoralis Major
Subclavius

Sternum:

Elevation
Sternocleidomastoid

Arm at the Shoulder Joint:

Flexion
Deltoid (anterior deltoid)
Pectoralis Major (clavicular head)
Coracobrachialis
Biceps Brachii (entire muscle)

Extension
Deltoid (posterior deltoid)
Latissimus Dorsi
Teres Major
Triceps Brachii (long head)
Pectoralis Major (sternocostal head)

Abduction
Deltoid (entire muscle)
Supraspinatus
Biceps Brachii (long head)
Pectoralis Major (clavicular head above 90°)

Adduction
Pectoralis Major
Latissimus Dorsi
Teres Major
Coracobrachialis
Biceps Brachii (short head)
Triceps Brachii (long head)
Teres Minor

SCAPULA/ARM – continued

Arm at the Shoulder Joint continued:

Lateral Rotation
- Deltoid(posterior deltoid)
- Infraspinatus
- Teres Minor

Medial Rotation
- Deltoid (anterior deltoid)
- Pectoralis Major
- Latissimus Dorsi
- Teres Major
- Subscapularis

Horizontal Flexion
- Anterior Deltoid
- Coracobrachialis
- Biceps Brachii
- Pectoralis Major

Horizontal Extension
- Posterior Deltoid
- Infraspinatus
- Teres Minor
- Supraspinatus
- Triceps Brachii (long head)

FOREARM

Forearm at the Elbow Joint:

Flexion
- Brachialis
- Biceps Brachii (entire muscle)
- Brachioradialis
- Pronator Teres
- Flexor Carpi Radialis
- Palmaris Longus
- Flexor Carpi Ulnaris
- Flexor Digitorum Superficialis
- Flexor Pollicis Longus
- Extensor Carpi Radialis Longus
- Extensor Carpi Radialis Brevis

Extension
- Triceps Brachii (entire muscle)
- Anconeus
- Extensor Digitorum
- Extensor Digiti Minimi
- Extensor Carpi Ulnaris

Forearm at the Radioulnar Joints:

Pronation
- Pronator Quadratus
- Pronator Teres
- Brachioradialis
- Flexor Carpi Radialis
- Palmaris Longus
- Extensor Carpi Radialis Longus

Supination
- Supinator
- Biceps Brachii (entire muscle)
- Brachioradialis
- Abductor Pollicis Longus
- Extensor Pollicis Brevis
- Extensor Pollicis Longus
- Extensor Indicis

HAND

Hand at the Wrist Joint:

Flexion
- Flexor Carpi Radialis
- Palmaris Longus
- Flexor Carpi Ulnaris
- Flexor Digitorum Superficialis
- Flexor Digitorum Profundus
- Flexor Pollicis Longus
- Abductor Pollicis Longus

Extension
- Extensor Carpi Radialis Longus
- Extensor Carpi Radialis Brevis
- Extensor Digitorum
- Extensor Digiti Minimi
- Extensor Carpi Ulnaris
- Extensor Pollicis Longus
- Extensor Indicis

Radial Deviation (Abduction)
- Extensor Carpi Radialis Longus
- Extensor Carpi Radialis Brevis
- Flexor Carpi Radialis
- Abductor Pollicis Longus
- Extensor Pollicis Brevis
- Extensor Pollicis Longus

Ulnar Deviation (Adduction)
- Flexor Carpi Ulnaris
- Extensor Carpi Ulnaris

Thumb - 1st Metacarpal - at the Carpometacarpal Joint:

Flexion
- Flexor Pollicis Longus
- Flexor Pollicis Brevis
- Opponens Pollicis
- Adductor Pollicis

Extension
- Extensor Pollicis Longus
- Extensor Pollicis Brevis
- Abductor Pollicis Longus
- Abductor Pollicis Brevis

Abduction
- Abductor Pollicis Longus
- Abductor Pollicis Brevis
- Extensor Pollicis Brevis
- Flexor Pollicis Brevis

Adduction
- Adductor Pollicis
- Opponens Pollicis

Medial Rotation
- Opponens Pollicis

Lateral Rotation
- Abductor Pollicis Longus
- Extensor Pollicis Brevis
- Extensor Pollicis Longus

Opposition
- Opponens Pollicis

Thumb - Proximal Phalanx - at the Metacarpophalangeal Joint:

Flexion
- Flexor Pollicis Longus
- Flexor Pollicis Brevis
- Adductor Pollicis
- Abductor Pollicis Brevis

Extension
- Extensor Pollicis Longus
- Extensor Pollicis Brevis

Thumb - Distal Phalanx - at the Interphalangeal Joint:

Flexion
- Flexor Pollicis Longus

Extension
- Extensor Pollicis Longus
- Adductor Pollicis
- Abductor Pollicis Brevis

HAND – continued

Finger #5 at the Carpometacarpal Joint:

Flexion
Opponens Digiti Minimi

Adduction
Opponens Digiti Minimi

Medial Rotation
Extensor Digitorum
Extensor Digiti Minimi

Lateral Rotation
Opponens Digiti Minimi

Opposition
Opponens Digiti Minimi

Fingers #2-5 - Proximal Phalanx - at the Metacarpophalangeal Joint:

Flexion
Flexor Digitorum Superficialis
Flexor Digitorum Profundus
Flexor Digiti Minimi Manus (5th finger only)
Lumbricals Manus
Palmar Interossei (fingers #2, 4 and 5 only)
Dorsal Interossei Manus (fingers #2-4 only)

Extension
Extensor Digitorum
Extensor Indicis (2nd finger only)
Extensor Digiti Minimi (5th finger only)

Abduction
Dorsal Interossei Manus (fingers #2-4 only)
Abductor Digiti Minimi Manus (5th finger only)

Adduction
Palmar Interossei (fingers #2, 4, and 5 only)
Extensor Indicis (2nd finger only)

Fingers #2-5 - Middle Phalanx - at the Proximal Interphalangeal Joint:

Flexion
Flexor Digitorum Superficialis
Flexor Digitorum Profundus

Extension
Extensor Digitorum
Extensor Indicis (2nd finger only)
Extensor Digiti Minimi (5th finger only)
Abductor Digiti Minimi Manus (5th finger only)
Lumbricals Manus
Palmar Interossei (fingers #2, 4 and 5 only)
Dorsal Interossei Manus (fingers #2-4 only)

Fingers #2-5 - Distal Phalanx - at the Distal Interphalangeal Joint:

Flexion
Flexor Digitorum Profundus

Extension
Extensor Digitorum
Extensor Indicis (2nd finger only)
Lumbricals Manus
Extensor Digiti Minimi (5th finger only)
Abductor Digiti Minimi Manus (5th finger only)
Palmar Interossei (fingers #2, 4 and 5 only)
Dorsal Interossei Manus (fingers #2-4 only)

Other Hand Actions:

Wrinkling the Skin of the Palm
Palmaris Brevis
Palmaris Longus

APPENDIX E – SOFT TISSUE ATTACHMENTS

The following attachments of skeletal muscles of the human body are all attachments into soft tissues: deep muscular fascia, aponeuroses, tendons of other muscles, joint capsules, etc. All these soft tissues are composed of fibrous fascia, which is a type of connective tissue. If these attachments were already stated in the individual muscle layout pages, it is noted.

The intent in providing these attachments is not to create another level of attachments that must be memorized, but rather to provide specific reference information that may be useful when working a particular area. Further, looking over this material is useful toward gaining an appreciation of how fibrous fascia truly creates a web that connects all structures of our body together!

PART ONE – THE AXIAL BODY

HEAD CHAPTER

Note: Only the muscles of mastication are covered in this appendix since the other muscles of the head primarily attach into soft tissue and these attachments are covered in the head chapter.

Temporalis: Superiorly, the temporalis has fibers that attach into the deep surface of the temporal fascia (as noted in the miscellaneous section).

Lateral Pterygoid: Laterally, the lateral pterygoid attaches into the articular capsule and the disc of the temporomandibular joint (T.M.J., as noted in the attachment section).

NECK CHAPTER

Trapezius: Medially, the trapezius attaches to the nuchal ligament (as noted in the attachment section) and the supraspinous ligament between C7 and T12. The occipital attachment also adheres to the skin of the scalp.

Splenius Capitis: Medially, the splenius capitis attaches to the nuchal ligament (as noted in the attachment section) and the supraspinous ligament between C7 and T4.

Levator Scapulae: Inferiorly, the levator scapulae attaches into the fascial sheath of the serratus anterior.

Rectus Capitis Posterior Minor: Superiorly, the rectus capitis posterior minor has some fibers that attach into the dura mater (as noted in the miscellaneous section).

Platysma: Inferiorly, the platysma attaches into the fascia of the pectoral and deltoid regions (as noted in the attachment section). The platysma also blends with the contralateral platysma in the midline (as noted in the miscellaneous section). Superiorly, the platysma attaches into the subcutaneous fascia of the lower face (as noted in the attachment section) and into many of the muscles of facial expression located in the lower face (as noted in the miscellaneous section).

Sternohyoid: Inferiorly, the sternohyoid attaches into the posterior sternoclavicular ligament.

Mylohyoid: The two mylohyoid muscles meet (and attach into) each other in the midline forming a median fibrous raphe (as noted in the miscellaneous section).

TRUNK CHAPTER

Latissimus Dorsi: Medially, the latissimus dorsi attaches into the thoracolumbar fascia (as noted in the attachment section). The latissimus dorsi also interdigitates with the external abdominal oblique (as noted in the relationship to other musculoskeletal structures section).

Rhomboids Major and Minor: The rhomboid major attaches into the supraspinous ligament of T2-T5 medially. The rhomboid minor attaches into the lower nuchal ligament (as noted in the attachment section). The rhomboid minor and serratus anterior are covered with fascia that adheres them to each other.

Serratus Anterior: Anteriorly, the serratus anterior has attachments into the fascia that covers the external intercostals between ribs #1-9.

Serratus Posterior Superior: Medially, the serratus posterior superior has fibers that attach into the lower nuchal ligament (as noted in the attachment section) and the supraspinous ligament between C7 and T3.

Serratus Posterior Inferior: Medially, the serratus posterior inferior has fibers that attach into the supraspinous ligament between T11 and L3.

Erector Spinae: Medially, the erector spinae attaches to the thoracolumbar fascia and the supraspinous ligaments of the lower thoracic and lumbar spine.

Transversospinalis: Inferiorly, the multifidi of the transversospinalis attach into the sacro-iliac ligament (as noted in the attachment section) and also into the aponeurosis of the erector spinae musculature.

Quadratus Lumborum: Inferiorly, the quadratus lumborum has fibers that attach into the iliolumbar ligament (as noted in the attachment section).

Pectoralis Major: Inferomedially, the pectoralis major has fibers that attach into the aponeurosis of the external abdominal oblique (as noted in the attachment section). Distally on the arm, it has fibers that converge into the deep fascia of the arm.

Pectoralis Minor:	Inferiorly, the pectoralis minor has fibers that arise from the fascia that covers the external intercostals between ribs #3-5. The pectoralis minor will often have fibers that attach into the coracoacromial ligament or even the coracohumeral ligament.
External Intercostal:	In the posterior thorax, the external intercostal has fibers that attach into the superior costotransverse ligaments.
Internal Intercostal:	In the posterior thorax, the internal intercostal has fibers that attach into the superior costotransverse ligaments. In the anterior thorax, the internal intercostals have fibers that attach into the fascia between the external and internal intercostal muscles.
Transversus Thoracis:	The most inferior fibers of the transversus thoracic are contiguous and blend into the most superior fibers of the transversus abdominis.
Rectus Abdominis:	Inferiorly, the rectus abdominis blends into the contralateral rectus abdominis and also attaches into the ligamentous fibers of the pubic symphysis joint.
External Abdominal Oblique:	Laterally, the external abdominal oblique interdigitates with the serratus anterior and the latissimus dorsi (as noted in the relationship to other musculoskeletal structures section). Medially, the aponeurosis of the external oblique meets the aponeurosis of the contralateral external abdominal oblique at the linea alba (as noted in the miscellaneous section).
Internal Abdominal Oblique:	Posteroinferiorly, the internal abdominal oblique arises from the thoracolumbar fascia; anteroinferiorly, it attaches into the inguinal ligament (as noted in the attachment section). Medially, the internal abdominal oblique attaches into the aponeurosis of the transversus abdominis and into the linea alba.
Transversus Abdominis:	Posteriorly, the transversus abdominis attaches into the thoracolumbar fascia; anteroinferiorly, it attaches into the inguinal ligament (as noted in the attachment section). Superiorly, the transversus abdominis interdigitates with the diaphragm and the transversus thoracis (as noted in the miscellaneous section). Medially, the fibers of the transversus abdominis merge with the fibers of the internal abdominal oblique and end at the linea alba.
Diaphragm:	The diaphragm interdigitates with the transversus abdominis (as noted in the miscellaneous section). The two crura of the diaphragm attach into the discs between L1 and L3 and blend with the anterior longitudinal ligament of the upper lumbar spine.

PART TWO – THE LOWER EXTREMITY

PELVIS CHAPTER

Psoas Major:	Proximally, the psoas major attaches into the discs of T12 –L5 (as noted in the attachment section) and into arches of tendinous tissue located between the attachments of the psoas major onto the vertebrae.
Iliacus:	Proximally, the iliacus has fibers that attach into the anterior sacro-iliac and iliolumbar ligaments as well as a few fibers that attach into the joint capsule of the hip joint. Distally, the iliacus actually attaches into the distal tendon of the psoas major (as noted in the miscellaneous section).
Psoas Minor:	Proximally, the psoas minor attaches into the T12-L1 disc (as noted in the attachment section). Distally, the psoas minor has fibers that attach into the deep iliac fascia.
Gluteus Maximus:	Proximally, the gluteus maximus attaches into the sacrotuberous ligament, the thoracolumbar fascia and the fascia overlying the gluteus medius. Distally, the gluteus maximus attaches into the iliotibial band. (This is all noted in the attachment section.)
Gluteus Medius:	Proximally, the gluteus medius attaches into the thick fascia that overlies it.
Gluteus Minimus:	Distally, the gluteus minimus has some fibers that attach into the capsule of the hip joint.
Piriformis:	Proximally, the piriformis has fibers that attach into the capsule of the sacro-iliac joint and usually has fibers that attach into the sacrotuberous ligament.
Obturator Internus:	Proximally, the obturator internus attaches into the obturator membrane (as noted in the attachment section) and the deep obturator fascia that covers the muscle.
Obturator Externus:	Proximally, the obturator externus attaches into the obturator membrane (as noted in the attachment section).

THIGH CHAPTER

Tensor Fasciae Latae:	Proximally, the tensor fasciae latae has fibers that arise from the deep fascia of the thigh (the "fascia latae"). Distally, the tensor fasciae latae attaches into the iliotibial band (as noted in the attachment section).
Sartorius:	Distally, the sartorius has fibers that attach into the capsule of the knee joint and the deep fascia of the medial leg.
Rectus Femoris:	Proximally, the reflected tendon of the rectus femoris has fibers that arise from the capsule of the hip joint.
Vastus Lateralis:	Proximally, the vastus lateralis has fibers that arise from the deep surface of the aponeurosis that covers it, as well as a few fibers that arise from the distal tendon of the gluteus maximus and the lateral intermuscular septum of the thigh that separates the vastus lateralis from the short head of the biceps femoris. Distally, the vastus lateralis has fibers that blend into the capsule of the knee joint and the iliotibial band.
Vastus Medialis:	Proximally, the vastus medialis has fibers that arise from the tendons of the adductor longus and adductor magnus and the medial intermuscular septum of the thigh. Distally, the vastus medialis has fibers that blend into the capsule of the knee joint.
Vastus Intermedius:	Proximally, the vastus intermedius has fibers that arise from the lateral intermuscular septum of the thigh.
Articularis Genus:	The distal attachment of the articularis genus is into the capsule of the knee joint (as noted in the attachment section).
Pectineus:	Proximally, the pectineus also has fibers that arise from the fascia that covers it anteriorly.

LEG CHAPTER

Tibialis Anterior:	Proximally, the tibialis anterior attaches into the interosseus membrane (as noted in the attachment section), the intermuscular septum between the tibialis anterior and the extensor digitorum longus, and the deep surface of the deep fascia of the leg (also known as the *fascia cruris*).

Extensor Digitorum Longus:	Proximally, the extensor digitorum longus attaches into the interosseus membrane (as noted in the attachment section), the intermuscular septum between the extensor digitorum longus and the tibialis anterior, the anterior crural intermuscular septum and the deep surface of the fascia of the leg (also known as the fascia cruris). Distally, the attachment of the extensor digitorum longus onto the toes broadens out to create the dorsal digital expansion (as noted in the attachment section).
Fibularis Tertius:	Proximally, the fibularis tertius attaches into the interosseus membrane (as noted in the attachment section) and the anterior crural intermuscular septum.
Fibularis Longus:	Proximally, the fibularis longus has fibers that arise from the deep surface of the deep fascia of the leg (also known as the fascia cruris) and the anterior and posterior crural intermuscular septa.
Fibularis Brevis:	Proximally, the fibularis brevis has fibers that arise from the anterior and posterior crural intermuscular septa.
Gastrocnemius:	Both heads of the gastrocnemius have fibers that arise from the joint capsule of the knee (as noted in the attachment section) as well as from the anterior surface of the aponeurosis that covers its proximal attachments.
Soleus:	Proximally, the soleus has fibers that arise from the posterior surface of a fibrous band that runs between the tibia and the fibula.
Plantaris:	Proximally, the plantaris has fibers that arise from the oblique popliteal ligament.
Popliteus:	Proximally, the popliteus arises from the lateral meniscus of the knee (as noted in the miscellaneous section) as well as the arcuate popliteal ligament and the fibrous capsule of the knee joint adjacent to the lateral meniscus.
Tibialis Posterior:	Proximally, the tibialis posterior attaches into the interosseus membrane (as noted in the attachment section), intermuscular fascia that separates the tibialis posterior from adjacent muscles and from deep transverse fascia of the leg.
Flexor Digitorum Longus:	Proximally, the flexor digitorum longus has fibers that arise from the fascia that overlies the tibialis posterior.
Flexor Hallucis Longus:	Proximally, the flexor hallucis longus has fibers that arise from the interosseus membrane (as noted in the attachment section), the posterior crural intermuscular septum and the fascia that overlies the tibialis posterior.

FOOT CHAPTER

Extensor Digitorum Brevis:	Proximally, the extensor digitorum brevis has fibers that arise from the interosseus talocalcaneal ligament and the inferior extensor retinaculum. Distally, the extensor digitorum brevis attaches into the lateral side of the distal tendons of the extensor digitorum longus (as noted in the attachment section).
Extensor Hallucis Brevis:	Proximally, the extensor hallucis brevis has fibers that arise from the interosseus talocalcaneal ligament and the inferior extensor retinaculum.
Abductor Hallucis:	Proximally, the abductor hallucis attaches into the flexor retinaculum and the plantar fascia (as noted in the attachment section), and the intermuscular septum located between this muscle and the flexor digitorum brevis.
Abductor Digiti Minimi Pedis:	Proximally, the abductor digiti minimi pedis attaches into the plantar fascia (as noted in the attachment section) and the intermuscular septum located between this muscle and the flexor digitorum brevis.
Flexor Digitorum Brevis:	Proximally, the flexor digitorum brevis attaches into the plantar fascia (as noted in the attachment section) and the intermuscular septum located between it and adjacent muscles.
Quadratus Plantae:	Proximally, the quadratus plantae has fibers that arise from the long plantar ligament.
Lumbricals Pedis:	Proximally, the lumbricals pedis arise from the distal tendons of the flexor digitorum longus (as noted in the attachment section). Distally, the lumbricals pedis attach into the dorsal digital expansion of the toes (as noted in the attachment section).
Flexor Hallucis Brevis:	Proximally, the flexor hallucis brevis has fibers that arise from the middle band of the medial intermuscular septum of the foot.
Flexor Digiti Minimi Pedis:	Proximally, the flexor digiti minimi pedis has fibers that arise from the distal tendon (specifically the sheath) of the fibularis longus (as noted in the attachment section).
Adductor Hallucis:	Proximally, the oblique head of the adductor hallucis has fibers that arise from the distal tendon (specifically the sheath) of the fibularis longus (as noted in the attachment section). The transverse head has fibers that arise from the plantar metatarsophalangeal ligaments of the 3rd, 4th and 5th toes (as noted in the attachment section) and from the deep transverse metatarsal ligaments between them.

Plantar Interossei: Distally, the plantar interossei attach into the dorsal digital expansions of the toes (as noted in the attachment section).

Dorsal Interossei Pedis: Distally, the dorsal interossei pedis attach into the dorsal digital expansions of the toes (as noted in the attachment section).

PART THREE – THE UPPER EXTREMITY

SCAPULA/ARM CHAPTER

Supraspinatus: The distal tendon of the supraspinatus also attaches into the capsule of the glenohumeral joint, which is deep to it (as noted in the miscellaneous section).

Infraspinatus: The proximal attachment of the infraspinatus has fibers that arise from the deep fibers of the overlying infraspinatus fascia. The distal tendon of the infraspinatus also attaches into the capsule of the glenohumeral joint, which is deep to it (as noted in the miscellaneous section).

Teres Minor: The distal tendon of the teres minor also attaches into the capsule of the glenohumeral joint, which is deep to it (as noted in the miscellaneous section).

Subscapularis: The proximal attachment of the subscapularis has fibers that arise from adjacent intermuscular septa and an aponeurosis that covers and separates the subscapularis from the teres major and the long head of the triceps brachii. The distal tendon of the subscapularis also attaches into the capsule of the glenohumeral joint, which is deep to it (as noted in the miscellaneous section).

Teres Major: The proximal attachment of the teres major has fibers that arise from a fibrous septum that separates it from the teres minor and the infraspinatus.

Deltoid: The distal tendon of the deltoid gives off fibers that attach into the deep brachial fascia of the arm and reach to the deep antebrachial fascia of the forearm.

Biceps Brachii: The bicipital aponeurosis attaches into the deep antebrachial fascia of the forearm, overlying the common flexor tendon (as noted in the attachment section).

Brachialis: The proximal attachment of the brachialis also arises from the medial and lateral intermuscular septa of the arm.

Triceps Brachii: The long head of the triceps brachii attaches proximally into the capsule of the glenohumeral joint, which is deep to it. The lateral head of the triceps brachii attaches proximally into the lateral intermuscular septum of the arm. The medial head of the triceps brachii attaches proximally into the medial intermuscular septum of the arm and blends with the deep antebrachial fascia distally.

FOREARM CHAPTER

Pronator Teres: Proximally, the humeral head of the pronator teres has fibers that arise from adjacent intermuscular septa and the deep antebrachial fascia.

Flexor Carpi Radialis: Proximally, the flexor carpi radialis has fibers that arise from adjacent intermuscular septa and the deep antebrachial fascia.

Palmaris Longus: Proximally, the palmaris longus has fibers that arise from adjacent intermuscular septa and the deep antebrachial fascia. Distally, the palmaris longus attaches into the palmar aponeurosis and the flexor retinaculum (as noted in the attachment section).

Flexor Carpi Ulnaris: Proximally, the ulnar head of the flexor carpi ulnaris has fibers that arise from adjacent intermuscular septa. Distally, the flexor carpi ulnaris may blend into the flexor retinaculum.

Flexor Digitorum Superficialis: Proximally, the humeral head of the flexor digitorum superficialis has fibers that arise from the ulnar collateral ligament of the elbow and adjacent intermuscular septa.

Brachioradialis: Proximally, the brachioradialis has fibers that arise from the lateral intermuscular septum of the arm.

Flexor Digitorum Profundus: Proximally, the flexor digitorum profundus attaches into the interosseus membrane (as noted in the attachment section). Proximally, the flexor digitorum profundus also has fibers that arise from an aponeurosis it shares with the flexor carpi ulnaris and the extensor carpi ulnaris.

Flexor Pollicis Longus: Proximally, the flexor pollicis longus attaches into the interosseus membrane (as noted in the attachment section).

Pronator Quadratus: The pronator quadratus has fibers that attach into a thick aponeurosis near its ulnar attachment.

Extensor Carpi Radialis Longus: Proximally, the extensor carpi radialis longus has fibers that arise from the lateral intermuscular septum of the arm.

Extensor Carpi Radialis Brevis: Proximally, the extensor carpi radialis brevis has fibers that arise from the radial collateral ligament of the elbow joint, a thick aponeurosis that covers it and adjacent intermuscular septa.

Extensor Digitorum: Proximally, the extensor digitorum has fibers that arise from adjacent intermuscular septa and the deep antebrachial fascia. Distally, the attachment of the extensor digitorum onto the fingers broadens out to create the dorsal digital expansion (as noted in the attachment section).

Extensor Digiti Minimi: Proximally, the extensor digiti minimi has fibers that arise from adjacent intermuscular septa. Distally, the extensor digiti minimi attaches into the ulnar side of the distal tendon of the extensor digitorum that goes to the little finger (as noted in the attachment section).

Extensor Carpi Ulnaris: Proximally, the extensor carpi ulnaris has fibers that arise from deep antebrachial fascia and an aponeurosis it shares with the flexor carpi ulnaris and the flexor digitorum profundus.

Supinator: Proximally, the supinator has fibers that arise from the annular ligament, the radial collateral ligament of the elbow and an aponeurosis that covers it.

Abductor Pollicis Longus: Proximally, the abductor pollicis longus attaches into the interosseus membrane (as noted in the attachment section).

Extensor Pollicis Brevis: Proximally, the extensor pollicis brevis attaches into the interosseus membrane (as noted in the attachment section).

Extensor Pollicis Longus: Proximally, the extensor pollicis longus attaches into the interosseus membrane (as noted in the attachment section). Distally, the attachment of the extensor pollicis longus onto the thumb broadens out to create the dorsal digital expansion of the thumb (as noted in the attachment section).

Extensor Indicis: Proximally, the extensor indicis attaches into the interosseus membrane (as noted in the attachment section). Distally, the extensor indicis attaches into the ulnar side of the distal tendon of the extensor digitorum that goes to the index finger (as noted in the attachment section).

HAND CHAPTER

Palmaris Brevis: Laterally, the palmaris brevis attaches into the flexor retinaculum and the palmar aponeurosis. Medially, the palmaris brevis attaches into the dermis of the ulnar border of the hand (as noted in the attachment section).

Abductor Pollicis Brevis:	Proximally, the abductor pollicis brevis attaches into the flexor retinaculum (as noted in the attachment section) and into the tendon of the abductor pollicis longus. Distally, the abductor pollicis brevis attaches into the dorsal digital expansion of the thumb (as noted in the attachment section).
Flexor Pollicis Brevis:	Proximally, the flexor pollicis brevis attaches into the flexor retinaculum (as noted in the attachment section).
Opponens Pollicis:	Proximally, the opponens pollicis attaches into the flexor retinaculum (as noted in the attachment section).
Abductor Digiti Minimi Manus:	Proximally, the abductor digiti minimi manus attaches into the distal tendon of the flexor carpi ulnaris (as noted in the attachment section) and the pisohamate ligament. Distally, the abductor digiti minimi attaches into the dorsal digital expansion of the little finger (as noted in the attachment section).
Flexor Digiti Minimi Manus:	Proximally, the flexor digiti minimi manus attaches into the flexor retinaculum (as noted in the attachment section).
Opponens Digiti Minimi:	Proximally, the opponens digiti minimi attaches into the flexor retinaculum (as noted in the attachment section).
Adductor Pollicis:	Medially, the adductor pollicis attaches into the carpal palmar ligaments and the sheath of the tendon of the flexor carpi radialis. Distally, the adductor pollicis attaches into the dorsal digital expansion of the thumb (as noted in the attachment section).
Lumbricals Manus:	Proximally, the lumbricals manus arise from the distal tendons of the flexor digitorum profundus (as noted in the attachment section). Distally, the lumbricals manus attach into the dorsal digital expansion of the fingers (as noted in the attachment section).
Palmar Interossei:	Distally, the palmar interossei attach into the dorsal digital expansion of the fingers (as noted in the attachment section).
Dorsal Interossei Manus:	Distally, the dorsal interossei manus attach into the dorsal digital expansion of the fingers (as noted in the attachment section). The first dorsal interosseus manus also has fibers that attach into the capsule of the 2nd metacarpophalangeal joint.

APPENDIX F – OTHER SKELETAL MUSCLES OF THE BODY

I. OTHER MUSCLES OF THE ABDOMEN

Below are two muscles of the abdomen that are not considered separately in the trunk chapter of this manual.

Cremaster: The cremaster is developed and present in males only. It attaches from the inguinal ligament down to the pubic bone. Along the way, its fibers drop down to attach into the spermatic cord that connects with the testes. When the cremaster contracts, it pulls the testes superiorly toward the abdomen, thus regulating the temperature of the testes. Although the cremaster muscle is striated, it is usually not under voluntary control. The cremaster is innervated by a branch of the genitofemoral nerve.

Pyramidalis: The pyramidalis is a small muscle that attaches from the anterior pubic bone inferiorly, to the linea alba superiorly (approximately midway between the umbilicus and the pubis). The pyramidalis is located superficially to the rectus abdominis muscle and within the rectus sheath. This muscle is broad inferiorly and pointed superiorly. It is shaped like a pyramid, hence its name. When the pyramidalis contracts, it exerts a compressive force upon the abdomen. (Compression against the abdomen plays an important role in expiration, expulsion of abdominal contents during vomiting and expulsion of feces from the intestines and urine from the bladder.) However, given its small size, the pyramidalis is considered to be functionally unimportant. The pyramidalis is variable and often absent. The pyramidalis is innervated by the subcostal nerve, which is the ventral ramus of T12.

ANTERIOR VIEWS OF THE OTHER MUSCLES OF THE ABDOMEN

SUPERIOR

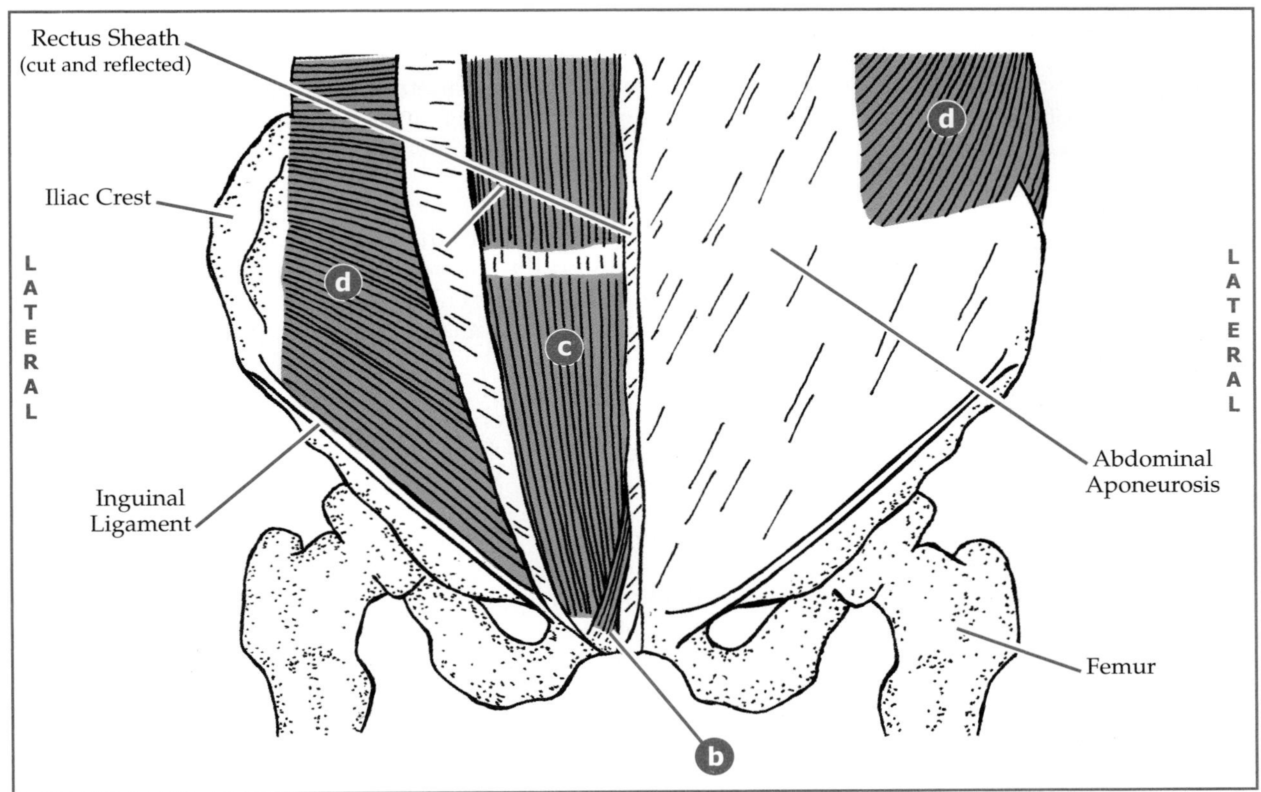

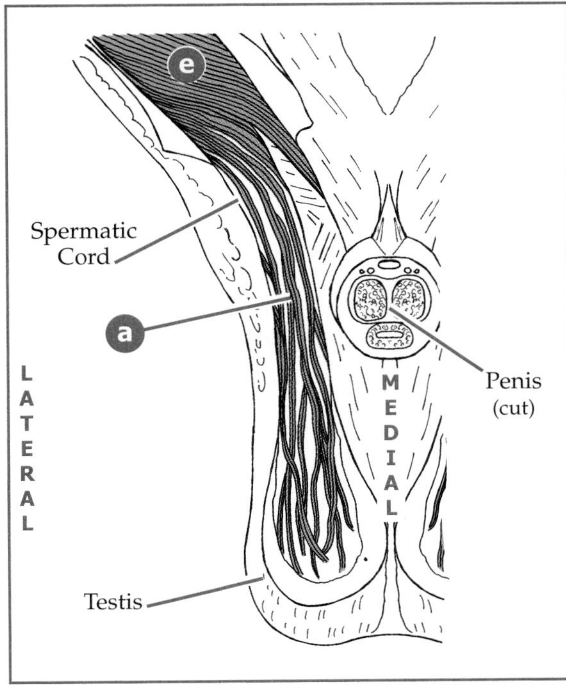

a. **Cremaster**
b. **Pyramidalis**
c. Rectus Abdominis
d. External Abdominal Oblique
e. Internal Abdominal Oblique

INFERIOR

II. MUSCLES OF THE PERINEUM

The perineum (the floor of the pelvis) is the region of the body that is bounded by the genitals anteriorly, the anus posteriorly, and the thighs laterally. All the muscles of the perineum are innervated by branches of either the pudendal nerve or branches of the pudendal plexus.

Levator Ani: The levator ani is a broad flat muscle located in the perineum, surrounding the anus. Contraction of the levator ani elevates the perineum around the anus and constricts the anus, thus stopping defecation from occurring. This muscle must relax to permit expulsion of fecal matter from the colon.

Coccygeus: The coccygeus is a flat triangular muscle that lies next to the levator ani. The coccygeus attaches to the ischial spine, sacrospinous ligament, coccyx and the sacrum. The function of the coccygeus is the same as the levator ani; the cocccygeus elevates the perineum around the anus and constricts the anus, thus stopping defecation from occurring. This muscle must relax to permit expulsion of fecal matter from the colon.

External Anal Sphincter: The external anal sphincter has an external and an internal part. It surrounds the most inferior part of the anus. Contraction of this muscle closes the anus to stop defecation from occurring.

Bulbospongiosus: The bulbospongiosus is a midline muscle located anterior to the rectum. In the male, the bulbospongiosus is primarily concerned with emptying the urethra at the end of urination and also assists with penile erection. In the female, the bulbospongiosus is primarily concerned with constriction of the vaginal orifice and assists erection of the clitoris.

Ischiocavernosus: In the male, the ischiocavernosus attaches to the underside of the penis and is primarily concerned with assisting penile erection. In the female, the ischiocavernosus attaches to the clitoris and is concerned with assisting clitoral erection.

Superficial and Deep Transverse Perinei: These muscles run transversely across the perineum. Their action is to pull on and thereby tether, i.e., fixate, the central tendon of the perineum. (The central tendon of the perineum, also known as the *perineal body*, is a fibromuscular node in the midline of the perineum. Other muscles attach into this structure; therefore, if it is fixated, the pull of these other muscles becomes more efficient.) Since the deep transverse perineal muscle surrounds the vagina, it can also assist in closing down the vagina.

Sphincter Urethrae: The sphincter urethrae surrounds the proximal urethra and the neck of the bladder. When it contracts, it prohibits the passage of urine (or sperm), thus aiding in the continence of urine (or sperm). The sphincter urethrae must be relaxed during urination. It may be contracted to expel the final drops of urine (or sperm).

Compressor Urethrae: The compressor urethra is only present in females. It is similar to the sphincter urethrae in that it surrounds the urethra. Therefore, its function is the same as the sphincter urethrae; it acts to prohibit the passage of urine through the urethra or to expel the last few drops of urine from the urethra.

Sphincter Urethrovaginalis: The sphincter urethrovaginalis is only present in females. It surrounds the vagina as well as the urethra. Its contraction aids in closing down the vagina as well as continence of urine.

VIEWS OF THE MUSCLES OF THE PERINEUM

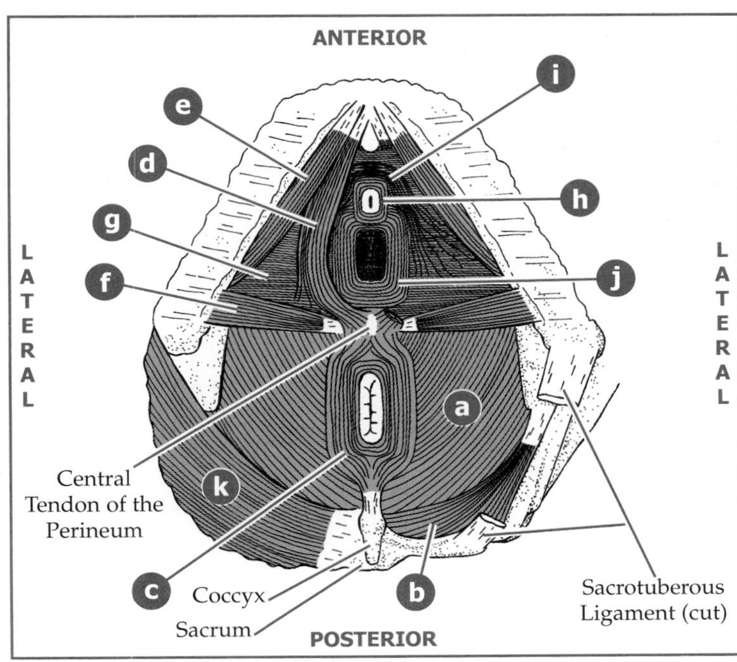

Superior View of the Female Perineum

a. **Levator Ani**
b. **Coccygeus**
c. **External Anal Sphincter**
d. **Bulbospongiosus**
e. **Ischiocavernosus**
f. **Superficial Transverse Perineal**
g. **Deep Transverse Perineal**
h. **Sphincter Urethrae**
i. **Compressor Urethrae**
j. **Sphincter Urethrovaginalis**
k. Gluteus Maximus

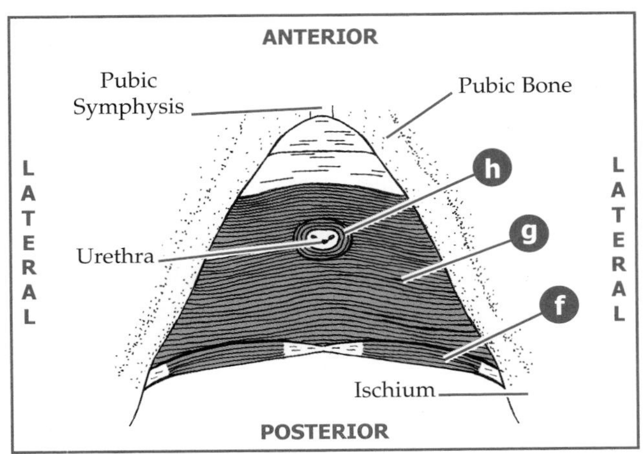

Superior View of the Male Perineum (Deep)

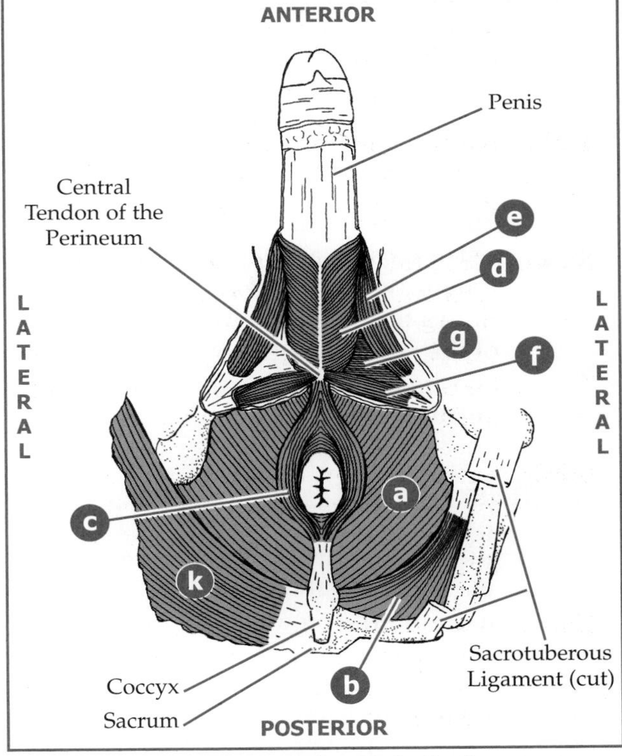

Superior View of the Male Perineum

III. MUSCLES OF THE TONGUE

The tongue is a structure whose surface is covered with a mucous membrane. However, the body of the tongue is composed primarily of skeletal muscle tissue.

There are nine muscles of the tongue, divisible into extrinsic and intrinsic muscle groups. The extrinsic muscles connect the tongue to neighboring structures, whereas the intrinsic muscles are wholly located within the tongue. All the extrinsic and intrinsic muscles of the tongue are innervated by the hypoglossal nerve (CN XII) except for the palatoglossus, which is innervated by the pharyngeal plexus.

EXTRINSIC MUSCLES OF THE TONGUE:

Genioglossus: The genioglossus attaches anteriorly to the internal surface of the mandible. Its fibers then run posteriorly to attach into the hyoid bone and superiorly to attach into the center of the tongue. When the genioglossus contracts, it depresses the tongue, especially the center of the tongue, making the dorsum of the tongue concave from side to side. Furthermore, the fibers of the genioglossus can protract the tongue and its anterior fibers can retract the tongue.

Hyoglossus: The hyoglossus is a thin, quadrilateral-shaped muscle that attaches from the hyoid bone inferiorly to attach into the sides of the tongue. When the hyoglossus contracts, it depresses the tongue. There are some fibers of the hyoglossus that are separated from the rest of the muscle by the genioglossus. These fibers are often given a separate name, the *chondroglossus*. The chondroglossus has the same action as the rest of the hyoglossus, depression of the tongue.

Styloglossus: The styloglossus attaches from the styloid process of the temporal bone posteriorly and superiorly to the tongue. When the styloglossus contracts, it retracts and elevates the tongue.

Palatoglossus: The palatoglossus, along with its overlying mucosa, forms the palatoglossal arch. The palatoglossus attaches from the soft palate superiorly to the tongue inferiorly. With regard to the tongue, when the palatoglossus contracts, it elevates the posterior tongue. The palatoglossus also draws the palatoglossal arch toward the opposite-sided palatoglossal arch, resulting in narrowing of the fauces (see the palatoglossus in the "Muscles of the Palate" section on page 736). Given its attachment into the palate, the palatoglossus is also considered to be a muscle of the palate. The palatoglossus is also known as the *glossopalatinus*.

INTRINSIC MUSCLES OF THE TONGUE:

The tongue is primarily made up of muscular tissue, in particular the following four intrinsic muscles of the tongue. Each of these four intrinsic muscles is found bilaterally. The intrinsic muscles of the tongue, acting alone or in combination with each other, give the tongue its shape and highly varied mobility, which is necessary for the action of speech and its digestive function.

Superior Longitudinal Muscle: The superior longitudinal muscle of the tongue runs from anterior to posterior in the superior aspect of the tongue. When the superior longitudinal muscle contracts, it shortens the tongue and elevates the apex (tip) and the sides of the tongue, making the dorsum of the tongue concave.

Inferior Longitudinal Muscle: The inferior longitudinal muscle of the tongue runs from anterior to posterior in the inferior aspect of the tongue. The inferior longitudinal muscle also attaches into the hyoid bone, thus anchoring the tongue to bone. When the inferior longitudinal muscle contracts, it shortens the tongue and depresses the apex (tip) and the sides of the tongue, making the dorsum of the tongue concave.

Transverse Muscle: The transverse muscle of the tongue runs transversely (left to right) across the tongue. When the transverse muscle contracts, it narrows and elongates the tongue.

Vertical Muscle: The vertical muscle of the tongue runs vertically (superior to inferior) within the tongue. When the vertical muscle contracts, it flattens and widens the tongue.

VIEWS OF THE MUSCLES OF THE TONGUE

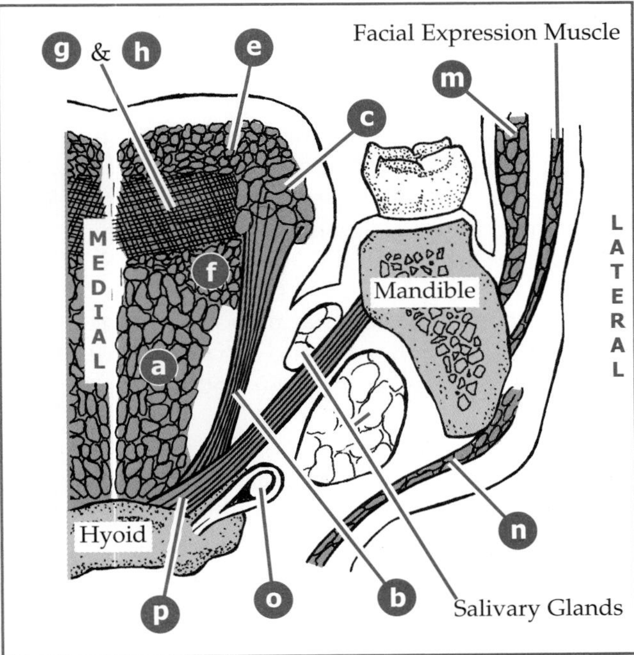

Anterior View (Frontal Plane Section) of the Tongue

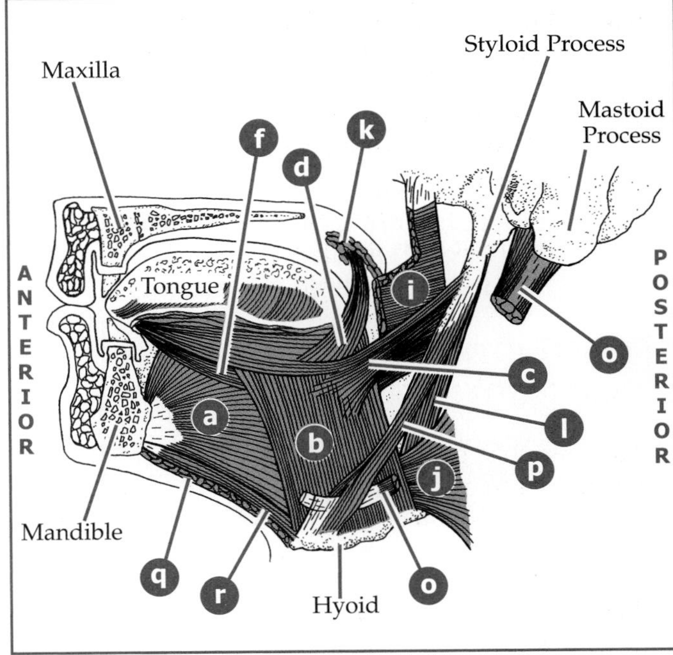

Lateral View (Sagittal Plane Section) of the Tongue

a. **Genioglossus**
b. **Hyoglossus**
c. **Styloglossus**
d. **Palatoglossus**
e. **Superior Longitudinal Muscle**
f. **Inferior Longitudinal Muscle**
g. **Transverse Muscle**
h. **Vertical Muscle**
i. Superior Pharyngeal Constrictor
j. Middle Pharyngeal Constrictor
k. Palatopharyngeus
l. Stylopharyngeus
m. Buccinator
n. Platysma
o. Digastric
p. Stylohyoid
q. Mylohyoid
r. Geniohyoid

IV. MUSCLES OF THE PALATE

The palate is the roof of the oral cavity. The palate is divisible into two regions: the hard palate anteriorly (formed by the maxillary bones and the palatine bones) and the soft palate posteriorly. The soft palate is a flap of soft tissue located between the oropharynx and the nasopharynx. The muscles of the palate are associated with the soft palate. There are five muscles of the palate, all of which are innervated by the pharyngeal plexus except the tensor veli palatini, which is innervated by the trigeminal nerve (CN V).

Levator Veli Palatini: The levator veli palatini is a small cylindrical muscle that attaches from the temporal bone superiorly and posteriorly, to the posterior aspect of the soft palate. When the levator veli palatini contracts, it elevates and retracts (and makes rigid) the posterior aspect of the soft palate. These actions are important during swallowing because in so doing, the levator veli palatini causes the soft palate to close off the oropharynx from the nasopharynx so that food is forced inferiorly toward the esophagus.

Tensor Veli Palatini: The tensor veli palatini is a thin, triangular-shaped muscle that attaches from the sphenoid bone superiorly and laterally, to the anterior aspect of the soft palate. When the tensor veli palatini contracts, it tenses the soft palate, causing the auditory tube (also known as the eustachian tube) to open. This action usually occurs during swallowing and yawning and is important because it allows the pressure in the middle ear cavity to equalize with the outside air pressure (barometric pressure). Note: the increased rigidity of the soft palate can help with its closure of the oropharynx from the nasopharynx during swallowing (see the levator veli palatini above).

Musculus Uvulae: The musculus uvulae is a small muscle that attaches from the palatine bone superiorly and posteriorly, to the uvula. When the musculus uvulae contracts, it elevates and retracts the uvula. This action is important in aiding the soft palate to close the oropharynx from the nasopharynx during swallowing (see the levator veli palatini).

Palatoglossus: The palatoglossus, along with its overlying mucosa, forms the palatoglossal arch. The palatoglossus attaches from the tongue inferiorly to the soft palate superiorly. When the palatoglossus contracts, it draws the palatoglossal arch toward the opposite-sided palatoglossal arch. This action results in narrowing the fauces (the opening from the oral cavity into the oropharynx), which is important during chewing. The palatoglossus also elevates the tongue, which further aids in narrowing the fauces. The palatoglossus is also considered to be a muscle of the tongue, given its attachment into the tongue and its ability to move it. The palatoglossus is also known as the *glossopalatinus*.

Palatopharyngeus: The palatopharyngeus, along with its overlying mucosa, forms the palatopharyngeal arch. The palatopharyngeus has two layers, an anterior layer and a posterior layer, that arise from the soft palate and are separated from each other by the levator veli palatini. These two layers unite in the posterolateral soft palate and then run through the wall of the pharynx, eventually attaching into the thyroid cartilage. When the palatopharyngeus contracts, it protracts the palatopharyngeal arch and draws the palatopharyngeal arch toward the opposite-sided palatopharyngeal arch. This movement of the palatopharyngeal arch results in narrowing the fauces (the opening from the oral cavity into the oropharynx), which is important during chewing. The palatopharyngeus also elevates the pharynx, an action that is important during swallowing. The palatopharyngeus is also considered to be a muscle of the pharynx, given its attachment into the pharynx and its ability to move the pharynx.

VIEW OF THE MUSCLES OF THE PALATE

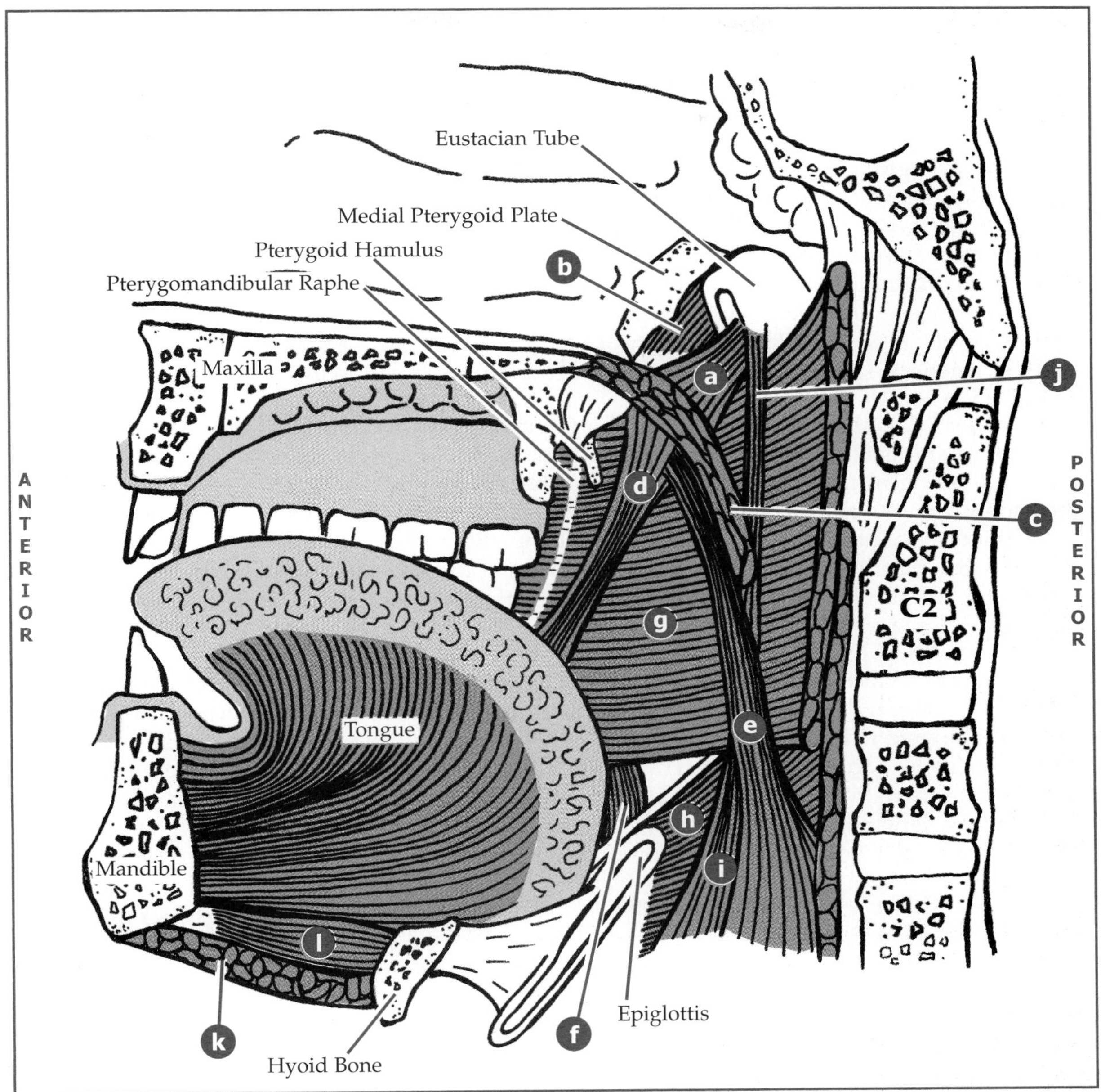

Medial View (Sagittal Plane Section) of the Muscles of the Palate

a. **Levator Veli Palatini**	g. Superior Pharyngeal Constrictor
b. **Tensor Veli Palatini**	h. Middle Pharyngeal Constrictor
c. **Musculusus Uvulae**	i. Stylopharyngeus
d. **Palatoglossus**	j. Salpingopharyngeus
e. **Palatopharyngeus**	k. Mylohyoid
f. Hyoglossus	l. Geniohyoid

V. MUSCLES OF THE PHARYNX

The pharynx (or in lay terms, the throat) is a musculomembranous tube that extends from the cranium all the way to the sixth cervical vertebra. The pharynx is divided into three sections: the nasopharynx, the oropharynx and the laryngopharynx. There are six muscles of the pharynx, all of which are innervated by the pharyngeal plexus except the stylopharyngeus, which is innervated by the glossopharyngeal nerve (CN IX).

Superior Pharyngeal Constrictor: The superior pharyngeal constrictor is located directly superior to the middle pharyngeal constrictor. The superior pharyngeal constrictor is a quadrilateral-shaped sheet of muscle that is considered to have four parts: the pterygopharyngeal part (named for its attachment onto the pterygoid portion of the sphenoid bone), the buccopharyngeal part (named for its attachment into the pterygomandibular raphe of the cheek), the mylopharyngeal part (named for its attachment onto the mylohyoid line of the mandible) and the glossopharyngeal part (named for its attachment into the lateral tongue). All these parts run posteriorly to attach into the posterior median raphe (posterior midline) of the pharynx. When the superior pharyngeal constrictor contracts, it constricts the pharynx, creating a general sphincteric and peristaltic action during swallowing.

Middle Pharyngeal Constrictor: The middle pharyngeal constrictor is located directly inferior to the superior pharyngeal constrictor and directly superior to the inferior pharyngeal constrictor. The middle pharyngeal constrictor is a fan-shaped sheet of muscle that is considered to have two parts: the chondropharyngeal part (attaching to the hyoid bone and the stylohyoid ligament) and the ceratopharyngeal part (attaching to the hyoid bone). Both of these parts run posteriorly to attach into the posterior median raphe (posterior midline) of the pharynx. When the middle pharyngeal constrictor contracts, it constricts the pharynx, creating a general sphincteric and peristaltic action during swallowing.

Inferior Pharyngeal Constrictor: The inferior pharyngeal constrictor is located directly inferior to the middle pharyngeal constrictor. The inferior pharyngeal constrictor is a fan-shaped sheet of muscle that is considered to have two parts: the cricopharyngeal part (named for its attachment onto the cricoid cartilage) and the thyropharyngeal part (named for its attachment onto the thyroid cartilage). Both of these parts run posteriorly to attach into the posterior median raphe (posterior midline) of the pharynx. When the inferior pharyngeal constrictor contracts, it constricts the pharynx, creating a general sphincteric and peristaltic action during swallowing.

Stylopharyngeus: The stylopharyngeus is a long, slender muscle that attaches from the styloid process of the temporal bone to the lateral wall of the pharynx. When it contracts, it elevates the pharynx during speech and swallowing.

Salpingopharyngeus: The salpingopharyngeus is a long, slender muscle. The salpingopharyngeus attaches into the cartilage of the auditory tube (also known as the *eustachian tube*) superiorly. It then runs inferiorly and blends into the palatopharyngeus. When the salpingopharyngeus contracts, it elevates the pharynx. This action is important during swallowing.

Palatopharyngeus: The palatopharyngeus, along with its overlying mucosa, forms the palatopharyngeal arch. The palatopharyngeus has two layers, an anterior layer and a posterior layer, that arise from the soft palate and are separated from each other by the levator veli palatini. These two layers unite in the posterolateral soft palate and then run through the wall of the pharynx, eventually attaching into the thyroid cartilage. When the palatopharyngeus contracts, it elevates the pharynx, an action important during swallowing. The palatopharyngeus also protracts the palatopharyngeal arch and draws the palatopharyngeal arch toward the opposite-sided palatopharyngeal arch. This movement of the palatopharyngeal arch results in narrowing the fauces (the fauces is the opening from the oral cavity into the oropharynx), which is important during chewing. Given its attachment into the palate, the palatopharyngeus is also considered to be a muscle of the palate.

VIEW OF THE MUSCLES OF THE PHARYNX

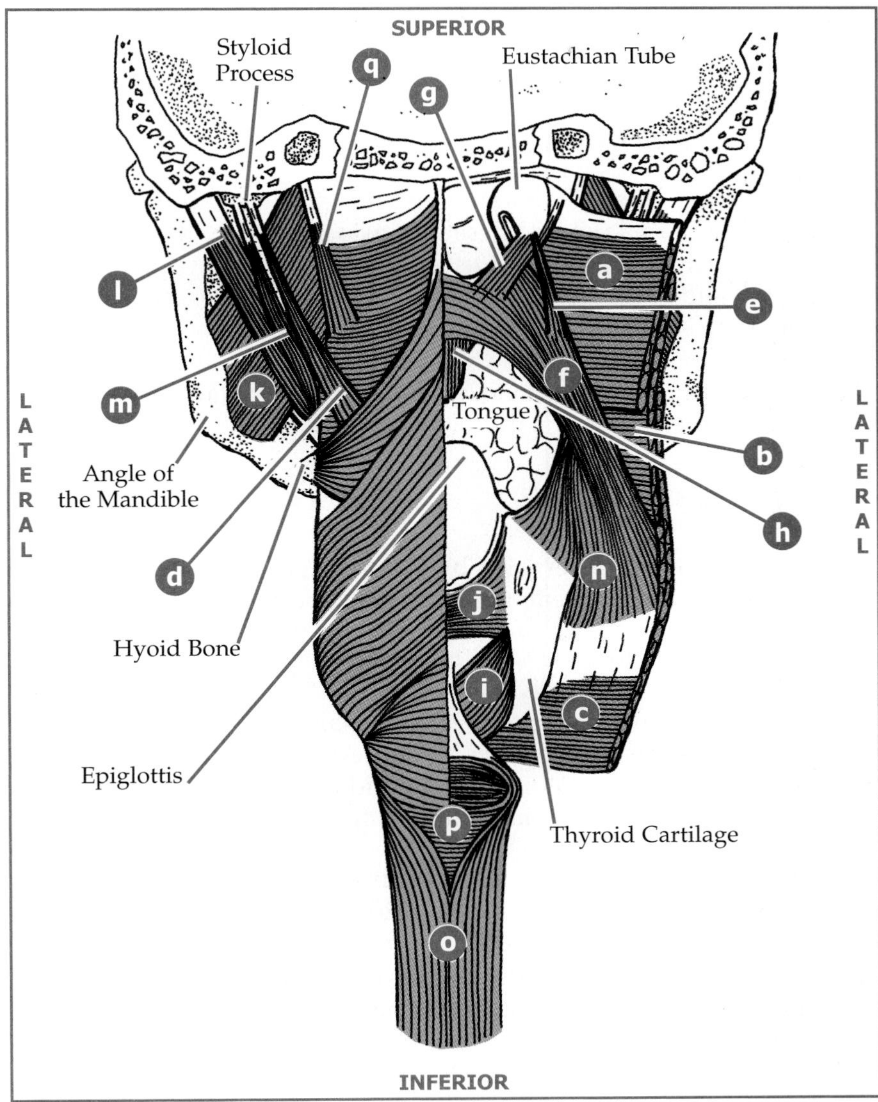

Posterior View of the Pharynx (opened up on the right side)

a. **Superior Pharyngeal Constrictor**
b. **Middle Pharyngeal Constrictor**
c. **Inferior Pharyngeal Constrictor**
d. **Stylopharyngeus**
e. **Salpingopharyngeus**
f. **Palatopharyngeus**
g. Levator Veli Palatini
h. Musculus Uvulae
i. Posterior Cricoarytenoid
j. Transverse and Oblique Arytenoids
k. Medial Pterygoid
l. Digastric
m. Stylohyoid
n. Longitudinal Pharyngeal Muscle
o. Longitudinal Esophageal Muscle
p. Circular Esophageal Muscle
q. Accessory Muscle Bundle from Temporal Bone

VI. MUSCLES OF THE LARYNX

The larynx is an enlargement of the airway between the pharynx and the trachea. The larynx contains the thyroid, cricoid, arytenoid and corniculate cartilages, as well as the vocal folds of tissue responsible for phonation (the process of making sounds). The larynx also contains a number of extrinsic and intrinsic muscles. The extrinsic muscles connect the larynx to neighboring structures whereas the intrinsic muscles are wholly located within the larynx.

EXTRINSIC MUSCLES OF THE LARYNX:

The extrinsic muscles, as a group, all attach into the thyroid cartilage and move the larynx superiorly and inferiorly during phonation and swallowing. These extrinsic muscles of the larynx have been considered elsewhere in this book. The extrinsic laryngeal muscles are the: sternothyroid and the thyrohyoid of the hyoid muscle group (see pages 149 and 151); the thyropharyngeus and the cricopharyngeus of the inferior pharyngeal constrictor, and the stylopharyngeus, salpingopharyngeus and the palatopharyngeus, all of the pharyngeal muscle group (see pages 738-9). Other muscles that do not attach directly into the thyroid cartilage, but attach, instead, into the hyoid bone, may also move the larynx indirectly due to the hyoid's strong connective tissue attachments into the thyroid cartilage.

INTRINSIC MUSCLES OF THE LARYNX:

The intrinsic muscles of the larynx are innervated by the recurrent laryngeal nerve except for the cricothyroid, which is innervated by the external laryngeal branch of the superior laryngeal nerve.

Cricothyroid: The cricothyroid has two parts, an oblique part and a straight part, that attach to the cricoid cartilage inferiorly and run posteriorly, superiorly and laterally. However, the oblique part runs primarily posteriorly and the straight part runs primarily superiorly. When the cricoid cartilage is fixed and the cricothyroid contracts, it depresses and anteriorly tilts the thyroid cartilage; this action tenses the vocal cords during phonation. When the thyroid cartilage is fixed and the cricothyroid contracts, it elevates and posteriorly tilts the cricoid cartilage; this action is important during swallowing.

Posterior Cricoarytenoid: The posterior cricoarytenoids run from the cricoid cartilage inferiorly to the arytenoid cartilages superiorly on the posterior side. (More specifically, the posterior cricoarytenoids attach from the posterior cricoid cartilage inferiorly, to the arytenoid cartilages anteriorly, superiorly and laterally.) When the posterior cricoarytenoids contract, they pull the arytenoid cartilages posteriorly, thereby stretching and tensing the vocal cords. The posterior cricoarytenoids can also rotate the arytenoid cartilages in such a manner that the rima glottides (the opening between the vocal folds) opens. Both of these actions are important during phonation.

Lateral Cricoarytenoid: The lateral cricoarytenoids run from the cricoid cartilage inferiorly to the arytenoid cartilages superiorly on the lateral side. (More specifically, the lateral cricoarytenoids attach from the lateral cricoid cartilage inferiorly, to the arytenoid cartilages posteriorly and superiorly.) When the lateral arytenoids contract, they rotate the arytenoid cartilages in such a manner that the rima glottides (the opening between the vocal folds) closes. This action is important during phonation.

Transverse Arytenoid: The transverse arytenoid is a single unpaired muscle that runs transversely across the posterior larynx from one arytenoid cartilage to the other. When the transverse arytenoid contracts, it pulls the vocal folds closer toward each other, thereby decreasing the size of the rima glottides (the opening between the vocal folds). This action is important during phonation.

Oblique Arytenoid: The oblique arytenoids are slender muscles that cross each other and lie superficial to the transverse arytenoid muscle at the posterior thyroid cartilage. The aryepiglottic muscles are actually the most anterior continuation of the oblique arytenoid muscles. When the oblique arytenoids contract, they pull the vocal folds closer toward each other, thereby decreasing the size of the rima glottides (the opening between the vocal folds). This action is important during phonation.

Thyroarytenoid: The thyroarytenoid muscles lie medial to the lateral walls of the thyroid cartilage, parallel to the vocal folds. The thyroarytenoid muscles attach to the thyroid cartilage anteriorly and run posteriorly (and also superolaterally) to attach to the arytenoid cartilages. The most inferior and deeper fibers of the thyroarytenoids are considered to be the vocalis muscles. Other fibers of the thyroarytenoids continue into the epiglottis; these fibers are considered to be the thyroepiglottis muscles. Sometimes small muscles, the superior thyroarytenoids, lying on the lateral surface of the thyroarytenoids are present. When the thyroarytenoids contract, they pull the arytenoid cartilages anteriorly toward the thyroid cartilage, thereby shortening and relaxing the vocal folds. The thyroarytenoids also rotate the arytenoid cartilages in such a manner that the rima glottides (the opening between the vocal folds) closes. Both of these actions are important during phonation. The vocalis portions of the thyroarytenoids relax only the posterior portion of the vocal folds (with the anterior portion staying tense); this affects vocal pitch.

VIEWS OF THE MUSCLES OF LARYNX

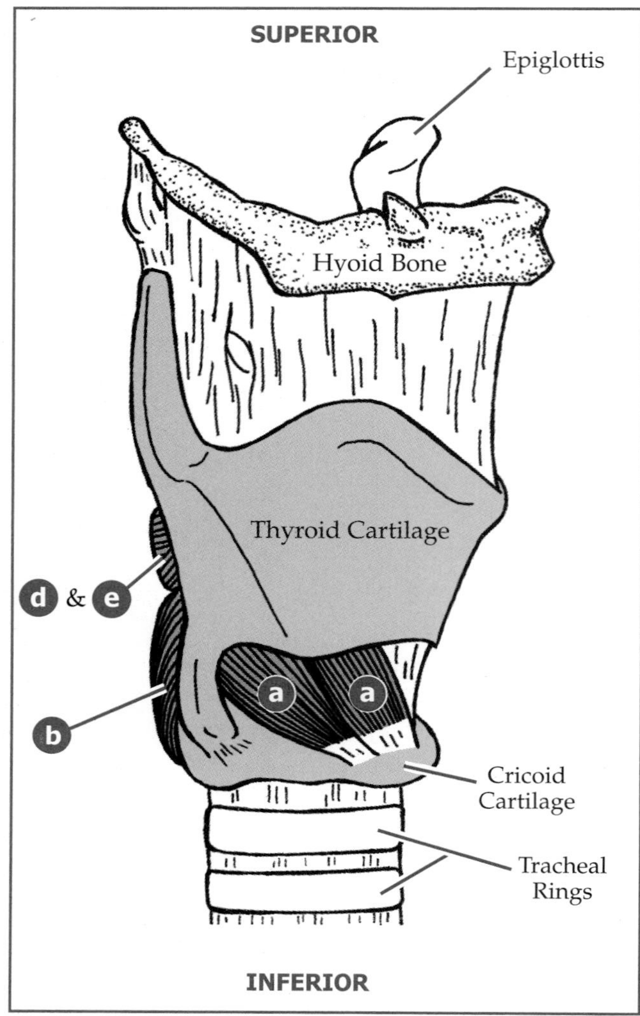

Lateral View of the Larynx

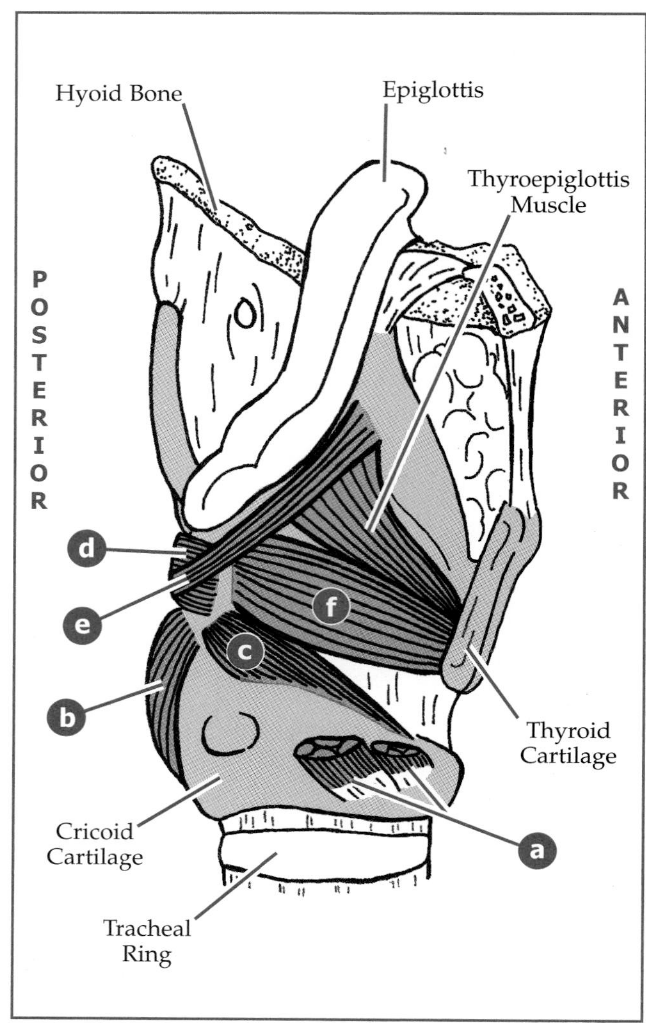

Lateral View of the Larynx (Dissected)

a. **Cricothyroid**
b. **Posterior Cricoarytenoid**
c. **Lateral Cricoarytenoid**
d. **Transverse Arytenoid**
e. **Oblique Arytenoid**
f. **Thyroarytenoid**

VIEWS OF THE MUSCLES OF THE LARYNX

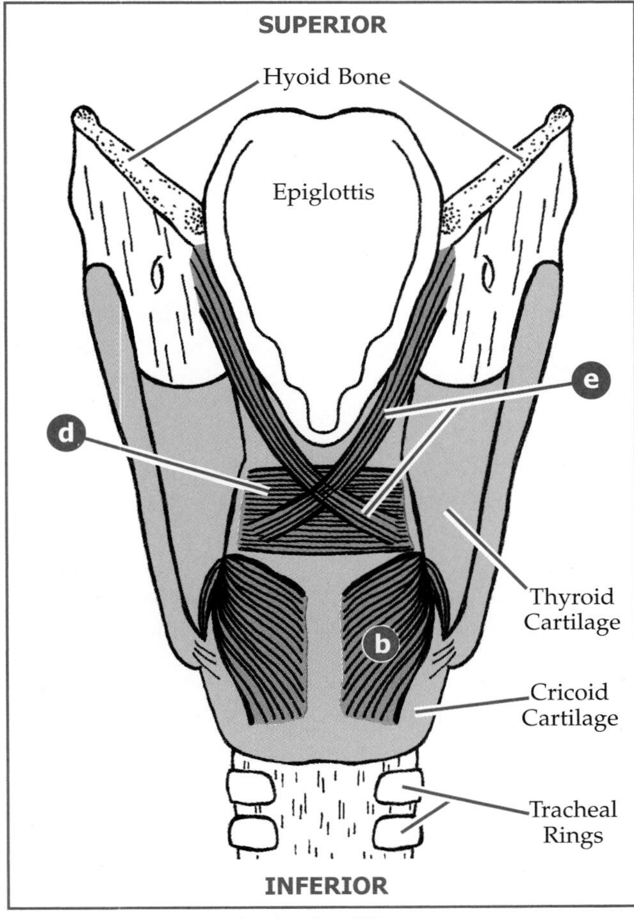

Posterior View of the Larynx

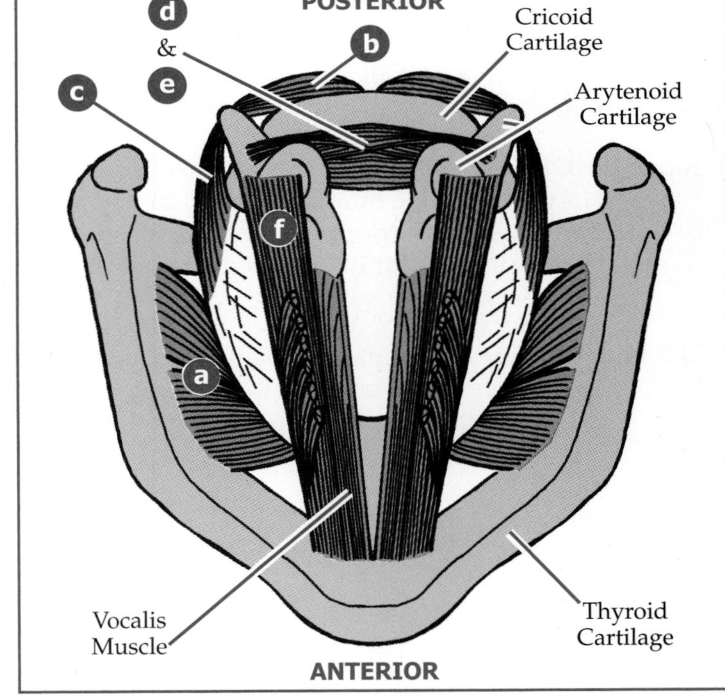

Superior View of the Larynx

a. **Cricothyroid**
b. **Posterior Cricoarytenoid**
c. **Lateral Cricoarytenoid**
d. **Transverse Arytenoid**
e. **Oblique Arytenoid**
f. **Thyroarytenoid**

VII. EXTRINSIC MUSCLES OF THE EYE

The extrinsic muscles of the eye are muscles that attach onto the eyeball. When they contract, they move the eyeball, allowing us to change where we look. There are six extrinsic muscles of the eye, all of which are innervated by the oculomotor nerve (CN III) except the lateral rectus and the superior oblique. The lateral rectus is innervated by the abducens nerve (CN VI) because this muscle abducts the eyeball; the superior oblique is innervated by the trochlear nerve (CN IV) because its tendon's line of pull is changed by going around the trochlea.

Superior Rectus: The superior rectus attaches from the common annular tendon to the anterosuperior aspect of the sclera of the eyeball, just posterior to the margin of the cornea. When the superior rectus muscle contracts, it elevates the eyeball so that you look up. The superior rectus can also adduct and medially rotate (perform intorsion) of the eyeball.

Inferior Rectus: The inferior rectus attaches from the common annular tendon to the anteroinferior aspect of the sclera of the eyeball, just posterior to the margin of the cornea. When the inferior rectus muscle contracts, it depresses the eyeball so that you look down. The inferior rectus can also adduct and laterally rotate (perform extorsion) of the eyeball.

Medial Rectus: The medial rectus attaches from the common annular tendon to the anteromedial aspect of the sclera of the eyeball, just posterior to the margin of the cornea. When the medial rectus muscle contracts, it adducts the eyeball so that you look medially.

Lateral Rectus: The lateral rectus attaches from the common annular tendon to the anterolateral aspect of the sclera of the eyeball, just posterior to the margin of the cornea. When the lateral rectus muscle contracts, it abducts the eyeball so that you look laterally.

Superior Oblique: The superior oblique begins its attachment posteriorly just superior to the optic foramen. However, its line of pull is altered by the fact that it then passes around the trochlea superior to the eyeball. The superior oblique attaches onto the posterolateral aspect of the sclera of the eyeball. When the superior oblique contracts, it depresses and abducts the eyeball so that you look down and laterally.

Inferior Oblique: The inferior oblique begins its attachment onto the floor of the orbit. It then attaches onto the posterolateral sclera of the eyeball. When the inferior oblique contracts, it elevates and abducts the eyeball so that you look up and laterally.

VIEWS OF THE EXTRINSIC MUSCLES OF THE RIGHT EYE

- a. **Superior Rectus**
- b. **Inferior Rectus**
- c. **Medial Rectus**
- d. **Lateral Rectus**
- e. **Superior Oblique**
- f. **Inferior Oblique**
- g. Levator Palpebrae Superioris

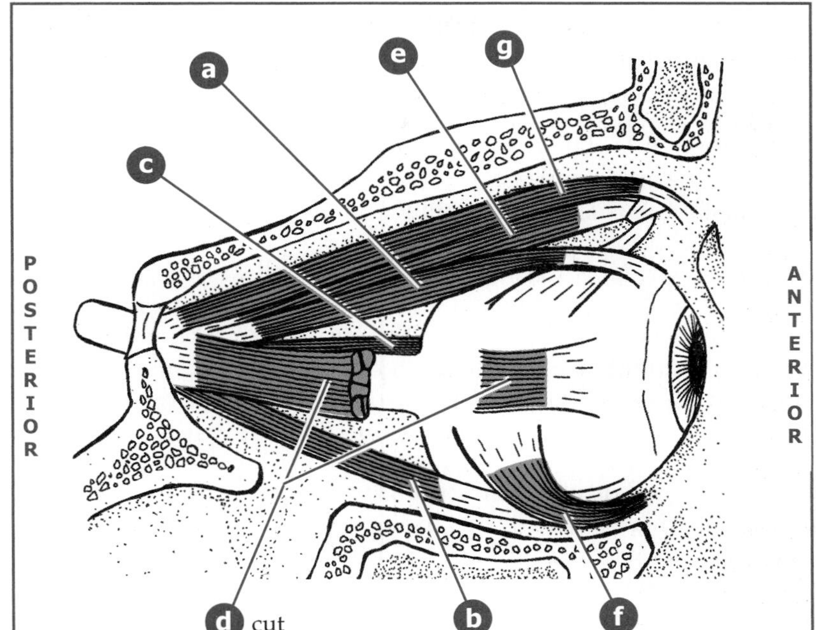

Lateral View of the Right Eye

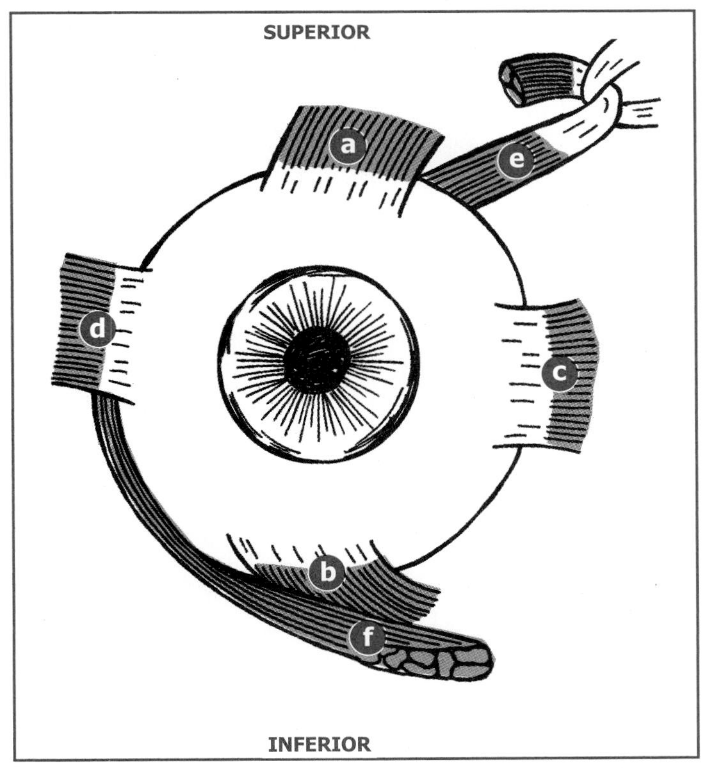

Anterior View of the Right Eye

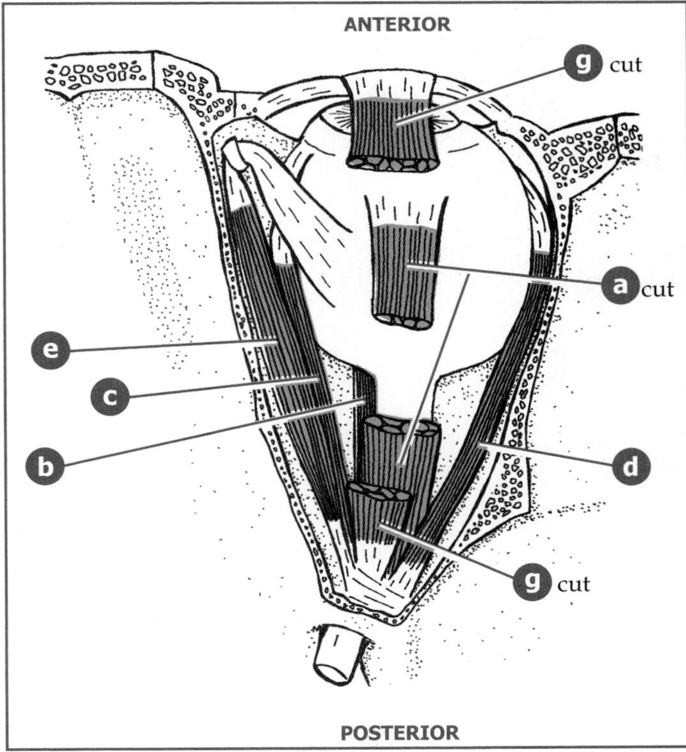

Superior View of the Right Eye

VIII. MUSCLES OF THE TYMPANIC CAVITY

The tympanic cavity is located within the temporal bone of the cranium. Located within the tympanic cavity (middle ear cavity) are three small bones (the auditory ossicles) that transmit vibrations from the tympanic membrane (the eardrum) to the inner ear.

There are also two small muscles located in the tympanic cavity. Their actions are similar in that when they contract, they function to dampen vibrations, which results in decreased transmission of sound waves from the tympanic membrane to the inner ear. The tensor tympani is innervated by a branch of the trigeminal nerve (CN V) and the stapedius is innervated by a branch of the facial nerve (CN VII).

Tensor Tympani: The tensor tympani is a very small muscle located in the middle ear cavity. The tensor tympani attaches onto the malleus, which is one of the auditory ossicles. (The other attachment of the tensor tympani is the cartilage of the eustachian tube, the temporal bone and the sphenoid bone.) In response to an intense sound, the tensor tympani contracts and pulls on the malleus, causing the tympanic membrane to tighten. When the tympanic membrane tightens, its ability to vibrate decreases. This results in decreased transmission of sound waves from the tympanic membrane to the inner ear.

Stapedius: The stapedius is a very small muscle located in the middle ear cavity. The stapedius attaches onto the stapes, which is one of the auditory ossicles. (The other attachment of the stapedius is the temporal bone.) In response to an intense sound, the stapedius contracts and pulls on the stapes, causing vibrations of the stapes to decrease. This results in decreased transmission of sound waves from the tympanic membrane to the inner ear. The stapedius is the smallest skeletal muscle in the human body. (More trivia: The stapedius also holds the distinction of being perhaps the only skeletal muscle of the human body that is under no conscious volitional control at all.)

VIEW OF THE MUSCLES OF THE TYMPANIC CAVITY

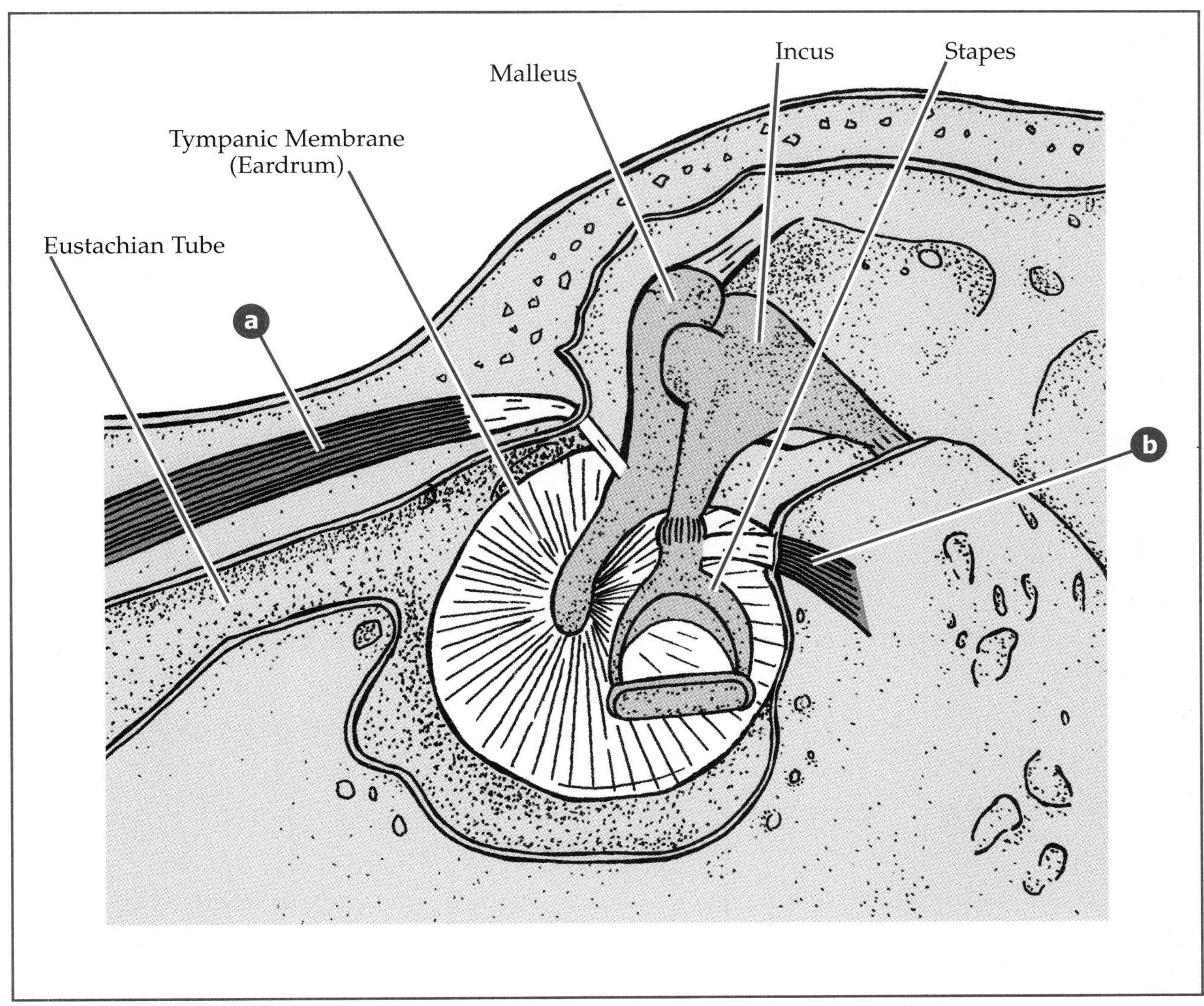

Medial View
of the Tympanic Cavity
(within the Temporal Bone)

a. Tensor Tympani
b. Stapedius

APPENDIX G – PALPATION GUIDELINES

Although a specific method for palpating each muscle has been provided, it must be emphasized that most muscles can be palpated in a number of ways. The essential information that must be known in order to palpate a muscle is the attachments and the actions of the muscle in question. The attachments must be known in order for you to know where to place your palpating fingers. If the muscle being palpated were superficial and easily distinguishable from adjacent muscles, this would be enough. However, most muscles are not so easily palpated. Therefore, we must use the knowledge of the muscle's action(s) to make the muscle contract so that it will become palpably firmer and easier to distinguish from adjacent musculature.

Sometimes, even when a muscle contracts to perform an action, it is still not readily distinguishable from adjacent musculature. Therefore, the next step would be to resist the muscle from doing its action so that it will contract harder and be even more palpable.

Certain situations exist that require one further step. When you are palpating a muscle, there may be a second muscle next to or superficial to the muscle that you want to palpate. This may interfere with your ability to palpate the desired muscle because this second muscle also contracts when the muscle that you want to palpate contracts. To eliminate this second muscle from interfering with your palpation, you need to get this second muscle to relax. What must be done is to have the client actively perform an action that is antagonistic to one of the actions of this second muscle. Doing this will trigger a neurological reflex called, *reciprocal inhibition,* that will inhibit this second muscle from contracting.

The following is a summarization of the steps that you should follow when you want to palpate a muscle:

1. Know the attachments of the muscle in question and place your palpating hand on the muscle you want to palpate.
2. If necessary, ask the client to actively perform one or more of the actions of the muscle you want to palpate to make it contract.
3. If further contraction of the muscle is necessary, resist the client from performing the action(s) of the muscle.
4. If there is a nearby or superficial second muscle that does the same action as the muscle you want to palpate, it will also contract and may interfere with your ability to palpate. To distinguish the muscle that you are palpating, have the client actively perform an action that is opposite to another action of the second muscle. This will cause a neurological reflex called *reciprocal inhibition* and will cause the second interfering muscle to relax.

Keep in mind:

1. It is usually best to palpate with the pads of the fingers because they are the most sensitive to touch.
2. Less can be more regarding palpatory pressure. Deeper pressure can be both uncomfortable for the client and can decrease your palpatory sensitivity. Ideally, your pressure should be *gentle but firm.*
3. When you ask a client to actively contract a muscle so that you can palpate it (whether you resist this contraction or not), do not have the client sustain the isometric contraction for too long. It may cause fatigue or injury to the client.
4. It is often helpful to ask the client to relax and contract repeatedly the muscle that you want to palpate. In this way, you can better feel the muscle when it first engages to contract.

5. When you resist an active movement on the part of the client, always try to place your hand that is resisting the client's joint action as close as possible to the joint that is being moved. Otherwise, the client may unconsciously contract other muscles that will make palpation of the muscle you want to palpate more difficult.

6. When you resist a client's contraction, your goal is not to actually move the client's body part, but rather to keep the client from moving the body part as he/she contracts. It is not a struggle to see who is stronger. Although a strong contraction is sometimes desired, a client will often recruit other muscles if you resist too strongly, which might cloud your ability to clearly feel the muscle you want to palpate. A milder contraction can be just as helpful and will certainly be less fatiguing and more efficient.

7. Be aware that reciprocal inhibition is not a guarantee that the muscle you are targeting to relax will relax completely. Sometimes the body's desire to contract the muscle you want to relax will overcome the reflex of reciprocal inhibition. This will especially be true if the force of contraction is greater.

8. If a client is ticklish, have the client place his/her hand over your palpating hand. This will often lessen or eliminate their ticklishness. Being ticklish is an oversensitivity due to a sense of intrusion upon one's space (you cannot tickle yourself). By having the clients's hand over your hand, that sense of intrusion is eliminated is diminished

EXAMPLE: THE HAMSTRINGS

The following is an example of the steps that one might follow to palpate the proximal attachments of the hamstring muscles.

1. **Know the attachments to place your hand:** Knowing the attachments of the hamstrings tells you to place your palpating hand just distal to the ischial tuberosity.

2. **Know the action(s) to make the muscle contract:** Since the hamstring's proximal attachment is deep to the gluteus maximus, simple palpation by step one alone will be difficult. Therefore, using your knowledge of the action(s) of the hamstrings, ask the client to actively perform extension of the thigh at the hip joint. This will cause the hamstrings to contract and be more clearly palpable.

3. **Add resistance:** If further contraction of the hamstrings is desired, you might place your non-palpating hand on the client's distal posterior thigh and add some resistance to the client's active thigh extension at the hip joint.

4. **Use Reciprocal Inhibition:** Given that the gluteus maximus is superficial to the ischial tuberosity attachment of the hamstrings and that the gluteus maximus is also an extensor of the thigh at the hip joint, the gluteus maximus will also contract with active extension of the thigh at the hip joint. This will impede your ability to palpate the hamstrings. Therefore, ask your client to actively medially rotate the thigh while extending the thigh at the hip joint. Since the gluteus maximus is a lateral rotator of the thigh at the hip joint, having the client medially rotate the thigh will cause the gluteus maximus to relax due to reciprocal inhibition. You will now be able to clearly palpate the ischial tuberosity attachment of the hamstrings!

Not every case will require all of these steps to be done. However, when a muscle is difficult to palpate, this is the order of steps you would follow to be able to palpate and clearly distinguish the muscle that you want to palpate from the adjacent muscles.

The beauty of understanding and applying these steps is that memorization of muscle palpation can be eliminated. Armed with the knowledge of a muscle's attachments and actions and these simple steps, you now have the ability to creatively figure out how to palpate any muscle in the human body! ☺

APPENDIX H – OVERVIEW OF INNERVATION

This overview is divided into three parts, the axial body, the upper extremity and the lower extremity, and is not meant to be comprehensive of the entire nervous system. Rather, it supplies the context information for innervation to skeletal muscles mentioned in the body of this book. It must be emphasized that there is variation in every anatomical system of the human body, including the nervous system. The innervation to skeletal muscles can vary from one individual to another.

THE NERVOUS SYSTEM:

Anatomically, the nervous system can be divided into two parts: the central nervous system and the peripheral nervous system. The central nervous system is made up of the brain and spinal cord (i.e., the two structures of the nervous system that are located in the "center" of the body). The peripheral nervous system is made up of all the cranial and spinal nerves that enter/exit from the central nervous system (i.e., the structures of the nervous system that are located "peripherally"). There are 12 pairs of cranial nerves that arise directly from the brain. There are 31 pairs of spinal nerves that arise from the spinal cord.

Physiologically, the nervous system is made up of nerve cells (neurons) that either carry sensory messages, motor messages or integrative messages (between sensory and motor neurons). All innervation to skeletal muscles of the body is motor innervation and arises from either cranial nerves and/or spinal nerves.

CRANIAL NERVE ORGANIZATION:

The names of the twelve pairs of cranial nerves are as follows:

- CN I - the olfactory nerve
- CN II - the optic nerve
- CN III - the oculomotor nerve
- CN IV - the trochlear nerve
- CN V - the trigeminal nerve
- CN VI - the abducens nerve
- CN VII - the facial nerve
- CN VIII - the acoustic (vestibulocochlear) nerve
- CN IX - the glossopharyngeal nerve
- CN X - the vagus nerve
- CN XI - the spinal accessory (accessory) nerve
- CN XII - the hypoglossal nerve

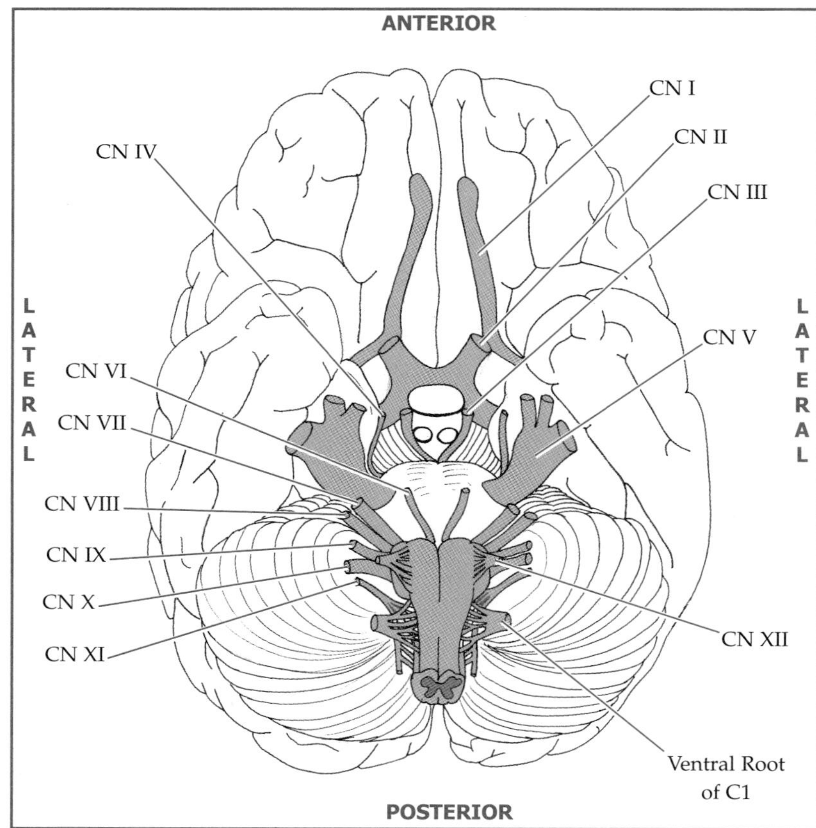

Inferior View of the Brain – The Cranial Nerves

SPINAL NERVE ORGANIZATION:

The 31 pairs of spinal nerves are named according to the level of the spine where they are located. The spinal nerves are subdivided as follows:

8 pairs of cervical nerves
12 pairs of the thoracic nerves
5 pairs of lumbar nerves
5 pairs of sacral nerves
1 pair of coccygeal nerves

The 1st cervical nerve exits the spine superior to C1, between C1 and the occiput. The spinal nerves of C2 through C7 exit the spine superior to the same named vertebra. The C8 spinal nerve exits the spine between C7 and T1. The spinal nerves of T1 through L5 exit the spine inferior to the same named vertebra. A spinal nerve exits the spinal cord and divides into a dorsal ramus (dorsal branch) and a ventral ramus (ventral branch). The dorsal rami (the plural of ramus is rami) travel posteriorly and innervate posterior muscles of the axial body. The ventral rami travel anteriorly and innervate anterior (and lateral) muscles of the axial body and the muscles of the lower and upper extremities. The dorsal ramus of C1 is located in the suboccipital region and known as the *suboccipital nerve*. The ventral rami of T1-T11 travel between the ribs and are known as *intercostal nerves*. The ventral ramus of T12 travels inferiorly to the 12th rib and is known as the *subcostal nerve*.

Dorsal rami of spinal nerves stay independent from one another and innervate structures that are located approximately at their segmental level. Ventral rami of spinal nerves in the thoracic region act in a similar manner. However, cervical, lumbar, sacral and coccygeal ventral rami are different in that they combine with other spinal ventral rami to form plexuses.

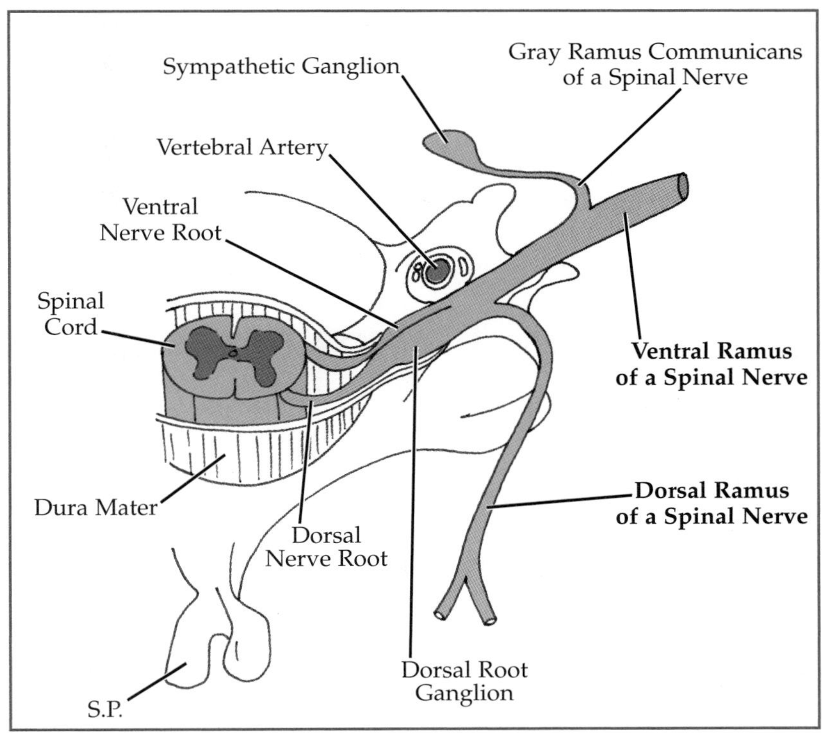

Cross Section View of the Spinal Cord – Spinal Nerve Diagram

PLEXUSES:

A nerve plexus is a network of nerves that join together. There are five plexuses in the human body: the cervical plexus, brachial plexus, lumbar plexus, sacral plexus and the coccygeal plexus. The lumbar and sacral plexuses intermix with each other and are often grouped together as the lumbosacral plexus. Although there is always some variability that exists, the plexuses are made up of the following spinal nerve ventral rami: the cervical plexus is made up of the ventral rami of C1-C4; the brachial plexus is made up of the ventral rami of C5-T1; the lumbar plexus is made up of the ventral rami of L1-L4; the sacral plexus is made up of the ventral rami of L4-S3; and the coccygeal plexus is made up of the ventral rami of S4, S5 and the coccygeal nerve. Only the plexuses and branches of the plexuses that contribute to innervation of the skeletal muscles located in the body of this book will be discussed.

PART I – OVERVIEW OF INNERVATION TO THE AXIAL BODY

The muscles of the axial body are innervated by both cranial nerves and spinal nerves. The cranial nerves that contribute to innervation of muscles of the axial body are the ***oculomotor nerve***, the ***trigeminal nerve***, the ***facial nerve***, the ***spinal accessory nerve*** and the ***hypoglossal nerve***. The ***trigeminal nerve*** has three divisions: the ***mandibular nerve***, the maxillary nerve and the opthalmic nerve. The mandibular nerve has an ***anterior trunk*** and a ***posterior trunk***; the ***medial pterygoid nerve*** also arises from the mandibular nerve. The ***lateral pterygoid nerve*** and ***deep temporal branches*** arise from the anterior trunk of the trigeminal nerve. The ***inferior alveolar nerve*** arises from the posterior trunk of the trigeminal nerve and gives rise to the ***mylohyoid branch***. The ***facial nerve*** gives rise to the ***posterior auricular nerve***, ***temporal branches***, ***zygomatic branches***, ***superior buccal branches***, a ***mandibular branch*** and a ***cervical branch***.

Spinal nerve ***dorsal rami*** and ***ventral rami*** contribute to innervation of muscles of the axial body. More specifically, the ***suboccipital nerve***, ***intercostal nerves*** and the ***subcostal nerve*** innervate axial muscles.

The plexuses that contribute innervation to muscles of the axial body are the ***cervical plexus***, the ***brachial plexus*** and the ***lumbar plexus***. The ***cervical plexus*** gives rise to the ***phrenic nerve*** that travels down through the thoracic cavity to innervate the diaphragm. There is also a loop of two branches of the cervical plexus that join together; this loop is called the ***ansa cervicalis***. The ***brachial plexus*** is primarily concerned with providing innervation to the upper extremity. (Brachium is the latin word for arm.) However, the following branches of the brachial plexus provide innervation to muscles listed in the axial body in this book: the ***thoracodorsal nerve***, the ***dorsal scapular nerve***, the ***long thoracic nerve***, ***medial pectoral nerves***, ***lateral pectoral nerves***, and a ***branch to the subclavius***.

PART II – OVERVIEW OF INNERVATION TO THE LOWER EXTREMITY

The muscles of the lower extremity are innervated by branches of the ***lumbar plexus***, the ***sacral plexus***, and the ***lumbosacral plexus***. Further, some muscles of the anterior pelvis are innervated directly by spinal nerve ventral rami.

Branches of the lumbosacral plexus innervate most of the deep lateral rotators of the thigh. Two major branches of the ***lumbar plexus*** are the ***femoral nerve*** and the ***obturator nerve***. The ***femoral nerve*** enters and innervates muscles of the anterior thigh. The ***obturator nerve*** enters and innervates muscles of the medial thigh. From the ***sacral plexus*** arise the ***superior gluteal nerve*** and the ***inferior gluteal nerve***, which innervate muscles of the pelvis and proximal anterolateral thigh. The other major nerve of the sacral plexus is the ***sciatic nerve***, the largest nerve in the human body. The sciatic nerve and its branches innervate the muscles of the posterior thigh and all muscles distal to the knee (i.e., all muscles of the leg and the foot). The sciatic nerve exits the pelvis between the piriformis and superior gemellus. It then enters and innervates the muscles of the posterior thigh. Just proximal to the knee, the sciatic nerve divides into the ***tibial nerve*** and the ***common fibular nerve***.

The tibial nerve enters and innervates the muscles of the posterior compartment of the leg. Posterior to the medial malleolus, the tibial nerve gives rise to its two terminal branches, the ***medial plantar nerve*** and the ***lateral plantar nerve***. The medial and lateral plantar nerves enter and innervate muscles in the plantar foot.

The common fibular nerve enters the anterior leg near the head of the fibula. It then divides into the ***superficial fibular nerve*** and the ***deep fibular nerve***. The ***superficial fibular nerve*** enters and innervates the muscles of the lateral compartment of the leg. The ***deep fibular nerve*** enters and innervates the muscles of the anterior compartment of the leg. The deep fibular nerve splits at the anterior ankle to form its terminal branches, which enter and innervate muscles of the dorsum of the foot.

PART III – OVERVIEW OF INNERVATION TO THE UPPER EXTREMITY

The muscles of the upper extremity are innervated by branches of the ***brachial plexus***. The major branches of the brachial plexus are the ***median nerve***, the ***radial nerve***, the ***ulnar nerve***, the ***musculocutaneous nerve***, the ***axillary nerve***, the ***suprascapular nerve*** and the ***upper and lower subscapular nerves***.

The median nerve travels through the anteromedial arm and the middle of the anterior forearm to enter the anterior hand. In the anterior forearm, the median nerve gives rise to the ***anterior interosseus nerve***. The radial nerve travels through the posterior arm and forearm and enters the posterior hand. In the posterior forearm, the radial nerve gives rise to the ***posterior interosseus nerve*** (also known as the deep branch of the radial nerve). The ulnar nerve travels through the anteromedial arm, then crosses the elbow on the medial side between the medial epicondyle of the humerus and the olecranon process of the ulna. (The ulnar nerve at this location is called the "funny bone.") The ulnar nerve continues down the anterior forearm on the ulnar side and enters the anterior hand on the ulnar side. The musculocutaneous nerve is located in the anterior arm. The axillary nerve is located in the axillary region. The suprascapular nerve travels superior to the scapula to enter the supraspinous fossa and then the infraspinous fossa. The upper and lower subscapular nerves travel to the anterior (subscapular) side of the scapula.

VIEWS OF THE CERVICAL AND BRACHIAL PLEXUSES

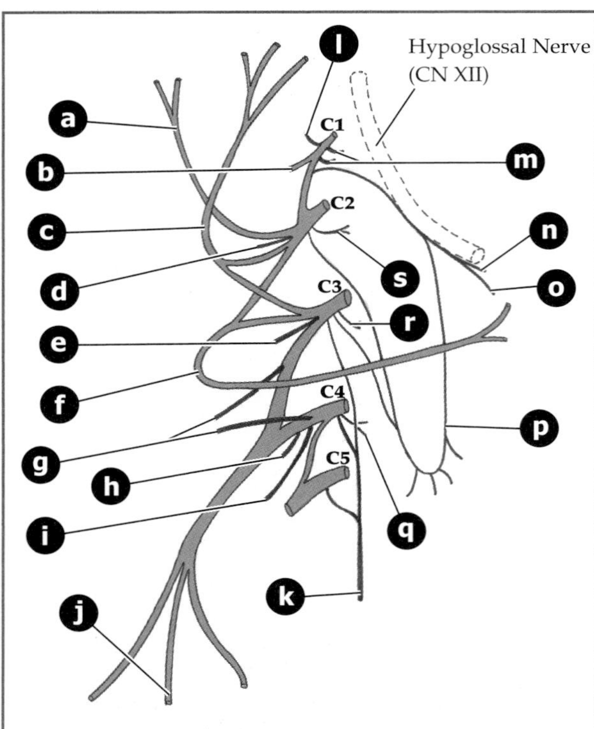

The Cervical Plexus

- a. **Lesser Occipital Nerve**
- b. **to the Vagus Nerve**
- c. **Greater Auricular Nerve**
- d. **to Sternocleidomastoid**
- e. **to Levator Scapulae**
- f. Transverse Cutaneous Nerve of the Neck
- g. **to Trapezius**
- h. **to Levator Scapulae**
- i. **to Middle Scalene**
- j. **Supraclavicular Nerve**
- k. **Phrenic Nerve**
- l. **to Rectus Lateralis**
- m. **to Rectus Capitis Anterior and Longus Capitis**
- n. **to Geniohyoid**
- o. **to Thyrohyoid**
- p. **Ansa Cervicalis**
- q. **to Longus Colli**
- r. **to Longus Capitis, Longus Colli and Middle Scalene**
- s. **to Longus Capitis and Longus Colli**

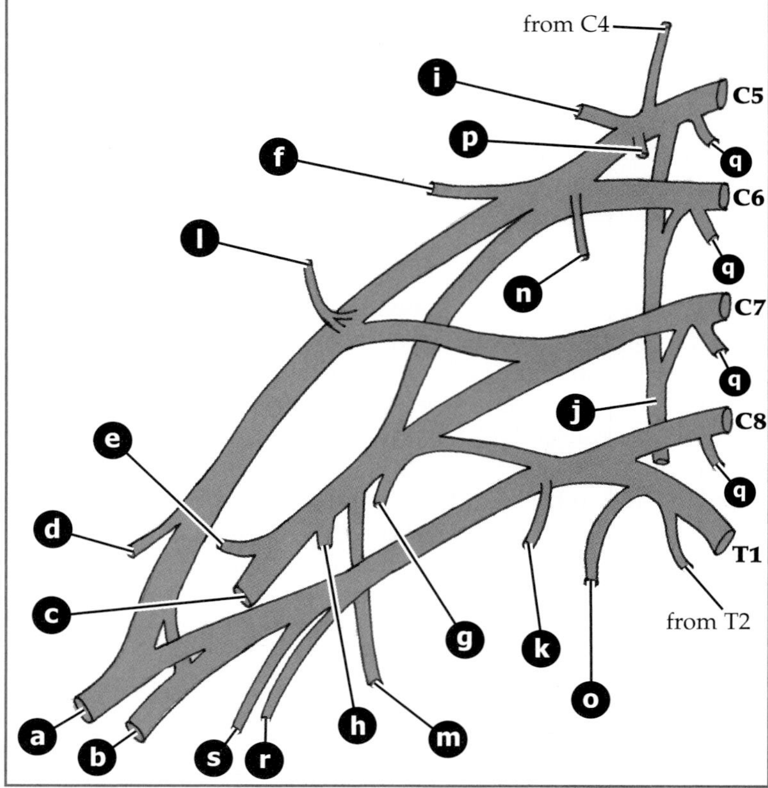

The Brachial Plexus

- a. **Median Nerve**
- b. **Ulnar Nerve**
- c. **Radial Nerve**
- d. **Musculocutaneous Nerve**
- e. **Axillary Nerve**
- f. **Suprascapular Nerve**
- g. **Upper Subscapular Nerve**
- h. **Lower Subscapular Nerve**
- i. **Dorsal Scapular Nerve**
- j. **Long Thoracic Nerve**
- k. **Medial Pectoral Nerve**
- l. **Lateral Pectoral Nerve**
- m. **Thoracodorsal Nerve**
- n. **Nerve to Subclavius**
- o. **First Intercostal Nerve**
- p. **to the Phrenic Nerve**
- q. **Nerve to Scalenes**
- r. Medial Brachial Cutaneous Nerve
- s. Medial Antebrachial Cutaneous Nerve

VIEWS OF THE LUMBAR, SACRAL AND COCCYGEAL PLEXUSES

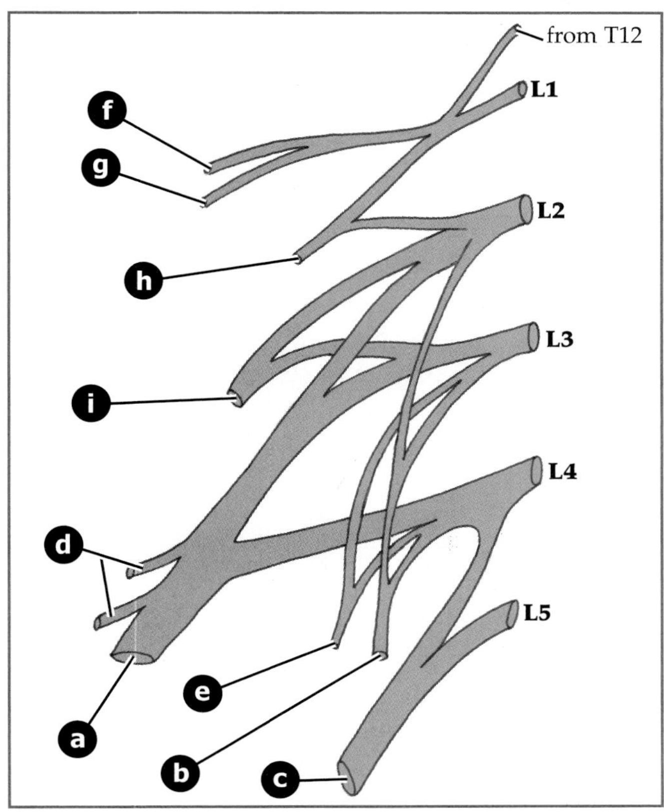

The Lumbar Plexus

a. **Femoral Nerve**
b. **Obturator Nerve**
c. **Lumbosacral Trunk**
d. **To Psoas and Iliacus (Iliopsoas)**
e. **Accessory Obturator Nerve**
f. **Iliohypogastric Nerve**
g. **Ilio-inguinal**
h. **Genitofemoral**
i. Lateral Cutaneous Nerve of the Thigh

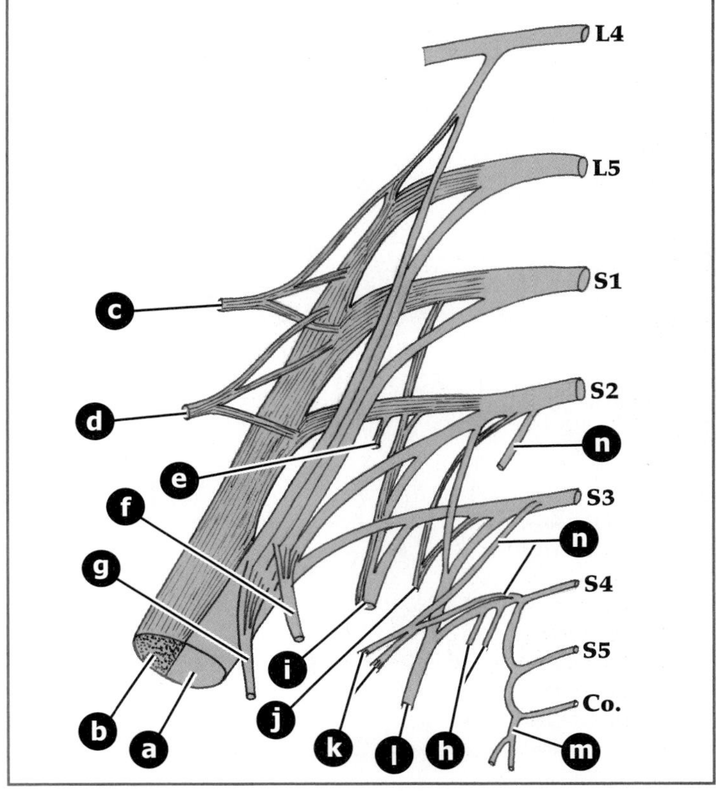

The Sacral and Coccygeal Plexuses

a. **Tibial Nerve of the Sciatic Nerve**
b. **Common Fibular Nerve of the Sciatic Nerve**
c. **Superior Gluteal Nerve**
d. **Inferior Gluteal Nerve**
e. **to Piriformis**
f. **to Superior Gemellus and Obturator Internus**
g. **to Inferior Gemellus and Quadratus Femoris**
h. **to Levator Ani, Coccygeous and External Anal Sphincter**
i. Posterior Femoral Cutaneous Nerve
j. Perforating Cutaneous Nerve
k. Pelvic Splanchnic Nerves
l. Pudendal Nerve
m. Anococcygeal Nerves
n. Visceral Branches

VIEWS OF INNERVATION TO THE RIGHT LOWER EXTREMITY

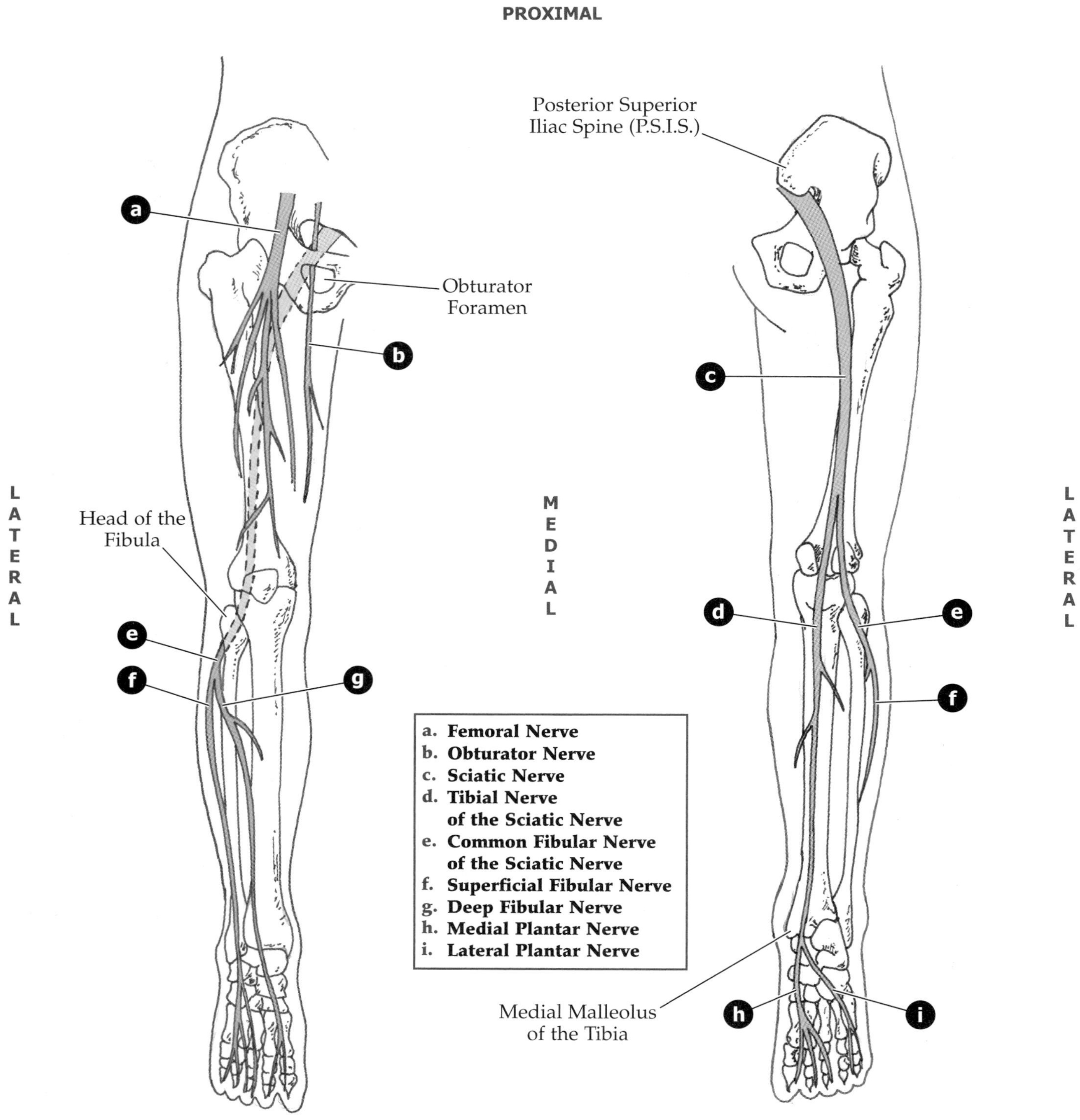

PROXIMAL

Posterior Superior Iliac Spine (P.S.I.S.)

Obturator Foramen

LATERAL

Head of the Fibula

MEDIAL

LATERAL

a. **Femoral Nerve**
b. **Obturator Nerve**
c. **Sciatic Nerve**
d. **Tibial Nerve of the Sciatic Nerve**
e. **Common Fibular Nerve of the Sciatic Nerve**
f. **Superficial Fibular Nerve**
g. **Deep Fibular Nerve**
h. **Medial Plantar Nerve**
i. **Lateral Plantar Nerve**

Medial Malleolus of the Tibia

DISTAL

Anterior View of the Lower Extremity

Posterior View of the Lower Extremity

ANTERIOR VIEW OF INNERVATION TO THE RIGHT UPPER EXTREMITY

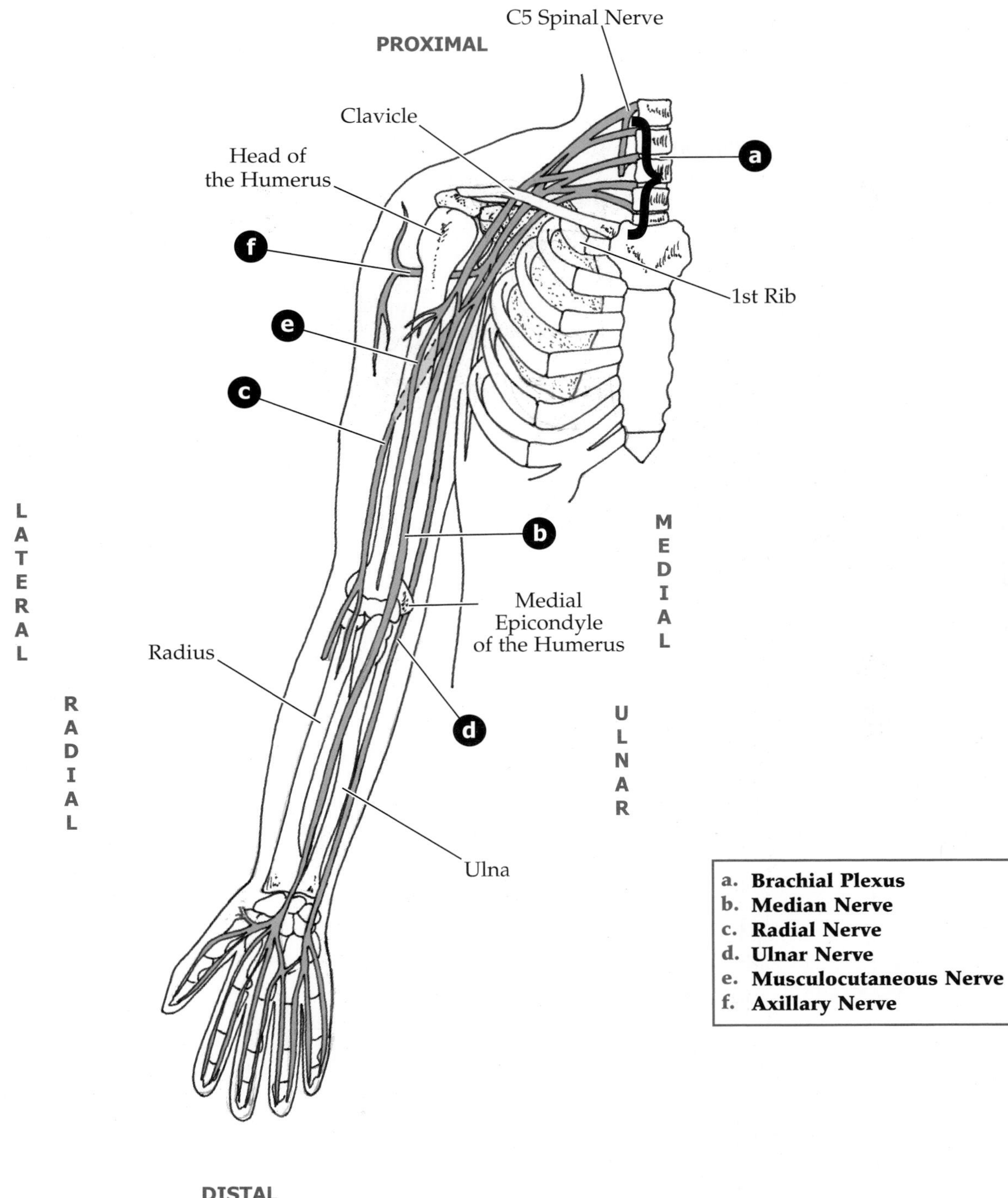

a. **Brachial Plexus**
b. **Median Nerve**
c. **Radial Nerve**
d. **Ulnar Nerve**
e. **Musculocutaneous Nerve**
f. **Axillary Nerve**

NERVOUS SYSTEM
MAJOR SOURCES OF INNERVATION

MAJOR SOURCES OF INNERVATION TO BODY PARTS OF THE LOWER EXTREMITY

Pelvis:	anterior:	branches of the lumbar plexus
	posterior:	superior and inferior gluteal nerves
Thigh:	anterior:	femoral nerve
	posterior:	sciatic nerve
	medial:	obturator nerve
Leg:	anterior:	deep fibular nerve
	posterior:	tibial nerve
	lateral:	superficial fibular nerve
Foot:	dorsal:	deep fibular nerve
	plantar:	medial and lateral plantar nerves

MAJOR SOURCES OF INNERVATION TO BODY PARTS OF THE UPPER EXTREMITY

Scapula:	anterior:	upper and lower subscapular nerves
	posterior:	suprascapular nerve
	axillary region:	axillary nerve
Arm:	anterior:	musculocutaneous nerve
	posterior:	radial nerve
Forearm:	anterior:	median nerve
	posterior:	radial nerve
Hand:	thenar eminence:	median nerve
	hypothenar eminence:	ulnar nerve
	central compartment:	ulnar nerve

LIST OF NERVES - BY BODY PART

LOWER EXTREMITY

Pelvis: branches of the lumbar plexus:
- femoral nerve
- obturator nerve

branches of the lumbosacral plexus:
- superior gluteal nerve
- inferior gluteal nerve

Thigh: branches of the lumbar plexus:
- femoral nerve
- obturator nerve

branches of the lumbosacral plexus:
- superior gluteal nerve
- sciatic nerve
- tibial nerve
- common fibular nerve

Leg: branches of the sciatic nerve:
- tibial nerve
- common fibular nerve
- superficial fibular nerve
- deep fibular nerve

Foot: branches of sciatic nerve:
- tibial nerve
- medial plantar nerve
- lateral plantar nerve
- deep fibular nerve branches

UPPER EXTREMITY

Scapula: branches of the brachial plexus:
- suprascapular nerve
- upper and lower subscapular nerves

Axilla: branches of the brachial plexus:
- axillary nerve

Arm: branches of the brachial plexus:
- musculocutaneous nerve
- radial nerve

Forearm: branches of the brachial plexus:
- median nerve
- anterior interosseus nerve
- radial nerve
- posterior interosseus nerve
- ulnar nerve

Hand: branches of brachial plexus:
- median nerve
- ulnar nerve

AXIAL BODY

Head: cranial nerves:
- oculomotor nerve (CN III)
- trigeminal nerve (CN V)
- facial nerve (CN VII)

Neck: cranial nerves:
- trigeminal nerve (CN V)
- facial nerve (CN VII)
- spinal accessory nerve (CN XI)
- hypoglossal nerve (CN XII)

cervical spinal nerves:
- dorsal rami
- ventral rami
- suboccipital nerve

branches of the cervical plexus:
- ansa cervicalis

branch of the brachial plexus:
- dorsal scapular nerve

Trunk: spinal nerves:
- dorsal rami
- ventral rami
- intercostal nerves

branch of the cervical plexus:
- phrenic nerve

branches of the brachial plexus:
- dorsal scapular nerve
- thoracodorsal nerve
- long thoracic nerve
- medial pectoral nerves
- lateral pectoral nerves
- nerve to subclavius

branch of the lumbar plexus:
- nerve to quadratus lumborum

APPENDIX I – OVERVIEW OF ARTERIAL SUPPLY

This overview is divided into three parts, the axial body, the upper extremity and the lower extremity, and is not meant to be comprehensive of the entire arterial system. Rather, it supplies the context information for arterial supply to skeletal muscles mentioned in the body of this book. It must be emphasized that while there is variation in every anatomical system of the human body, variation especially occurs in the arterial system. The arterial supply to skeletal muscles can vary tremendously from one individual to another. The frequent anastamostes between vessels opens the door to the primary source of arterial supply to a muscle coming from what would normally be considered a "less important" artery.

PART I – OVERVIEW OF ARTERIAL SUPPLY TO THE AXIAL BODY

The Aorta: Arterial supply to the tissues of the body (except the lungs) originates from the left ventricle via the ***aorta***. The aorta has three parts: the ascending aorta, the arch of the aorta and the descending aorta. The ascending aorta and the arch of the aorta are located in the thoracic cavity. The descending aorta begins in the thoracic cavity and then pierces the diaphragm to enter the abdominal cavity where it ends by dividing into the right and left common iliac arteries.

The Branches of the Arch of the Aorta: There are three major branches off the arch of the aorta: the left common carotid artery and the left subclavian artery, both of which are located on the left side of the body, and the brachiocephalic trunk, located on the right side of the body. The brachiocephalic trunk gives rise to the right common carotid and the right subclavian arteries. (Hence, the arterial supply directly off the arch of the aorta is not initially symmetrical.) Each common carotid artery splits to form internal and external carotid arteries.

The External Carotid Artery: The external carotid artery has eight branches. They are the ***superior thyroid***, ***ascending pharyngeal***, ***lingual***, ***facial***, ***occipital***, ***posterior auricular***, ***superficial temporal*** and ***maxillary*** arteries.

The ***superior thyroid artery*** arises anteriorly just inferior to the hyoid bone and travels to the anterior neck. The ***ascending pharyngeal artery*** arises posteriorly from the origin of the external carotid and travels to the base of the cranium. The ***lingual artery*** also arises from the external carotid anteriorly, at the level of the hyoid bone, and travels to the tongue and floor of the mouth. The ***facial artery*** arises from the external carotid artery slightly superior to the hyoid bone and supplies the mandibular area and the lower face. The ***occipital artery*** branches off the external carotid artery posteriorly and travels to the occipital region. There is a branch of the occipital artery called the ***descending branch of the occipital artery*** that is found in the suboccipital region. The ***posterior auricular artery*** also branches off the external carotid artery posteriorly and travels to the scalp posterior to the ear. The ***superficial temporal artery*** is one of the two terminal branches of the external carotid artery. It supplies the region of the scalp that overlies the temporal and frontal bones. Additionally, a branch of the superficial temporal artery named the ***transverse facial artery*** supplies the lateral face. The ***maxillary artery*** is the other terminal branch of the external carotid artery and branches off anteriorly to supply deeper parts of the face. One branch of the maxillary artery is the ***infraorbital artery***, which travels to the eye socket and the region of the face inferior to the eye; another branch of the maxillary artery is the ***inferior alveolar artery***, which travels to the mandibular region.

The Internal Carotid Artery: The internal carotid artery enters the cranial cavity to supply blood to the brain. One branch of the internal carotid artery is the ***ophthalmic artery***, which enters the eye socket. Two branches of the ophthalmic artery are the ***supratrochlear artery*** and the ***supraorbital artery***.

The Subclavian Artery: The subclavian artery has five branches: the ***vertebral***, ***internal thoracic***, thyrocervical, ***costocervical*** and ***dorsal scapular*** arteries. The ***vertebral artery*** arises posteriorly from the subclavian to travel through the transverse foramina of cervical vertebrae and ends in the suboccipital region. Along its course, the vertebral artery gives off ***muscular branches***. The ***internal thoracic artery*** branches from the subclavian and descends within the thoracic cavity. It gives off the ***pericardiacophrenic artery*** and the ***anterior intercostal arteries*** and ultimately divides into its two terminal branches, the ***musculophrenic artery*** and the ***superior epigastric artery***. The thyrocervical trunk arises anteriorly from the inferior subclavian and divides almost immediately into the ***inferior thyroid artery***, suprascapular artery and the superficial cervical artery; another branch of the thyrocervical trunk is the ***transverse cervical artery***. The inferior thyroid artery of the thyrocervical trunk gives off the ***ascending cervical artery***. The ***costocervical trunk*** arises from the subclavian and soon divides into the superior intercostal artery and the ***deep cervical artery***. The ***dorsal scapular artery*** travels to the posterior trunk where it descends between the scapula and the spinal column. (Note: The dorsal scapular artery may arise from the costocervical trunk instead of arising directly from the subclavian artery.)

The Axillary Artery: At the outer border of the first rib, the subclavian artery becomes the axillary artery. The axillary artery has six branches. They are the ***superior thoracic***, ***thoracoacromial***, ***lateral thoracic***, ***subscapular*** and the ***anterior and posterior circumflex humeral arteries***.

The ***thoracoacromial trunk*** has a ***pectoral branch***, a ***clavicular branch***, an acromial branch and a ***deltoid branch***. The lateral thoracic artery travels through the anterolateral chest. The ***subscapular artery*** is the largest of the axillary branches and it gives off a number of branches, one of which is the ***thoracodorsal artery***. The axillary artery ends at the distal border of the tendon of the teres major, where it becomes the brachial artery.

The Descending Aorta: The descending aorta gives off the ***superior phrenic artery***, ***posterior intercostal arteries*** and the ***subcostal artery*** (also known as the 12th intercostal artery) in the thoracic region and the ***inferior phrenic artery*** and ***lumbar arteries*** in the abdominal region. The descending aorta ends in the abdominal cavity by dividing into the left and right common iliac arteries. Each common iliac then divides into an external and internal iliac artery.

The External Iliac Artery: Just before passing deep to the inguinal ligament, the external iliac artery gives off the ***inferior epigastric artery*** and the ***deep circumflex iliac artery***.

The Internal Iliac Artery: The internal iliac artery has an anterior and posterior trunk. Arising from its posterior trunk is the ***iliolumbar artery***.

MAJOR SOURCES OF ARTERIAL SUPPLY TO THE AXIAL BODY

Head: Arterial supply to the head originates either directly or indirectly from branches from the internal and external carotid arteries. Five of the eight branches of the external carotid artery (facial, occipital, posterior auricular, superficial temporal and maxillary) are pertinent to the head chapter of this book.

Neck: Arterial supply to the muscles of the neck originates either directly or indirectly from branches of the external carotid, subclavian and the posterior intercostal arteries. Seven of the eight branches of the external carotid artery (superior thyroid, ascending pharyngeal, lingual, facial, occipital, posterior auricular and maxillary) are pertinent to the neck chapter of this book.

Trunk: The arterial supply to muscles of the trunk is varied. Most of the muscles of the posterior trunk receive some or all of their arterial supply from dorsal branches of posterior intercostal arteries. Descending arteries that arise from the subclavian and/or axillary arteries supply superior segments of posterior trunk muscles. Dorsal branches of lumbar arteries supply inferior segments of posterior trunk muscles. Generally, the chest is supplied by anterior and posterior intercostal arteries, and the muscles of the anterior abdominal wall are supplied by the superior and inferior epigastric arteries and the posterior intercostal and subcostal arteries.

LATERAL VIEW OF ARTERIAL SUPPLY TO THE AXIAL BODY

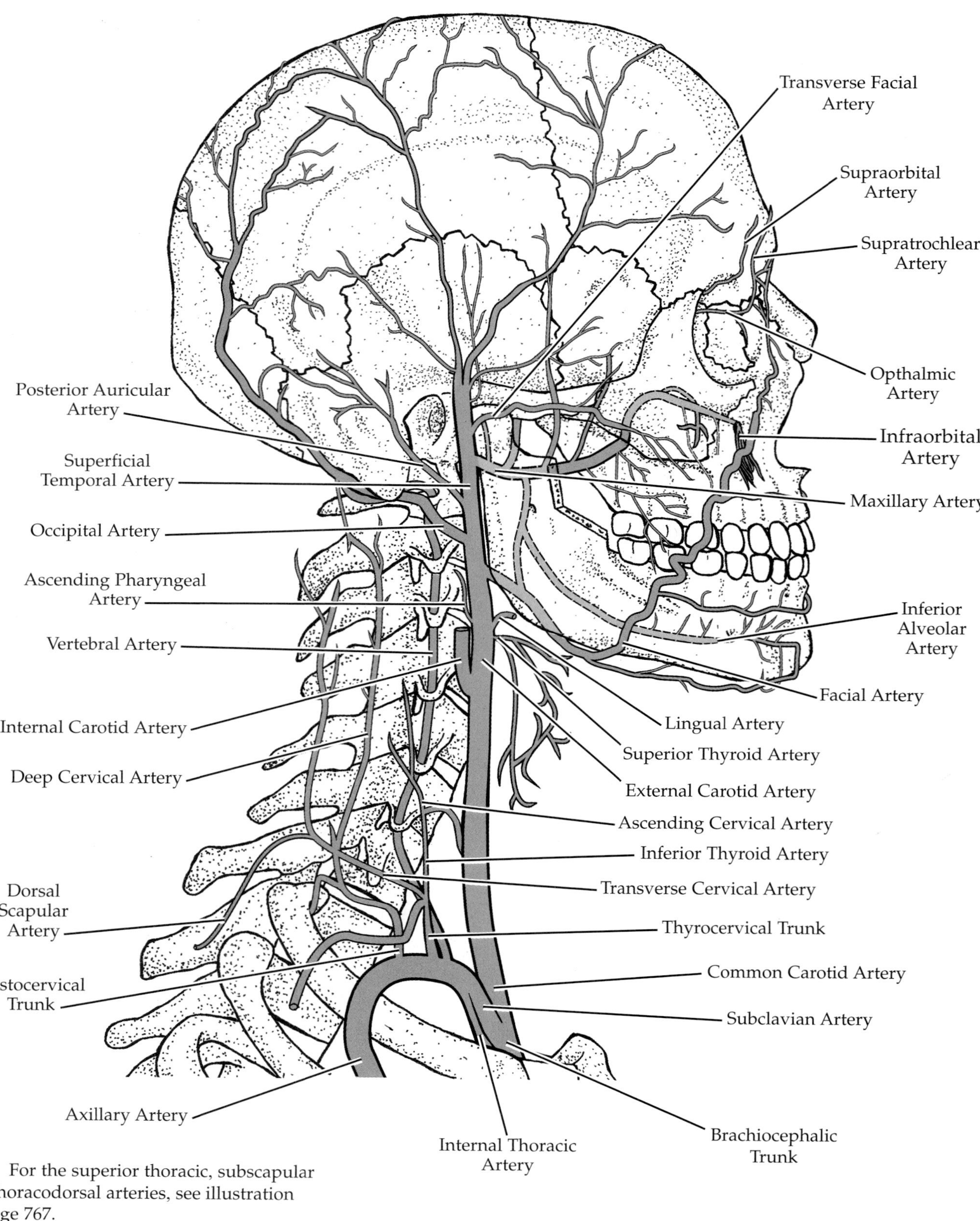

Note: For the superior thoracic, subscapular and thoracodorsal arteries, see illustration on page 767.

ANTERIOR VIEW OF ARTERIAL SUPPLY TO THE AXIAL BODY

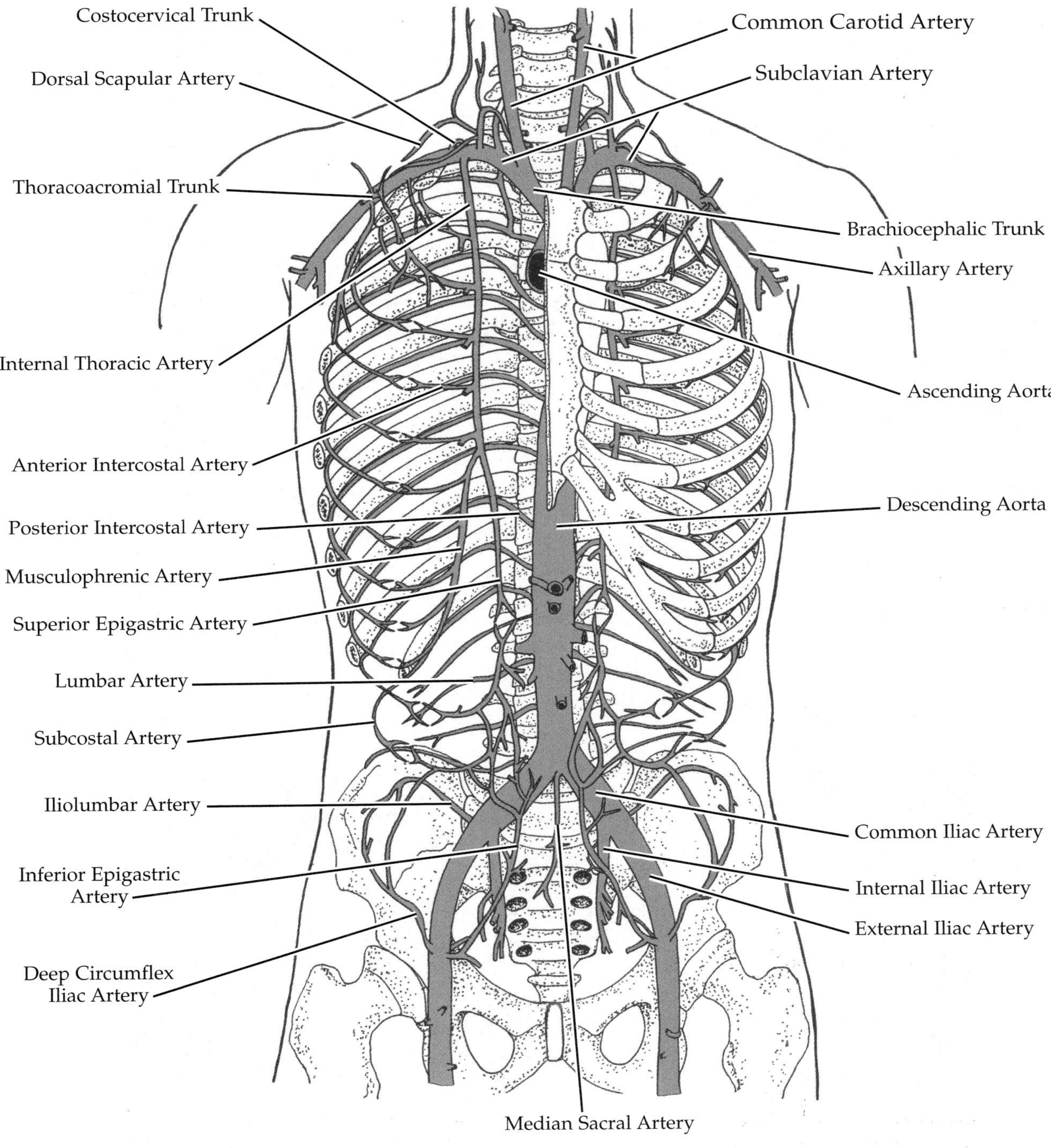

Note: The pericardiacophrenic and superior and inferior phrenic arteries are not shown.

PART II – OVERVIEW OF ARTERIAL SUPPLY TO THE LOWER EXTREMITY

Trunk/Pelvis: Within the abdomen, the descending aorta gives off ***lumbar arteries*** and the ***median sacral artery***; the median sacral artery gives off its own small branch, the ***arteria lumbalis ima***. The aorta divides into right and left ***common iliac arteries*** at approximately the L4 vertebral level. Within the pelvis, each common iliac artery then divides into an ***internal iliac artery*** and an ***external iliac artery***. The internal iliac artery primarily feeds arterial supply to the structures of the pelvis but also gives arterial supply to some structures of the proximal thigh. Branches of the internal iliac artery include the ***superior gluteal artery***, the ***inferior gluteal artery***, the ***obturator artery*** and the ***iliolumbar artery***. Each external iliac artery descends through the pelvis and then passes deep to the inguinal ligament.

Thigh: When the external iliac passes deep to the inguinal ligament, it enters the anterior thigh and becomes the ***femoral artery***. The femoral artery and its branches provide arterial supply to nearly the entire lower extremity. Within the thigh, the femoral artery gives rise to the ***deep femoral artery*** (also known as the profunda femoris artery). The deep femoral artery gives rise to ***perforating branches of the deep femoral artery***, which pass into the posterior thigh. The main trunk of the femoral artery continues to descend within the anterior thigh. In the distal thigh, the femoral artery passes through the adductor hiatus and enters the popliteal region (distal posterior thigh), posterior to the knee; here, its name changes to the popliteal artery. In this region, the ***popliteal artery*** gives off ***sural branches of the popliteal artery***. (Note: The obturator artery from the pelvis also exits the pelvis and enters the medial thigh, where it helps supply much of the medial and posterior thigh musculature.)

Leg: The popliteal artery continues into the posterior leg. At the inferior border of the popliteus muscle, the popliteal artery divides into its terminal branches, the ***anterior tibial artery*** and the ***posterior tibial artery***. Almost immediately, the posterior tibial artery gives off the ***fibular artery***. The posterior tibial artery continues to descend through the posterior compartment of the leg. The anterior tibial artery enters the anterior compartment of the leg and descends through the anterior compartment to the ankle.

Foot: The anterior tibial artery enters the dorsum of the foot and becomes the ***dorsalis pedis artery***. As the posterior tibial artery enters the plantar surface of the foot on the medial side, it bifurcates into its two terminal branches, the ***medial plantar artery*** and the ***lateral plantar artery***. Within the plantar compartment of the foot, the ***plantar arch*** is formed by an anastomosis between the lateral plantar artery and the continuation of the dorsalis pedis artery from the dorsum of the foot.

MAJOR SOURCES OF ARTERIAL SUPPLY TO BODY PARTS OF THE LOWER EXTREMITY

Pelvis:		branches of the internal and external iliac arteries
Thigh:	anterior:	femoral and deep femoral arteries
	posterior:	deep femoral and popliteal arteries
	medial:	femoral, deep femoral and obturator arteries
Leg:	anterior:	anterior tibial artery
	posterior:	posterior tibial artery
	lateral:	fibular artery
Foot:	dorsal:	dorsalis pedis artery
	plantar:	medial and lateral plantar arteries and the plantar arch

ANTERIOR VIEW OF ARTERIAL SUPPLY TO THE RIGHT LOWER EXTREMITY

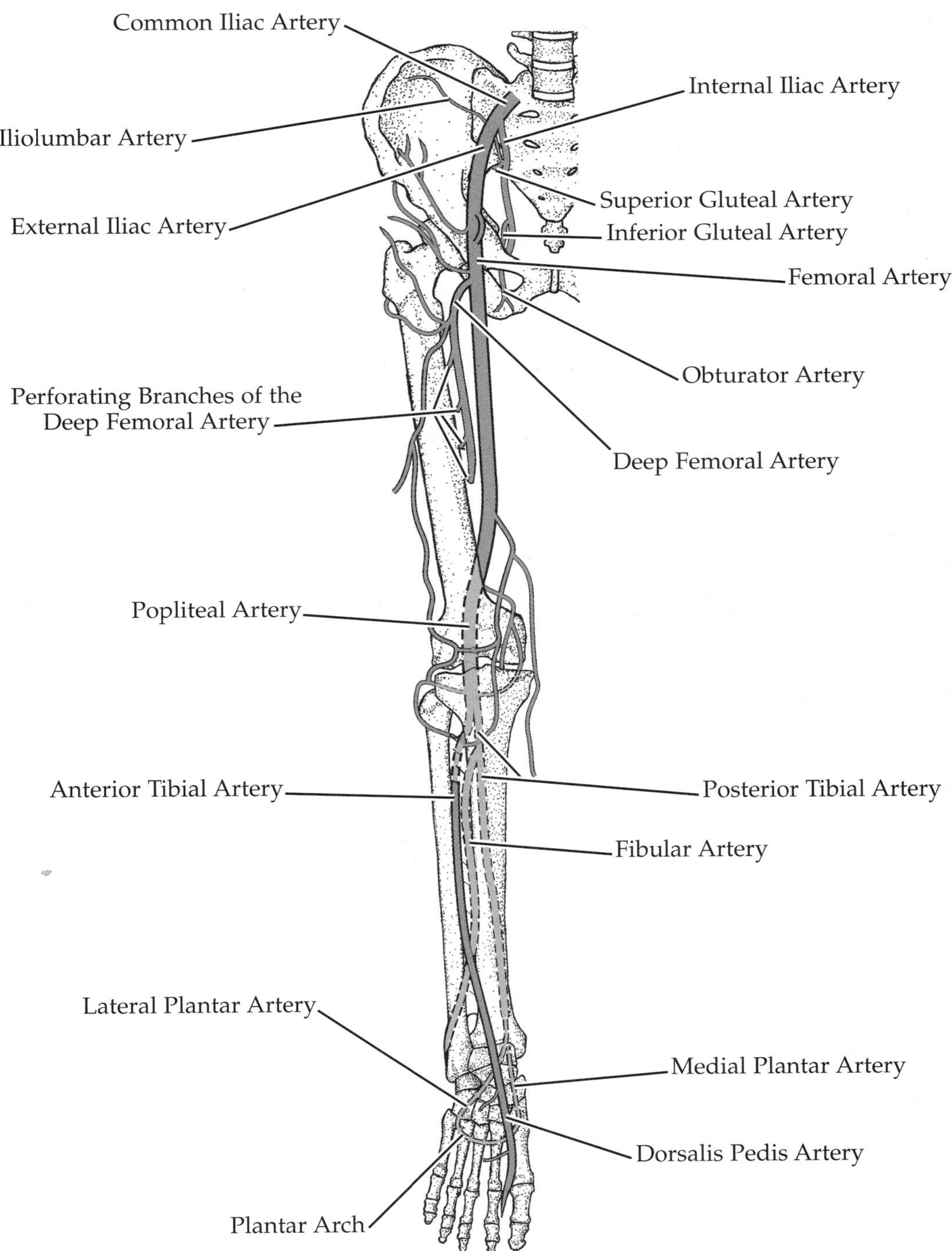

Note: For the lumbar arteries and the median sacral artery, see illustration on page 763. The arteria lumbalis ima is not shown.

PART III – OVERVIEW OF ARTERIAL SUPPLY TO THE UPPER EXTREMITY

Trunk/Axillary Region: In the trunk, the subclavian artery passes superiorly to the 1st rib. The subclavian artery gives off a branch called the thyrocervical trunk, which then divides to form the ***suprascapular artery*** (and the transverse cervical and inferior thyroid arteries) and another branch called the ***dorsal scapular artery***.

In the axillary region, at the lateral border of the 1st rib, each subclavian artery becomes the axillary artery. The axillary artery gives off 1) the ***thoracoacromial trunk***, 2) the ***lateral thoracic artery***, 3) the subscapular artery, which divides to form the ***thoracodorsal artery*** and the ***circumflex scapular artery***, 4) the ***anterior circumflex humeral artery*** and 5) the ***posterior circumflex humeral artery***.

Arm: The axillary artery enters the arm, passing anterior to the tendon of the teres major muscle. At the inferior border of the teres major, the axillary artery becomes the ***brachial artery***. In the anteromedial arm, the brachial artery gives off the ***deep brachial artery***.

Forearm: The brachial artery crosses the elbow joint anteriorly to enter the forearm and immediately divides into its terminal branches, the ***radial artery*** and the ***ulnar artery***. Near the ulnar tuberosity, the ulnar artery gives off a large branch called the common interosseus artery; the common interosseus artery then divides into three branches: the ***interosseus recurrent artery***, the ***anterior interosseus artery*** and the ***posterior interosseus artery***. The anterior interosseus artery travels down the anterior forearm and sends ***perforating branches*** into the deeper musculature of the distal anterior forearm. The posterior interosseus artery and the interosseus recurrent artery pass into the posterior forearm where the posterior interosseus artery then travels down the posterior forearm and the interosseus recurrent artery travels up to the posterior elbow region. The radial and ulnar arteries continue traveling down the anterior forearm as well and pass into the hand.

Hand: In the hand, the radial and ulnar arteries form two anastomosing arches, the ***superficial palmar arterial arch*** and the ***deep palmar arterial arch***. The superficial palmar arterial arch is supplied primarily by the ulnar artery, which anastomoses with the superficial palmar branch of the radial artery. The deep palmar arterial arch is supplied primarily by the radial artery (by anastomosing with the deep palmar branch of the ulnar artery).

MAJOR SOURCES OF ARTERIAL SUPPLY TO BODY PARTS OF THE UPPER EXTREMITY

Trunk/Axillary region:		anastomoses of the branches of the subclavian and axillary arteries
Arm:	anterior:	brachial artery
	posterior:	deep brachial artery
Forearm:	anterior/ulnar side:	ulnar artery
	anterior/radial side:	radial artery
	posterior:	posterior interosseus artery
Hand:	thenar eminence:	radial artery
	hypothenar eminence:	ulnar artery
	central compartment:	radial and ulnar arteries

ANTERIOR VIEW OF ARTERIAL SUPPLY TO THE RIGHT UPPER EXTREMITY

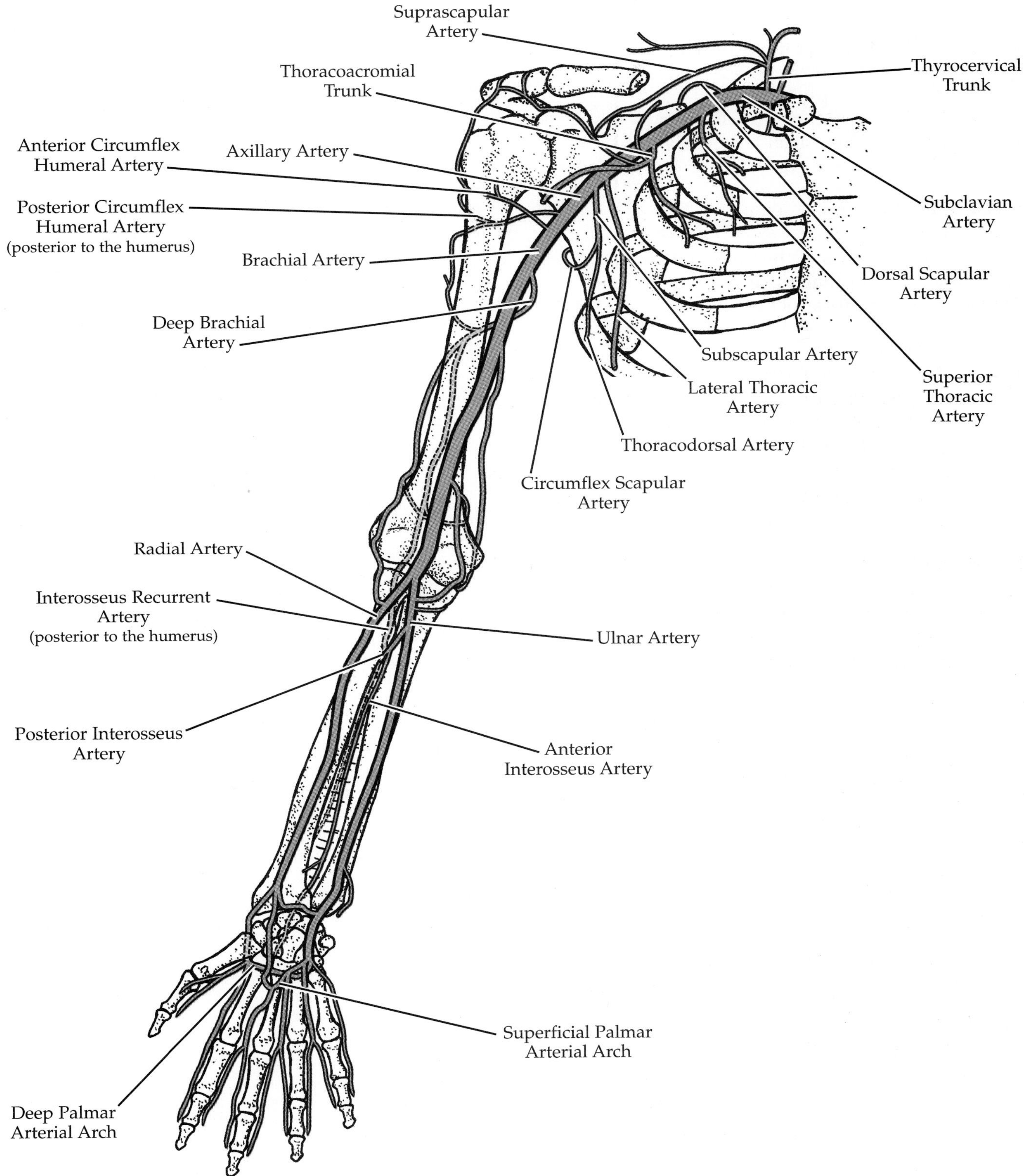
Suprascapular Artery
Thyrocervical Trunk
Thoracoacromial Trunk
Anterior Circumflex Humeral Artery
Axillary Artery
Posterior Circumflex Humeral Artery (posterior to the humerus)
Subclavian Artery
Brachial Artery
Dorsal Scapular Artery
Deep Brachial Artery
Subscapular Artery
Superior Thoracic Artery
Lateral Thoracic Artery
Thoracodorsal Artery
Circumflex Scapular Artery
Radial Artery
Interosseus Recurrent Artery (posterior to the humerus)
Ulnar Artery
Posterior Interosseus Artery
Anterior Interosseus Artery
Superficial Palmar Arterial Arch
Deep Palmar Arterial Arch

LIST OF ARTERIES - BY BODY PART

AXIAL BODY

Head:

branches of the external carotid artery:
- facial artery
- occipital artery
- posterior auricular artery
- superficial temporal artery
- transverse facial artery
- maxillary artery
- infraorbital artery

branches of the internal carotid artery:
- opthalmic artery
- supratrochlear artery
- supraorbital artery

Neck:

branches of the external carotid artery:
- superior thyroid artery
- ascending pharyngeal artery
- lingual artery
- facial artery
- occipital artery
- descending branch of the occipital artery
- posterior auricular artery
- maxillary artery
- inferior alveolar artery

branches of the subclavian artery:
- vertebral artery
  - muscular branches
- internal thoracic artery
- thyrocervical trunk
- transverse cervical artery
- inferior thyroid artery
- ascending cervical artery
- costocervical trunk
- deep cervical artery
- dorsal scapular artery

branches of the aorta:
- posterior intercostal arteries
- dorsal branches

Trunk:

branch of the external carotid artery:
- occipital artery

branches of the subclavian artery:
- internal thoracic artery
- pericardiacophrenic artery
- anterior intercostal arteries
- musculophrenic artery
- superior epigastric artery
- costocervical trunk
- deep cervical artery
- dorsal scapular artery

branches of the axillary artery:
- superior thoracic artery
- thoracoacromial trunk
  - pectoral branch
  - clavicular branch
- lateral thoracic artery
- subscapular artery
- thoracodorsal artery

branches of the aorta:
- superior phrenic artery
- posterior intercostal arteries
  - dorsal branches
- subcostal artery
  - dorsal branch
- inferior phrenic artery
- lumbar arteries
  - dorsal branches

branches of the external iliac artery:
- inferior epigastric artery
- deep circumflex iliac artery

branch of the internal iliac artery:
- iliolumbar artery

LIST OF ARTERIES - BY BODY PART

LOWER EXTREMITY

Pelvis: branches of the aorta:
- median sacral artery
  - arteria lumbalis ima

branches of the internal iliac artery:
- superior gluteal artery
- inferior gluteal artery
- obturator artery

Thigh: femoral artery and its branches:
- femoral artery
- deep femoral artery
  - perforating branches
- popliteal artery
  - sural branches

Leg: branches of the popliteal artery:
- anterior tibial artery
- posterior tibial artery
- fibular artery

Foot: branches of the anterior and posterior tibial arteries:
- dorsalis pedis artery
- medial plantar artery
- lateral plantar artery
- plantar arch

UPPER EXTREMITY

Trunk: branches of the subclavian artery:
- suprascapular artery
- dorsal scapular artery

Axillary Region: branches of the axillary artery:
- thoracoacromial trunk
  - deltoid branch
- lateral thoracic artery
- thoracodorsal artery
- circumflex scapular artery
- anterior circumflex humeral artery
- posterior circumflex humeral artery

Arm: brachial artery and its branches:
- brachial artery
- deep brachial artery

Forearm: radial and ulnar arteries and their branches:
- radial artery
- ulnar artery
- interosseus recurrent artery
- anterior interosseus artery
  - perforating branches
- posterior interosseus artery

Hand: branches and anastomoses of the radial and ulnar arteries:
- superficial palmar arterial arch
- deep palmar arterial arch
- superficial palmar branch of the radial artery

APPENDIX J – MNEMONICS

Although I am a firm believer that the best way to learn material is by truly understanding it, I do realize that when one is first confronted with a tremendous amount of new material to digest, little gimmicks here and there can be of use. Towards that end, I am including this appendix of mnemonics and other such helpful learning aids.

Some may be helpful to you, others not. I recommend that you don't try to memorize too many of these. Rather, use a few of them here and there when you need a little extra help. ☺

PART ONE – THE AXIAL BODY

HEAD CHAPTER

Muscles of the Scalp:

Old **T**oupees **A**lways **M**ove
Occipitofrontalis, **T**emporalis, **A**uricularis **M**uscles
Over **T**ime **A**ccumulates **M**oney
Occipitofrontalis, **T**emporalis, **A**uricularis **M**uscles

Facial Expression Muscles of the Eye:

Only **O**ne **L**olli **P**op **S**tarts **C**hildren **S**ucking
Orbicularis **O**culi, **L**evator **P**alpebrae **S**uperioris, **C**orrugator **S**upercilii
Openly **O**gling **L**ets **P**eople **S**ee **C**learly **S**ometimes
Orbicularis **O**culi, **L**evator **P**alpebrae **S**uperioris, **C**orrugator **S**upercilii

Facial Expression Muscles of the Nose:

Play **N**ow, **D**on't **S**tudy **N**ow.
Procerus, **N**asalis, **D**epressor **S**epti **N**asi
Pink **N**oses **D**o **S**weetly **N**uzzle
Procerus, **N**asalis, **D**epressor **S**epti **N**asi

Muscles of Mastication:

Tiny **M**ice **M**ake **P**retty **L**ittle **P**awprints.
Temporalis, **M**asseter, **M**edial **P**terygoid, **L**ateral **P**terygoid

Masking **T**ape **M**akes **P**ainting **L**ines **P**erfect.
Masseter, **T**emporalis, **M**edial **P**terygoid, **L**ateral **P**terygoid

NECK CHAPTER

Suboccipital Muscles:

Roger **Ca**n **P**lay **M**elodies.	**R**ectus **Ca**pitis **P**osterior **M**ajor
Roger **Ca**n **P**lay **M**usic.	**R**ectus **Ca**pitis **P**osterior **M**inor
Oscar **Ca**n **S**wim.	**O**bliquus **Ca**pitis **S**uperior
Oscar **Ca**n **I**ceskate.	**O**bliquus **Ca**pitis **I**nferior

Infrahyoid Muscles:

Super **S**onic **T**ake **O**ff.

Sternohyoid, **S**ternothyroid, **T**hyrohyoid, **O**mohyoid

Suprahyoid Muscles:

Don't **S**wallow **M**y **G**um!

Digastric, **S**tylohyoid, **M**ylohyoid, **G**eniohyoid

Prevertebral Muscles:

Last **C**all! **L**ast **C**hance! **R**eally **C**ool **A**rtwork, **R**eally **C**ool **L**andscapes!

Longus **C**olli, **L**ongus **C**apitis, **R**ectus **C**apitis **A**nterior, **R**ectus **C**apitis **L**ateralis

---

TRUNK CHAPTER

Erector Spinae Subdivisions (lateral to medial):

I Love **Spin**ach.

Iliocostalis, **Lo**ngissimus, **Spin**alis

Transversospinalis Subdivisions (superficial to deep):

Sometimes **S**cared **M**en **R**etreat.

Semi**S**pinalis, **M**ultifidus, **R**otatores

Transversospinalis Subdivisions (superficial to deep):

Try **S**melling **M**ore **R**oses.

Transversospinalis: **S**emispinalis, **M**ultifidus, **R**otatores

Muscles of the Anterior Abdomen:

(Not in any particular order)

TIRE (Think "spare tire" around the abdomen.)

Transversus Abdominis
Internal Abdominal Oblique
Rectus Abdominis
External Abdominal oblique

External Abdominal Oblique actions
(All actions are of the trunk except the last one):

Frank **C**an **R**un **L**ike **F**reddy **C**an.

Flexion, **C**ontralateral **R**otation, **L**ateral **F**lexion, **C**ompression (of the abdominal contents)

Diaphragm Innervation (the spinal roots of the phrenic nerve):

"C3, 4, 5 keeps the diaphragm alive!"

Serratus Anterior Innervation:

"**SALT**"

Serratus **A**nterior – **L**ong **T**horacic (nerve)

LAtissimus Dorsi – Distal Attachment:

"The LADY between two MAJORS"

On the humerus, the **Latissimus Dorsi (Lady)** is between the Teres **Major** and the Pectoralis **Major**.

PART TWO – THE LOWER EXTREMITY

PELVIS CHAPTER

Lateral Rotators of the Hip (from superior to inferior):

"**P**lay **G**olf **O**r **G**o **O**n **Q**uaaludes."

Piriformis, **G**emellus Superior, **O**bturator Internus, **G**emellus Inferior, **O**bturator Externus, **Q**uadratus Femoris

---

THIGH CHAPTER

Pes Anserine Muscles (anterior to posterior):

Pretty **A**rt **S**hows **G**ood **S**ense.

Pes **A**nserine: **S**artorius, **G**racilis, **S**emitendinosus

Pes Anserine Muscles (anterior to posterior):

Sensitive **G**uys **S**mile **T**enderly.

Sartorius, **G**racilis, **S**emiten**d**inosus

Adductor Muscle Group:
(pectineus and gracilis and then the three "adductors" are in superficial to deep order)

Pretty **G**irls **L**ove **B**ig **M**uscles.

Pectineus, **G**racilis, (Adductor) **L**ongus, (Adductor) **B**revis, (Adductor) **M**agnus

Listed by pelvic attachment from anterior to posterior:

People **L**ove **G**etting **B**ack **M**oney. OR **P**etty **L**ittle **G**ripes **B**other **M**om.

Pectineus, (Adductor) Longus, Gracilis, (Adductor) Brevis, (Adductor) Magnus

Adductor Magnus Innervation:

"AM SO!"

Adductor **M**agnus innervated by the **S**ciatic and **O**bturator Nerves

Hamstring Muscles:

(Lateral to medial and then superficial to deep for all three):

Hurray! **B**ob **F**inally **S**aved **S**am!

Hamstrings: **B**iceps **F**emoris, **S**emitendinosus, **S**emimembranosus

Big **F**ables **S**ometimes **T**ell **S**illy **M**orals.

Biceps **F**emoris, **S**emi**T**endinosus, **S**emi**M**embranosus

Bitter **F**emales **S**end **T**ense **S**ounding **M**essages.

Biceps **F**emoris, **S**emi**T**endinosus, **S**emi**M**embranosus

Quadriceps Group:

Robert's **F**amily: **V**ery **M**usical, **V**ery **I**nteresting, **V**ery **L**oud!

Rectus **F**emoris, **V**astus **M**edialis, **V**astus **I**ntermedius, **V**astus **L**ateralis

---

LEG CHAPTER

Anterior Leg Muscles:

To **An** **E**xciting **D**estination, **L**ong **E**xpected **H**oliday, **L**eave **F**or **T**ahiti!

Tibialis **An**terior, **E**xtensor **D**igitorum **L**ongus, **E**xtensor **H**allucis **L**ongus, **F**ibularis **T**ertius

Lateral Leg Muscles:

Feet **L**ove **F**uzzy **B**ooties

Fibularis **L**ongus, **F**ibularis **B**revis

Quadriceps Surae Muscles:

Guys **S**hould **P**ay!

Gastrocnemius, **S**oleus, **P**lantaris

Deep Posterior Leg Muscles:
(their distal tendons all cross directly posterior to the medial malleolus of the tibia):

"**T**om, **D**ick and **H**arry"

Tibialis Posterior, Flexor **D**igitorum Longus, Flexor **H**allucis Longus

---

FOOT CHAPTER

Muscles of the Dorsum of the Foot:

Each **D**ay **B**egin **E**xercising **H**ealthy **B**odies.

Extensor **D**igitorum **B**revis, **E**xtensor **H**allucis **B**revis

Every **D**ay **B**ert **E**xamines **H**is **B**oots

Extensor **D**igitorum **B**revis, **E**xtensor **H**allucis **B**revis

Plantar Muscles of the Foot - Layer I

Able **H**ospital **A**ides **D**iligently **M**ake **P**atients' **F**luffy **D**own **B**eds.

Abductor **H**allucis, **A**bductor **D**igiti **M**inimi **P**edis, **F**lexor **D**igitorum **B**revis

Plantar Muscles of the Foot - Layer II

Quiet **P**lease **L**oud **P**eople!

Quadratus **P**lantae, **L**umbricals **P**edis

Plantar Muscles of the Foot - Layer III

Five **H**andsome **B**rothers **F**ind **D**ivine **M**aidens **P**leasant **A**nd **H**appy!

Flexor **H**allucis **B**revis, **F**lexor **D**igiti **M**inimi **P**edis, **A**dductor **H**allucis

Plantar Muscles of the Foot - Layer IV

Put **I**t **D**own **I**zzi!

Plantar **I**nterossei, **D**orsal **I**nterossei

PART THREE – THE UPPER EXTREMITY

SCAPULA/ARM CHAPTER

Rotator Cuff Group of Muscles:

SITS muscles: **S**upraspinatus, **I**nfraspinatus, **T**eres Minor, **S**ubscapularis

or

Soup **I**n **T**he **M**idget's **S**ubmarine.

Supraspinatus, **I**nfraspinatus, **T**eres **M**inor, **S**ubscapularis

Flexors of the Forearm at the Elbow Joint:

"3 "**B**"s **B**end the el**B**ow."

Brachialis, **B**iceps Brachii, **B**rachioradialis

Flexors of the Arm at the Shoulder Joint:

Please **M**ake **A**nother **D**ashing **C**omment, **B**ig **B**oy!

Pectoralis **M**ajor, **A**nterior **D**eltoid, **C**oracobrachialis, **B**iceps **B**rachii

Biceps Brachii's Major Actions:

(the first two actions are of the forearm, the last action is of the arm)

Felix **S**crubs **F**aucets.

Flexion, **S**upination, **F**lexion

FOREARM CHAPTER

Supination of the Forearm – Position

(if your elbow joint is first flexed to 90° degrees):

SUPination is to turn the palm**s** **UP**. - or - You **SUP**inate and turn your palms up to hold a bowl of **SOUP**.

Supination of the Forearm – Action

"*Righty Tighty, Lefty Loosey*"

Supination of the forearm is a stronger motion than pronation of the forearm: Since more people are right-handed and it takes more force to tighten a screw than to loosen it, screws were designed to be tightened with supination to the right by a right-handed person.

Radial Group of Forearm Muscles:

Because	**B**rachioradialis
Every	**E**xtensor
Child	**C**arpi
Receives	**R**adialis
Love	**L**ongus
Every	**E**xtensor
Child	**C**arpi
Relates	**R**adialis
Better	**B**revis

Humeral Epicondylar "common" tendon attachments:
The common flexor tendon attaches medially; the common extensor tendon attaches laterally.

FM radio – **E**asy **L**istening music

Flexors **M**edial – **E**xtensors **L**ateral

Wrist Flexors – Superficial Group:
(lateral to medial):

Five **C**ats **R**an **P**ast **L**ucy's **F**avorite **C**rystal **U**nicorn.

Flexor **C**arpi **R**adialis, **P**almaris **L**ongus, Flexor **C**arpi **U**lnaris

Wrist Extensors – Superficial Group:
(lateral to medial):

Every **C**hild **R**espects **L**ove, **E**very **C**hild **R**espects **B**ravery, **E**very **C**hild **U**nderstands.

Extensor **C**arpi **R**adialis **L**ongus, **E**xtensor **C**arpi **R**adialis **B**revis, **E**xtensor **C**arpi **U**lnaris

Common Flexor Tendon Muscles:
(lateral to medial):

People **T**hink **F**ancy **C**ars **R**epresent **P**rosperity, **L**ike **F**ine **C**lothing. **U**sually **F**inances **D**ictate **S**pending

Pronator **T**eres, **F**lexor **C**arpi **R**adialis, **P**almaris **L**ongus, **F**lexor **C**arpi **U**lnaris, **F**lexor **D**igitorum **S**uperficialis.

Common Extensor Tendon Muscles
(lateral to medial):

Every **C**hild **R**eally **B**enefits **E**ach **D**ay, **E**ducation **D**oes **M**ake **E**very **C**hild **U**nderstand.

Extensor **C**arpi **R**adialis **B**revis, **E**xtensor **D**igitorum, **E**xtensor **D**igiti, **M**inimi, **E**xtensor **C**arpi **U**lnaris

Anterior Forearm Deep Muscles:

Fancying **D**an's **P**ropensity **F**or **P**assion, **L**ucy **P**roposed **Q**uickly.

Flexor **D**igitorum **P**rofundus, **F**lexor **P**ollicis **L**ongus, **P**ronator **Q**uadratus

Posterior Forearm Deep Muscles:

Some **A**thletes **P**refer **L**earning **E**xercise **P**rograms **B**efore **E**xercise **P**roduces **L**ong-term **E**xcruciating **I**njuries.

Supinator, **A**bductor **P**ollicis **L**ongus, **E**xtensor **P**ollicis **B**revis, **E**xtensor **P**ollicis **L**ongus, **E**xtensor **I**ndicis

---

HAND CHAPTER

Carpal Bones:
(lateral to medial, proximal row, then distal row):

Some **L**overs **T**ry **P**ositions That **T**hey **C**an't **H**andle.

Scaphoid, **L**unate, **T**riquetrum, **P**isiform – **T**rapezium, **T**rapezoid, **C**apitate, **H**amate

Thenar Group of Muscles:

A Perfect **B**oy **F**riend **P**leases **B**y **O**ffering **P**resents!

Abductor **P**ollicis **B**revis, **F**lexor **P**ollicis **B**revis, **O**pponens **P**ollicis

Hypothenar Group of Muscles:
(spoken with an old-time New York City gangster accent):

Find **D**a **M**oney **M**ugsy	**F**lexor **D**igiti **M**inimi **M**anus
And **B**ring **D**a **M**oney **M**ugsy	**AB**ductor **D**igiti **M**inimi **M**anus
On **D**is **M**onday!	**O**pponens **D**igiti **M**inimi

Central Compartment Muscles:

Algebra **P**leases **L**izzy's **M**ath **P**rofessor, **I**t **D**oesn't **I**nterest **M**e!

Adductor **P**ollicis, **L**umbricals **M**anus, **P**almar **I**nterossei, **D**orsal **I**nterossei **M**anus

Finger Flexors:
(flexor digitorum superficialis and the flexor digitorum profundus distal attachments) - it rhymes:

"Superficialis Splits in two, Permits Profundus Passing through."

Lumbricals Manus' actions of the fingers:

Think of the shape of the letter "**L.**"
(The lumbricals manus flex the metacarpophalangeal joint and extend the interphalangeal joints creating a right angle, creating the shape of the letter "L".)

Interossei Muscles' Actions Upon the Digits of the Hand and the Feet:

PAD - DAB
Palmar **AD**duct – **D**orsal **AB**duct
Plantar **AD**duct – **D**orsal **AB**duct

TERMINOLOGY

INTRODUCTION TO LOCATION AND MOVEMENT TERMINOLOGY

Location Terminology: Location terminology is the terminology of describing the relative location of a static point on the body or a structure of the body. Examples of location terminology might be: the sternum is anterior to the spinal column or the arm is lateral to the trunk. An analogy can be drawn to a geographical map. On a map, a point may be defined as being located north of another point. Just as north/south and east/west define the directions on a map of the earth, the human body can also be mapped with location terminology that defines the location of a point on the human body. These location terms always come in pairs such as anterior/posterior or superior/inferior, each term of the pair being the opposite of the other. Also, these terms are often combined into one word. For example, a point or structure may be stated as being anteromedial to another point, meaning it is both anterior to the other point and medial to the other point. This is similar in concept to stating geographically that a location is northwest of another location.

Movement Terminology: Movement terminology is the terminology of describing dynamic movements of a body part. Examples of movement terminology might be: flexion of the arm at the shoulder joint, or abduction of the thigh at the hip joint. Movement terminology is dependent upon location terminology. For example, since flexion of the arm at the shoulder joint is defined as being an anterior movement of the arm at the shoulder joint, it is necessary to first understand the location term "anterior" before the movement term "flexion" can truly be understood. Therefore, movement terms build upon location terms to determine the direction of a movement instead of describing the static location of a point. Using the analogy to geographical terms, a person can be described as moving north (i.e., in a northerly direction). Similar to directional terminology, movement terminology also comes in pairs in which each term of the pair is the opposite of the other. For example, flexion/extension is a pair of movement terms; right rotation/left rotation is another pair of movement terms. To be complete when using a movement term, the body part that is moving and the joint at which the movement is occurring should also be named. For example, instead of saying "flexion of the elbow joint" or "flexion of the forearm," the complete description of the movement would be "flexion of the forearm at the elbow joint." Unlike location terminology, movement terms are never combined into one word. If a person moves his/her arm in a direction that is a combination of both flexion and abduction at the shoulder joint, it is said that the person flexed and abducted the arm at the shoulder joint.

Anatomical Position: Anatomical position is the position in which a person is facing forward with the upper and lower extremities fully extended, the palms facing forward and the feet together (see Appendix A, page 678). Anatomical position is important because it is the position in which location terms such as anterior/posterior are defined. Given that movement terminology is based upon location terminology, anatomical position is ultimately the foundation for movement terminology as well. Whenever a movement term is to be applied, it is important to mentally place the person into anatomical position and then name the movement that the body part has undergone relative to that position. However, it must be emphasized that although movement terminology is originally defined relative to anatomical position, movements do not need to begin from anatomical position, and in fact, rarely do.

Planes of the Body: There are three cardinal planes that divide the body (see Appendix A, page 679). It is important to know the three cardinal planes because joint movements occur within these planes. For example, when we say that flexion of the arm at the shoulder joint is an anterior movement of the arm, it is helpful to understand that this anterior movement occurs within the sagittal plane; when we say that abduction of the thigh at the hip joint is a movement laterally away from the midline, it is helpful to understand that this lateral movement occurs within the frontal plane. The three cardinal planes are the sagittal, frontal and transverse planes. Any plane that is not perfectly one of these three cardinal planes is called an *oblique plane*. Hence, an oblique plane is a combination of two or more of the three cardinal planes.

Sagittal Plane: A sagittal plane is a plane that divides the body into left and right portions.

Frontal Plane: A frontal plane is a plane that divides the body into anterior and posterior portions. A frontal plane may also be called a *coronal plane*.

Transverse Plane: A transverse plane is a plane that divides the body into superior and inferior (or proximal and distal) portions.

LOCATION TERMINOLOGY PAIRS

Anterior/Posterior are used throughout the entire body.

Anterior: Toward the front. The term *ventral* is sometimes used for anterior.

Posterior: Toward the back. The term *dorsal* is sometimes used for posterior.

Medial/Lateral are used throughout the entire body.

Medial: Toward the midline of the body (the mid-sagittal plane).

Lateral: Away from the midline of the body, i.e., toward the side.

Superior/Inferior are used to name points on the axial body only.

Superior: Toward the head.

Inferior: Away from the head.

Proximal/Distal are used to name points on the appendicular body only.

Proximal: Toward the axial body.

Distal: Farther away (more distant) from the axial body.

Superficial/Deep are used throughout the entire body.

Superficial: Toward the surface of the body.

Deep: Away from the surface of the body.

Note: Superficial and Deep are not absolute terms as the others are. When using the terms superficial and deep, it should always be stated from which perspective one is viewing the body. A point or structure that is deep from one perspective may be superficial from another perspective.

Radial/Ulnar are used only in the forearm and sometimes in the hand.

Radial: Toward the radius.

Ulnar: Toward the ulna.

Note: Radial is equivalent to lateral; ulnar is equivalent to medial.

Note: Because of the angulation between the leg and the foot, it is difficult to directly relate plantar and dorsal to other location terminology pairs.

Fibular/Tibial are used in the leg only.

Fibular: Toward the fibula.

Tibial: Toward the tibia.

Note: Fibular is equivalent to lateral; tibial is equivalent to medial.

Palmar/Dorsal are used in the hand only.

Palmar: Toward the palm.

Dorsal: Away from the palm (toward the dorsum of the hand).

Note: Palmar is equivalent to anterior; dorsal is equivalent to posterior.

Plantar/Dorsal are used in the foot only.

Plantar: Toward the plantar surface of the foot.

Dorsal: Away from the plantar surface of the foot (toward the dorsum of the foot).

Note: Because of the angulation between the leg and the foot, it is difficult to directly relate plantar and dorsal to other location terminology pairs.

MOVEMENT TERMINOLOGY PAIRS

(For illustrations of these movements, see Appendix B.)

Flexion/Extension

Flexion: Flexion is a movement of a body part anteriorly in the sagittal plane (except from the knee joint and farther distally, wherein flexion is a posterior movement within the sagittal plane). Flexion occurs in both the axial body and the appendicular body. The opposite of flexion is extension. (A way to remember flexion is that when a person sleeps in a fetal position, all the joints of the body are usually fully flexed.)

Extension: Extension is a movement of a body part posteriorly in the sagittal plane (except from the knee joint and farther distally, wherein extension is an anterior movement within the sagittal plane). Extension occurs in both the axial body and the appendicular body. The opposite of extension is flexion.

Abduction/Adduction

Abduction: Abduction is a movement of an appendicular body part laterally away from the midline of the body in the frontal plane. Abduction occurs in the appendicular body only. The opposite of abduction is adduction.

Adduction: Adduction is a movement of an appendicular body part toward the midline of the body in the frontal plane. Adduction occurs in the appendicular body only. The opposite of adduction is abduction.

Note: When the arm is abducting at the shoulder joint beyond 90°, one may be tempted to say that the arm is now returning back toward the midline as it continues to abduct and consequently name the continued movement as adduction. However, the name of this continued movement is still abduction. A similar case exists with adduction of the arm at the shoulder joint and adduction of the thigh at the hip joint; the body part may cross the midline at a certain point and may seem to now be moving away from the midline on the other side of the body. However, the name of this continued movement is still adduction.

Right Lateral Flexion/Left Lateral Flexion

Right Lateral Flexion: Right lateral flexion is a movement of an axial body part to the right side within the frontal plane. Right lateral flexion occurs in the axial body only. The opposite of right lateral flexion is left lateral flexion.

Left Lateral Flexion: Left lateral flexion is a movement of an axial body part to the left side within the frontal plane. Left lateral flexion occurs in the axial body only. The opposite of left lateral flexion is right lateral flexion.

Lateral Rotation/Medial Rotation

Lateral Rotation: Lateral rotation is a movement of an appendicular body part within the transverse plane wherein the anterior surface of the body part rotates to face the midline. Lateral rotation occurs in the appendicular body only. The opposite of lateral rotation is medial rotation.

Medial Rotation: Medial rotation is a movement of an appendicular body part within the transverse plane wherein the anterior surface of the body part rotates to face away from the midline (i.e., toward the side). Medial rotation occurs in the appendicular body only. The opposite of medial rotation is lateral rotation.

Right Rotation/Left Rotation

Right Rotation: Right rotation is a movement of an axial body part within the transverse plane wherein the anterior surface of the body part rotates to face the right side. Right rotation occurs in the axial body only. The opposite of right rotation is left rotation.

Left Rotation: Left rotation is a movement of an axial body part within the transverse plane wherein the anterior surface of the body part rotates to face the left side. Left rotation occurs in the axial body only. The opposite of left rotation is right rotation

Note: The terms contralateral rotation and ipsilateral rotation are often used in conjunction with muscles that produce right or left rotation of an axial body part. An ipsilateral rotator is a muscle that rotates an axial body part toward the same side of the body that the muscle is located; hence, a muscle of the right side of the body that causes right rotation of an axial body part would be an ipsilateral rotator. A contralateral rotator is a muscle that rotates an axial body part toward the opposite side of the body from the side that the muscle is located; hence, a muscle on the right side of the body that causes left rotation of an axial body part would be a contralateral rotator.

Elevation/Depression

Elevation: Elevation is a movement wherein the body part moves superiorly, i.e., elevates. The opposite of elevation is depression.

Depression: depression is a movement wherein the body part moves inferiorly, i.e., down. The opposite of depression is elevation.

Note: Examples of body parts that are described as elevating and depressing are the mandible, hyoid bone, thyroid cartilage, scapula, clavicle and the pelvis.

Protraction/Retraction

Protraction: Protraction is a movement of a body part wherein the body part moves anteriorly. The opposite of protraction is retraction.

Retraction: Retraction is a movement of a body part wherein the body part moves posteriorly (to retract something is to take it back). The opposite of retraction is protraction.

Note: Examples of body parts that are described as protracting and retracting are the mandible, scapula and the clavicle.

Pronation/Supination

Pronation: Pronation is a movement of the forearm wherein the radius moves relative to the ulna; the proximal radius (the head of the radius) medially rotates and the distal radius swings anteriorly and medially around the ulna, resulting in these two bones being crossed. The opposite of pronation is supination.

Supination: Supination is a movement of the forearm wherein the radius moves relative to the ulna; the proximal radius (the head of the radius) laterally rotates and the distal radius swings anteriorly and laterally around the ulna, resulting in these two bones lying parallel. The opposite of supination is pronation.

Note: Pronation and supination of the forearm do not occur at the elbow joint; they occur at the proximal and distal radioulnar joints. The terms pronation and supination are also applied to a movement between tarsal bones (primarily the subtalar joint between the talus and the calcaneus).

Inversion/Eversion

Inversion: Inversion is a movement of the foot wherein the plantar surface of the foot faces medially. The opposite of inversion is eversion.

Eversion: Eversion is a movement of the foot wherein the plantar surface of the foot faces laterally. The opposite of eversion is inversion.

Note: Inversion and Eversion of the foot do not occur at the ankle joint; they occur at the tarsal joints (primarily the subtalar joint between the talus and the calcaneus).

Dorsiflexion/Plantarflexion

Dorsiflexion: Dorsiflexion is a movement of the foot wherein the foot moves superiorly, i.e., in a dorsal direction. The opposite of dorsiflexion is plantarflexion.

Plantarflexion: Plantarflexion is a movement of the foot wherein the foot moves inferiorly, i.e., in a plantar direction. The opposite of plantarflexion is dorsiflexion.

Note: If the terms flexion and extension are to be related to dorsiflexion and plantarflexion, then dorsiflexion is equivalent to extension and plantarflexion is equivalent to flexion.

Abduction/Adduction of the Fingers

Abduction of the fingers is a movement of the fingers away from the midline of the hand, which is an imaginary line through the 3rd finger.

Adduction of the fingers is a movement of the fingers toward the imaginary midline of the hand.

Note: The 3rd finger, being the midline, can only do radial or ulnar abduction (it cannot adduct).

Flexion/Extension and Abduction/Adduction of the Thumb

The named movements of flexion/extension and abduction/adduction of the thumb are unusual in that flexion and extension occur in the frontal plane, and abduction and adduction occur in the sagittal plane. This is because embryologically the thumb rotates 90° to allow for opposition of the thumb against the other fingers.

Opposition/Reposition of the Thumb

Opposition of the thumb is actually not an action, but rather is three actions that occur together. These three actions are flexion, adduction and medial rotation of the (metacarpal of the) thumb at the carpometacarpal joint. The opposite of opposition is reposition.

Reposition of the thumb is a return from opposition to anatomical position and is a combination of extension, abduction and lateral rotation of the thumb at the carpometacarpal joint. The opposite of reposition is opposition.

Note: The little finger (finger #5) can also do opposition and reposition.

Abduction/Adduction of the Toes

Abduction of the toes is a movement of the toes away from the midline of the foot, which is an imaginary line through the 2nd toe.

Adduction of the toes is a movement of the toes toward the imaginary midline of the foot.

Note: The 2nd toe, being the midline, can only do tibial or fibular abduction (it cannot adduct).

Upward Rotation/Downward Rotation of the Scapula

Upward Rotation of the scapula is a movement of the scapula that orients the glenoid fossa of the scapula superiorly. The opposite of upward rotation is downward rotation.

Downward Rotation of the scapula is a movement of the scapula that orients the glenoid fossa of the scapula inferiorly. The opposite of downward rotation is upward rotation.

Note: Upward and Downward Rotation of the scapula are movements that usually cannot be isolated and performed by themselves. They are necessary as "coupled actions" that accompany certain humeral movements. The clavicle can also upwardly and downwardly rotate at the sternoclavicular joint

Horizontal Flexion/Horizontal Extension

Horizontal Flexion: Horizontal flexion is a movement wherein the arm or the thigh begins in a horizontal position (for example, abducted to 90° and then moves anteriorly. Because this anterior movement also involves the arm or thigh moving medially, horizontal flexion is also known as horizontal adduction.

Horizontal Extension: Horizontal extension is a movement wherein the arm or the thigh begins in a horizontal position (for example, abducted to 90° and then moves posteriorly. Because this posterior movement also involves the arm or thigh moving away from the midline of the body anteriorly, horizontal extension is also known as horizontal abduction.

Hyperextension: Hyperextension is a term that is used widely to describe extension beyond neutral or anatomical position. This book does not employ this terminology because it is not a consistent use of the prefix "hyper." Usually, the prefix "hyper" denotes an excessive amount of whatever follows it. Therefore, hyperextension should mean an excessive (more than usual or more than healthy) amount of extension. However, there is nothing unusual or unhealthy about extending a body part beyond neutral or anatomical position. Further, if hyperextension is used to describe extension beyond neutral, then it follows that terms such as hyperflexion, hyperabduction and hyperadduction should be used to describe these actions beyond neutral or anatomical position, but these terms do not exist. However, given the widespread prevalence of the term hyperextension for this context, it is important to be aware of this usage of the term.

Circumduction: Circumduction is not an action. Rather, circumduction is a sequence of four actions carried out one after the other. For example, if the arm sequentially flexes, abducts, extends and then adducts at the shoulder joint, then the distal arm or the hand will be observed to carve out a square. If the person carries out these movements in such a manner that the corners are rounded out, then the distal arm or hand will be observed to carve out a circle. This impression leads many people to erroneously name this set of actions as rotation (of all the actions involved in circumduction, it is ironic that rotation is not even one of them). It is worth pointing out that true rotation involves a body part rotating about an axis that is located through the center of its bone. Therefore, with rotation, the bone does not actually change location within space. With circumduction, the actual position of the bone in space clearly changes.

MUSCLE ATTACHMENT TERMINOLOGIES

Physiological Terminology: The terminology for naming a muscle's attachments has traditionally been to use the terms *origin* and *insertion*. Origin has classically been defined as the attachment of the muscle that is more fixed, and insertion has been defined as the attachment of the muscle that is more mobile. For example, the humeral attachment of the brachialis is usually fixed, so it is called the origin; the ulnar attachment usually moves, so it is called the insertion. The problem with this terminology is that it can create an impression in the student's mind that one attachment of a muscle is always fixed and that the other attachment always moves. It should always be kept in mind that (except in a few rare cases) either attachment of a muscle can be fixed and either attachment of the muscle can move. In the case of the brachialis, the ulnar attachment can easily be fixed and the humeral attachment can move. This situation occurs whenever the body is being pulled toward the arm, for example, when a pull-up is done. Origin and insertion terminology is a physiological description of a muscle's attachments because it names an attachment based upon whether or not it moves (i.e., what it does, physiology).

Anatomical Terminology: An alternative method for naming a muscle's attachments is simply to name the location of the muscle's attachments using location terminology. Describing the attachments of the brachialis, the humeral attachment would be called the proximal attachment and the ulnar attachment would be called the distal attachment. This method of naming a muscle's attachments is an anatomical description because it names the anatomical locations of the attachments. This book employs this simpler anatomical terminology. For those who are accustomed to the origin/insertion terminology, the first attachment listed for each muscle is typically described as the origin.

REVERSE ACTION

A reverse action is an action of the muscle in which the attachment that is usually designated as the origin moves and the attachment usually designated as the insertion stays fixed (see illustrations in Appendix C, page 702).

APPENDIX L – LEARNING HOW MUSCLES FUNCTION

A BRIEF SKETCH OF THE BIG PICTURE OF LEARNING HOW MUSCLES FUNCTION

The basics of muscle structure and function:

A muscle attaches, via its tendons, from one bone to another bone. In so doing, a muscle crosses the joint that is located between the two bones (see figure 1).

When a muscle contracts, it attempts to shorten toward its center. If the muscle is successful in shortening toward its center, then the two bones that it is attached to will have a force exerted upon them that will pull them toward each other (see figure 2).

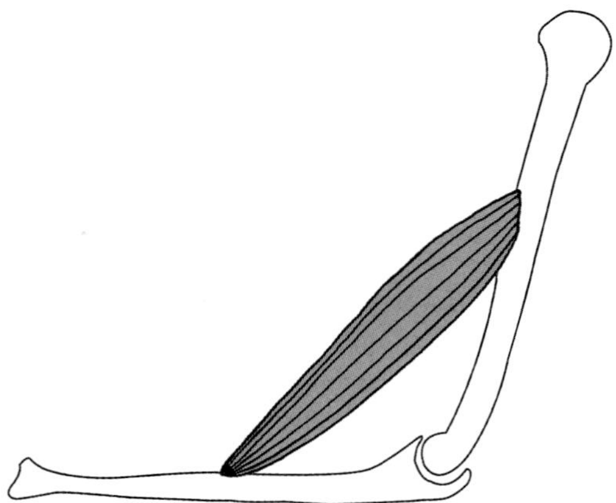

Figure 1: The location of a muscle is shown; it attaches from one bone to another bone and crosses the joint that is located between the two bones.

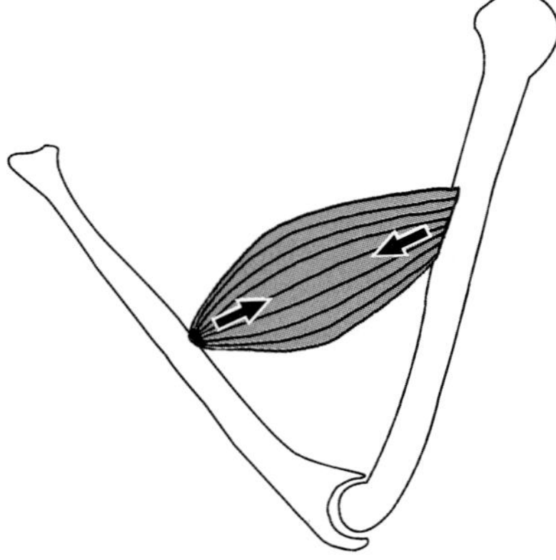

Figure 2: A muscle is shown contracting and shortening (a concentric contraction).

Since the bony attachments of the muscle are within body parts, if the muscle moves a bone, then the body part that the bone is within is moved. In this way, muscles can cause movement of parts of the body. When a muscle contracts and shortens as described here, this type of contraction is called a concentric contraction and the muscle that is concentrically contracting is called a "mover".

It is worth noting that whether or not a muscle is successful in shortening toward its center is determined by the strength of the pulling force of the muscle compared to the force necessary to actually move one or both body parts that the muscle is attached to. The force necessary to move a body part is usually the force necessary to move the weight of the body part. However, other forces may be involved.

What happens when a muscle concentrically contracts?:

Assuming that a muscle contracts with sufficient strength to shorten toward its center, lets look at the possible scenarios that can occur. If we call one of the attachments of the muscle "Bone A" and the other attachment of the muscle "Bone B", then we see that there are three possible scenarios: (see Figure 3).

1) "Bone A" will be pulled toward "Bone B".

2) "Bone B" will be pulled toward "Bone A".

3) Both "Bone A" and "Bone B" will be pulled toward each other.

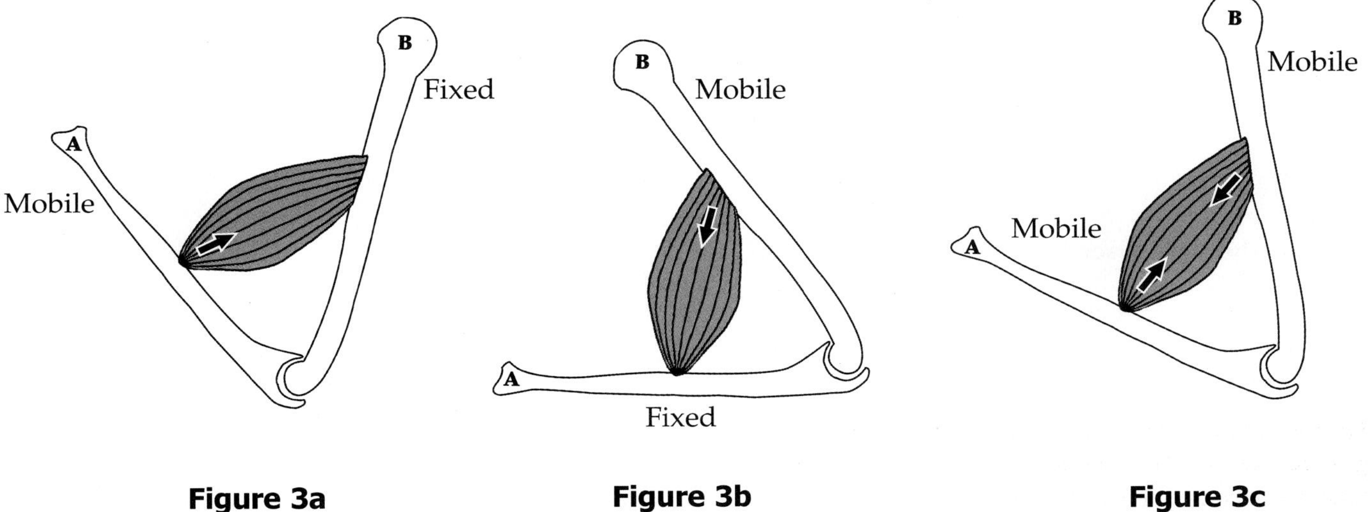

Figure 3: The three scenarios of a muscle concentrically contracting are shown.
In figure 3a, "Bone A" moves toward "Bone B".
In figure 3b, "Bone B" moves toward "Bone A".
In figure 3c, "Bone A" and "Bone B" both move toward each other.

In this manner, a muscle creates a joint action. To fully describe this joint action, we must state which body part has moved and we also must state at which joint the movement has occurred.

As an example to illustrate these concepts, lets look at the brachialis muscle. One attachment of the brachialis is onto the humerus of the arm and the other attachment of the brachialis is onto the ulna of the forearm. In attaching to the arm and the forearm, the brachialis crosses the elbow joint that is located between these two body parts (see figure 4).

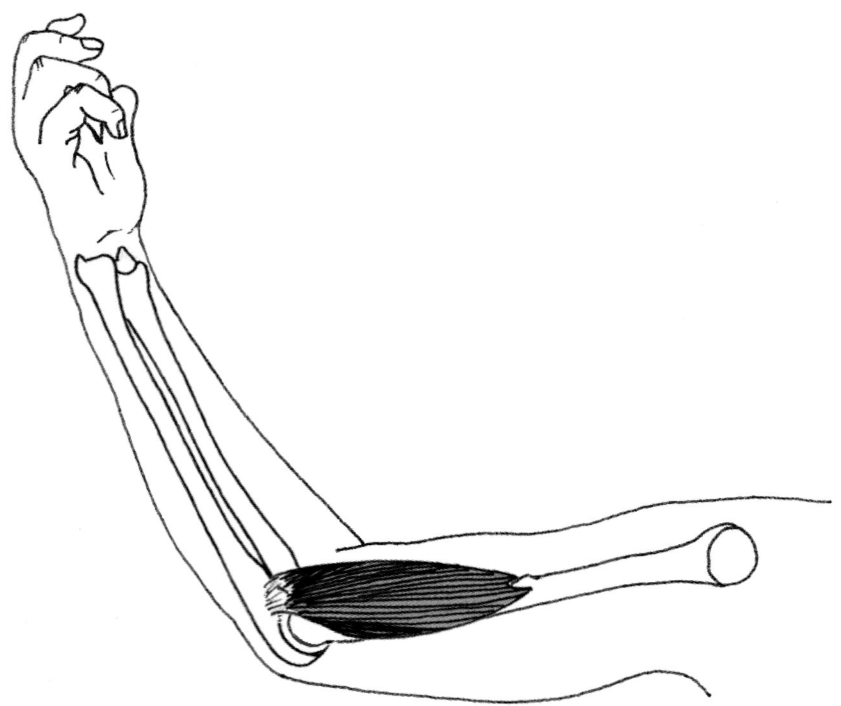

Figure 4. The right brachialis muscle at rest (medial view).

When the brachialis contracts, it attempts to shorten toward its center and exerts a pulling force upon the forearm and the arm.

Scenario 1: The usual result of the brachialis contracting is that the forearm will be pulled toward the arm. This is because the forearm is lighter than the arm and therefore would be likely to move before the arm would. (Additionally, if the arm were to move, the trunk would have to move as well, which makes it even less likely that the arm will be the attachment that will move.) To fully describe this action, we call it flexion of the forearm at the elbow joint (see figure 5a). In this scenario, the arm is the attachment that is fixed and the forearm is the attachment that is mobile.

Scenario 2: However, it is possible for the arm to move toward the forearm. If the forearm were to be fixed in place, perhaps because the hand is holding on to an immovable object, then the arm would have to move instead. This action is called flexion of the arm at the elbow joint (see figure 5b). In this scenario, the forearm is the attachment that is fixed and the arm is the attachment that is mobile. This scenario can be called a "reverse action" because the attachment that is usually fixed, the arm, is now mobile, and the attachment that is usually mobile, the forearm, is now fixed.

Scenario 3: Since the contraction of the brachialis exerts a pulling force upon the forearm and the arm, it is possible for both of these bones to move. When this occurs, there are two actions: flexion of the forearm at the elbow joint and flexion of the arm at the elbow joint (see figure 5c). In this case, both bones are mobile and neither one is fixed.

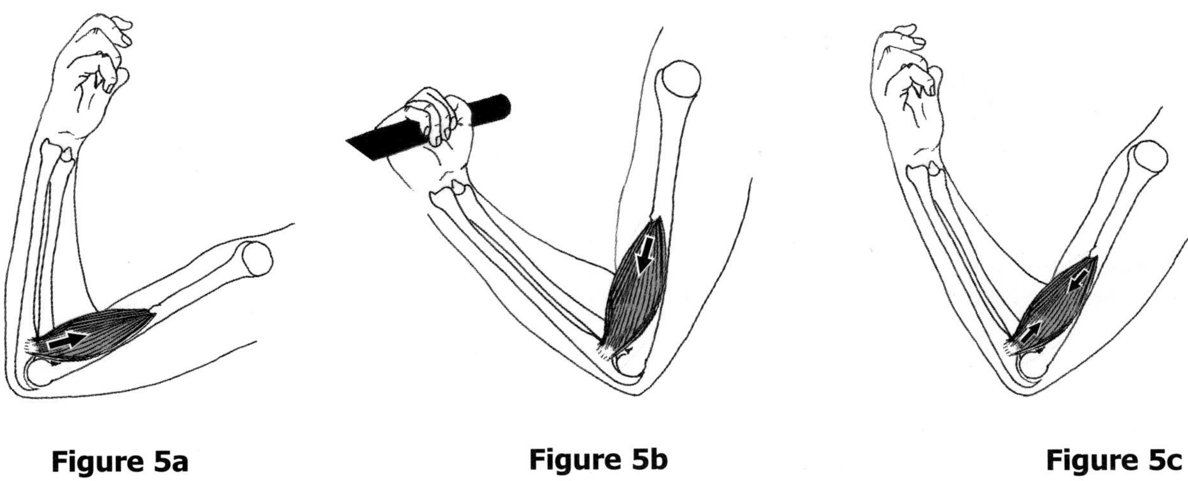

Figure 5a **Figure 5b** **Figure 5c**

Figure 5: The three scenarios that can result from a concentric contraction of the brachialis muscle.

Figure 5a: Flexion of the forearm at the elbow joint. The arm is fixed and the forearm is mobile, moving toward the arm.

Figure 5b: Flexion of the arm at the elbow joint. The forearm is fixed (in our illustration, the hand is holding onto an immovable bar) and the arm is mobile, moving toward the forearm.

Figure 5c: Flexion of the forearm and the arm at the elbow joint. Neither attachment is fixed so both are mobile, moving toward each other.

It is important to realize that the brachialis does not intend nor choose which attachment will move, or if both attachments will move. When a muscle contracts, it merely exerts a pulling force toward its center. Which attachment moves is determined by other factors. The relative weight of the body parts is the most common factor. However, another common determinant is when the central nervous system directs another muscle in the body to contract that may stop or "fix" one of the attachments of our mover muscle. (If this occurs, this second muscle that contracts to fix a body part would be called a "fixator" or "stabilizer" muscle.) It follows that if one attachment is fixed, then the other attachment would be mobile.

Beginning the process of learning muscles:

Essentially, when learning about muscles, there are two major aspects that must be learned: the attachments and actions of the muscle.

Generally speaking, attachments of a muscle must be memorized. However, there are times when clues are given about the attachments of a muscle by the muscle's name. For example, the name coracobrachialis tells us that the coracobrachialis muscle has one attachment on the coracoid process of the scapula and that its other attachment is on the brachium, i.e., the humerus. Similarly, the name zygomaticus major tells us that this muscle attaches onto the zygomatic bone (and that there must be another muscle called the zygomaticus minor).

Unlike muscle attachments, muscle actions do not have to be memorized. Instead, by understanding the simple concept that a muscle pulls at its attachments to move a body part, the action or actions of a muscle can be reasoned out.

5 Step Approach to Learning Muscles:

When first confronted with having to study and learn about a muscle, I recommend the following approach:

1. Look at the name of the muscle to see if it gives you any "free information" that saves you from having to memorize attachments or actions of the muscle.
2. Learn the general location of the muscle well enough to be able to visualize the muscle on your body. At this point, you need only know it well enough to know: 1) which joint it crosses, 2) where it crosses the joint, and 3) how it crosses the joint, i.e., what direction its fibers are running.
3. Use this general knowledge of the muscle's location to figure out the actions of the muscle.
4. Go back and learn (memorize, if necessary) the specific attachments of the muscle.
5. Now look at the relationship of this muscle to other muscles (and other soft tissue structures) of the body. Look at the following: Is this muscle superficial or deep? And, what other muscles (and other soft tissue structures) are located near this muscle?

Figuring Out a Muscle's Actions:

Once you have a general familiarity with a muscle's location on your body, then it is time to begin the process of reasoning out the actions of the muscle. The most important thing that you must look at is:

the direction of the muscle fibers relative to the joint that it crosses.

By doing this, you can see:

the line of pull of the muscle relative to the joint.

This line of pull will determine the actions of the muscle, i.e., how the contraction of the muscle will cause the body parts to move at that joint.

The approach that I like to have my students follow is to ask the following three questions of themselves:

1: What joint does the muscle cross?

2: Where does the muscle cross the joint?

3: How does the muscle cross the joint?

Step 1 – What joint does the muscle cross?:

I always recommend to my students that the first step in figuring out the actions of a muscle is to simply know what joint it crosses. The following rule applies: *If a muscle crosses a joint, then it will have an action at that joint.* For example, if we look at the coracobrachialis, knowing that it crosses the shoulder joint tells us that it must have an action at the shoulder joint. We may not know what the exact action of the coracobrachialis is yet, but at least we now know at what joint it has its actions. To figure out exactly what these actions are, we need to look at the next two questions. (It is worth pointing out that the converse of this rule is also true, that is: *if a muscle does not cross a joint, then it will not have an action at that joint.*)

Steps 2 and 3: – Where does the muscle cross the joint? and How does the muscle cross the joint?:

These two questions must be looked at together. The "where" of a muscle crossing a joint is whether it crosses the joint anteriorly, posteriorly, medially or laterally. It is helpful to place a muscle into one of these broad groups because the following general rules apply: muscles that cross a joint anteriorly will usually flex a body part at that joint; muscles that cross a joint posteriorly will usually extend a body part at that joint; muscles that cross a joint laterally will usually abduct or laterally flex a body part at that joint, and muscles that cross a joint medially will usually adduct a body part at that joint. The "how" of a muscle crossing a joint is whether it crosses the joint with its fibers running vertically or horizontally. This is also very important.

To illustrate this idea, lets look at the pectoralis major muscle. The pectoralis major has two parts, a clavicular head and a sternocostal head. The "where" of these two heads of the pectoralis major crossing the shoulder joint is the same, that is, they both cross the shoulder joint anteriorly. But the "how" of these two heads crossing the shoulder joint is very different. The clavicular head crosses the shoulder joint with its fibers running vertically, therefore it flexes the arm at the shoulder joint (because it pulls the arm upward in the sagittal plane, which is flexion). However, the sternocostal head crosses the shoulder joint with its fibers running horizontally, therefore it adducts the arm at the shoulder joint (because it pulls the arm from lateral to medial in the frontal plane, which is adduction).

With a muscle that has a horizontal direction to its fibers, there is another factor that must be considered when looking at "how" this muscle crosses the joint. That is whether the muscle attaches to the first place on the bone that it reaches, or whether the muscle wraps around the bone before attaching to it. Muscles that run horizontally (in the transverse plane) and wrap around the bone before attaching to it create a rotation action when they contract and pull on the attachment. For example, the sternocostal head of the pectoralis major does not attach to the first point on the humerus that it reaches. Instead, it continues to wrap around the shaft of the humerus to attach onto the lateral lip of the bicipital groove of the humerus. When the sternocostal head pulls, it medially rotates the arm at the shoulder joint.

In essence, by asking the three questions: What joint does a muscle cross?, Where does the muscle cross the joint?, and How does the muscle cross the joint?, we are trying to determine the direction of the muscle fibers relative to the joint. Determining this will give us the line of pull of the muscle relative to the joint and that will give us the actions of the muscle, saving us the trouble of having to memorize this information!

A Visual and Kinesthetic Approach to Learning a Muscle's Actions:

An excellent method for learning the actions of a muscle is to place a shoelace (or string or rubber band) on your body in the same location that the muscle is located. Make sure that you have the shoelace running in the same direction as the direction of the fibers of the muscle. You may even tie the shoelace around the body parts that are the attachments of the muscle if it is not uncomfortable. Pull one of the ends of the shoelace toward the center of the shoelace to see the action that the shoelace/muscle has upon that body part's attachment; pull the other end of the shoelace toward the center of the shoelace to see the action that the shoelace/muscle has upon the other body part's attachment.

By placing the shoestring on your body, you are simulating the direction of the muscle's fibers relative to the joint. By pulling on the shoestring, you are simulating the line of pull of the muscle relative to the joint. The resultant movements that occur are the actions that the muscle would have. This is an excellent approach to both visually see the actions of a muscle and to kinesthetically experience the actions of a muscle. This method is an excellent way to learn all muscle actions, and can be especially helpful for determining rotation actions, which are sometimes a little more difficult to see without a visual and kinesthetic aid such as this.

BIBLIOGRAPHY

Books (listed by title)

A.D.A.M. Student Atlas of Anatomy by Todd R. Olson
Published by Williams & Wilkins, Baltimore, MD (1996)

Anatomy: A Regional Atlas of the Human Body (2nd and 4th Editions) by Carmine D. Clemente
Published by Urban & Schwarzenberg, Baltimore, MD (1981, 1997)

Anatomy of Movement by Blandine Calaise-Germaine
Published by Eastland Press, Seattle, WA (1991)

Atlas of Human Anatomy by Frank H. Netter
Published by Ciba-Geigy Corporation, Summit, NJ (1989)

Atlas of Radiological Anatomy by Jamie Weir and Peter Abrahams
Published by Pitman Medical Publishing Co., Kent, England (1978)

Atlas of Skeletal Muscles (2nd Edition) by Robert J. Stone and Judith A. Stone
Published by Wm. C. Brown Publishers, Guilford, CT (1997)

The Body Moveable by David Gorman
Published by Ampersand Press, Guelph, Ontario (1981)

Brunnstrom's Clinical Kinesiology (5th Edition)
Published by F.A. Davis Company, Philadelphia, PA (1996)

Cassell's Latin English Dictionary
Published by Macmillan Publishing Co., New York, NY (1963)

Clinically Oriented Anatomy by Keith L. Moore
Published by Williams & Wilkins, Baltimore, MD (1980)

Color Atlas of Anatomy by R.M.H. McMinn and R.T. Hutchings
Published by Year Book Medical Publishers, Chicago, IL (1977)

Essential Clinical Anatomy by Keith L. Moore and Anne M. R. Agur
Published by Williams & Wilkins, Baltimore, MD (1995)

Essentials of Exercise Physiology by William D. McArdle, Frank I. Katch and Victor L. Katch
Published by Williams & Wilkins, Baltimore, MD (1991)

Essentials of Human Anatomy (9th Edition) by William E. Burkel
Published by Oxford University Press, New York, NY (1994)

The Extremities (4th Edition) by John H. Warfel
Published by Lea & Febiger, Philadelphia, PA (1974)

Grant's Dissector (9th Edition) by Eberhardt K. Sauerland
Published by Williams & Wilkins, Baltimore, MD (1984)

Gray's Anatomy (37th and 38th Editions)
Published by Churchill Livingstone, New York, NY (1989, 1995)

The Head, Neck, and Trunk (4th Edition) by John H. Warfel
Published by Lea & Febiger, Philadelphia, PA (1973)

Hole's Essentials of Human Anatomy and Physiology (6th Edition)
Published by WCB McGraw-Hill, New York, NY (1998)

Illustrated Essentials of Musculoskeletal Anatomy (2nd and 3rd Editions) by Kay W. Sieg and Sandra P. Adams
Published by Megabooks, Gainesville, FL (1985, 1996)

Job's Body: A Handbook for Bodywork by Deane Juhan
Published by Station Hill Press, Barrytown, NY (1987)

Joint Structure & Function: A Comprehensive Analysis (2nd Edition) by Cynthia C. and Pamela K. Levangie
Published by F.A. Davis Company, Philadelphia, PA (1992)

Kinesiology: Scientific Basis of Human Motion (8th Edition) by Kathryn Luttgens, Helga Deutsch and Nancy Hamilton
Published by WCB Brown & Benchmark, Madison, WI (1992)

Learning Human Anatomy: A Laboratory Text and Workbook (2nd Edition) by Julia F. Guy
Published by Prentice Hall, Upper Saddle River, NJ (1998)

Living Anatomy (2nd Edition) by Joseph E. Donnelly
Published by Human Kinetics, Champaign, IL (1990)

Muscles, Testing, and Function (4th Edition) by Florence P. Kendall, Elizabeth K. McCreary and Patricia G. Provance
Published by Williams & Wilkins, Baltimore, MD (1993)

Myofascial Pain and Dysfunction: The Trigger Point Manual (Volumes I & II) by Janet G. Travell and David G. Simons
Published by Williams & Wilkins, Baltimore, MD (1983)

Neuromechanics of Human Movement (3rd Edition) by Roger M. Enoka, PhD
Published by Human Kinetics, Champaign, IL (2002)

Physical Examination of the Spine and Extremities by Stanley Hoppenfeld
Published by Appleton-Century-Crofts, New York, NY (1976)

The Physiology of the Joints (Volume III) by I.A. Kapandji
Published by Churchill Livingstone, New York, NY (1974)

Review of Gross Anatomy (4th Edition) by Ben Pansky
Published by Macmillan Publishing Co., New York, NY (1979)

Stedman's Concise Medical Dictionary for the Health Professions – Illustrated (4th Edition)
Published by Lippincott Williams & Wilkins, New York, NY (2001)

Structure and Function of the Musculoskeletal System by James Watkins
Published by Human Kinetics, Champaign, IL (1999)

Taber's Cyclopedic Medical Dictionary (13th Edition)
Published by F.A. Davis Company, Philadelphia, PA (1977)

Trail Guide to the Body (1st and 2nd Editions) by Andrew Biel
Published by Books of Discovery, Boulder, CO (1997, 2001)

Videos

Acland's Video Atlas of Human Anatomy (Tapes 1-5) by Robert D. Acland
Lippincott Williams & Wilkins, Baltimore, MD (2000)

A

B

C

D

E

F

G

H

I

J

K

L

M

Q

R

S

T

U

V

W

Z

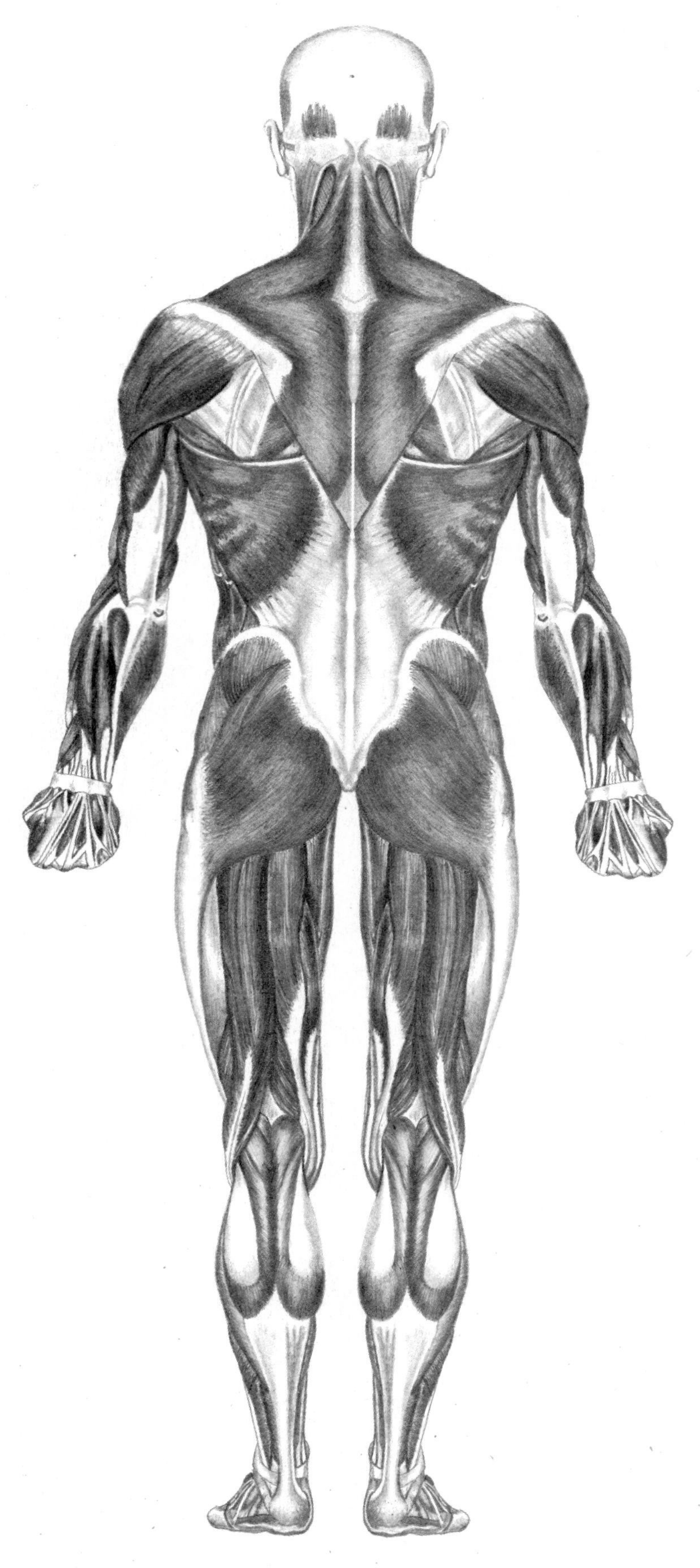

The Muscular System Manual
The Skeletal Muscles of the Human Body